Common haematology values

Haemoglobin	men:	130–180g/L	p324
	women:	115–160g/L	p324
Mean cell volume, MCV		76–96fL	↓p326; ↑p332
Platelets		150–400 × 10^9/L	p364
White cells (total)		4–11 × 10^9/L	p330
neutrophils		2.0–7.5 × 10^9/L	p330
lymphocytes		1.0–4.5 × 10^9/L	p330
eosinophils		0.04–0.4 × 10^9/L	p330

Blood gases

pH	7.35–7.45	p670
P_aO_2	>10.6kPa	p670
P_aCO_2	4.7–6kPa	p670
Base excess	±2mmol/L	p670

U&Es (urea and electrolytes)

Sodium	135–145mmol/L	p672
Potassium	3.5–5.3mmol/L	p674
Creatinine	70–100μmol/L	p298–301
Urea	2.5–6.7mmol/L	p298–301
eGFR	>60	p669

LFTs (liver function tests)

Bilirubin	3–17μmol/L	p272, p274
Alanine aminotransferase, ALT	5–35IU/L	p272, p274
Aspartate transaminase, AST	5–35IU/L	p272, p274
Alkaline phosphatase, ALP	30–130IU/L (*non-pregnant adults*)	p272, p274
Albumin	35–50g/L	p686

Cardiac enzymes

Troponin T	<99th percentile of upper reference limit: value depends on local assay	p119

Other biochemical values

Cholesterol	<5mmol/L	p690
Triglycerides	Fasting: 0.5–2.3mmol/L	p690
Amylase	0–180 IU/dL	p636
C-reactive protein, CRP	<10mg/L	p686
Corrected calcium	2.12–2.60mmol/L	p676
Glucose, fasting	3.5–5.5mmol/L	p206
Thyroid stimulating hormone, TSH	0.5–4.2mU/L	p216

For all other reference intervals, see p750–7

He moved	N. 48
all the brightest gems	N. 24
faster and faster towards the	N. 18
ever-growing bucket of lost hopes; had there been just one more year	N. 14
of peace the battalion would have made a floating system of perpetual drainage.	N. 12
A silent fall of immense snow came near oily remains of the recently eaten supper on the table.	N. 10
We drove on in our old sunless walnut. Presently classical eggs ticked in the new afternoon shadows.	N. 8
We were instructed by my cousin Jasper not to exercise by country house visiting unless accompanied by thirteen geese or gangsters.	N. 6
The modern American did not prevail over the pair of redundant bronze puppies. The worn-out principle is a bad omen which I am never glad to ransom in August.	N. 5

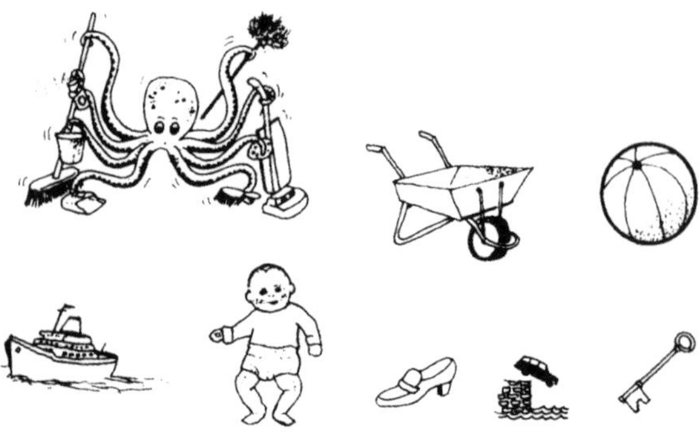

Reading tests Hold this chart (well-illuminated) 30cm away, and record the smallest type read (eg N12 left eye, N6 right eye, spectacles worn) or object named accurately.

Contents

Each chapter's contents are detailed on its first page

Preface to the tenth edition

This is the first edition of the book without either of the original authors—Tony Hope and Murray Longmore. Both have now moved on to do other things, and enjoy a well-earned rest from authorship. In this book, I am joined by a Nephrologist, Gastroenterologist, and trainees destined for careers in Cardiology, Dermatology, and General Practice. Five physicians, each with very different interests and approaches, yet bringing their own knowledge, expertise, and styles. When combined with that of our specialist and junior readers, I hope this creates a book that is greater than the sum of its parts, yet true to the original concept and ethos of the original authors. Life and medicine have moved on in the 30 years since the first edition was published, but medicine and science are largely iterative; true novel 'ground-breaking' or 'practice-changing' discoveries are rare, to quote Isaac Newton: '*If I have seen further, it is by standing on the shoulders of giants*'. Therefore, when we set about writing this edition we drew inspiration from the original book and its authors; updating, adding, and clarifying, but trying to retain the unique feel and perspective that the *OHCM* has provided to generations of trainees and clinicians.

IBW, 2017

Preface to the first edition

We wrote this book not because we know so much, but because we know we remember so little...the problem is not simply the quantity of information, but the diversity of places from which it is dispensed. Trailing eagerly behind the surgeon, the student is admonished never to forget alcohol withdrawal as a cause of post-operative confusion. The scrap of paper on which this is written spends a month in the pocket before being lost for ever in the laundry. At different times, and in inconvenient places, a number of other causes may be presented to the student. Not only are these causes and aphorisms never brought together, but when, as a surgical house officer, the former student faces a confused patient, none is to hand.

We aim to encourage the doctor to enjoy his patients: in doing so we believe he will prosper in the practice of medicine. For a long time now, house officers have been encouraged to adopt monstrous proportions in order to straddle the diverse pinnacles of clinical science and clinical experience. We hope that this book will make this endeavour a little easier by moving a cumulative memory burden from the mind into the pocket, and by removing some of the fears that are naturally felt when starting a career in medicine, thereby freely allowing the doctor's clinical acumen to grow by the slow accretion of many, many days and nights.

RA Hope and JM Longmore, 1985

Acknowledgements

Heart-felt thanks to our advisers on specific sections—each is acknowledged on the chapter's first page. Thanks also to our junior readers, Charles Badu-Boateng, Clare Coggins, and Luke Walls. We especially thank all our mentors and teachers, and patients who provide our inspiration and remind us that one never stops learning. We acknowledge the Department of Radiology at both the Leeds Teaching Hospitals NHS Trust and the Norfolk and Norwich University Hospital for their kind help in providing many images, particularly Dr Edmund Godfrey, whose tireless hunt for perfect images has improved so many chapters.

Readers' comments These have formed a vital part of our endeavour to provide an accurate, comprehensive, and up-to-date text. We sincerely thank the many students, doctors, and other health professionals who have found the time and the generosity to write to us on our Reader's Comments Cards, in editions past, or, in more recent times, via the web. These have now become so numerous for past editions that they cannot all be listed. See http://www.oup.com/uk/academic/series/oxhmed/links for a full list, and our very heart-felt tokens of thanks.

Symbols and abbreviations

► ...... this fact or idea is important

►► ...... don't dawdle!—prompt action saves lives

[1] ...... reference

♂:♀ ...... male-to-female ratio. ♂:♀=2:1 means twice as common in males

∴ ...... therefore

~ ...... approximately

–ve ...... negative (+ve is positive)

↑↓ ...... increased or decreased

↔ ...... normal (eg serum level)

1° ...... primary

2° ...... secondary

Δ ...... diagnosis

ΔΔ ...... differential diagnosis

A:CR ...... albumin to creatinine ratio (mg/mmol)

A_2 ...... aortic component of the 2nd heart sound

Ab ...... antibody

ABC ...... airway, breathing, and circulation

ABG ...... arterial blood gas: P_aO_2, P_aCO_2, pH, HCO_3

ABPA ...... allergic bronchopulmonary aspergillosis

ACE-i ...... angiotensin-converting enzyme inhibitor

ACS ...... acute coronary syndrome

ACTH ...... adrenocorticotrophic hormone

ADH ...... antidiuretic hormone

AF ...... atrial fibrillation

AFB ...... acid-fast bacillus

Ag ...... antigen

AIDS ...... acquired immunodeficiency syndrome

AKI ...... acute kidney injury

ALL ...... acute lymphoblastic leukaemia

ALP ...... alkaline phosphatase

AMA ...... antimitochondrial antibody

AMP ...... adenosine monophosphate

ANA ...... antinuclear antibody

ANCA ...... antineutrophil cytoplasmic antibody

APTT ...... activated partial thromboplastin time

AR ...... aortic regurgitation

ARB ...... angiotensin II receptor 'blocker' (antagonist)

ARDS ...... acute respiratory distress syndrome

ART ...... antiretroviral therapy

AS ...... aortic stenosis

ASD ...... atrial septal defect

AST ...... aspartate transaminase

ATN ...... acute tubular necrosis

ATP ...... adenosine triphosphate

AV ...... atrioventricular

AVM ...... arteriovenous malformation(s)

AXR ...... abdominal x-ray (plain)

Ba ...... barium

BAL ...... bronchoalveolar lavage

bd ...... bis die (Latin for twice a day)

BKA ...... below-knee amputation

BNF ...... *British National Formulary*

BNP ...... brain natriuretic peptide

BP ...... blood pressure

BPH ...... benign prostatic hyperplasia

bpm ...... beats per minute

ca ...... cancer

CABG ...... coronary artery bypass graft

CAMP ...... cyclic adenosine monophosphate (AMP)

CAPD ...... continuous ambulatory peritoneal dialysis

CCF ...... congestive cardiac failure (ie left and right heart failure)

CCU ...... coronary care unit

CDT ...... *Clostridium difficile* toxin

CHB ...... complete heart block

CHD ...... coronary heart disease

CI ...... contraindications

CK ...... creatine (phospho)kinase

CKD ...... chronic kidney disease

CLL ...... chronic lymphocytic leukaemia

CML ...... chronic myeloid leukaemia

CMV ...... cytomegalovirus

CNS ...... central nervous system

COC ...... combined oral contraceptive pill

COPD ...... chronic obstructive pulmonary disease

CPAP ...... continuous positive airway pressure

CPR ...... cardiopulmonary resuscitation

CRP ...... c-reactive protein

CSF ...... cerebrospinal fluid

CT ...... computed tomography

CVA ...... cerebrovascular accident

CVP ...... central venous pressure

CVS ...... cardiovascular system

CXR ...... chest x-ray

d ...... day(s); also expressed as /7; months are /12

DC ...... direct current

DIC ...... disseminated intravascular coagulation

DIP ...... distal interphalangeal

dL ...... decilitre

DM ...... diabetes mellitus

DOAC ...... direct oral anticoagulant

DU ...... duodenal ulcer

D&V ...... diarrhoea and vomiting

DVT ...... deep venous thrombosis

DXT ...... deep radiotherapy

EBV ...... Epstein-Barr virus

ECG ...... electrocardiogram

Echo ...... echocardiogram

EDTA ...... ethylene diamine tetra-acetic acid (anticoagulant coating, eg in FBC bottles)

EEG ...... electroencephalogram

eGFR ...... estimated glomerular filtration rate (in mL/min/1.73m^2)

ELISA ...... enzyme-linked immunosorbent assay

EM ...... electron microscope

EMG ...... electromyogram

ENT ...... ear, nose, and throat

ERCP ...... endoscopic retrograde cholangiopancreatography

ESR ...... erythrocyte sedimentation rate

ESRF ...... end-stage renal failure

EUA ...... examination under anaesthesia

FBC ...... full blood count

FDP ...... fibrin degradation products

FEV_1 ...... forced expiratory volume in 1st sec

F_iO_2 ...... partial pressure of O_2 in inspired air

FFP ...... fresh frozen plasma

FSH ...... follicle-stimulating hormone

FVC ...... forced vital capacity

g ...... gram

G6PD ...... glucose-6-phosphate dehydrogenase

GA ...... general anaesthetic

GCS ...... Glasgow Coma Scale

GFR ...... glomerular filtration rate

GGT ...... gamma-glutamyl transferase

GH ...... growth hormone

GI ...... gastrointestinal

GN ...... glomerulonephritis

GP ...... general practitioner

GPA ...... granulomatosis with polyangiitis (formerly Wegener's granulomatosis)

GTN ...... glyceryl trinitrate

GTT ...... glucose tolerance test

GU(M) ...... genitourinary (medicine)

h ...... hour

HAV ...... hepatitis A virus

Hb ...... haemoglobin

HbA1c ...... glycated haemoglobin

HBsAg ...... hepatitis B surface antigen

HBV ...... hepatitis B virus

HCC ...... hepatocellular cancer

HCM ...... hypertrophic obstructive cardiomyopathy

Hct ...... haematocrit

HCV ...... hepatitis C virus

HDV ...... hepatitis D virus

HDL ...... high-density lipoprotein

HHT ...... hereditary haemorrhagic telangiectasia

HIV ...... human immunodeficiency virus

HLA ...... human leucocyte antigen

HONK ...... hyperosmolar non-ketotic (coma)

HPV ...... human papillomavirus

HRT ...... hormone replacement therapy

HSP ...... Henoch-Schönlein purpura

HSV ...... herpes simplex virus

HUS ...... haemolytic uraemic syndrome

IBD ...... inflammatory bowel disease

IBW ...... ideal body weight

ICD ...... implantable cardiac defibrillator

ICP ...... intracranial pressure

IC(T)U ...... intensive care unit

IDDM ...... insulin-dependent diabetes mellitus

IFN-α ...... interferon alpha

IE ...... infective endocarditis

Ig ...... immunoglobulin

IHD ...... ischaemic heart disease

IM ...... intramuscular

INR ...... international normalized ratio

IP ...... interphalangeal

IPPV ...... intermittent positive pressure ventilation

ITP ...... idiopathic thrombocytopenic purpura

IU ...... international unit

IVC ...... inferior vena cava

IV(I) ...... intravenous (infusion)

IVU ...... intravenous urography

JVP ...... jugular venous pressure

K ...... potassium

kg ...... kilogram

KPa ...... kiloPascal

L ...... litre

LAD ...... left axis deviation on the ECG

LBBB ...... left bundle branch block

LDH ...... lactate dehydrogenase

LDL ...... low-density lipoprotein

LFT ...... liver function test

LH ....luteinizing hormone
LIF ....left iliac fossa
LKKS ....liver, kidney (R), kidney (L), spleen
LMN .....lower motor neuron
LMWH ..low-molecular-weight heparin
LOC ......loss of consciousness
LP ....lumbar puncture
LUQ ......left upper quadrant
LV ....left ventricle of the heart
LVF ....left ventricular failure
LVH ......left ventricular hypertrophy
MAI .....*Mycobacterium avium intracellulare*
MALT ...mucosa-associated lymphoid tissue
mane ..morning (from Latin)
MAOI ...monoamine oxidase inhibitor
MAP .....mean arterial pressure
MC&S ...microscopy, culture, and sensitivity
mcg ....microgram
MCP .....metacarpo-phalangeal
MCV .....mean cell volume
MDMA ..3,4-methylenedioxymethamphetamine
ME ....myalgic encephalomyelitis
mg ......milligram
MI ....myocardial infarction
min(s) minute(s)
mL ....millilitre
mmHg millimetres of mercury
MND .....motor neuron disease
MR ....modified release or mitral regurgitation
MRCP ...magnetic resonance cholangiopancreatography
MRI ......magnetic resonance imaging
MRSA ...meticillin-resistant *Staph. aureus*
MS ....multiple sclerosis
MSM ....men who have sex with men
MSU .....midstream urine
N&V .....nausea and/or vomiting
NAD .....nothing abnormal detected
NBM .....nil by mouth
ND ....notifiable disease
NEWS ..National Early Warning Score
ng ....nanogram
NG ....nasogastric
NHS .....National Health Service (UK)
NICE ....National Institute for Health and Care Excellence, http://www.nice.org.uk
NIDDM .non-insulin-dependent diabetes mellitus
NMDA ..*N*-methyl-D-aspartate
NNT .....number needed to treat
nocte ..at night
NR ....normal range (=reference interval)
NSAID ..non-steroidal anti-inflammatory drug
OCP ......oral contraceptive pill
od ....omni die (Latin for once daily)
OGD .....oesophagogastroduodenoscopy
OGTT ....oral glucose tolerance test
OHCS ....*Oxford Handbook of Clinical Specialties*
om ......omni mane (in the morning)
on ....omni nocte (at night)
OPD ......outpatients department
OT ....occupational therapist
P:CR .....protein to creatinine ratio (mg/mmol)
P_2 ....pulmonary component of 2nd heart sound
P_aCO_2 ...partial pressure of CO_2 in arterial blood
PAN ......polyarteritis nodosa
P_aO_2 .....partial pressure of O_2 in arterial blood
PBC ......primary biliary cirrhosis
PCR ......polymerase chain reaction
PCV ......packed cell volume
PE ....pulmonary embolism
PEEP ....positive end-expiratory pressure
PEF(R) ..peak expiratory flow (rate)
PERLA ..pupils equal and reactive to light and accommodation
PET ......positron emission tomography
PID ......pelvic inflammatory disease
PIP ....proximal interphalangeal (joint)
PMH .....past medical history
PND .....paroxysmal nocturnal dyspnoea
PO ....per os (by mouth)
PPI ....proton pump inhibitor, eg omeprazole
PR ....per rectum (by the rectum)
PRL ......prolactin
PRN ......pro re nata (Latin for as required)
PRV ......polycythaemia rubra vera
PSA ......prostate-specific antigen
PTH ......parathyroid hormone
PTT ......prothrombin time
PUO ......pyrexia of unknown origin
PV ....per vaginam (by the vagina, eg pessary)
PVD ......peripheral vascular disease
QDS ......quater die sumendus; take 4 times daily
qqh .....quarta quaque hora: take every 4h
R ....right
RA ....rheumatoid arthritis
RAD .....right axis deviation on the ECG
RBBB ...right bundle branch block
RBC ......red blood cell
RCT ......randomized controlled trial
RDW ....red cell distribution width
RFT ......respiratory function tests
Rh ....Rhesus status
RIF ....right iliac fossa
RRT ......renal replacement therapy
RUQ .....right upper quadrant
RV ....right ventricle of heart
RVF ......right ventricular failure
RVH ......right ventricular hypertrophy
℞ ....recipe (Latin for treat with)
s/sec ...second(s)
S_1, S_2 ....first and second heart sounds
SBE ......subacute bacterial endocarditis
SC ....subcutaneous
SD ....standard deviation
SE ....side-effect(s)
SIADH ..syndrome of inappropriate anti-diuretic hormone secretion
SL ....sublingual
SLE ......systemic lupus erythematosus
SOB ......short of breath
SOBOE .short of breath on exertion
SpO_2 ....peripheral oxygen saturation (%)
SR ....slow-release
stat ....statim (immediately; as initial dose)
STD/I ...sexually transmitted disease/infection
SVC ......superior vena cava
SVT ......supraventricular tachycardia
T° ....temperature
*t*½ ....biological half-life
T_3 ....tri-iodothyronine
T_4 ....thyroxine
TB ....tuberculosis
TDS ......ter die sumendus (take 3 times a day)
TFT ......thyroid function test (eg TSH)
TIA ......transient ischaemic attack
TIBC ....total iron-binding capacity
TPN ......total parenteral nutrition
TPR ......temperature, pulse, and respirations count
TRH ......thyrotropin-releasing hormone
TSH ......thyroid-stimulating hormone
TTP ......thrombotic thrombocytopenic purpura
U ....units
UC ....ulcerative colitis
U&E .....urea and electrolytes and creatinine
UMN .....upper motor neuron
URT(I) ..upper respiratory tract (infection)
US(S) ....ultrasound (scan)
UTI ......urinary tract infection
VDRL ....Venereal Diseases Research Laboratory
VE ....ventricular extrasystole
VF ....ventricular fibrillation
VHF ......viral haemorrahgic fever
VMA ....vanillylmandelic acid (HMMA)
V/Q ....ventilation/perfusion scan
VRE ......vancomycin resistant enterococci
VSD ......ventricular-septal defect
VT ....ventricular tachycardia
VTE ......venous thromboembolism
WBC ....white blood cell
WCC ....white blood cell count
wk(s) ..week(s)
yr(s) ...year(s)
ZN ....Ziehl-Neelsen stain, eg for mycobacteria

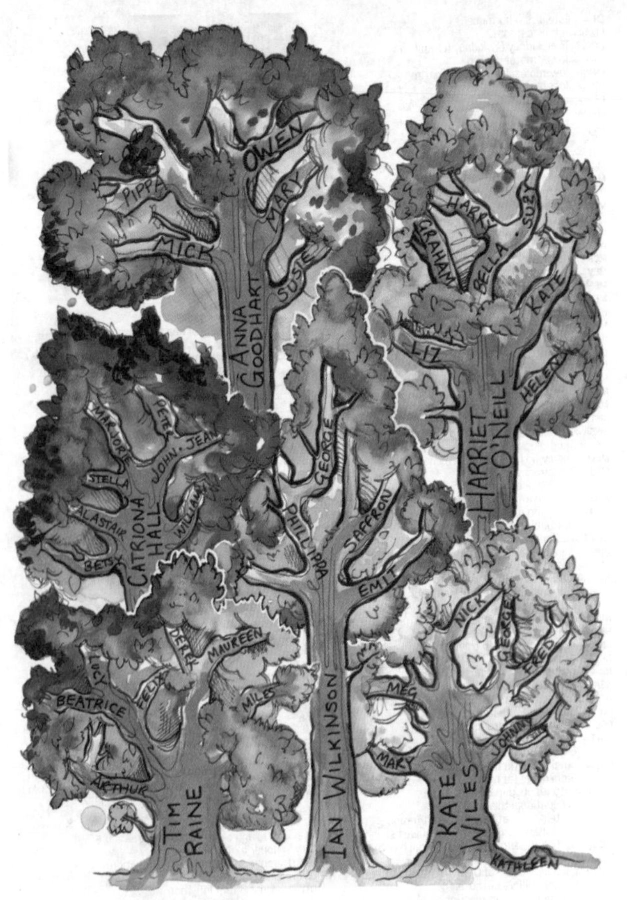

OWEN
PIPPA
MARY
MICK
SUSIE
ANNA GOODHART
HARRY
SUZY
GRAHAM
BELLA
KATE
LIZ
HELEN
HARRIET O'NEILL
MARJORIE
PETE
JOHN
STELLA
ALASTAIR
WILLIAM
BETSY
CATRIONA HALL
GEORGE
PHILLIPPA
SAFFRON
EMIT
MAUREEN
LUCY
FELIX
BEATRICE
MILES
ARTHUR
TIM RAINE
IAN WILKINSON
NICK
GEORGE
FRED
MEG
MARY
JOHNNY
KATE WILES
KATHLEEN

'He who studies medicine without books sails an unchartered sea, but he who studies medicine without patients does not go to sea at all'

William Osler 1849–1919

The word 'patient' occurs frequently throughout this book.
Do not skim over it lightly.
Rather pause and doff your metaphorical cap, offering due respect to those who by the opening up of their lives to you, become your true teachers.
Without your patients, you are a technician with a useless skill.
With them, you are a doctor.

1 Thinking about medicine

Contents

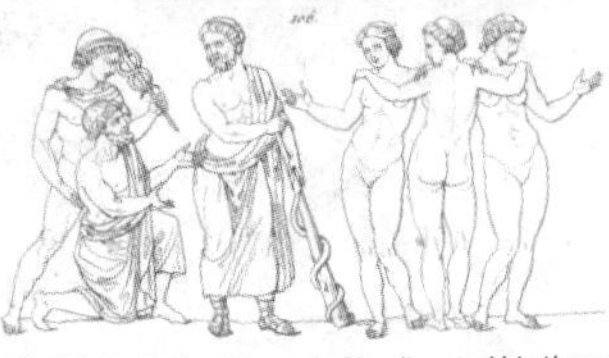

Fig 1.1 Asclepius, the god of healing and his three daughters, Meditrina (medicine), Hygieia (hygiene), and Panacea (healing). The staff and single snake of Asclepius should not be confused with the twin snakes and caduceus of Hermes, the deified trickster and god of commerce, who is viewed with disdain.

Plate from Aubin L Millin, *Galerie Mythologique* (1811)

We thank Dr Kate Mansfield, our Specialist Reader, for her contribution to this chapter.

The Hippocratic oath ~4th century BC

I swear by Apollo the physician and Asclepius and Hygieia and Panacea and all the gods and goddesses, making them my witnesses, that I will fulfil according to my ability and judgement this oath and this covenant.

To hold him who has taught me this art as equal to my parents and to live my life in partnership with him, and if he is in need of money to give him a share of mine, and to regard his offspring as equal to my own brethren and to teach them this art, if they desire to learn it, without fee and covenant. I will impart it by precept, by lecture and by all other manner of teaching, not only to my own sons but also to the sons of him who has taught me, and to disciples bound by covenant and oath according to the law of physicians, but to none other.

The regimen I shall adopt shall be to the benefit of the patients to the best of my power and judgement, not for their injury or any wrongful purpose.

I will not give a deadly drug to anyone though it be asked of me, nor will I lead the way in such counsel.[1] And likewise I will not give a woman a pessary to procure abortion.[2] But I will keep my life and my art in purity and holiness. I will not use the knife,[3] not even, verily, on sufferers of stone but I will give place to such as are craftsmen therein.

Whatsoever house I enter, I will enter for the benefit of the sick, refraining from all voluntary wrongdoing and corruption, especially seduction of male or female, bond or free.

Whatsoever things I see or hear concerning the life of men, in my attendance on the sick, or even apart from my attendance, which ought not to be blabbed abroad, I will keep silence on them, counting such things to be as religious secrets.

If I fulfil this oath and do not violate it, may it be granted to me to enjoy life and art alike, with good repute for all time to come; but may the contrary befall me if I transgress and violate my oath.

The endurance of the Hippocratic oath

Paternalistic, irrelevant, inadequate, and possibly plagiarized from the followers of Pythagoras of Samos; it is argued that the Hippocratic oath has failed to evolve into anything more than a right of passage for physicians. Is it adequate to address the scientific, political, social, and economic realities that exist for doctors today? Certainly, medical training without a fee appears to have been confined to history. Yet it remains one of the oldest binding documents in history and its principles of commitment, ethics, justice, professionalism, and confidentiality transcend time.

The absence of autonomy as a fundamental tenet of modern medical care can be debated. But just as anatomy and physiology have been added to the doctor's repertoire since Hippocrates, omissions should not undermine the oath as a paradigm of self-regulation amongst a group of specialists committed to an ideal. And do not forget that illness may represent a temporary loss of autonomy caused by fear, vulnerability, and a subjective weighting of present versus future. It could be argued that Hippocratic paternalism is, in fact, required to restore autonomy. Contemporary versions of the oath often fail to make doctors accountable for keeping to any aspect of the pledge. And beware the oath that is nothing more than historic ritual without accountability, for then it can be superseded by personal, political, social, or economic priorities:

'In Auschwitz, doctors presided over the murder of most of the one million victims.... [They] did not recall being especially aware in Auschwitz of their Hippocratic oath, and were not surprisingly, uncomfortable discussing it...The oath of loyalty to Hitler...was much more real to them.'

Robert Jay Lifton, *The Nazi Doctors*.

1 This is unlikely to be a commentary on euthanasia (easeful death) as the oath predates the word. Rather, it is believed to allude to the common practice of using doctors as political assassins.
2 Abortion by oral methods was legal in ancient Greece. The oath cautions only against the use of pessaries as a potential source of lethal infection.
3 The oath does not disavow surgery, merely asks the physician to cede to others with expertise.

Medical care

Advice for doctors

- Do not blame the sick for being sick.
- Seek to discover your patient's wishes and comply with them.
- Learn.
- Work for your patients, not your consultant.
- Respect opinions.
- Treat a patient, not a disease.
- Admit a person, not a diagnosis.
- Spend time with the bereaved; help them to shed tears.
- Give the patient (and yourself) time: for questions, to reflect, and to allow healing.
- Give patients the benefit of the doubt.
- Be optimistic.
- Be kind to yourself: you are not an inexhaustible resource.
- Question your conscience.
- Tell the truth.
- Recognize that the scientific approach may be finite, but experience and empathy are limitless.

Medicine and the stars

Decision and *intervention* are the essence of action, *reflection* and *conjecture* are the essence of thought; the essence of medicine is combining these in the service of others. We offer our ideals to stimulate thought and action: like the stars, ideals are hard to reach, but they are used for navigation. Orion (fig 1.2) is our star of choice. His constellation is visible across the globe so he links our readers everywhere, and he will remain recognizable long after other constellations have distorted.

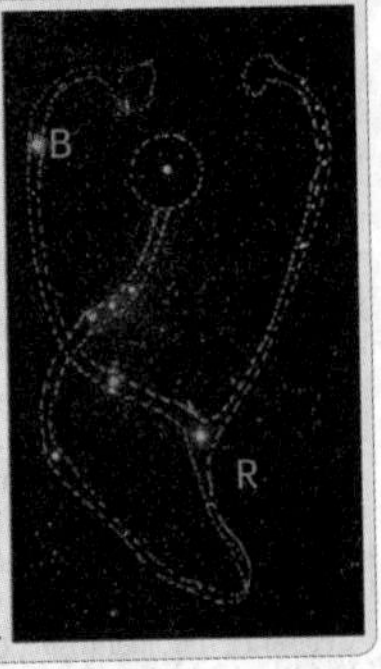

Fig 1.2 The constellation of Orion has three superb stars: *Bellatrix* (the stethoscope's bell), *Betelgeuse* (B), and *Rigel* (R). The three stars at the crossover (Orion's Belt) are Alnitak, Alnilam, and Mintaka.

The National Health Service

'The resources of medical skill and the apparatus of healing shall be placed at the disposal of the patient, without charge, when he or she needs them; that medical treatment and care should be a communal responsibility, that they should be made available to rich and poor alike in accordance with medical need and by no other criteria...Society becomes more wholesome, more serene, and spiritually healthier, if it knows that its citizens have at the back of their consciousness the knowledge that not only themselves, but all their fellows, have access, when ill, to the best that medical skill can provide...You can always 'pass by on the other side'. That may be sound economics. It could not be worse morals.'

Aneurin Bevan, *In Place of Fear*, 1952.

In 2014, the Commonwealth Fund presented an overview of international healthcare systems examining financing, governance, healthcare quality, efficiency, evidence-based practice, and innovation. In a scoring system of 11 nations across 11 categories, the NHS came first overall, at less than half the cost per head spent in the USA.[1] The King's Fund debunks the myth that the NHS is unaffordable in the modern era,[2] although funding remains a political choice. Bevan prophesied, 'The NHS will last as long as there are folk left with the faith to fight for it.' Guard it well.

QALYs and resource rationing

'There is a good deal of hit and miss about general medicine. It is a profession where exact measurement is not easy and the absence of it opens the mind to endless conjecture as to the efficacy of this or that form of treatment.'

Aneurin Bevan, *In Place of Fear*, 1952.

A QALY is a quality-adjusted life year. One year of healthy life expectancy = 1 QALY, whereas 1 year of unhealthy life expectancy is worth <1 QALY, the precise value falling with progressively worsening quality of life. If an intervention means that you are likely to live for 8 years in perfect health then that intervention would have a QALY value of 8. If a new drug improves your quality of life from 0.5 to 0.7 for 25 years, then it has a QALY value of (0.7 – 0.5)×25=5. Based on the price of the intervention, the cost of 1 QALY can be calculated. Healthcare priorities can then be weighted towards low cost QALYs. The National Institute for Health and Care Excellence (NICE) considers that interventions for which 1 QALY=<£30 000 are cost-effective. However, as a practical application of utilitarian theory, QALYs remain open to criticism (table 1.1). Remember that although for a clinician, time is unambiguous and quantifiable, time experienced by patients is more like literature than science: a minute might be a chapter, a year a single sentence.[3]

Table 1.1 The advantages and disadvantages of QALYs

Advantages	Disadvantages
Transparent societal decision making	Focuses on slice (disease), not pie (health)
Common unit for different interventions	Based on a value judgement that living longer is a measure of success
Allows cost-effectiveness analysis	Quality of life assessment comes from general public, not those with disease
Allows international comparison	Potentially ageist—the elderly always have less 'life expectancy' to gain
	Focus on outcomes, not process ie care, compassion

The inverse care law, equity, and distributive justice:

The inverse care law states that the availability of good medical care varies inversely with the need for it. This arises due to poorer quality services, barriers to service access, and external disadvantage. By focusing on the benefit gained from an intervention, the QALY system treats everyone as equal. But is this really equality? Distributive justice is the distribution of 'goods' so that those who are worst off become better off. In healthcare terms, this means allocation of resources to those in greatest need, regardless of QALYs.

Compassion

The importance of compassion[4,5] in medicine is undisputed. It is an emotional response to negativity or suffering that motivates a desire to help. It is more than 'pity', which has connotations of inferiority; and different from 'empathy', which is a vicarious experience of the emotional state of another. It requires imaginative indwelling into another's condition. The fictional Jules Henri experiences a loss of sense of the second person; another person's despair alters his perception of the world so that they are '*connected in some universal, though unseen, pattern of humanity*'.[4] With compassion, the pain of another is '*intensified by the imagination and prolonged by a hundred echoes*'.[5] Compassion cannot be taught; it requires engagement with suffering, cultural understanding, and a mutuality, rather than paternalism. Adverse political, excessively mechanical, and managerial environments discourage its expression. When compassion (what is felt) is difficult, etiquette (what is done) must not fail: reflection, empathy, respectfulness, attention, and manners count: '*For I could never even have prayed for this: that you would have pity on me and endure my agonies and stay with me and help me*'.[6]

4 Sebastian Faulkes, *Human Traces*, 2005.
5 Milan Kundera, *The Unbearable Lightness of Being*, 1984.
6 *Philoctetes* by Sophocles 409 BC (translation Phillips and Clay, 2003).

How to formulate a diagnosis

Diagnosing by recognition: For students, this is the most irritating method. You spend an hour asking all the wrong questions, and in waltzes a doctor who names the disease before you have even finished taking the pulse. This doctor has simply recognized the illness like he recognizes an old friend (or enemy).

Diagnosing by probability: Over our clinical lives we build up a personal database of diagnoses and associated pitfalls. We unconsciously run each new 'case' through this continuously developing probabilistic algorithm with increasing speed and effortlessness.

Diagnosing by reasoning: Like Sherlock Holmes, we must exclude each differential, and the diagnosis is what remains. This is dependent on the quality of the differential and presupposes methods for *absolutely* excluding diseases. All tests are statistical rather than absolute (5% of the population lie outside the 'normal' range), which is why this method remains, like Sherlock Holmes, fictional at best.

Diagnosing by watching and waiting: The dangers and expense of exhaustive tests may be obviated by the skilful use of time.

Diagnosing by selective doubting: Diagnosis relies on clinical signs and investigative tests. Yet there are no hard signs or perfect tests. When diagnosis is difficult, try doubting the signs, then doubting the tests. But the game of medicine is unplayable if you doubt everything: so doubt selectively.

Diagnosis by iteration and reiteration: A brief history suggests looking for a few signs, which leads to further questions and a few tests. As the process reiterates, various diagnostic possibilities crop up, leading to further questions and further tests. And so history taking and diagnosing never end.

A razor, a dictum, and a bludgeon

Consider three wise men:[6]

Occam's razor: Entia non sunt multiplicanda praeter necessitatem translates as 'entities must not be multiplied unnecessarily'. The physician should therefore seek to achieve diagnostic parsimony and find a single disease to explain all symptoms, rather than proffer two or three unrelated diagnoses.

Hickam's dictum: Patients can have as many diagnoses as they damn well please. Signs and symptoms may be due to more than one pathology. Indeed, a patient is statistically more likely to have two common diagnoses than one unifying rare condition.

Crabtree's bludgeon: No set of mutually inconsistent observations can exist for which some human intellect cannot conceive a coherent explanation however complicated. This acts as a reminder that physicians prefer Occam to Hickam: a unifying diagnosis is a much more pleasing thing. Confirmation bias then ensues as we look for supporting information to fit with our unifying theory. Remember to test the validity of your diagnosis, no matter how pleasing it may seem.

Heuristic pitfalls

Heuristics are the cognitive shortcuts which allow quick decision-making by focusing on relevant predictors. Be aware of them so you can be vigilant of their traps.[7]

Representativeness: Diagnosis is driven by the 'classic case'. Do not forget the atypical variant.

Availability: The diseases that we remember, or treated most recently, carry more weight in our diagnostic hierarchy. Question whether this more readily available information is truly relevant.

Overconfidence: Are you overestimating how much you know and how well you know it? Probably.

Bias: The hunt for, and recall of, clinical information that fits with our expectations. Can you disprove your own diagnostic hypothesis?

Illusory correlation: Associated events are presumed to be causal. But was it treatment or time that cured the patient?

OXFORD HANDBOOK OF CLINICAL MEDICINE

TENTH EDITION

Ian B. Wilkinson

Tim Raine

Kate Wiles

Anna Goodhart

Catriona Hall

Harriet O'Neill

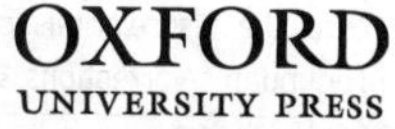

Oxford University Press, Great Clarendon Street, Oxford OX2 6DP

Oxford University Press is a department of the University of Oxford. It furthers the University's objective of excellence in research, scholarship, and education by publishing worldwide. Oxford is a registered trade mark of Oxford University Press in the UK and in certain other countries.

Published in the United States by Oxford University Press Inc., New York

First published 1985 (RA Hope & JM Longmore)
Second edition 1989
Third edition 1993
Fourth edition 1998
Fifth edition 2001 (JM Longmore & IB Wilkinson)
Sixth edition 2004
Seventh edition 2007
Eighth edition 2010
Ninth edition 2014
Tenth edition 2017 (IB Wilkinson, T Raine & K Wiles)

Translations:

Chinese	French	Hungarian	Polish	Russian
Czech	German	Indonesian	Portuguese	Spanish
Estonian	Greek	Italian	Romanian	

British Library Cataloguing in Publication Data
Data available

Library of Congress Control Number: 2017939060

Typeset by GreenGate Publishing Services, Tonbridge, UK; printed in China by C&C Offset Printing Co. Ltd.

ISBN 978-0-19-968990-3

Impression 2

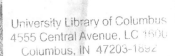

Drugs

Except where otherwise stated, recommendations are for the **non-pregnant adult** who is **not breastfeeding** and who has reasonable **renal and hepatic function.**

We have made every effort to check this text, but it is still possible that drug or other errors have been missed. OUP makes no representation, express or implied, that doses are correct. Readers are urged to check with the most up to date product information, codes of conduct, and safety regulations. The authors and the publishers do not accept responsibility or legal liability for any errors in the text, or for the misuse or misapplication of material in this work.

For updates/corrections, see **http://www.oup.co.uk/academic/series/oxhmed/updates/**

Being wrong

It is always possible to be wrong[8] because you remain unaware of it while it is happening. Such error-blindness is why 'I *am* wrong' is a statement of impossibility. Once you are aware that you are wrong, you are no longer wrong, and can therefore only declare 'I *was* wrong'. It is also the reason that fallibility must be accepted as a universally human phenomenon. Conversely, certainty is the conviction that we cannot be wrong because our biases and beliefs must be grounded in fact. Certainty produces the comforting illusion that the world (and medicine) is knowable. But be cautious of certainty for it involves a shift in perspective inwards, towards our own convictions. This means that other people's stories can cease to matter to us. Certainty becomes lethal to empathy.

In order to determine how and why mistakes are made, error must be acknowledged and accepted. Defensiveness is bad for progress. 'I was wrong, *but...*' is rarely an open and honest analysis of error that will facilitate different and better action in the future. It is only with close scrutiny of mistakes that you can see the possibility of change at the core of error. And yet, medical practice is littered with examples of resistance to disclosure, and reward for the concealment of error. This must change.[4] Remember error blindness and protect your whistle-blowers. Listen. It is an act of humility that acknowledges the position of others, and the possibility of error in yourself. Knowledge persists only until it can be disproved. Better to aspire to the *aporia* of Socrates:

> *'At first, he didn't know...just as he doesn't yet know the answer now either; but he still thought he knew the answer then, and he was answering confidently, as if he had knowledge. He didn't think he was stuck before, but now he appreciates that he is stuck...At any rate, it would seem that we've increased his chances of finding out the truth of the matter, because now, given his lack of knowledge, he'll be glad to undertake the investigation...Do you think he'd have tried to enquire or learn about this matter when he thought he knew it (even though he didn't), until he'd become bogged down and stuck, and had come to appreciate his ignorance and to long for knowledge?'*

Plato: *Meno and other dialogues*, 402 BC; Waterfield translation, 2005.

Medicine, error, and the humanities

Error provides a link between medicine and the humanities. Both strive to bridge the gap between ourselves and the world. Medicine attempts to do this in an objective manner, using disproved hypotheses (error) to progress towards a 'truth'. Art, however, accepts the unknown, and celebrates transience and subjectivity. By seeing the world through someone else's eyes, art teaches us empathy. It is at the point where art and medicine collide that doctors can re-attach themselves to the human race and feel those emotions that motivate or terrify our patients. 'Unknowing' drives medical theory, but also stories and pictures. And these are the hallmark of our highest endeavours.

> *'We all know that Art is not truth. Art is a lie that makes us realise the truth, at least the truth that is given to us to understand.'*

Pablo Picasso in *Picasso Speaks*, 1923.

Duty of candour

In a world in which a 'mistake' can be redefined as a 'complication', it is easy to conceal error behind a veil of technical language. In 2014, a professional duty of candour became statutory in England for incidents that cause death, severe or moderate harm, or prolonged psychological harm. As soon as practicable, the patient must be told in person what happened, given details of further enquiries, and offered an apology. But this should not lead to the proffering of a 'tick-box' apology of questionable value. Be reassured that an apology is not an admission of liability. Risks and imperfections are inherent to medicine and you have the freedom to be sorry whenever they occur. Focus not on legislation, but on transparency and learning. The ethics of forgiveness require a complete response in which the patient's voice is placed at the heart of the process.[9]

Bedside manner and communication skills

A good bedside manner is dynamic. It develops in the light of a patient's needs and is grounded in honesty, humour, and humility, in the presence of human weakness. But it is fragile: 'It is unsettling to find how little it takes to defeat success in medicine... You do not imagine that a mere matter of etiquette could foil you. But the social dimension turns out to be as essential as the scientific... How each interaction is negotiated can determine whether a doctor is trusted, whether a patient is heard, whether the right diagnosis is made, the right treatment given. But in this realm there are no perfect formulas.' (Atul Gawande, *Better: A Surgeon's Notes on Performance*, 2008)

A patient may not care how much you know, until they know how much you care. Without care and trust, there can be little healing. Pre-set formulas offer, at best, a guide:

Introduce yourself every time you see a patient, giving your name and your role.

> *'Introductions are about making a human connection between one human being who is suffering and vulnerable, and another human being who wishes to help. They begin therapeutic relationships and can instantly build trust'*
>
> Kate Granger, hellomynameis.org.uk, #hellomynameis

Be friendly. Smile. Sit down. Take an interest in the patient and ask an unscripted question. Use the patient's name more than once.

Listen. Do not be the average physician who interrupts after 20–30 seconds.

> *'Look wise, say nothing, and grunt. Speech was given to conceal thought.'*
>
> William Osler (1849–1919).

Increase the wait-time between listening and speaking. The patient may say more.

Pay attention to the non-verbal. Observe gestures, body language, and eye contact. Be aware of your own.

Explain. Consider written or drawn explanations. When appropriate, include relatives in discussions to assist in understanding and recall.

Adapt your language. An explanation in fluent medicalese may mean nothing to your patient.

Clarify understanding. 'Acute', 'chronic', 'dizzy', 'jaundice', 'shock', 'malignant', 'remission': do these words have the same meaning for both you and your patient?

Be polite. It requires no talent.

> *'Politeness is prudence and consequently rudeness is folly. To make enemies by being...unnecessarily rude is as crazy as setting one's house on fire.'*
>
> Arthur Schopenhauer (1788–1860).

Address silent fears. Give patients a chance to raise their concerns: 'What are you worried this might be?', 'Some people worry about...., does that worry you?'

Consider the patient's disease model. Patients may have their own explanations for their symptoms. Acknowledge their theories and, if appropriate, make an effort to explain why you think them unlikely.

> *'A physician is obligated to consider more than a diseased organ, more even than the whole man - he must view the man in his world.'*
>
> Harvey Cushing (1869–1939).

Keep the patient informed. Explain your working diagnosis and relate this to their understanding, beliefs, and concerns. Let them know what will happen next, and the likely timing. 'Soon' may mean a month to a doctor, but a day to a patient. Apologize for any delay.

Summarize. Is there anything you have missed?

Communication, partnership, and health promotion are improved when doctors are trained to **KEPe Warm**:[10]

- **K**nowing—the patient's history, social talk.
- **E**ncouraging—back-channelling (hmmm, aahh).
- **P**hysically **e**ngaging—hand gestures, appropriate contact, lean in to the patient.
- **Warm** up—cooler, professional but supportive at the start of the consultation, making sure to avoid dominance, patronizing, and non-verbal cut-offs (ie turning away from the patient) at the end.

Asking questions

Open questions 'How are you?', 'How does it feel?' The direction a patient chooses offers valuable information. 'Tell me about the vomit.' 'It was dark.' 'How dark?' 'Dark bits in it.' 'Like...?' 'Like bits of soil in it.' This information is gold, although it is not cast in the form of coffee grounds.

Patient-centred questions Patients may have their own ideas about what is causing their symptoms, how they impact, and what should be done. This is ever truer as patients frequently consult Dr Google before their GP. Unless their ideas, concerns, and expectations are elucidated, your patient may never be fully satisfied with you, or able to be fully involved in their own care.

Considering the whole Humans are not self-sufficient units; we are complex relational beings, constantly reacting to events, environments, and each other. To understand your patient's concerns you must understand their context: home-life, work, dreams, fears. Information from family and friends can be very helpful for identifying triggering and exacerbating factors, and elucidating the true underlying cause. A headache caused by anxiety is best treated not with analgesics, but by helping the patient access support.

Silence and echoes Often the most valuable details are the most difficult to verbalize. Help your patients express such thoughts by giving them time: if you interrogate a robin, he will fly away; treelike silence may bring him to your hand.

> '*Trade Secret: the best diagnosticians in medicine are not internists, but patients. If only the doctor would sit down, shut up, and listen, the patient will eventually tell him the diagnosis.*'
>
> Oscar London, *Kill as Few Patients as Possible*, 1987.

Whilst powerful, silence should not be oppressive—try echoing the last words said to encourage your patient to continue vocalizing a particular thought.

Try to avoid

Closed questions: These permit no opportunity to deny assumptions. 'Have you had hip pain since your fall?' 'Yes, doctor.' Investigations are requested even though the same hip pain was also present for many years before the fall!

Questions suggesting the answer: 'Was the vomit black—like coffee grounds?' 'Yes, like coffee grounds, doctor.' The doctor's expectations and hurry to get the evidence into a pre-decided format have so tarnished the story as to make it useless.

Shared decision-making: no decision about me, without me

Shared decision-making aims to place patients' needs, wishes, and preferences at the centre of clinical decision-making.

- *Support* patients to articulate their understanding of their condition.
- *Inform* patients about their condition, treatment options, benefits, and risk.
- Make decisions based on *mutual understanding*.

Consider asking not, 'What is the matter?' but, 'What matters to you?'.

Consider also your tendency towards libertarian paternalism or 'nudge'. This is when information is given in such a way as to encourage individuals to make a particular choice that is felt to be in their best interests, and to correct apparent 'reasoning failure' in the patient. This is done by *framing* the information in either a positive or negative light depending on your view and how you might wish to sway your audience. Consider the following statements made about a new drug which offers 96% survival compared to 94% with an older drug:

- More people survive if they take this drug.
- This new drug reduces mortality by a third.
- This new drug benefits only 2% of patients.
- There may be unknown side-effects to the new drug.

How do you choose?

Prescribing drugs

►Consult the *BNF* or *BNF for Children* or similar before giving any drug with which you are not thoroughly familiar.

►Check the patient's allergy status and make all reasonable attempts to qualify the reaction (table 1.2). The burden of iatrogenic hospital admission and avoidable drug-related deaths is real. Equally, do not deny life-saving treatment based on a mild and predictable reaction.

►Check drug interactions meticulously.

Table 1.2 Drug reactions

Type of reaction	Examples
True allergy	Anaphylaxis: oedema, urticaria, wheeze (p794–5)
Side-effect	All medications have side-effects. The most common are rash, itch, nausea, diarrhoea, lethargy, and headache
Increased effect/ toxicity	Due to inter-individual variance. Dosage regimen normally corrects for this but beware states of altered drug clearance such as liver and renal (p305) impairment
Drug interaction	Reaction due to drugs used in combination, eg azathioprine and allopurinol, erythromycin and warfarin

Remember *primum non nocere*: first do no harm. The more minor the illness, the more weight this carries. Overall, doctors have a tendency to prescribe too much rather than too little.

Consider the following when prescribing any medication:

1 The *underlying pathology*. Do not let the amelioration of symptoms lead to failure of investigation and diagnosis.
2 Is this prescription according to *best evidence*?
3 *Drug reactions.* All medications come with risks, potential side-effects, inconvenience to the patient, and expense.
4 Is the patient taking *other medications*?
5 *Alternatives to medication*. Does the patient really need or want medication? Are you giving medication out of a sense of needing to do something, or because you genuinely feel it will help the patient? Is it more appropriate to offer information, reassurance, or lifestyle modification?
6 Is there a risk of *overdose or addiction*?
7 Can you *assist* the patient? Once per day is better than four times. How easy is it to open the bottle? Is there an intervention that can help with medicine management, eg a multi-compartment compliance aid, patient counselling, an IT solution such as a smartphone app?
8 *Future planning.* How are you going to decide whether the medication has worked? What are the indications to continue, stop, or change the prescribed regimen?

In appreciation of pain

Pain is often seen as an unequivocally bad thing, and certainly many patients dream of a life without pain. However, without pain we are vulnerable to ourselves and our behaviours, and risk ignorance of underlying conditions.

While most children quickly learn not to touch boiling water as their own body disciplines their behaviour with the punishment of pain; children born with congenital insensitivity to pain (CIPA) can burn themselves, break bones, and tear skin without feeling any immediate ill effect. Their health is constantly at risk from unconsciously self-mutilating behaviours and unnoticed trauma. CIPA is very rare but examples of the human tendency for self-damage without the protective factor of pain are common. Have you ever bitten your tongue or cheek after a dental anaesthetic? Patients with diabetic neuropathy risk osteomyelitis and arthropathy in their pain-free feet.

If you receive a message of bad news, you do not solve the problem by hiding the message. Listen to the pain as well as making the patient comfortable.

Compliance and concordance

Compliance embodies the imbalance of power between doctor and patient: the doctor knows best and the patient's only responsibility is to comply with that monopoly of medical knowledge. Devaluing of patients and ethically dubious, the term 'compliance' has been relegated from modern prescribing practice. Concordance is now king: a prescribing agreement that incorporates the beliefs and wishes of the patient.

Only 50–70% of patients take medicines as prescribed to them. This leads to concern over wasted resources and avoidable illness. Interventions that increase concordance are promoted using the mnemonic: **Educating Patients Enhances Care Received**

- **E**xplanation: discuss the benefits and risks of taking and not-taking medication. Some patients will prefer not to be treated and, if the patient has capacity and understands the risks, such a decision should be respected.
- **P**roblems: talk through the patient's experience of their treatment—have they suffered side-effects which have prompted non-concordance?
- **E**xpectations: discuss what they should expect from their treatment. This is important especially in the treatment of silent conditions where there is no symptomatic benefit, eg antihypertensive treatment.
- **C**apability: talk through the medication regimen with them and consider ways to reduce its complexity.
- **R**einforcement: reproduce your discussion in written form for the patient to take home. Check how they are managing their medications when you next see them.

But remember that there is little evidence that increasing information improves concordance. And if concordance is increased solely by the 'education' of the patient then it starts to look a lot like compliance.[11] A truly shared agreement will not always 'comply' or 'concord' with the prescriber. The capacity of the informed individual to consent or not, means that in some cases, concordance looks more like informed divergence.

The placebo effect

The placebo effect is a well-recognized phenomenon whereby patients improve after undergoing therapy that is believed by clinicians to have no direct effect on the pathophysiology of their disease. The nature of the therapy (pills, rituals, massages) matters less than whether the patient believes the therapy will help.

Examples of the placebo effect in modern medicine include participants in the placebo arm of a clinical trial who see dramatic improvements in their refractory illness, and patients in severe pain who assume the saline flush prior to their IV morphine is opioid and reporting relief of pain before the morphine has been administered. It is likely that much of the symptomatic relief experienced from 'active' medicines in fact results from a placebo effect.

The complementary therapy industry has many ingenious ways of utilizing the placebo effect. These can give great benefits to patients, often with minimal risk; but there remains the potential for significant harm, both financially and by dissuading patients from seeking necessary medical help.

Why evolution has given us bodies with a degree of self-healing ability in response to a belief that healing will happen, and not in response to a desire for healing, is unclear. Perhaps the belief that a solution is underway 'snoozes' the internal alarm systems that are designed to tell us there is a problem, and so improve the symptoms that result from the body's perception of harm.

Many patients who receive therapies are unaware of their intended effects, thus missing out on the narrative that may give them an expectation of improvement. Try to find time to discuss with your patients the story of how you hope treatment will address their problems.

Surviving life on the wards

The ward round

- All entries on the patient record must have: date, time, the name of the clinician leading the interaction, the clinical findings and plan, your signature, printed name, and contact details. Make sure the patient details are at the top of every side of paper. Write legibly—this may save more than the patient.
- A problem list will help you structure your thoughts and guide others.
- **BODEX: B**lood results, **O**bservations, **D**rug chart, **E**CG, **X**-rays. Look at these. If you think there is something of concern, make sure someone else looks at them too.
- Document what information has been given to the patient and relatives.

Handover

- Make sure you know when and where to attend.
- Make sure you understand what you need to do and why. 'Check blood results' or 'Review warning score' is not enough. Better to: 'Check potassium in 4 hours and discuss with a senior if it remains >6.0mmol/L'.

On call

- Write it down.
- The ABCDE approach (p779) to a sick patient is never wrong.
- Try and establish the clinical context of tasks you are asked to do. Prioritize and let staff know when you are likely to get to them.
- Learn the national early warning score (NEWS) (p892, fig A1).
- Smile, even when talking by phone. Be polite.
- Eat and drink, preferably with your team.

Making a referral

- Have the clinical notes, observation chart, drug chart, and investigation results to hand. Read them before you call.
- Use **SBAR: S**itutation (who you are, who the patient is, the reason for the call), **B**ackground, **A**ssessment of the patient now, **R**equest.
- Anticipate: urine dip for the nephrologist, PR exam for the gastroenterologist.

Living with blood spattered armour

With the going down of the sun we can momentarily cheer ourselves up by the thought that we are one day nearer to the end of life on earth—and our responsibility for the unending tide of illness that floods into our corridors, and seeps into our wards and consulting rooms. Of course you may have many other quiet satisfactions, but if not, read on and wink with us as we hear some fool telling us that our aim should be to produce the greatest health and happiness for the greatest number. When we hear this, we don't expect cheering from the tattered ranks of on-call doctors; rather, our ears detect a decimated groan, because these men and women know that there is something at stake in on-call doctoring far more elemental than health or happiness: namely survival.

Within the first weeks, however brightly your armour shone, it will now be smeared and spattered, if not with blood, then with the fallout from the many decisions that were taken without sufficient care and attention. *Force majeure* on the part of Nature and the exigencies of ward life have, we are suddenly stunned to realize, taught us to be second-rate; for to insist on being first-rate in all areas is to sign a death warrant for ourselves and our patients. Don't keep re-polishing your armour, for perfectionism does not survive untarnished in our clinical world. Rather, to flourish, furnish your mind and nourish your body. Regular food makes midnight groans less intrusive. Drink plenty: doctors are more likely to be oliguric than their patients. And do not voluntarily deny yourself the restorative power of sleep, for it is our natural state, in which we were first created, and we only wake to feed our dreams.

We cannot prepare you for finding out that you are not at ease with the person you are becoming, and neither would we dream of imposing a specific regimen of exercise, diet, and mental fitness. Finding out what can lead you through adversity is the art of living.

On being busy: Corrigan's secret door

Dr Corrigan of Dublin was:

> *'tall, erect, of commanding figure...He had the countenance of an intellectual... and his face "beamed with kindness"...In temperament his distinguishing traits were kindness and tenderness towards the sick, and the ability to make a bold decision.'*
>
> E. O'Brien, *Conscience and Conflict: A Biography of Sir Dominic Corrigan* 1802–1880, 1983

Was he busy? At the start of his professional life he was advised that the best way to get business was to pretend to have it. It was suggested that a note marked 'Immediate and pressing' should be ostentatiously handed to him at the dinner table, but always at a suitable time so as not to miss the best food. Such advice was not taken. Corrigan aspired to hard work and taught his students the value of 'never doing nothing'. The city in which he practised had a 'degree of filth, stench and darkness, inconceivable by those who have not experienced them', and 'not enough hospital beds to care for the great numbers in need.' And so the story of a secret door, made in his consulting room, to escape the ever growing queue of eager patients.

In times of chaos, filled with competing, urgent, simultaneous demands, excessive paperwork, too few beds, effort-reward imbalance, personal sacrifice, and despair; we all need Corrigan to take us by the shadow of our hand, and walk with us through a secret door into a calm inner world. Our metaphorical door has five parts:

1. However lonely you feel, you are not usually alone. Do not pride yourself on not asking for help. If a decision is a hard one, share it with a colleague.
2. Take any chance you get to sit down and rest. Have a cup of tea with other members of staff, or with a friendly patient (patients are sources of renewal, not just devourers of your energies).
3. Do not miss meals. If there is no time to go to the canteen, ensure that food is put aside for you to eat when you can: hard work and sleeplessness are twice as bad when you are hungry.
4. Avoid making work for yourself. It is too easy for doctors, trapped in their image of excessive work, and blackmailed by misplaced guilt, to remain on the wards re-clerking patients, re-writing notes, or re-checking results at an hour when the priority should be caring for themselves.
5. Look to the future. Plan for a good time after a bad rota.

The origins of the story of Corrigan's secret door are unknown. It may never have existed other than in these hallowed pages. But when the legend becomes fact, print the legend.[7]

Resilience and coping

'Burnout' is common in clinical medicine. It is a syndrome of lost enthusiasm, reduced empathy, increased cynicism, and a decrease in the meaningfulness of work. Coping styles and resilience can protect doctors and better equip them to meet, and learn from, the challenges of clinical practice:[12]

- Self-directedness correlates strongly with resilience. A personal sense of responsibility allows learning from mistakes and moving on.
- Cooperativeness is the ability to work with opinions and behaviours different to your own, preventing them becoming a source of stress.
- Clinicians who are low in harm avoidance are better able to accept uncertainty and a degree of risk. This facilitates decision-making as it is unclouded by anxiety and pessimism about potential problems. Supervised experience outside your comfort zone may help you deal better with uncertainty.
- Be persistent but set realistic goals. Perfectionism can be detrimental.
- Task-orientated coping occurs when a situation is seen as changeable. This is associated with less burnout than emotion-orientated coping when situations are considered unchangeable: don't just do something, stand there.
- Be self-aware. Development or modification of your personality traits may reduce your vulnerability.

7 *The Man Who Shot Liberty Valance*, 1962: Ransom Stoddard (Jimmy Stewart) becomes a legend after killing Liberty Valance in a duel. It does not matter that the real shooter was Tom Doniphon (John Wayne) all along.

The wisdom of death

Death is nature's cruel master stroke, allowing genotypes space to try new phenotypes. The time comes in the life of every organism when it is better to start from scratch, rather than carry on with the weight and muddle of endless accretions. Our bodies and minds are the perishable phenotypes on the wave of our genes. But our genes are not really *our* genes. It is we who belong to them for a few decades. And death is nature's great insult, that she should prefer to put all her eggs in the basket of a defenceless, incompetent neonate; rather than in the tried and tested custody of our own superb minds. But as our neurofibrils begin to tangle, and that neonate walks to a wisdom that eludes us, we are forced to give nature credit for her daring idea. Of course, nature, in her careless way, can get it wrong: people often die in the wrong order and one of our chief roles is to prevent this misordering of deaths, not the phenomenon of death itself. With that exception, we must admit that dying is a brilliant idea, and one that it is most unlikely we would ever have devised ourselves.

Diagnosing dying

Would you be surprised if your patient were to die in the next few days, weeks, or months? If the answer is 'no' then end-of-life choices, decisions, and care should be addressed.

Consider: decline in functional performance, eg in bed or chair >50% of day, increasing dependence, weight of co-morbidity, unstable or deteriorating symptom burden, decreased treatment response, weight loss >10% in 6 months, crisis admissions, serum albumin <25g/L, sentinel event, eg fall, transfer to nursing home.

Diagnosing death

Death[13] is the irreversible loss of the essential characteristics which are necessary for the existence of a human being.

Death following cessation of cardiorespiratory function:

►Simultaneous and irreversible onset of apnoea, absence of circulation, and unconsciousness.

Cardiorespiratory arrest is confirmed by observation of the following:

- Absence of central pulse on palpation.
- Absence of heart sounds on auscultation.
- After 5 minutes of cardiorespiratory arrest absence of brainstem activity is confirmed by the absence of pupillary responses to light, an absent corneal reflex, and no motor response to supra-orbital pressure.

The time of death is the time at which these criteria are fulfilled.

Brainstem death:

►Brainstem pathology causing irreversible damage to its integrative functions including neural control of cardiorespiratory function and consciousness.

Diagnosed by an absence of brainstem reflexes:

- No pupil light response.
- No corneal reflex (blink to touch).
- Absent oculovestibular reflexes (no eye movements seen with injection of ice-cold water into each external auditory meatus, tympanic membranes visualized).
- No motor response to stimulation within the cranial nerve distribution (supra-orbital pressure).
- No cough/gag reflex.
- No respiratory response to hypercarbia: oxgenation is maintained (SpO_2>85%) but ventilation is reduced to achieve $P_aCO_2 \geq 6.0$kPa with pH ≤7.40. No respiratory response is seen within 5 minutes and P_aCO_2 rises by >0.5kPa.

Diagnosis is made by two competent doctors registered for >5 years testing together completely and successfully on two separate occasions.

Managing death

Death may be regarded as a medical failure rather than an inevitable consequence of life. But when medical treatments can no longer offer a cure, and a patient enters the end of life, active management of death is vital. Remember that the focus of medicine is narrow and concerned more with the repair of health, rather than the sustenance of the soul. This medical imperative may fail in its duty to make life-in-death better. Priorities at the end of life include freedom from pain, achieving a sense of completeness, being treated as a whole person, and finding peace with God.[14]

Swift death due to a catastrophic event is rare. Most death is the end product of a struggle with long-term, progressive disease: cancer, COPD, vascular disease, neurological deterioration, frailty, or dementia. Although death is inevitable, prognostication is difficult and inaccurate with remarkable variation in time to death. The patient in front of you may be the median, mean, or on the 99th centile. Dare to hope, but prepare for the worst. Prioritize preferences and aim to meet individual needs.[15]

- Seek help from experienced members of staff including palliative care teams.
- Elicit needs: physiological, psychological, social, and spiritual. Discuss fears.
- Establish the wishes of the patient. What trade-offs are they willing to accept, eg treatment toxicity for potential time gained? What is unacceptable to them?
- Consider the views of those important to the patient.
- Hydration: give support to allow the dying to drink, offer mouth care. Consider clinically assisted hydration (parenteral, enteral, intravenous) according to wishes and if distressing signs/symptoms of dehydration are possible. Stop according to wishes and harm.
- Manage pain promptly and effectively. Treat any reversible causes of pain.
- Consider a syringe pump if symptom control medications are required more than twice in 24 hours (see p536).
- Anticipate likely symptoms: the PRN side of the drug chart should cover all possibilities (see p536).

Death may or may not come with peace and acceptance. Patients may rage mightily against the dying of the light. Bear witness for them: listen and hold their hand.

Organ donation

Over 6000 people are waiting for an organ transplant in the UK and approximately 1000 people in need of a transplant will die each year (see p308).

Any patient who is a potential donor can be referred to a specialist organ donation service. That service will provide advice as to suitability for transplantation and will coordinate the approach to families. They are contactable 24 hours a day and their details will be held in your A&E and/or ITU departments.

Organs can be retrieved from:

- *donor after brainstem death* or heart-beating donor.
- *donor after cardiac death* or non-heart-beating donor. Includes death following unsuccessful CPR and patients for whom death is inevitable but do not meet the criteria for brainstem death.

There are two legislative frameworks for organ donation:

- *Opt-in.* Donors give their explicit consent
- *Opt-out.* Anyone who has not actively refused consent is a donor.

The association between an opt-out system and higher organ donation rates is complicated by the presence of multiple cofounding factors. Non-legislative change including national coordination, support and training of clinicians, routine discussion as part of end-of-life care, and efficient organ retrieval also increase donation rates. The ethics of presumed consent should also be considered: the absence of an objection would not be an acceptable substitute for informed consent in other areas of clinical practice.

In the UK, although consent for transplantation rests with the deceased, if the patient's family or representative cannot support donation then it will not go ahead. Register your decision on the NHS Organ Donor Register (https://www.organdonation.nhs.uk/register-to-donate/register-your-details/) and more importantly, let your family know your wishes.

Medical ethics

'Our clinical practice is steered by ethical principles. They guide the decisions we make in our clinics and ward rounds, what we tell our patients, and what we omit to tell them.' Tony Lopez, *Journal of Royal Society of Medicine* 2001;94:603–4.

In the silences of our consultations it is we who are under the microscope, and we cannot escape our destiny in the sphere of ethics. To give us courage in this enterprise, we can recall the law of the aviator and seagull: it is only by facing the prevailing wind that we can become airborne, and achieve a new vantage point from which to survey our world. We hope for moral perception: to be able to visualize the morally salient features of a situation. For without this, ethical issues may float past never to be resolved. Be alert to words which may carry hidden assumptions: 'futility', 'consent', 'best interests'.[16] Consider **WIGWAM** in your routine patient review:

- **W**ishes of the patient: are they known or unknown?
- **I**ssues of confidentiality/disclosure.
- **G**oals of care: are they clear? Whose are they: yours or the patient's?
- **W**ants: to decline treatment or discharge against advice.
- **A**rguments between family/friends/doctors.
- **M**oney: concerns of the patient, concerns of the healthcare provider.

Ethical frameworks

Offer structure, comprehensiveness, and transparency in deliberation.[16,17]

Four principles

Autonomy: Self governance: the ability of a patient to make a choice based on their own values and beliefs. *Beneficence:* The obligation to benefit patients. Links with autonomy as benefit is dependent upon the view of the patient. *Non-maleficence:* Do not harm. Or more appropriately, do no overall harm: you should stick a needle into someone when they need dialysis. *Justice:* A collection of obligations including legality, human rights, fairness, and resource distribution.

Four quadrants method

Medical indications: Identify the clinical problem, treatment options, goals of treatment, and likelihood of success. *Patient preferences:* What is the patient's autonomous decision? (And is the patient capable of making one? If not, look for previously expressed wishes from advanced directives, family, friends, GP.) *Quality of life:* How will the proposed treatment affect quality of life? This is subjective: recognize your own biases and accommodate those of the patient. *Contextual factors:* The wider context: legal, cultural, religious, familial, and anything else that may impact.

These frameworks describe individual voices within the ethics choir. Sometimes there is a beautiful harmony, but how should you act when there is discordance? There is no hierarchy within the frameworks. Each component is binding unless it is trumped by a stronger principle. How you weigh up and balance the ethical components of a situation is not easy, but it should be clear and justified. Know the patient. Consult others, especially those who hold different opinions to yourself. Can you adequately defend your decision to the patient? Their family? Your consultant? Another consultant? A lawyer? If an investigative journalist were to sit on a sulcus of yours, having full knowledge of all thoughts and actions, would he be composing vitriol for tomorrow's newspapers? If so, can you answer him, point for point?

Beyond the ethical framework

To force an ethical problem to fit a framework may be inadequate, reductionistic, and inconsistent.[18] It is potentially biased towards Western culture, discounts the non-autonomous, and is vulnerable to poorly considered emphasis and error. 'Doing' ethics can become a check-list exercise where thinking is lost. But doctors are not moral philosophers. They are clinicians. A framework therefore provides a starting point from which to work. It is the toe which tests the water of moral deliberation. Be aware of the cultural setting of your dilemma and consider carefully the weight of synthesis. Be prepared to wade deeper if needed. But acknowledge that moral wisdom may well be out of your depth.

Psychiatry on medical and surgical wards

'Body and soul cannot be separated for purposes of treatment, for they are one and indivisible. Sick minds must be healed as well as sick bodies.' C Jeff Miller, 1931.

Mental state examination: ASEPTIC

- **A**ppearance and behaviour: dress, hygiene, eye contact, rapport.
- **S**peech: volume, rate, tone.
- **E**motion: mood (subjective and objective), affect (how mood is expressed with behaviour—appropriate or incongruent?).
- **P**erception: hallucinations—auditory (in the second or third person)?, visual?
- **T**hought:
  - Form: block, insertion, broadcast, flight of ideas, knight's move.
  - Content: delusions, obsessions, phobias, preoccupations, *self-harm, suicide.*
- **I**nsight: ask the patient why they have presented today.
- **C**ognition: orientation, registration, recall, concentration, knowledge.

Do not be afraid to ask about suicidal thoughts and plans. Remove yourself from the situation if you feel threatened.

Depression

Two questions can be used to identify depression:[19]

1. *During the last month, have you been bothered by feeling down, depressed, or hopeless?*
2. *During the last month, have you often been bothered by having little interest or pleasure in doing things?*

If a person answers 'yes' to either question they should undergo mental health assessment including a risk assessment of self-harm and suicide. Appropriate treatments include psychosocial intervention (guided self-help, cognitive behavioural therapy, structured physical activity) and medication. Treatment choice depends on disease severity, previous psychiatric history, response to treatment, and patient preference. If medication is indicated, a generic SSRI should be considered first line after consideration of GI bleeding risk, drug interactions, toxicity, overdose, and discontinuation symptoms. The full effect of medication is gradual, over 4–6 weeks.

Capacity

The Mental Capacity Act (MCA) 2005 has a two-stage test for lack of capacity:

1. There is an impairment or disturbed functioning of the mind.
2. The patient is unable to make a decision.

Decision-making is impaired if the patient is unable to: *understand* the relevant information, *retain* it for long enough to make a decision, *weigh up* the information, *communicate* their decision. Capacity is decision-specific not patient-specific. When treatment is proposed to those who lack capacity, a capacity advocate should be provided. Even patients without capacity should be as involved as possible in decision-making.

Mental Health Act (MHA) and common law

A patient can be detained under common law (subject to a test of reasonableness) or under the MHA, only if they lack capacity to remain informally and are a danger to themselves or others. You will have more experience in verbal and non-verbal communication, than in detention under the MHA, so use these skills first to try and de-escalate the situation. If rapid tranquillization is needed, be familiar with dosage, side-effects, and the need for ongoing observation. If there is no history to guide choice of medication, intramuscular lorazepam can be used.[20]

Doctors and mental health

Suicide rates are three times higher in doctors compared to the general population. Up to 7% of doctors will have a substance abuse problem within their lifetime. Do not ignore feeling low, poor concentration, and reduced energy levels. Do not self-diagnose and manage. Avoid 'corridor consultations'. Trust your GP. Seek support:

- British Medical Association: www.bma.org.uk/doctorsfordoctors.
- Doctors' Support Network: www.dsn.org.uk.
- Doctors' Support Line: 0844 395 3010.
- Sick Doctors Trust: www.sick-doctors-trust.co.uk.

'To know how to grow old is the master-work of wisdom, and one of the most difficult chapters in the great art of living.' Henri Amiel, *Journal Intime*, 21 Sept 1874.

Ageing is an inevitable and irreversible decline in organ function that occurs with time, in the absence of injury or illness, and despite the existence of complex pathways of maintenance and repair.

Healthy ageing is the maintenance of physical and mental abilities that enable well-being and independence in older age.

►Do not presume ageing. Look for preventable and reversible pathology. Old age does not cause disease (although it can increase vulnerability and recovery time).

►Look for ways to reduce disability and support older people in their own homes.

Differences in the evaluation of the older person

1 *Multiple pathologies:* Elderly patients have, on average, six diagnosable disorders. Effects may be multiplicative. Treatment must be integrated.
2 *Multiple aetiologies:* One problem may have several causes, eg falls. Treating each alone may do little good, treating all may be of great benefit.
3 *Non-specific/atypical presentation:* Delirium, dizziness, falls, mobility problems, weight loss, and incontinence can be due to disorders in more than one organ system. Typical signs and symptoms may be absent. Ask about functional decline in activities of daily living—this may be the only symptom.
4 *Missed or delayed diagnosis:* The older person may decline quickly if treatment is delayed. Complications are common. Use a collateral history: what is the patient usually like?
5 *Pharmacy and polypharmacy:* NSAIDs, anticoagulants, anti-parkinson drugs, hypoglycaemic drugs, and psychoactive drugs can pose a particular risk in the older patient. Double check for interactions. Consider body weight, liver and renal function—drug doses may need to be modified. The STOPP/START criteria detail >100 potentially inappropriate prescriptions and prescribing omissions relevant to the older patient.[21]
6 *Prolonged recovery time:* Anticipate and plan for this. Don't forget nutrition.
7 *Rehabilitation and social factors:* Essential for healthy ageing.

A quick ward assessment of the older person

History: In addition to routine elements, include function in activities of daily living, continence, and social support. Ask if there is an advanced care directive and nominated proxy healthcare decision maker.

Examination:

- Appearance and affect: hygiene, nutrition, hydration. Briefly assess mood.
- Senses: vision, hearing, assess swallowing with 20mL of water.
- Cognition: brief screening test, eg AMTS (p64), 2-step command.
- Pulse and blood pressure: lying/sitting *and* standing.
- Peripheral neurological exam: tone, power, wasting, active range of movement.
- Other periphery: pulses, oedema, skin integrity, pressure areas.
- Walking: stand patient, balance, transfers, observe gait (be ready to assist).
- Other systems: CV, respiratory, abdomen (don't forget to palpate for bladder).[22]

Falls

50% aged >80 will fall at least once per year. Falls[23] lead to injury, pain, distress, loss of confidence, loss of independence, and mortality. Cost to the NHS is £2.3bn/year.

- History: frequency, context and circumstances, severity, injuries.
- Multifactorial risk assessment: gait, balance, muscle strength, osteoporosis risk, perceived functional ability, fear of falls, vision, cognition, neurological examination, continence, home and hazards, cardiovascular examination, medication review.
- Interventions: strength and balance training, home hazard intervention, correct vision, modification/withdrawal of medication (cardiovascular, psychotropic), integrated management of contributing morbidities. Consider barriers to change, eg fear, patient preference.

The pregnant woman

►Pre-existing conditions and non-obstetric disease cause more maternal deaths in the UK than obstetric complications.[24]

►Pregnant women should receive the same investigations and treatment as non-pregnant patients, with avoidance of harm/potential harm to the fetus whenever possible.

►Most mistakes made in the medical management of pregnant women are due to acts of omission caused by inappropriate weighting of risk and benefit.

Physiological changes in pregnancy

Clinical assessment in pregnancy requires knowledge of the physiological changes associated with the gravid state. Expected changes and guidance on when to investigate for possible underlying pathology is given in **table 1.3**

Table 1.3 Physiology and pathology in pregnancy

System	Normal pregnancy	Consider pathology
Cardiovascular	↓BP before 20 weeks' gestation	Diastolic BP >80mmHg in 1st trimester
	↑Heart rate	Sustained tachycardia >100/min
Respiratory	Compensated respiratory alkalosis	Serum bicarbonate <18mmol/L
	No change in PEFR	Decrease in PEFR
	↑Respiratory rate by 10%	Respiratory rate >20/min
Renal	↑GFR and creatinine clearance	Creatinine >85µmol/L (eGFR not valid in pregnancy)
	↑Protein excretion	Protein:creatinine ratio >30mg/mmol
Endocrine	Altered glucose handling	Fasting glucose >5.0mmol/L
Haematology	Haemodilution	Hb <10.5g/dL, platelets <100x10^9/L

Radiology

If the uterus is positioned outside the imaging field of view, the radiation dose to the conceptus is minimal. Exposure from the following investigations is well below the threshold of risk to the fetus:

- Plain radiograph: chest, extremities, spine.
- CT: head, chest (but consider radiation to maternal breast in pregnancy/lactation).

Ultrasound and MRI are preferentially used when imaging the abdomen.

►Reassure your pregnant patient that a chest x-ray is safe. It is the equivalent of 3 days of background radiation. Do not presume it is not required—how else will you pick up the widened mediastinum as a cause for her chest pain?

Drugs

For drugs prescribed in pregnancy, benefit must be balanced against risk (**table 1.4**). For information on drugs in lactation see: https://toxnet.nlm.nih.gov/newtoxnet/lactmed.htm.

Table 1.4 Drugs in pregnancy

Considered safe	Contraindicated
Penicillins	Tetracycline/doxycycline
Macrolides	Ciprofloxacin
Low-molecular-weight heparin	Trimethoprim (1st trimester)
Aspirin	NSAIDs (3rd trimester)
Labetalol	ACE-i
Nifedipine	ARA
Adenosine	Mycophenolate
Prednisolone	Warfarin
Treatment for asthma: salbutamol, ipratropium, aminophylline, leukotriene antagonists	Live vaccines (MMR, BCG, Varicella)

Sepsis

►►Do not underestimate sepsis in pregnancy. Septic shock can be rapid. ***Do not ignore tachypnoea.*** All pregnant women should receive the influenza vaccine.

'The work of epidemiology is related to unanswered questions, but also to unquestioned answers.' Patricia Buffler, North American Congress of Epidemiology, 2011.

► Who, what, when, where, why, and how?

Epidemiology is the study of the distribution of clinical phenomena in populations. It analyses disease in terms of host, agent, and environment (the 'epidemiologist's triad'). It elucidates risks and mechanisms for the development of disease, and reveals potential targets for disease prevention and treatment. Epidemiology does not look at the individual patient, but examines a defined population. How applicable its findings are depend upon how well the ***sample*** population mirrors the ***study*** population, which must, in turn, mirror the ***target*** population. Does your patient fit in this 'target'? If 'yes', then the epidemiological findings may be applicable.

Measures of disease frequency

Incidence proportion is the number of new cases of disease as a proportion of the population. Synonyms include probability of disease, cumulative incidence, risk.

Incidence rate is the number of new cases per unit of person-time, ie one person observed for 5 years contributes 5 person-years of follow-up.

Prevalence is the number of cases that exist at a given time (point prevalence) or time-frame (period prevalence), divided by the total population being studied. For example, the lifetime prevalence of hiccups is ~100% and incidence is millions/year. However, the point prevalence at 3am may be 0 if no one is actually having hiccups.

Comparisons of outcome frequency

Differences in outcome rates between populations point to an ***association*** between the outcome and factors distinguishing the populations (eg a smoking population compared to a non-smoking population). Challenges arise as populations tend to differ from each other in many ways, so it may not be clear which factor(s) affect outcome frequency. This leads to ***confounding***. For example, we might find that heart disease is more common in those who use walking sticks. But we cannot conclude that walking sticks cause heart disease as age is a confounding factor: age is causal, not walking sticks.

Ways of accounting for associations: *A* may cause *B* (antacids cause cancer), *B* may cause *A* (cancer causes antacid use), a 3rd unknown agent *X* (eg age) may cause *A* and *B*, or the association may be a chance finding. When considering the options, it is useful to bear in mind the Bradford Hill 'criteria' for causation (NB he did not claim any were essential):

1 Consistency of findings: among different populations, studies, time periods.
2 Temporality: the effect must occur after the cause.
3 Biological gradient: a dose response whereby more exposure = more effect.
4 Specificity: exposure causes a single outcome (smoking does not conform!).
5 Strength of association: strong associations are more likely to be causal.
6 Biological plausibility: there is a mechanism linking cause and effect.
7 Coherence: the relationship is supported by current disease knowledge.
8 Experiment: does removal of exposure reduce outcome frequency?

Epidemiological studies

Studies should be designed to give an adequate answer to a specific research question. Samples need to be representative and of sufficient size to answer the question.

Ecological studies: Outcome rates are examined in different populations, eg trend over time, geographically distinct groups, social class. Populations rather than individuals are the unit of study.

Longitudinal (cohort) studies: Subjects are followed over time with measurement of exposure and outcome.

Case-control studies: Patients with the outcome of interest are identified and past exposure is assessed in comparison to 'controls' who did not develop the outcome. Cases and controls should be adequately matched for other factors that may affect outcome, or these differences should be corrected for (mathematical assumption).

Experimental studies: Exposure is allocated to a study group and compared to those who are not exposed, eg randomized controlled trials.

Randomized controlled trials

In a randomized controlled trial (RCT), participants are allocated to an intervention/exposure (eg new drug treatment) or no intervention (eg placebo, standard care) by a process which equates to the flip of a coin, ie all participants have an equal chance of being in either arm of the study. The aim is to minimize bias and attempt to get at the truth as to whether the intervention is any good or not. Both groups are followed up and analysed against predefined end-points.

Randomizing Done with the aim of eliminating the effects of non-studied factors. With randomization (and sufficient study size) the two arms of the study will be identical (on average), with the exception of the intervention of interest.

Blinding There is a risk that factors during the trial may affect the outcome, eg participant or clinician optimism if they know the patient is on active treatment, or an unwillingness to expose more severe disease to placebo. If the subject does not know which intervention they are having, the trial is single-blind. Ideally, the experimenter should not know either, and the study should be double-blind.

►In a good trial, the blind lead the blind.

Journal club: how good is this RCT?

- Does the study answer a useful question? Does it add to current literature: bigger, better, different target population?
- Does the target population in the study include your patient(s)? Check the inclusion and exclusion criteria including age and comorbidity.
- Is the intervention well described so it can be replicated in clinical practice?
- Was the sample size big enough to detect an effect? Can you find a sample size calculation? Watch out for sub-group analyses for which the sample size was not calculated.
- Were outcome measures predefined?
- Is randomization adequate? Look at the baseline data for each group—are there significant differences? Are any parameters of interest (that might affect outcome) not included?
- Who was blinded and how blind were they?
- Are statistical methods reported and appropriate? There should be a measure of the effect size and its precision (confidence interval, see p20).
- Is the effect clinically significant? Watch out for surrogate end-points which do not directly measure benefit, harm, or the treatment response of interest.
- How long was the follow-up? Was it long enough to determine outcome?
- How complete was the follow-up? How many patients were left at the end of the follow-up period? Were those who left the study included in the analysis (intention-to-treat)?[25]

When a randomized controlled trial might not be the best method

- Generating new ideas beyond current paradigms (case reports).
- Researching causes of illnesses and prognoses (cohort studies).
- Evaluating diagnostic tests (cohort study and decision model).
- Where the researcher has no idea of the effective dose of a drug (dose-ranging adaptive design).
- When recruiting of patients would be impossible or unethical.
- When personalized medicine is the aim, eg treatments matched to patients' biomarker profiles (adaptive design, cohort study).

►In the end, all randomized trials have to submit to the ultimate test when the statistical collides with the personal: 'Will this treatment help me?', 'Will this procedure help you?' No randomized trial is complete until real-life decisions taken in the light of its findings are scrutinized. Remember Osler: *'no two individuals react alike and behave alike under the abnormal conditions which we know as disease. This is the fundamental difficulty of the physician'.* Do not ask for definitive trials: everything is provisional.

'When you can measure what you are speaking about, and express it in numbers, you know something about it; but when you cannot measure it, when you cannot express it in numbers, your knowledge is of a meagre and unsatisfactory kind.'

Lord Kelvin, 1883.

Comparison measures

Comparisons between 'exposed' and 'unexposed' populations are made in terms of the risk or likelihood of an outcome This can be appreciated by plotting a 2×2 table (table 1.5).

Table 1.5 2×2 table analysis

	Outcome		
Exposure	**Event**	**No event**	**Total**
Yes	70	20	90
No	120	450	570
Total	190	470	

- *Absolute risk difference (attributable risk)* = disease frequency in exposed minus the disease frequency in unexposed. Example (table 1.5): (70/90) – (120/570) = 0.57 ∴ exposure increases risk by 57%.
- *Relative risk* = ratio of outcome in exposed population compared to unexposed. Relative risk of 1 means risk is same in both populations. Relative risk >1 means exposure increases risk. Relative risk <1 means exposure lessens risk, eg vaccination. Example (table 1.5): (70/90)÷(120/570) = 3.69 ∴ risk is 3.69 × higher with exposure.
- *Odds ratio* = ratio of the probability of an outcome occurring compared to the probability of an outcome not occurring. Example (table 1.5): (70/20)÷(120/450) = 13.13 ∴ odds of outcome are 13.13 × higher with exposure.

Relative risk is easier to interpret than odds ratio but relies on a meaningful prevalence/incidence. For the individual, absolute risk difference may be most relevant.

P-values and confidence intervals

In a study of two groups (eg new treatment versus placebo), it is possible that there is no difference (ie new treatment has no benefit). This is the *null hypothesis*. A p-value measures the strength of evidence in relation to the null hypothesis:
- Low p-value: data unlikely if null hypothesis is true.
- High p-value: data likely is null hypothesis is true.

A p-value is not the probability that your results occurred by chance, and it cannot tell you how good a study is. There will be many assumptions in the statistical model. Look at the details: have confounding or bias affected the result? *Do not consider p <0.05 as 'statistically significant'*: a small p-value just flags the data as unusual.[26] You need to question why and decide if this is clinically important.

Confidence intervals (CI) give a guide to the effect size and direction (eg benefit/harm). They give a margin of error that indicates the amount of uncertainty in the statistical estimate.

Assessing validity

The validity of a test which dichotomizes study participants can be assessed by examining the results from the test against a standard reference (or outcome: did the participant actually have the disease?) (see table 1.6).

Sensitivity TP/(TP + FN) = of those with the condition, how many test positive? A sensitive test is able to correctly identify those with the disease.

Specificity TN/(TN + FP) = of those who do not have the condition, how many test negative? A specific test is able to correctly identify those without a disease.

'Do they have abdominal pain?' as a test for appendicitis will have ↑sensitivity (most cases have pain), but ↓specificity (many patients with pain do not have appendicitis).

Positive predictive value (TP/(TP + FP) indicates how likely it is that someone with a positive test result has the condition.

Negative predictive value (TN/(TN + FN) indicates how likely it is that someone with a negative test result does not have the condition. When you receive a test result, you need to know how likely it is to be correct.

Table 1.6 Table of possible test results

Test result	Patient has condition	Patient does not have condition
Positive	True positive (TP)	False positive (FP)
Negative	False negative (FN)	True negative (TN)

Number needed to treat

Number needed to treat (NNT) is a useful way of reporting the results of randomized clinical trials. It is the reciprocal of the absolute risk difference: 1 ÷ ARR.

A large treatment effect means that fewer patients need to receive treatment in order for one to benefit. It is specific to the chosen comparator (eg placebo or usual care), the measured outcome (eg death, blood pressure fall), and the duration of treatment follow-up used in the study. Look carefully at the details of the question that the NNT is attempting to quantify.

- Advantages: easily calculated, single numerical value for efficacy, can be used to examine harm (becomes the number needed to harm).
- Disadvantages: confidence intervals are difficult when the differences between treatments are not significant.

The doctor as a gambler

Yes or No? Your tutor asks whether Gobble's disease is commoner in women or men. You have no idea, and make a guess. What is the chance of getting it right? Common sense decrees that you have a 50:50 chance. Sod's law predicts that whatever you guess, you will always be wrong. Somewhere between the two is Damon Runyon's view that 'all life is 6 to 5 against': Will you pick the right answer? Perhaps, but don't bet on it!

New or existing disease? Suppose singultus is a rare symptom of Gobble's disease (seen in 5% of patients), but that it is a very common symptom of Kobble's disease (seen in 90%). If we have a man whom we already know has Gobble's disease, who goes on to develop singultus, is it more likely to be due to Kobble's, rather than Gobble's disease? The answer is usually no: it is generally the case that most symptoms are due to a disease that is already known, and do not imply a new disease (Occam's razor, p4). The 'odds ratio' makes this clearer, ie the ratio of [the probability of the symptom, given the known disease] to [the probability of the symptom due to new disease × the probability of developing the new disease]. Usually this is vastly in favour of the symptom being due to the old disease, because of the prior odds of the two diseases. This will work until Kobble's disease increases in prevalence so as to increase the odds of a second disease (then Hickam trumps Occam, p4).

How to play the odds It is distasteful to think that doctors can gamble with patients' lives. It is also distasteful to think of serious diseases being 'missed', and invasive procedures being done unnecessarily. Yet we do not have an evidence base or an experience base which can tell us definitively which cough or lethargy or sore toe is just 'one of those things', and which is the result of undiagnosed cancer or HIV or osteomyelitis. And so we gamble.

Medicine is not for pessimists—almost anything can be made to seem fatal, so that a pessimistic doctor would never get any sleep at night due to worry about the meaning of their patients' symptoms. Medicine is not for blind optimists either, who too easily embrace a fool's paradise of false reassurance. Rather, medicine is for informed gamblers: gamblers who are happy to use subtle clues to change their outlook from pessimism to optimism and vice versa. Sometimes the gambling is scientific, rational, methodical, and reproducible (odds ratio); sometimes it instinctual, due to clinical intuition (vital but ill-defined).

Of course, gambling inevitably results in losses, and in medicine the chips are not just financial. They betoken the health of your patient, your reputation, and your confidence. Perhaps the hardest part of medicine is the inevitability of making mistakes whilst attempting to help (see 'Being wrong', p5). But do not worry about gambling: gambling is your job. If you cannot gamble, you cannot walk the thin line between successfully addressing health needs, and causing over-medicalization (p23). But try hard to assemble sufficient evidence to maximize the chances of being lucky. Lucky gambling is a requisite for successful doctoring and the casino of medical practice celebrates the card counter. But the cardinal clinical virtue is courage: without it we would not follow our hunches and take justified risks.

Evidence-based medicine (EBM)

EBM is the conscientious and judicious use of current, best research evidence to optimize management plans and integrate them with patients' values by:

1 Asking answerable questions.
2 Finding the best information.
3 Appraising the information for quality, validity, and relevance.
4 Dialogue to find out what the patient wants.
5 Applying data to patient care.
6 Evaluation.

The amount of evidence

More than 2 million new biomedical papers are published each year including >20 000 new randomized trials. Patients benefit directly from a tiny fraction of these papers. How do we find them?

- A hierarchy of evidence (fig 1.3) is used to identify the best research available to answer our question.
- Specialist EBM journals, eg *Evidence-based Medicine*, appraise published information for quality, relevance, and interest on our behalf.
- The Cochrane Collaboration gathers and summarizes best evidence, free from commercial sponsorship and conflicts of interest. >37 000 researchers from 130 countries contribute.

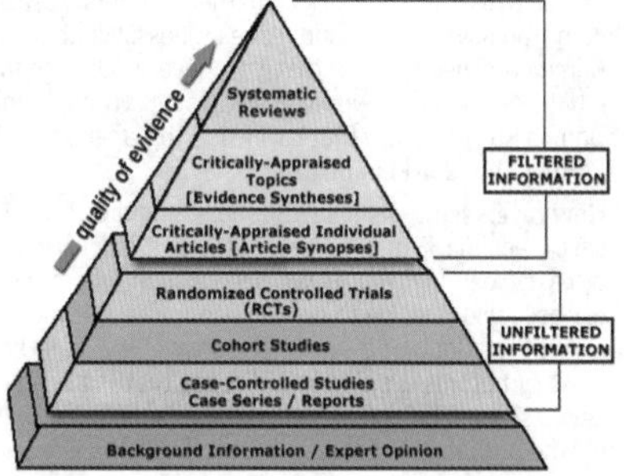

Fig 1.3 Hierarchy of evidence.
EBM Pyramid and EBM Page Generator, copyright 2006 Trustees of Dartmouth College and Yale University.

Problems:

- The concept of scientific rigour is opaque. What do we want? The science, the rigour, the truth, or what will be most useful to patients? These may overlap, but they are not the same. Can average cohort results inform clinical decisions on an individual level (especially in the context of comorbidity)?
- Can we really appraise ALL the evidence?[27] We are hindered by publication bias. Around half of all clinical trials remain unpublished. See www.alltrials.net for the campaign to register all trials, and ensure methods and summary results are available.
- Evidence can be expensive. Who paid the bill and what is their vested interest?
- Is the result clinically significant? What is the level of benefit to the individual, as opposed to the population? Is the EBM tail wagging the clinical dog?
- How is our innate hierarchy of evidence constructed? Do we maintain the same standard of the evidence for all changes to our practice?
- Have you checked the correspondence columns in journals from which winning papers are extracted? It may take years for unforeseen flaws to surface.
- There is a danger that by always asking, 'What is the evidence?', we will divert resources from hard-to-prove areas (eg psychosocial interventions).
- EBM is never 100% up to date and reworking meta-analyses takes time and money. Specialists may ostensibly reject a new trial due to a tiny flaw, when the real dread is that it might flip their once-perfect formulation.
- EBM lies uncomfortably in a world of clinical intuition and instinctual premonition. Yet these instincts may be vital.
- If EBM is prescriptive, patient choice declines. Does our zeal for EBM make us arrogant, mechanical, and defensive? Where is the shared decision-making (p7)?
- By focusing on answerable questions, EBM can distract us from our patients' unanswerable questions; questions that still require time and acknowledgement.

►The practice of EBM must be informed by clinical judgement and compassion.

Medicalization

Using Illness as a Metaphor,[8] Susan Sontag describes two kingdoms: that of the well, and that of the sick. She describes our dual citizenship, and the use of a passport to travel from one kingdom to the other. But medicalization blurs this distinction. The boundary between the 'Kingdom of the Sick' and the 'Kingdom of Well' is lost and there is an anschluss of healthy people annexed into the potentially predatory and frightening kingdom of the sick from which there may well be no escape.

'Too much medicine' occurs as a result of:

- *Overdiagnosis*: Labelling an (asymptomatic) person as 'sick' despite the fact that subsequent treatment, lifestyle advice, or monitoring provides no benefit to their outcome (and potentially causes harm), eg non-progressive breast cancer.
- *Overdetection:* Increasingly sensitive tests identify pathology that is indolent or non-progressive, eg subsegmental pulmonary emboli diagnosed on CT angiography.
- *Overdefiniton:* Expansion of disease definitions or lowering of disease thresholds, eg an eGFR diagnosis of chronic kidney disease now means that 1 in 8 adults are labelled with the disease, many of whom will never progress to symptomatic kidney failure; 15% of pregnant women now have subclinical hypothyroidism without evidence that thyroxine replacement is beneficial (2016).
- *Disease mongering:* The creation of pseudodiseases which pose no threat to health, eg restless legs, sexual health dysfunction, multiple chemical sensitivity.
- *Overutilization:* Healthcare practice that provides no net benefit, eg routine MRI for lower back pain.
- *Overtreatment:* Treatment that is of no benefit (and may cause harm), eg antibiotics for viral infections, polypill for the population.

Too much medicine arises from the fear of missing a diagnosis, and concern about avoidable morbidity or mortality. A punitive society means there is a perceived need for more tests, to seek more certainty. But certainty is the holy grail of myth and legend. The individual patient is a unique set of symptoms, stoicism, experience, and need. And by the nature of life, all cure can only ever be temporary.

Choosing wisely

CHOOSING WISELY is an initiative to change doctors' practice away from interventions that are not:

- supported by evidence
- free from harm
- truly necessary (including duplicative tests).

The top 5-10 interventions that should not be used routinely are given for each specialty. Search for those relevant to your current post at: www.choosingwisely.org/doctor-patient-lists/.

Screening

Consider medicalization when screening for disease. Remember all screening programmes do harm, some do good. The Wilson criteria for screening lists the important features necessary for a screening programme and the mnemonic **IATROGENIC** reminds of our pressing duty to do no harm:

1. The condition screened for should be an **i**mportant one.
2. There should be an **a**cceptable treatment for the disease.
3. Diagnostic and **t**reatment facilities should be available.
4. A **r**ecognizable latent or early symptomatic stage is required.
5. **O**pinions on who to treat must be agreed.
6. The test must be **g**ood: high discriminatory power, valid, and reproducible with safety **g**uaranteed.
7. The **e**xamination must be acceptable to the patient.
8. The untreated **n**atural history of the disease must be known.
9. It should be **i**nexpensive.
10. Screening must be **c**ontinuous (ie not a 'one-off' affair).

8 Susan Sontag, *Illness as a Metaphor*, 1978

2 History and examination

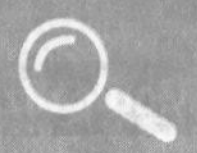

Contents

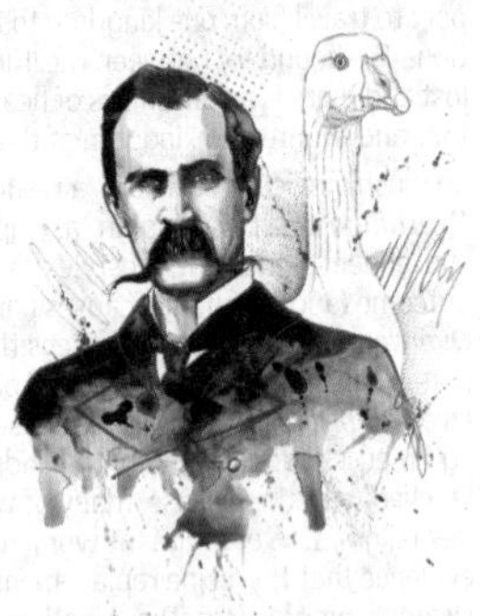

Fig 2.1 William Osler (1849-1919) was a great medical educationalist who loved practical jokes. He introduced many novelties to the classroom, including, on one occasion, a gaggle of geese. We can all identify with his geese, because these birds show exceptional learning ability and resilience.

Osler did not agree with gavage, a method whereby geese (and medical students) are forcibly stuffed by funnel to fatten them for the delight of gluttons. We are too familiar with the three Rs of medical education: Ram→Remember→Regurgitate, a sequence that turns once-bright medical students into tearful wrecks. Luckily in the realm of History & Examination we can flee the library and alight at the bedside, bearing in mind another of Osler's aphorisms: 'He who studies medicine without books sails an uncharted sea, but he who studies medicine without patients does not go to sea at all.'

We thank Dr Petra Sulentic, our Specialist Reader, for her contribution to this chapter.

Advice and experience

1 The way to learn physical signs is at the bedside, with guidance from a senior doctor or an experienced colleague. This chapter is not a substitute for this process: it is simply an aide-memoire both on the wards and when preparing for exams.

2 We ask questions to get information to help with differential diagnosis. But we also ask questions to find out about the lives our patients live so that we can respect them as individuals. The patient is likely to notice and reciprocate this respect, and the rapport that you build with your patient in this way is a key component to diagnosing and managing their disease.

3 Patients (and diseases) rarely read textbooks, so don't be surprised that some symptoms are ambiguous, and others meaningless. Get good at recognizing patterns, but not so good that you create them when none exist. We all fall into this trap!

4 Signs can be easy to detect, or subtle. Some will be found by all the new medical students, others require experienced ears or eyes. Remember, *you can be a fine doctor without being able to elicit every sign.*[1] However, finding signs and putting together the clues they give us to find a diagnosis is one of the best parts of being a doctor. It is also essential that we learn those signs that highlight diseases we should never miss. However, in an exam, if you cannot find a sign, never be tempted to make up something you think should be there. If the examiner is pushing you to describe something you cannot see, be honest and admit you cannot see it. Learning is a lifelong process, and nobody becomes a consultant overnight.

Developing your own routine

While on the acute medical or surgical take you will 'clerk' countless numbers of patients. This involves taking a full history: history-taking may seem deceptively easy, as if the patient knew the hard facts and the only problem was extracting them; but what a patient says is a mixture of hearsay ('She said I looked very pale'), innuendo ('You know, doctor, *down below*'), legend ('I suppose I bit my tongue; it was a real fit, you know'), exaggeration ('I didn't sleep a wink'), and improbabilities ('The Pope put a transmitter in my brain'). The great skill (and pleasure) in taking a history lies not in ignoring these garbled messages, but in making sense of them. Next you will likely perform all the core examinations (cardiovascular, respiratory, abdominal, and neurological) and any relevant additional ones (eg breast, thyroid, peripheral vascular). No two doctors will have identical examination techniques. Relish this variation as it helps you craft your own routine.

An insightful student

Having a template for the all-important history and examination is no more than a rough guide and you must flesh it out with your own learning. We start out nervous of missing some question or sign, but what we should really be nervous about is losing our humanity in the hurly-burly of a time-pressed interview. Here is how one student put some flesh on the bones—for a man in a wheelchair: she asked all about the presenting complaint, and how it fitted in with his CNS condition and life at home—and then found out that his daughter had had a nervous breakdown at the start of his illness, 5 years ago. 'How is she now?' she asked. 'Fine—I've got two lovely grandchildren...Jim is just learning to walk...' 'Oh...you must be so *busy*!' the student said with a joyful smile. This man had not been busy for 5 years, and was fed up with his passive dependency. The thought of being busy again made his face light up—and when the student left he rose up out of his wheelchair to shake her by the hand, a movement we doctors thought was impossible. Jim and his grandfather were learning to walk, but this student was up and running—far ahead of her teachers.

Taking a good history is an art and an essential skill: 80% of diagnoses should be made on history alone, with the signs you elicit adding an extra 10% and tests only giving the final 5% or so. Do not rely on signs or investigations for your diagnosis, but use them rather to confirm what you suspected. Try to put the patient at ease: a good rapport may relieve distress. Introduce yourself and check whether the patient is comfortable. Be conversational rather than interrogative. Start with open questions, allow the patient to tell their story, but if they stray off topic, gently steer them back towards the important points.

Presenting complaint (PC) Open questions: 'Why have you come to see me today?' Record the patient's own words rather than medical terms.

History of presenting complaint (HPC) When did it start? What was the first thing noticed? Progress since then. Ever had it before? 'SOCRATES' questions: **s**ite; **o**nset (gradual, sudden); **c**haracter; **r**adiation; **a**ssociations (eg nausea, sweating); **t**iming of pain/duration; **e**xacerbating and alleviating factors; **s**everity (eg scale of 1-10, compared with worst ever previous pain). *Direct questioning* (to narrow list of possible diagnoses). Specific or 'closed' questions about the differential diagnoses you have in mind (+risk factors, eg travel—p414) and a review of the relevant system.

Past medical history (PMH) Ever in hospital? Illnesses? Operations? Ask specifically about MIJTHREADS: **MI**, **j**aundice, **T**B, **h**igh BP, **r**heumatic fever, **e**pilepsy, **a**sthma, **d**iabetes, **s**troke, anaesthetic problems.

Drug history (DH) Any tablets, injections, 'over-the-counter' drugs, herbal remedies, oral contraceptives? Ask about *allergies* and what the patient experienced, eg may be an intolerance (nausea, diarrhoea), or may have been a minor reaction of sensitization (eg rash and wheeze) before full-blown anaphylaxis.

Social history (SH) Probe without prying. 'Who else is there at home?' Job. Marital status. Spouse's job and health. Housing—any stairs at home? Who visits—relatives, neighbours, GP, nurse? Are there any dependants at home? Mobility—any walking aids needed? Who does the cooking and shopping? What can the patient not do because of the illness? Ask about occupation, hobbies, sport, exercise, and ethnic origin.

The social history is all too often seen as a dispensable adjunct but vital clues may be missed about the quality of life and it is too late to ask when the surgeon's hand is deep in the belly and they are wondering how radical a procedure to perform. Utilize the GP's knowledge of the patient: they may have known them and/or their family for decades. He or she may even hold a 'living will' or advance directive if they cannot speak for themselves. Tactfully ask about *alcohol, tobacco, and recreational drugs*. How much? How long? When stopped? 1 unit = 8g of ethanol = 1 spirits measure = 1/2 glass of wine = 1/3 pint of beer. The CAGE questionnaire is a useful screening test for alcoholism (p281). Quantify smoking in terms of **pack-years**: 20 cigarettes/day for 1 year equals 1 pack-year. We all like to present ourselves well, so be inclined to double stated quantities (Holt's 'law').

Family history (FH) Areas of the family history may need detailed questioning, eg to determine if there is a significant family history of heart disease you need to ask about the health of the patient's grandfathers and male siblings, smoking, tendency to hypertension, hyperlipidaemia, and claudication before they were 60 years old, as well as ascertaining the cause of death. Ask about TB, diabetes, and other relevant diseases. Draw a family tree (see BOX). ►*Be tactful when asking about a family history of malignancy.*

Systemic enquiry (See p30.) Helps uncover undeclared symptoms. Some of this may already have been incorporated into the history.

► Always enquire, without sounding robotic, if your patient has any *ideas* of what the problem might be, if he/she has any particular *concerns* or *expectations*, and give him/her an opportunity to *ask you questions* or *tell you anything you may have missed*.

► Don't hesitate to review the history later: recollections change (as you will find, often on the post-take ward round when the Consultant is asking the questions!).

Drawing family trees to reveal dominantly inherited disease

Advances in genetics are touching all branches of medicine. It is increasingly important for doctors to identify patients at high risk of genetic disease, and to make appropriate referrals. The key skill is drawing a family tree to help you structure a family history as follows:

1 Start with your patient. Draw a square for a male and a circle for a female. Add a small arrow (see fig 2.2) to show that this person is the *propositus* (the person through whom the family tree is ascertained).

2 Add your patient's parents, brothers, and sisters. Record basic information only, eg age, and if alive and well (a&w). If dead, note age and cause of death, and pass an oblique stroke through that person's symbol.

3 Ask the key question 'Has anybody else in your family had a similar problem as yourself?', eg heart attack/angina/stroke/cancer. Ask only about the family of diseases that relate to your patient's main problem. Do not record a potted medical history for each family member: time is too short.

4 Extend the family tree upwards to include grandparents. If you haven't revealed a problem by now, *go no further*—you are unlikely to miss important familial disease. If your patient is elderly it may be impossible to obtain good information about grandparents. If so, fill out the family tree with your patient's uncles and aunts on both the mother's and father's sides.

5 Shade those in the family tree affected by the disease. ● = an affected female; ■ = an affected male. This helps to show any genetic problem and, if there is one, will help demonstrate the pattern of inheritance.

6 If you have identified a familial susceptibility, or your patient has a recognized genetic disease, extend the family tree down to include children, to identify others who may be at risk and who may benefit from screening. ►You should find out who is pregnant in the family, or may soon be, and arrange appropriate genetic counselling (*OHCS* p154). Refer for genetics opinion.

The family tree (fig 2.2) shows these ideas at work and indicates that there is evidence for genetic risk of colon cancer, meriting referral to a geneticist. N.B: use a different approach in paediatrics, and for autosomal or sex-linked disease. Ask if parents are related (consanguinity ↑risk of recessive diseases).

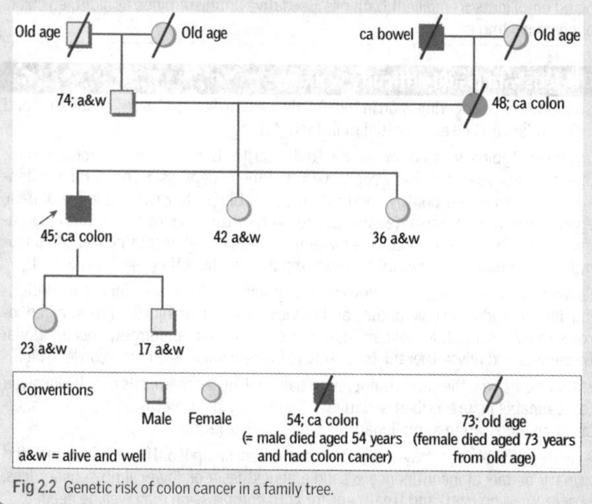

Fig 2.2 Genetic risk of colon cancer in a family tree.

Acknowlegement

The box in this section owes much to Dr Helen Firth, who we thank.

Symptoms are features which patients report. *Physical signs* are elicited at the bedside. Together, they constitute the features of the condition in that patient. Their evolution over time and interaction with the physical, psychological, and social spheres comprise the natural history of any disease. Throughout this chapter, we discuss symptoms in isolation and attempt to classify them into a 'system' or present them in the following BOXES as 'non-specific'. This is unnatural but a good first step in learning how to diagnose. All doctors have to know about symptoms and their relief. Part of becoming a good doctor is learning to link symptoms together, to identify those that may be normal, and those that are worrying. There are many online tools and books that can help with this, but there is no substitute for experience. If you aren't sure, ask a specialist in that area for advice.

The following are common 'non-specific' presentations.

Itch

Itching (pruritus) Common and, if chronic, most unpleasant.

Table 2.1 Aetiology of pruritus

Local causes	Systemic (do FBC, ESR, glucose, LFT, U&E, ferritin, TFT)	
Eczema, atopy, urticaria	Liver disease (bile salts, eg PBC)	Old age; pregnancy
Scabies	Uraemia (eg CKD)	Drugs (eg morphine)
Lichen planus	Malignancy (eg lymphoma)	Diabetes mellitus
Dermatitis herpetiformis	Polycythaemia rubra vera	Thyroid disease
Spinal cord tumours (rare)	Iron deficiency anaemia	HIV infection

Questions: Wheals (urticaria)? Worse at night? Others affected (scabies)? What provokes it? After a bath ≈ polycythaemia rubra vera (p366). Exposure, eg to animals (atopy?) or fibre glass (irritant eczema?).

See table 2.1. Look for *local causes:* Scabies burrows in finger webs, lice on hair shafts, knee and elbow blisters (dermatitis herpetiformis). *Systemic:* Splenomegaly, nodes, jaundice, flushed face, or thyroid signs? ℞: Treat causes; try soothing bland emollients ± emollient bath oils ± sedative antihistamines at night, eg chlorphenamine 4mg PO.

'Off-legs'—falls and difficulty walking

Common causes of admission in the elderly, and can lead to loss of confidence and independence. Causes are often multifactorial:

Intrinsic: Typically osteo- or rheumatoid arthritis, but remember fractured neck of femur, CNS disease, ↓ vision, cognitive impairment, depression, postural hypotension, peripheral neuropathy, medication (eg antihypertensives, sedatives), pain, eg arthritis, parkinsonism (eg drugs: prochlorperazine, neuroleptics, metoclopramide), muscle weakness (consider vitamin D deficiency), incontinence, UTI, pneumonia, anaemia, hypothyroidism, renal impairment, hypothermia, and alcohol.

Environment: Poor lighting, uneven walking surface. Treatment includes addressing injuries, reducing risk factors, and reducing the risk of injury, eg treat osteoporosis (p682). A multidisciplinary multifactorial approach alongside occupational therapists and physiotherapists is likely to be beneficial. See gait disorders, p467.

If there is ataxia, the cause is not always alcohol: other chemicals may be involved (eg cannabis or prescribed sedatives). There may be a metastatic or non-metastatic manifestation of malignancy, or a cerebellar lesion.

► Bilateral weak legs may suggest a cord lesion: see p466. If there is associated urinary or faecal incontinence ± saddle anaesthesia or lower limb sensory loss, urgent imaging (MRI) and treatment for cord compression may well be needed.

Fatigue

So common that it is a variant of normality. Only 1 in 400 episodes of fatigue leads to visiting the doctor. ►Don't miss depression (p15). Even if depressed, still rule out common treatable causes—eg anaemia, hypothyroidism, diabetes. After history and examination: FBC, ESR, U&E, plasma glucose, TFT, ± CXR. Follow up to see what develops, and to address emotional problems. Take a sleep history.

Fevers, rigors, sweats

While some night sweating is common in anxiety, drenching sweats requiring changes of night-clothes are a more ominous symptom associated with infection (eg TB, brucellosis), lymphoproliferative disease, or other malignancies. Patterns of fever may be relevant (see p442).

Rigors are uncontrolled paroxysms of shivering which occur as a patient's temperature rises rapidly.

Sweating excessively (hyperhidrosis) may be primary (eg hidradenitis suppurativa may be very distressing to the patient)—or secondary to fever, pain or anxiety (cold & sweaty) or a systemic condition: the menopause, hyperthyroidism (warm & sweaty), acromegaly, malignancy, phaeochromocytoma, amyloidosis, or neuroleptic malignant syndrome (+hyperthermia). Or it may reflect gabapentin or opiate withdrawal, or a cholinergic or parasympathomimetic side-effect (amitriptyline, bethanechol, distigmine, spider bites)—also hormonal drugs, eg levothyroxine, gonadorelin or somatostatin analogues, vasopressin, and ephedrine. Also amiodarone, ciprofloxacin, levodopa, lisinopril, rivastigmine, ritonavir, pioglitazone, venlafaxine. At the bedside: ask about all drugs, examine all over for nodes; any signs of hyperthyroidism? Any splenomegaly? Test the urine; do T°, ESR, TSH, FBC, & blood culture. ℞: Antiperspirants (aluminium chloride 20%=Driclor®), sympathectomy, or iontophoresis may be tried.

Insomnia

This is trivial—until we ourselves have a few sleepless nights. Then sleep becomes the most desirable thing imaginable, and bestowing it the best thing we can do, like relieving pain. But don't give drugs without looking for a cause.

- ***Self-limiting:*** Jet lag; stress; shift work; in hospital. We need less sleep as we age.
- ***Psychic:*** Depression; anxiety; mania; grief; psychomotor agitation/psychosis.
- ***Organic:*** Drugs (many; eg caffeine; mefloquine; nicotine withdrawal); nocturia; alcohol; pain (eg acid reflux—worse on lying down); itch; tinnitus; asthma; dystonias; obstructive sleep apnoea (p194); dementia; restless leg syndrome (p698, check ferritin). Rarer: encephalitis (eg West Nile virus) and encephalopathy (Whipple's; pellagra; HIV; prion diseases, eg CJD, p696, and fatal familial insomnia).

℞ ***Sleep hygiene.*** No daytime naps; don't turn in till you feel sleepy; regular bedtime routines. Keep a room for sleep; don't eat or work in it (not viable for much of the world). Less caffeine, nicotine, late exercise (but sexual activity may give excellent torpor!), and alcohol (its abuse causes paradoxical pro-adrenergic tremor and insomnia). Try monitoring quality with a sleep diary (unless already overobsessive). Music and relaxation may make sleep more restorative and augment personal resources.

Hypnotic drugs. Give for a few nights only (addictive and cause daytime somnolence ± rebound insomnia on stopping). Warn about driving/machine use. Example: zopiclone 3.75–7.5mg. ***Obstructive sleep apnoea***, p194. ***Parasomnias***, ***sleep paralysis***, etc. *OHCS* p371. ***Narcolepsy***, p700.

Systemic enquiry

Just as skilled acrobats are happy to work without safety nets, so experienced clinicians may operate without the functional enquiry. But to do this you must be experienced enough to understand all the nuances of the presenting complaint.

General questions

May be the most significant, eg in TB, endocrine problems, or cancer:

- Weight loss.
- Night sweats.
- Any lumps.
- Fatigue/malaise/lethargy.
- Sleeping pattern.[1]
- Appetite.
- Fevers.
- Itch or rash.
- Recent trauma.

Cardiorespiratory symptoms

- Chest pain (p94).
- Exertional dyspnoea (=breathlessness): quantify exercise tolerance and how it has changed, eg stairs climbed, or distance walked, before onset of breathlessness.
- Paroxysmal nocturnal dyspnoea (PND). Orthopnoea, ie breathlessness on lying flat (a symptom of left ventricular failure): quantify in terms of number of pillows the patient must sleep on to prevent dyspnoea.
- Oedema: ankles, legs, lower back (dependent areas).
- Palpitations (awareness of heartbeats): can they tap out the rhythm?
- Cough: sputum, haemoptysis (coughing up blood).
- Wheeze.

Gastrointestinal symptoms

- Abdominal pain (constant or colicky, sharp or dull; site; radiation; duration; onset; severity; relationship to eating and bowel action; alleviating or exacerbating, or associated features).
- Other questions—think of symptoms throughout the GI tract, from mouth to anus:
  - Swallowing (p250).
  - Indigestion (p252).
  - Nausea/vomiting; blood? (p250).
  - Bowel habit (p258 & p260).
  - Stool: colour, consistency, blood, mucus; difficulty flushing away (p266); tenesmus or urgency.

Tenesmus is the feeling of incomplete evacuation of the bowels (eg due to a tumour or irritable bowel syndrome). ***Haematemesis*** is vomiting blood. ***Melaena*** is altered (black) blood passed PR (p256), with a characteristic offensive smell and tar like appearance.

Genitourinary symptoms

- Incontinence (stress or urge, p648).
- Dysuria (painful micturition).
- Urinary abnormalities: colour? Haematuria (streaks or pink urine?) Frothy?
- Nocturia (needing to micturate at night).
- Frequency (frequent micturition) or polyuria (the frequent passing of large volumes of urine).
- Hesitancy (difficulty starting micturition).
- Terminal dribbling.
- Vaginal discharge (colour, odour); pain on intercourse (dyspareunia) (p412).
- Menses: frequency, regularity, heavy or light, duration, painful? First day of last menstrual period (LMP). Number of pregnancies and births. Menarche. Menopause. Any chance of pregnancy now?

1 Too sleepy? Think of myxoedema or narcolepsy. Early waking? Think of depression. Being woken by pain is always a serious sign.► For the significance of the other questions listed here, see Chapter 3.

Neurological symptoms

- *Special senses:* sight, hearing, smell, and taste.
- Seizures, faints, 'funny turns'.
- Headache.
- 'Pins and needles' (paraesthesiae) or numbness.
- Limb weakness ('Are your arms and legs weaker than normal?'), poor balance.
- Speech problems (p86).
- Sphincter disturbance.
- Higher mental function and psychiatric symptoms (p86–p89). The important thing is to assess function: what the patient can and cannot do at home, work, etc.

Musculoskeletal symptoms

- Pain, stiffness, swelling of joints.
- Diurnal variation in symptoms (ie worse in mornings).
- Functional deficit.
- Signs of systemic disease: rashes, mouth ulcers, nasal stuffiness, malaise, and constitutional symptoms.

Thyroid symptoms

- *Hyperthyroidism:* Prefers cold weather, bad tempered, sweaty, diarrhoea, oligomenorrhoea, ↓weight (though often ↑appetite), tremor, palpitations, visual problems.
- *Hypothyroidism:* Depressed, slow, tired, thin hair, croaky voice, heavy periods, constipation, dry skin, prefers warm weather.

Physical examination

The physical examination is not so much an extension of the history, but more of the first investigation, to confirm, exclude, define, or show the progress of the provisional diagnosis as revealed in the history. Even in the emergency department where the history may be brief, eg 'trauma', the examination is to confirm a fracture, or to decide that a fracture is less likely. The examination sheds further light on the history. As you get better, your physical examination gets briefer. Establish your own routine—practice is the key.

End of the bed

- Look at the patient—are they well or in extremis? What makes you think this? Are they in pain? If so, does it make them lie still (eg peritonitis) or writhe about (eg colic)? What is the pattern of breathing: laboured; rapid; shallow; irregular; distressed? Are they obese or cachectic? Is their behaviour appropriate? Can you detect any unusual *smell*, eg hepatic fetor (p274), cigarettes, alcohol?
- Also take a moment to look around the bed for other clues, eg inhalers, insulin administration kit, walking aids, etc.

Face and body habitus

- Does the patient's appearance suggest any particular diseases, eg acromegaly, thyrotoxicosis, myxoedema, Cushing's syndrome, or hypopituitarism? See p202.
- Is there an abnormal distribution of body hair (eg bearded ♀, or hairless ♂) suggestive of endocrine disease?
- Is there anything about the patient to trigger thoughts about Paget's disease, Marfan's, myotonia, or Parkinson's syndrome? Look for rashes, eg the malar flush of mitral disease and the butterfly rash of SLE.

Peripheral stigmata of disease

Specific signs are associated with different diseases: consider the nails (koilonychia = iron deficiency), subcutaneous nodules (rheumatoid, neurofibroma?), and look for lymph nodes (cervical, axillary, inguinal). See specific systems for features to assess for, but for all systems consider:

Skin colour:

- Blue/purple = cyanosis (can also be central only, p34).
- Yellow = jaundice (yellow skin can also be caused by uraemia, pernicious anaemia, carotenaemia—check the sclera: if they are also yellow it is jaundice).
- Pallor: this is non-specific; anaemia is assessed from the palmar skin creases (when spread) and conjunctivae (fig 8.3)—usually pale if Hb <80-90g/L: you cannot conclude anything from normal conjunctival colour, but if they are pale, the patient is probably anaemic.
- Hyperpigmentation: Addison's, haemochromatosis (slate-grey) and amiodarone, gold, silver, and minocycline therapy.

Charts:

- Temperature: varies during the day; a morning oral temperature >37.2°C or evening >37.7°C constitutes a fever.[3] Rectal temperatures are generally 0.6°C above oral temperatures. Remember that temperatures are generally lower in elderly patients and therefore fevers may not be as pronounced.[4] A core temperature <35°C indicates hypothermia; special low-reading thermometers may be required.
- Blood pressure and pulse—trends are more important than one-off values; repeat if concerned.
- Urine: check urinalysis and input/output charts if available.

Fluid status When admitting an unwell patient, don't forget to assess their hydration, check skin turgor and mucous membranes, look for sunken eyes, and check capillary refill (if well perfused <2s) and JVP.

Unexplained signs and symptoms: how to refer for an opinion

►*When you don't know: ask. If you are wondering if you should ask: ask.*

Frequently, the skills needed for diagnosis or treatment will lie beyond the team you are working for, so, during ward rounds, agree who should be asked for an opinion. You will be left with the job of making the arrangements, so check before your senior leaves exactly what their question is. Don't be intimidated, but follow these simple rules:

- Know the history and examination findings (ideally your own), and have the patient's notes, observations, recent test results, and drug charts to hand (table 2.2).
- At the outset, state if you are just looking for advice or if you are asking if the patient could be seen. Make it clear exactly what the question is that you want addressed, allowing the listener to focus their thoughts and ask relevant questions.
- Give the patient's age and run through a *brief* history including relevant past medical history. If you would like the patient to be seen, give warning if they will be leaving the ward for a test at a particular time.
- The visiting doctor may be unfamiliar with your ward. When he or she arrives introduce yourself, get the notes and charts, and give your contact details in case they have further questions.

Table 2.2 Referring for a specialist opinion

Team	Key questions
Anaesthetics	Previous anaesthetic? Reaction? Last ate/drank?
Cardiology	Known IHD? BP? ECG findings? Echo findings? Murmurs? Troponin? Temperature/possibility of endocarditis? (ESR, microscopic haematuria, etc. p150)
Dermatology	Site, onset, and appearance of rash? Drugs? Systemic disease? History of atopy?
Endocrinology	Diabetes: blood glucose, usual insulin regimen, complications. Other: blood results? Stable/unstable—eg Addisonian crisis. Usual steroid dose?
Gastroenterology/ Hepatology	Bleeding: Rockall score (p257)? Shock? Diarrhoea: blood? Foreign travel? Frequency per day? Liver disease: signs of decompensation (p274)? Ascites? Encephalopathy grade?
Gynaecology/ Obstetrics	LMP? Possibility of pregnancy? Previous pregnancies? Vaginal discharge? Hormonal contraceptives? STIs?
Haematology	Blood results? Splenomegaly? Fever? Lymphadenopathy? Bleeding: anticoagulants? Clotting results?
Infectious diseases/ Microbiology	Possible source? Antibiotics (current/recent/previous)? Foreign travel? Risk factors for HIV?
Nephrology	Creatinine (current, old)? Clotting? Urine output? Potassium? BP? Fluid status? Drugs? Known renal disease?
Neurology/Stroke	Neurological examination?* CT/MRI scan findings?
Radiology	See p720. Contrast or not? Creatinine? Clotting? Cannula *in situ*? Metallic implants?
Respiratory	O_2 sats? Respiratory rate? ABG? CXR? Inhalers/nebs? Home O_2? Respiratory support, eg NIV/CPAP?
Surgery (general)	Pain? Scan findings? Acutely unwell? Clotting?
Urology	History of LUTS (lower urinary tract symptoms) p642? Catheter? Haematuria? History of stones? Scan findings (ultrasound, CT)?

*You would be amazed at how many people refer to neurology/stroke without having done a neurological examination! Don't be one of them...

The following signs are not specific to a particular system:

Cyanosis
Dusky blue skin (*peripheral*—of the fingers) or mucosae (*central*—of the tongue), representing 50g/L of Hb in its reduced (hence hypoxic) form, it occurs more readily in polycythaemia than anaemia.

Causes:

- *Lung disease* with inadequate oxygen transfer, eg luminal obstruction, asthma, COPD, pneumonia, PE, pulmonary oedema—may be correctable by ↑ inspired O_2.
- *Congenital cyanotic heart disease*, where there is a mixture, eg transposition of the great arteries or right-to-left shunt (eg VSD with Eisenmenger's syndrome; see p156)—cyanosis is *not* reversed by increasing inspired oxygen.
- *Rare causes*—methaemoglobinaemia, a congenital or acquired red cell disorder.

►Acute cyanosis is an emergency. Is there asthma, an inhaled foreign body, a pneumothorax (p749, fig 1) or pulmonary oedema? See p814.

Peripheral cyanosis will occur in causes of central cyanosis, but may also be induced by changes in the peripheral and cutaneous vascular systems in patients with normal oxygen saturations. It occurs in the cold, in hypovolaemia, and in arterial disease, and is, therefore, not a specific sign.

Pallor
May be racial or familial—or from anaemia, shock/faints, Stokes-Adams attack (p460, pale first, then flushing), hypothyroidism, hypopituitarism, and albinism.

Anaemia is haemoglobin concentration <130g/L in men and <120g/L in non-pregnant women (p324). It may be assessed from the conjunctivae and skin creases. Koilonychia and stomatitis (p32) suggest iron deficiency. Anaemia with jaundice suggests haemolysis. ►►If pallor just one limb or digit, think of emboli.

Skin discolouration
Generalized hyperpigmentation may be genetic (racial) or due to radiation; ↑ACTH (cross-reacts with melanin receptors, eg Addison's disease (p226), Nelson's syndrome (p76), ectopic ACTH in bronchial carcinoma); chronic kidney disease (↑urea, p302); malabsorption; chloasma (seen in pregnancy or with the oral contraceptive pill); biliary cirrhosis; haemochromatosis ('bronzed diabetes'); carotenaemia; or drugs (eg chlorpromazine, busulfan, amiodarone, gold).

Obesity
Defined by the World Health Organization as a BMI of over 30kg/m^2. A higher waist to hip ratio, indicating central fat distribution, is commoner in ♂ and is associated with greater health risks, which include type 2 diabetes mellitus, IHD, dyslipidaemia, ↑BP, osteoarthritis of weight-bearing joints, and cancer (breast and bowel); see p206. The majority of cases are not due to specific metabolic disorders. Lifestyle change is key to treatment, to increase energy expenditure and reduce intake (p244). Medication ± surgery may be considered if the patient fulfils strict criteria (BMI of 40 kg/m^2 or more, or between 35 kg/m^2 and 40 kg/m^2 and other significant disease that could improve with weight loss, non-surgical measures have been tried and failed, patient receives intensive management in a tier 3 service, and fit for anaesthesia and surgery). Conditions associated with obesity include: genetic (Prader-Willi syndrome, Lawrence-Moon syndrome), hypothyroidism, Cushing's syndrome, and hypothalamic damage (eg tumour or trauma → damage to satiety regions).

Lymphadenopathy

Causes of lymphadenopathy are either reactive or infiltrative:

Reactive:

Infective:

- Bacterial: eg pyogenic, TB, brucella, syphilis.
- Viral: EBV, HIV, CMV, infectious hepatitis.
- Others: toxoplasmosis, trypanosomiasis.

Non-infective: sarcoidosis, amyloidosis, berylliosis, connective tissue disease (eg rheumatoid, SLE), dermatological (eczema, psoriasis), drugs (eg phenytoin).

Infiltrative:

Benign histiocytosis—*OHCS* p644, lipoidoses.

Malignant:

- *Haematological*: lymphoma or leukaemia: ALL, CLL, AML (p356).
- *Metastatic carcinoma*: from breast, lung, bowel, prostate, kidney, or head and neck cancers.

Oedema

(See p579.)

Pitting oedema: Fluid can either be squeezed out of the veins (increased hydrostatic pressure, eg DVT, right heart failure) or diffuse out because of reduced oncotic pressure (low plasma proteins, eg cirrhosis, nephrotic syndrome, protein-losing enteropathy) leading to an osmotic gradient with the tissues (fig 2.9, p39, p579). The cause of oedema is still not completely understood.[5]

Periorbital oedema: Oedema around the face has a very different differential; the eyelid skin is very thin so periorbital oedema is usually the first sign—think of allergies (contact dermatitis, eg from eye make-up, stings), angioedema (can be hereditary), infection (►orbital cellulitis can be life-threatening, refer to hospital immediately if concerned, other infections include EBV and sinusitis); if there is proptosis (p219) think Graves' disease, connective tissue diseases (eg dermatomyositis, SLE, sarcoid, amyloid); and many others. Assess for systemic disease before putting it down to allergies.

Non-pitting oedema: Ie non-indentable, is lymphoedema due to poor lymphatic drainage. Can be due to radiotherapy, malignant infiltration, infection, filariasis, or rarely primary lymphoedema (Milroy's syndrome p706).

Weight loss

Weight loss can be both a symptom (ie reported by the patient) and a sign (identified by physician). A feature of chronic disease, depression, malnutrition, malignancy, chronic infections (eg TB, HIV/enteropathic AIDS), diabetes mellitus, and hyperthyroidism (typically in the presence of increased appetite). Severe generalized muscle wasting is also seen as part of a number of degenerative neurological diseases and in cardiac failure (cardiac cachexia), although in the latter, right heart failure may not make weight loss a major complaint. Do not forget anorexia nervosa (*OHCS* p382) as an underlying cause of weight loss.

Rule out treatable causes, eg diabetes is easy to diagnose—TB can be very hard. For example, the CXR may look like cancer so don't forget to send bronchoscopy samples for ZN stain and TB culture. Unintentional weight loss should always ring alarm bells, so assess patients carefully.

Cachexia

General muscle wasting from *famine*, or ↓*eating* (dementia; stroke; MND, p506; anorexia nervosa), *malabsorption* (enteropathic AIDS/slim disease/*Cryptosporidium*; Whipple's) or ↑*catabolism* (neoplasia; CCF; TB; chronic kidney disease; ↑leptin).[6]

Table 2.3 Presenting symptoms and questions to ask

Presenting symptoms	Direct questions
Chest pain (see pp94–5 and p784)	**S**ite? Central? **O**nset? (Sudden? What was the patient doing?) **C**haracter? Ask patient to describe pain (Crushing? Heavy?). **R**adiation? Ask specifically if moves to arm, neck, or jaw? **A**ssociations? Ask specifically about shortness of breath, nausea, sweating. **T**iming? Duration? **E**xacerbating and alleviating factors? Worse with respiration or movement (less likely to be angina)? Relieved by GTN? Worse on inspiration and better when sitting forwards (pericarditis)? **S**everity: out of 10? Is patient known to have angina or chest pain; better/worse/same as usual pain; is it more frequent? Decreasing exercise tolerance? NB: 'heartburn' more likely if 'burning', onset after eating/drinking, worse lying flat, or associated with dysphagia.
Palpitations	'Ever aware of your own heartbeat'? When and how did it start/stop? Duration? Onset sudden/gradual? Associated with blackout (how long)? Chest pain? Dyspnoea? Food related (eg caffeine)? Regular fast palpitations may reflect paroxysmal supraventricular tachycardia (SVT) or ventricular tachycardia (VT). Irregular fast palpitations are likely to be paroxysmal AF, or atrial flutter with variable block. Dropped or missed beats related to rest, recumbency, or eating are likely to be atrial or ventricular ectopics. Regular pounding may be due to anxiety. Slow palpitations are likely to be due to drugs such as β-blockers, or bigeminus (fig 3.34, p129). Reassurance is vital and can be therapeutic. Check a TSH and consider a 24h ECG (Holter monitor, p125). An event recorder, if available, is better than 24h ECGs.
Dyspnoea (see p52, and p782)	Duration? At rest? On exertion? Determine exercise tolerance (and any other reason for limitation, eg arthritis). NYHA classification (p135)? Worse when lying flat, how many pillows does the patient sleep with (orthopnoea)? Does the patient ever wake up in the night gasping for breath (paroxysmal nocturnal dyspnoea), and how often? Any ankle swelling?
Dizziness/ blackouts (see pp460–3)	*Dizziness* is a loose term, so try to clarify if your patient means: did patient lose consciousness, and for how long (short duration suggests cardiac while longer duration suggests a neurological cause)? Any warning (*pre-syncope*)? What was patient doing at the time? Sudden/ gradual? Associated symptoms? Any residual symptoms, eg confusion? How long did it take for patient to return to 'normal'? Tongue biting (pp460–1), seizure, incontinence? Witnessed? Memory loss pre/post event? *Vertigo* (p462), the illusion of rotation of either the patient or their surroundings ± difficulty walking/standing, patients may fall over. *Imbalance*, a difficulty in walking straight but without vertigo, from peripheral nerve, posterior column, cerebellar, or other central pathway failure. *Faintness* ie 'light-headedness', seen in anaemia, ↓BP, postural hypotension, hypoglycaemia, carotid sinus hypersensitivity, and epilepsy.
Claudication	SOCRATES? Foot/calf/thigh/buttock? 'Claudication distance', ie how long can patient walk before onset of pain? Rest pain?

Screen for presenting symptoms (table 2.3) before proceeding to past history:

Past history

Ask specifically about: angina, any previous heart attack or stroke, rheumatic fever, diabetes, hypertension, hypercholesterolaemia, previous tests/procedures (ECG, angiograms, angioplasty/stents, echocardiogram, cardiac scintigraphy, coronary artery bypass grafts (CABGs)).

Drug history

Particularly note aspirin/GTN/β-blocker/diuretic/ACE-i/digoxin/statin/anticoagulant use.

Family history

Enquire specifically if any 1st-degree relatives having cardiovascular events (especially if <60yrs).

Social history

Smoking, impact of symptoms on daily life, alcohol (clarify number of units), hobbies, exercise.

Ischaemic heart disease risk factors

- Hypertension.
- Smoking.
- Diabetes mellitus.
- Family history (1st-degree relative <60yrs old with IHD).
- Hyperlipidaemia.

The cardiovascular system: examination 1

Introduce yourself, obtain consent to examine, and position the patient appropriately: lying on a bed, sitting up at 45°. Expose them to the waist (for female patients, delay until examining the praecordium). Explain what you are doing throughout.

1 General inspection
- Assess general state (ill/well)
- Look for clues (oxygen, GTN spray)
- Colour (pale, cyanosed, flushed)
- Short of breath?
- Scars on chest wall (fig 2.3)?

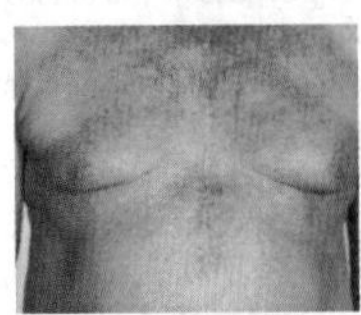

Fig 2.3 CABG scar.

↓

2 Hands
- *Temperature:* Capillary refill time
- *Inspect:*
  Skin: tobacco staining, peripheral cyanosis (fig 2.4), tendon xanthomata, *Janeway lesions*, *Osler's nodes* (signs of infective endocarditis)
  Nails: clubbing, splinter haemorrhages, nail bed pulsation (*Quincke's sign* of aortic regurgitation)

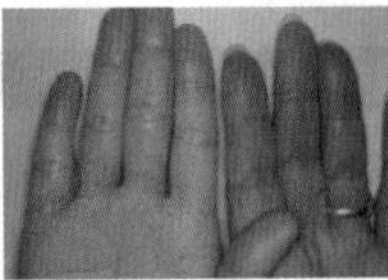

Fig 2.4 Peripheral cyanosis.
Reproduced from Ball G, *et al.* (eds). *Oxford Textbook of Vasculitis* (2014), with permission from Oxford University Press.

↓

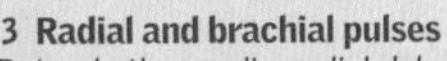

3 Radial and brachial pulses
- *Radial:* Rate, rhythm; radio-radial delay (palpate pulse bilaterally simultaneously), radiofemoral delay (palpate ipsilateral pulses simultaneously), collapsing pulse (identify radial pulse (fig 2.5), then wrap your fingers around wrist. Before elevating arm from the elbow check for pain in arm/shoulder. Lift arm straight up: collapsing pulse, felt as 'waterhammer' pulsation.
- *Brachial:* (Just medial to tendinous insertion of biceps.) Waveform character.

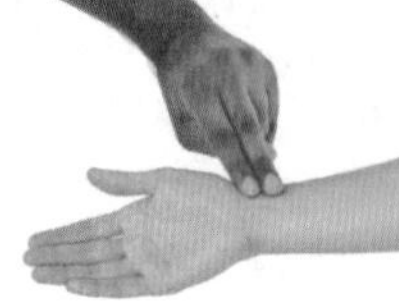

Fig 2.5 Radial pulse.
Reproduced from Thomas J, *et al.* (eds). *Oxford Handbook of Clinical Examination and Practical Skills* (2014), with permission from Oxford University Press.

↓

4 Blood pressure
- Hyper- or hypotensive?
- Pulse pressure (wide = aortic regurgitation, arteriosclerosis, narrow = aortic stenosis, dry)

↓

5 Neck
- *JVP:* Ask patient to turn head to the left and look at the supraclavicular fossa (see fig 2.6 and p43). Comment on the height of the JVP and waveform. Press on the abdomen to check the abdomino-jugular reflex.
- *Carotid pulse:* inspect (visible carotid = *Corrigan's sign* of aortic regurgitation), and palpate volume and character on one side then the other.

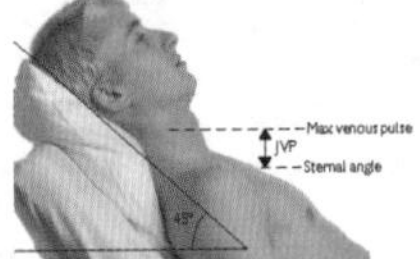

Fig 2.6 The JVP.
Reproduced from Thomas J, *et al.* (eds). *Oxford Handbook of Clinical Examination and Practical Skills* (2014), with permission from Oxford University Press.

6 Face

- *Colour:* Pale, flushed, central cyanosis
- *Features:* Corneal/senile arcus (fig 2.7), xanthelasma (see fig 2.29, p60)
- Pallor of the conjunctiva (anaemia)
- Malar flush (mitral stenosis)
- Dental hygiene

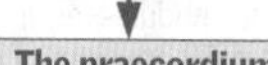

7 The praecordium

Inspect:

- *Scars*—midline sternotomy, lateral thoracotomy (mitral stenosis valvotomy).

Palpate:

- *Apex beat (lowermost lateral pulsation)*—usually 5th intercostal space in mid-clavicular line; measure position by counting intercostal spaces (sternal notch = 2nd intercostal space). Undisplaced/displaced? *Character:* impalpable (?dextrocardia/COPD), tapping (palpable S_1), double impulse, sustained/strong. Count rate if pulse irregular (AF, p130).
- *'Heaves' and 'thrills'*—place the heel of the hand flat on chest to left then right of sternum. *Heave*: sustained, thrusting usually felt at left sternal edge (= right ventricular enlargement). *Thrill*: palpable murmur felt as a vibration beneath your hand.

Auscultate: (palpate carotid pulse simultaneously)

- *Apex (mitral area)*—listen with bell and diaphragm. Identify *1st* and *2nd heart sounds*: are they normal? Listen for *added sounds* (p44) and *murmurs* (p46); with the diaphragm listen for a *pansystolic murmur* radiating to the axilla—*mitral regurgitation* (see fig 2.8).
- At apex with bell, ask the patient to 'Roll over onto your left side, breathe out, and hold it there' (*a rumbling mid-diastolic murmur—mitral stenosis*).
- *Lower left sternal edge (tricuspid area)* and pulmonary area (left of manubrium in the 2nd intercostal space): if suspect right-sided mumur, listen with patient's breath held in inspiration.
- *Right of manubrium in 2nd intercostal space (aortic area)—ejection systolic murmur* radiating to the carotids—*aortic stenosis*.
- Sit the patient up and listen at the lower left sternal edge with patient held in expiration (*early diastolic murmur: aortic regurgitation*?).

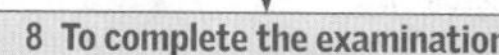

8 To complete the examination

- Palpate for *sacral and ankle oedema* (fig 2.9).
- Auscultate the *lung bases* for inspiratory crackles.
- Examine the abdomen for a *pulsatile liver* and *aortic aneurysm*.
- Check peripheral pulses, observation chart for temperature and O_2 sats, dip urine, perform fundoscopy.

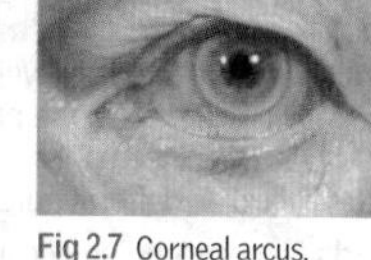

Fig 2.7 Corneal arcus.

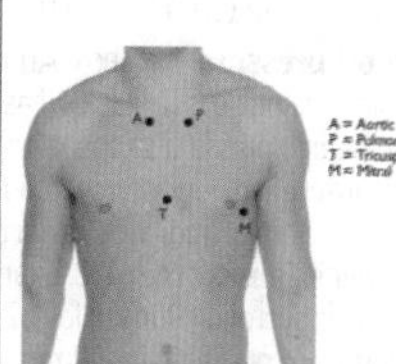

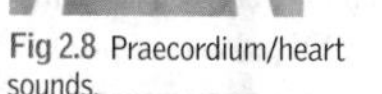

Fig 2.8 Praecordium/heart sounds.

Reproduced from Thomas J, *et al.* (eds). *Oxford Handbook of Clinical Examination and Practical Skills* (2014), with permission from Oxford University Press.

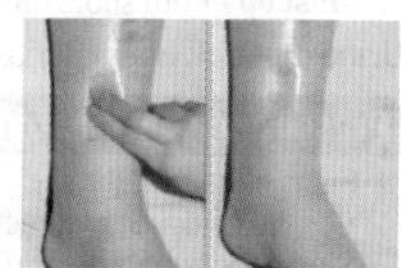

Fig 2.9 Pitting oedema, apply firm pressure for a few seconds.

The cardiovascular system: examination 2

General inspection Ill or well? In pain? Dyspnoeic? Are they pale, cold, and clammy? Can you hear the click of a prosthetic valve? Inspect for *scars*: median sternotomy (CABG; valve replacement; congenital heart disease). Inspect for any pacemakers/ internal cardiac defibrillators (ICDs). Look around the bed for oxygen and GTN spray.

Hands Finger clubbing occurs in congenital cyanotic heart disease and endocarditis. Splinter haemorrhages, Osler's nodes (tender nodules, eg in finger pulps) and Janeway lesions (red macules on palms, fig 3.38, p151) are signs of infective endocarditis. If found, examine the fundi for Roth's spots (retinal infarcts, p560). Are there nail fold infarcts (vasculitis, p556) or nailbed capillary pulsation (Quincke's sign in aortic regurgitation)? Is there arachnodactyly (Marfan's) or polydactyly (ASD)? Are there tendon xanthomata (see BOX 'Hyperlipidaemia')?

Pulse See p42. Feel for *radio-femoral delay* (coarctation of the aorta) and *radio-radial delay* (eg from aortic arch aneurysm).

Blood pressure (see BOX 'An unusual BP measurement') *Systolic* BP is the pressure at which the pulse is first heard as on cuff deflation (Korotkoff sounds); the *diastolic* is when the heart sounds disappear or become muffled (eg in the young). The *pulse pressure* is the difference between systolic and diastolic pressures. It is narrow in aortic stenosis and hypovolaemia, and wide in aortic regurgitation, arteriosclerosis, and septic shock. Defining hypertension: see p138. Examine the fundi for hypertensive changes (p138). *Shock* may occur if systolic <90mmHg (p790). *Postural hypotension* is defined as a drop in systolic >20mmHg or diastolic >10mmHg on standing for 3–5 min (see BOX 'Postural hypotension').

Carotid pulse (See p42.)

Jugular venous pressure (See p43.)

Face Is there corneal arcus (fig 2.7, p39) or xanthelasma (fig 2.29, p60, signifying dyslipidaemia, p690)? Is there a malar flush (mitral stenosis, low cardiac output)? Are there signs of Graves' disease, eg bulging eyes (exophthalmos) or goitre—p218)? Is the face dysmorphic, eg Down's syndrome, Marfan's syndrome (p706)—or Turner's, Noonan's, or Williams syndromes (p149)?

Praecordium Palpate the *apex beat*. Normal position: 5th intercostal space in the mid-clavicular line. Is it displaced laterally? Is it abnormal in nature: *heaving* (caused by outflow obstruction, eg aortic stenosis or systemic hypertension), *thrusting* (caused by volume overload, eg mitral or aortic incompetence), *tapping* (mitral stenosis, essentially a palpable 1st heart sound), *diffuse* (LV failure, dilated cardiomyopathy) or *double impulse* (H(O)CM, p152)? Is there dextrocardia? Feel for *left parasternal heave* (RV enlargement, eg in pulmonary stenosis, cor pulmonale, ASD) or *thrills* (transmitted murmurs).

Auscultating the heart Also auscultate for *bruits* over the carotids and elsewhere, particularly if there is inequality between pulses or absence of a pulse. Causes: atherosclerosis (elderly), vasculitis (young, p556).

Lungs Examine the bases for creps & pleural effusions, indicative of cardiac failure.

Oedema Examine the ankles, legs, sacrum, and torso for pitting oedema. (You may prefer to examine ankles while standing at the foot of the bed as it is a good early clue that there may be further pathology to be found.)

Abdomen Hepatomegaly and ascites in right-sided heart failure; pulsatile hepatomegaly with tricuspid regurgitation; splenomegaly with infective endocarditis.

Fundoscopy Roth spots (infective endocarditis).

Urine dipstick Haematuria.

Presenting your findings

1 Signs of heart failure?
2 Clinical evidence of infective endocarditis?
3 Sinus/abnormal rhythm?
4 Heart sounds normal, abnormal, or additional?
5 Murmurs?

An unusual BP measurement

Don't interpret a BP value in isolation (p138). We cannot diagnose hypertension (or hypotension) on one BP reading. Take into account pain, the 'white coat' effect (BP higher in a medical setting), and equipment. Getting cuff size right is vital. ►*Optimal cuff width is 40% of the arm circumference*. If you suspect a BP reading to be anomalous, check the equipment and review the observation chart for previous readings and other vital signs. Consider taking a manual reading with a different set yourself.

Often a quiet chat will bring the BP down (yours and your patient's: keep your ears open, and the patient may reveal some new tangential but vital fact that the official history glossed over). Many things affect BP readings from background noise to how much you touch the patient. If ↑BP, eg ≳150/90, check both arms. If the systolic difference is >20mmHg, consider peripheral vascular disease, and if the patient could have a thoracic aortic aneurysm or coarctation (rare). NB: right arm diastolic is normally 2.4–5mmHg higher than left.

Postural hypotension

This is an important cause of falls and faints in the elderly. It is defined as a drop in systolic BP >20mmHg or diastolic >10mmHg after standing for 3min vs lying.
Causes: Hypovolaemia (early sign); drugs, eg nitrates, diuretics, antihypertensives, antipsychotics; Addison's (p226); hypopituitarism (↓ACTH); autonomic neuropathy (p505, DM, multisystem atrophy, p494); after a marathon run (peripheral resistance is low for some hours); idiopathic.
Treatment:

- Lie down if feeling faint.
- Stand slowly (with escape route: don't move away from the chair too soon!).
- Consider referral to a 'falls clinic', where special equipment is available for monitoring patient under various tilts.
- Manage autonomic neuropathy, p505.
- ↑Water and salt ingestion can help (eg 150mmol Na^+/d), but Na^+ has its problems.
- Physical measures: leg crossing, squatting, elastic compression stockings (check dorsalis pedis pulse is present), and careful exercise may help.
- If post-prandial dizziness, eat little and often; ↓carbohydrate and alcohol intake.
- Head-up tilt of the bed at night ↑renin release, so ↓fluid loss and ↑standing BP.
- 1st-line drugs: fludrocortisone (retains fluid) 50mcg/d; go up to 300mcg/24h PO only if tolerated. Monitor weight; beware if CCF, renal impairment, or ↓albumin as fludrocortisone worsens oedema.
- 2nd-line drugs: sympathomimetics, eg midodrine (not always available) or ephedrine; pyridostigmine (eg if detrusor under-activity too).
- If these fail, turn things on their head and ask: *is this really supine hypertension?*

Hyperlipidaemia

Xanthomata are localized deposits of fat under the skin, occurring over joints, tendons, hands, and feet. *Xanthelasma* refers to xanthoma on the eyelid (p691, fig 14.13). *Corneal arcus* (fig 2.7, p39) is a crescentic-shaped opacity at the periphery of the cornea. Common in those over 60yrs, can be normal, but may represent hyperlipidaemia, especially in those under this age.

Top tips

The hand can be used as a manometer to estimate JVP/CVP if you cannot see the neck properly (eg central line *in situ*). Hold the hand palm down below the level of the heart until the veins dilate (patient must be warm!), then lift slowly, keeping the arm horizontal. The veins should empty as the hand is raised. Empty veins below the level of the heart suggests a low CVP, if they remain full it suggests a normal/high CVP.

Pulses

►Assess the radial pulse to determine rate and rhythm. *Character and volume* are best assessed at the brachial or carotid arteries. A *collapsing pulse* may also be felt at the radial artery when the patient's arm is elevated above their head. See fig 2.10.

Rate Is the pulse fast (≳100bpm, p126) or slow (≲60bpm, p124)?

Rhythm An irregularly irregular pulse occurs in AF or multiple ectopics. A regularly irregular pulse occurs in 2° heart block and ventricular bigeminus.

Character and volume

- *Bounding pulses* are caused by CO_2 retention, liver failure, and sepsis.
- *Small volume pulses* occur in aortic stenosis, shock, and pericardial effusion.
- *Collapsing ('waterhammer') pulses* are caused by aortic incompetence, AV malformations, and a patent ductus arteriosus.
- *Anacrotic (slow-rising) pulses* occur in aortic stenosis.
- *Bisferiens pulses* occur in combined aortic stenosis and regurgitation.
- *Pulsus alternans* (alternating strong and weak beats) suggests LVF, cardiomyopathy, or aortic stenosis.
- *Jerky pulses* occur in H(O)CM.
- *Pulsus paradoxus* (systolic pressure weakens in inspiration by >10mmHg) occurs in severe asthma, pericardial constriction, or cardiac tamponade.

Peripheral pulses (See p36.) See p771 for arterial blood gas (ABG) sampling.

Waterhammer pulse

The waterhammer was a popular toy that consisted of a vacuum tube half-filled with water. On inversion, the whoosh of water produced an intriguing hammer-blow as it rushed from end to end. This is the alternative name for Corrigan's collapsing pulse—ie one in which the upstroke is abrupt and steep, whose peak is reached early and with abnormal force—before a rapid downstroke (as blood whooshes back into the left ventricle through an incompetent aortic valve).

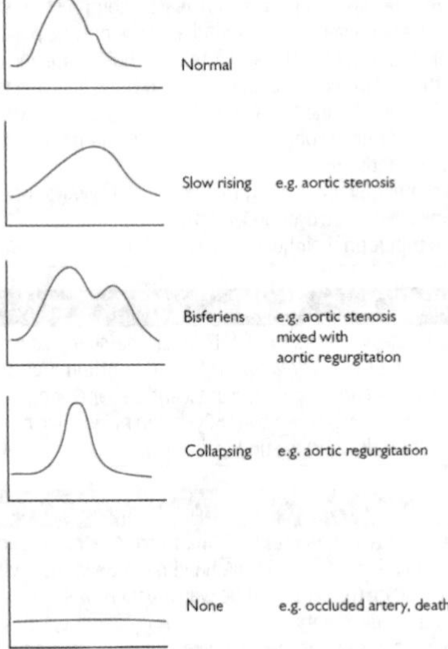

Fig 2.10 Arterial pulse waveforms.

History and examination

The jugular venous pressure (JVP)

The internal jugular vein acts as a capricious manometer of right atrial pressure. Observe the *height* and the *waveform* of the pulse. JVP observations are often difficult. so do not be downhearted if the skill seems to elude you. Examine necks, and the patterns you see may slowly start to make sense—see fig 2.11 for the local venous anatomy. Concomitantly palpate the arterial pulse to help decipher patterns.

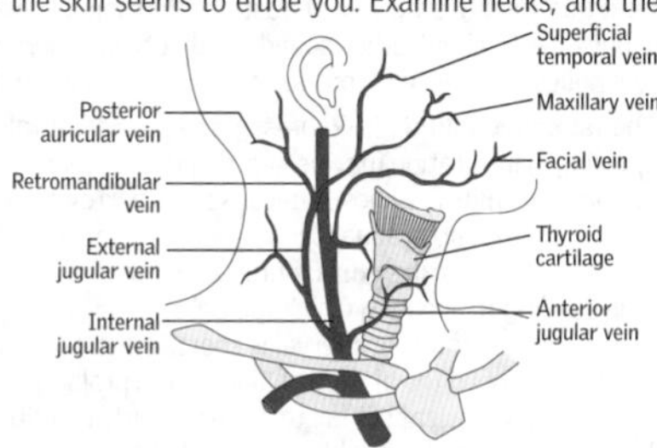

Fig 2.11 The jugular venous system.

The height

Observe the patient at 45°, with their head turned slightly to the left and neck relaxed. Good lighting and correct positioning are key. Look for the right internal jugular vein as it passes just medial to the clavicular head of the sternocleidomastoid up behind the angle of the jaw to the earlobes. The JVP is assessed by measuring the vertical height from the manubriosternal angle (*not* the sternal notch) to the top of the pulse. Pressure at zero (at the sternal angle) is 5cm, so add the height of the JVP with 5cm to obtain the right heart filling pressure in cm of water. A pressure above 9cm (4cm above the sternal angle at 45°) is elevated.

Is the pulse venous (and not arterial)?

- Usually impalpable, and obliterated by finger pressure on the vessel.
- Rises transiently with pressure on abdomen (*abdominojugular reflux*)[2] or on liver (*hepatojugular reflux*), and alters with posture and respiration (disappears when patient sits from lying flat).
- Usually has a double pulse for every arterial pulse. See fig 2.12.

Abnormalities of the JVP

- *Raised JVP with normal waveform:* Fluid overload, right heart failure.
- *Fixed raised JVP with absent pulsation:* SVC obstruction (p528).
- *Large a wave:* Pulmonary hypertension, pulmonary stenosis.
- *Cannon a wave:* When the right atrium contracts against a closed tricuspid valve, large 'cannon' a waves result. *Causes*—complete heart block, single chamber ventricular pacing, ventricular arrhythmias/ectopics.
- *Absent a wave:* Atrial fibrillation.
- *Large v waves:* Tricuspid regurgitation—look for earlobe movement.
- *Constrictive pericarditis:* High plateau of JVP (which rises on inspiration—Kussmaul's sign) with deep x and y descents.
- *Absent JVP:* When lying flat, the jugular vein should be filled. If there is reduced circulatory volume (eg dehydration, haemorrhage) the JVP may be absent.

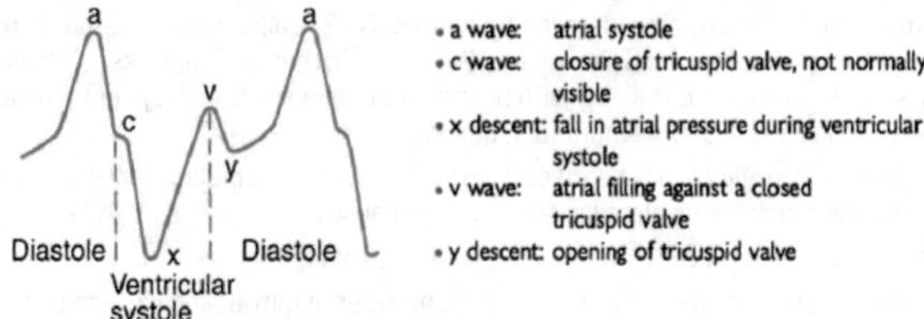

Fig 2.12 The jugular venous pressure wave. The JVP drops as the x descent during ventricular systole because the right atrium is no longer contracting. This means that the pressure in the right atrium is dropping and this is reflected by the JVP.

After *Clinical Examination*, Macleod, Churchill and *Aids to Undergraduate Medicine*, J Burton, Churchill.

2 This sign was first described by Pasteur in 1885 in the context of tricuspid incompetence.

The heart sounds

►Listen systematically: sounds then murmurs. While listening, palpate the carotid artery: S_1 is synchronous with the upstroke.

Heart sounds See fig 2.13. The 1st and 2nd sounds are usually clear. Confident pronouncements about other sounds and soft murmurs may be difficult. Even senior colleagues disagree with one another about the more difficult sounds and murmurs.

The 1st heart sound (S_1) Represents closure of mitral (M_1) and tricuspid (T_1) valves. Splitting in inspiration may be heard and is normal.

- *Loud* S_1 In mitral stenosis, because the narrowed valve orifice limits ventricular filling, there is no gradual decrease in flow towards the end of diastole. The valves are, therefore, at their maximum excursion at the end of diastole, and so shut rapidly leading to a loud S_1 (the 'tapping' apex). S_1 is also loud if diastolic filling time is shortened, eg if the PR interval is short, and in tachycardia.
- *Soft* S_1 occurs if the diastolic filling time is prolonged, eg prolonged PR interval, or if the mitral valve leaflets fail to close properly (ie mitral incompetence).

The intensity of S_1 is variable in AV block, AF, and nodal or ventricular tachycardia.

The 2nd heart sound (S_2) Represents aortic (A_2) and pulmonary valve (P_2) closure. The most important abnormality of A_2 is softening in aortic stenosis.

- A_2 is said to be loud in tachycardia, hypertension, and transposition, but this is probably not a useful clinical entity.
- P_2 is loud in pulmonary hypertension and soft in pulmonary stenosis.
- *Splitting of* S_2 in inspiration is normal and is mainly due to the variation of right heart venous return with respiration, delaying the pulmonary component.
  - *Wide splitting* occurs in right bundle branch block (BBB), pulmonary stenosis, deep inspiration, mitral regurgitation, and VSD.
  - *Wide fixed splitting* occurs in atrial septal defect (ASD).
  - *Reversed splitting* (ie A_2 following P_2, with splitting increasing on expiration) occurs in left bundle branch block, aortic stenosis, PDA (patent ductus arteriosus), and right ventricular pacing.
  - A single S_2 occurs in Fallot's tetralogy, severe aortic or pulmonary stenosis, pulmonary atresia, Eisenmenger's syndrome (p156), large VSD, or hypertension.

NB: splitting and P_2 are heard best in the pulmonary area.

Additional sounds

3rd heart sound (S_3) may occur just after S_2. It is low pitched and best heard with the bell of the stethoscope. S_3 is pathological over the age of 30yrs. A loud S_3 occurs in a dilated left ventricle with rapid ventricular filling (mitral regurgitation, VSD) or poor LV function (post MI, dilated cardiomyopathy). In constrictive pericarditis or restrictive cardiomyopathy it occurs early and is more high pitched ('pericardial knock').

4th heart sound (S_4) occurs just before S_1. Always abnormal, it represents atrial contraction against a ventricle made stiff by any cause, eg aortic stenosis or hypertensive heart disease.

Triple and gallop rhythms A 3rd or 4th heart sound occurring with a sinus tachycardia may give the impression of galloping hooves. An S_3 gallop has the same rhythm as '*Ken*-tucky', whereas an S_4 gallop has the same rhythm as 'Tenne-*ssee*'. When S_3 and S_4 occur in a tachycardia, eg with pulmonary embolism, they may summate and appear as a single sound, a summation gallop.

An ejection systolic click is heard early in systole with bicuspid aortic valves, and if ↑BP. The right heart equivalent lesions may also cause clicks.

Mid-systolic clicks occur in mitral valve prolapse (p144).

An opening snap precedes the mid-diastolic murmur of mitral (and tricuspid) stenosis. It indicates a pliable (non-calcified) valve.

Prosthetic sounds are caused by non-biological valves, on opening and closing: *rumbling sounds* ≈ ball and cage valves (eg Starr-Edwards); *single clicks* ≈ tilting disc valve (eg single disc: Bjork Shiley; bileaflet: St Jude—often quieter). Prosthetic mitral valve clicks occur in time with S_1, aortic valve clicks in time with S_2.

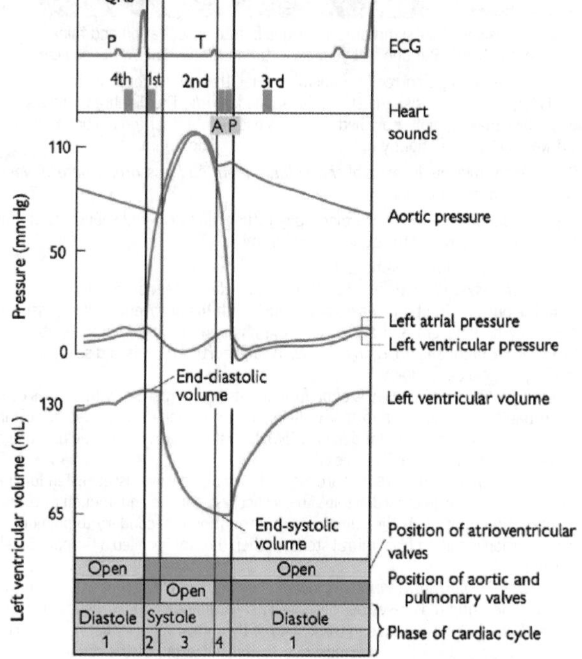

Fig 2.13 The cardiac cycle.

Cardiac murmurs

►Always consider other symptoms and signs before auscultation and think: 'What do I expect to hear?' But don't let your expectations determine what you hear.

►Use the stethoscope correctly: remember that the bell is good for low-pitched sounds (eg mitral stenosis) and should be applied *gently*. The diaphragm filters out low pitches, making higher-pitched murmurs easier to detect (eg aortic regurgitation). NB: a bell applied tightly to the skin becomes a diaphragm.

►Consider any murmur in terms of *character, timing, loudness, area where loudest, radiation*, and *accentuating manoeuvres*.

►When in doubt, rely on echocardiography rather than disputed sounds. (But still enjoy trying to figure out the clinical conundrum!)

Character and timing (See fig 2.14.)

- *An ejection-systolic murmur* (*ESM*, crescendo-decrescendo) usually originates from the outflow tract and waxes and wanes with the intraventricular pressures. ESMs may be innocent and are common in children and high-output states (eg tachycardia, pregnancy). Organic causes include aortic stenosis and sclerosis, pulmonary stenosis, and H(O)CM.
- *A pansystolic murmur (PSM)* is of uniform intensity and merges with S_2. It is usually organic and occurs in mitral or tricuspid regurgitation (S_1 may also be soft in these), or a ventricular septal defect (p156). Mitral valve prolapse may produce a late systolic murmur ± midsystolic click.
- *Early diastolic murmurs (EDMS)* are high pitched and easily missed: listen for the 'absence of silence' in early diastole. An EDM occurs in aortic and, though rare, pulmonary regurgitation. If the pulmonary regurgitation is secondary to pulmonary hypertension resulting from mitral stenosis, then the EDM is called a Graham Steell murmur.
- *Mid-diastolic murmurs (MDMS)* are low pitched and rumbling. They occur in mitral stenosis (accentuated presystolically if heart still in sinus rhythm), rheumatic fever (Carey Coombs' murmur: due to thickening of the mitral valve leaflets), and aortic regurgitation (Austin Flint murmur: due to the fluttering of the anterior mitral valve cusp caused by the regurgitant stream).

Intensity All murmurs are graded on a scale of 1-6 (see table 2.4), though in practice diastolic murmurs, being less loud, are only graded 1-4. Intensity is a poor guide to the severity of a lesion—an ESM may be inaudible in severe aortic stenosis.

Area where loudest Though an unreliable sign, mitral murmurs tend to be loudest over the apex, in contrast to the area of greatest intensity from lesions of the aortic (right 2nd intercostal space), pulmonary (left 2nd intercostal space), and tricuspid (lower left sternal edge) valves.

Radiation The ESM of aortic stenosis classically radiates to the carotids, in contrast to the PSM of mitral regurgitation, which radiates to the axilla.

Accentuating manoeuvres

- *Movements* that bring the relevant part of the heart closer to the stethoscope accentuate murmurs (eg leaning forward for aortic regurgitation, left lateral position for mitral stenosis).
- *Expiration* increases blood flow to the left side of the heart and therefore accentuates left-sided murmurs. *Inspiration* has the opposite effect.
- *Valsalva manoeuvre* (forced expiration against a closed glottis) decreases systemic venous return, accentuating mitral valve prolapse and H(O)CM, but softening mitral regurgitation and aortic stenosis. *Squatting* has exactly the opposite effect. *Exercise* accentuates the murmur of mitral stenosis.

Non-valvular murmurs *A pericardial friction rub* may be heard in pericarditis. It is a superficial scratching sound, not confined to systole or diastole. *Continuous murmurs* are present throughout the cardiac cycle and may occur with a patent ductus arteriosus, arteriovenous fistula, or ruptured sinus of Valsalva.

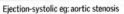

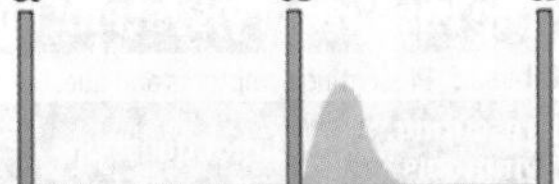
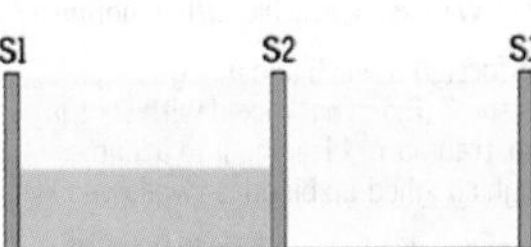
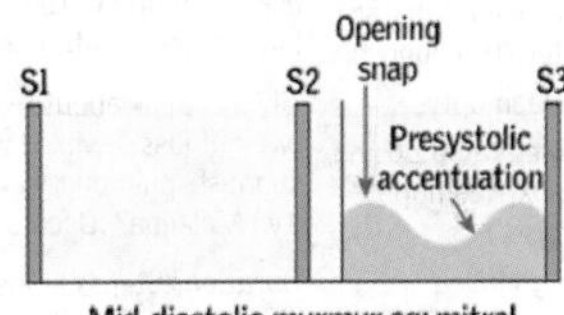

Fig 2.14 Typical waveforms of common heart murmurs.

Grading intensity of heart murmurs

►The following grading is commonly used for murmurs—systolic murmurs from 1 to 6 and diastolic murmurs from 1 to 4, never being clinically >4/6.

Table 2.4 Grading of heart murmurs.

Grade	Description
1/6	Very soft, only heard after listening for a while
2/6	Soft, but detectable immediately
3/6	Clearly audible, but no thrill palpable
4/6	Clearly audible, palpable thrill
5/6	Audible with stethoscope only partially touching chest
6/6	Can be heard without placing stethoscope on chest

Prosthetic valve murmurs

Prosthetic valves: Created either from synthetic material (mechanical prosthesis) or from biological tissue (bioprosthesis). The choice of prosthesis is determined by the anticipated longevity of the patient and the patient's ability to tolerate anticoagulation. Three mechanical valve designs exist: the caged ball valve, the tilting disc (single leaflet) valve, and the bileaflet valve. Tissue valves are made from porcine valves or bovine pericardium.

Prosthetic aortic valves: All types produce a degree of outflow obstruction and thus have an ESM. The intensity of this murmur increases as the valve fails. Ball and cage valves (eg Starr-Edwards) and tissue valves *do* close completely in diastole and so any diastolic murmur implies valve failure.

Prosthetic mitral valves: Ball and cage valves project into the left ventricle and can cause a low-intensity ESM as they interfere with the ejected stream. Tissue valves and bileaflet valves can have a low-intensity diastolic murmur. Consider any systolic murmur of loud intensity to be a sign of regurgitation and ∴ failure.

Eponymous signs of aortic regurgitation

- de Musset's sign—head nodding in time with the pulse.
- Müller's sign—systolic pulsations of the uvula.
- Corrigan's sign—visible carotid pulsations.
- Quincke's sign—capillary nailbed pulsation in the fingers.
- Traube's sign—'pistol shot' femorals, a booming sound heard over the femorals.
- Duroziez's sign—to and fro diastolic murmur heard when compressing the femorals proximally with the stethoscope.

The respiratory system: history

Table 2.5 Presenting symptoms and questions to ask

Presenting symptoms	Direct questions
Cough (see BOX 'Characteristic coughs')	Duration? Character (eg barking/hollow/dry)? Nocturnal (≈asthma, ask about other atopic symptoms, ie eczema, hay fever)? Exacerbating factors? Sputum (colour? How much?). Any blood/haemoptysis?
Haemoptysis (see table 2.6 and BOX 'Haemoptysis')	Always think about TB (recent foreign travel?) and malignancy (weight loss?). Mixed with sputum? (Blood not mixed with sputum suggests pulmonary embolism, trauma, or bleeding into a lung cavity.) Melaena? (Occurs if enough coughed-up blood is swallowed.)
Dyspnoea (see table 2.7 and BOX 'Dyspnoea' and p782)	Duration? Steps climbed/distance walked before onset? NYHA classification (p135)? Diurnal variation (≈asthma)? Ask specifically about circumstances in which dyspnoea occurs (eg occupational allergen exposure).
Hoarseness (OHCS p568)	Eg due to laryngitis, recurrent laryngeal nerve palsy, Singer's nodules, or laryngeal tumour.
Wheeze (p52)	
Fever/night sweats (p29)	
Chest pain (p94 & p784)	SOCRATES (see p36), usually 'pleuritic' if respiratory (ie worse on inspiration?).
Stridor (see BOX 'Stridor')	

History Ask about current symptoms (table 2.5) and past history: pneumonia/bronchitis; TB; atopy[3] (asthma/eczema/hay fever); previous CXR abnormalities; lung surgery; myopathy; neurological disorders. Connective tissue disorders, eg rheumatoid, SLE.

Drug history Respiratory drugs (eg steroids, bronchodilators)? Any other drugs, especially with respiratory SE (eg ACE inhibitors, cytotoxics, β-blockers, amiodarone)?

Family history Atopy?[3] Emphysema? TB?

Social history Quantify smoking in 'pack-years' (20 cigarettes/day for 1 year = 1 pack-year). Occupational exposure (farming, mining, asbestos) has possible compensatory implications. Pets at home (eg birds)? Recent travel/TB contacts?

Stridor

Inspiratory sound due to partial obstruction of upper airways. Obstruction may be due to something *within the lumen* (eg foreign body, tumour, bilateral vocal cord palsy), *within the wall* (eg oedema from anaphylaxis, laryngospasm, tumour, croup, acute epiglottitis, amyloidosis), or *extrinsic* (eg goitre, oesophagus, lymphadenopathy, post-op stridor, after neck surgery). It's an emergency (►►p772) if gas exchange is compromised. NB: wheeze is an *expiratory* sound.

Characteristic coughs

Coughing is relatively non-specific, resulting from irritation anywhere from the pharynx to the lungs. The character of a cough may, however, give clues as to the underlying cause:

- *Loud, brassy coughing* suggests pressure on the trachea, eg by a tumour.
- *Hollow, 'bovine' coughing* is associated with recurrent laryngeal nerve palsy.
- *Barking coughs* occur in croup.
- *Chronic cough* Think of pertussis, TB, foreign body, asthma (eg nocturnal).
- *Dry, chronic coughing* may occur following acid irritation of the lungs in oesophageal reflux, and as a side-effect of ACE inhibitors.

►Do not ignore a change in character of a chronic cough; it may signify a new problem, eg infection, malignancy.

3 Atopy implies predisposition to, or concurrence of, asthma, hay fever and eczema with production of specific IgE on exposure to common allergens (eg house dust mite, grass, cats).

Haemoptysis

Blood is *coughed* up, eg frothy, *alkaline*, and bright red, often in a context of known chest disease (*vomited* blood is acidic and dark).

Table 2.6 Respiratory causes of haemoptysis.

1 Infective	TB; bronchiectasis; bronchitis; pneumonia; lung abscess; COPD; fungi (eg aspergillosis); viruses (from pneumonitis, cryoglobulinaemia, eg with hepatitis viruses, HIV-associated pneumocystosis, or MAI, p400). Helminths: paragonimiasis; hydatid (p435); schistosomiasis.
2 Neoplastic	Primary or secondary.
3 Vascular	Lung infarction (PE); vasculitis (ANCA-associated; RA; SLE); hereditary haemorrhagic telangiectasia; AV malformation; capillaritis.
4 Parenchymal	Diffuse interstitial fibrosis; sarcoidosis; haemosiderosis; Goodpasture's syndrome; cystic fibrosis.
5 Pulmonary hypertension	Idiopathic, thromboembolic, congenital cyanotic heart disease (p156), pulmonary fibrosis, bronchiectasis.
6 Coagulopathies	Any—eg thrombocytopenia, p344; DIC; warfarin excess.
7 Trauma/foreign body	Eg post-intubation, or an eroding implanted defibrillator.
8 Pseudo-haemoptysis	Munchausen's (p706); aspirated haematemesis; red pigment (prodigiosin) from *Serratia marcescens (Gram-negative bacteria)* in sputum.[7]

Rare causes refuse to be classified neatly: vascular causes may have infective origins, eg hydatid cyst may count as a foreign body, *and* infection, *and* vascular if it fistulates with the aorta; ditto for infected (mycotic) aneurysm rupture, or TB aortitis. Infective causes entailing coagulopathy: dengue; leptospirosis. In monthly haemoptysis, think of lung endometriosis.

℞: Haemoptysis may need treating in its own right, if massive (eg trauma, TB, hydatid cyst, cancer, AV malformation): call chest team, consider interventional radiology input (danger is drowning: lobe resection, endobronchial tamponade, or arterial embolization may be needed). Set up IVI, do CXR, blood gases, FBC, INR/APTT, crossmatch. If distressing, give *prompt* IV morphine, eg if inoperable malignancy.

Dyspnoea

Subjective sensation of shortness of breath, often exacerbated by exertion.

- *Lung*—airway and interstitial disease. May be hard to separate from cardiac causes; asthma may wake patient, and cause early morning dyspnoea & wheeze.
- *Cardiac*—eg ischaemic heart disease or left ventricular failure (LVF), mitral stenosis, of any cause. LVF is associated with *orthopnoea* (dyspnoea worse on lying; 'How many pillows?') and *paroxysmal nocturnal dyspnoea* (PND; dyspnoea waking one up). Other features include ankle oedema, lung crepitations, and ↑JVP.
- *Anatomical*—eg diseases of the chest wall, muscles, pleura. Ascites can cause breathlessness by splinting the diaphragm, restricting its movement.
- *Others* ►Any shocked patient may also be dyspnoeic (p790 & p607)—dyspnoea may be shock's presenting feature. Also anaemia or metabolic acidosis causing respiratory compensation, eg ketoacidosis, aspirin poisoning. Look for other clues—dyspnoea at rest *unassociated with exertion,* may be psychogenic: prolonged hyperventilation causes respiratory alkalosis. This causes a fall in ionized calcium leading to apparent hypocalcaemia. Features include peripheral and perioral paraesthesiae ± carpopedal spasm. Speed of onset helps diagnosis:

Table 2.7 Aetiology of dyspnoea by timing of onset.

Acute	Subacute	Chronic
Foreign body	Asthma	COPD and chronic parenchymal diseases
Pneumothorax (p749, fig 16.43)	Parenchymal disease, eg alveolitis pneumonia	Non-respiratory causes, eg cardiac failure, anaemia
Pulmonary embolus	Effusion	
Acute pulmonary oedema	Psychogenic	
Psychogenic		

The respiratory system: examination 1

Begin by introducing yourself, obtaining consent to examine and position the patient appropriately: lying on a bed, sitting up at 45°. Expose them to the waist (for female patients, delay until examining the chest). Explain what you are doing throughout.

1 General inspection

- Assess general state (ill/well/cachexic)
- Look for clues (oxygen, inhalers, nebulizers, venturi mask)
- Colour (pale, cyanosed (fig 2.15), flushed)
- Short of breath? Accessory muscle use?
- Scars on chest wall?

Ask the patient to take a deep breath in, watch chest movement and symmetry, any coughing?

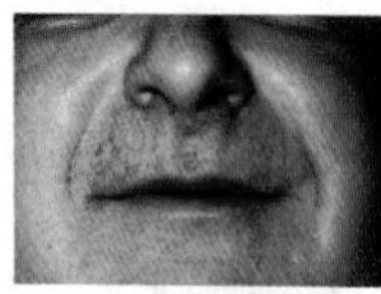
Fig 2.15 Cyanosis.

2 Hands

- *Inspect:*
  Tobacco staining (fig 2.16), peripheral cyanosis, clubbing, signs of systemic disease (systemic sclerosis, rheumatoid arthritis)
- *Asterixis:*
  Ask the patient to hold their hands out and cock their wrists back

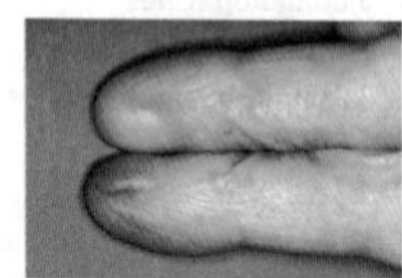
Fig 2.16 Tar stains.

3 Arms

- Time pulse rate, with fingers still on the pulse, check respiratory rate (this can increase if the patient is aware you are timing it)—and pattern (p53)
- Bounding pulse (CO_2 retention)?
- Check blood pressure

4 Neck

- *Trachea:* Feel in sternal notch (fig 2.17, deviated?), assess cricosternal distance in finger-breadths and feel for tracheal tug
- *Lymphadenopathy:* From behind with patient sat forward palpate lymph nodes of head and neck
- *JVP:* Raised in cor pulmonale, fixed and raised in superior vena cava obstruction

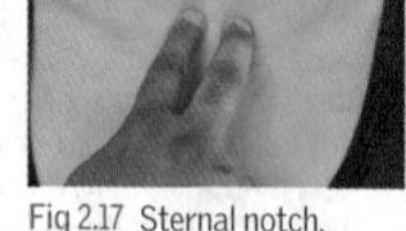
Fig 2.17 Sternal notch.
Reproduced from Thomas *et al.* (eds), *Oxford Handbook of Clinical Examination and Practical Skills* (2014) with permission from Oxford University Press.

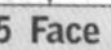

5 Face

- *Inspect:* For signs of Horner's (fig 2.18), conjunctival pallor, central cyanosis (ask patient to stick out tongue), pursed lip breathing

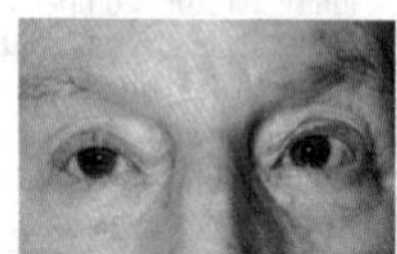
Fig 2.18 Horner's syndrome.

6 Front of chest

- *Apex beat.*
- *Expansion:* Ask patient to 'breathe all the way out', place hands as in fig 2.19, 'now a deep breath in', and note distance of thumbs to midline, is expansion equal? Repeat with hands laid on upper chest.
- *Tactile vocal fremitus:* Palpate the chest wall with your fingertips and ask the patient to repeat '99', each time they feel your hand, comparing right to left. This is rarely used.
- *Percussion:* Percuss over different respiratory segments, comparing right and left (see fig 2.21, p53).
- *Auscultation:* Ask patient to 'take steady breaths in and out through your mouth' and listen with diaphragm from apices to bases, comparing right and left (see table 2.8, p52).
- *Vocal resonance:* Repeat auscultation, asking patient to repeat '99' each time they feel the stethoscope. If marked ↑resonance heard, repeat with asking patient to whisper '99'; if clearly heard this is termed 'whispering pectoriloquy' and is a sensitive sign for consolidation. Outside of exams, the choice of vocal resonance or tactile vocal fremitus is a personal preference. Many clinicians prefer vocal resonance as it provides more information than tactile vocal fremitus.

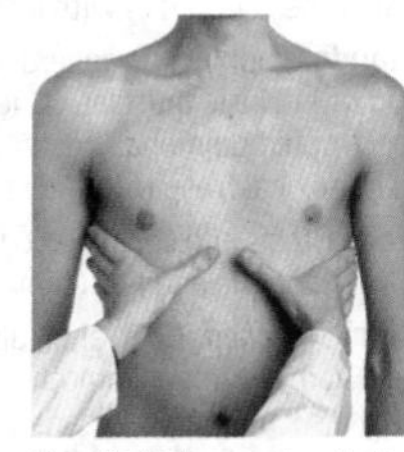

Fig 2.19 Placement of the hands for testing chest expansion: anchor with the fingers and leave the thumbs free-floating.

7 Back of chest

- *Expansion*
- *Tactile vocal fremitus*
- *Percussion*
- *Auscultation*
- *Vocal resonance*

8 To complete the examination

- Palpate for *sacral and ankle oedema* (fig 2.20)
- Check peripheral pulses, observation chart for temperature and O_2 sats
- Examine the sputum pot and check PEFR

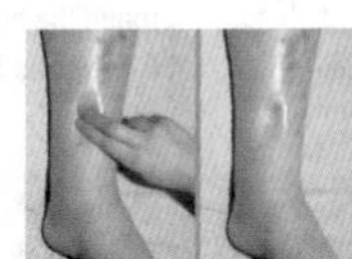

Fig 2.20 Ankle oedema.

Top tips

- Whispering pectoriloquy is a classic and specific sign of consolidation.
- If you don't adequately expose the chest you may miss small scars, eg from video thoracoscopy.
- If you see Horner's syndrome, check for wasting of the small muscles of the hand; see p702 and p708.

The respiratory system: examination 2

General inspection 'Comfortable at rest' or unwell? Cachectic? *Respiratory distress*? (if high negative intrathoracic pressures are needed to generate air entry). Stridor? *Respiratory rate, breathing pattern* (see BOX 'Breathing patterns'). Look for *chest wall and spine deformities* (see p55). Inspect for *scars* of past surgery, chest drains, or radiotherapy (skin thickening, tattoos for radiotherapy). *Chest wall movement:* symmetrical? (if not, pathology on restricted side). Paradoxical respiration? (abdomen sucked in with inspiration; seen in diaphragmatic paralysis, see p502).

Hands Clubbing, peripheral cyanosis, tar stains, fine tremor (β-agonist use), wasting of intrinsic muscles (T1 lesions, eg Pancoast's tumour, p708). Tender wrists (hypertrophic pulmonary osteoarthropathy—cancer). Asterixis (CO_2 retention). Pulse: paradoxical (respiratory distress), bounding (CO_2 retention).

Face Ptosis and constricted pupil (Horner's syndrome, eg Pancoast's tumour, p708)? Bluish tongue and lips (central cyanosis, p34)? Conjunctival pallor (anaemia)?

Neck *Trachea:* Central or displaced? (towards collapse or away from large pleural effusion/tension pneumothorax; slight deviation to right is normal). Cricosternal distance <3cm is hyperexpansion. *Tracheal tug:* descent of trachea with inspiration (severe airflow limitation). *Lymphadenopathy:* TB/Ca? *JVP:* ↑ in cor pulmonale.

Palpation *Apex beat:* Impalpable? (COPD/pleural effusion/dextrocardia?) *Expansion:* <5cm on deep inspiration is abnormal. Symmetry? *Tactile vocal fremitus:* ↑ implies consolidation.

Percussion *Dull percussion note:* Collapse, consolidation, fibrosis, pleural thickening, or pleural effusion (*'stony dull'*). *Cardiac dullness* usually detectable over the left side. *Liver dullness* usually extends up to 5th rib, right mid-clavicular line; below this, resonant chest is a sign of lung hyperexpansion (eg asthma, COPD). *Hyper-resonant percussion note:* Pneumothorax or hyperinflation (COPD).

Table 2.8 Auscultation

Breath sounds	Description	Pathology
Vesicular	Rustling quality	Normal
Bronchial breathing	Harsh with gap between inspiration and expiration. Increased *vocal resonance* and whispering pectoriloquy	Consolidation, localized fibrosis, above pleural/percardial effusion (Ewart's sign, p154)
Diminished breath sounds	Difficult to hear	Pleural effusion, pleural thickening, pneumothorax, bronchial obstruction, asthma, or COPD
Silent chest	Inaudible breath sounds	Life-threatening asthma
Wheeze (rhonchi)	Air expired through narrow airways	
	• Monophonic (single note, partial obstruction one airway)	• Tumour occluding airway
	• Polyphonic (multiple notes, widespread airway narrowing)	• Asthma, cardiac wheeze (LVF)
Crackles (crepitations)	Reopening of small airways on inspiration	
	• Fine and late in inspiration	• Pulmonary oedema
	• Coarse and mid inspiratory	• Bronchiectasis
	• Early inspiratory	• Small airway disease
	• Late/pan inspiratory	• Alveolar disease
	• Disappear post cough	• Insignificant
Pleural rub	Movement of visceral pleura over parietal when both are roughened (eg due to inflammatory exudate)	• Pneumonia • Pulmonary infarction
Pneumothorax click	Shallow left pneumothorax between layers of parietal pleura overlying heart, heard during cardiac systole	

⚠ Signs of respiratory distress

- Tachypnoea.
- Nasal flaring.
- Tracheal tug (pulling of thyroid cartilage towards sternal notch in inspiration).
- Use of accessory muscles (sternocleidomastoid, platysma, infrahyoid).
- Intercostal, subcostal, and sternal recession.
- Pulsus paradoxus (p42).

Breathing patterns

Hyperventilation: Tachypnoea (ie >20 breaths/min) or *deep* (hyperpnoea, ie ↑tidal volume). Hyperpnoea is not unpleasant, unlike dyspnoea. It may cause respiratory alkalosis, hence paraesthesiae ± muscle spasm (↓Ca^{2+}). The main cause is anxiety: associated dizziness, chest tightness/pain, palpitations, and panic. Rare causes: response to metabolic acidosis; brainstem lesions.

- *Kussmaul respiration* is deep, sighing breaths in severe metabolic acidosis (blowing off CO_2), eg diabetic or alcoholic ketoacidosis, renal impairment.
- *Neurogenic hyperventilation* is produced by pontine lesions.
- The *hyperventilation syndrome* involves panic attacks associated with hyperventilation, palpitations, dizziness, faintness, tinnitus, alarming chest pain/tightness, perioral and peripheral tingling (plasma ↓Ca^{2+}). Treatment: relaxation techniques and breathing into a paper bag (↑inspired CO_2 corrects the alkalosis). NB: the anxious patient in A&E with hyperventilation and a respiratory alkalosis may actually be presenting with an aspirin overdose (p844).

Cheyne–Stokes breathing: Breaths get deeper and deeper, then shallower (±episodic apnoea) in cycles. *Causes*—brainstem lesions or compression (stroke, ↑ICP). If the cycle is long (eg 3min), the cause may be a long lung-to-brain circulation time (eg in chronic pulmonary oedema or ↓cardiac output). It is enhanced by opioids.

Sputum examination

Further examination—sputum, temperature charts, O_2 sats, PEFR: Inspect sputum and send suspicious sputum for microscopy (Gram stain and auramine/ZN stain, if indicated), culture, and cytology.

- *Black carbon specks* suggests smoking: commonest cause of increased sputum.
- *Yellow/green sputum* suggests infection, eg bronchiectasis, pneumonia.
- *Pink frothy sputum* suggests pulmonary oedema.
- *Bloody sputum (haemoptysis)* may be due to malignancy, TB, infection, or trauma, and requires investigation for these causes. See p49.
- *Clear sputum* is probably saliva.

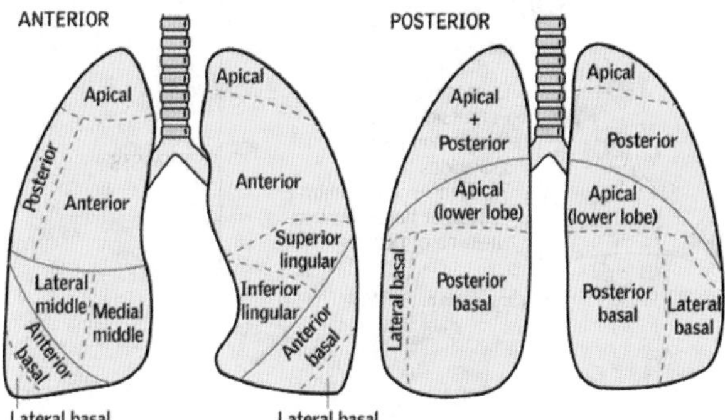

Fig 2.21 The respiratory segments supplied by the segmental bronchi.

Some physical signs (fig 2.22).

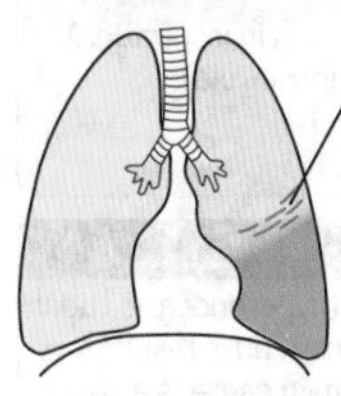

(There may be bronchial breathing at the top of an effusion)

Expansion: ↓
Percussion: ↓ (stony dull)
Air entry: ↓
Vocal resonance: ↓
Trachea + mediastinum central (shift away from affected side only with massive effusions ≥1000mL)

} PLEURAL EFFUSION

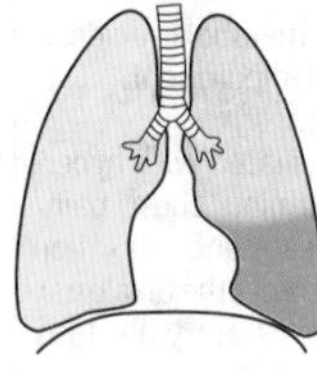

Expansion ↓
Percussion note ↓
Vocal resonance ↑
Bronchial breathing ± coarse crackles (with whispering pectoriloquy)
Trachea + mediastinum central

} CONSOLIDATION

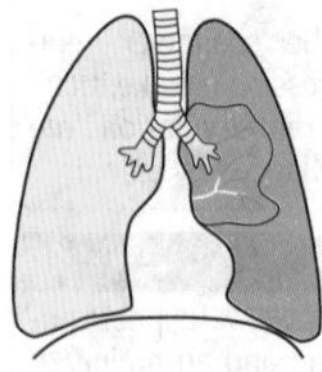

Expansion ↓
Percussion note ↑
Breath sounds ↓
Trachea + mediastinum shift towards the affected side

} SPONTANEOUS PNEUMOTHORAX/ EXTENSIVE COLLAPSE (ΔΔ LOBECTOMY/ PNEUMONECTOMY)

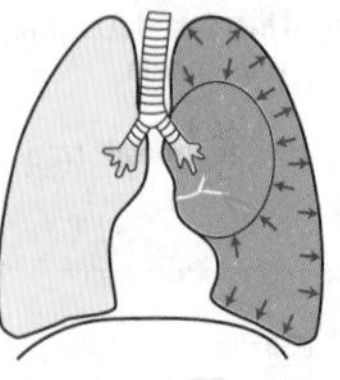

Expansion ↓
Percussion note ↑
Breath sounds ↓
Trachea + mediastinum shift away from the affected side

} TENSION PNEUMOTHORAX (See fig 16.43, p749 for chest x-ray image)

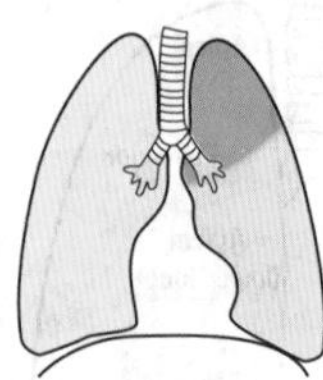

Expansion ↓
Percussion note ↓
Breath sounds bronchial ± crackles
Trachea + mediastinum central or pulled towards the area of fibrosis

} FIBROSIS

Fig 2.22 Physical signs on chest examination.

Chest deformities

- *Barrel chest:* ↑AP diameter, tracheal descent and chest expansion ↓, seen in chronic hyperinflation (eg asthma/COPD).
- *Pigeon chest (pectus carinatum):* See fig 2.23.
- *Funnel chest (pectus excavatum):* Developmental defect involving local sternum depression (lower end). See fig 2.24.
- *Kyphosis:* 'Humpback' from ↑AP thoracic spine curvature.
- *Scoliosis:* Lateral curvature (*OHCS* p674); all of these may cause a restrictive ventilatory defect.

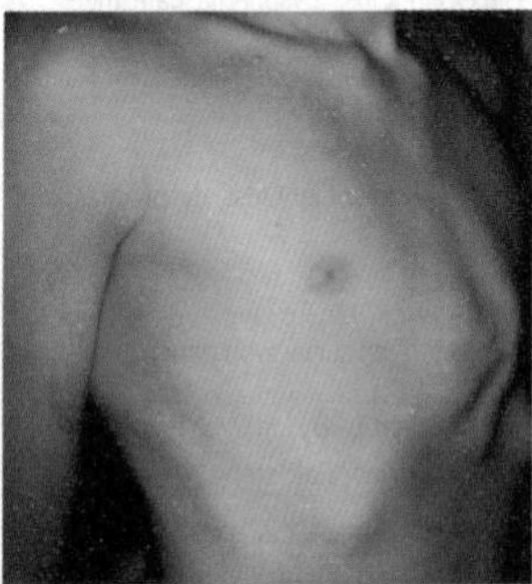

Fig 2.23 Pectus carinatum (pigeon chest). Prominent sternum, from lung hyperinflation while the bony thorax is still developing, eg in chronic childhood asthma. Often seen with *Harrison's sulcus*, a groove deformity caused by indrawing of lower ribs at the diaphragm attachment site. This usually has little functional significance in terms of respiration but can have significant psychological effects: see BOX.

Image courtesy of Prof Eric Fonkalsrud.

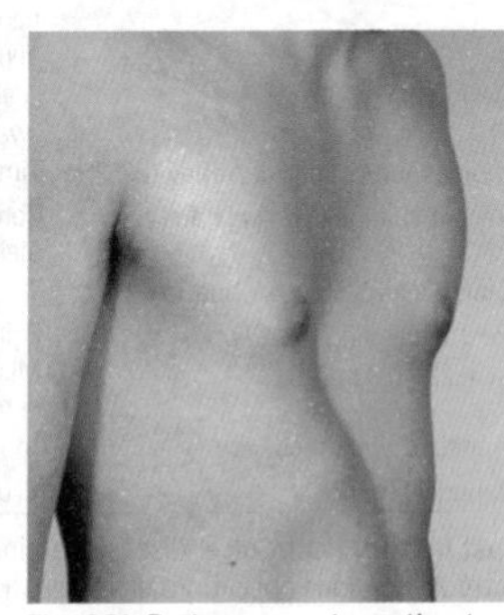

Fig 2.24 Pectus excavatum; the term for funnel or sunken chest. It is often asymptomatic, but may cause displacement of the heart to the left, and restricted ventilatory capacity ± mild air-trapping. Associations: scoliosis; Marfan's; Ehlers-Danlos syndrome.

Image courtesy of Prof Eric Fonkalsrud.

Herr Minty and his pigeon chest

Chest wall deformities such as pectus excavatum are quite common, often appearing during adolescent growth spurts. Exercise intolerance is the main symptom (from heart compression—consider CXR/CT). Indications for surgical correction (rarely needed): ≥2: a severe, symptomatic deformity; progression of deformity; paradoxical respiratory chest wall motion; pectus index >3.25 on CT; cardiac or lung compression; restrictive spirometry; cardiac pathology that might be from compression of the heart.

Psychological effects are interesting and not to be dismissed as their effects may be greater than any physical effects.[8] Because these people hate exposing their chests they may become introverted, and never learn to swim, so don't let them sink without trace. Be sympathetic, and remember Herr Minty, who inaugurated Graham Greene's *theory of compensation*: wherever a defect exists we must look for a compensating perfection to account for how the defect survives. In Minty's case, although 'crooked and yellow and pigeon-chested he had his deep refuge, the inexhaustible ingenuity of his mind.'

See table 2.9 for direct questions to ask regarding presenting symptoms.

Table 2.9 Presenting symptoms and questions to ask

Presenting symptoms	Direct questions
Abdominal pain (see p57 and p606)	SOCRATES (p36)
Distension (see p57)	
Nausea, vomiting (see table 2.10) Haematemesis (pp256-7)	Timing? Relation to meals? Amount? Content (liquid, solid, bile, blood)? Frequency? Fresh (bright red)/dark/'coffee grounds'? Consider neoplasia (weight loss, dysphagia, pain, melaena?), NSAIDs/warfarin? Surgery? Smoking?
Dysphagia (p250)	Level? Onset? Intermittent? Progressive? Painful swallow (*odynophagia*)?
Indigestion/dyspepsia/reflux (p252)	Timing (relation to meals)?
Recent change in bowel habit	Consider neoplasia (weight loss, dysphagia, pain, melaena?)
Diarrhoea (p258), constipation (p260)	
Rectal bleeding (p629) or melaena (p246)	Pain on defecation? Mucus? Fresh/dark/black? Mixed with stool/on surface/on paper/in the pan?
Appetite, weight change	Intentional? Quantify. Dysphagia? Pain?
Jaundice (p272)	Pruritus? Dark urine? Pale stools?

Past history Peptic ulcer disease, carcinoma, jaundice, hepatitis, blood transfusions, tattoos, previous operations, last menstrual period (LMP), dietary changes.

Drug history Especially steroids, NSAIDs, antibiotics, anticoagulants (eg clopidogrel with SSRI—see BOX 'SSRIs and upper GI bleeding risk').

Family history Irritable bowel syndrome (IBS), inflammatory bowel disease (IBD), peptic ulcer disease, polyps, cancer, jaundice.

Social history Smoking, alcohol (quantify units/week), recreational drug use, travel history, tropical illnesses, contact with jaundiced persons, occupational exposures, sexual history, blood transfusions, surgery over-seas.

Vomiting History is vital. Associated symptoms and past medical history often indicate cause (table 2.10). Examine for dehydration, distension, tenderness, abdominal mass, succussion splash in children (pyloric stenosis), or tinkling bowel sounds (intestinal obstruction).

Table 2.10 Causes of vomiting

Gastrointestinal	CNS	Metabolic/endocrine
• Gastroenteritis	• Meningitis/encephalitis	• Uraemia
• Peptic ulceration	• Migraine	• Hypercalcaemia
• Pyloric stenosis	• ↑Intracranial pressure	• Hyponatraemia
• Intestinal obstruction	• Brainstem lesions	• Pregnancy
• Paralytic ileus	• Motion sickness	• Diabetic ketoacidosis
• Acute cholecystitis	• Ménière's disease	• Addison's disease
• Acute pancreatitis	• Labyrinthitis	
Alcohol and drugs	**Psychiatric**	**Others***
• Antibiotics	• Self-induced	• Myocardial infarction
• Opiates	• Psychogenic	• Autonomic neuropathy
• Cytotoxics	• Bulimia nervosa	• Sepsis (UTI; meningitis)
• Digoxin		

How to remember the chief non-GI causes of vomiting?* Try **ABCDEFGHI: **A**cute kidney injury **A**ddison's disease; **B**rain (eg ↑ICP); **C**ardiac (myocardial infarct); **D**iabetic ketoacidosis; **E**ars (eg labyrinthitis, Ménière's disease); **F**oreign substances (alcohol; drugs, eg opiates); **G**ravidity (eg hyperemesis gravidarum); **H**ypercalcaemia/**H**yponatraemia; **I**nfection (eg UTI, meningitis).

Abdominal pain

Character depends on underlying cause. Examples: irritation of the mucosa (acute gastritis), smooth muscle spasm (acute enterocolitis), capsular stretching (liver congestion in CCF), peritoneal inflammation (acute appendicitis), and direct splanchnic nerve stimulation (retroperitoneal extension of tumour). The *character* (constant or colicky, sharp or dull), *duration*, and *frequency* depend on the mechanism of production. The *location* and *distribution* of referred pain depend on the anatomical site. *Time of occurrence* and *aggravating* or *relieving factors* such as meals, defecation, and sleep also have special significance related to the underlying disease process. The site of the pain may provide a clue:

- *Epigastric:* Pancreatitis, gastritis/duodenitis, peptic ulcer, gallbladder disease, aortic aneurysm.
- *Left upper quadrant:* Peptic ulcer, gastric or colonic (splenic flexure) cancer, splenic rupture, subphrenic or perinephric abscess, renal (colic, pyelonephritis).
- *Right upper quadrant:* Cholecystitis, biliary colic, hepatitis, peptic ulcer, colonic cancer (hepatic flexure), renal (colic, pyelonephritis), subphrenic/perinephric abscess.
- *Loin:* (lateral ⅓ of back between thorax and pelvis—merges with the flank, p565) Renal colic, pyelonephritis, renal tumour, perinephric abscess, pain referred from vertebral column. Causes of *flank pain* are similar (see index for fuller list).
- *Left iliac fossa:* Diverticulitis, volvulus, colon cancer, pelvic abscess, inflammatory bowel disease, hip pathology, renal colic, urinary tract infection (UTI), cancer in undescended testis; zoster—wait for the rash! (p454). *Gynae:* torsion of ovarian cyst, salpingitis, ectopic pregnancy.
- *Right iliac fossa pain:* All causes of left iliac fossa pain plus appendicitis and Crohn's ileitis, but usually excluding diverticulitis.
- *Pelvic: Urological:* UTI, retention, stones. *Gynae:* menstruation, pregnancy, endometriosis (*OHCS* p288), salpingitis, endometritis (*OHCS* p274), ovarian cyst torsion.
- *Generalized:* Gastroenteritis, irritable bowel syndrome, peritonitis, constipation.
- *Central:* Mesenteric ischaemia, abdominal aneurysm, pancreatitis.

Remember referred pain: Myocardial infarct → epigastrium; pleural pathology.

Abdominal distension (masses and the 'famous five' Fs)

Enid Blyton's Famous Five characters can generally solve any crime or diagnostic problem using 1950s methodologies steeped in endless school holidays, copious confection-laden midnight feasts, and lashings of homemade ginger beer.

Let's give them the problem of abdominal distension. The sweets and drinks used by the Famous Five actually contribute to the distension itself: **f**at, **f**luid, **f**aeces, **f**latus, and **f**etus. If you think it far-fetched to implicate ginger beer in the genesis of fetuses, note that because it was homemade, like the fun, there was no limit to its intoxicating powers in those long-gone vintage summers. The point is to think to ask 'When was your last period?' *whenever* confronted by a distended abdomen.

Flatus will be resonant on percussion. Fluid will be dull, and can be from ascites (eg from malignancy or cirrhosis: look for shifting dullness), distended bladder (cannot get below it) or an aortic aneurysm (expansile). Masses can be pelvic (think of uterine fibroids or ovarian pathology) or tumours from colon, stomach, pancreas, liver, or kidney. Also see causes of *ascites with portal hypertension* (p604), *hepatomegaly* (p61), *splenomegaly*, and *other abdominal masses* (p604).

SSRIs and upper GI bleeding risk

SSRIs have been associated with an increased risk of bleeding.[9] SSRIs are thought to increase gastric acidity and serotonin is thought to play a role in platelet aggregation. This may lead to an increased risk of ulcers and bleeding, particularly when co-prescribed with anticoagulants and drugs affecting intestinal lining (eg NSAIDs). NICE[10] recommends cautious concomitant use of SSRIs with anticoagulants or NSAIDs and recommends gastroprotection (eg PPI) for older patients taking NSAIDS or aspirin.

Faecal incontinence

This is common in the elderly. Do your best to help, and get social services involved if concerned. Continence depends on many factors—mental function, stool (volume and consistency), anatomy (sphincter function, rectal distensibility, anorectal sensation and reflexes). Defects in any area can cause loss of faecal continence.

Causes: Often multifactorial. Is it passive faecal soiling or urgency-related stool loss? Consider the following:

- *Sphincter dysfunction:*
  - Vaginal delivery is the commonest cause due to sphincter tears or pudendal nerve damage.
  - Surgical trauma, eg following procedures for fistulas, haemorrhoids, fissures.
- *Impaired sensation*—diabetes, MS, dementia, any spinal cord lesions (►►consider cord compression if acute faecal incontinence).
- *Faecal impaction*—overflow diarrhoea, extremely common, especially in the elderly, and very easily treated.
- *Idiopathic*—although there is often no clear cause found, especially in elderly women, this is usually multifactorial, including a combination of poor sphincter tone and pudendal damage leading to poor sensation.

Assessment:

►Do PR (overflow incontinence? poor tone?) and assess neurological function of legs, particularly checking sensation.

Refer to a specialist (esp. if rectal prolapse, anal sphincter injury, lumbar disc disease, or alarm symptoms for colon ca exist). Consider anorectal manometry, pelvic ultrasound or MRI, and pudendal nerve testing may be needed.

Treat according to cause and to promote dignity:

►Never let your own embarrassment stop you from offering help. Knowledge and behaviour are key factors:

- Ensure toilet is in easy reach. Plan trips in the knowledge of toilet locations.
- Obey call-to-stool impulses (esp. after meal, ie the gastro-colic reflex).
- Ensure access to latest continence aids and advice on use, refer to continence nurse specialist for assessment.
- Pelvic floor rehabilitation: eg can help faecal incontinence, squeeze pressure, and maximal tolerated volume.
- Loperamide 2-4mg 45min before social engagements may prevent accidents outside home. An anal cotton plug may help isolated internal sphincter weakness. Skin care. Support agencies.

If all sensible measures fail, try a brake-and-accelerator approach: enemas to empty the rectum (twice weekly) and codeine phosphate, eg 15mg/12h, on non-enema days to constipate. It's not a cure, but makes the incontinence manageable.

Flatulence

Normally, 400-1300mL of gas is expelled PR in 8-20 discrete (or indiscrete) episodes per day. If this, with any eructation (belching) or distension, seems excessive to the patient, they may complain of flatulence. Eructation occurs in hiatus hernia—but most patients with 'flatulence' have no GI disease. Air swallowing (aerophagy) is the main cause of flatus; here N_2 is the chief gas. If flatus is mostly methane, H_2 and CO_2, then fermentation by bowel bacteria is the cause, and reducing carbohydrate intake (eg less lactose and wheat) may help.

Tenesmus

This is a sensation in the rectum of incomplete emptying *after* defecation. It's common in irritable bowel syndrome (p266), but can be caused by tumours.

Regurgitation

Gastric and oesophageal contents are regurgitated effortlessly into the mouth—without contraction of abdominal muscles and diaphragm (so distinguishing it from true vomiting). It may be worse on lying flat, and can cause cough and nocturnal asthma. Regurgitation is rarely preceded by nausea, and when due to gastro-oesophageal reflux, it is often associated with heartburn. An oesophageal pouch may cause regurgitation. Very high GI obstructions (eg gastric volvulus, p611) cause non-productive retching rather than true regurgitation.

Steatorrhoea

These are pale stools that are difficult to flush, and are caused by malabsorption of fat in the small intestine and hence greater fat content in the stool.

Causes: Ileal disease (eg Crohn's or ileal resection), pancreatic disease, and obstructive jaundice (due to ↓excretion of bile salts from the gallbladder).

Dyspepsia

Dyspepsia and indigestion (p252) are broad terms. Dyspepsia is defined as one or more of post-prandial fullness, early satiety (unable to finish meal), and/or epigastric or retrosternal pain or burning. 'Indigestion' reported by the patient can refer to dyspepsia, bloating, nausea, and vomiting. Try to find out exactly what your patient means and when these symptoms occur in relation to meals, eg the classic symptoms of peptic ulcers occur 2–5 hours after a meal and on an empty stomach. Look for alarm symptoms (see p248); these have high negative predictive value. If all patients with dyspepsia undergo endoscopy, <33% have clinically significant findings.[11] Myocardial infaction may present as 'indigestion'.

Halitosis

Halitosis (fetor oris, oral malodour) results from gingivitis (rarely severe enough to cause Vincent's angina, p712), metabolic activity of bacteria in plaque, or sulfide-yielding food putrefaction, eg in gingival pockets and tonsillar crypts. Patients can often be anxious and convinced of halitosis when it is not present (and vice versa!).

Contributory factors:

Smoking, drugs (disulfiram; isosorbide), lung disease, hangovers.

℞:

Try to eliminate anaerobes:

- Good dental hygiene, dental floss, tongue scraping.
- 0.2% aqueous chlorhexidine gluconate.

The very common halitosis arising from the tongue's dorsum is secondary to over-populated volatile sulfur compound-producing bacteria. Locally retained bacteria metabolize sulfur-containing amino acids to yield volatile (∴ smelly) hydrogen sulfide and methylmercaptane, which perpetuate periodontal disease. At night and between meals, conditions are optimal for odour production—so eating regularly may help. Treat by mechanical cleansing/scraping using tongue brushes or scrapes plus mouthwashes. Oral care products containing metal ions, especially Zn, inhibit odour formation, it is thought, because of affinity of the metal ion to sulfur. It is possible to measure the level of volatile sulfur-containing compounds in the air in the mouth directly by means of a portable sulfide monitor.

Examination of the abdomen

Begin by introducing yourself, obtaining consent to examine, and position the patient appropriately; lie the patient down as flat as possible, ideally exposing from 'nipples to knees'. In practice, keep the groin covered and examine separately for hernias, etc.

1 General inspection

- Assess general state (ill/well/cachexic)
- Clues (vomit bowl, stoma bags, catheter, urine colour)
- Colour (pale, jaundiced, uraemic)
- Body mass index?
- Scars on the abdomen? Stomas (fig 2.25)?

Ask the patient to lift their head off the bed, or cough, looking for bulges, distension or pain.

↓

2 Hands

- *Inspect:* Clubbing, koilonychia, leuconychia, Muehrcke's lines, palmar erythema, Dupuytren's contracture (fig 2.26), pigmentation of the palmer creases
- *Asterixis:* (See p50)

↓

3 Arms

- Check pulse and blood pressure
- Look in the distribution of the SVC (arms, upper chest, upper back) for spider naevi (fig 2.27)
- Check for track marks, bruising, pigmentation, scratch marks, arterio-venous fistulae (see p303 for signs seen in patients with chronic kidney disease)

↓

4 Neck

- Examine cervical and supraclavicular lymph nodes (see fig 2.28)
- JVP raised in fluid overload (renal dysfunction, liver dysfunction), tricuspid regurgitation (may cause pulsatile hepatomegaly)
- Scars from tunnelled haemodialysis lines (see p303) or other central venous access

↓

5 Face

- *Skin and eyes:* Jaundice, conjunctival pallor, Kayser–Fleischer rings, xanthelasma (see fig 2.29), sunken eyes (dehydration)
- *Mouth:* Angular stomatitis, pigmentation, telangiectasia, ulcers, glossitis

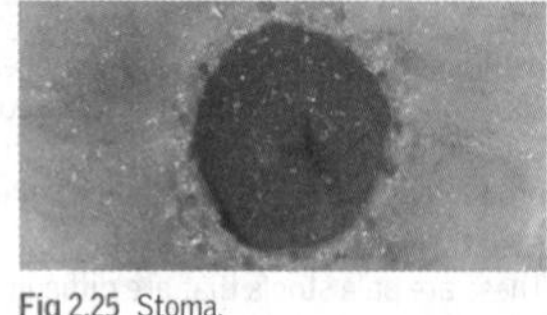

Fig 2.25 Stoma.

Reproduced from MacKay G, *et al.* (eds). *Oxford Specialist Handbook of Colorectal Surgery* (2010), with permission from Oxford University Press.

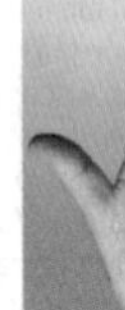

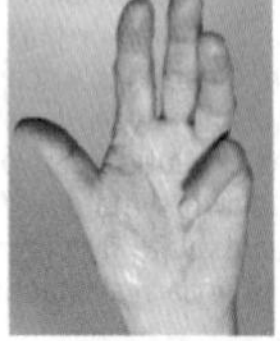

Fig 2.26 Dupuytren's contracture.

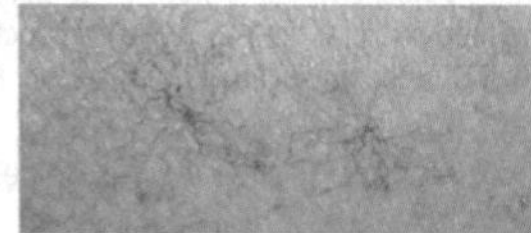

Fig 2.27 Spider naevi.

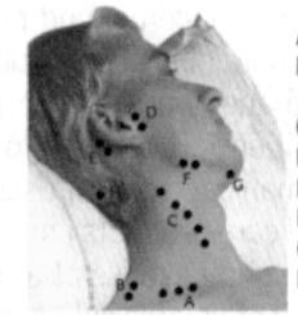

Fig 2.28 Cervical and supraclavicular nodes.

Reproduced from Thomas J, *et al.* (eds). *Oxford Handbook of Clinical Examination and Practical Skills* (2014), with permission from Oxford University Press.

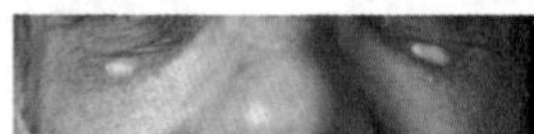

Fig 2.29 Xanthelasma.

6 Abdomen

Inspection:

- Scars—previous surgery, transplant, stoma
- Visible masses, hernias, or pulsation of AAA
- Visible veins suggesting portal hypertension
- Gynaecomastia, hair loss, acanthosis nigricans

Palpation:

Squat by the bed so that the patient's abdomen is at your eye level. Ask if there is any pain and examine this part last. Watch the patient's face for signs of discomfort. Palpate the entire abdomen (see p565):

- *Light palpation*—if this elicits pain, check for *rebound tenderness*. Any involuntary tension in muscles ('*guarding*')? See p606.
- *Deep palpation*—to detect masses.
- *Liver*—using the radial border of the index finger aligned with the costal margin start palpation from the RIF. Press down and ask patient to take a deep breath. Continue upwards towards the costal margin until you feel the liver edge.
- *Spleen*—start palpation in RIF and work towards the left costal margin asking the patient to take a deep breath in and feeling for edge of the spleen.
- *Kidneys*—for each kidney: place one hand behind patient's loin, press down on the abdomen with your other hand and 'ballot' the kidney up with your lower hand against your upper hand (fig 2.30). Unless slim or pathology present, may not be palpable.
- *Aorta*—palpate midline above umbilicus, is it expansile? (fig 2.49, p79).

Percussion:

- *Liver*—percuss to map upper & lower border of liver.
- *Spleen*—percuss from border of spleen as palpated, around to mid-axillary line.
- *Bladder*—if enlarged, suprapubic region will be dull.
- *Ascites—shifting dullness:* percuss centrally to laterally until dull, keep your finger at the dull spot and ask patient to lean onto opposite side. If the dullness was fluid, this will now have moved by gravity and the previously dull area will be resonant.

Auscultation:

- *Bowel sounds*—listen just below the umbilicus.
- *Bruits*—listen over aorta and renal arteries (either side of midline above umbilicus).

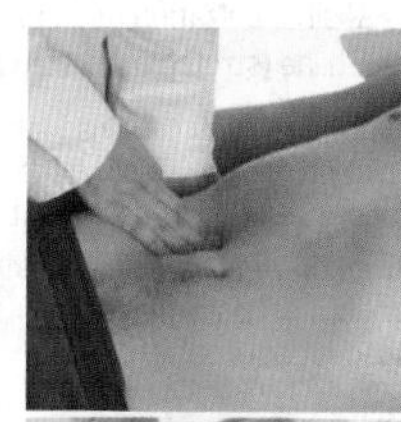

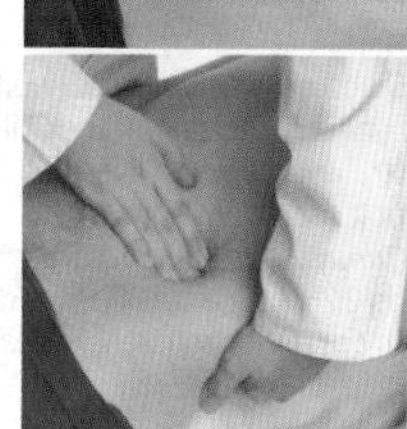

Fig 2.30 Ballottement of the kidneys.

Reproduced from Thomas J, *et al.* (eds). *Oxford Handbook of Clinical Examination and Practical Skills* (2007), with permission from Oxford University Press.

7 To complete the examination

- Palpate for *ankle oedema*, examine the *hernial orifices*, *external genitalia*, and perform a rectal examination. Check the observation chart and dipstick urine.

Top tips

- If you think there is a spleen tip, roll the patient onto their right side and feel again. This tips the spleen forward and allows you to percuss around to the back.
- Check the back for spider naevi, even if the chest appears clear (look for nephrectomy scars as you do this).
- Light palpation really should be light, to check for tenderness and very large masses, watching the patient's face throughout.
- If you suspect voluntary guarding, use the diaphragm of your stethoscope to assist with palpation and distract the patient who will think you are auscultating!

Inspection

Does your patient appear comfortable or in distress? Look for abnormal contours/distension. Tattoos? Cushingoid appearance may suggest steroid use post-transplant or IBD. *Inspect* (and smell) for signs of chronic liver disease:

- Hepatic fetor on breath (p274).
- Purpura (purple-stained skin, p344).
- Spider naevi (fig 2.27, p60).
- Asterixis.
- Gynaecomastia.
- Scratch marks.
- Palmar erythema.
- Clubbing (rare).
- Muscle wasting.
- Jaundice.

Look for signs of malignancy (cachexia, masses), anaemia, jaundice, Virchow's node. From the end of the bed inspect the abdomen for:

- Visible pulsation (aneurysm, p654).
- Striae (stretch marks, eg pregnancy).
- Peristalsis.
- Distension.
- Scars.
- Genitalia.
- Masses.
- Herniae.

If abdominal wall veins look dilated, assess *direction of flow*. In inferior vena caval (IVC) obstruction, below the umbilicus blood flows up; in portal hypertension (*caput medusae*), flow radiates out from the umbilicus.

The cough test: While looking at the face, ask the patient to cough. If this causes abdominal pain, flinching, or a protective movement of hands towards the abdomen, suspect peritonitis.

Hands

Clubbing, *leuconychia* (whitening of the nails due to hypoalbuminaemia), *koilonychia* ('spooning' of the nails due to iron, B_{12}, or folate deficiency), *Muehrcke's lines* (transverse white lines due to hypoalbuminaemia), *blue lunulae* (bluish discolouration seen in Wilson's disease). *Palmar erythema* (chronic liver disease, pregnancy), *Dupuytren's contracture* (thickening and fibrous contraction of palmar fascia (see fig 2.26, p60; alcoholic liver disease)). *Hepatic flap/asterixis* (hepatic encephalopathy, uraemia from renal disease), check pulse and respiratory rate (infection/sepsis?), palpate for AV fistulae in the forearm (haemodialysis access in renal failure).

Face

Assess for jaundice, anaemia, xanthelasma (PBC, chronic obstruction), *Kayser-Fleischer rings* (green-yellow ring at corneal margin seen in Wilson's disease). Inspect mouth for angular stomatitis (thiamine, B_{12}, iron deficiency), pigmentation (Peutz-Jeghers syndrome, p709, fig 15.14), telangiectasia (Osler-Weber-Rendu syndrome/hereditary haemorrhagic telangiectasia, p709, fig 15.12), ulcers (IBD), glossitis (iron, B_{12}, or folate deficiency).

Cervical lymph nodes

Palpate for enlarged left supraclavicular lymph node (*Virchow's node/Troisier's sign*) (gastric carcinoma?).

Abdomen

Inspect: Look around to the flanks for nephrectomy scars.

Palpate: Note any masses, tenderness, guarding (involuntary tensing of abdominal muscles—pain or fear of it), or rebound tenderness (greater pain on removing hand than on gently depressing abdomen—peritoneal inflammation); Rovsing's sign (appendicitis, p608); Murphy's sign (cholecystitis, p634). *Palpating the liver:* Assess size (see BOX 'Causes of hepatomegaly'), regularity, smoothness, and tenderness. Pulsatile (tricuspid regurgitation)? *The scratch test* is another way to find the lower liver edge (if it is below the costal margin): start with diaphragm of stethoscope at right costal margin. Gently scratch the abdominal wall, starting in the right lower quadrant, working towards the liver edge. A sharp increase in transmission of the scratch is heard when the border of the liver is reached. *Palpating the spleen:* If suspect splenomegaly but cannot detect it, assess patient in the right lateral position with your left hand pulling forwards from behind the rib cage. *Palpating the kidneys:* See fig 2.30, p61. May be non palpable unless slim. Enlarged? Nodular? *Palpating the aorta:* Normally palpable transmitted pulsation in thin individuals.

Percussion

Confirm the lower border and define the upper border of the liver and spleen (dull in the mid-axillary line in the 10th intercostal space). Percuss all regions of abdomen. If this induces pain, there may be peritoneal inflammation below (eg an inflamed appendix). Some experts percuss first, before palpation, because even anxious patients do not expect this to hurt—so, if it does hurt, this is a very valuable sign. Percuss for the shifting dullness of ascites (p61 & p604) but ultrasound is a more reliable way of detecting ascites.

Auscultation

Bowel sounds: absence implies ileus; they are enhanced and tinkling in bowel obstruction. Listen for bruits in the aorta, renal and femoral arteries.

Further examination Check for hernias (p612), perform a PR examination see BOX 'Examination of the rectum and anus'.

Examination of the rectum and anus

►It is necessary to have a chaperone present for the examination. Explain what you are about to do. Make sure curtains are pulled. Have the patient lie on their left side, with knees brought up towards the chest. Use gloves and lubricant. Part the buttocks and *inspect the anus*: •A gaping anus suggests a neuropathy or megarectum. •Symmetry (a tender unilateral bulge suggests an abscess). •Prolapsed piles. •A subanodermal clot may peep out. •Prolapsed rectum (descent of >3cm when asked to strain, as if to pass a motion). •Anodermatitis (from frequent soiling). The anocutaneous reflex tests sensory and motor innervation—on lightly stroking the anal skin, does the external sphincter briefly contract?

Press your index finger against the side of the anus. Ask the patient to breathe deeply and insert your finger slowly. Feel for masses (haemorrhoids are not palpable) or impacted stool. Twist your arm so that the pad of your finger is feeling anteriorly. Feel for the cervix or prostate. Note consistency, size, and symmetry of the prostate. If there is faecal incontinence or concern about the spinal cord, ask the patient to squeeze your finger and note the tone. This is best done with your finger pad facing posteriorly. Note stool or blood on the glove and test for occult blood.

Wipe the anus. Consider proctoscopy (for the anus) or sigmoidoscopy (which mainly inspects the rectum).

Causes of hepatomegaly

(For hepatosplenomegaly, see p604.)

Malignancy: Metastatic or primary (usually craggy, irregular edge).

Hepatic congestion: Right heart failure—may be pulsatile in tricuspid incompetence, hepatic vein thrombosis (Budd-Chiari syndrome, p696).

Anatomical: Riedel's lobe (normal variant).

Infection: Infectious mononucleosis (glandular fever), hepatitis viruses, malaria, schistosomiasis, amoebic abscess, hydatid cyst.

Haematological: Leukaemia, lymphoma, myeloproliferative disorders (eg myelofibrosis), sickle-cell disease, haemolytic anaemias.

Others: Fatty liver, porphyria, amyloidosis, glycogen storage disorders.

Splenomegaly

• Abnormally large spleen.

Causes: See p604. If **m**assive, think of: chronic **m**yeloid leukaemia, **m**yelofibrosis, **m**alaria (or leishmaniasis).

Features of the spleen differentiating it from an enlarged kidney

• Cannot get above it (ribs overlie the upper border of the spleen).
• Dull to percussion (kidney is usually resonant because of overlying bowel).
• Moves towards RIF with inspiration (kidney tends to move downwards).
• May have palpable notch on its medial side.

The neurological system: history

History This should be taken from the patient and if possible from a close friend or relative as well for corroboration/discrepancies. The patient's memory, perception, or speech may be affected by the disorder, making the history difficult to obtain. Note the progression of the symptoms and signs: gradual deterioration (eg tumour) vs intermittent exacerbations (eg multiple sclerosis) vs rapid onset (eg stroke). Ask about age, occupation, and ethnic origin. Right- or left-hand dominant?

Presenting symptoms

- *Headache:* (p456 & p780.) Different to usual headaches? Acute/chronic? Speed of onset? Single/recurrent? Unilateral/bilateral? Associated symptoms (eg aura with migraine, p458)? Any meningism (p822)? Worse on waking (↑ICP)? Decreased conscious level? ►Take a 'worst-ever' headache very seriously. (See p749.)
- *Muscle weakness:* (p466.) Speed of onset? Muscle groups affected? Sensory loss? Any sphincter disturbance? Loss of balance? Associated spinal/root pain?
- *Visual disturbance:* (*OHCS* p410.) eg blurring, double vision (diplopia), photophobia, visual loss. Speed of onset? Any preceding symptoms? Pain in eye?
- *Change in other senses:* Hearing (p464), smell, taste? Abnormalities are not always due to neurological disease, consider ENT disease.
- *Dizziness:* (p462.) Illusion of surroundings moving (vertigo)? Hearing loss/tinnitus? Any loss of consciousness? Positional?
- *Speech disturbance:* (p86.) Difficulty in expression, articulation, or comprehension (can be difficult to determine)? Sudden onset or gradual?
- *Dysphagia:* (p250.) Solids and/or liquids? Intermittent or constant? Difficulty in coordination? Painful (odynophagia)?
- *Fits/faints/'funny turns'/involuntary movements:* (p468.) Frequency? Duration? Mode of onset? Preceding aura? Loss of consciousness? Tongue biting? Incontinence? Any residual weakness/confusion? Family history?
- *Abnormal sensations:* Eg numbness, 'pins & needles' (paraesthesiae), pain, odd sensations. Distribution? Speed of onset? Associated weakness?
- *Tremor:* (p65.) Rapid or slow? Present at rest? Worse on deliberate movement? Taking β-agonists? Any thyroid problems? Any family history? Fasciculations?

Cognitive state If there is any doubt about the patient's cognition, cognitive testing should be undertaken. There are a number of tools including MMSE (subject to strict copyright), GPCOG, TYM, and 6-CIT. The Abbreviated Mental Test Score (AMTS) is a commonly used screening questionnaire for cognitive impairment:[12]

1. Tell patient an address to recall at the end (eg 42 West Street)
2. Age
3. Time (to nearest hour)
4. What year is it?
5. Recognize 2 people (eg doctor & nurse)
6. Date of birth
7. Dates of the Second World War
8. Name of current monarch/prime minister
9. Where are you now? (Which hospital?)
10. Count backwards from 20 to 1

A score of ≤6 suggests poor cognition, acute (delirium), or chronic (dementia). AMTS correlates well with the more detailed Mini-Mental State Examination (MMSE™) NB: deaf, dysphasic, depressed, and uncooperative patients, as well as those who do not understand English, will also get low scores.[13]

Past medical history Ask about meningitis/encephalitis, head/spine trauma, seizures, previous operations, risk factors for vascular disease (p470, AF, hypertension, hyperlipidaemia, diabetes, smoking), and recent travel, especially exotic destinations. Is there any chance that the patient is pregnant (eclampsia, *OHCS* p48)?

Drug history Any anticonvulsant/antipsychotic/antidepressant medication? Any psychotropic drugs (eg ecstasy)? Any medication with neurological side-effects (eg isoniazid which can cause a peripheral neuropathy)?

Social and family history What can the patient do/not do, ie activities of daily living (ADLs)? What's the Barthel Index score? Any family history of neurological or psychiatric disease? Any consanguinity? Consider sexual history, eg syphilis.

Cramp

This is painful muscle spasm. Leg cramps are common at night or after heavy exercise, and in patients with renal impairment or on dialysis. Cramp can signify salt depletion, and rarely: muscle ischaemia (claudication, DM), myopathy (McArdle, p704), or dystonia (writer's cramp, p469). Forearm cramps suggest motor neuron disease. Night cramps may respond to quinine bisulfate 300mg at night PO.

Drugs causing cramp: Diuretics (? from ↓K^+), domperidone, salbutamol/terbutaline IVI, ACE-i, telmisartan, celecoxib, lacidipine, ergot alkaloids, levothyroxine.

Paraesthesiae

'Pins and needles', numbness/tingling, which can hurt or 'burn' (dysaesthesia).

Causes:

Metabolic, ↓Ca^{2+} (perioral); ↑P_aCO_2; myxoedema; neurotoxins (tick bite; sting). *Vascular,* ►►arterial emboli; Raynaud's; DVT; high plasma viscosity. *Antibody-mediated,* paraneoplastic; SLE; ITP. *Infection,* rare: Lyme; rabies. *Drugs,* ACE-i. *Brain,* thalamic/parietal lesions. *Cord,* MS; myelitis/HIV; ↓B_{12}; ►►lumbar fracture. *Plexopathy/mononeuropathy,* see p502, cervical rib; carpal tunnel; sciatica. *Peripheral neuropathy,* glove & stocking, p504, eg DM; CKD. If *paroxysmal,* migraine; epilepsy; phaeochromocytoma. If *wandering,* take travel history, consider infection, eg strongyloides.

Tremor

Tremor is rhythmic oscillation of limbs, trunk, head, or tongue. Three types:

1 *Resting tremor*—worst at rest—eg from parkinsonism (±bradykinesia and rigidity; tremor is more resistant to treatment than other symptoms). It is usually a slow tremor (frequency of 3–5Hz), typically 'pill-rolling' of the thumb over a finger.
2 *Postural tremor*—worst if arms are outstretched. Typically *rapid* (8–12Hz). May be exaggerated physiological tremor (eg anxiety, hyperthyroidism, alcohol, drugs), due to brain damage (eg Wilson's disease, syphilis) or *benign essential tremor* (BET). This is often familial (autosomal dominant) tremor of arms and head presenting at any age. Cogwheeling may occur but there is no bradykinesia. It is suppressed by alcohol, and patients may self-medicate rather than admit problems. Rarely progressive (unless onset is unilateral). Propranolol (40–80mg/8–12h PO) can help, but not in all patients.
3 *Intention tremor*—worst on movement, seen in cerebellar disease, with past-pointing and dysdiadochokinesis (see p499). No effective drug has been found.

Facial pain

CNS causes: Migraine, trigeminal, or glossopharyngeal neuralgia (p457) or from any other pain-sensitive structure in the head or neck. *Post-herpetic neuralgia:* nasty burning-and-stabbing pain involves dermatomal areas affected by shingles (p404); it may affect cranial nerves V and VII in the face. It all too often becomes chronic and intractable (skin affected is exquisitely sensitive). Treatment is hard. Always give strong psychological support. Transcutaneous nerve stimulation, capsaicin ointment, and infiltrating local anaesthetic are tried. Neuropathic pain agents, such as amitriptyline, eg 10-25mg/24h at night, or gabapentin (p504) may help. NB: famciclovir or valaciclovir given in acute shingles may ↓ duration of neuralgia.[14]

Vascular and non-neurological causes:

- *Neck*—cervical disc pathology.
- *Bone/sinuses*—sinusitis; neoplasia.
- *Eye*—glaucoma; iritis; orbital cellulitis; eye strain; AVM.
- *Temporomandibular joint*—arthritis or idiopathic dysfunction (common).
- *Teeth/gums*—caries; broken teeth; abscess; malocclusion.
- *Ear*—otitis media; otitis externa.
- *Vascular/vasculitis*—arteriovenous fistula; aneurysm; or AVM at the cerebellopontine angle; giant cell arteritis; SLE.

Neurological examination of the upper limbs

The neurological system is usually the most daunting examination, so learn at the bedside from a senior colleague, preferably a neurologist. Keep practising. Be aware that books present ideal situations: often one or more signs are equivocal or even contrary to expectation; consider signs in the context of the history and try re-examining the patient, as signs may evolve over time. The only essential point is to distinguish whether weakness is upper (UMN) or lower (LMN) motor neuron (p446). Position the patient comfortably, sitting up at 45° and with arms exposed. The order of examination should be Inspection, Tone, Power, Reflexes, Coordination, Sensation (fig 2.31).

1 General inspection

Abnormal posturing, asymmetry, abnormal movements (fasciculation/tremor/dystonia/athetosis), muscle wasting (especially small muscles of the hand)—symmetrical/asymmetrical? Local/general?

↓

2 Tone

Ask patient to 'relax/go floppy like a rag-doll'. Ask if patient has any pain in hands/arm/shoulder before passively flexing and extending limb while also pronating and supinating the forearm. Any spasticity or rigidity?

↓

3 Power

Direct patient to adopt each position and follow commands while you as the examiner stabilize the joint above and resist movements as appropriate to grade power (see BOX 'Muscle weakness grading' on p446). Test each muscle group bilaterally before moving on to the next position. See p452-3 for myotomes.

- 'Shrug your shoulders and don't let me push down; push your arms out to the side against me; try to pull them back in.'
- 'Hold your arms up like this and pull me towards you, now push me away.'
- 'Hold your hand out flat, don't let me push it down; now don't let me push it up.'
- Offer the patient two (crossed) fingers of yours and ask them to 'squeeze my fingers.'
- Ask patient to 'spread your fingers and stop me pushing them back together', then hand the patient a piece of paper to grip between two fingers. You as the examiner should grip the paper with your corresponding fingers while asking patient to 'grip the paper and don't let me pull it away.'

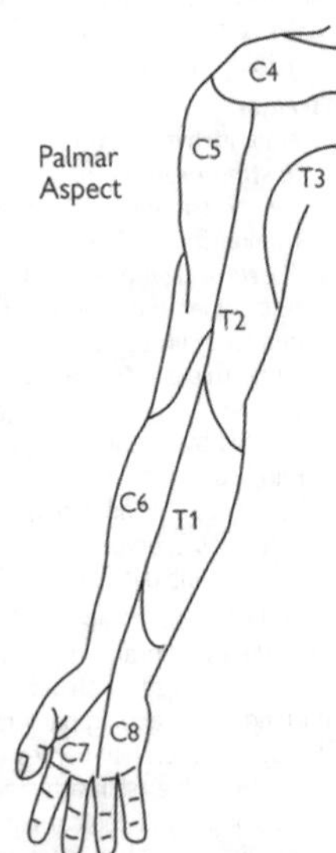

4 Reflexes

For each reflex, test right, then left and compare. If absent, attempt to elicit with 'reinforcement' by asking patient to clench their teeth on a count of three, at which time you strike (Jendrassik manoeuvre). Are reflexes absent/present (with reinforcement)/normal/brisk/exaggerated? •*Biceps* (C5,6) •*Triceps* (C7) •*Supinator* (C6).

↓

5 Coordination

Holding your finger in front of the patient instruct 'touch my finger then your nose...as fast as you can'. Look for intention tremor, and 'past pointing'.

- *Test for dysdiadokokinesis:* ask patient to repeatedly pronate and supinate forearm, tapping hands each time. Test both limbs. You may have to demonstrate. Failure to perform rapidly alternating movements is dysdiadokokinesis.
- *Test for pronator drift:* with patient's eyes closed and arms outstretched, tap down on their up-facing palms and look for a failure to maintain supination.

↓

6 Sensation

- *Light touch:* Use cotton wool, touch (not rub) it to sternum first—'this is what it should feel like, tell me where you feel it and if it feels different'. Proceed to test with cotton wool in all dermatomes (see p454), comparing left and right.
- *Pin prick:* Repeat as above using a neurological pin, asking patient to tell you if it feels sharp or dull.
- *Temperature:* Repeat as above, alternating hot and cold probes. Can the patient tell hot from cold?
- *Vibration:* Using a 128Hz tuning fork (128 vibrate!) confirm with patient that they 'can feel a buzzing' when you place the tuning fork on their sternum. Proceed to test at the most distal bony prominence and move proximally by placing the buzzing fork on the bony prominence, then stopping it with your fingers. Ask the patient to tell you when the buzzing stops.
- *Proprioception:* With the patient's eyes closed grasp distal phalanx of the index finger at the sides, not on top. Stabilize the rest of the finger. Flex and extend the joint, stopping at intervals to ask whether the finger tip is up or down.

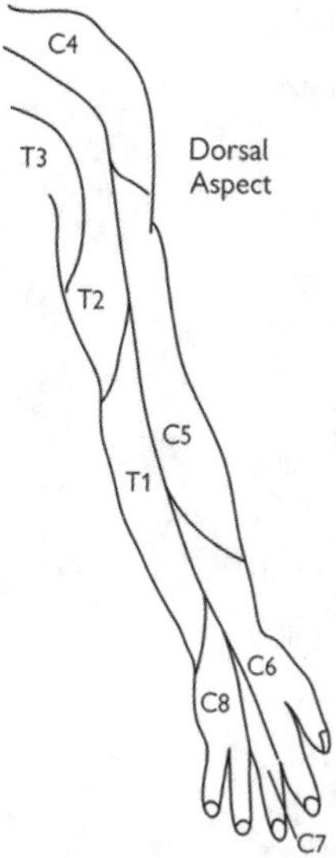

C4
T3
Dorsal Aspect
T2
C5
T1
C6
C8
C7

Fig 2.31 Sensory dermatomes.
Reproduced from Harrison (ed) *Revision Notes for MCEM Part A* (2011), with permission from Oxford University Press.

Top tips

- Use the tendon hammer like a pendulum, let it drop, don't grip it too tightly.
- Ensure you are testing light touch, not stroke sensation.

Neurological examination of the lower limbs

If the patient is able, begin your examination by asking the patient to remove their lower garments down to underwear, and to walk across the room. Gait analysis (p467) gives you more information than any other test. If they aren't able to walk, start with them lying down, legs fully exposed. Then, Inspection, Tone, Reflexes, Power, Coordination, Sensation (fig 2.32).

1 General inspection and gait

Gait: Ask patient to walk a few metres, turn, and walk back to you. Note use of walking aids, symmetry, size of paces, arm swing. Ask patient to 'walk heel-to-toe as if on a tightrope' to exaggerate any instability. Ask patient to walk on tiptoes, then on heels. Inability to walk on tiptoes indicates S1 or gastrocnemius lesion. Inability to walk on heels indicates L4,5 lesion or foot drop.

Romberg's test: Ask patient to stand unaided with arms by their sides and close their eyes (be ready to support them). If they sway/lose balance the test is positive and indicates posterior column disease/sensory ataxia.

Inspect: Abnormal posturing, muscle wasting, fasciculation (LMN lesion?), deformities of the foot (eg pes cavus of *Friedreich's ataxia* or *Charcot-Marie-Tooth disease*). Is one leg smaller than the other (*old polio, infantile hemiplegia*)?

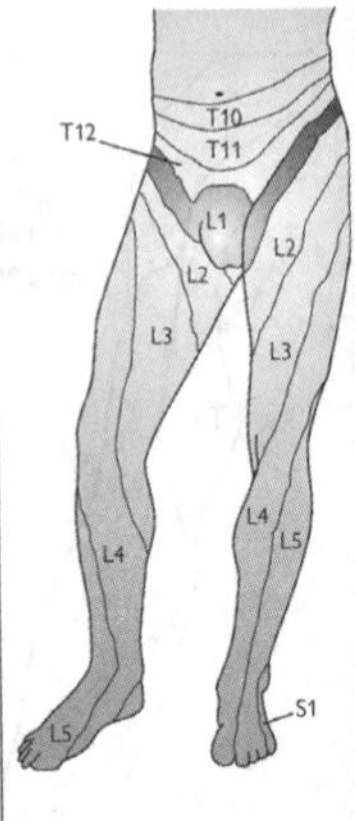

2 Tone

Ask patient to 'relax/go floppy like a rag-doll'. Ask if they have any pain in feet/legs/hips before passively flexing and extending each limb while also internally and externally rotating. Hold the patient's knee and roll it from side to side. Put your hand behind the knee and raise it quickly. The heel should lift slightly from the bed if tone is normal. Any spasticity/rigidity?

Clonus: Plantar flex the foot then quickly dorsiflex and hold. More than 3 'beats' of plantar flexion is sustained clonus and is abnormal. Clonus can also be elicited at the patella with rapid downward movement of patella. Hypertonia and clonus suggest an upper motor neuron lesion.

3 Reflexes

For each reflex, test right, then left and compare. If absent, attempt to elicit with 'reinforcement'. Decide whether reflexes are absent/present (with reinforcement)/normal/brisk/exaggerated.

- *Knee:* (L3,4.) Strike on the patella tendon, just below the patella.
- *Ankle:* (L5,S1.) Several accepted methods; ideally ask the patient to slightly bend the knee, then drop it laterally, grasp the foot and dorsiflex, then strike the Achilles tendon. If hip pain limits mobility, dorsiflex the foot with a straight leg and strike your hand, feeling for an ankle jerk.
- *Plantar reflexes:* (L5, S1, S2.) Stroke the patient's sole with an orange stick or similar. The normal reflex is downward movement of the great toe. *Babinski's sign* is positive if there is dorsiflexion of the great toe (this is abnormal (upper motor neuron lesion) if patient age >6 months).

4 Power

Direct patient to adopt position and follow the following commands while you as the examiner resist movements as appropriate to grade power (p446). Test each muscle group bilaterally before moving on to the next position. See pp452-3 for myotomes.

- *Hip flexion:* 'Keeping your leg straight, can you lift your leg off the bed, don't let me push it down.'
- *Hip extension:* 'And now using your leg, push my hand into the bed.'
- *Hip abduction:* Position hands on outer thighs—'push your legs out to the sides.'
- *Hip adduction:* Position hands on inner thighs—'and push your legs together.'
- *Knee flexion and extension:* 'Bend your knee and bring your heel to your bottom, don't let me pull it away... and now kick out against me and push me away.'
- *Ankle plantar flexion:* With your hand on the underside of the patient's foot ask them to 'bend your foot down, pushing my hand away.'
- *Ankle dorsiflexion:* Put your hand on the dorsum of the foot and ask them to 'lift up your foot, point your toes at the ceiling, don't let me push your foot down.'

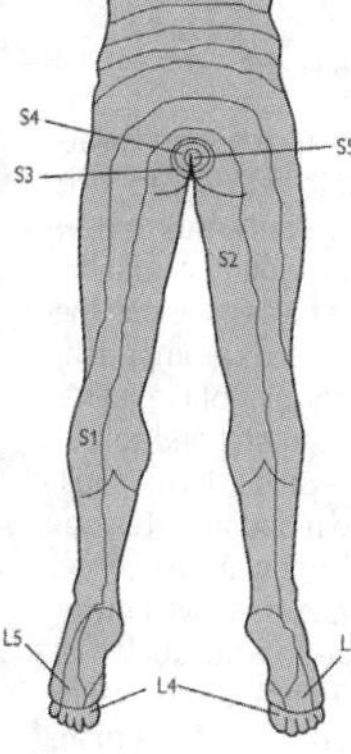

Fig 2.32 Dermatomes of lower limb.

Reproduced from Harrison (ed) *Revision Notes for MCEM Part A* (2011), with permission from Oxford University Press.

5 Coordination

Heel-shin test: Using your finger on the patient's shin to demonstrate, instruct patient to 'put your heel just below your knee then run it smoothly down your shin, lift it up and place it back on your knee, now run it down again', etc. Repeat on the other side. Also, fast alternate foot tapping onto examiners's hands with patient lying down.

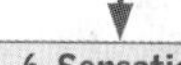

6 Sensation

As upper limbs (p67).

- *Light touch:* Lower limb dermatomes (p454).
- *Pin prick*
- *Temperature*
- *Vibration*
- *Joint position sense:* With the patient's eyes closed grasp distal phalanx of the great toe at the sides. Stabilize the rest of the toe. Move the joint up and tell patient 'this is up', and down, saying 'this is down'. Flex and extend the joint, stopping at intervals to ask whether the toe is up or down.

Top tips

- If you are limited for time, gait is the most useful test to start with.
- Make sure you test each muscle group individually by stabilizing above the joint you are testing.
- Test vibration by putting a buzzing tuning fork on the bony part of a joint (most distal point) with the patient's eyes closed then ask them to tell you when the buzzing stops (pinch the tuning fork to stop it) to distinguish vibration from pressure sensation.

Cranial nerve names
I olfactory
II optic
III oculomotor
IV trochlear
V1 ophthalmic division
V2 maxillary division
V3 mandibular division
VI abducens
VII facial
VIII vestibulocochlear
IX glossopharyngeal
X vagus
XI accessory
XII hypoglossal

Approach to examining the cranial nerves Where is the lesion? Think systematically. Is it in the brainstem (eg MS) or outside, pressing on the brainstem? Is it the neuromuscular junction (myasthenia) or the muscles (eg a dystrophy)? Cranial nerves may be affected singly or in groups. ►Face the patient (helps spot asymmetry). For causes of lesions see BOX 'Causes of cranial nerve lesions'.

- *I: Smell*—test ability of each nostril (separately) to distinguish familiar smells, eg coffee.
- *II: Acuity*—test each eye separately, and its correctability with glasses or pin-hole; use Snellen chart, or the one inside the cover of this book. *Visual fields*—compare with your own fields or formally via perimetry testing. Any losses/inattention? Sites of lesions: *OHCS* p428. *Pupils* (p72)—size, shape, symmetry, reaction to light (direct and consensual) or accommodation. Swinging light test for relative afferent pupillary defect. *Ophthalmoscopy* (*OHCS*, p414)—best learnt from an ophthalmologist and dilating drops help! Darken the room, warn the patient you will need to get close to their face. Focus the lens on the optic disc (pale? swollen?). Follow vessels outwards to view each quadrant. If the view is obscured, examine the red reflex, with your focus on the margin of the pupil, to look for a cataract. Try to get a view of the fovea by asking the patient to look directly at the ophthalmoscope ►Pathology here needs prompt ophthalmic review. If in doubt, ask for slit lamp examination or photography of the retina.
- *III*[P]*, IV, & VI*—eye movements. Ask the patient to keep their head still and follow your finger as you trace an imaginary 'H'. *IIIrd nerve palsy*—ptosis, large pupil, eye down and out. *IVth nerve palsy*—diplopia on looking down and in (often noticed on descending stairs)—head tilting compensates for this (ocular torticollis). *VIth nerve palsy*—horizontal diplopia on looking out. *Nystagmus* is involuntary, often jerky, eye oscillations. Horizontal nystagmus is often due to a vestibular lesion (acute: nystagmus away from lesion; chronic: towards lesion), or cerebellar lesion (unilateral lesions cause nystagmus towards the affected side). If it is more in whichever eye is abducting, MS may be the cause (internuclear ophthalmoplegia, see fig 2.34). If also deafness/tinnitus, suspect a peripheral cause (eg VIIIth nerve lesion, barotrauma, Ménière's, p462). If it varies with head position, suspect benign positional vertigo (p462). If it is up-and-down, ask a neurologist to review—upbeat nystagmus classically occurs with lesions in the midbrain or at the base of the 4th ventricle, downbeat nystagmus in foramen magnum lesions. Nystagmus lasting ≤2 beats is normal, as is nystagmus at the extremes of gaze.
- *V: Motor palsy*—'Open your mouth'; jaw deviates to side of lesion, muscles of mastication (temporalis, masseter and pterygoids). *Sensory*—check all three divisions. Consider corneal reflex (lost first).
- *VII:*[P] *Facial nerve lesions* cause droop and weakness. As the forehead has bilateral representation in the brain, only the lower two-thirds is affected in UMN lesions, but all of one side of the face in LMN lesions. Ask to 'raise your eyebrows', 'show me your teeth', 'puff out your cheeks'. Test taste with salt/sweet solutions (supplies anterior two-thirds of tongue).
- *VIII: Hearing*—p464. Ask to repeat a number whispered in an ear while you block the other. Perform Weber's and Rinne's tests (p464). *Balance/vertigo*—p462.
- *IX*[P] *& X:*[P] *Gag reflex*—ask the patient to say 'Ah'. Xth nerve lesions also cause the palate to be pulled to the normal side on saying 'Ah', uvula deviates away. Ask them to swallow a sip of water. Consider gag reflex—touch the back of the soft palate with an orange stick. The afferent arm of the reflex involves IX; the efferent arm involves X.
- *XI: Trapezii*—'Shrug your shoulders' against resistance. *Sternocleidomastoid*: 'Turn your head to the left/right' against resistance.
- *XII: Tongue movement*—the tongue deviates to the side of the lesion.

Causes of cranial nerve lesions

Any cranial nerve may be affected by diabetes mellitus; stroke; MS; tumours; sarcoidosis; vasculitis (p556), eg PAN (p556), SLE (p554); syphilis. Chronic meningitis (malignant, TB, or fungal) tends to pick off the lower cranial nerves one by one.

- *I:* Trauma; respiratory tract infection; meningitis; frontal lobe tumour.
- *II:* Field defects may start as small areas of visual loss (scotomas, eg in glaucoma). *Monocular blindness*—lesions of one eye or optic nerve eg MS, giant cell arteritis. *Bilateral blindness*[4]—any cause of mononeuritis, eg diabetes, MS; rarely methanol, neurosyphilis. *Field defects—bitemporal hemianopia*—optic chiasm compression, eg pituitary adenoma, craniopharyngioma, internal carotid artery aneurysm (fig 10.3, p451). *Homonymous hemianopia*—affects half the visual field contralateral to the lesion in each eye. Lesions lie beyond the chiasm in the tracts, radiation, or occipital cortex, eg stroke, abscess, tumour. *Optic neuritis* (pain on moving eye, loss of central vision, relative afferent pupillary defect, disc swelling from papillitis[5])—*causes* demyelination (eg MS); rarely sinusitis, syphilis, collagen vascular disorders. *Ischaemic papillopathy*—swelling of optic disc due to stenosis of the posterior ciliary artery (eg in giant cell arteritis). *Papilloedema* (bilaterally swollen discs, fig 12.20, p560)—most commonly ↑ICP (tumour, abscess, encephalitis, hydrocephalus, idiopathic intracranial hypertension); rarer: retro-orbital lesion (eg cavernous sinus thrombosis, p480). *Optic atrophy* (pale optic discs and reduced acuity)—MS; frontal tumours; Friedreich's ataxia; retinitis pigmentosa; syphilis; glaucoma; Leber's optic atrophy; chronic optic nerve compression.
- *III:*[c] *Alone*[c]—'medical' causes (pupillary sparing): diabetes; HTN; giant cell arteritis; syphilis; idiopathic. 'Surgical' causes (early pupil involvement due to external compression of nerve damaging parasympathetic fibres): posterior communicating artery aneurysm (+ surgery) ↑ICP (if uncal herniation through the tentorium compresses the nerve); tumours.
- *IV:*[c] *Alone*—rare and usually due to trauma to the orbit.
- *V:*[c] *Sensory*—trigeminal neuralgia (pain but no sensory loss, p457); herpes zoster, nasopharyngeal cancer, acoustic neuroma (p462). *Motor*—rare.
- *VI:*[c] *Alone*—MS, Wernicke's encephalopathy, false localizing sign in ↑ICP, pontine stroke (presents with fixed small pupils ± quadriparesis).
- *VII: LMN*—Bell's palsy (p500), polio, otitis media, skull fracture; cerebellopontine angle tumours, eg acoustic neuroma, malignant parotid tumours, herpes zoster (Ramsay Hunt syndrome p501, *OHCS* p652). *UMN*—(spares the forehead, because of its bilateral cortical representation), stroke, tumour.
- *VIII:* (p462 & p464.) Noise damage, Paget's disease, Ménière's disease, herpes zoster, acoustic neuroma, brainstem CVA, drugs (eg aminoglycosides).
- *IX, X, XI:* Trauma, brainstem lesions, neck tumours.
- *XII:* Rare. Polio, syringomyelia, tumour, stroke, bulbar palsy, trauma, TB.

Groups of cranial nerves:

VIII, then *V, VI, IX,* & *X*: cerebellopontine angle tumours, eg acoustic neuroma (p462; facial weakness is not a prominent sign). *III, IV* & *VI*: stroke, tumours, Wernicke's encephalopathy; aneurysms, MS. *III, IV,* V_a, & *VI*: cavernous sinus thrombosis, superior orbital fissure lesions (Tolosa-Hunt syndrome, *OHCS* p654). *IX, X,* & *XI*: jugular foramen lesion. ΔΔ: myasthenia gravis, muscular dystrophy, myotonic dystrophy, mononeuritis multiplex (p502).

Top tips

If the patient is able to shake their head, there is no meningism.

4 Remember the commonest cause of monocular or binocular blindness is not a cranial nerve lesion but a problem with the eye itself (cataracts, retinal problems). Neurological disorders more commonly cause loss of part of the visual field.

5 Unilateral disc swelling = papillitis, bilateral papillitis/disc swelling = papilloedema. Check both eyes!

c= structures passing through the cavernous sinus; see BOX 'Psychiatric symptoms', p89. NB: V_a is the only division of V to do so.

P= Remember that these cranial nerves carry parasympathetic fibres. Sympathetic fibres originate from the thoracic chain and run with the arterial supply to distribute about the body (see also *OHCS*, fig 9.6, p621).

Cranial nerve lesions of the eye

Pupillary abnormalities

Key questions: •Equal, central, circular, dilated, or constricted? •React to light, directly and consensually? •Constrict normally on convergence/accommodation?

Irregular pupils: Anterior uveitis (iritis), trauma to the eye, syphilis.

Dilated pupils: CN III lesions (►inc. ↑ICP, p830) and mydriatic drugs. *Always ask: is this pupil dilated, or is it the other that is constricted?*

Constricted pupils: Old age, sympathetic nerve damage (Horner's, p702, and ptosis, p73), opiates, miotics (pilocarpine drops for glaucoma), pontine damage.

Unequal pupils (anisocoria): May be due to unilateral lesion, eye-drops, eye surgery, syphilis, or Holmes-Adie pupil. Some inequality is normal.

Light reaction: Test: cover one eye and shine light into the other obliquely. Both pupils should constrict, one by direct, other by consensual light reflex (fig 2.33). The lesion site is deduced by knowing the pathway: from the retina the message passes up the optic nerve (CNII) to the superior colliculus (midbrain) and thence to the CNIII nuclei on both sides. The IIIrd cranial nerve causes pupillary constriction. If a light in one eye causes only contralateral constriction, the defect is 'efferent', as the afferent pathways from the retina being stimulated must be intact. Test for *relative afferent pupillary defect:* move torch quickly from pupil to pupil. If there has been incomplete damage to the afferent pathway, the affected pupil will paradoxically dilate when light is moved from the normal eye to the abnormal eye. This is because, in the face of reduced afferent input from the affected eye, the consensual pupillary relaxation response from the normal eye predominates. This is the *Marcus Gunn sign*, and may occur after apparent complete recovery from the initial lesion.

Reaction to accommodation/convergence: If the patient first looks at a distant object and then at the examiner's finger held a few inches away, the eyes will converge and the pupils constrict. Afferent fibres in each optic nerve pass to the lateral geniculate bodies. Impulses then pass to the pre-tectal nucleus and then to the parasympathetic nuclei of the IIIrd cranial nerves, causing pupillary constriction.

- *Holmes-Adie (myotonic) pupil:* The affected pupil is normally moderately dilated and is poorly reactive to light, if at all. It is slowly reactive to accommodation; wait and watch carefully: it may eventually constrict more than a normal pupil. It is often associated with diminished or absent ankle and knee reflexes, in which case the Holmes-Adie syndrome is present. Usually a benign incidental finding. Rare causes: Lyme disease, syphilis, parvovirus B19, HSV, autoimmunity. ♀>♂.
- *Argyll Robertson pupil:* This occurs in neurosyphilis. The pupil is constricted and unreactive to light, but reacts to accommodation. Other possible causes: Lyme disease; HIV; zoster; diabetes mellitus; sarcoidosis; MS; paraneoplastic; $\downarrow B_{12}$. The iris may be patchily atrophied, irregular, and depigmented. The lesion site is not *always* near the Edinger-Westphal nucleus or even in the midbrain. Pseudo-Argyll Robertson pupils occur in Parinaud's syndrome (p708).
- *Hutchinson pupil:* This is the sequence of events resulting from rapidly rising unilateral intracranial pressure (eg in intracerebral haemorrhage). The pupil on the side of the lesion first constricts then widely dilates. The other pupil then goes through the same sequence. ►See p830.

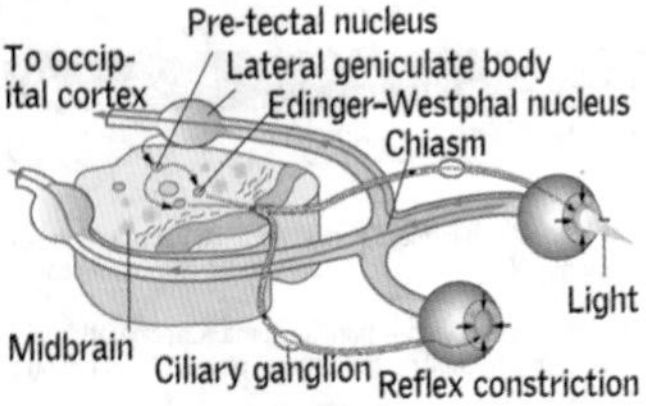

Fig 2.33 Light reflex. Action potentials go along optic nerve (red), traversing optic chiasm, passing synapses at pre-tectal nucleus, *en route* to Edinger-Westphal nuclei of CNIII. These send fibres to *both* irises' ciliary muscles (so *both* pupils constrict) via *ciliary ganglion* (also relays accommodation and corneal sensation, and gets sympathetic roots from C8-T2, carrying fibres to dilate pupil).

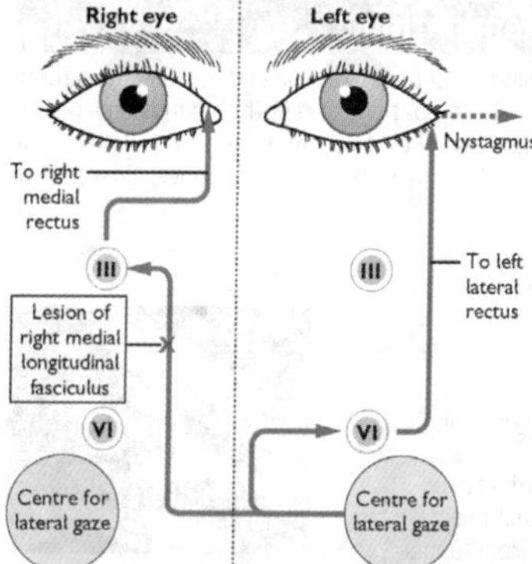

Fig 2.34 Internuclear ophthalmoplegia (INO) and its causes. To produce synchronous eye movements, cranial nerves III, IV, and VI communicate through medial longitudinal fasciculus in midbrain. In INO, a lesion disrupts communication, causing weakness in adduction of the ipsilateral eye with nystagmus of the contralateral eye *only when abducting*. There may be incomplete or slow abduction of the ipsilateral eye during lateral gaze. Convergence is preserved. *Causes* MS or vascular (rarely: HIV; syphilis; Lyme disease; brainstem tumours; phenothiazine toxicity).

Ptosis

Drooping of the upper eyelid. Best observed with patient sitting up, with head held by examiner. Oculomotor nerve (CN III) innervates main muscle concerned (levator palpebrae), but nerves from the cervical sympathetic chain innervate superior tarsal muscle, and a lesion of these nerves causes mild ptosis which can be overcome on looking up. *Causes:*

1. CN III lesions cause unilateral *complete* ptosis: look for other evidence of a CN III lesion: ophthalmoplegia with 'down and out' deviation of the eye, pupil dilated and unreactive to light or accommodation. If eye pain too, suspect infiltration (eg by lymphoma or sarcoidosis). If ↑T° or ↓consciousness, suspect infection (any tick bites?).
2. Sympathetic paralysis usually causes unilateral partial ptosis. Look for other evidence of a sympathetic lesion, as in Horner's syndrome (p702): constricted pupil = *miosis*, lack of sweating on same side of the face (=*anhidrosis*).
3. Myopathy, eg dystrophia myotonica, myasthenia gravis (cause bilateral partial ptosis).
4. Congenital; usually partial and without other CNS signs.

Visual loss

►Get ophthalmology help. See *OHCS* p434–p455. Consider:

- Is the eye red? (*Glaucoma*, *uveitis* p561.)
- Pain? *Giant cell arteritis*: severe temporal headache, jaw claudication, scalp tenderness, ↑ESR: ► urgent steroids (p556). *Optic neuritis*: eg in MS.
- Is the cornea cloudy: *corneal ulcer* (*OHCS* p435), *glaucoma* (*OHCS* p433)?
- Is there a contact lens problem (*infection*)?
- Any flashes/floaters? (*TIA*, *migraine*, *retinal detachment*?)
- Is there a visual field problem (*stroke*, *space-occupying lesion*, *glaucoma*)?
- Are there any focal CNS signs?
- Any valvular heart disease/carotid bruits (*emboli*)? Hyperlipidaemia (p690)?
- Is there a relative afferent pupillary defect (p72)?
- Any past history of trauma, migraine, hypertension, cerebrovascular disease, MS, diabetes or connective tissue disease?
- Any distant signs: eg *HIV* (causes retinitis), *SLE*, *sarcoidosis*?

Sudden: • Acute glaucoma • Retinal detachment • Vitreous haemorrhage (eg in diabetic proliferative retinopathy) • Central retinal artery or vein occlusion • Migraine • CNS: TIA (amaurosis fugax), stroke, space-occupying lesion • Optic neuritis (eg MS) • Temporal arteritis • Drugs: quinine/methanol • Pituitary apoplexy.

Gradual: • Optic atrophy • Chronic glaucoma • Cataracts • Macular degeneration • Tobacco amblyopia.

Musculoskeletal hand examination 1

Begin by introducing yourself, obtaining consent to examine and position the patient appropriately. Expose the arms, then ask the patient to rest their hands on a pillow. Start by examining the dorsal surface and then turn the hands over. Always ask about pain or tender areas. Follow the 'look, ask the patient to move, then feel' to avoid causing pain.

Skin

On both the palm and the dorsum start by inspecting the skin for:

1 *Colour*—pigmentation of creases, jaundice, palmar erythema (fig 2.44).
2 *Consistency*—tight (sclerodactyly), thick (DM, acromegaly) (fig 2.39).
3 *Characteristic lesions*—pulp infarcts, rashes, purpura, spider naevi, telangiectasia, tophi (fig 2.35), scars (eg carpal tunnel release).

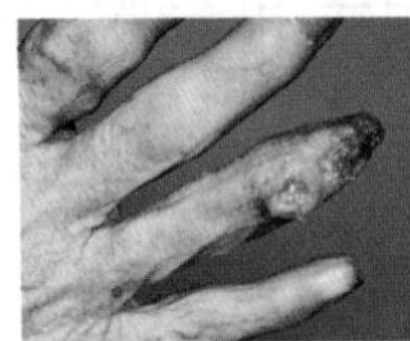

Fig 2.35 Gouty tophi.

Nails

Look for the same skin changes as the palm, plus tendon xanthomata, plaques, and joint replacement scars, and examine the nails for:

- Pitting and onycholysis (p76).
- Clubbing (p77).
- Nail fold infarcts and splinter haemorrhages.
- Other lesions, eg Beau's lines (fig 2.41, p76), koilonychia, leuconychia (fig 2.36).

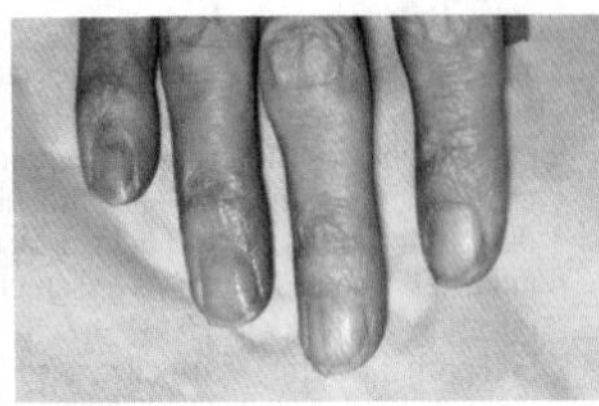

Fig 2.36 Leuconychia.

Muscles

Examine the muscles for wasting and fasciculations; on the dorsal surface look for wasting, particularly of dorsal interossei. On the palm look particularly at the thenar and hypothenar eminences.

- Thenar wasting (fig 2.37) = median nerve lesion.
- Generalized wasting, particularly of the interossei on the dorsum, but sparing of the thenar eminence = ulnar nerve lesion.

Also look for *Dupuytren's* contracture and perform *Tinel's test* (percuss over the distal skin crease of the wrist). *Phalen's test* (patient holds dorsal surfaces of both hands together for 60 seconds). Both tests are positive if tingling reported, suggesting carpal tunnel syndrome.

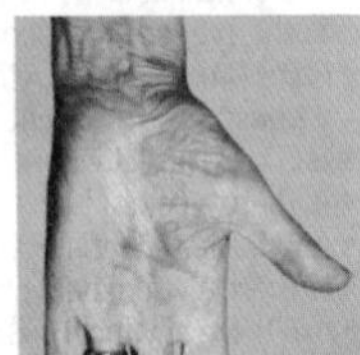

Fig 2.37 Thenar wasting.

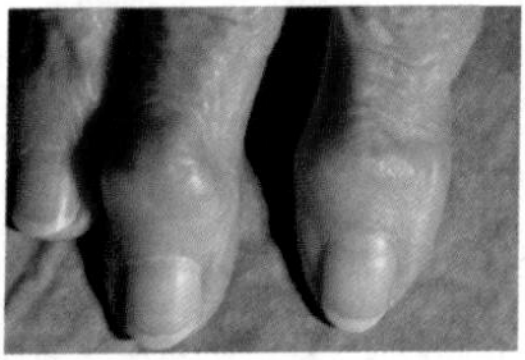

Fig 2.38 Osteoarthritis.

Joints

Examine for acute inflammation (swollen, red joints) as well as the characteristic deformities of chronic arthritis, eg rheumatoid, osteoarthritis (fig 2.38).

- Ulnar deviation at the wrist.
- Z deformity of the thumb.
- Swan-neck (flexed DIP, hyperextended PIP—fig 12.2, p540).
- Boutonnière (hyperextended DIP, flexed PIP).
- Heberden's nodes (DIP joints, p77).
- Bouchard's nodes (PIP joints).

↓

Move and feel

By this point, you should know the likely diagnosis, so assess neurological function looking at power, function, and sensation:

- *Wrist and forearm*: Extension (prayer position) and flexion (reverse prayer), supination and pronation. Look at the elbows.
- *Small muscles*: Pincer grip, power grip (squeeze my two fingers), abduction of the thumb, abduction (spread your fingers), and adduction (grip this piece of paper between your fingers) of the fingers. NB *Froment's sign* = flexion of the thumb during grip as ulnar nerve lesion prevents adduction (p453).
- *Function*: Write a sentence, undo a button, pick up a coin.
- *Sensation*: Test little finger (ulnar), index finger (median), and anatomical snuffbox (radial) using light touch/pinprick.

When you have clinched the diagnosis and functional status, examine each joint, palpating for tenderness, effusions, and crepitus. Test sensation (see p67) and examine the elbows. Consider examination of upper limbs and face.

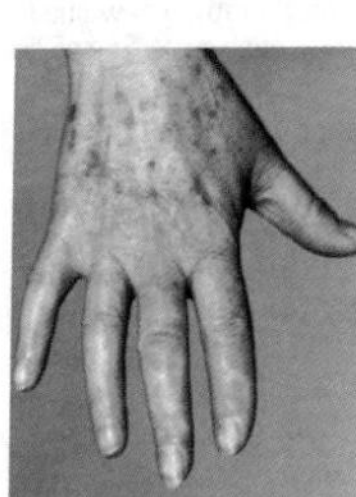

Fig 2.39 Sclerosis.

Top tips

- Cross your fingers before the patient grips them, it hurts less!
- Don't forget to palpate the radial pulse.
- Don't forget to look at the elbows for plaques of psoriasis and rheumatoid nodules.

Musculoskeletal hand examination 2

The hands can give you a wealth of information about a patient. Shaking hands can tell you about thyroid disease (warm, sweaty, tremor), anxiety (cold, sweaty), and neurological disease (myotonic dystrophy patients have difficulty relaxing their grip, a weak grip may suggest muscle wasting or peripheral neuropathy). The nails and skin can inform about systemic disease:

Nail abnormalities

- *Koilonychia* (spoon-shaped nails, fig 2.40) suggests iron deficiency, haemochromatosis, infection (eg fungal), endocrine disorders (eg acromegaly, hypothyroidism), or malnutrition.
- *Onycholysis* (detachment of the nail from the nail-bed) is seen with hyperthyroidism, fungal infection, and psoriasis.
- *Beau's lines* (fig 2.41) are transverse furrows from temporary arrest of nail growth at times of biological stress: severe infection. Nails grow at ~0.1mm/d, the furrow's distance from the cuticle allows dating of the stress.
- *Mees' lines* are single white transverse bands classically seen in arsenic poisoning, chronic kidney disease, and carbon monoxide poisoning among others.
- *Muehrcke's lines* are paired white parallel transverse bands (without furrowing of the nail itself, distinguishing them from Beau's lines) seen, eg, in chronic hypoalbuminaemia, Hodgkin's disease, pellagra (p268), chronic kidney disease.
- *Terry's nails*: Proximal portion of nail is white/pink, nail tip is red/brown (causes include cirrhosis, chronic kidney disease, congestive cardiac failure).
- *Pitting* is seen in psoriasis and alopecia areata.
- *Splinter haemorrhages* (fig 2.42) are fine longitudinal haemorrhagic streaks (under the nails), which in the febrile patient may suggest infective endocarditis. They may be microemboli, or be normal—eg due to gardening.
- *Nail-fold infarcts:* Embolic, typically seen in vasculitic disorders (OHCS, p452).
- *Nail clubbing* See p77.
- *Chronic paronychia* is a chronic infection of the nail-fold and presents as a painful swollen nail with intermittent discharge (fig 2.43).

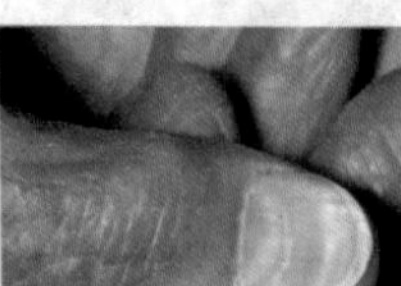

Fig 2.40 Koilonychia.

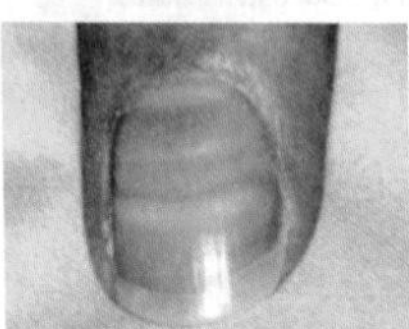

Fig 2.41 Beau's lines, here due to chemotherapy, a new line is seen with each cycle. See p525.

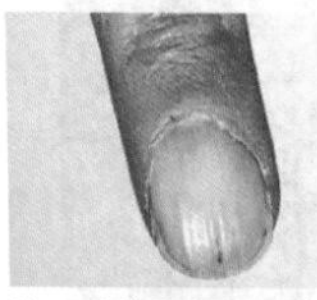

Fig 2.42 Splinter haemorrhages.

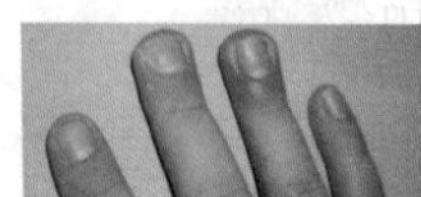

Fig 2.43 Paronychia.

Skin changes

- *Palmar erythema* (fig 2.44) is associated with cirrhosis, pregnancy, hyperthyroidism, rheumatoid arthritis, polycythaemia; also chronic liver disease—via ↓inactivation of vasoactive endotoxins by the liver. Also chemotherapy-induced palmar/plantar erythrodysaesthesia.
- *Pallor* of the palmar creases suggests anaemia.
- *Pigmentation* of the palmar creases is normal in people of African-Caribbean or Asian origin but is also seen in Addison's disease and Nelson's syndrome (increased ACTH after removal of the adrenal glands in Cushing's disease).[15]
- *Gottron's papules* (purple rash on the knuckles) with dilated end-capillary loops at the nail fold suggests dermatomyositis (p552).

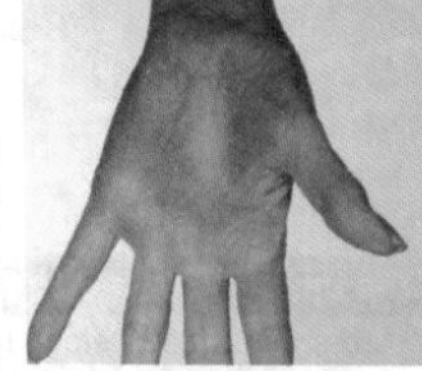

Fig 2.44 Palmar erythema.

Nodules and contractures

- Dupuytren's contracture (see fig 2.26, p60) fibrosis and contracture of palmar fascia, p698) is seen in liver disease, trauma, epilepsy, and ageing.
- Look for Heberden's (DIP) fig 2.45 and Bouchard's (PIP) 'nodes'—osteophytes (bone over-growth at a joint) seen with osteoarthritis.

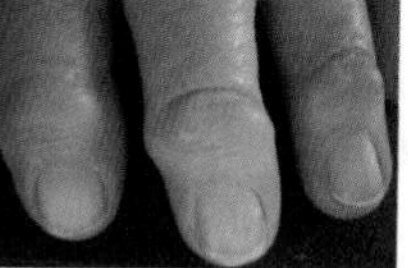

Fig 2.45 Heberden's (DIP).
Reproduced from Watts *et al.* (eds) *Oxford Textbook of Rheumatology* (2013), with permission from Oxford University Press.

Clubbing

Fingernails (± toenails) have increased curvature in all directions and loss of the angle between nail and nail fold and feel boggy (figs 2.46, 2.47). Pathogenesis is unclear although the platelet theory was developed in 1987.[16] Megakaryocytes are normally fragmented into platelets in the lungs, and the original theory was that any disruption to normal pulmonary circulation (inflammation, cancer, cardiac right-to-left shunting) would allow large megakaryocytes into the systemic circulation. They become lodged in the capillaries of the fingers and toes, releasing platelet-derived growth factor and vascular endothelial growth factor, which lead to tissue growth, vascular permeability, and recruitment of inflammatory cells. Evidence showing platelet microthrombi in clubbed fingers, and high levels of PDGF and VEGF in patients with hypertrophic osteoarthropathy, support the theory. This does not explain the changes in patients with unilateral clubbing, usually seen in neurological disorders.

Causes

Thoracic:
- Bronchial cancer (clubbing is twice as common in women); usually *not* small cell cancer
- Chronic lung suppuration:
  - Empyema, abscess
  - Bronchiectasis
  - Cystic fibrosis
- Fibrosing alveolitis
- Mesothelioma
- TB.

GI:
- Inflammatory bowel disease (especially Crohn's)
- Cirrhosis
- GI lymphoma
- Malabsorption, eg coeliac.

Rare:
- Familial
- Thyroid acropachy (p562).

Cardiovascular:
- Cyanotic congenital heart disease
- Endocarditis
- Atrial myxoma
- Aneurysms
- Infected grafts.

Unilateral clubbing:
- Hemiplegia
- Vascular lesions, eg upper-limb artery aneurysm, Takayasu's arteritis, brachial arteriovenous malformations (including iatrogenic— haemodialysis fistulas).

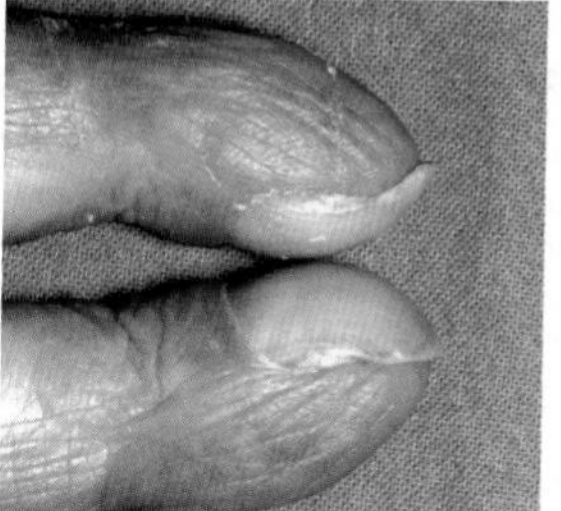

Fig 2.46 Finger clubbing.

(a)

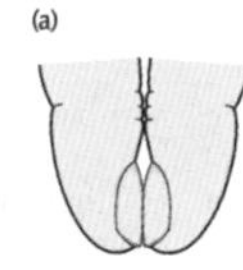

The dorsal aspect of 2 fingers, side by side with the nails touching. Normally, you should see a kite-shaped gap. If not, there is clubbing.

(b)

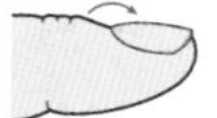

(c)

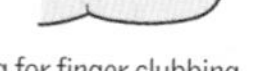

Fig 2.47 Testing for finger clubbing.

The peripheral vascular system: examination

Arterial

►►If limb is pale, pulseless, painful, paralysed, paraesthetic, and 'perishingly cold' this is acute ischaemia and is a surgical emergency (see p595 and p657).

1 *Inspection:* Look for scars of previous surgery and signs of peripheral arterial disease; loss of hair, pallor, shiny skin, cyanosis, dry skin, scaling, deformed toenails, ulcers, gangrene. Be sure to inspect the pressure points, ie between the toes and under the heel.

2 *Palpation:* Skin temperature will be cool in peripheral arterial disease. Is there a level above which it is warm? Delayed capillary refill (>2s) also indicates arterial disease. Are peripheral pulses palpable or not? 'If you cannot count it, you are not feeling it.' Note down on a quick stick-man diagram where they become palpable. Check for atrial fibrillation or other arrhythmias, as these can be the cause of embolic disease. Palpate for an enlarged abdominal aorta and attempt to assess size. (Though don't press too firmly!) ►►An expansile pulsatile mass in the presence of abdominal symptoms is a ruptured aneurysm until proven otherwise.

3 *Auscultation:* The presence of bruits suggests arterial disease. Listen over the major arteries—carotids, abdominal aorta, renal arteries, iliac femorals.

4 *Special tests: Buerger's angle* is that above the horizontal plane which leads to development of pallor (<20° indicates severe ischaemia). *Buerger's sign* is the sequential change in colour from white to pink, upon return to the dependent position; if the limbs become flushed red (reactive hyperaemia) this is indicative of more severe disease.

5 *Complete your examination:* measure ABPI (p656), US Doppler assessment, and a neurological examination of the lower limbs.

Venous

(See also p658.)

1 *Inspection:* Look for any varicosities and decide whether they are the long saphenous vein (medial), short saphenous vein (posterior lateral, below the knee), or from the calf perforators (usually few varicosities but commonly show skin changes). Ulcers around the medial malleolus are more suggestive of venous disease, whereas those at the pressure points suggest arterial pathology. Brown haemosiderin deposits result from venous hypertension. There may also be atrophy and loss of skin elasticity (lipodermatosclerosis) in venous disease.

2 *Palpation:* Warm varicose veins may indicate infection. Are they tender? Firm, tender varicosities suggests thrombosis. Palpate the saphenofemoral junction (SFJ) for a saphena varix which displays a cough impulse. Similarly, incompetence at the saphenopopliteal junction (SPJ) may be felt as a cough impulse. If ulceration is present, it is prudent to palpate the arterial pulses to rule out arterial disease.

3 *Tap test:* A transmitted percussion impulse from the lower limit of the varicose vein to the saphenofemoral junction demonstrates incompetence of superficial valves.

4 *Auscultation:* Bruits over the varicosities means there is an arteriovenous malformation.

5 *Doppler:* Test for the level of reflux. On squeezing the leg distal to placement of the probe you should only hear one 'whoosh' if the valves are competent at the level of probe placement.

6 *Trendelenburg's test* assesses if the SFJ valve is competent. Doppler USS has largely consigned this and other examination methods (eg *Tourniquet* and *Perthes' test*) to the history books.

7 *Complete examination:* examine the abdomen, pelvis in females, and external genitalia in males (for masses).

Arterial

1 **General inspection** Introduction, consent, patient sitting back at 45°. Inspect skin (hair loss, etc.). Look between toes and lift up heels to inspect for ulcers.

2 **Palpation**
- *Temperature:* Bilaterally in thighs, legs, and feet.
- *Capillary refill:* Press/squeeze great toe until blanches, release, and measure time for colour to return (normal <2s).
- *Peripheral pulses: Radial, brachial* (medial to biceps tendon), *carotid, femoral* (mid-inguinal point), *popliteal* (flex patient's knees slightly, press into centre of popliteal fossa; fig 2.48), *posterior tibial* (just posterior & inferior to medial malleolus) and *dorsalis pedis* (between bases of 1st & 2nd metatarsals, lateral to extensor hallucis longus); assess whether palpable bilaterally. Detect rate and rhythm. For brachial and carotid, determine volume and character.
- *Abdominal aorta:* Palpate midline above umbilicus; position fingers either side of outermost palpable margins (fig 2.49).

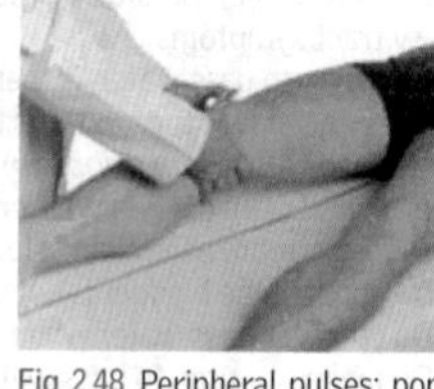

Fig 2.48 Peripheral pulses: popliteal.

Reproduced from Thomas J, *et al.* (eds). *Oxford Handbook of Clinical Examination and Practical Skills* (2014), with permission from Oxford University Press.

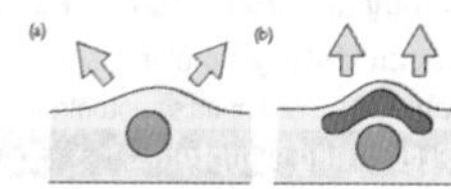

Fig 2.49 Pulses: abdominal aorta. (a) Expansile (aneurysm?) (b) Transmitted.

Reproduced from Thomas J, *et al.* (eds). *Oxford Handbook of Clinical Examination and Practical Skills* (2014), with permission from Oxford University Press.

3 **Auscultation** for carotid, femoral, renal iliac, and aortic bruits.

4 **Special tests**
Buerger's test: Lift both legs to 45° above the horizontal, supporting at heels. Allow a minute for legs to become pale. If they do, ask patient to sit up and swing around to lower legs to ground—observe colour change.

5 **Complete examination**
Doppler probe to detect pulses and measure ankle-brachial pressure index; conduct neurological examination of lower limbs.

Venous

1 **Inspection** Introduction, consent. Inspect, initially with patient standing, for varicosities and skin changes.

2 **Palpation** •*Temperature* of varicosities. •Ask patient to cough while you *palpate for impulse at* SFJ *and* SPJ.

3 **Tap test** Percuss lower limit of varicosity and feel for impulse at SFJ.

4 **Auscultation** Listen for bruits over any varicosities.

5 **Doppler** Place probe over SFJ, squeeze calf and listen. Repeat with probe at SPJ.

6 **Tourniquet test** Elevate leg and massage veins to empty varicosities. Apply tourniquet to upper thigh. Ask patient to stand. If not controlled, repeat, placing tourniquet below knee.

7 **Finish with examinations** of abdomen; rectum; pelvis (♀); genitals (♂).

The genitourinary system: history

See table 2.11 for direct questions to ask regarding presenting symptoms.

Detecting outflow obstruction (See 'Irritative or obstructive bladder symptoms' later in topic.) Eg prostatic hyperplasia; stricture; stone. Ask about *LUTS* (lower urinary tract symptoms).

- On trying to pass water, is there delay before you start? (*Hesitancy*)
- Does the flow stop and start? Do you go on dribbling when you think you've stopped? (*Terminal dribbling*)
- Is your stream getting weaker? (*Poor stream*)
- Is your stream painful and slow/'drop-by-drop'? (eg from bladder stone)
- Do you feel the bladder is not empty after passing water?[i]
- Do you ever pass water when you do not want to? (*Incontinence*—p648)
- On feeling an urge to pass water, do you have to go at once? (*Urgency*)[i]
- Do you urinate often at night? (*Nocturia*)[i] In the day? (*Frequency*)[i] How often?

Past history Renal colic, urinary tract infection, diabetes, ↑BP, gout, analgesic use (p318), previous operations.

Drug history Anticholinergics, prophylactic antibiotics.

Family history Prostate carcinoma? Renal disease?

Social history Smoking, sexual history.

Table 2.11 Presenting symptoms and questions to ask

Presenting symptoms	Direct questions
Dysuria	Pain: SOCRATES (p36). Fever? Sexual history. Abnormal-looking urine? Previous problems.
Lower urinary tract symptoms (LUTS)	
Loin/scrotal pain	Must rule out testicular torsion (p652).
Haematuria (p293 and p647)	
Urethral/vaginal discharge (p413)	
Sex problems; dyspareunia (OHCS p310)	
Menses (OHCS p250)	Ask about menarche, menopause, length of periods, amount, pain? Intermenstrual loss? 1st day of last menstrual period (LMP)?

Dysuria

Be sure you mean the same as your patient and colleagues, as dysuria refers to both painful micturition ('*uralgia*') and difficult micturition (*voiding difficulty*, p81). Uralgia is typically from urethral, bladder, or vaginal inflammation (UTI; perfumed bath products, spermicides, urethral syndrome, p300). If postmenopausal, look for a urethral caruncle—fleshy outgrowth of distal urethral mucosa, ≤1cm, typically originating from the posterior urethral lip. Also think of prostatitis, STI/urethritis (p413), vaginitis, and vulvitis. *Rare causes:* Stones, urethral lesions (eg carcinoma, lymphoma, papilloma), post-partum complications (eg retained products of conception).

Voiding difficulty is a sign of outflow obstruction, eg from an enlarged prostate, or urethral stricture (commonly post-traumatic, post-gonococcal). Other features: straining to void, poor stream, urinary retention, and incontinence. *Strangury* is urethral pain, usually referred from the bladder base, causing a constant distressing desire to urinate even if there is little urine to void. *Causes:* Stones, catheters, cystitis, prostatitis, bladder neoplasia, rarely: bladder endometriosis, schistosomiasis.

Frequency

Aim to differentiate ↑urine production (eg diabetes mellitus and insipidus, polydipsia, diuretics, alcohol, renal tubular disease, adrenal insufficiency) from frequent passage of small amounts of urine (eg in cystitis, urethritis, neurogenic bladder), or bladder compression or outflow obstruction (pregnancy, bladder tumour, enlarged prostate).

[i] = irritative (or 'filling') symptoms: they can be caused by, for example, UTI, as well as obstructions.

Oliguria/anuria

Oliguria is defined as a urine output of <400mL/24h or <0.5mL/kg/h and can be a sign of shock (eg post-op, p576) or acute kidney injury: causes: p298. *Anuria* is defined as <50mL/24h. In a catheterized patient with sudden anuria consider catheter blockage, with slow decline of oliguria to anuria renal dysfunction is more likely.

Polyuria

Increased urine volume, eg >3L/24h. *Causes:* Over-enthusiastic IV fluid therapy; diabetes mellitus & insipidus (diabetes is Greek for fountain);↑Ca^{2+}; psychogenic polydipsia/PIP syndrome (p240); polyuric phase of recovering acute tubular necrosis.

Irritative or obstructive bladder symptoms

(See also p642.) Symptoms of prostate enlargement are miscalled 'prostatism'; it is better to talk about *irritative* or *obstructive bladder* symptoms, as bladder neck obstruction or a stricture may be the cause.

1. *Irritative bladder symptoms:* Urgency, dysuria, frequency, nocturia[6] (the last two are also associated with causes of *polyuria*).
2. *Obstructive symptoms:* Reduced size and force of urinary stream, hesitancy and interruption of stream during voiding and terminal dribbling—the usual cause is enlargement of the prostate (prostatic hyperplasia), but other causes include a urethral stricture, tumour, urethral valves, or bladder neck contracture. The maximum flow rate of urine is normally ~18-30mL/s.

Terminal dribbling

Dribbling at the end of urination, often seen in conjunction with incontinence following incomplete urination, associated with prostatism.

Urinary changes

Cloudy urine suggests pus (UTI) but is often normal phosphate precipitation in an alkaline urine. *Pneumaturia* (bubbles in urine as it is passed). Occurs with UTI due to gas-forming organisms or may signal an enterovesical (bowel-bladder) fistula from diverticulitis, Crohn's disease or neoplastic disease of the bowel. *Nocturia* occurs with 'irritative bladder', diabetes mellitus, UTI, and reversed diurnal rhythm (seen in renal and cardiac failure). *Haematuria* (RBC in urine) is due to neoplasia or glomerulonephritis (p310) until proven otherwise. Rule out UTI.

Voiding difficulty

This includes poor flow, straining to void, hesitancy, intermittent stream, incontinence (eg overflow), retention (acute or chronic), incomplete emptying (±UTI from residual urine). ►*Remember faecal impaction as a cause of retention with overflow.* ***Causes:*** *Obstructive:* prostatic hyperplasia, early oedema after bladder neck repair, uterine prolapse, retroverted gravid uterus, fibroids, ovarian cysts, urethral foreign body, ectopic ureterocele, bladder polyp, or cancer. *Bladder overdistension*—eg after epidural for childbirth. *Detrusor weakness or myopathy* causes incomplete emptying + dribbling overflow incontinence (do cystometry/electromyography; causes include neurological disease and interstitial cystitis (*OHCS* p306); it may lead to a contracted bladder, eg requiring substitution enterocystoplasty). *Drugs:* epidural anaesthesia; tricyclics, anticholinergics. *CNS:* suprapontine (stroke); cord lesions (cord injury, multiple sclerosis); peripheral nerve (prolapsed disc, diabetic or other neuropathy); or reflex, due to pain (eg with herpes infections).

6 In the elderly, nocturia (1-2/night) may be 'normal' because of: **i)** loss of ability to concentrate urine; **ii)** peripheral oedema fluid returns to the circulation at night; **iii)** circadian rhythms may be lost; **iv)** less sleep is needed and waking may be interpreted as a need to void (a conditioned Pavlovian response).

The breast: history

See table 2.12 for direct questions to ask regarding presenting symptoms.

Table 2.12 Presenting symptoms and questions to ask

Presenting symptoms	Direct questions
Breast lump	Previous lumps? Family history? Pain? Nipple discharge? Nipple inversion? Skin changes? Change in size related to menstrual cycle? Number of pregnancies? First/last/latest period? Postnatal? Breast feeding? Drugs (eg HRT)? Consider metastatic disease (weight loss, breathlessness, back pain, abdominal mass?)
Breast pain (see BOX 'Breast pain')	SOCRATES (p36). Bilateral/unilateral? Rule out cardiac chest pain (p94 & p784). History of trauma? Any mass? Related to menstrual cycle?
Nipple discharge (see BOX 'Nipple discharge')	Amount? Nature (colour? consistency? any blood?)

Past history Any previous lumps and/or malignancies. Previous mammograms, clinical examinations of the breast, USS, fine-needle aspirate (FNA)/core biopsies.

Drug history Ask specifically about HRT and the Pill.

Family history See p520.

Social history Try to gain an impression of support network if suspect malignancy.

Breast pain

Is it premenstrual (*cyclical mastalgia*, *OHCS* p254)? Breast cancer (refer, eg, for mammography if needed)? If non-malignant and non-cyclical, think of:

- Tietze's syndrome (costochondritis plus swelling of the costal cartilage)
- Bornholm disease/Devil's grip (Coxsackie B virus, causing chest and abdominal pain, which may be mistaken for cardiac pain or an acute surgical abdomen. It resolves within ~2 weeks)
- angina
- gallstones
- lung disease
- thoracic outlet syndrome
- oestrogens/HRT.

If none of the above, wearing a firm bra all day may help, as may NSAIDs.

Nipple discharge

Causes: Duct ectasia (green/brown/red, often multiple ducts and bilateral), intraductal papilloma/adenoma/carcinoma (bloody discharge, often single duct), lactation. *Management:* Diagnose the cause (mammogram, ultrasound, ductogram); then treat appropriately. Cessation of smoking reduces discharge from duct ectasia. Microdochectomy/total duct excision can be considered if other measures fail, though may give no improvement in symptoms.

With thanks to Dr Simon Vann Jones for his contribution to this page.

1 **Inspection** Assess size and shape of any masses as well as overlying surface. Which quadrant (see fig 2.51)? Note skin involvement; ulceration, dimpling (*peau d'orange*), and nipple inversion/discharge.

2 **Palpation of the breast** Confirm size, and shape of any lump. Is it fixed/tethered to skin or underlying structures (see BOX 2 'Palpation')? Is it fluctuant/compressible/hard? Temperature? Tender? Mobile (more likely to be fibroadenoma)?

3 **Palpation of the axilla for lymph nodes** Metastatic spread? Ipsilateral/bilateral? Matted? Fixed?

4 **Further examination** Examine abdomen for hepatomegaly, spine for tenderness, lungs (metastatic spread).

1 General inspection

►*Always have a chaperone present when examining the breast.*

Introduction, consent, position patient sitting at edge of bed with hands by her side, expose to waist. Inspect both breasts for obvious masses, contour anomalies, asymmetry, scars, ulceration, skin changes, eg *peau d'orange* (orange peel appearance resulting from oedema). Look for nipple inversion and nipple discharge. Ask her to 'press hands on hips' and then 'hands on head' to accentuate any asymmetrical changes. While patient has her hands raised inspect axillae for any masses as well as inspecting under the breasts.

2 Palpation of the breast

Position patient sitting back at 45° with hand behind head (ie right hand behind head when examining the right breast—see fig 2.50). Ask patient if she has any pain or discharge. Examine painful areas last and then ask her to express any discharge. Examine each breast with the 'normal' side first. Examine each quadrant in turn as well as the axillary tail of Spence (fig 2.51) or use a concentric spiral method (fig 2.52) using a flat hand to roll breast against underlying chest wall. Define any lumps/lumpy areas. If you discover a lump, to examine for fixity to the pectoral muscles ask the patient to push against your hand with her arm outstretched.

3 Palpation of the axilla

Examine both axillae. When examining right axilla, hold the patient's right arm with your right hand and examine axilla with left hand.

Five sets of axillary nodes:

i) apical (palpate against glenohumeral joint)
ii) anterior (palpate against pectoralis major)
iii) central (palpate against lateral chest wall)
iv) posterior (palpate against latissimus dorsi)
v) medial (palpate against humerus).

4 Further examination

Complete examination by palpating down spine for tenderness, examining abdomen for hepatomegaly, and lungs for signs of metastases. Thank patient and wash hands.

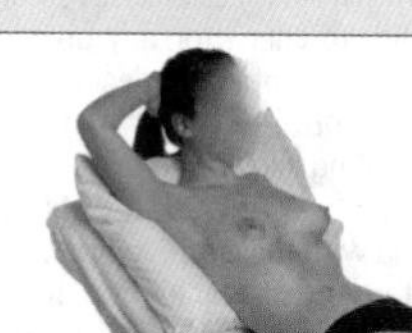

Fig 2.50 Correct patient position for breast examination.

Reproduced from Thomas J, *et al. Oxford Handbook of Clinical Examination and Practical Skills* (2014), with permission from Oxford University Press.

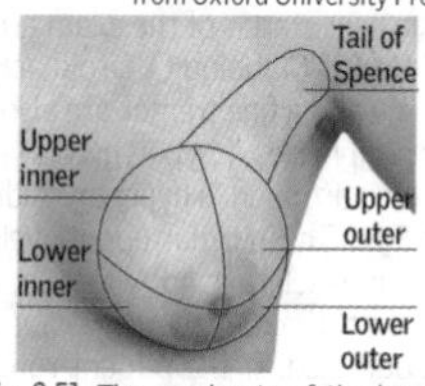

Fig 2.51 The quadrants of the breast with the axillary tail of Spence.

Reproduced from Thomas J, *et al. Oxford Handbook of Clinical Examination and Practical Skills* (2014), with permission from Oxford University Press.

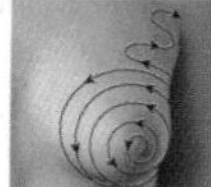
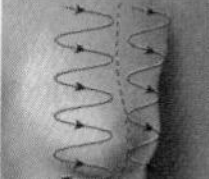

Fig 2.52 Methods for systematic breast palpation.

Reproduced from Thomas J, *et al. Oxford Handbook of Clinical Examination and Practical Skills* (2014), with permission from Oxford University Press.

The thyroid: examination

For symptoms of thyroid disease see p218 & p220. See also lumps in the neck, p598-600.

1 **Inspection** The key questions to ask oneself when presented with a lump in the neck are: Is this lump thyroid related or not? What is the patient's thyroid status? Inspect the neck; the normal thyroid is usually neither visible nor palpable. A midline swelling should raise your suspicion of thyroid pathology. Look for scars (eg collar incision from previous thyroid surgery). Examine the face for signs of hypothyroidism (puffiness, pallor, dry flaky skin, xanthelasma, corneal arcus, balding, loss of lateral third of eyebrow) as well as overall body habitus. Assess the patient's demeanour; do they appear anxious, nervous, agitated, fidgety (hyperthyroid)? Or slow and lethargic (hypothyroid)?

2 **Swallow test** Only goitres (p600), thyroglossal cysts (p598) and in some cases lymph nodes should move up on swallowing.

3 **Tongue protrusion test** A thyroglossal cyst will move up on tongue protrusion.

4 **Palpation** (By this stage of the examination if the evidence is in favour of the lump not rising from the thyroid it is acceptable to examine the lump like any other (p594); assess site, size, shape, smoothness (consistency), surface (contour/edge/colour), and surroundings, as well as transilluminance, fixation/tethering, fluctuance/compressibility, temperature, tenderness and whether it is pulsatile.) If a thyroid mass is suspected, standing behind the patient provides an opportunity to check for any proptosis (hyperthyroidism). Proceed to palpate each lobe, attempting to decide whether any lump is *solitary or multiple*, *nodular or smooth/diffuse* as well as site, size, etc. Repeating the swallow test while palpating allows you to confirm the early finding, but also attempt to 'get below the lump'. If there is a distinct inferior border under which you can place your hand with the entire lump above it then the goitre is unlikely to have retrosternal extension. Examining for 'spread' to the lymph nodes is particularly important if you suspect a thyroid malignancy (p600). Complete palpation by assessing if the presence of the lump has caused the trachea to deviate from the midline.

5 **Percussion** A retrosternal goitre will produce a dull percussion note when the sternum is percussed.

6 **Auscultation** A bruit in a smooth thyroid goitre is suggestive of Graves' disease (p218).

The next stages of the exam are to examine the systemic signs of thyroid status.

7 **Hands** Clubbing ('thyroid acropachy') is seen in Graves' disease. Palmar erythema and a fine tremor are also signs of thyrotoxicosis. Assess temperature (warm peripheries if hyperthyroid) and the radial pulse; tachycardia and atrial fibrillation are seen in hyperthyroidism, while bradycardia is seen in hypothyroidism.

8 **Eyes** The 'normal' upper eyelid should always cover the upper eye such that the white sclera is not visible between the lid and the iris. In hyperthyroidism with exophthalmus there is proptosis as well as lid retraction and 'lid lag' may also be detected. If the patient reports double vision when eye movements are being tested this indicates ophthalmoplegia of hyperthyroidism.

9 Asking the patient to stand allows you to assess whether there is any proximal myopathy (hypothyroidism). Look for pretibial myxoedema (brown swelling of the lower leg above the lateral malleoli in Graves' disease). Finally, test the reflexes; these will be slow relaxing in hypothyroidism and brisk in hyperthyroidism.

10 Thank the patient and consider whether the lump is a goitre, and if so whether it is single/multiple, diffuse/nodular, as well as the patient's thyroid status. Decide on a diagnosis (p600).

1 Inspection
Introduction, consent, position patient sitting on a chair (with space behind), adequately expose neck. Inspect from front and sides for any obvious goitres or swellings, scars, signs of hypo-/hyperthyroidism.

↓

2 Swallow test
Standing in front of the patient ask them to 'sip water...hold in your mouth...and swallow' to see if any midline swelling moves up on swallowing.

↓

3 Tongue protrusion test
Ask patient to 'stick out your tongue'. Does the lump move up? (Thyroglossal cyst.)

↓ *If evidence favours lump not arising from thyroid, examine lump like any other (p594)*

4 Palpation
Stand behind the patient.
- *Proptosis:* (p219.) While standing behind the patient ask them to tilt their head back slightly; this will give you a better view to assess any proptosis than when assessing the other aspects of eye pathology from front on, as in **8**)
- *The thyroid gland:* Ask the patient 'any pain?' Place middle 3 fingers of either hand along midline below chin and 'walk down' to thyroid, 2 finger breadths below the cricoid on both sides. Assess any enlargement/ nodules
- *Swallow test:* Repeat as before, now palpating; attempt to 'get under' the lump
- *Lymph nodes:* Examine lymph nodes of head and neck (p60). Stand in front of the patient
- *Trachea:* Palpate for tracheal deviation from the midline.

↓

5 Percussion
Percuss the sternum for dullness of retrosternal extension of a goitre.

↓

6 Auscultation
Listen over the goitre for a bruit.

↓

7 Hands
- *Inspect:* For thyroid acropachy (clubbing) and palmar erythema
- *Temperature*
- *Pulse:* Rate and rhythm
- *Fine tremor:* Ask patient to 'hold hands out', place sheet of paper over outstretched hands to help.

↓

8 Eyes
- *Exophthalmos:* Inspect for lid retraction and proptosis (p219)
- *Lid lag:* Ask patient to 'look down following finger' as you move your finger from a point above the eye to below
- *Eye movements:* Ask patient to follow your finger, keeping their head still, as you make an 'H' shape. Any double vision?

↓

9 Completion
Ask patient to stand up from the chair to assess for proximal myopathy, look for pretibial myxoedema, test ankle reflexes (ask patient to face away from you with knee resting on chair). Thank patient and wash hands.

Speech and higher mental function

►Have mercy on those with dysphasia: it is one of the most debilitating neurological conditions, and the more frustrating when cognitive function is intact.

Dysphasia Impairment of language caused by brain damage.

Assessment:

1 If speech is fluent, grammatical, and meaningful, dysphasia is unlikely.
2 *Comprehension:* can the patient follow one-, two-, and several-step commands (touch your ear, stand up, then close the door)?
3 *Repetition:* can the patient repeat a sentence? Eg British Constitution.
4 *Naming:* can they name common and uncommon things (eg parts of a watch)?
5 *Reading and writing:* normal? They are usually affected like speech in dysphasia. If normal, the patient is unlikely to be aphasic—could they be mute?

Classification:

- *Broca's (expressive) anterior dysphasia*—non-fluent speech produced with effort and frustration with malformed words, eg 'spoot' for 'spoon' (or 'that thing'). Reading and writing are impaired but comprehension is relatively intact. Patients understand questions and attempt to convey meaningful answers. *Site of lesion:* infero-lateral dominant frontal lobe (see BOX 'Problems with classifying dysphasias').
- *Wernicke's (receptive) posterior dysphasia*—empty, fluent speech, like talking ragtime with phonemic ('flush' for 'brush') and semantic ('comb' for 'brush') paraphasias/neologisms (may be mistaken for psychotic speech). The patient is oblivious of errors. Reading, writing, *and* comprehension are impaired (replies are inappropriate). *Site of lesion:* posterior superior dominant temporal lobe.
- *Conduction aphasia*—(traffic between Broca's and Wernicke's area is interrupted.) Repetition is impaired; comprehension and fluency less so.
- *Nominal dysphasia*—naming is affected in all dysphasias, but in nominal dysphasia, objects cannot be named but other aspects of speech are normal. This occurs with posterior dominant temporoparietal lesions.

►Mixed dysphasias are common. Discriminating features take time to emerge after an acute brain injury. Speech therapy is important, but may not help.

Dysarthria Difficulty with articulation due to incoordination or weakness of the musculature of speech. Language is normal (see earlier in topic).

- *Assessment:* Ask to repeat 'British Constitution' or 'baby hippopotamus'.
- *Cerebellar disease:* Ataxia speech muscles cause slurring (as if drunk) and speech irregular in volume and staccato in quality.
- *Extrapyramidal disease:* Soft, indistinct, and monotonous speech.
- *Pseudobulbar palsy:* (p507) Spastic dysarthria (*upper motor neuron*). Speech is slow, indistinct, nasal and effortful ('hot potato' voice from bilateral hemispheric lesions, MND (p506), or severe MS).
- *Bulbar palsy: Lower motor neuron* (eg facial nerve palsy, Guillain-Barré, MND, p506)—any associated palatal paralysis gives speech a nasal character.

Dysphonia Difficulty with speech volume due to weakness of respiratory muscles or vocal cords (myasthenia, p512; Guillain-Barré syndrome, p702). It may be precipitated in myasthenia by asking the patient to count to 100. Parkinson's gives a mixed picture of dysarthria and dysphonia.

Dyspraxia Poor performance of complex movements despite ability to do each individual component. Test by asking the patient to copy unfamiliar hand positions, or mime an object's use, eg a comb. The term 'dyspraxia' is used in three other ways:

- *Dressing dyspraxia:* The patient is unsure of the orientation of clothes on his body. Test by pulling one sleeve of a sweater inside out before asking the patient to put it back on (mostly non-dominant hemisphere lesions).
- *Constructional dyspraxia:* Difficulty in assembling objects or drawing, eg a five-pointed star (non-dominant hemisphere lesions, hepatic encephalopathy).
- *Gait dyspraxia:* More common in the elderly; seen with bilateral frontal lesions, lesions in the posterior temporal region, and hydrocephalus.

Assessing higher mental function: a practical guide

Start by reassuring the patient 'I know this may be difficult...' and try to engage in conversation; asking questions that need to phrase to answer (ie not just yes/no). This tests fluency and reception, understanding, and allows assessment of articulation, eg 'How did you travel here today?', 'I came by bus'. Then assess dysphasia by asking: 'What is this' eg pen (tests for nominal dysphasia), repeat 'British Constitution' (tests for conduction dysphasia and dysarthria). Then ask patient to follow one-, two-, and three-step commands ensuring these 'cross the midline', eg make a fist with your right hand then extend your right index finger and touch your left ear.

Problems with classifying dysphasias

The classical model of language comprehension occurring in Wernicke's area and language expression in Broca's area is too simple. Functional MRI studies show old ideas that processing of abstract words is confined to the left hemisphere whereas concrete words are processed on the right are too simplistic.[7] It may be better to think of a mosaic of language centres in the brain with more or less specialized functions. There is evidence that tool-naming is handled differently and in a different area to fruit-naming. There are also individual differences in the anatomy of these mosaics. This is depressing for those who want a rigid classification of aphasia, but a source of hope to those who have had a stroke: recovery may be better than neuroimaging leads us to believe.

Movement disorders

Symptoms of movement disorders

Athetosis is due to a lesion in the putamen, causing slow sinuous writhing movements in the hands, which are present at rest. *Pseudoathetosis* refers to athetoid movements in patients with severe proprioceptive loss.

Chorea means *dance* (hence 'choreography')—a flow of jerky movements, flitting from one limb to another (each seemingly a fragment of a normal movement). Distinguish from athetosis/pseudoathetosis (above-mentioned), and hemiballismus (p468). *Causes:* Basal ganglia lesion (stroke, Huntington's, p702); streptococci (Sydenham's chorea; St Vitus' dance, p142); SLE (p554); Wilson's (p285); neonatal kernicterus; polycythaemia (p366); neuroacanthocytosis (genetic, with acanthocytes in peripheral blood, chorea, oro-facial dyskinesia, and axonal neuropathy); hyperthyroidism (p218); drugs (levodopa, oral contraceptives/HRT, chlorpromazine, cocaine—'*crack dancing*'). The early stages of chorea may be detected by feeling fluctuations in muscle tension while the patient grips your finger.

℞: Dopamine antagonists, eg tetrabenazine 12.5mg/12h (/24h if elderly) PO; increase, eg to 25mg/8h PO; max 200mg/d.

Hemiballismus is uncontrolled unilateral flailing movements of proximal limb joints caused by contralateral subthalamic lesions. See p468.

Cerebellar signs

Speech: Slurred/ataxic/staccato. *Eye movements:* Nystagmus. *Tone and power:* Hypotonia and reduced power. *Coordination:* Finger-to-nose test; test for dysdiadochokinesis, p499. *Gait:* Broad based, patients fall to the side of the lesion. *Romberg's test:* ask patient to stand with eyes closed. If he/she loses balance, the test is positive and a sign of posterior column disease. Cerebellar disease is Romberg negative.

(**DASHING**: **D**ysdiadochokinesis, **A**taxia, **S**lurred speech, **H**ypotonia and reduced power, **I**ntention tremor, **N**ystagmus, broad based **G**ait.)

7 While abstract words activate a sub-region of the left inferior frontal gyrus more strongly than concrete words, specific activity for concrete words can also be observed in the left basal temporal cortex.

Psychiatric assessment

Introduce yourself, ask a few factual questions (precise name, age, job, and who is at home). These may help your patient to relax, but be careful that you do not touch on a nerve, eg if job recently lost, marriage recently ended so living alone.

Presenting problem Ask for the main problems that have led to this consultation. Sit back and listen. Don't worry whether the information is in a convenient form or not—this is an opportunity for the patient to come out with worries, ideas, and preoccupations unsullied by your expectations. After >3–5min it is often good to aim to have a list of all the problems (each sketched only briefly). Read them back to the patient and ask if there are any more. Then ask about:

History of presenting problem For each problem obtain details, both current state and history of onset, precipitating factors, and effects on life.

Check of major psychiatric symptoms Check those that have not yet been covered: *depression*—low mood, anhedonia (inability to feel pleasure), thoughts of worthlessness/hopelessness, sleep disturbance with early morning waking, loss of weight and appetite. Ask specifically about *suicidal thoughts and plans:* 'Have you ever been so low that you thought of harming yourself?', 'What thoughts have you had?' Check for hypomanic and manic features which can be missed in a patient presenting as depressed. *Hallucinations* ('Have you ever heard voices or seen things when there hasn't been anyone or anything there?') and *delusions* ('Have you ever had any thoughts or beliefs that have struck you afterwards as bizarre?'); *anxiety* and *avoidance behaviour* (eg avoiding shopping because of anxiety or phobias); *obsessional thoughts* and *compulsive behaviour*, *eating disorders*, *alcohol* (see p281 for alcohol screening tests) and *other drugs*.

Present circumstances Housing, finance, work, relationships, friends.

Family history Ask about health, personality, and occupation of parents and siblings, and the *family's medical and psychiatric history*.

Background history Try to understand the context of the presenting problem.
- *Biography:* Relationships with family and peers as a child; school and work record; sexual relationships and current relationships; and family. Previous ways of dealing with stress and whether there have been problems and symptoms similar to the presenting ones.
- *Premorbid personality:* Mood, character, hobbies, attitudes, and beliefs.

Past medical and psychiatric history Establish any past or present co-morbidities.

Mental state examination This is the state *now*, at the time of interview.
Appearance: Clothing, glasses, headwear? Unkempt/normal/meticulous?
Observable behaviour: Eg excessive slowness, signs of anxiety, gesture, gaze or avoiding gaze, tears, laughter, pauses (while listening to voices?), attitude (eg withdrawn).
Mode of speech: Include the rate, eg retarded or gabbling (pressure of speech), rhythm, and tone of speech.
Mood: Note thoughts about harming self or others. Gauge your own responses to the patient. The laughter and grand ideas of manic patients are contagious, as to a lesser extent is the expression of thoughts from a depressed person.
Thoughts: Content: eg about himself, his own body, about other people, and the future, any suicidal ideation? Note abnormal beliefs (delusions), eg that thoughts are overheard, and abnormal ideas (eg persecutory, grandiose). *Form:* flight of ideas? Knight's move thinking? (See BOX 'Psychiatric symptoms'.)
Unusual experiences or hallucinations: Note modality, eg visual, auditory.
Cognition: Orientated in time, place, and person? *Short-term memory*: give a name and address and test recall after 5min. Draw the face of a clock (requires good frontal and parietal function). *Long-term memory*: current affairs recall. Name of current political leaders (p64). This tests many other CNS functions, not just memory.
Concentration: Months of the year backwards.
Insight: Does the patient think they are unwell? Do they think you can help?

Psychiatric symptoms

There are many different ways to think about psychiatric symptoms. One simple approach can be to consider negative and positive symptoms. ***Negative symptoms*** involve the absence of a behaviour, thought, feeling, or sensation (eg lack of appetite, apathy, and blunted emotions in depression), whereas ***positive symptoms*** involve their presence when not normally expected (eg thought insertion, ie 'Someone is putting thoughts into my head'). Understanding the difference between psychosis and neurosis is vital. ***Psychosis*** entails a thought disorder (eg thought insertion, thought broadcasting) ± delusions (abnormal beliefs which are held to despite all reasoning, and which run counter to the patient's cultural background) and abnormal perceptions (eg hallucinations). ***Neurosis*** entails insight—if there are intrusive ideas or odd experiential phenomena, the person knows that they are false or illusory (and may be triggered by stress, etc.).

Disorders of thought include ***flight of ideas***, in which the speech races through themes, switching whimsically or through associations, eg 'clang' association: 'Yesterday I went down to the local shop. I didn't hop (*clang*), but I walked. Kangaroos hop, don't they? My friend Joey wasn't there, though...'. ***Knight's move*** is an unexpected change in the direction of speech or conversation (akin to the lateral component of the move of the knight's piece in chess) and ***neologism*** is the formation of new words. They may be normal or indicate an organic brain condition or a psychosis.

Many psychiatric symptoms in isolation, to a lesser degree of severity, or even in a different culture, may well be considered part of 'normal' behaviour. For example, a vision from a religious figure may be considered normal, whereas one from an alien may not. Consider your patient in their cultural and religious context. As with so many aspects of medicine, in psychiatry there is a vast spectrum of behaviour, thought, and perception, at least one extreme of which is considered to be 'abnormal'. It is in part our challenge to attempt to interpret these symptoms with relevance, insight, and impartiality so that we may best benefit our patients and not form opinions that are set in stone. On acute medical wards psychiatric symptoms are often due to stress, drug or alcohol withdrawal, U&E imbalance, or medication. When in doubt, ask a psychiatrist to help.

►Beware of simplistic formulations, eg *If you talk to God, you are praying. If God talks to you, you have schizophrenia* (Dr Thomas Szasz). It is not the auditory phenomenon that makes the diagnosis of psychosis: what matters is what the patient believes about the phenomenon, and whether they are associated with a thought disorder or a delusion.

Method and order for routine examination

1 Look at the patient. Healthy, unwell, or *in extremis*? This vital skill improves with practice. ►*Beware those who are sicker than they look*, eg cardiogenic shock; cord compression; non-accidental injury.
2 Pulse, BP, RR, O_2 sats, T°.
3 Examine nails, hands, conjunctivae (anaemia), and sclerae (jaundice). Consider: Paget's, acromegaly, endocrine disease (thyroid, pituitary, or adrenal hypo- or hyper-function), body hair, abnormal pigmentation, skin.
4 Examine mouth and tongue (cyanosed; smooth; furred; beefy, eg rhomboid area denuded of papillae by *Candida*, after prolonged steroid inhaler use).
5 Examine the neck from behind: lymph nodes, goitre.
6 Make sure the patient is at 45° to begin CVS examination in the neck: JVP; feel for character and volume of carotid pulse.
7 The praecordium. Look for abnormal pulsations. Feel the apex beat (character; position). Any parasternal heave or thrill? Auscultate (bell and diaphragm) apex in the left lateral position, then the other three areas (p39) and carotids. Sit the patient forward: listen during expiration.
8 While sitting forward, look for sacral oedema.
9 Respiratory examination with the patient at 90°. Observe (and count) RR; note posterior chest wall movement. Assess chest expansion, percuss and auscultate.
10 Sit the patient back. Feel the trachea. Inspect again. Assess expansion of the anterior chest. Percuss and auscultate again.
11 Examine axillae and breasts, if indicated (chaperone for *all* intimate examinations).
12 Lie patient flat (1 pillow) to inspect, palpate, percuss, and auscultate abdomen.
13 Look at the legs: swellings, perfusion, pulses, or oedema? Pitting? What level?
14 CNS exam: *Cranial nerves*: pupil responses; fundi; visual fields; visual acuity. Consider corneal reflexes. 'Open your mouth; stick your tongue out; screw up your eyes; show me your teeth; raise your eyebrows.' *Limbs (most signs are due to central not peripheral nerve lesions)*: look for wasting and fasciculation. Test tone in all limbs. 'Hold your hands out with your palms towards the ceiling and fingers wide. Now shut your eyes.' Watch for pronator drift. 'Keep your eyes shut and touch your nose with each index finger.' 'Lift your leg straight in the air. Keep it there. Put your heel on the opposite knee (eyes shut) and run it up your own shin.' You have now tested power, coordination, and joint position sense. Tuning fork on toes and index fingers to assess vibration sense.
15 Examine gait and speech. Any abnormalities of higher mental function?
16 Consider rectal and vaginal examination (chaperone essential).
17 Examine the urine with dipstick if appropriate.

►In general, go into detail where you find (or suspect) something to be wrong.

This page intentionally blank

3 Cardiovascular medicine

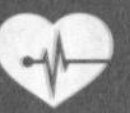

Contents

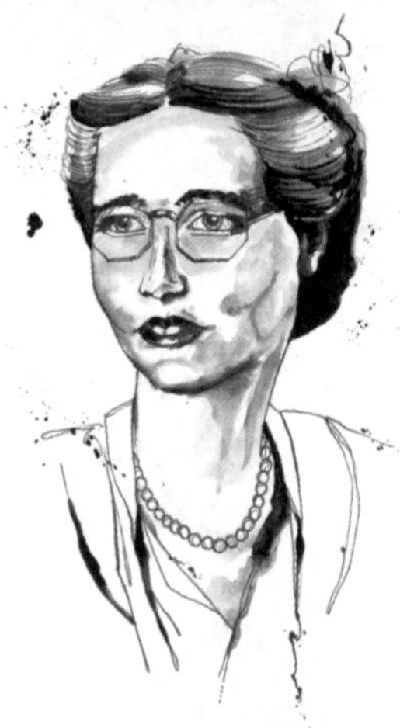

Fig 3.1 Helen Taussig (1898-1986) battled dyslexia, deafness, and a male-dominated world to become a leading cardiologist. She noticed that 'blue babies' with a patent ductus arteriosus (PDA) tended to survive longer than those without. This was because many blue babies have congenital obstruction to pulmonary blood flow (eg pulmonary stenosis in tetralogy of Fallot, p157) and PDAs increase blood flow to the lungs, reducing cyanosis. She devised the Blalock-Taussig shunt which creates a passage from the subclavian or carotid artery to one of the pulmonary arteries, mimicing a PDA. This dramatically improved survival in babies with tetralogy of Fallot.

One of the joys of cardiology is how often solutions already exist in nature and much of our intervention involves trying to mimic circumstances that can occur naturally. Hence, a good grasp of the underlying physiology is essential for understanding clinical cardiology; as well as interesting to pursue in its own right.

We thank Dr Parag Gajendragadkar, our Specialist Reader, for his contribution to this chapter.

Cardiovascular health

Ischaemic heart disease (IHD) is the most common cause of death worldwide. Encouraging cardiovascular health is not *only* about preventing IHD: health entails the ability to *exercise*, and enjoying vigorous activity (within reason!) is one of the best ways of achieving health, not just because the heart likes it (↓BP, ↑'good' high-density lipoprotein (HDL))—it can prevent osteoporosis, improve glucose tolerance, and augment immune function (eg in cancer and if HIV+ve). People who improve *and maintain* their fitness live longer: ►*age-adjusted mortality from all causes is reduced by >40%.* Avoiding obesity helps too, but weight loss per se is only useful in reducing cardiovascular risk and the risk of developing diabetes when combined with regular exercise. Moderate alcohol drinking may also promote cardiovascular health.

Hypertension is the chief risk factor for cardiovascular mortality, followed by smoking. Giving up smoking, even after many years, does bring benefit. *Simple advice works*. Most smokers want to give up. Just because smoking advice does *not always* work, do not stop giving it. Ask about smoking in consultations—especially those regarding smoking-related diseases.

- *Ensure advice is congruent* with the patient's beliefs about smoking.
- Getting patients to enumerate the advantages of giving up ↑ motivation.
- Invite the patient to choose a date (when there will be few stresses) on which he or she will become a non-smoker.
- Suggest throwing away all accessories (cigarettes, pipes, ash trays, lighters, matches) in advance; inform friends of the new change; practise saying 'no' to their offers of 'just one little cigarette'.
- *Nicotine gum*, chewed intermittently to limit nicotine release: ≥ ten 2mg sticks may be needed/day. Transdermal nicotine patches may be easier. A dose increase at 1wk can help. Written advice offers no added benefit to advice from nurses. Always offer follow-up.
- *Varenicline* is an oral selective nicotine receptor partial agonist. Start 1wk before target stop date and gradually increase the dose. *SEs:* appetite change; dry mouth; taste disturbance; headache; drowsiness; dizziness; sleep disorders; abnormal dreams; depression; suicidal thoughts; panic; dysarthria.
- *Bupropion* (=amfebutamone) is said to ↑ quit rate to 30% at 1yr vs 16% with patches and 15.6% for placebo (patches + bupropion: 35.5%):[1] consider if the above fails. *Warn of SEs:* seizures (risk <1:1000), insomnia, headache.

Lipids and diabetes (pp690, 206) are the other major *modifiable* risk factors. The QRISK2 score (www.qrisk.org) is used in the UK to integrate a patient's different cardiovascular risk factors in order to predict future cardiovascular health.[2] It can be used as part of a consultation on lifestyle factors to show patients that addressing certain risk factors (eg smoking, BP) will reduce their risk of MIs and strokes.

►Apply preventive measures such as healthy eating (p244) *early* in life to maximize impact, when there are most years to save, and before bad habits get ingrained.

The randomized trial

Cardiovascular medicine has an unrivalled treasure house of randomized trials. One of the chief pleasures of cardiovascular medicine lies in integrating these with clinical reasoning in a humane way. After a cardiac event, a protocol may 'mandate' statins, aspirin, β-blockers, ACE-i (p114), and a target BP and LDL cholesterol that makes your patient feel dreadful. What to do? Inform, negotiate, and compromise. Never reject your patient because of lack of compliance with your over-exacting regimens. Keep smiling, keep communicating, and keep up to date: the latest data may show that your patient was right all along.[3]

Chest pain ►Cardiac-sounding chest pain may have no serious cause, but always think 'Could this be a myocardial infarction (MI), dissecting aortic aneurysm, pericarditis, or pulmonary embolism?'.

Character: Constricting suggests angina, oesophageal spasm, or anxiety; a sharp pain may be from the pleura, pericardium, or chest wall. A prolonged (>½h), dull, central crushing pain or pressure suggests MI.

Radiation: To shoulder, either or both arms, or neck/jaw suggests cardiac ischaemia. The pain of aortic dissection (p654) is classically instantaneous, tearing, and interscapular, but may be retrosternal. Epigastric pain may be cardiac.

Precipitants: Pain associated with cold, exercise, palpitations, or emotion suggests cardiac pain or anxiety; if brought on by food, lying flat, hot drinks, or alcohol, consider oesophageal spasm/disease (but meals can also cause angina).

Relieving factors: If pain is relieved within minutes by rest or glyceryl trinitrate (GTN), suspect angina (GTN relieves oesophageal spasm more slowly). If antacids help, suspect GI causes. Pericarditic pain improves on leaning forward.

Associations: Dyspnoea occurs with cardiac pain, pulmonary emboli, pleurisy, or anxiety. MI may cause nausea, vomiting, or sweating. Angina is caused by coronary artery disease—and also by aortic stenosis, hypertrophic cardiomyopathy (HCM), paroxysmal supraventricular tachycardia (SVT)—and can be exacerbated by anaemia. Chest pain with tenderness suggests self-limiting Tietze's syndrome.[1] Odd neurological symptoms and atypical chest pain—think aortic dissection.

Pleuritic pain: Pain exacerbated by inspiration. Implies inflammation of the pleura from pulmonary infection, inflammation, or infarction. It causes us to 'catch our breath'. *ΔΔ*: musculoskeletal pain;[1] fractured rib (pain on respiration, exacerbated by gentle pressure on the sternum); subdiaphragmatic pathology (eg gallstones).

►►*Chest pain & acutely unwell* (see p784) • Admit • Check pulse, BP in both arms (unequal in aortic dissection p654), JVP, heart sounds; examine legs for DVT • Give O_2 • IV line • Relieve pain (eg 5–10mg IV morphine) • Cardiac monitor • 12-lead ECG • CXR • Arterial blood gas (ABG) *Famous traps:* Aortic dissection; zoster (p404); ruptured oesophagus; cardiac tamponade (p154); opiate addiction.

Dyspnoea May be from LVF, PE, any respiratory cause, anaemia, pain, or anxiety. *Severity:* ►►Emergency presentations: p782. Ask about shortness of breath at rest, on exertion, and on lying flat; has their exercise tolerance changed? *Associations:* Specific symptoms associated with heart failure are orthopnoea (ask about number of pillows used at night), paroxysmal nocturnal dyspnoea (waking up at night gasping for breath, p49), and peripheral oedema. Pulmonary embolism is associated with acute onset of dyspnoea and pleuritic chest pain; ask about risk factors for DVT.

Palpitation(s) May be due to ectopics, sinus tachycardia, AF, SVT, VT, thyrotoxicosis, anxiety, and rarely phaeochromocytoma. See p36. *History:* Characterize: do they mean their heart was beating fast, hard, or irregularly? Ask about previous episodes, precipitating/relieving factors, duration of symptoms, associated chest pain, dyspnoea, dizziness, or collapse. Did the patient check their pulse?

Syncope May reflect cardiac or CNS events. Vasovagal 'faints' are common (pulse↓, pupils dilated). The history from an observer is invaluable in diagnosis. *Prodromal symptoms:* Chest pain, palpitations, or dyspnoea point to a cardiac cause, eg arrhythmia. Aura, headache, dysarthria, and limb weakness indicate CNS causes. *During the episode:* Was there a pulse? Limb jerking, tongue biting, or urinary incontinence? NB: hypoxia from lack of cerebral perfusion may cause seizures. *Recovery:* Was this rapid (arrhythmia) or prolonged, with drowsiness (seizure)?

1 25% of non-cardiac chest pain is *musculoskeletal:* look for pain on specific postures or activity. Aim to reproduce the pain by movement and, sometimes, palpation over the structure causing it. Focal injection of local anaesthetic helps diagnostically and is therapeutic. *Tietze's syndrome:* self-limiting costochondritis ± costosternal joint swelling. Causes: idiopathic; microtrauma; infection; psoriatic/rheumatoid arthritis. ℞: NSAIDs or steroid injections. Tenderness is also caused by: fibrositis, lymphoma, chondrosarcoma, myeloma, metastases, rib TB. Imaging: bone scintigraphy; CT.

Chest pain from the patient's perspective

On acute wards we are always hearing questions such as 'Is your pain sharp or dull?', followed by an equivocal answer. The doctor goes on: 'Sharp like a knife—or dull and crushing?' The doctor is getting irritated because the patient must know the answer but is not saying it. A true story paves the way to being less inquisitorial and having a more creative understanding of the nature of symptoms.

A patient came to a previous *OHCM* author saying 'Last night I dreamed I had a pain in my chest. Now I've woken up, and I'm not sure—have I got chest pain, doctor? What do you think?' How odd it is to be asked to examine a patient to exclude a symptom, not a disease. (It turned out that she did have serious chest pathology.) Odd, until one realizes that symptoms are often half-formed, and it is our role to give them a local habitation and a name. Dialogue can transform a symptom from 'airy nothingness' to a fact.[2]

Patients often avoid using the word 'pain' to describe ischaemia: 'wind', 'tightening', 'pressure', 'burning', or 'a lump in the throat' (angina means to choke) may be used. They may say 'sharp' to communicate severity, and not character. So be as vague in your questioning as your patient is in their answers. 'Tell me some more about what you are feeling (long pause) ... as if someone was doing what to you?' 'Sitting on me' or 'like a hotness' might be the response (suggesting cardiac ischaemia). Do not ask 'Does it go into your left arm'. Try 'Is there anything else about it?' (pause) ... 'Does it go anywhere?' Note down your patient's exact words.

A good history, taking account of these features, is the best way to stratify patients likely to have cardiac pain. If the history is non-specific, there are no risk factors for cardiovascular diseases, and ECG and plasma troponin T (p118) are normal 6-12h after the onset of pain, discharge will probably be OK.[4] When in doubt, get help. Features making cardiac pain unlikely:

- Stabbing, shooting pain.
- Pain lasting <30s, however intense.
- Well-localized, left sub-mammary pain ('In my heart, doctor').
- Pains of continually varying location.
- Youth.

Do not feel that you must diagnose every pain. Chest pain with no cause is common, even after extensive tests. Some patients have a 'chronic pain syndrome' similar to post-herpetic neuralgia. Typically, this responds to a tricyclic, eg low-dose amitriptyline at night (this dose does not imply any depression).

Avoid being that doctor who triumphantly tells a patient that they are fine and can go home, only to be met by a glare, as the disabling pain the patient presented with is no better than when they arrived. Take time to explain why you do not believe the pain is a result of dangerous pathology; to give advice on pain control and 'red flags'; and to reassure the patient that their problem is likely to resolve with time.

2 Dialogue-transformed symptoms explain one of the junior doctor's main vexations: when patients retell symptoms to a consultant in the light of day, they bear no resemblance to what you originally heard. But do not be vexed: your dialogue may have helped the patient far more than any ward round.

ECG—a methodical approach

Reading an ECG

►First confirm the patient's name and age, and the ECG date. Then (see fig 3.3):

- *Rate:* At usual speed (25mm/s) each 'big square' is 0.2s; each 'small square' is 0.04s. To calculate the rate, divide 300 by the number of big squares between two consecutive R waves (table 3.1). The normal rate is 60–100bpm.
- *Rhythm:* If cycles are not clearly regular, use the 'card method': lay a card along the ECG, marking positions of three successive R waves. Slide the card to and fro to check that all intervals are equal. If they are not, note if:
  - there is slight but regular lengthening and then shortening (with respiration)—sinus arrhythmia, common in the young
  - there are different rates which are multiples of each other—varying block
  - it is 100% irregular—atrial fibrillation (AF) or ventricular fibrillation (VF).

  Sinus rhythm is characterized by a P wave followed by a QRS complex. AF has no discernible P waves and QRS complexes are irregularly irregular. Atrial flutter (p130, fig 3.35 p131) has a 'sawtooth' baseline of atrial depolarization (~300/min) and regular QRS complexes. Ventricular rhythm has QRS complexes >0.12s with P waves following them or absent (fig 3.12, p106).
- *Axis:* The overall direction of depolarization across the patient's anterior chest; this is the sum of all the ventricular electrical forces during ventricular depolarization. See BOX 'Determining the ECG axis'. Left axis deviation can result from left anterior hemiblock, inferior MI, VT from a left ventricular focus, WPW, LVH. Right axis deviation can result from RVH, PE, anterolateral MI, WPW and left posterior hemiblock.
- *P wave:* Normally precedes each QRS complex, and upright in II, III, & aVF but inverted in aVR. Absent P wave: AF, P hidden due to junctional or ventricular rhythm. P mitrale: bifid P wave, indicates left atrial hypertrophy. P pulmonale: peaked P wave, indicates right atrial hypertrophy. Pseudo-P-pulmonale seen if ↑K⁺.
- *PR interval:* Measure from start of P wave to start of QRS. Normal range: 0.12–0.2s (3–5 small squares). A prolonged PR interval implies delayed AV conduction (1st degree heart block). A short PR interval implies unusually fast AV conduction down an accessory pathway, eg WPW (see fig 3.37, p133). See heart block, p98.

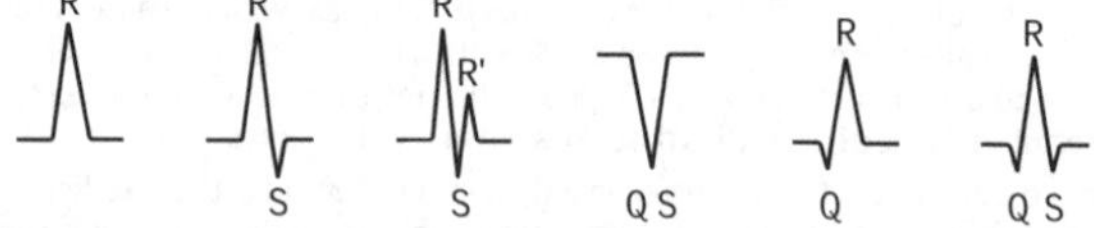

Fig 3.2 'QRS' complexes. If the first deflection from the isoelectric line is negative, it is a Q wave. Any positive deflection is an R wave. Any negative deflection after an R is an S.

- *QRS complex:* See fig 3.2. Normal duration: <0.12s. QRS >0.12s suggests ventricular conduction defects, eg a bundle branch block (pp99, 100), metabolic disturbance, or ventricular origin (eg ventricular ectopic). High-amplitude QRS complexes suggest ventricular hypertrophy (p100). Normal Q waves are <0.04s wide and <2mm deep; they are often seen in leads I, aVL, V_5, and V_6 and reflect normal septal depolarization. Pathological Q waves (deep and wide) may occur within a few hours of an acute MI.
- *QT interval:* Measure from start of QRS to end of T wave. It varies with rate. The corrected QT interval (QT^c) is the QT interval divided by the square root of the R-R interval, ie $QT^c = QT/\sqrt{RR}$. Normal QT^c: 0.38–0.42s. For causes of prolonged QT interval see p711. Long QT can lead to VT and sudden death.
- *ST segment:* Usually isoelectric. Planar elevation (>1mm) or depression (>0.5mm) usually implies infarction (p119, figs 3.9, 3.10, pp103–4) or ischaemia, respectively.
- *T wave:* Normally inverted in aVR, V_1, and occasionally V_2. Normal if inverted in isolation in lead III. Abnormal if inverted in I, II, and V_4–V_6. Peaked in hyperkalaemia (fig 14.4, p675) and flattened in hypokalaemia.
- *J wave:* See p849. The J point is where the S wave finishes and ST segment starts. A J wave is a notch at this point. Seen in hypothermia, SAH, and ↑Ca^{2+}.

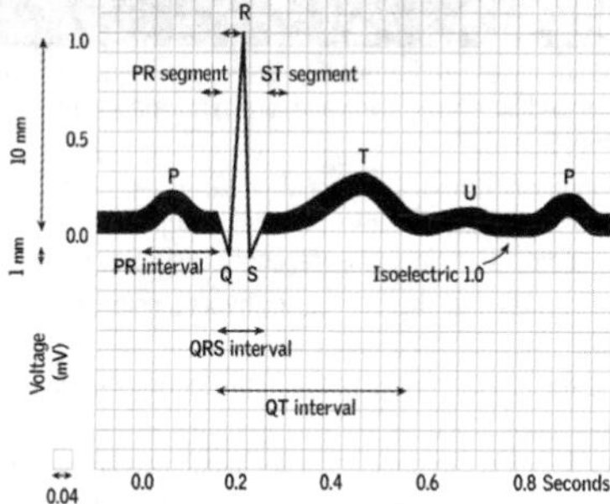

Fig 3.3 Schematic diagram of a normal ECG trace.

Calculating the heart rate

Divide 300 by the number of big squares per R-R interval (assumes the UK standard ECG speed of 25mm/s, elsewhere 50mm/s may be used: don't be confused!).

Table 3.1 Calculating heart rate from the R-R interval.

R-R duration (s)	Big squares	Rate (per min)
0.2	1	300
0.6	3	100
1.0	5	60
1.4	7	43

Determining the ECG axis

Each 'lead' on the 12-lead ECG represents electrical activity along a particular plane (see fig 3.4).

The axis lies at 90° to the direction of the lead in which the isoelectric (equally +ve and −ve) QRS complex is found. For example, if the QRS is isoelectric in lead II (+60°), the axis is either:

+60° − 90° = −30°, or
+60° + 90° = +150°.

If the QRS is more positive than negative in lead I (0°) then the axis must be −30°, and vice versa.

HEAD
aVR −150°
−90°
aVL −30°
RIGHT
±180°
I 0°
LEFT
+120° III
II +60°
aVF
+90°
FEET

Fig 3.4 The planes represented by the limb 'leads'.

In practice, the exact axis matters little; what you need to be able to recognize is whether the axis is normal (−30° to +90°), left-deviated (<−30°), or right deviated (>+90°). There are many ways of doing this. If the QRS in lead I (0°) is predominantly positive (the R wave is taller than the S wave is deep), the axis must be between −90° and +90°. If lead II (+60°) is mostly positive, the axis must be between −30° and +150°. So if both I and II are positive, the axis must be between −30° and +90°—the normal range. When II is negative, the axis is likely to be left-deviated (<−30°) and when I is negative, the axis is likely to be right-deviated (>+90°). One way of remembering this is:

Lovers **L**eaving—**L**eft axis deviation—the QRS complexes in I and II point away from each other.

Lovers **R**eturning—**R**ight axis deviation—the QRS complexes in I and III ± II point towards each other (fig 3.11).

ECG—abnormalities

Sinus tachycardia All impulses are initiated in the sinoatrial node ('sinus rhythm') hence all QRSs are preceeded by a normal P wave with a normal PR interval. Tachycardia means rate >100bpm. See p127.

Sinus bradycardia Sinus rhythm at a rate <60bpm. *Causes:* Physical fitness, vasovagal attacks, sick sinus syndrome, drugs (β-blockers, digoxin, amiodarone), hypothyroidism, hypothermia, ↑intracranial pressure, cholestasis. See p122.

AF (ECG p125) Common causes: IHD, thyrotoxicosis, hypertension, obesity, heart failure, alcohol. See p130.

Heart block (HB) (See fig 3.5.) Disrupted passage of electrical impulse through the AV node.

1st-degree HB: The PR interval is prolonged and unchanging; no missed beats.

2nd-degree HB: Mobitz I: The PR interval becomes longer and longer until a QRS is missed, the pattern then resets. This is Wenckebach phenomenon.

2nd-degree HB: Mobitz II: QRSs are regularly missed. eg P - QRS - P - - P - QRS - P - - this would be Mobitz II with 2:1 block (2P:1QRS). This is a dangerous rhythm as it may progress to complete heart block.

1st- and 2nd-degree HB may be caused by: normal variant, athletes, sick sinus syndrome, IHD (esp inferior MI), acute myocarditis, drugs (digoxin, β-blockers).

3rd-degree HB: Complete heart block: No impulses are passed from atria to ventricles so P waves and QRSs appear independently of each other. As tissue distal to the AVN paces slowly, the patient becomes very bradycardic, and may develop haemodynamic compromise. Urgent treatment is required. Causes: IHD (esp inferior MI), idiopathic (fibrosis), congenital, aortic valve calcification, cardiac surgery/trauma, digoxin toxicity, infiltration (abscesses, granulomas, tumours, parasites).

ST elevation Normal variant (high take-off), acute MI (STEMI), Prinzmetal's angina (p708), acute pericarditis (saddle-shaped), left ventricular aneurysm.

ST depression Normal variant (upward sloping), digoxin toxicity (downward sloping), ischaemic (horizontal): angina, NSTEMI, acute posterior MI (ST depression in V_1–V_3).

T inversion In V_1–V_3: normal (black patients and children), right bundle branch block (RBBB), RV strain (eg secondary to PE). In V_2–V_5: anterior ischaemia, HCM, subarachnoid haemorrhage, lithium. In V_4–V_6 and aVL: lateral ischaemia, LVH, left bundle branch block (LBBB). In II, III and aVF: inferior ischaemia.

NB: ST- and T-wave changes are often non-specific, and must be interpreted in the light of the clinical context.

Myocardial infarction (See p118 and fig 3.21; example ECGs figs 3.9, 3.10)
- Within hours, the T wave may become peaked and ST segments may begin to rise.
- Within 24h, the T wave inverts. ST elevation rarely persists, unless a left ventricular aneurysm develops. T-wave inversion may or may not persist.
- Within a few days, pathological Q waves begin to form. Q waves usually persist, but may resolve in 10% of patients.
- The location of these changes indicates the ischaemic area location, see table 3.2.

Pulmonary embolism (fig 3.11) ECG findings may include: sinus tachycardia (commonest), RBBB (p100), right ventricular strain pattern (R-axis deviation, dominant R wave and T-wave inversion/ST depression in V_1 and V_2.). Rarely, the '$S_I Q_{III} T_{III}$' pattern occurs: deep S waves in I, pathological Q waves in III, inverted T waves in III.

Metabolic abnormalities *Digoxin effect:* Down-sloping ST depression and inverted T wave in V_5–V_6 ('reversed tick', see fig 3.19). In digoxin toxicity, any arrhythmia may occur (ventricular ectopics and nodal bradycardia are common). *Hyperkalaemia:* Tall, tented T wave, widened QRS, absent P waves, 'sine wave' appearance (see fig 14.4, p675). *Hypokalaemia:* Small T waves, prominent U waves, peaked P waves. *Hypercalcaemia:* Short QT interval. *Hypocalcaemia:* Long QT interval, small T waves. See p711 for causes of long QT intervals.

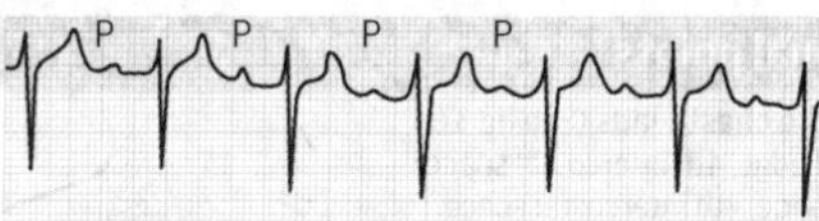

First degree AV block. P-R interval = 0.28s.

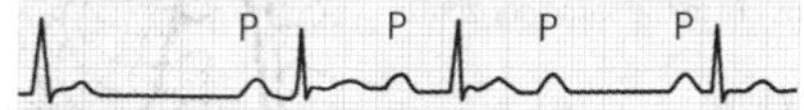

Mobitz type I (Wenckebach) AV block. With each successive QRS, the P-R interval increases until there is a non-conducted P wave.

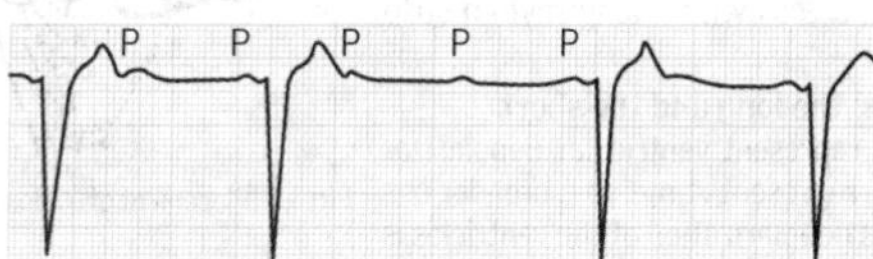

Mobitz type II AV block. Ratio of AV conduction varies from 2:1 to 3:1.

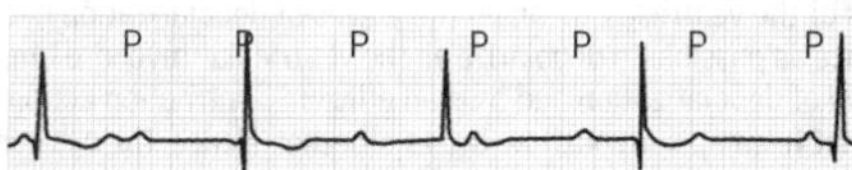

Complete AV block with narrow ventricular complex.
There is no relation between atrial and the slower ventricular activity.

Fig 3.5 Rhythm strips of heart blocks.

Location, location, location

When considering rate and rhythm, your findings should be the same in all leads, albeit clearer in some than others. Other ECG features may vary lead by lead, both in terms of what is 'normal' and in what a change indicates. For example, ST elevation in leads II, III, and aVF suggests an inferior MI requiring immediate treatment, likely PCI to the right coronary artery, see table 3.2. ST elevation across *all* leads, however, suggests instead pericarditis which necessitates entirely different management (p154). An R wave taller than the S is deep (R dominance) is normal in V_5 and V_6 but may suggest right ventricular strain or posterior MI if seen in V_1 and V_2.

Table 3.2 ECG territories

ECG leads	Heart territory	Coronary artery
I, aVL, V_4–V_6	Lateral	Circumflex
V_{1-3}	Anterioseptal	Left anterior descending
II, III, aVF	Inferior	Right coronary artery in 80% Circumflex in 20%: 'left dominant'
V_{7-9}	Posterior	Circumflex

Following a *posterior MI*, the standard 12-lead ECG will not show Q waves, ST elevation or hyperacute T waves. Instead, you may find these changes but 'upside-down' in V_1–V_3: prominent R waves, flat ST depression, and T-wave inversion. If you record V_7–V_9 leads, you may find the classic ST elevation pattern and so confirm posterior MI. See fig 3.24.

The 'upside-down' changes seen in posterior MI are called *'reciprocal changes'*: changes that appear when 'looking' at ischaemic myocardium from the other side of the heart. These can arise with MIs in other locations (fig 3.9). They are particularly important in posterior MI as they may be the only changes on the 12-lead ECG. ►See fig 3.9, 3.10, 3.24 for example ECGs. See fig 3.18 for coronary artery anatomy.

Where to place the chest leads (See fig 3.6.)

V_1: Right sternal edge, 4th intercostal space.
V_2: Left sternal edge, 4th intercostal space.
V_3: Half-way between V_2 and V_4.
V_4: 5th intercostal space, mid-clavicular line; all subsequent leads are in the same horizontal plane as V_4.
V_5: Anterior axillary line.
V_6: Mid-axillary line (V_7: posterior axillary line).

Good skin preparation (clean with non-alcoholic wipe, shave if hairy, etc.) will improve ECG quality. Finish 12-lead ECGs with a long rhythm strip in lead II.

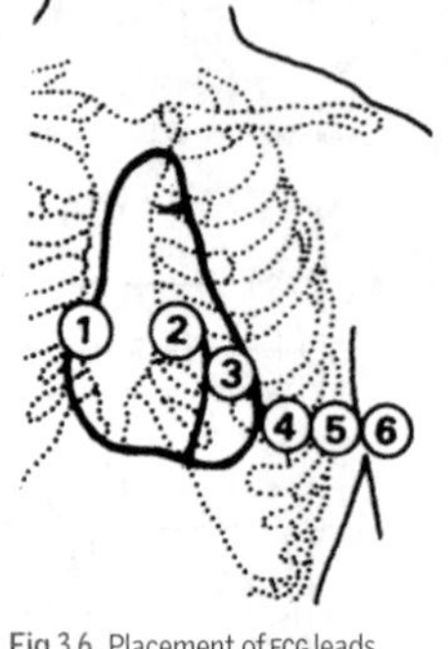

Fig 3.6 Placement of ECG leads.

QRS complexes: the long and the short

QRS complexes represent ventricular depolarization, and width represents time, so a broader QRS complex means depolarization of the ventricles is taking longer. Normally, a wave of depolarization reaches the ventricles via the specialist conduction pathways—the bundles of His. This delivers the electrical activity to certain points of the ventricles, meaning the waves of depolarization need travel as short a distance as possible to depolarize all the ventricular myocardium. This allows rapid spread of depolarization and thus an efficient contraction action as both ventricles contract from apex to outflow tracts together. Hence, the QRS complex is narrow (<120ms).

Ventricular depolarization takes longer when depolarization is not initiated in this pattern. For example, if it originates in the ventricles (eg ventricular ectopics, VT) or if one or more branches of the bundles of His are blocked—bundle branch blocks—meaning depolarization is initiated in one ventricle but not the other, so it has to travel the long (in time and space) path from one ventricle to the other.

Ventricular depolarization also takes longer if all conduction is slowed. This may happen in some electrolyte imbalances, eg hyperkalaemia.

Right bundle branch block: (p102, fig 3.8) QRS >0.12s, 'RSR' pattern in V_1; dominant R in V_1; inverted T waves in V_1–V_3 or V_4; wide, slurred S wave in V_6. Causes: normal variant (isolated RBBB), pulmonary embolism, cor pulmonale.

Left bundle branch block: (p101, fig 3.7) QRS >0.12s, 'M' pattern in V_5, dominant S in V_1, inverted T waves in I, aVL, V_5–V_6. Causes: IHD, hypertension, cardiomyopathy, idiopathic fibrosis. ►NB: if there is LBBB, no comment can be made on the ST segment or T wave. ►►New LBBB may represent a STEMI, see p798.

Bifascicular block: The combination of RBBB and left bundle hemiblock, manifest as an axis deviation, eg left axis deviation in the case of left anterior hemiblock.

Trifascicular block: Bifascicular block plus 1st-degree HB. ►May need pacing (p132).

Suspect *left ventricular hypertrophy* (LVH) if the R wave in V_6 is >25mm or the sum of the S wave in V_1 and the R wave in V_6 is >35mm (see fig 3.41).

Suspect *right ventricular hypertrophy* (RVH) if dominant R wave in V_1, T wave inversion in V_1–V_3 or V_4, deep S wave in V_6, right axis deviation.

Other causes of dominant R wave in V_1: RBBB, posterior MI, type A WPW syndrome (p133).

Causes of low-voltage QRS complex: (QRS <5mm in all limb leads.) Hypothyroidism, chronic obstructive pulmonary disease (COPD), ↑haematocrit (intracardiac blood resistivity is related to haematocrit), changes in chest wall impedance (eg in renal failure & subcutaneous emphysema but not obesity), pulmonary embolism, bundle branch block, carcinoid heart disease, myocarditis, cardiac amyloid, doxorubicin cardiotoxicity, and other heart muscle diseases, pericardial effusion, pericarditis.[5]

See lifeinthefastlane.com for excellent ECG tutorials, cases, and examples.

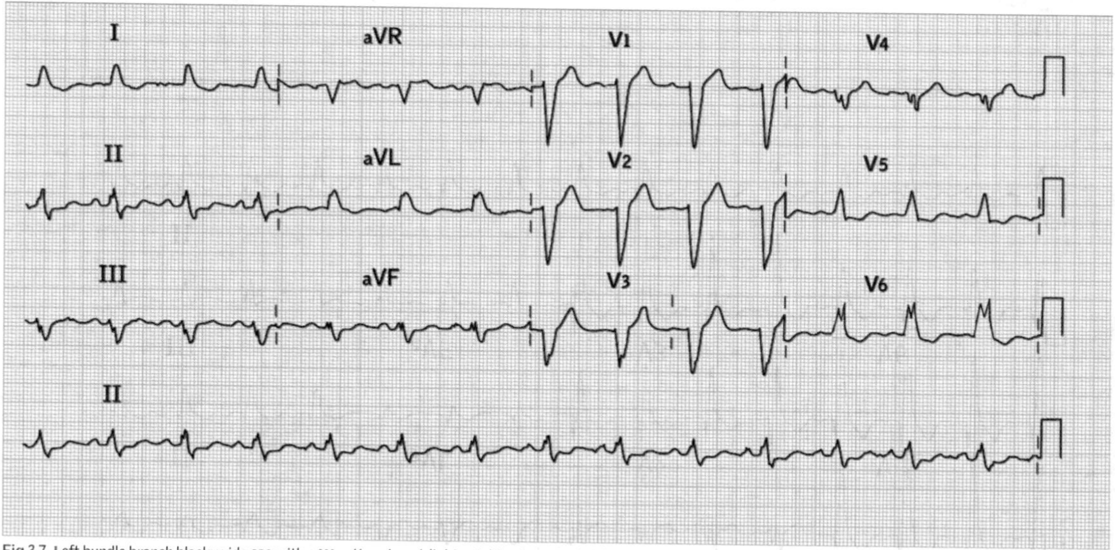

Fig 3.7 Left bundle branch block: wide QRS with a **W** pattern in V_1 (slight notching in upstroke of S wave—clearer in V_3) and the **M** pattern in V_6. **W**i**LL**ia**M** = **L**BBB.

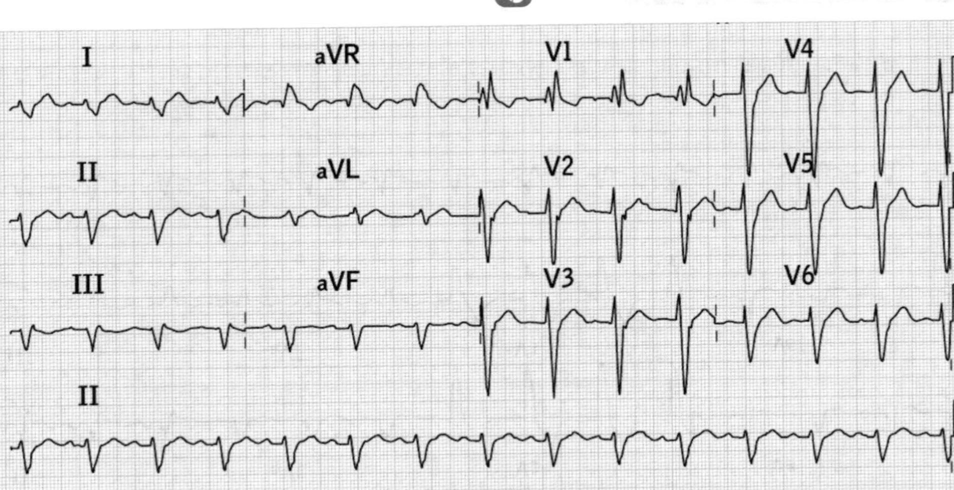

Fig 3.8 Right bundle branch block—broad QRS, M pattern in V_1 and sloped S wave (with the eye of faith, a 'W' shape) in V_5. MaRRoW = RBBB.

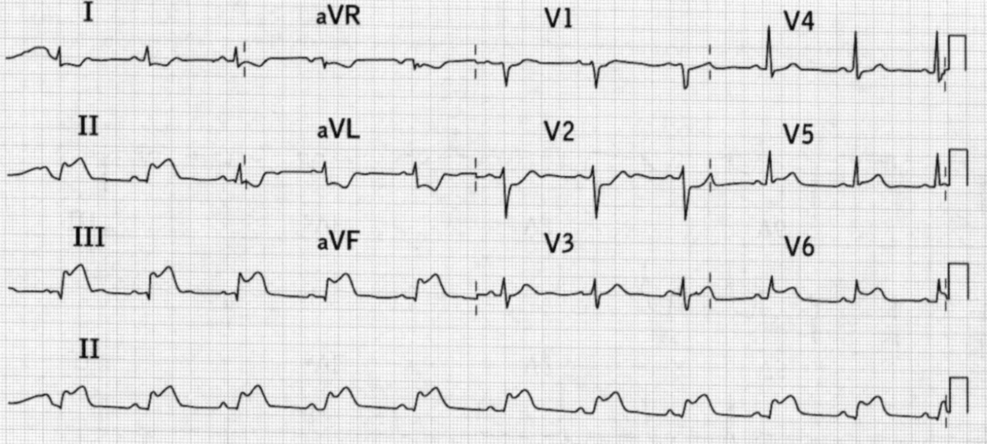

Fig 3.9 Acute infero-lateral myocardial infarction: marked ST elevation in the inferior leads (II, III, aVF), but also in V_5 and V_6, indicating lateral involvement. There is a 'reciprocal change' of ST-segment depression in leads I and aVL; this is often seen with a large inferior myocardial infarction.

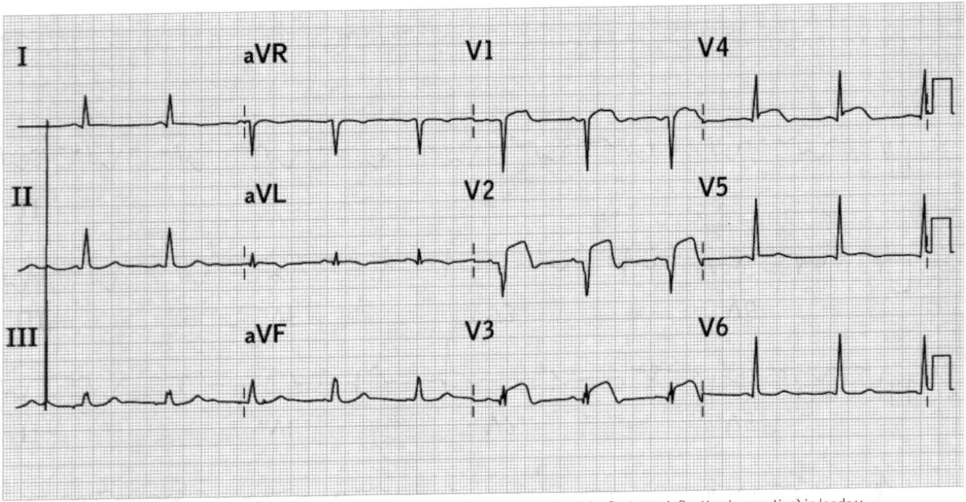

I aVR V1 V4

II aVL V2 V5

III aVF V3 V6

Fig 3.10 Acute anterior myocardial infarction—ST segment elevation and evolving Q waves (the first QRS deflection is negative) in leads V_{1-4}.

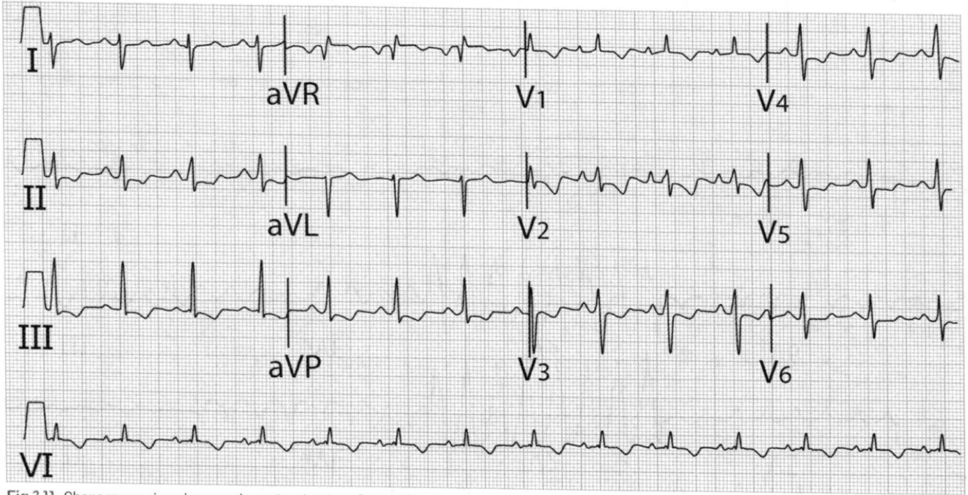

Fig 3.11 Changes seen in pulmonary hypertension (eg after a PE).

- Right axis deviation (QRS more negative than positive in lead I);
- Positive QRS complexes ('dominant R waves') in V_1 and V_2 suggesting right ventricular hypertrophy;
- ST depression and T-wave inversion in the right precordial leads (V_{1-3}) suggesting right ventricular strain;
- Peaked P waves (P pulmonale) suggesting right atrial hypertrophy.

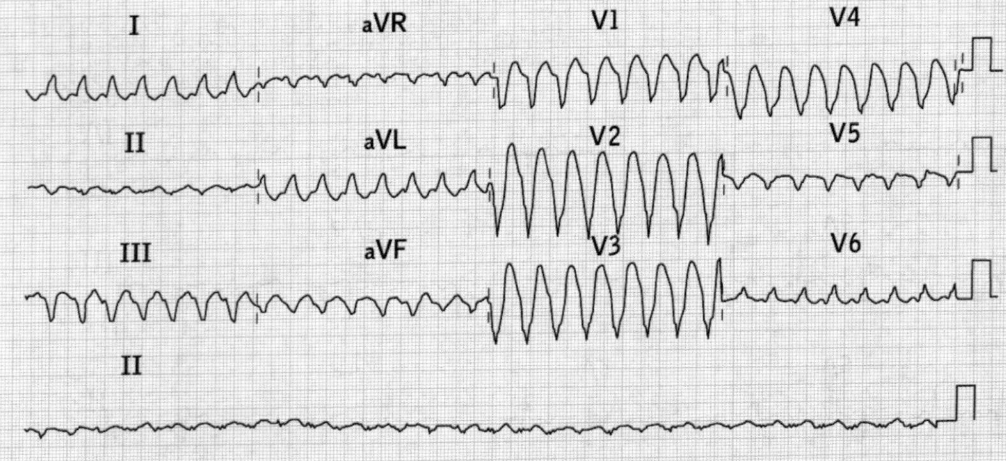

Fig 3.12 Ventricular tachycardia—regular broad complex tachycardiac indicating a likely ventricular origin for the rhythm.

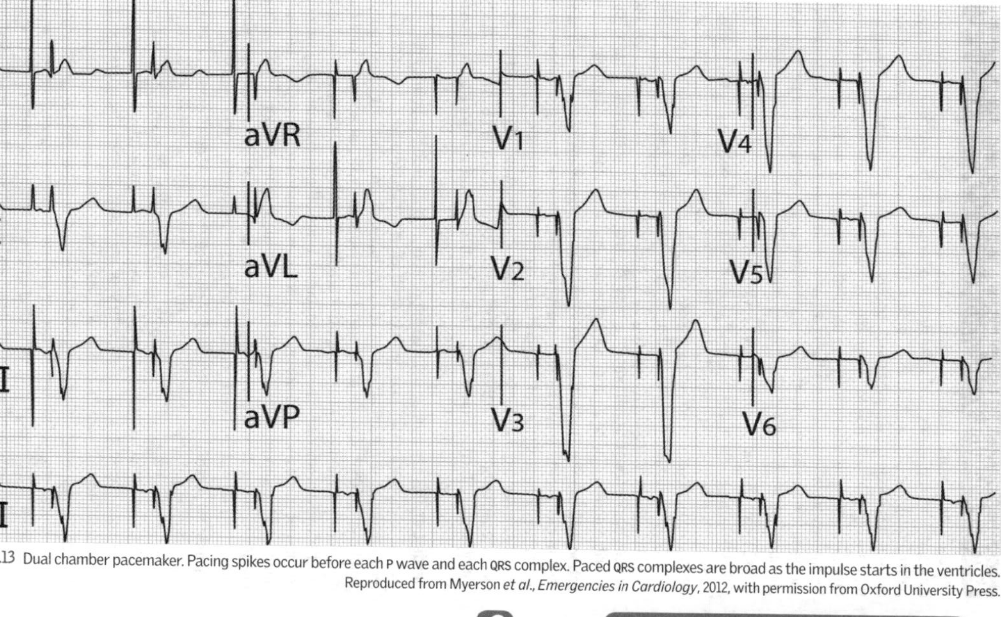

Fig 3.13 Dual chamber pacemaker. Pacing spikes occur before each P wave and each QRS complex. Paced QRS complexes are broad as the impulse starts in the ventricles.
Reproduced from Myerson *et al.*, *Emergencies in Cardiology*, 2012, with permission from Oxford University Press.

Cardiac imaging

There are many heart conditions associated with structural defects, eg valve defects, congenital heart diseases, and some muscle disorders (eg hypertrophic cardiomyopathy (HCM)). Whilst clues to these can sometimes be found on history, examination, and ECG, it is imaging that gives the diagnosis. Imaging is also helpful for conditions that are not primarily due to deformities but which affect the way the heart functions. For example, after an MI the affected territory may be hypokinetic. Stress techniques allow us to observe the heart at rest and then under stress, comparing the perfusion and function in the two states. Cardiac MRI is a rapidly expanding area although not yet available in all major hospitals.

Chest X-ray The humble chest X-ray provides just a snapshot of the heart and little detail but can be an important source of information and is often the only immediately accessible imaging modality for a new or newly unwell patient. An enlarged heart (cardiothoracic ratio >0.5) suggests congestive heart failure; signs of pulmonary oedema suggest decompensated heart failure (see fig 3.38); a globular heart may indicate pericardial effusion (fig 3.14); metal wires and valves will show up, evidencing previous cardiothoracic surgery; dextrocardia may explain a bizarre ECG; and rib notching may be an important clue in coarctation of the aorta (p156).

Echocardiography This is the workhorse of cardiological imaging. Ultrasound is used to give real-time images of the moving heart. This can be transthoracic (TTE) or transoesophageal (TOE), at rest, during exercise, or after infusion of a pharmacological stressor (eg dobutamine). If the patient is too unwell to be moved, an echo machine can be brought to them and continuous TOE imaging may be used as a guide during surgery. Increasingly pocket-sized echo machines are used for a quick assessment of an unwell patient, to be followed by a formal scan later. See p110.

Cardiac CT This can provide detailed information about cardiac structure and function. CT angiography (fig 3.15) permits contrast-enhanced imaging of coronary arteries during a single breath hold with very low radiation doses. It can diagnose significant (>50%) stenosis in coronary artery disease with an accuracy of 89%. CT coronary angiography has a negative predictive value of >99%, which makes it an effective non-invasive alternative to routine transcatheter coronary angiography to rule out coronary artery disease.[6] Medications are often given to slow the heart down and the imaging may be 'gated', meaning the scanner is programmed to take images at times corresponding to certain points on the patient's ECG. This allows characterization of the heart at different points in the cardiac cycle. See p740.

Cardiac MR A radiation-free method of characterizing cardiac structure and function including viability of myocardium. By varying the settings, different defects can be found. MR is the first-choice imaging method to look at diseases that directly affect the myocardium (fig 3.16). Nowadays, pacemakers are available which are safe for MR scanning—check MR safety with your cardiac technicians before requesting MR for patients with pacemakers *in situ*. See p740.

Nuclear imaging Perfusion is assessed at rest and with exercise- or pharmacologically-induced stress. This test is particularly useful for assessing whether myocardium distal to a blockage is viable and so whether stenting or CABG will be of value. If hypoperfusion is 'fixed', ie present at rest and under stress, the hypoperfused area is probably scar tissue and so non-viable. If hypoperfusion is 'reversible' at rest, the myocardium may benefit from improved blood supply. See p741.

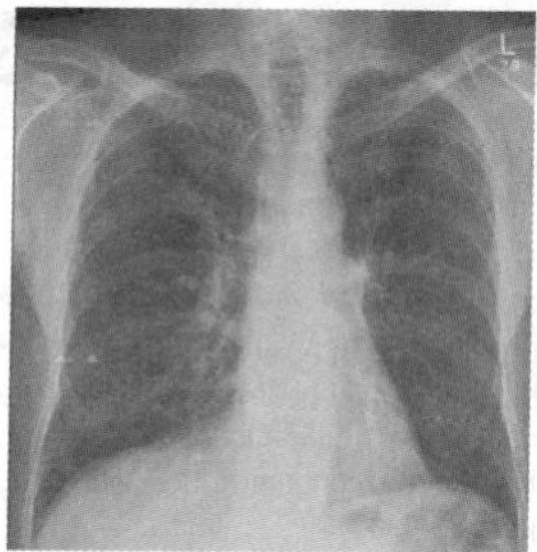

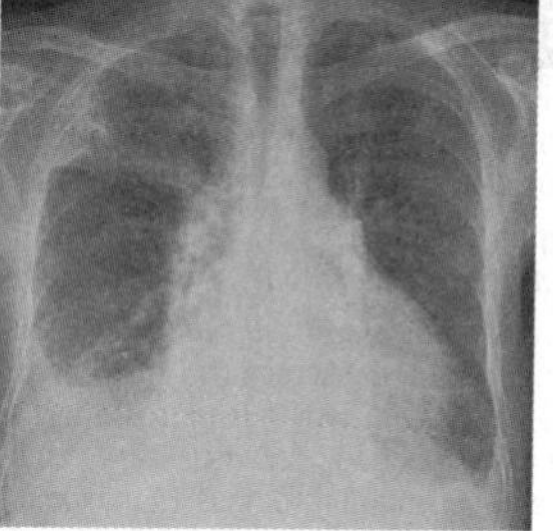

Fig 3.14 Two chest x-rays of the same patient, the one on the right was taken 6 months after the one on the left. On the later image, a pericardial effusion has expanded the cardiac shadow and given it a 'globular' shape.

Reproduced from Leeson, *Cardiovascular Imaging*, 2011, with permission from Oxford University Press.

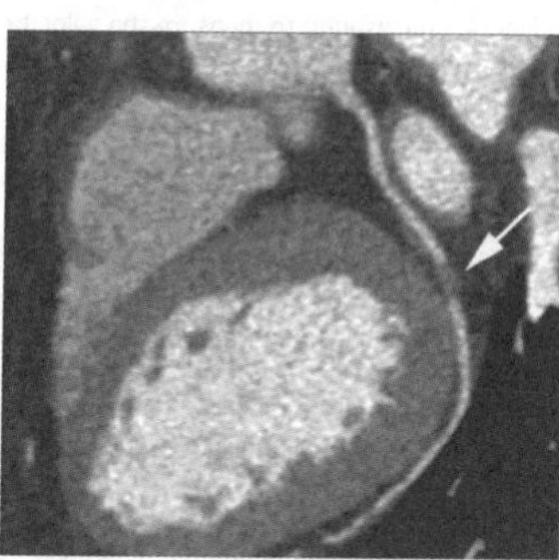

Fig 3.15 Cardiac CT demonstrating coronary artery stenosis.

Reproduced from Camm *et al.*, *ESC Textbook of Cardiovascular Medicine*, 2009, with permission from Oxford University Press.

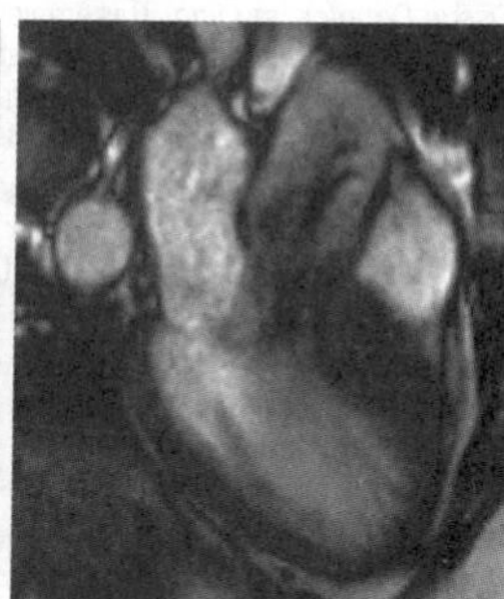

Fig 3.16 Cardiac MR image demonstrating the asymmetrical left ventricular wall thickening typical of hypertrophic cardiomyopathy.

Reproduced from Myerson *et al.*, *Cardiovascular Magnetic Resonance*, 2013, with permission from Oxford University Press.

Echocardiography

This non-invasive technique uses the differing ability of various structures within the heart to reflect ultrasound waves. It not only demonstrates anatomy but also provides a continuous display of the functioning heart throughout its cycle.

Types of scan

M-mode (motion mode): A single-dimension image.

Two-dimensional (real time): A 2D, fan-shaped image of a segment of the heart is produced on the screen (fig 3.17); the moving image may be 'frozen'. Several views are possible, including long axis, short axis, 4-chamber, and subcostal. 2D echocardiography is good for visualizing conditions such as: congenital heart disease, LV aneurysm, mural thrombus, LA myxoma, septal defects.

3D echocardiography: Now possible with matrix array probes, and is termed 4D (3D + time) if the images are moving.

Doppler and colour-flow echocardiography: Different coloured jets illustrate flow and gradients across valves and septal defects (p156) (Doppler effect, p736).

Tissue Doppler imaging: This employs Doppler ultrasound to measure the velocity of myocardial segments over the cardiac cycle. It is particularly useful for assessing longitudinal motion—and hence long-axis ventricular function, which is a sensitive marker of systolic and diastolic heart failure.

Transoesophageal echocardiography (TOE): More sensitive than transthoracic echocardiography (TTE) as the transducer is nearer to the heart. Indications: diagnosing aortic dissections; assessing prosthetic valves; finding cardiac source of emboli, and IE/SBE. Contraindicated in oesophageal disease and cervical spine instability.

Stress echocardiography: Used to evaluate ventricular function, ejection fraction, myocardial thickening, regional wall motion pre- and post-exercise, and to characterize valvular lesions. Dobutamine or dipyridamole may be used if the patient cannot exercise. Inexpensive and as sensitive/specific as a thallium scan (p741).

Uses of echocardiography

Quantification of global LV function: Heart failure may be due to systolic or diastolic ventricular impairment (or both). Echo helps by measuring end-diastolic volume. If this is large, systolic dysfunction is the likely cause. If small, diastolic. Pure forms of diastolic dysfunction are rare. Differentiation is important because vasodilators are less useful in diastolic dysfunction as a high ventricular filling pressure is required.

Echo is also useful for detecting focal and global hypokinesia, LV aneurysm, mural thrombus, and LVH (echo is 5–10 times more sensitive than ECG in detecting this).

Estimating right heart haemodynamics: Doppler studies of pulmonary artery flow and tricuspid regurgitation allow evaluation of RV function and pressures.

Valve disease: The technique of choice for measuring pressure gradients and valve orifice areas in stenotic lesions. Detecting valvular regurgitation and estimating its significance is less accurate. Evaluating function of prosthetic valves is another role.

Congenital heart disease: Establishing the presence of lesions, and significance.

Endocarditis: Vegetations may not be seen if <2mm in size. TTE with colour Doppler is best for aortic regurgitation (AR). TOE is useful for visualizing mitral valve vegetations, leaflet perforation, or looking for an aortic root abscess.

Pericardial effusion: Best diagnosed by echo. Fluid may first accumulate between the posterior pericardium and the left ventricle, then anterior to both ventricles and anterior and lateral to the right atrium. There may be paradoxical septal motion.

HCM: (p152) Echo features include asymmetrical septal hypertrophy, small LV cavity, dilated left atrium, and systolic anterior motion of the mitral valve.

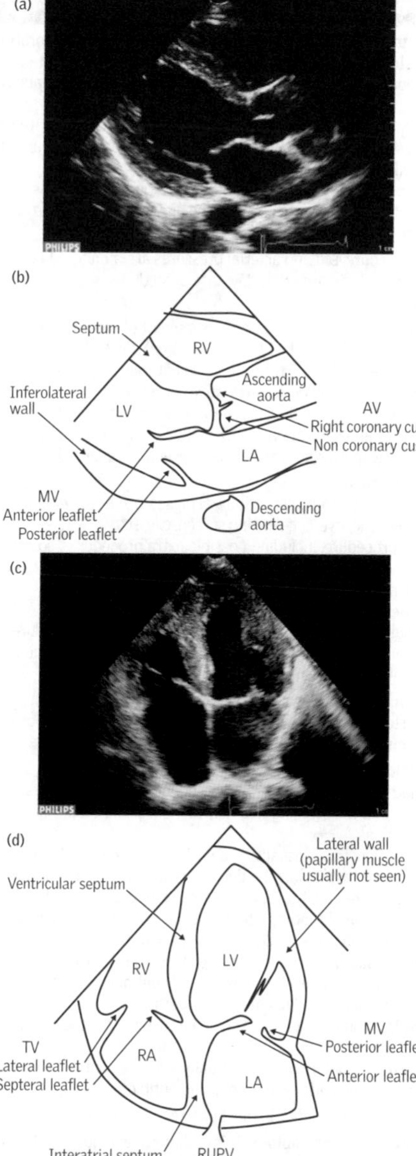

Fig 3.17 Echo images. (a) A normal heart seen with the parasternal long-axis view. (b) Diagram of what can be seen in (a). (c) A normal heart seen in apical four-chamber view. (d) Diagram of what can be seen in (c).

Cardiac catheterization

This involves the insertion of a catheter into the heart via the femoral or radial artery or venous system, and manipulating it within the heart and great vessels to:

- Inject radiopaque contrast medium to image cardiac anatomy and blood flow, see fig 3.18a.
- Perform angioplasty (ballooning and stenting), valvuloplasty (eg transcatheter aortic valve implantation (TAVI, fig 3.45)), cardiac biopsies, transcatheter septal defect closure.
- Perform electrophysiology studies and radiofrequency ablations.
- Sample blood to assess oxygen saturation and measure pressures.
- Perform intravascular ultrasound or echocardiography.

During the procedure, ECG and arterial pressures are monitored continuously. In the UK, the majority are performed as day-case procedures.

Indications

- Coronary artery disease: diagnostic (assessment of coronary vessels and graft patency); therapeutic (angioplasty, stent insertion), fig 3.18b.
- Valvular disease: diagnostic (pressures indicate severity); therapeutic valvuloplasty (if the patient is too ill or declines valve surgery).
- Congenital heart disease: diagnostic (assessment of severity of lesions by measuring pressures and saturations); therapeutic (balloon dilatation or septostomy).
- Other: cardiomyopathy; pericardial disease; endomyocardial biopsy.

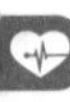

Pre-procedure checks

- Brief history/examination; NB: peripheral pulses, bruits, aneurysms.
- Investigations: FBC, U&E, LFT, clotting screen, CXR, ECG.
- Consent for procedure, including possible extra procedures, eg consent for angioplasty if planning to do angiography as you may find a lesion that needs stenting. Explain reason for procedure and possible complications.
- IV access, ideally in the left hand.
- Patient should be nil by mouth (NBM) from 6h before the procedure.
- Patients should take all their morning drugs (and pre-medication if needed)—but withhold oral hypoglycaemics.

Post-procedure checks

- Pulse, BP, arterial puncture site (for bruising or swelling), foot pulses.
- Investigations: FBC and clotting (if suspected blood loss), ECG.

Complications

- Haemorrhage: apply firm pressure over puncture site. If you suspect a false aneurysm, ultrasound the swelling and consider surgical repair. Haematomas are high risk for infections.
- Contrast reaction: this is usually mild with modern contrast agents.
- Loss of peripheral pulse: may be due to dissection, thrombosis, or arterial spasm. Occurs in <1% of brachial catheterizations. Rare with femoral catheterization.
- Angina: may occur during or after cardiac catheterization. Usually responds to sublingual GTN; if not, give analgesia and IV nitrates.
- Arrhythmias: usually transient. Manage along standard lines.
- Pericardial effusion: suspect if unexplained continued chest pain. May need drain depending on severity and haemodynamic status.
- Pericardial tamponade: rare, but should be suspected if the patient becomes hypotensive and anuric. ΔΔ Urgent pericardial drain.
- Infection: post-catheter pyrexia is usually due to a contrast reaction. If it persists for >24h, take blood cultures before giving antibiotics.

Mortality <1 in 1000 patients, in most centres.

Intracardiac electrophysiology This catheter technique can determine types and origins of arrhythmias, and locate and ablate problem areas, eg aberrant pathways in WPW or arrhythmogenic foci. Arrhythmias may be induced, and the effectiveness of control by drugs assessed.

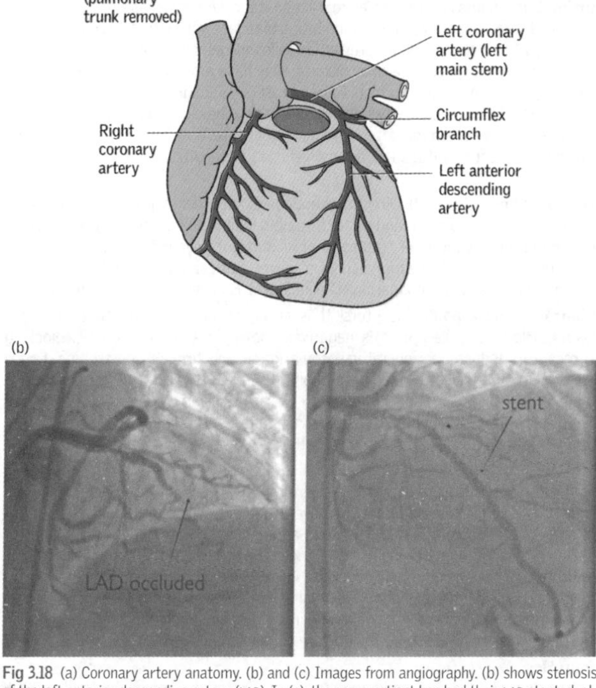

Fig 3.18 (a) Coronary artery anatomy. (b) and (c) Images from angiography. (b) shows stenosis of the left anterior descending artery (LAD). In (c), the same patient has had their LAD stented, allowing contrast to flow freely through to the distal vessel. The stenting is a type of angioplasty (a procedure to widen the lumen of a blood vessel); in the context of coronary arteries, it is called PCI (percutaneous coronary intervention). PPCI (primary PCI) is PCI performed acutely for a patient with acute coronary syndrome (ACS), see p120.

Antiplatelet drugs Aspirin irreversibly acetylates cyclo-oxygenase, preventing production of thromboxane A_2, thereby inhibiting platelet aggregation. Used in low dose (eg 75mg/24h PO) for secondary prevention following MI, TIA/stroke, and for patients with angina or peripheral vascular disease. May have a role in primary prevention.[7] ADP receptor antagonists (eg clopidogrel, prasugrel, ticagrelor) also block platelet aggregation, but may cause less gastric irritation. They have a role if truly intolerant of aspirin; with aspirin after coronary stent insertion; and in acute coronary syndrome. Glycoprotein IIb/IIIa antagonists (eg tirofiban) have a role in unstable angina/MI.[8]

Anticoagulants See p350. Direct oral anticoagulants (DOACs, previously NOACs), eg Xa inhibitors (eg apixaban) and direct thrombin inhibitors (dabigatran), are increasingly replacing warfarin[9] for treatment of AF and clots, see p350. Warfarin remains the anticoagulant of choice for mechanical valves. Anticoagulants used in ACS include treatment dose LMWH, fondaparinux (Xa inhibitor), & bivalirudin (thrombin inhibitor).

β-blockers Block β-adrenoceptors, thus antagonizing the sympathetic nervous system. Blocking β_1-receptors is negatively inotropic and chronotropic; blocking β_2-receptors induces peripheral vasoconstriction and bronchoconstriction. Drugs vary in their β_1/β_2 selectivity (eg propranolol is non-selective, and bisoprolol relatively β_1 selective), but this does not seem to alter their clinical efficacy. *Uses:* Angina, hypertension, antidysrhythmic, post MI (↓mortality), heart failure (with caution). *CI:* Severe asthma/COPD, heart block. *SEs:* Lethargy, erectile dysfunction, ↓joie de vivre, nightmares, headache.

ACE inhibitors These are used in hypertension (HT), heart failure, and post-MI. First dose HT is a concern in patients with severe CCF and malignant HT. In CCF patients, reduce diuretic dose initially and use long-acting ACE-i. Monitor U&E when starting or raising ACE-i dose, a creatinine rise of >20% is concerning. If the patient starts ACE-i prior to discharge, ask the GP to check U&E in 1-2 weeks. If renal function deteriorates markedly, consider investigating for renal artery stenosis. The risk to the kidneys is greater when the patient is unwell. Hold in AKI and hyperkalaemia; avoid starting if the patient is dehydrated. *SEs:* Include dry cough and urticaria.

Diuretics

- *Loop diuretics* (eg furosemide) are used in heart failure, and inhibit the Na/2Cl/K co-transporter. *SEs:* dehydration, ↓Na^+,↓K^+, ↓Ca^{2+}, ototoxic
- *Thiazides* and thiazide-like diuretics are used in hypertension (eg indapamide) and heart failure (eg metolazone). *SE:* ↓K^+, ↑Ca^{2+}, ↓Mg^{2+}, ↑urate (±gout), impotence (NB: small doses, eg chlortalidone 25mg/24h rarely cause significant SEs)
- *Potassium-sparing diuretics*: aldosterone antagonists (eg spironolactone, eplerenone) directly block aldosterone receptors; amiloride blocks the epithelial sodium channel in the distal convoluted tubules.

Vasodilators Used in heart failure, IHD, and hypertension. Nitrates (p116) preferentially dilate veins and the large arteries, ↓ filling pressure (pre-load), while hydralazine (often used with nitrates) primarily dilates the resistance vessels, thus ↓ BP (after-load). Prazosin (an α-blocker) dilates arteries and veins.

Calcium antagonists These ↓ cell entry of Ca^{2+} via voltage-sensitive channels in smooth muscle, thereby promoting coronary and peripheral vasodilation and reducing myocardial oxygen consumption. All current drugs block L-type Ca^{2+} channels. However, their effects differ because of differential binding properties.

- The *dihydropyridines*, eg nifedipine, amlodipine, are mainly peripheral vasodilators (also dilate coronary arteries) and cause a reflex tachycardia, so are often used with a β-blocker. They are used mainly in hypertension and angina.
- The *non-dihydropyridines*—verapamil and diltiazem—also slow conduction at the AV and SA nodes and may be used to treat hypertension, angina, and dysrhythmias. ⚠ Don't give non-dihydropyridines with β-blockers (risk of severe bradycardia ± LVF).

SEs: Flushes, headache, ankle oedema (diuretic unresponsive), ↓LV function, gingival hypertrophy. *CI:* Heart block.

Digoxin Blocks the Na^+/K^+ pump. It is used to slow the pulse in fast AF (p130; aim for ≤100). As it is a weak +ve inotrope, its role in heart failure in sinus rhythm may be best reserved if symptomatic despite optimal ACE-i therapy;[10] here there is little benefit vis-à-vis mortality (but admissions for worsening CCF are ↓ by ~25%).[11] Elderly people are at ↑risk of toxicity: use lower doses. Measure plasma levels >6h post-dose (p756). Typical dose: 500mcg stat PO, repeated after 12h, then 125mcg (if elderly) to 250mcg/d PO OD (62.5mcg/d is almost never enough). IV dose: 0.75–1mg in 0.9% NaCl over 2h. ↑Toxicity risk if: ↓K^+, ↓Mg^{2+}, or ↑Ca^{2+}. $t_{1/2} \approx$ 36h. If on digoxin, use less energy in cardioversion (start at 5J). ►If on amiodarone, halve the dose of digoxin. *SEs:* Any arrhythmia (supraventricular tachycardia with AV block is suggestive), nausea, ↓appetite, yellow vision, confusion, gynaecomastia. If toxicity is suspected, do an ECG (fig 3.19), digoxin levels, and check K^+, Mg^{2+}, and Ca^{2+}. If toxicity is confirmed, stop digoxin, correct electrolyte imbalances, treat arrhythmias, and consider IV DigiFab® (p842). *CIs:* HCM; WPW syndrome (p133).

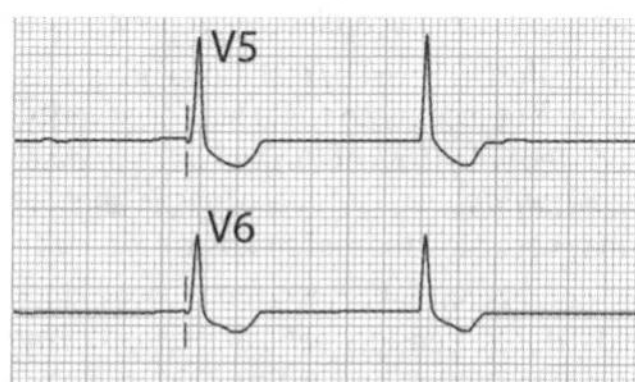

Fig 3.19 This ECG shows the classic 'reverse tick' of digoxin toxicity: downsloping ST wave with rapid upstroke back to isoelectric line. The bradycardia is also suggestive of digoxin toxicity.

Sodium channel blockers Class I anti-arrhythmics. Procainamide (1a) and lidocaine (1b) can be used to terminate VT. NB QT interval may be prolonged. Flecainide (1c) is useful for AF cardioversion in patients without contraindications, and for arrhythmia prophylaxis in patients with WPW or troublesome paroxysmal AF. *CIs:* Heart failure, IHD, valve disease, and heart block.

Amiodarone A class III anti-arrhythmic. Amiodarone prolongs the cardiac action potential, reducing the potential for tachyarrhythmias. Used in both supra-ventricular and ventricular tachycardias, including during cardiac arrest. Broad range of side effects incl. thyroid disease, liver disease, pulmonary fibrosis and peripheral neuropathy. Monitor TFTs and LFTs every 6 months.

Ivabradine Blocks the pacemaker 'funny current', slowing pulse rate without significantly dropping blood pressure. Used in angina, heart failure, and (off-licence) in autonomic tachycardia syndromes. *CIs:* Acute MI, bradycardia, long QT syndrome, shock. Many drug interactions, including with calcium antagonists.

Statins Statins (eg simvastatin, p690) inhibit the enzyme HMG-COA reductase, which causes *de novo* synthesis of cholesterol in the liver. This increases LDL receptor expression by hepatocytes leading to ↓circulating LDL cholesterol. More effective if given at night, but optimum dose and target plasma cholesterol are unknown. *SEs:* Muscle aches, abdominal discomfort, ↑transaminases (eg ALT), ↑CK, myositis, rarely rhabdomyolysis (more common if used with fibrates). Statins are generally well tolerated. There are currently ~3 million people taking statins in England, which saves ~10 000 lives a year. See also hyperlipidaemia, pp690–1, fig 14.13.

Anti-anginal drugs p116. **Antihypertensives** p140.

Drugs that slow conduction through the atrioventricular node

Drugs that slow conduction through the atrioventricular node (AVN) include digoxin, verapamil, and adenosine. Uses include cardioverting AVNRT and diagnosing atrial tachycardias.

Drugs that slow AVN conduction should be avoided in patients with aberrant pathways (eg WPW) as blocking the AVN can increase conduction via the alternative pathways. AVN blockers are contraindicated in patients with or at risk of VT, eg those with long QT syndrome.

Angina pectoris

►If ACS is a possible diagnosis (including unstable angina), see pp798–801.

Angina[12] is symptomatic reversible myocardial ischaemia. Features:

1 Constricting/heavy discomfort to the chest, jaw, neck, shoulders, or arms.
2 Symptoms brought on by exertion.
3 Symptoms relieved within 5min by rest or GTN.

All 3 features = ***typical angina***; 2 features = ***atypical angina***; 0–1 features = ***non-anginal chest pain***.

Other precipitants: emotion, cold weather, and heavy meals. *Associated symptoms:* dyspnoea, nausea, sweatiness, faintness. *Features that make angina less likely:* pain that is continuous, pleuritic or worse with swallowing; pain associated with palpitations, dizziness or tingling.

Causes Atheroma. Rarely: anaemia; coronary artery spasm; AS; tachyarrhythmias; HCM; arteritis/small vessel disease (microvascular angina/cardiac syndrome X).

Types of angina *Stable angina:* Induced by effort, relieved by rest. Good prognosis. ***Unstable angina:*** (Crescendo angina.) Angina of increasing frequency or severity; occurs on minimal exertion or at rest; associated with ↑↑risk of MI. ***Decubitus angina:*** Precipitated by lying flat. ***Variant (Prinzmetal) angina:*** (BOX 'Vasospastic angina') Caused by coronary artery spasm (rare; may coexist with fixed stenoses).

Tests *ECG* usually normal, but may show ST depression; flat or inverted T waves; signs of past MI. ***Blood tests:*** FBC, U&E, TFTs, lipids, HbA1c. Consider *echo* and *chest x-ray*. ***Further investigations*** are usually necessary to confirm an IHD diagnosis—see BOX.

Management

Address exacerbating factors: Anaemia, tachycardia (eg fast AF), thyrotoxicosis.

Secondary prevention of cardiovascular disease:

- Stop smoking; exercise; dietary advice; optimize hypertension and diabetes control.
- 75mg aspirin daily if not contraindicated.
- Address hyperlipidaemia—see p690.
- Consider ACE inhibitors, eg if diabetic.

PRN symptom relief: Glyceryl trinitrate (GTN) spray or sublingual tabs. Advise the patient to repeat the dose if the pain has not gone after 5min and to call an ambulance if the pain is still present 5min after the second dose. SE: headaches, BP↓.

Anti-anginal medication: (p114) First line: β-blocker and/or calcium channel blocker (►do not combine β-blockers with non-dihydropyridine calcium antagonists). If these fail to control symptoms or are not tolerated, trial other agents.

- *β-blockers:* eg atenolol 50mg BD or bisoprolol 5–10mg OD.
- *Calcium antagonists:* amlodipine—start at 5mg OD; diltiazem—dose depends on formulation.
- *Long-acting nitrates:* eg isosorbide mononitrate—starting regimen depends on formulation. Alternatives: GTN skin patches. SEs: headaches, ↓BP.
- *Ivabradine:* reduces heart rate with minimal impact on BP. Patient must be in sinus rhythm. Start with 5mg BD (2.5mg in elderly).
- *Ranolazine:* inhibits late Na^+ current. Start at 375mg BD. Caution if heart failure, elderly, weight <60kg or prolonged QT interval.
- *Nicorandil:* a K^+ channel activator. Start with 5–10mg BD. CI: acute pulmonary oedema, severe hypotension, hypovolaemia, LV failure.

Revascularization: Considered when optimal medical therapy proves inadequate.

- *Percutaneous coronary intervention (PCI):* (p112) a balloon is inflated inside the stenosed vessel, opening the lumen. A stent is usually inserted to reduce the risk of re-stenosis. Dual antiplatelet therapy (DAPT; usually aspirin and clopidogel) is recommended for at least 12 months after stent insertion to reduce the risk of in-stent thrombosis. Specialist advice should be sought regarding antiplatelets if the patient has a high bleeding risk or requires surgery.
- *CABG:* (p123) compared to PCI, patients undergoing CABG are less likely to need repeat revascularization and those with multivessel disease can expect better outcomes. However, CABG is open heart surgery and so recovery is slower and the patient is left with two large wounds (sternal and vein harvesting).

Investigating patients with ? stable angina

Investigations for ischaemic heart disease (IHD) include:

- Exercise ECG—assess for ischaemic ECG changes.
- Angiography—either using cardiac CT with contrast, or transcatheter angiography (more invasive but can be combined with stenting, p112).
- Functional imaging (see p108): myocardial perfusion scintigraphy, stress echo (echo whilst undergoing exercise or receiving dobutamine), cardiac MRI.

NICE recommend the following investigations when considering stable angina.[13]

Typical angina in a patient with previously proven IHD:

Treat as stable angina; if further confirmation is required, use non-invasive testing, eg exercise ECG.

Typical and atypical angina:

CT angiography, fig 3.20. If inconclusive, use functional imaging as 2nd line and transcatheter angiography as 3rd line.

Non-anginal chest pain:

Does the patient have ischaemic changes on 12 lead ECG?

- Yes: investigate as per typical and atypical angina
- No: no further investigations for IHD at this point (unless high clinical suspicion of IHD for other reasons—discuss with a specialist). Ensure alternative chest pain diagnoses are adequately explored.

These are guidelines and must be interpreted within the clinical context.

Further investigations:

If the patient has typical angina but few risk factors for IHD, be sure to look for possible precipitating or exacerbating factors, for example severe anaemia or cardiomyopathy.

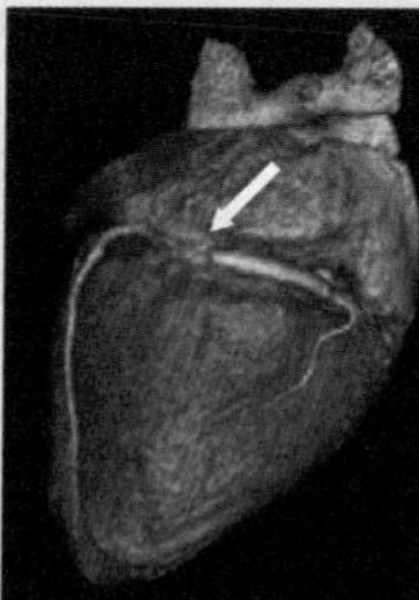

Fig 3.20 CT angiogram data has been used to construct this 3D image. The white arrow points to an obstruction of the right coronary artery

Reprinted from *Journal of the American College of Cardiology*, 52(3), MM Henneman *et al.*, Noninvasive Evaluation With Multislice Computed Tomography in Suspected Acute Coronary Syndrome, 216–22, 2008, with permission from Elsevier.

Vasospastic angina (Prinzmetal angina)

Angina due to coronary artery spasm, which can occur even in normal coronary arteries. The pain usually occurs during rest and resolves rapidly with short-acting nitrates (eg GTN spray). ECG during pain shows ST segment elevation.

Risks and triggers: Smoking increases risk but hypertension and hypercholesterolaemia do not. Probable triggers include cocaine, amphetamine, marijuana, low magnesium, and artery instrumentation (eg during angiography).

Treatment: Avoid triggers. Correct low magnesium. Stop smoking. PRN GTN. Calcium channel blockers ± long-acting nitrates. Avoid non-selective β-blockers, aspirin, and triptans. Prognosis is usually very good.

Acute coronary syndromes (ACS)

Definitions *ACS* includes unstable angina and myocardial infarctions (MIs). These share a common underlying pathology—plaque rupture, thrombosis, and inflammation. However, ACS may rarely be due to emboli, coronary spasm, or vasculitis (p556) in normal coronary arteries. ***Myocardial infarction*** means there is myocardial cell death, releasing troponin. ***Ischaemia*** means a lack of blood supply, ±cell death. MIs have troponin rises, unstable angina does not. An MI may be a ***STEMI***—ACS with ST-segment elevation (may only be present in V_7–V_9 if posterior STEMI) or new-onset LBBB; or an ***NSTEMI***—trop-positive ACS without ST-segment elevation—the ECG may show ST depression, T-wave inversion, non-specific changes, or be normal. The degree of irreversible myocyte death varies, and significant necrosis can occur without ST elevation.

Risk factors Non-modifiable: age, ♂ gender, family history of IHD (MI in 1st-degree relative <55yrs). Modifiable: smoking, hypertension, DM, hyperlipidaemia, obesity, sedentary lifestyle, cocaine use. Controversial risk factors include: stress, type A personality, LVH, fibrinogen↑, hyperinsulinaemia, ↑homocysteine levels, ACE genotype.

Incidence 5/1000 per annum (UK) for ST-segment elevation (declining in UK & USA).

Diagnosis An increase in cardiac biomarkers (eg troponin) and either: symptoms of ischaemia, ECG changes of new ischaemia, development of pathological Q waves, new loss of myocardium, or regional wall motion abnormalities on imaging.

Symptoms Acute central chest pain, lasting >20min, often associated with nausea, sweatiness, dyspnoea, palpitations. ACS without chest pain is called 'silent'; mostly seen in elderly and diabetic patients. Silent MIs may present with: syncope, pulmonary oedema, epigastric pain and vomiting, post-operative hypotension or oliguria, acute confusional state, stroke, and diabetic hyperglycaemic states.

Signs Distress, anxiety, pallor, sweatiness, pulse ↑ or ↓, BP ↑ or ↓, 4th heart sound. There may be signs of heart failure (↑JVP, 3rd heart sound, basal crepitations) or a pansystolic murmur (papillary muscle dysfunction/rupture, VSD). Low-grade fever may be present. Later, a pericardial friction rub or peripheral oedema may develop.

Tests *ECG:* (See fig 3.21.) STEMI: classically, hyperacute (tall) T waves, ST elevation, or new LBBB occur within hours. T-wave inversion and pathological Q waves follow over hours to days (p98). NSTEMI/unstable angina: ST depression, T wave inversion, non-specific changes, or normal. ►In 20% of MI, the ECG may be normal initially. Paced ECGs and ECGs with chronic bundle branch block are unhelpful for diagnosing NSTEMIs[14] and may hinder STEMI[15] diagnosis; in these cases, clinical assessment and troponin levels are especially important. *CXR:* Look for cardiomegaly, pulmonary oedema, or a widened mediastinum. Don't routinely delay treatment whilst waiting for a CXR. *Blood:* FBC, U&E, glucose, lipids, cardiac enzymes. *Cardiac enzymes:* (See BOX 'Troponin'.) Cardiac troponin levels (T and I) are the most sensitive and specific markers of myocardial necrosis. Different hospitals use different assays: check the required timing of troponin blood samples where you work (eg two samples 3h apart). Other cardiac enzymes (see fig 3.22) are sensitive but less specific; their role in ACS diagnosis is decreasing as troponin testing improves. *Echo:* Regional wall abnormalities.

Differential diagnosis (p94.) Stable angina, pericarditis, myocarditis, Takotsubo cardiomyopathy (p145), aortic dissection (p655), PE, oesophageal reflux/spasm, pneumothorax, musculoskeletal pain, pancreatitis.

Management See p120, pp798–801.

Mortality 50% of deaths occur within 2h of onset of symptoms. Up to 7% die before discharge. Worse prognosis if: elderly, LV failure, and ST changes.[16]

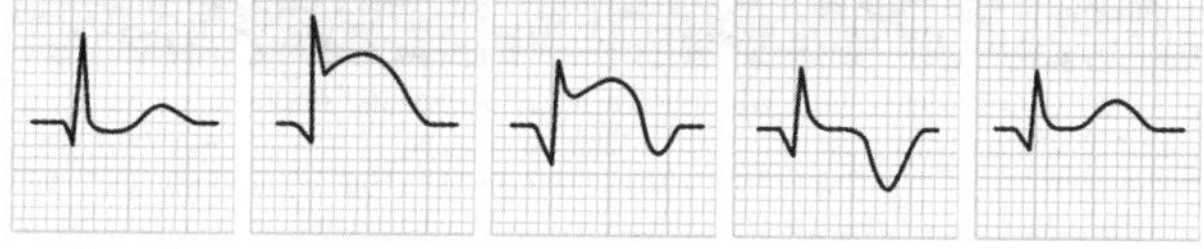

Fig 3.21 Sequential ECG changes following acute MI.

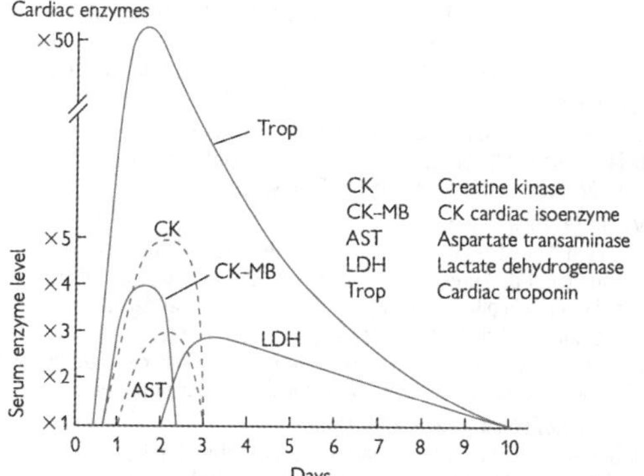

Fig 3.22 Enzyme changes following acute MI. Increasingly, high-sensitivity troponins are used alone for routine investigation of ACS.

Troponin

Troponins are proteins involved in cardiac and skeletal muscle contraction (fig 3.23). When myocardial cells are damaged, troponins are released and enter the bloodstream. The levels of troponin in the blood can therefore help with diagnosing myocardial damage. Troponins I and T are most specific to the heart.

Troponin levels are most commonly measured when ACS is suspected. In this circumstance, one would expect troponin levels to rise in the hours following the insult (fig 3.22). Troponin levels can be high with other causes of myocardial damage, for example myocarditis, pericarditis, and ventricular strain. With these conditions, the troponin levels are likely to change little hour by hour as the insults are ongoing. Discrete episodes of tachyarrhythmias may cause troponin rises similar to in ACS. Troponin levels can also be raised iatrogenically, eg following CPR, DC cardioversion, ablation therapy.

A troponin rise may have a non-cardiac aetiology. This can be indirectly related to the heart, eg a massive PE causing right ventricular strain, or have no clear cardiac connection, eg subarachnoid haemorrhage, burns, or sepsis. A common cause of consistently elevated troponin is renal failure. Hence, when measuring troponin, change in level is often more important than the level itself.

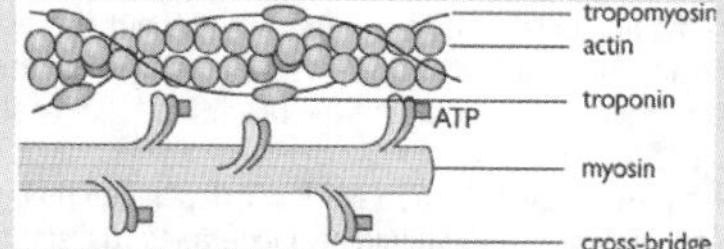

Fig 3.23 Diagram of myocardial contraction unit. The troponin complex controls when the myosin heads can bind to the actin chain, shortening the muscle fibre.

ACS management depends on whether the ACS is 'ST elevated' or not:

1 ST elevated myocardial infarction (STEMI): this category includes ACS with ST elevation on ECG (fig 3.9) but also ACS with new LBBB (fig 3.7); and posterior MIs (fig 3.24) where ST elevation may only be seen with extra leads (V_7–V_9). Urgent revascularization is essential. ▸▸p796.

2 ACS without ST elevation: serial troponins are needed to differentiate non-ST elevated MIs (NSTEMIs) (trop rise) from unstable angina (no trop rise). ▸▸p798.

After the immediate actions described on pp796-9, treatment of ACS[17] focuses on managing symptoms, secondary prevention of further cardiovascular disease, revascularization (if not already undertaken), and addressing complications.

Symptom control

Manage chest pain with PRN GTN and opiates. If this proves insufficient, consider a GTN infusion (monitor BP, omit if recent sildenafil use). If pain is deteriorating, seek senior help. Manage symptomatic heart failure, p136.

Modify risk factors

- Patients should be strongly advised and helped to stop smoking (p93).
- Identify and treat diabetes mellitus, hypertension, and hyperlipidaemia.
- Advise a diet high in oily fish, fruit, vegetables, & fibre, and low in saturated fats.
- Encourage daily exercise. Refer to a cardiac rehab programme.
- Mental health: flag to the patient's GP if depression or anxiety are present—these are independently associated with poor cardiovascular outcomes.

Optimize cardioprotective medications

- Antiplatelets: aspirin (75mg OD) and a second antiplatelet agent (eg clopidogrel) for at least 12 months to ↓vascular events (eg MI, stroke). Consider adding a PPI (eg lansoprazole) for gastric protection.
- Anticoagulate, eg with fondaparinux, until discharge.
- β-blockade reduces myocardial oxygen demand. Start low and increase slowly, monitoring pulse and BP. If contraindicated, consider verapamil or diltiazem.
- ACE-i in patients with LV dysfunction, hypertension, or diabetes unless not tolerated (consider ARB). Titrate up slowly, monitoring renal function.
- High-dose statin, eg atorvastatin 80mg.
- Do an echo to assess LV function. Eplerenone improves outcomes in MI patients with heart failure (ejection fraction <40%).

Revascularization

- STEMI patients and very high-risk NSTEMI patients (eg haemodynamically unstable) should receive immediate angiography ± PCI. NSTEMI patients who are high risk (eg GRACE score >140) should have angiography within 24h; intermediate risk (eg GRACE 109–140) within 3d; low-risk patients may be considered for non-invasive testing.
- Patients with multivessel disease may be considered for CABG instead of PCI (p123).

Manage complications See p122.

Discharge Address any questions the patient has. Discuss 'red flag' symptoms and where to seek medical advice should they arise. Ensure the management plan is communicated to the patient's GP. Book clinic and cardiac rehab appointments.

General advice

- *Driving:*[18] drivers with group 1 licences (car and motorcycle) can resume driving 1wk after successful angioplasty, or 4wk after ACS without successful angioplasty, if their ejection fraction is >40%. Group 2 licence holders must inform the DVLA of their ACS and stop driving; depending on the results of functional tests, they may be able to restart after 6wk.
- *Work:* how soon a patient can return to work will depend on their clinical progress and the nature of their work. They should be encouraged to discuss speed of return ± changes in duties (eg to lighter work if manual labour) with their employer. Some occupations cannot be restarted post-MI: eg airline pilots & air traffic controllers. Drivers of public service or heavy goods vehicles will have to undergo functional testing (eg exercise test), as mentioned previously.

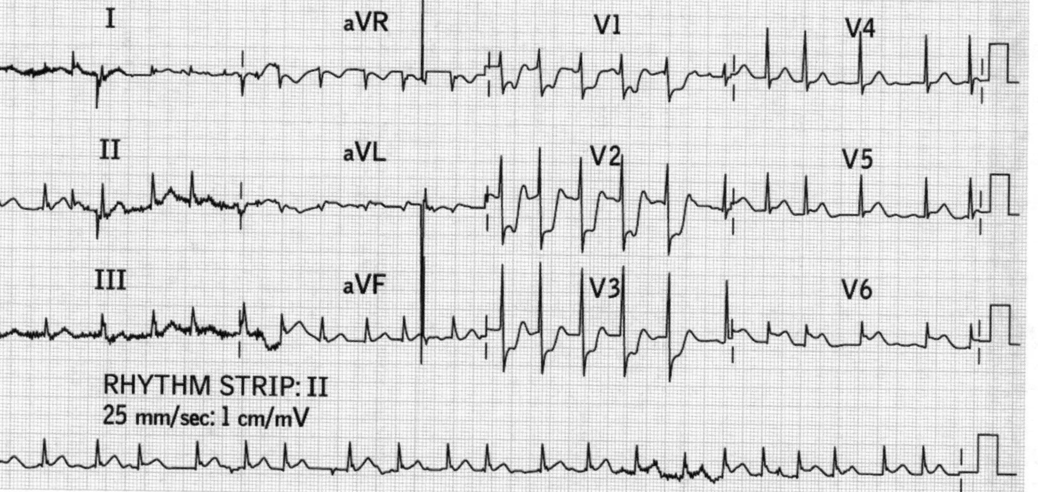

Fig 3.24 Acute postero-lateral MI. The posterior infarct is evidenced by the reciprocal changes seen in $V_{1\text{-}3}$: dominant R waves ('upside-down' pathological Q waves) and ST depression ('upside-down' ST elevation). If extra chest leads were added ($V_{7\text{-}9}$), we would see the classic ST elevation pattern, see p 98. The ST elevation in V_6 suggests lateral infarction. A blockage in the circumflex coronary artery could explain both the posterior and lateral changes.

Complications of MI

Cardiac arrest (See p894, fig A3.) **Cardiogenic shock** (p802.) **Left ventricular failure** (p136, p800, p802.)

Bradyarrhythmias *Sinus bradycardia:* See p808. Patients with inferior MIs may suffer atropine-unresponsive bradycardia due to infarction of nodal tissue. *1st-degree AV block:* Most commonly seen in inferior MI. Observe closely as approximately 40% develop higher degrees of AV block (in which case calcium channel blockers and β-blockers should be stopped). *Wenckebach phenomenon:* (Mobitz type I) Does not require pacing unless poorly tolerated. *Mobitz type II block:* Carries a high risk of developing sudden complete AV block; should be paced. *Complete AV block:* Usually resolves within a few days. Insert pacemaker (may not be necessary after inferior MI if narrow QRS, reasonably stable and pulse ≳40–50). *Bundle branch block:* MI complicated by trifascicular block or non-adjacent bifascicular disease (p132) should be paced.

Tachyarrhythmias NB: ↓K^+, hypoxia, and acidosis all predispose to arrhythmias and should be corrected. *Sinus tachycardia:* Can ↑ myocardial O_2 demand, treat causes (pain, hypoxia, sepsis, etc.) and add β-blocker if not contraindicated. *SVT:* p126. *AF or flutter:* If compromised, DC cardioversion. Otherwise, medical therapy as per p130. *Frequent PVCs* (premature ventricular complexes) and *non-sustained VT* (≥3 consecutive PVCs >100bpm and lasting <30s) are common after acute MI and are associated with increased risk of sudden death. Correct hypokalaemia and hypomagnesaemia and ensure the patient is on β-blockers, if not contraindicated.[19] *Sustained VT:* (Consecutive PVCs >100bpm and lasting >30s.) Treat with synchronized DC shock (if no pulse, treat as per advanced life support algorithm, see p894, fig A3). Use anti-arrhythmics only if VT recurrent and not controlled with shocks. Consider ablation +/or ICD. *Ventricular fibrillation:* 80% occurs within 12h. VF occuring after 48h usually indicates pump failure or cardiogenic shock. ℞: DC shock (see p894, fig A3), consider ICD.

Right ventricular failure (RVF)/infarction Presents with low cardiac output and ↑JVP. Fluid is key; avoid vasodilators (eg nitrates) and diuretics.[20] Inotropes are required in some cases.

Pericarditis Central chest pain, relieved by sitting forwards. ECG: saddle-shaped ST elevation, see fig 3.51, p155. Treatment: NSAIDs. Echo to check for effusion.

Systemic embolism May arise from LV mural thrombus. After large anterior MI, consider anticoagulation with warfarin for 3 months.

Cardiac tamponade (p802) Presents with low cardiac output, pulsus paradoxus, Kussmaul's sign,[3] muffled heart sounds. Diagnosis: echo. Treatment: pericardial aspiration (provides temporary relief, ▸▸see p773 for technique), surgery.

Mitral regurgitation May be mild (minor papillary muscle dysfunction) or severe (chordal or papillary muscle rupture secondary to ischaemia). Presentation: pulmonary oedema. Treat LVF (p800) and consider valve replacement.

Ventricular septal defect Presents with pansystolic murmur, ↑JVP, cardiac failure. Diagnosis: echo. Treatment: surgery. 50% mortality in first week.

Late malignant ventricular arrhythmias Occur 1–3wks post-MI and are the cardiologist's nightmare. Avoid hypokalaemia, the most easily avoidable cause. Consider 24h ECG monitoring prior to discharge if large MI.

Dressler's syndrome (p698) Recurrent pericarditis, pleural effusions, fever, anaemia, and ↑ESR 1–3wks post-MI. Treatment: consider NSAIDs; steroids if severe.

Left ventricular aneurysm This occurs late (4–6wks post-MI), and presents with LVF, angina, recurrent VT, or systemic embolism. ECG: persistent ST-segment elevation. Treatment: anticoagulate, consider excision.

3 **JVP rises during inspiration.** Adolf Kussmaul was a prominent 19th-century physician and the first to attempt gastroscopy. Inspired by a sword swallower he passed a rigid tube into the stomach, however light technology was limited and it was not until years later that gastroscopists could visualize the stomach.

Coronary artery bypass graft (CABG)

CABG is performed in left main stem disease; multi-vessel disease; multiple severe stenoses; patients unsuitable for angioplasty; failed angioplasty; refractory angina.

Indications for CABG—to improve survival:
- Left main stem disease.
- Triple-vessel disease involving proximal part of the left anterior descending.

Indications for CABG—to relieve symptoms:
- Angina unresponsive to drugs.
- Unstable angina (sometimes).
- If angioplasty is unsuccessful.

NB: when CABG and percutaneous coronary intervention (PCI, eg angioplasty) are both clinically valid options, NICE recommends that the availability of new stent technology should push the decision towards PCI. In practice, patients with single-vessel coronary artery disease and normal LV function usually undergo PCI, and those with triple-vessel disease and abnormal LV function more often undergo CABG.

Compared with PCI, CABG results in longer recovery time and length of inpatient stay. Recent RCTs indicate that early procedural mortality rates and 5-year survival rates are similar after PCI and CABG. Compared with PCI, CABG probably provides more complete long-term relief of angina in patients, and less repeated revascularization.

Procedure: The heart is usually stopped and blood pumped artificially by a machine outside the body (cardiac bypass). Minimally invasive thoracotomies not requiring this are well described,[21] but randomized trials are few. The patient's own saphenous vein or internal mammary artery is used as the graft. Several grafts may be placed. >50% of vein grafts close in 10yrs (low-dose aspirin helps prevent this). Internal mammary artery grafts last longer (but may cause chest-wall numbness).

On-pump or off-pump:
Seems to make little difference.[22]

After CABG: If angina persists or recurs (from poor graft run-off, distal disease, new atheroma, or graft occlusion) restart antianginal drugs, and consider angioplasty. Ensure optimal management of hypertension, diabetes, and hyperlipidaemia, and that smoking is addressed. Continue aspirin 75mg OD indefinitely; consider clopidogrel if aspirin contraindicated. Mood, sex, and intellectual problems[23] are common early. Rehabilitation helps:
- Exercise: walk→cycle→swim→jog.
- Drive at 1 month: no need to tell DVLA if non-HGV licences, p158.
- Return to work, eg at 3 months.

Arrhythmias—overview

Disturbances of cardiac rhythm (arrhythmias) are:

- common
- often benign (but may reflect underlying heart disease)
- often intermittent, causing diagnostic difficulty see BOX 'Continuous ECG monitoring'
- occasionally severe, causing cardiac compromise which may be fatal.

►►Emergency management: pp804-9.

Causes *Cardiac:* Ischaemic heart disease (IHD); structural changes, eg left atrial dilatation secondary to mitral regurgitation; cardiomyopathy; pericarditis; myocarditis; aberrant conduction pathways. *Non-cardiac:* Caffeine; smoking; alcohol; pneumonia; drugs (β_2-agonists, digoxin, L-dopa, tricyclics, doxorubicin); metabolic imbalance (K^+, Ca^{2+}, Mg^{2+}, hypoxia, hypercapnia, metabolic acidosis, thyroid disease); and phaeochromocytoma.

Presentation Palpitations, chest pain, presyncope/syncope, hypotension, or pulmonary oedema. Some arrhythmias may be asymptomatic, incidental findings, eg AF.

History Take a detailed history of palpitations (p36). Ask about precipitating factors, onset/offset, nature (fast or slow, regular or irregular), duration, associated symptoms (chest pain, dyspnoea, collapse). Review drug history. Ask about past medical history and family history of cardiac disease and sudden death. Syncope occuring during exercise is always concerning; the patient may have a condition predisposing them to sudden cardiac death (eg long QT syndrome).

Tests FBC, U&E, glucose, Ca^{2+}, Mg^{2+}, TSH, ECG: Look for signs of IHD, AF, short PR interval (WPW syndrome), long QT interval (metabolic imbalance, drugs, congenital), U waves (hypokalaemia). 24h ECG monitoring or other continuous ECG monitoring (see BOX 'Continuous ECG monitoring'). Echo to look for structural heart disease, eg mitral stenosis, HCM. Provocation tests: exercise ECG, cardiac catheterization ± electrophysiological studies may be needed.

►►*Narrow complex tachycardias:* See pp806-7, 126.

►►*Atrial fibrillation and flutter:* See pp806-7, 130.

►►*Broad complex tachycardias:* See pp804-5, 128.

►►*Bradycardia:* See p808 (causes and management of acute bradycardia) and p98 (heart block). Intermittent, self-resolving bradycardic episodes can cause significant problems (eg recurrent syncope). Continuous ECG monitoring (BOX 'Continuous ECG monitoring') will be needed to assist the diagnosis ±specialist tests (eg tilt table testing for reflex syncope). Seek out reversible causes, eg hypothyroidism or medications such as β-blockers. In some cases, no reversible cause is found and the intermittent bradycardia is sufficiently dangerous to warrant a permanent pacemaker (p132). See BOX, 'Sick sinus syndrome'.

Management Some arrhythmias can be managed *conservatively*, eg by reducing alcohol intake. Many arrhythmias respond to *medical* management with regular tablets or a 'pill in the pocket'. *Interventional* management may include pacemakers (p132), ablation (eg of accessory pathways or arrhythmogenic foci), or implantable cardioverter defibrillators (ICDs), eg in patients with ventricular arrhythmias post-MI and in those with congenital arrhythmogenic conditions (p133).

Continuous ECG monitoring

A simple 12-lead ECG only gives a snapshot of the heart's electrical activities. Many disorders, particularly the arrhythmias, come and go and so may be missed at the time of the ECG recording. If you feel you are missing a paroxysmal arrhythmia, there are many ways of recording the electrical activity over a longer period:

Telemetry: An inpatient wears ECG leads and the signals are shown on screens being watched by staff. Thus, if a dangerous arrhythmia occurs, help is immediately available. This is very resource intensive so reserved for those at high risk of dangerous arrhythmias, eg immediately post-STEMI.

Exercise ECGs: The patient exercises according to a standardized protocol (eg Bruce on a treadmill) and the BP and ECG are monitored, looking for ischaemic changes, arrhythmias, and features suggestive of arrhythmia risk, such as delta waves.

Holter monitors: The patient wears an ECG monitor which records their rhythm for 24h–7d whilst they go about their normal life, this is later analysed. These can also be used to pick up ST changes suggestive of ischaemia.

Loop recorders: These record only when activated by the patient—they cleverly save a small amount of ECG data before the event—useful if the arrhythmia causes loss of consciousness: the patient can press the button when they wake up. Loop recorders may be implanted just under the skin (eg Reveal® or the newer, injectable LINQ device), and are especially useful in patients with infrequent episodes as they can continually monitor for months or years awaiting an event (Fig 3.25).

Pacemakers and ICDs: These record details of cardiac electrical activity and device activity. This information can be useful for establishing an arrhythmic origin for symptoms.

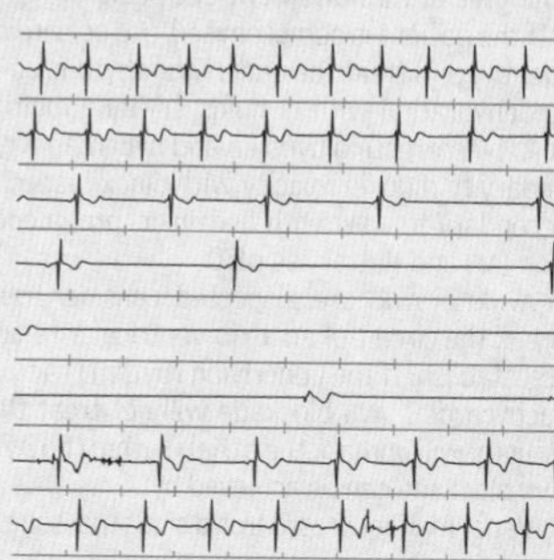

Fig 3.25 This is a recording from a loop recorder, each line follows on from the one above. This tracing was recorded at the time of a syncopal episode, it shows cardiac slowing then a 15sec pause: quite long enough to cause syncope! But not long enough to arrange a standard ECG, even if the patient were in hospital.

Reproduced from Camm *et al.*, *ESC Textbook of Cardiovascular Medicine*, 2009, with permission from Oxford University Press.

Sick sinus syndrome

Sick sinus syndrome is usually caused by sinus node fibrosis, typically in elderly patients. The sinus node becomes dysfunctional, in some cases slowing to the point of sinus bradycardia or sinus pauses, in others generating tachyarrhythmias such as atrial fibrillation and atrial tachycardia.

Symptoms: Syncope and pre-syncope, light-headedness, palpitations, breathlessness.

Management:

- Thromboembolism prophylaxis if episodes of AF are detected.
- Permanent pacemakers for patients with symptomatic bradycardia or sinus pauses.

Some patients develop a '*tachy brady syndrome*', suffering from alternating tachycardic and bradycardic rhythms. This can prove difficult to treat medically as treating one circumstance (eg tachycardia) increases the risk from the other. Pacing for bradycardic episodes in combination with rate-slowing medications for tachycardic episodes may be required if the patient is symptomatic or unstable.

Narrow complex tachycardia

Definition ECG shows rate of >100bpm and QRS complex duration of <120ms. Narrow QRS complexes occur when the ventricles are depolarized via the normal conduction pathways (fig 3.26).

Differential diagnosis

Regular narrow complex tachycardias: See fig 3.27.

Irregular narrow complex tachycardias:

- Normal variant: sinus arrhythmia (rate changes with inspiration/expiration); sinus rhythm with frequent ectopic beats.
- Atrial fibrillation (AF): p131, fig 3.35.
- Atrial flutter with variable block: eg P-P-P-QRS-P-P-QRS (3:1 block then 2:1 block). The atrial rhythm is regular but the ventricular rhythm (hence pulse) is irregular.
- Multifocal atrial tachycardia: like focal atrial tachycardia but there are multiple groups of atrial cells taking it in turns to initiate a cardiac cycle. P-wave morphology and P-P intervals vary. Usually associated with COPD.

Principles of management See p807.

►►If the patient is compromised, use DC cardioversion (p770).

- Identify and treat the underlying rhythm: eg treating sinus tachycardia secondary to dehydration with IV fluids; treating multifocal sinus tachycardia secondary to COPD by correcting hypoxia and hypercapnia; treating focal atrial tachycardia secondary to digoxin toxicity with digoxin-specific antibody fragments; treating AVRT secondary to WPW with flecainide, propafenone, or amiodarone; for atrial fibrillation (AF) and flutter see p130.
- If AVNRT or AVRT are suspected, consider transiently blocking the AVN. This should break the circuit of an atrio-ventricular re-entry rhythm, allowing sinus rhythm to re-establish. If the underlying rhythm is actually atrial in origin (eg flutter or atrial tachycardia), AVN blockade will not treat the rhythm but the paused ventricular activity will unmask the atrial rhythm (fig 3.28), aiding diagnosis and management. AVN blockade can be achieved by:
  1. Vagal manoeuvres: carotid sinus massage, Valsalva manoeuvre (eg blowing into a syringe).
  2. IV adenosine: see p806.
- In some cases, narrow complex tachyarrhythmias cause symptomatic episodes of sufficient severity and frequency to warrant more invasive treatment, eg ablation therapy for accessory pathways.

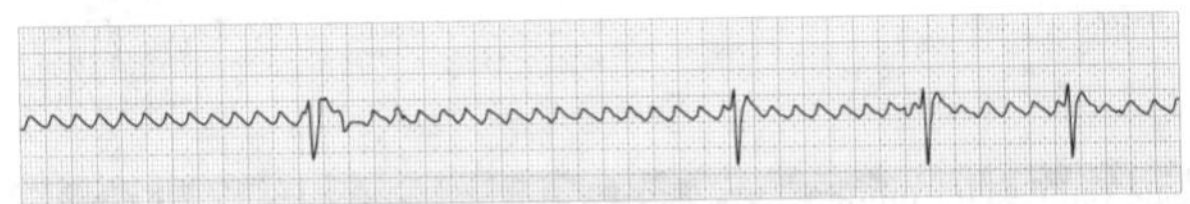

Fig 3.28 This patient was given adenosine for tachycardia thought to be due to AVRT or AVNRT. The adenosine has slowed the ventricular rate, revealing flutter waves (sawtooth appearance), disproving an AVRT/AVNRT diagnosis.

Image courtesy of Dr Ed Burns, www.lifeinthefastlane.com.

Holiday heart syndrome

Binge drinking in a person ***without*** any clinical evidence of heart disease may result in acute cardiac rhythm and/or conduction disturbances, which is called holiday heart syndrome (note that recreational use of marijuana may have similar effects). The most common rhythm disorders are supraventricular tachyarrhythmia and AF (consider this diagnosis in patients without structural heart disease who present with new-onset AF).

The prognosis is excellent, especially in young patients without structural heart disease. As holiday heart syndrome resolves rapidly by abstinence from alcohol use, advise all patients against the excessive use of alcohol in future.

Normal conduction

Normal conduction: initiated by the sinoatrial node (SAN), electrical activity spreads around the atria. The atrioventricular node (AVN) receives this activity, pauses, then passes it on, down the bundle of His which splits into left and right bundle branches. These cause depolarization of the ventricular myocardium from bottom (apex) to top (outflow tracts).

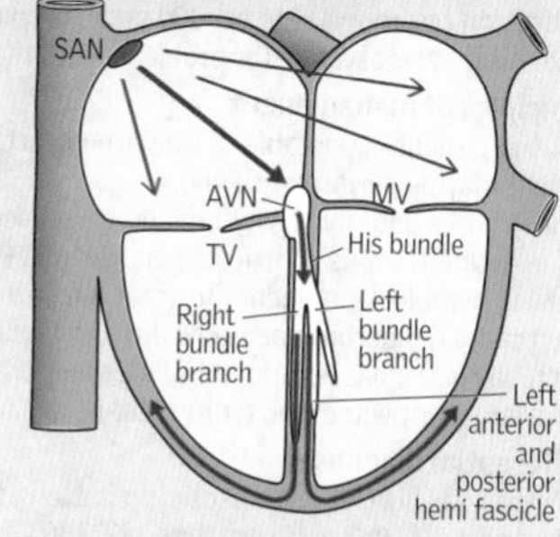

Fig 3.26 Normal conduction.

Regular rhythm tachycardia

See fig 3.27.

A. Sinus tachycardia: Conduction occurs as per fig 3.26 but impulses are initiated at a high frequency. Causes include infection, pain, exercise, anxiety, dehydration, bleed, systemic vasodilation (eg in sepsis), drugs (caffeine, nicotine, salbutamol), anaemia, fever, PE, hyperthyroidism, pregnancy, CO_2 retention, autonomic neuropathy (eg inappropriate sinus tachycardia).

B. Focal atrial tachycardia: A group of atrial cells act as a pacemaker, out-pacing the SAN. P-wave morphology (shape) is different to sinus.

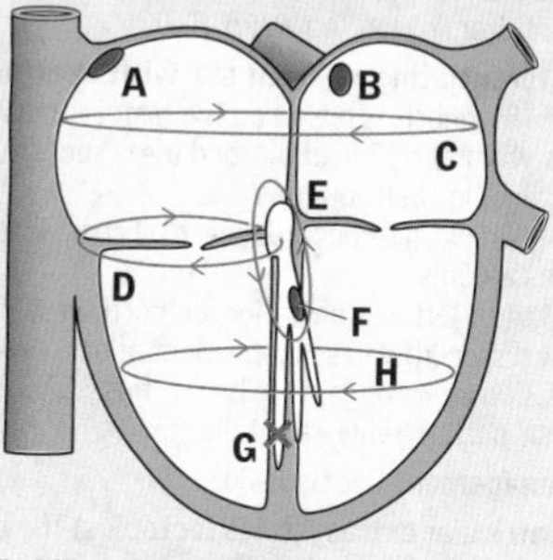

Fig 3.27 Regular tachycardias.

C. Atrial flutter: Electrical activity circles the atria 300 times per minute, giving a 'sawtooth' baseline, see fig 3.35. The AVN passes some of these impulses on, resulting in ventricular rates that are factors of 300 (150, 100, 75).

D. Atrioventricular re-entry tachycardia: (AVRT) An accessory pathway (eg in Wolff-Parkinson-White (WPW), p133) allows electrical activity from the ventricles to pass to the resting atrial myocytes, creating a circuit: atria-AVN-ventricles-accessory pathway-atria. This direction is called 'orthodromic' conduction and results in narrow QRS complexes as ventricular depolarization is triggered via the bundles of His. Conduction in the other direction is called 'antidromic' and results in broad QRS complexes.

E. Atrioventricular nodal re-entry tachycardia: (AVNRT) Circuits form within the AVN, causing narrow complex tachycardias. This is very common.

F. Junctional tachycardia: Cells in the AVN become the pacemaker, giving narrow QRS complexes as impulses reach the ventricles through the normal routes; P waves may be inverted and late.

G. Bundle branch block: Any of the above conditions can result in broad complex tachycardias if there is bundle branch block (see p100).

H. Ventricular tachycardia: (VT) This can result from circuits, similar to atrial flutter, or from focuses of rapidly-firing cells. The QRS is broad. When a circuit is in action and its plane rotates, the ECG shows broad complex tachycardia with regularly increasing and decreasing amplitudes; this is called *torsades de pointes*.

Broad complex tachycardia

Definition ECG shows rate of >100 and QRS complexes >120ms. If no clear QRS complexes, it is VF or asystole (or problems with the ECG machine or stickers).

Principles of management

▸▸If the patient is unstable or you are uncertain of what to do, get help fast—the patient may be periarrest (p804).

- Identify the underlying rhythm and treat accordingly.
- If in doubt, treat as ventricular tachycardia (VT)—the commonest cause.
- Giving AVN blocking agents to treat SVT with aberrancy when the patient is in VT can cause dangerous haemodynamic instability. Treating for VT when the patient is actually in SVT has less potential for deterioration.
- If WPW is suspected, avoid drugs that slow AV conduction—see p114.

Differential diagnosis

- Ventricular fibrillation—chaotic, no pattern, fig 3.29.
- Ventricular tachycardia (VT), figs 3.12, 3.30.
- *Torsade de pointes (polymorphic* VT*)*—VT with varying axis (see fig 3.31), may look like VF. ↑QT interval is a predisposing factor.
- Any cause of narrow complex tachycardias (p126) when in combination with bundle branch block or metabolic causes of broad QRS.
- Antidromic AVRT (eg WPW), p127.

Differentiating VT from SVT with aberrancy This may be difficult; seek expert help. Diagnosis is based on the history (IHD increases the likelihood of a ventricular arrhythmia), a 12-lead ECG, and the response (or lack thereof) to certain medications. ECG findings in favour of VT:

- +ve or −ve QRS concordance in all chest leads (ie all +ve (R) or all −ve (QS)).
- QRS >160ms.
- Marked left axis deviation, or 'northwest axis' (QRS positive in aVR).
- AV dissociation (Ps independent of QRSs) or 2:1 or 3:1 Mobitz II heart block.
- Fusion beats or capture beats (figs 3.32, 3.33).
- RSR' pattern where R is taller than R'. (R' taller than R suggests RBBB.)

Management See page 805.

Ventricular extrasystoles (ectopics) These are common and can be symptomatic—patients describe palpitations, a thumping sensation, or their heart 'missing a beat'. The pulse may feel irregular if there are frequent ectopics. On ECG, ventricular ectopics are broad QRS complexes; they may be single or occur in patterns:

- *Bigeminy*—ectopic every other beat, see fig 3.34. ECG machines may disregard the second QRS and so calculate the rate to be half the true value.
- *Trigeminy*—every third beat is an ectopic.
- *Couplet*—two ectopics together.
- *Triplet*—three ectopics together.

Occasional ventricular ectopics[24] in otherwise healthy people are extremely common and rarely significant. Frequent ectopics (>60/hour), particularly couplets and triplets, should prompt testing for underlying cardiac conditions. Post-MI, ventricular ectopics are associated with increased risk of dangerous arrhythmias. Pay attention to whether the ectopics all 'look' the same on the ECG suggesting a single focus (monomorphic) or may come from multiple foci (polymorphic). Causes and management can be different.

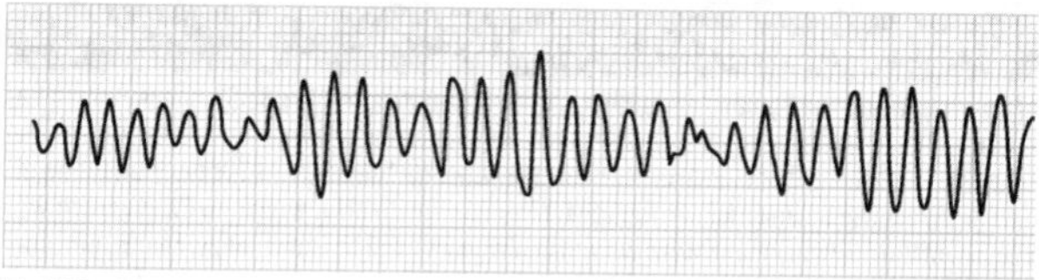

Fig 3.29 VF (p894).

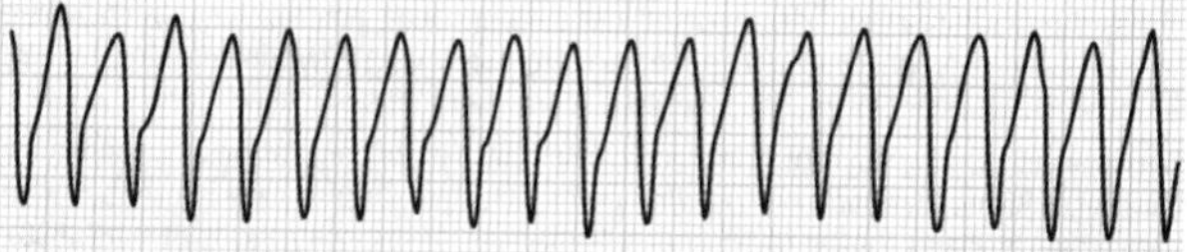

Fig 3.30 VT with a rate of 235/min.

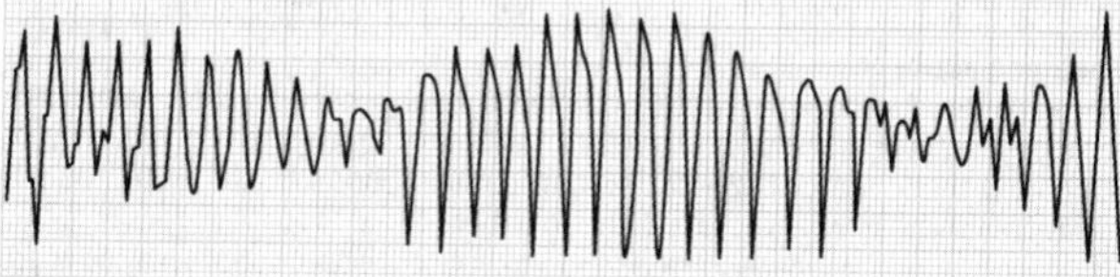

Fig 3.31 *Torsade de pointes* tachycardia.

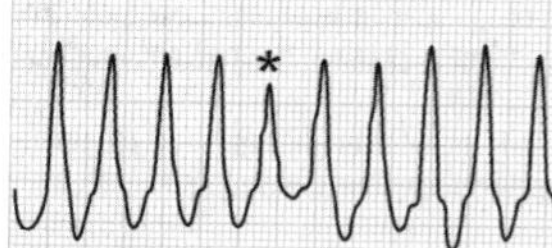

Fig 3.32 A fusion beat (*)—a 'normal beat' fuses with a VT complex creating an unusual complex.

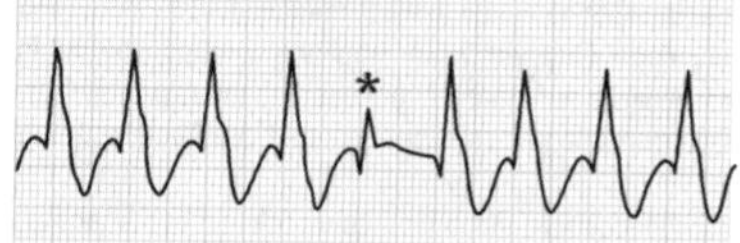

Fig 3.33 A capture beat (*)—a normal QRS amongst runs of VT. This would not be expected if the QRS breadth were down to bundle branch block or metabolic causes.

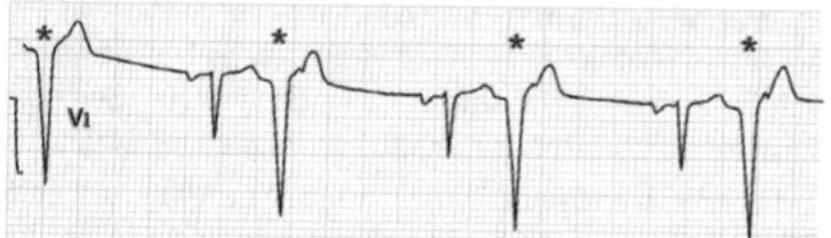

Fig 3.34 Bigeminy—a normal QRS is followed by a ventricular ectopic beat * then a compensatory pause, this pattern then repeats. The ectopic beats have the same morphology as each other so probably all share an origin.

Atrial fibrillation (AF) and flutter

AF[25] is a chaotic, irregular atrial rhythm at 300-600bpm (fig 3.35); the AV node responds intermittently, hence an irregular ventricular rhythm. Cardiac output drops by 10-20% as the ventricles aren't primed reliably by the atria. AF is common in the elderly (≤9%). The main risk is embolic stroke. Warfarin reduces this to 1%/yr from 4%. So, *do an ECG on everyone with an irregular pulse* (±24h ECG if dizzy, faints, palpitations, etc.). If AF started more than 48h ago, intracardiac clots may have formed, necessitating anticoagulation prior to cardioversion. see BOX 'Anticoagulation and AF'.

Causes Heart failure; hypertension; IHD (seen in 22% MI patients);[26] PE; mitral valve disease; pneumonia; hyperthyroidism; caffeine; alcohol; post-op; ↓K^+; ↓Mg^{2+}. *Rare causes:* Cardiomyopathy; constrictive pericarditis; sick sinus syndrome; lung cancer; endocarditis; haemochromatosis; sarcoid. 'Lone' AF means no cause found.

Symptoms May be asymptomatic or cause chest pain, palpitations, dyspnoea, or faintness. **Signs** *Irregularly irregular pulse*, the apical pulse rate is greater than the radial rate, and the 1st heart sound is of variable intensity; signs of LVF (p800). ►Examine the whole patient: AF is *often* associated with non-cardiac disease.

Tests *ECG* shows absent P waves, irregular QRS complexes, fig 3.35. *Blood tests:* U&E, cardiac enzymes, thyroid function tests. Echo to look for left atrial enlargement, mitral valve disease, poor LV function, and other structural abnormalities.

Managing acute AF

- If the patient has adverse signs (shock, myocardial ischaemia (chest pain or ECG changes), syncope, heart failure): ►►ABCDE, get senior input ►►DC cardioversion (synchronized shock, start at 120-150J) ± amiodarone if unsuccessful (p807); do not delay treatment in order to start anticoagulation.
- If the patient is stable & AF started <48h ago: rate or rhythm control may be tried. For rhythm control, DC cardiovert or give flecainide (CI: structural heart disease, IHD) or amiodarone. Start heparin in case cardioversion is delayed (see BOX 'Anticoagulation and AF').
- If the patient is stable & AF started >48h ago or unclear time of onset: rate control (eg with bisoprolol or diltiazem). If rhythm control is chosen, the patient must be anticoagulated for >3wks first.
- Correct electrolyte imbalances (K^+, Mg^{2+}, Ca^{2+}); ℞ associated illnesses (eg MI, pneumonia); and consider anticoagulation (see BOX 'Anticoagulation and AF').

Managing chronic AF

The main goals are rate control and anticoagulation. Rate control is at least as good as rhythm control,[27] but rhythm control may be appropriate if •symptomatic or CCF •younger •presenting for 1st time with lone AF •AF from a corrected precipitant (eg ↑↓U&E). *Anticoagulation:* See BOX 'Anticoagulation and AF'.

Rate control: β-blocker or rate-limiting Ca^{2+} blocker are 1st choice. If this fails, add digoxin (p115), then consider amiodarone. Digoxin as monotherapy in chronic AF is only acceptable in sedentary patients. ►Do not give β-blockers with verapamil. Aim for heart rate <90bpm at rest and 200 minus age (yrs) bpm on exertion. Avoid getting fixated on a target heart rate.

Rhythm control: Elective DC cardioversion: do echo first to check for intracardiac thrombi. If there is ↑risk of cardioversion failure (past failure, or past recurrence) give amiodarone for 4wks before the procedure and 12 months after. *Elective pharmacological cardioversion:* flecainide is 1st choice (CI if structural heart disease, eg scar tissue from MI: use IV amiodarone instead). In refractory cases, AVN ablation with pacing, pulmonary vein ablation, or the maze procedure may be considered.[28]

Paroxysmal AF: 'Pill in the pocket' (eg sotalol or flecainide PRN) may be tried if: infrequent AF, BP >100mmHg systolic, no past LV dysfunction. Anticoagulate (See BOX 'Anticoagulation and AF'). Consider ablation if symptomatic or frequent episodes.

Atrial flutter See pp130-1, fig 3.35. *Treatment:* Similar to AF regarding rate and rhythm control and the need for anticoagulation.[29] DC cardioversion is preferred to pharmacological cardioversion; start with 70-120J. IV amiodarone may be needed if rate control is proving difficult. Recurrence rates are high so radiofrequency ablation is often recommended for long-term management.

Anticoagulation and AF

Acute AF: Use heparin until a full risk assessment for emboli (see below) is made—eg AF started <48h ago and elective cardioversion is being planned. If >48h, ensure ≥3wks of therapeutic anticoagulation before elective cardioversion; NB trans-oesophageal-guided cardioversion is an option if urgent cardioversion is required. Use a DOAC (eg apixaban) or warfarin (target INR 2-3) if high risk of emboli (past ischaemic stroke, TIA, or emboli; ≥75yrs with ↑BP, DM; coronary or peripheral arterial disease; evidence of valve disease or ↓LV function/CCF—only do echo if unsure).[30] Use *no anticoagulation* if *stable* sinus rhythm has been restored, no risk factors for emboli, and AF recurrence unlikely (ie no failed cardioversions, no structural heart disease, no previous recurrences, no sustained AF for >1yr).

Chronic AF: Chronic AF may be paroxysmal (terminates in <7d but may recur), persistent (lasts >7d), or permanent (long-term, continuous AF, sinus rhythm not achievable despite treatment). In all cases, the need for anticoagulation should be assessed using the CHA_2DS_2-VASc score to assess embolic stroke risk (consider anticoagulation if score ♂ >0, ♀ >1), and balancing this against the risks of anticoagulation to the patient, assessed with the HAS-BLED score. Long-term anticoagulation should be with a DOAC (see p350) or warfarin.

CHA_2DS_2-VASc—**C**ongestive cardiac failure (1 point), **H**ypertension (1), **A**ge 65–74y (1), **A**ge >74y (2), **D**iabetes (1), previous **S**troke/TIA/thromboembolism (2), **Va**scular disease (1), **S**ex **C**ategory (1 if female). A score of 2 = an annual stroke risk of 2.2%. Online calculators can be helpful, eg www.mdcalc.com.

HAS-BLED—1 point for each of: • labile INR • age >65 • use of medications that can predispose to bleeding (eg NSAIDs, anti-platelets) • alcohol abuse • uncontrolled hypertension • history of, or predisposition to, major bleeding • renal disease • liver disease • stroke history.

Pre-excited AF

In pre-excited AF, accessory pathways capable of conducting at rapid rates (eg sometimes in WPW syndrome) pass erratic electrical activity from the atria to the ventricles, unfiltered by the AVN. ECGs will show irregular, broad QRS complexes at >200bpm. Ventricles cannot sustain this rate for long; the patient is at high risk of VT and VF.

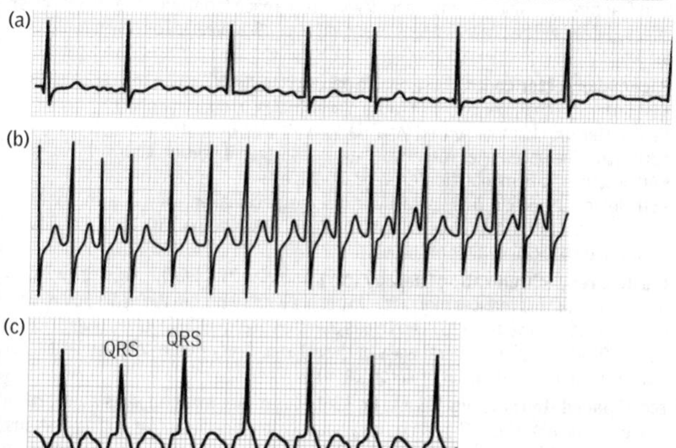

Fig 3.35 (a) AF: note the irregular spacing of QRS complexes and lack of P waves. (b) AF with a rapid ventricular response (sometimes referred to as 'fast AF'). No pattern to QRS complex spacing, and rate >100bpm. (c) Atrial flutter with 2:1 block (2 P waves for every 1 QRS complex). The P waves have the classic 'sawtooth' appearance. Alternate P waves are merged with the QRS complex.

Pacemakers

In normal circumstances the SAN plays the role of pacemaker. On occasion, other areas of myocardium will set the pace (see earlier in chapter). If the heart is not pacing itself fast enough, artificial pacing may be required. Options include 'percussion pacing'—fist strikes to the precordium, used only in periarrest situations; transcutaneous pacing—electrical stimulation via defibrillator pads (p770); temporary transvenous pacing (p776); and a subcutaneously implanted permanent pacemaker.

Indications for temporary cardiac pacing include

- Symptomatic bradycardia, unresponsive to atropine.
- After acute *anterior* MI, prophylactic pacing is required in:
  - complete AV block
  - Mobitz type I AV block (Wenckebach)
  - Mobitz type II AV block
  - non-adjacent bifascicular, or trifascicular block (p100).
- After *inferior* MI, pacing may not be needed in complete AV block if reasonably stable, rate is >40–50, and QRS complexes are narrow.
- Suppression of drug-resistant tachyarrhythmias by overdrive pacing, eg SVT, VT.
- Special situations: during general anaesthesia; during cardiac surgery; during electrophysiological studies; drug overdose (eg digoxin, β-blockers, verapamil).

►See p776 for further details and insertion technique.

Indications for a permanent pacemaker (PPM) include

- Complete AV block (Stokes-Adams attacks, asymptomatic, congenital).
- Mobitz type II AV block (p99).
- Persistent AV block after anterior MI.
- Symptomatic bradycardias (eg sick sinus syndrome, p125).
- Heart failure (cardiac resynchronization therapy).
- Drug-resistant tachyarrhythmias.

Pre-operative assessment Bloods (FBC, clotting screen, renal function), IV cannula, consent, antibiotics as per local protocol.

Post-operative management Prior to discharge, check wound for bleeding or haematoma; check lead positions and for pneumothorax on CXR; check pacemaker function. During 1st week, inspect for wound haematoma or dehiscence. Other problems: lead fracture or dislodgement; pacemaker interference (eg from patient's muscles); infected device. The battery needs changing every 5–10 years. For driving rules see p158.

Pacemaker letter codes These enable pacemaker identification (min is 3 letters):

- 1st letter the chamber paced (A=atria, V=ventricles, D=dual chamber).
- 2nd letter the chamber sensed (A=atria, V=ventricles, D=dual chamber, O=none).
- 3rd letter the pacemaker response (T=triggered, I=inhibited, D=dual).
- 4th letter (R=rate modulation, P=programmable, M=multiprogrammable).
- 5th letter (P means that in tachycardia the pacemaker will pace the patient. S means that in tachycardia the pacemaker shocks the patient. D=dual ability to pace and shock. O=neither of these).

Cardiac resynchronization therapy (CRT) Improves the synchronization of cardiac contraction and reduces mortality[31] in people with symptomatic heart failure who have an ejection fraction <35% and a QRS duration >120ms.[32] It involves biventricular pacing (both septal and lateral walls of the LV) and, if required, also an atrial lead. It may be combined with a defibrillator (CRT-D).

ECG of paced rhythms (fig 3.13 and fig 3.36). Pacemaker input appears as a vertical 'spike' on the ECG. This spike can be very small with modern bipolar pacing systems. Ventricular pacing usually has a broad QRS morphology (similar to LBBB). Systems are usually programmed 'on demand' so will only pace when necessary. Modern systems are generally very reliable but pacing spikes with no capture afterwards suggests a problem. Programming of devices is complicated so seek help early if concerned. Many pacemakers store intracardiac electrograms which can be accessed to correlate rhythm with any symptoms.

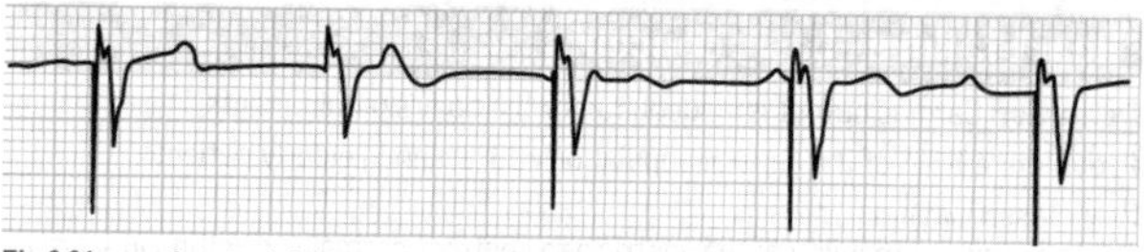

Fig 3.36 ECG of a paced rhythm.

Some pacemaker terms

Fusion beat: Union of native depolarization and pacemaker impulse.

Pseudofusion beat: The pacemaker impulse occurs just after cardiac depolarization, so it is ineffective, but it distorts the QRS morphology.

Pseudopseudofusion beat: If a DVI pacemaker gives an atrial spike within a native QRS complex, the atrial output is non-contributory.

Pacemaker syndrome: In single-chamber pacing, retrograde conduction to the atria, which then contract during ventricular systole. This leads to retrograde flow in pulmonary veins, and ↓cardiac output, dyspnoea, palpitations, malaise, and even syncope.

Pacemaker-mediated tachycardia: Retrograde conduction to the atrium is sensed by the pacemaker and ventricular pacing delivered in response. This again causes retrograde atrial conduction causing a repetitive sensing/pacing loop. This can be fixed by changing pacing programming parameters.

Congenital arrhythmogenic cardiac conditions

As well as the many acquired conditions that can predispose to arrhythmias (p125), there are a number of congenital conditions. These may be clinically silent until a fatal attack and are likely to be responsible for most cases of sudden adult death syndrome (SADS). They include:

WPW syndrome (Wolff-Parkinson-White; fig 3.37.) Caused by congenital accessory conduction pathway between atria and ventricles. Resting ECG shows short PR interval, wide QRS complex (due to slurred upstroke or 'delta wave') and ST-T changes. Two types: WPW type A (+ve δ wave in V_1), WPW type B (−ve δ wave in V_1). Tachycardia can be due to an AVRT or pre-excited AF/atrial flutter (p130). Management may include ablation of the accessory pathway.

LQTS (Long QT syndromes.) These are channelopathies that result in prolonged repolarization phases, predisposing the patient to ventricular arrhythmias; classically *torsades de pointes*. ►p804. Conditions associated with LQTS include Jervell and Lange-Nielsen syndrome (p702) and Romano-Ward syndrome (p710).

ARVC (Arrhythmogenic right ventricular cardiomyopathy.) RV myocardium is replaced with fibro-fatty material. Symptoms: palpitations and syncope during exercise. ECG changes include epsilon wave; T inversion and broad QRS in V_1–V_3.

Brugada Sodium channelopathy. Diagnosis: classic coved ST elevation in V_1–V_3 *plus* suggestive clinical history. ECG changes and arrhythmias can be precipitated by fever, medications (www.brugadadrugs.org), electrolyte imbalances, and ischaemia.

Many of these patients can be treated medically or conservatively but those at high risk may require an implantable cardiac defibrillator (ICD). Screening family members is important for picking up undiagnosed cases.

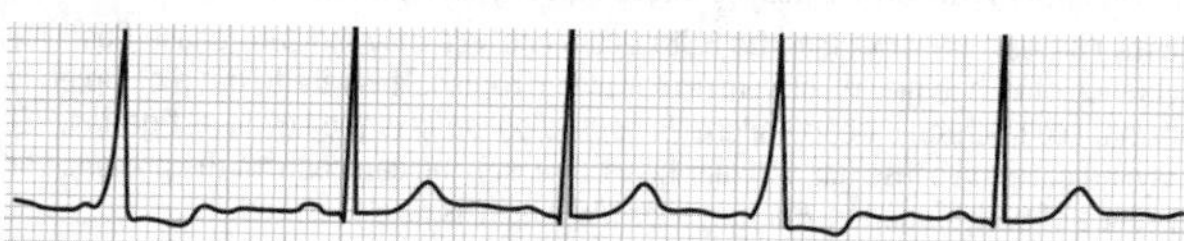

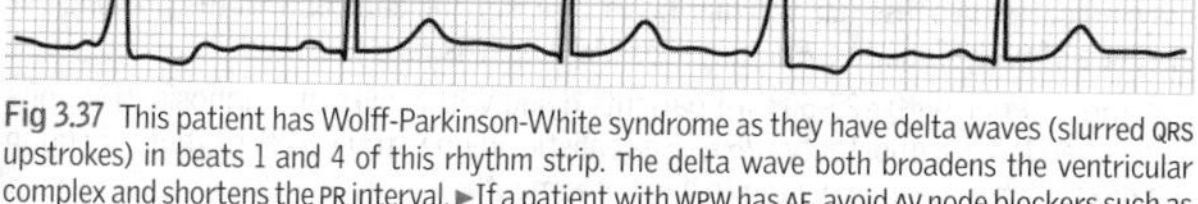

Fig 3.37 This patient has Wolff-Parkinson-White syndrome as they have delta waves (slurred QRS upstrokes) in beats 1 and 4 of this rhythm strip. The delta wave both broadens the ventricular complex and shortens the PR interval. ►If a patient with WPW has AF, avoid AV node blockers such as diltiazem, verapamil, and digoxin—but flecainide may be used.

Heart failure—basic concepts

Definition Cardiac output is inadequate for the body's requirements.[33]

Prevalence 1-3% of the general population; ~10% among elderly patients.[34]

Key classifications

Systolic failure: Inability of the ventricle to contract normally, resulting in ↓cardiac output. Ejection fraction (EF) is <40%. Causes: IHD, MI, cardiomyopathy.

Diastolic failure: Inability of the ventricle to relax and fill normally, causing ↑filling pressures. Typically EF is >50%, this is termed *HFpEF (heart failure with preserved EF).* Causes: ventricular hypertrophy, constrictive pericarditis, tamponade, restrictive cardiomyopathy, obesity. NB: systolic and diastolic failure pathophysiology often coexists.

Left ventricular failure (LVF): Symptoms: dyspnoea, poor exercise tolerance, fatigue, orthopnoea, paroxysmal nocturnal dyspnoea (PND), nocturnal cough (±pink frothy sputum), wheeze (cardiac 'asthma'), nocturia, cold peripheries, weight loss.

Right ventricular failure (RVF): Causes: LVF, pulmonary stenosis, lung disease (cor pulmonale, see p194). Symptoms: peripheral oedema (up to thighs, sacrum, abdominal wall), ascites, nausea, anorexia, facial engorgement, epistaxis.

LVF and RVF may occur independently, or together as *congestive cardiac failure* (CCF).

Acute heart failure: Often used exclusively to mean new-onset acute or decompensation of chronic heart failure characterized by pulmonary and/or peripheral oedema with or without signs of peripheral hypoperfusion. *Chronic heart failure:* Develops or progresses slowly. Venous congestion is common but arterial pressure is well maintained until very late.

Low-output heart failure: Cardiac output is ↓ and fails to ↑ normally with exertion. *Causes:*

- *Excessive preload:* eg mitral regurgitation or fluid overload (eg renal failure or too rapid IV infusions, particularly in the elderly and those with established HF).
- *Pump failure:* systolic and/or diastolic HF (see above), ↓heart rate (eg β-blockers, heart block, post MI), negatively inotropic drugs (eg most antiarrhythmic agents).
- *Chronic excessive afterload:* eg aortic stenosis, hypertension.

Excessive preload can cause ventricular dilatation, this exacerbates pump failure. *Excessive afterload* prompts ventricular muscle thickening (ventricular hypertrophy), resulting in stiff walls and diastolic dysfunction.

High-output heart failure: This is rare. Here, output is normal or increased in the face of ↑↑needs. Failure occurs when cardiac output fails to meet these needs. It will occur with a normal heart, but even earlier if there is heart disease. *Causes:* anaemia, pregnancy, hyperthyroidism, Paget's disease, arteriovenous malformation, beriberi. *Consequences:* initially features of RVF; later LVF becomes evident.

Diagnosis Requires symptoms of failure (see above) and objective evidence of cardiac dysfunction at rest. For CCF, use the *Framingham* criteria.[35]

Signs As described previously plus cyanosis, ↓BP, narrow pulse pressure, pulsus alternans, displaced apex (LV dilatation), RV heave (pulmonary hypertension), signs of valve diseases. Severity can be graded using the New York classification (see BOX).

Investigations According to NICE,[33] if ECG and B-type natriuretic peptide (BNP; p137) are normal, heart failure is unlikely, and an alternative diagnosis should be considered; if either is abnormal, then echocardiography (p110) is required.

Tests FBC; U&E; BNP; CXR (see fig 3.38); ECG; echo. *ECG* may indicate cause (look for evidence of ischaemia, MI, or ventricular hypertrophy). It is rare to get a completely normal ECG in chronic heart failure. *Echocardiography* is the key investigation.[36] It may indicate the cause (MI, valvular heart disease) and can confirm the presence or absence of LV dysfunction. *Endomyocardial biopsy* is rarely needed.

Prognosis Poor with ~25–50% of patients dying within 5yrs of diagnosis. If admission is needed, 5yr mortality ≈75%. Be realistic: in one study, 54% of those dying in the next 72h had been expected to live for >6months.[37]

New York classification of heart failure

I Heart disease present, but no undue dyspnoea from ordinary activity.
II Comfortable at rest; dyspnoea during ordinary activities.
III Less than ordinary activity causes dyspnoea, which is limiting.
IV Dyspnoea present at rest; all activity causes discomfort.

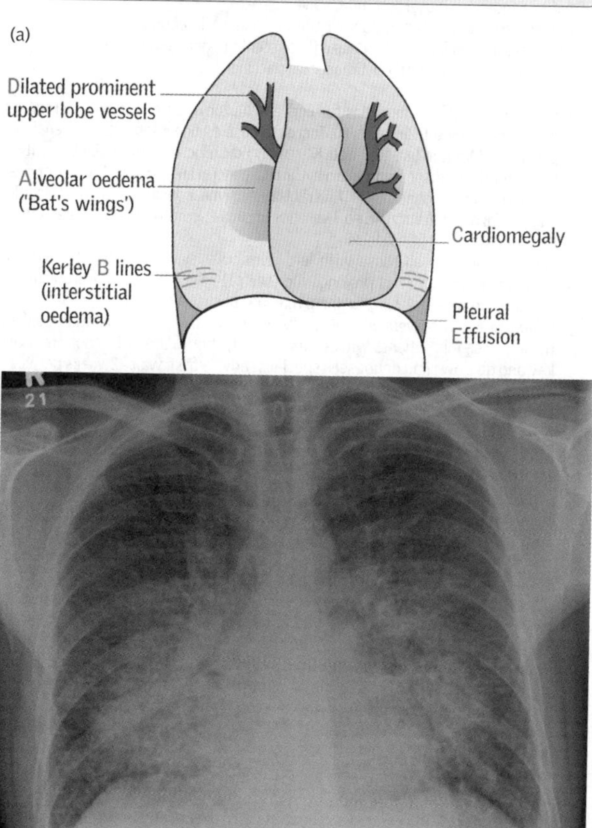

Fig 3.38 (a) The CXR in left ventricular failure. These features can be remembered as A B C D E. **A**lveolar oedema, classically this is perihilar 'bat's wing' shadowing. Kerley **B** lines—now known as septal lines. These are variously attributed to interstitial oedema and engorged peripheral lymphatics. **C**ardiomegaly—cardiothoracic ratio >50% on a PA film. **D**ilated prominent upper lobe veins (upper lobe diversion). Pleural **E**ffusions. Other features include peribronchial cuffing (thickened bronchial walls) and fluid in the fissures. (b) 'Bat's wing', peri-hilar pulmonary oedema indicating heart failure and fluid overload.

Heart failure—management

Acute heart failure ►►This is a medical emergency (p800).

Chronic heart failure ►Stop smoking. Stop drinking alcohol. Eat less salt. Optimize weight & nutrition.[33]

- Treat the cause (eg if dysrhythmias; valve disease).
- Treat exacerbating factors (anaemia, thyroid disease, infection, ↑BP).
- Avoid exacerbating factors, eg NSAIDs (fluid retention) and verapamil (−ve inotrope).
- Annual 'flu vaccine, one-off pneumococcal vaccine.
- Drugs:

 1 *Diuretics:* Give loop diuretics to relieve symptoms, eg furosemide 40mg/24h PO or bumetanide 1–2mg/24h PO. Increase dose as necessary. SE: K^+↓, renal impairment. Monitor U&E and add K^+-sparing diuretic (eg spironolactone) if K^+ <3.2mmol/L, predisposition to arrhythmias, concurrent digoxin therapy, or pre-existing K^+-losing conditions. If refractory oedema, consider adding a thiazide, eg metolazone 5–20mg/24h PO. Diuretics improve symptoms but studies showing mortality benefit are lacking.

 2 *ACE-i:* Consider in all those with left ventricular systolic dysfunction (LVSD); improves symptoms and prolongs life (see p114–5). If cough is a problem, an *angiotensin receptor blocker* (ARB) may be substituted. SE: ↑K^+.

 3 *β-blockers:* (eg carvedilol) ↓mortality in heart failure—benefit additional to those of ACE-i in patients with systolic dysfunction.[38] Use with caution: 'start low and go slow'; if in doubt seek specialist advice first; wait ≥2weeks between each dose increment. β-blocker therapy in patients hospitalized with decompensated heart failure is associated with lower post-discharge mortality risk and improved treatment rates.[39]

 4 *Mineralocorticoid receptor antagonists:* Spironolactone (25mg/24h PO) ↓mortality by 30% when added to conventional therapy.[40] Use in those still symptomatic despite optimal therapy as listed previously, and in post-MI patients with LVSD. Spironolactone is K^+-sparing, but there is little risk of significant hyperkalaemia, even when given with ACE-i. Nevertheless, U&E should be monitored, particularly if the patient has known CKD. Eplerenone is an alternative if spironolactone is not tolerated.

 5 *Digoxin:* Helps symptoms even in those with sinus rhythm, and should be considered for patients with LVSD who have signs or symptoms of heart failure while receiving standard therapy, including ACE-i and β-blockers, or in patients with AF. Dose example: 125mcg/24h PO if sinus rhythm. Monitor U&E; maintain K^+ at 4–5mmol/L as ↓K^+ risks digoxin toxicity, and vice versa. Digoxin levels: p756. Other inotropes are unhelpful in terms of outcome.

 6 *Vasodilators:* The combination of hydralazine (SE: drug-induced lupus) and isosorbide dinitrate should be used if intolerant of ACE-i and ARBs as it reduces mortality. It also reduces mortality when added to standard therapy (including ACE-i) in black patients with heart failure.[41]

Intractable heart failure Reassess the cause. Are they taking the drugs?—at maximum dose? Switching furosemide to bumetanide (one 5mg tab≈200mg furosemide) might help. Inpatient management may include:

- Minimal exertion; Na^+ & fluid restriction (1.5L/24h PO).
- Metolazone (as above) and IV furosemide (p800).
- Opiates and IV nitrates may relieve symptoms (p800).
- Weigh daily. Do frequent U&E (beware ↓K^+).
- Give DVT prophylaxis: heparin + TED stockings (p578).

In extremis: Try IV inotropes (p802; it may be difficult to wean patients off them).

Consider: Cardiac resynchronization (p132), LV assist device (BOX 'Pulseless patients'), or transplantation.

Palliative care Treat/prevent comorbidities (eg 'flu vaccination). Good nutrition (allow alcohol!). Involve GP: continuity of care and discussion of prognosis is much appreciated.[42] Dyspnoea, pain (from liver capsule stretching), nausea, constipation, and ↓mood all need tackling.[43] Opiates improve pain and dyspnoea. O_2 may help.

Pulseless patients

Left ventricular assist devices (LVADs) are increasingly used as bridging therapies for patients awaiting heart transplantation (fig 3.39). An internalized pump forces blood through tubing from the left ventricle to the aorta. To power the pump, the patient attaches the device to the mains electricity, and uses batteries when out and about. Patients with continuous (rather than pulsatile) flow LVADs have no pulse (fig 3.39c) and ascultation will reveal a loud, continuous, mechanical hum. If the patient collapses and there is no hum, resuscitation should include checking the LVAD power supply!

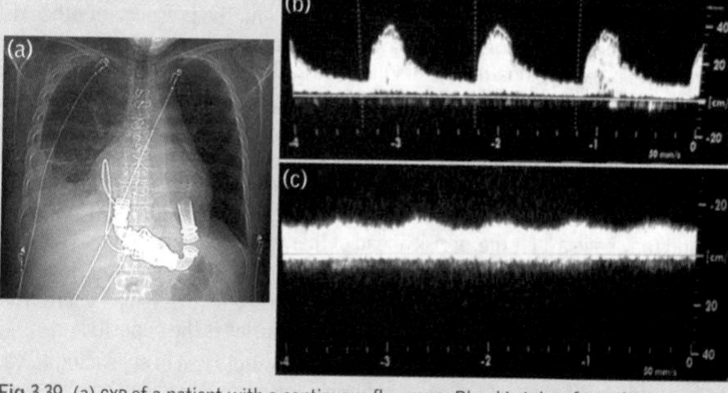

Fig 3.39 (a) CXR of a patient with a continuous flow LVAD. Blood is taken from the LV apex and pumped into the aorta. (b) Retinal flow velocity trace from a normal subject—large peaks in flow rate during systole. (c) Retinal flow velocity trace from a patient with an LVAD. The flow rate only slightly rises during systole as the flow from the LVAD is continuous.

Image in a) reproduced from Gardener *et al.*, *Heart Failure*, 2014, with permission from Oxford University Press. (b) and (c) courtesy of Barry McDonnell.

Natriuretic peptides

Secretory granules have long been known to exist in the atria, and if homogenized atrial tissue is injected into rats, their urine volume (and Na^+ excretion) rises; this is because of atrial natriuretic peptide (ANP). BNP is a similar hormone originally identified from pig brain (hence the B), but most BNP is secreted from ventricular myocardium. Plasma BNP is closely related to LV pressure and in MI and LV dysfunction, these hormones can be released in large quantities. Secretion is also increased by tachycardia, glucocorticoids, and thyroid hormones.

Role: ANP and BNP assist the stretched atria and ventricles by increasing GFR and decreasing renal Na^+ resorption, thereby reducing fluid load; and by relaxing smooth muscle, thereby decreasing preload.

BNP as a biomarker of heart failure: ↑BNP distinguishes heart failure from other causes of dyspnoea more accurately than other biomarkers and LV ejection fraction (sensitivity: >90%; specificity: 80–90%). The rises are greater with left than right heart failure and with systolic than diastolic dysfunction.

What BNP threshold for diagnosing heart failure: If BNP >100ng/L, this 'diagnoses' heart failure better than other clinical variables or clinical judgement (history, examination, and CXR). BNP can be used to 'rule out' heart failure if <50ng/L. A BNP >50ng/L does not exclude other coexisting diseases; conditions that can cause BNP rises include tachycardia, cardiac ischaemia, COPD, PE, renal disease, sepsis, hepatic cirrhosis, diabetes, and old age. Also, assays vary, so liaise with your lab.

Prognosis in heart failure: The higher the BNP, the higher the cardiovascular and all-cause mortality (independent of age, NYHA class, previous MI, and LV ejection fraction) and the greater the risk of sudden death. So, a patient whose symptoms are currently well controlled may benefit from more aggressive treatment if their BNP if persistently raised.

Hypertension

Hypertension[44] is the most important risk factor for premature death and CVD; causing ~50% of all vascular deaths (8×10^6/yr). Usually asymptomatic, so regular screening (eg 3-yrly) is a *vital* task—most preventable deaths are in areas without universal screening.[45]

Defining hypertension BP has a skewed normal distribution (p751) within the population, and risk is continuously related to BP, so it is impossible to define 'hypertension'.[46] We choose to select a value above which risk is significantly increased and the benefit of treatment is clear cut, see below. Don't rely on a single reading—assess over a period of time (how long depends on the BP and the presence of other risk factors or end-organ damage). Confirm with 24hr ambulatory BP monitoring (ABPM); or a week of home readings. NB: the diagnostic threshold is lower ~135/85mmHg.

Whom to treat All with BP ≥160/100mmHg (or ABPM ≥150/95mmHg). For those ≥140/90, the decision depends on the risk of coronary events, presence of diabetes, or end-organ damage; see fig 3.40.[44] The HYVET study showed that there is even substantial benefit in treating the over-80s.[47] Lower thresholds may be appropriate for young people—BP is on average lower in young people (eg 100–110/60–70 in 18-year-olds) and they have a 'lifetime' of risk ahead of them; but evidence to treat is lacking.

White-coat hypertension Refers to an elevated *clinic* pressure, but normal *ABPM* (day average <135/85). NICE says don't treat; but more likely to develop hypertension in future, and may have ↑risk of CVD. Masked hypertension is the opposite.

'Malignant' or accelerated phase hypertension: A rapid rise in BP leading to vascular damage (pathological hallmark is fibrinoid necrosis). Usually there is severe hypertension (eg systolic >200, diastolic>130mmHg) + bilateral retinal haemorrhages and exudates; papilloedema may or may not be present. Symptoms are common, eg headache ± visual disturbance. It requires urgent treatment, and may also precipitate acute kidney injury, heart failure, or encephalopathy, which are hypertensive emergencies. Untreated, 90% die in 1yr; treated, 70% survive 5yrs. It is more common in younger and in black subjects. Look hard for any underlying cause.

Primary or 'essential' hypertension: (Cause unknown.) ~95% of cases.

Secondary hypertension: ~5% of cases. Causes include:

- *Renal disease:* the most common secondary cause. 75% are from *intrinsic renal disease:* glomerulonephritis, polyarteritis nodosa (PAN), systemic sclerosis, chronic pyelonephritis, or polycystic kidneys. 25% are due to *renovascular disease*, most frequently atheromatous (elderly ♂ cigarette smokers, eg with peripheral vascular disease) or rarely fibromuscular dysplasia (young ♀).
- *Endocrine disease:* Cushing's (p224) and Conn's syndromes (p228), phaeochromocytoma (p228), acromegaly, hyperparathyroidism.
- *Others:* coarctation (p156), pregnancy (*OHCS* p48), liquorice, drugs: steroids, MAOI, oral contraceptive pill, cocaine, amphetamines.

Signs and symptoms Usually asymptomatic (except malignant hypertension, see earlier in topic). Headache is no more common than in the general population. Always examine the CVS fully and check for retinopathy. Are there features of an underlying cause (phaeochromocytoma, p228, etc.), signs of renal disease, radiofemoral delay, or weak femoral pulses (coarctation), renal bruits, palpable kidneys, or Cushing's syndrome? Look for end-organ damage: LVH, retinopathy and proteinuria—indicates severity and duration of hypertension and associated with a poorer prognosis.

Tests *To confirm diagnosis:* ABPM or home BP monitoring. *To help quantify overall risk:* Fasting glucose; cholesterol. *To look for end-organ damage:* ECG or echo (any LV hypertrophy? past MI?); urine analysis (protein, blood). *To 'exclude' secondary causes:* U&E (eg K^+↓ in Conn's); Ca^{2+} (↑ in hyperparathyroidism). *Special tests:* Renal ultrasound/arteriography (renal artery stenosis); 24h urinary meta-adrenaline (p228); urinary free cortisol (p225); renin; aldosterone; MR aorta (coarctation).

Grading hypertensive retinopathy

1 Tortuous arteries with thick shiny walls (silver or copper wiring, p560, fig 12.18).
2 AV nipping (narrowing where arteries cross veins, p560, fig 12.19).
3 Flame haemorrhages and cotton-wool spots.
4 Papilloedema, p560, fig 12.20.

Measuring BP with a sphygmomanometer

- Use the correct size cuff. The cuff width should be >40% of the arm circumference. The bladder should be centred over the brachial artery, and the cuff applied snugly. Support the arm in a horizontal position at mid-sternal level.
- Inflate the cuff while palpating the brachial artery, until the pulse disappears. This provides an estimate of systolic pressure.
- Inflate the cuff until 30mmHg above systolic pressure, then place stethoscope over the brachial artery. Deflate the cuff at 2mmHg/s.
- *Systolic pressure:* appearance of sustained repetitive tapping sounds (Korotkoff I).
- *Diastolic pressure:* usually the disappearance of sounds (Korotkoff V). However, in some individuals (eg pregnant women) sounds are present until the zero point. In this case, the muffling of sounds, Korotkoff IV, should be used. State which is used for a given reading. For children, see *OHCS* p157.
- For advice on using automated sphygmomanometers and a list of validated devices see http://www.bhsoc.org/latest-guidelines/how-to-measure-blood-pressure/

Managing suspected hypertension

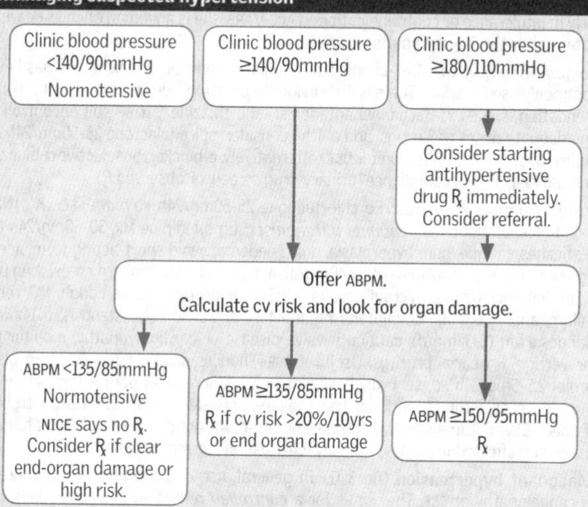

Fig 3.40 Managing suspected hypertension.

Target pressure is <140/90mmHg (150/90 if aged >80), but in diabetes mellitus aim for <130/80mmHg, and <125/75 if proteinuria. To quantify CV risk, see www.bhsoc.org. NB: CV threshold of 20% ≈ 15% for CHD alone. Examples of target (end-organ) damage: • LVH • PMH of MI or angina • PMH of stroke/TIA • Peripheral vascular disease • Renal failure.

Data source NICE CG127, https://www.nice.org.uk/guidance/cg127/resources/hypertension-in-adults-diagnosis-and-management-35109454941637.

Hypertension—management

Look for and treat underlying causes (eg renal disease, ↑alcohol: see p138). Drug therapy reduces the risk of CVD and death. Almost any adult over 50 would benefit from antihypertensives, whatever their starting BP.[48] Treatment is especially important if: BP is persistently ≥160/100mmHg or cardiovascular risk ↑ (10yr risk of vascular disease ≥20%), or existing vascular disease or target organ damage (eg brain, kidney, heart, retina) with BP >140/90mmHg. Essential hypertension is not 'curable' and long-term treatment is needed.

Treatment goal <140/90mmHg (<130/80 in diabetes, 150/90 if aged >80). Reduce blood pressure *slowly*; rapid reduction can be fatal, especially in the context of an acute stroke. These may fall—SPRINT[49] showed a target of 120/80 was beneficial.

Lifestyle changes ↓Concomitant risk factors: stop smoking; low-fat diet. Reduce alcohol and salt intake; increase exercise; reduce weight if obese.

Drugs The ALLHAT study suggests that adequate BP reduction is more important than the specific drug used.[50] However, β-blockers seem to be less effective than other drugs at reducing major cardiovascular events, particularly stroke. β-blockers and thiazides may increase the risk of new-onset diabetes, Ca^{2+}-channel blockers appear neutral, and ACE-i or ARB may reduce the risk.[44]

Monotherapy: If ≥55yrs, and in black patients of any age, 1st choice is a Ca^{2+}-channel antagonist or thiazide. If <55, 1st choice is ACE-i (or ARB if ACE-i intolerant, eg cough). β-blockers are not 1st line for hypertension, but consider in younger people, particularly if: intolerance or contraindication to ACE-i/ARB, she is a woman of child-bearing potential, or there is ↑sympathetic drive.

Combination ℞: ACE-i + Ca^{2+}-channel antagonist or diuretic is logical, and has been commonly used in trials. There is little evidence on using 3 drugs but current recommendation is ACE-i, Ca^{2+}-channel antagonist, and thiazide.[44] If BP still uncontrolled on adequate doses of 3 drugs, add a 4th—consider: spironolactone 25-50mg/24h or higher-dose thiazide, but monitor U&E. Alternatively, β-blocker, or selective α-blocker and get help. Check compliance (urinary drug screen, or observed ℞).

Drug examples *Thiazides:* Eg chlortalidone 25-50mg/24h PO *mané*. SE: ↓K^+, ↓Na^+, impotence. CI: gout. *Ca^{2+}-channel antagonists:* Eg nifedipine MR, 30-60mg/24h PO. SE: flushes, fatigue, gum hyperplasia, ankle oedema; avoid short-acting form. *ACE-i:* Eg lisinopril 10-40mg/24h PO (max 40mg/d). ACE-i may be 1st choice if co-existing LVF, or in diabetics (esp. if microalbuminuria, p314) or proteinuria. SE: cough, ↑K^+, renal failure, angio-oedema. CI: bilateral renal artery or aortic valve stenosis; p114. *ARB:* Candesartan (8-32mg/d); caution if valve disease or cardiomyopathy; monitor K^+. SE: vertigo, urticaria, pruritus. Useful if ACE-i induces cough. *β-blockers:* Eg bisoprolol 2.5-5mg/24h PO. SE: bronchospasm, heart failure, cold peripheries, lethargy, impotence. CI: asthma; caution in heart failure. Consider aspirin when BP controlled, if aged >55yrs. Add a *statin* if cholesterol raised. ►Most drugs take 4-8wks to gain maximum effect: don't assess efficacy with just one BP measurement.

Malignant hypertension (fig 3.41) In general, use oral therapy, unless there is encephalopathy or CCF. The aim is for a *controlled* reduction in BP over days, not hours. Avoid sudden drops in BP as cerebral autoregulation is poor (↑stroke risk). Bed rest; there is no ideal hypotensive, but atenolol or long-acting Ca^{2+} blockers may be used PO.

Encephalopathy: (Headache, focal CNS signs, seizures, coma.) Aim to reduce BP to ~110mmHg diastolic over 4h. Admit to monitored area. Insert intra-arterial line for pressure monitoring. Either IV labetalol (eg 50mg IV over 1min, repeated every 5min, max 200mg) or sodium nitroprusside infusion (0.5mcg/kg/min IVI titrated up to 8mcg/kg/min, eg 50mg in 1L glucose 5%; expect to give 100-200mL/h for a few hours only, to avoid cyanide risk).

►Never use sublingual nifedipine to reduce BP (rapid drop in BP may cause stroke).[51]

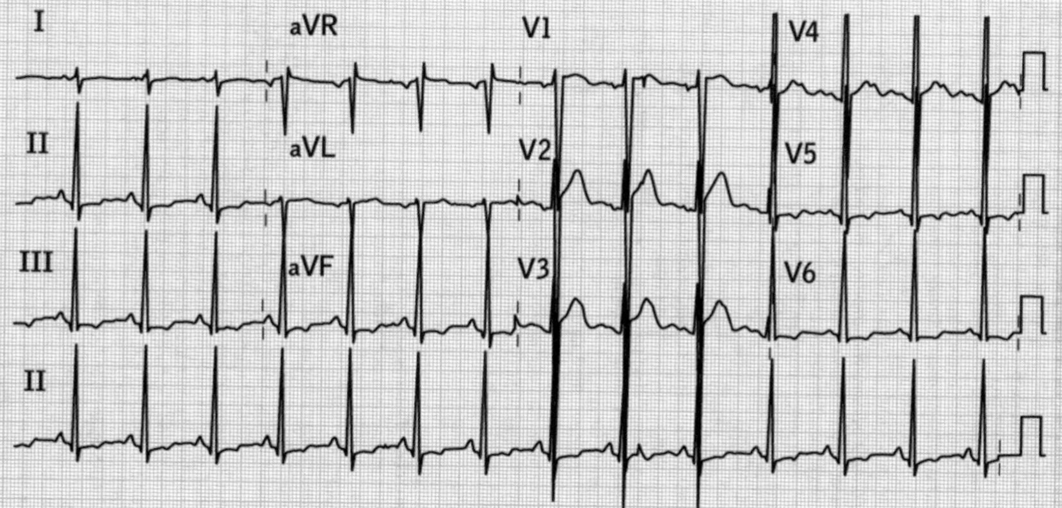

Fig 3.41 Left ventricular hypertrophy—this is from a patient with malignant hypertension—note the sum of the S-wave in V_2 and R-wave in V_6 is greater than 35mm.

Rheumatic fever (RF)

This systemic infection is still common in developing countries but increasingly rare in the West. Peak incidence: 5-15yrs. Tends to recur unless prevented. Pharyngeal infection with Lancefield group A β-haemolytic streptococci triggers rheumatic fever 2-4wks later, in the susceptible 2% of the population. An antibody to the carbohydrate cell wall of the streptococcus cross-reacts with valve tissue (antigenic mimicry) and may cause permanent damage to the heart valves.

Diagnosis Use the **revised Jones criteria** (may be over-rigorous). There must be evidence of recent strep infection plus 2 major criteria, or 1 major + 2 minor.

Evidence of group A β-haemolytic streptococcal infection:
- Positive throat culture (usually negative by the time RF symptoms appear).
- Rapid streptococcal antigen test +ve.
- Elevated or rising streptococcal antibody titre (eg anti-streptolysin O (ASO) or DNase B titre).
- Recent scarlet fever.

Major criteria:
- *Carditis:* tachycardia, murmurs (mitral or aortic regurgitation, Carey Coombs' murmur, p46), pericardial rub, CCF, cardiomegaly, conduction defects (45-70%). An apical systolic murmur may be the only sign.[52]
- *Arthritis:* a migratory, 'flitting' polyarthritis; usually affects larger joints (75%).
- *Subcutaneous nodules:* small, mobile, painless nodules on extensor surfaces of joints and spine (2-20%).
- *Erythema marginatum:* (fig 3.42) geographical-type rash with red, raised edges and clear centre; occurs mainly on trunk, thighs and arms in 2-10% (p562).
- *Sydenham's chorea (St Vitus' dance):* occurs late in 10%. Unilateral or bilateral involuntary semi-purposeful movements. May be preceded by emotional lability and uncharacteristic behaviour.

Minor criteria:
- Fever.
- Raised ESR or CRP.
- Arthralgia (but not if arthritis is one of the major criteria).
- Prolonged PR interval (but not if carditis is major criterion).
- Previous rheumatic fever.

Management
- Bed rest until CRP normal for 2wks (may be 3 months).
- Benzylpenicillin 0.6-1.2g IV stat, then phenoxymethylpenicillin 250-500mg 4 times daily PO for 10 days (if allergic to penicillin, give erythromycin or azithromycin for 10 days).
- Analgesia for carditis/arthritis: aspirin 100mg/kg/d PO in divided doses (max 4-8g/d) for 2d, then 70mg/kg/d for 6wks. Monitor salicylate level. Toxicity causes tinnitus, hyperventilation, and metabolic acidosis. Risk of Reye syndrome in children. Alternative: NSAIDs (p546). If moderate-to-severe carditis is present (cardiomegaly, CCF, or 3rd-degree heart block), add oral prednisolone to salicylate therapy. In case of heart failure, treat appropriately (p136), with severe valve disease, surgery may be required.
- Immobilize joints in severe arthritis.
- Haloperidol (0.5mg/8h PO) or diazepam for the chorea.

Prognosis 60% with carditis develop chronic rheumatic heart disease. This correlates with the severity of the carditis.[53] Acute attacks last an average of 3 months. Recurrence may be precipitated by further streptococcal infections, pregnancy, or use of the oral contraceptive pill. Cardiac sequelae affect mitral (70%), aortic (40%), tricuspid (10%), and pulmonary (2%) valves. Incompetent lesions develop during the attack, stenoses years later.

Secondary prophylaxis Penicillin V 250mg/12h PO. Alternatives: sulfadiazine 1g daily (0.5g if <30kg) or erythromycin 250mg twice daily (if penicillin allergic). Duration: If carditis+persistent valvular disease, continue at least until age of 40 (sometimes lifelong). If carditis but no valvular disease, continue for 10yrs. If there is no carditis, 5yrs of prophylaxis (until age of 21) is sufficient.

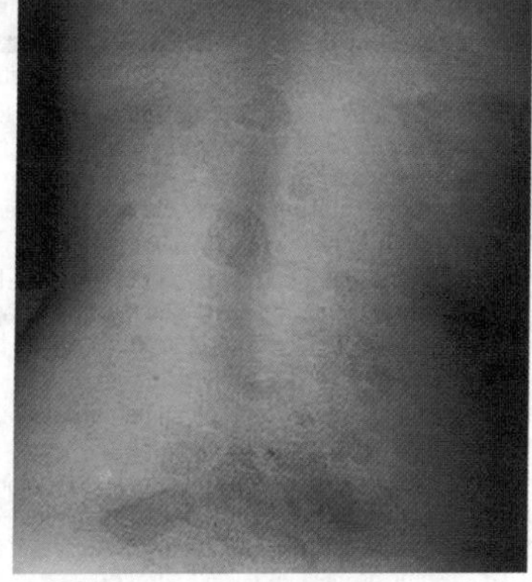

Fig 3.42 Erythema marginatum.
Image courtesy of Dr Maria Angelica Binotto.

Mitral valve disease

Mitral regurgitation (MR) Backflow through the mitral valve during systole.

Causes: Functional (LV dilatation); annular calcification (elderly); rheumatic fever; infective endocarditis; mitral valve prolapse; ruptured chordae tendinae; papillary muscle dysfunction/rupture (eg post-MI); connective tissue disorders (Ehlers-Danlos, Marfan's); cardiomyopathy; congenital (may be associated with other defects, eg ASD, AV canal); appetite suppressants (eg fenfluramine, phentermine).

Symptoms: Dyspnoea; fatigue; palpitations; symptoms of causative factor (eg fever). *Signs:* AF; displaced, hyperdynamic apex; pansystolic murmur at apex radiating to axilla; soft S_1; split S_2; loud P_2 (pulmonary hypertension). *Severity:* the more severe, the larger the left ventricle.

Tests: ECG: AF; P-mitrale if in sinus rhythm (may mean ↑left atrial size); LVH. *CXR:* big LA & LV; mitral valve calcification; pulmonary oedema.

Echocardiogram: To assess LV function and MR severity and aetiology (transoesophageal to assess severity and suitability for repair rather than replacement). *Cardiac catheterization* to confirm diagnosis, exclude other valve disease, and assess coronary artery disease (can combine CABG with valve surgery).

Management: Control rate if fast AF. Anticoagulate if: AF; history of embolism; prosthetic valve; additional mitral stenosis. Diuretics improve symptoms. Surgery[4] for deteriorating symptoms; aim to repair or replace the valve before LV is irreversibly impaired.

Mitral valve prolapse: Is the most common valvular abnormality (prevalence: ~5%). Occurs alone or with: ASD, patent ductus arteriosus, cardiomyopathy, Turner's syndrome, Marfan's syndrome, osteogenesis imperfecta, pseudoxanthoma elasticum, WPW (p133). *Symptoms:* Usually asymptomatic. May develop atypical chest pain, palpitations, and autonomic dysfunction symptoms. *Signs:* Mid-systolic click and/or a late systolic murmur. *Complications:* MR, cerebral emboli, arrhythmias, sudden death. *Tests: Echo* is diagnostic. *ECG* may show inferior T-wave inversion. *℞:* β-blockers may help palpitations and chest pain. Surgery if severe MR.

Mitral stenosis *Causes:* Rheumatic fever, congenital, mucopolysaccharidoses, endocardial fibroelastosis, malignant carcinoid (p271; rare), prosthetic valve.

Presentation: Normal mitral valve orifice area is ~4-6cm². Symptoms usually begin when the orifice becomes <2cm². Pulmonary hypertension causes dyspnoea, haemoptysis, chronic bronchitis-like picture; pressure from large left atrium on local structures causes hoarseness (recurrent laryngeal nerve), dysphagia (oesophagus), bronchial obstruction; also fatigue, palpitations, chest pain, systemic emboli, infective endocarditis (rare).

Signs: Malar flush on cheeks (due to ↓cardiac output); low-volume pulse; AF common (due to enlarged LA); tapping, non-displaced, apex beat (palpable S_1); RV heave. On auscultation: loud S_1; opening snap (pliable valve); rumbling mid-diastolic murmur (heard best in expiration, with patient on left side). Graham Steell murmur (p46) may occur. *Severity:* the more severe the stenosis, the longer the diastolic murmur, and the closer the opening snap is to S_2.

Tests: ECG: AF; P-mitrale; RVH; progressive RAD. CXR: left atrial enlargement (double shadow in right cardiac silhouette); pulmonary oedema; mitral valve calcification. *Echo* is diagnostic. Significant stenosis exists if the valve orifice is <1cm²/m² body surface area. Indications for *cardiac catheterization:* previous valvotomy; signs of other valve disease; angina; severe pulmonary hypertension; calcified mitral valve.

Management: If in AF, *rate control* (p130) *is crucial*; anticoagulate with warfarin (p350). Diuretics ↓ preload and pulmonary venous congestion. If this fails to control symptoms, balloon valvuloplasty (if pliable, non-calcified valve), open mitral valvotomy, or valve replacement.

4 In patients with severe symptoms for whom open surgery is too dangerous, consider transcatheter valve repair, eg with MitraClip®. This is only available in specialist centres.

What Becomes of the Broken Hearted?

'For who loveth extreamely, and feeleth not that passion to dissolve his hearte?
Who rejoyceth, and proveth not his heart dilated?
Who is moyled with heavinesse, or plunged with payne,
and perceiveth not his heart to bee coarcted?
Whom inflameth ire, and hath not heart-burning?
By these experiences, wee prove in our hearts the working of Passions,
and by the noyse of their tumult, wee understand the woorke of their presence'
Thomas Wright, *The Passions of the Minde in Generall,* 1604

From Aztec priests raising beating human hearts to the Sun-God, to heart metaphors in song lyrics today, ideas of links between the heart and human psychosocial self/soul/experience-of-being have pervaded the imaginative landscapes of cultures throughout time and place.

Some of these links relate to physiological changes associated with emotion-triggered adrenaline surges—'my heart raced', for example, is a phrase we relate to both physically and emotionally. Other heart-phrases result from poetic extrapolations of heart/self ideas and have no physiological explanation, eg 'he wears his heart on his sleeve'.

Evidence is building that heart/self interactions exist beyond metaphor and symptomatic 'flight-or-fight' responses. Affective disorders, certain personality types, and traumatic life-experiences increase the risk of cardiac disease, even when lifestyle factors are controlled for.[54-56] In 'broken heart syndrome' (Takotsubo cardiomyopathy), ventricular contraction morphology changes in response to emotional or physical stress (fig 3.43). It mimics a myocardial infarction in terms of clinical history, ECG changes, and troponin rises, but the prognosis and management may be quite different so accurate diagnosis is important.

As physicians, we often focus on explainable physical aspects of disease, but the physical and psychosocial are inconveniently related and both should be assessed to determine best management. Should an IHD sufferer be offered CBT alongside their statins? Could a grieving patient's 'MI' be Takotsubo cardiomyopathy? To answer these questions we must look beyond ECGs and troponin, to the 'heart-ache' of the literary and philosophical kinds.

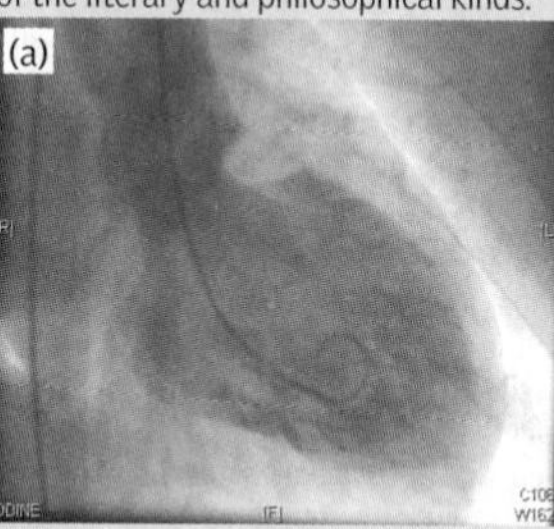

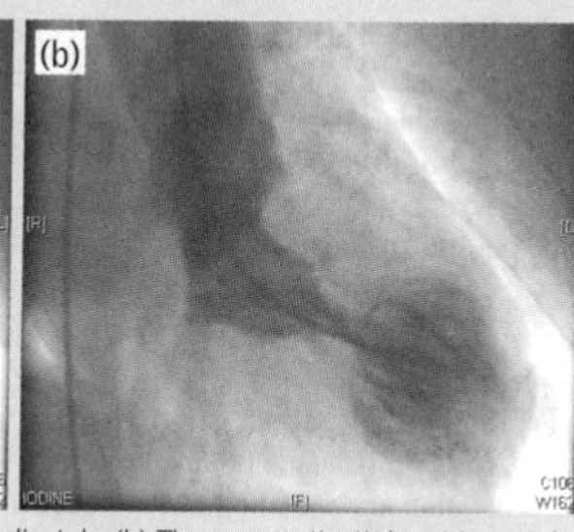

Fig 3.43 (a) Left ventriculogram of a heart in diastole. (b) The same patient's heart in systole. The apex is ballooning whilst the base contracts, causing inefficient pumping and a risk of rupture. This pattern is classic of Takotsubo cardiomyopathy.

Aortic valve disease

Aortic stenosis (AS) *Causes:* Senile calcification is the commonest.[57] Others: congenital (bicuspid valve, Williams syndrome, p149), rheumatic heart disease.

Presentation: Think of AS in any elderly person with chest pain, exertional dyspnoea, or syncope. The classic triad includes angina, syncope, and heart failure. Also: dyspnoea; dizziness; faints; systemic emboli if infective endocarditis; sudden death. *Signs:* Slow rising pulse with narrow pulse pressure (feel for diminished and delayed carotid upstroke—*parvus et tardus*); heaving, non-displaced apex beat; LV heave; aortic thrill; ejection systolic murmur (heard at the base, left sternal edge and the aortic area, radiates to the carotids). S_1 is usually normal. As stenosis worsens, A_2 is increasingly delayed, giving first a single S_2 and then reversed splitting. But this sign is rare. More common is a quiet A_2. In severe AS, A_2 may be inaudible (calcified valve). There may be an ejection click (pliable valve) or an S_4.

Tests: ECG: LVH with strain pattern; P-mitrale; LAD; poor R-wave progression; LBBB or complete AV block (calcified ring). *CXR:* LVH; calcified aortic valve (fig 3.44); post-stenotic dilatation of ascending aorta. *Echo:* diagnostic (p110). Doppler echo can estimate the gradient across valves: severe stenosis if peak gradient ≳40mmHg (but beware the poor left ventricle not able to generate gradient) and valve area <1cm^2. If the aortic jet velocity is >4m/s (or is increasing by >0.3m/s per yr) risk of complications is increased.[57] *Cardiac catheter* can assess: valve gradient; LV function; coronary artery disease; risks: emboli generation.

Differential diagnosis: Hypertrophic cardiomyopathy (HCM, p152); aortic sclerosis.

Management: If symptomatic, prognosis is poor without surgery: 2-3yr survival if angina/syncope; 1-2yr if cardiac failure. If moderate-to-severe and treated medically, mortality can be as high as 50% at 2yrs, therefore prompt valve replacement (p148) is usually recommended. In asymptomatic patients with severe AS and a deteriorating ECG, valve replacement is also recommended. If the patient is not medically fit for surgery, percutaneous valvuloplasty/replacement (TAVI = transcatheter aortic valve implantation) may be attempted (fig 3.45).

Aortic sclerosis Senile degeneration of the valve. There is an ejection systolic murmur; but no carotid radiation, and normal pulse (character and volume) and S_2.

Aortic regurgitation (AR) *Acute:* Infective endocarditis, ascending aortic dissection, chest trauma. *Chronic:* Congenital, connective tissue disorders (Marfan's syndrome, Ehlers-Danlos), rheumatic fever, Takayasu arteritis, rheumatoid arthritis, SLE, pseudoxanthoma elasticum, appetite suppressants (eg fenfluramine, phentermine), seronegative arthritides (ankylosing spondylitis, Reiter's syndrome, psoriatic arthropathy), hypertension, osteogenesis imperfecta, syphilitic aortitis.

Symptoms: Exertional dyspnoea, orthopnoea, and PND. Also: palpitations, angina, syncope, CCF. *Signs:* Collapsing (water-hammer) pulse (p42); wide pulse pressure; displaced, hyperdynamic apex beat; high-pitched early diastolic murmur (heard best in expiration, with patient sat forward). Eponyms: *Corrigan's sign:* carotid pulsation; *de Musset's sign:* head nodding with each heart beat; *Quincke's sign:* capillary pulsations in nail beds; *Duroziez's sign:* in the groin, a finger compressing the femoral artery 2cm proximal to the stethoscope gives a systolic murmur; if 2cm distal, it gives a diastolic murmur as blood flows backwards; *Traube's sign:* 'pistol shot' sound over femoral arteries; an *Austin Flint* murmur (p46) denotes *severe* AR.

Tests: ECG: LVH. *CXR:* cardiomegaly; dilated ascending aorta; pulmonary oedema. *Echo* is diagnostic. *Cardiac catheterization* to assess: severity of lesion; anatomy of aortic root; LV function; coronary artery disease; other valve disease.

Management: The main goal of medical therapy is to reduce systolic hypertension; ACE-i are helpful. Echo every 6-12 months to monitor. Indications for surgery: severe AR with enlarged ascending aorta, increasing symptoms, enlarging LV or deteriorating LV function on echo; or infective endocarditis refractory to medical therapy. Aim to replace the valve before significant LV dysfunction occurs. Predictors of poor post-operative survival: ejection fraction <50%, NYHA class III or IV (p135), duration of CCF >12 months.

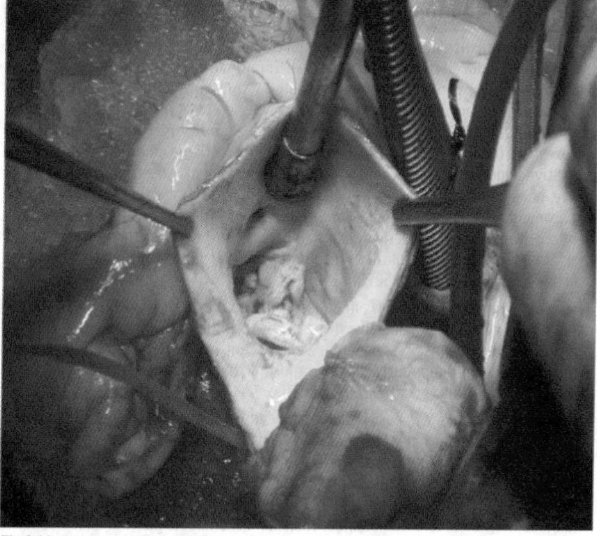

Fig 3.44 Severely calcified aortic valve.

Reproduced with permission from Hamid Reza Taghipour.

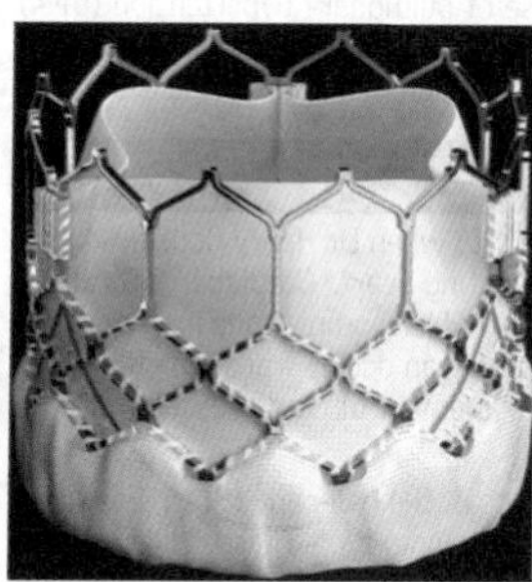

Fig 3.45 This is one of the two main types of transcatheter aortic valve implants: animal valve leaflets mounted on metal stents. This extraordinary stucture must be resilient against the movement of the heart walls and the powerful flow of blood; it must avoid obstructing forward flow of blood whilst providing a near-complete block to backflow; and it has surfaces of foreign material yet must avoid triggering clots or allowing microbial growth. On top of this, it must be able to fold down over a wire to allow safe passage through the arterial tree from the groin to the heart, before being opened out by an inflated balloon.

Image courtesy of Edwards Lifesciences LLC, Irvine, CA. Edwards, Edwards Lifesciences, Edwards SAPIEN, SAPIEN, SAPIEN XT and SAPIEN 3 are trademarks of Edwards Lifesciences Corporation.

Right heart valve disease

Tricuspid regurgitation *Causes:* Functional (RV dilatation; eg due to pulmonary hypertension induced by LV failure or PE); rheumatic fever; infective endocarditis (IV drug abuser[5]); carcinoid syndrome; congenital (eg ASD, AV canal, Ebstein's anomaly (downward displacement of the tricuspid valve—see *OHCS* p642)); drugs (eg ergot-derived dopamine agonists, p495; fenfluramine). *Symptoms:* Fatigue; hepatic pain on exertion (due to hepatic congestion); ascites; oedema and symptoms of the causative condition. *Signs:* Giant *v* waves and prominent *y* descent in JVP (p43); RV heave; pansystolic murmur, heard best at lower sternal edge in inspiration; pulsatile hepatomegaly; jaundice; ascites. *Management:* Drugs: diuretics for systemic congestion; drugs to treat underlying cause. Valve repair or replacement (~10% 30-day mortality). Tricuspid regurgitation resulting from myocardial dysfunction or dilatation has a mortality of up to 50% at 5 yrs.

Tricuspid stenosis *Causes:* Main cause is rheumatic fever, which almost always occurs with mitral or aortic valve disease. Also: congenital, infective endocarditis. *Symptoms:* Fatigue, ascites, oedema. *Signs:* Giant *a* wave and slow *y* descent in JVP (p43); opening snap, early diastolic murmur heard at the left sternal edge in inspiration. AF can also occur. *Diagnosis:* Echo. *Treatment:* Diuretics; surgical repair.

Pulmonary stenosis *Causes:* Usually congenital (Turner syndrome, Noonan syndrome, Williams syndrome, Fallot's tetralogy, rubella). Acquired causes: rheumatic fever, carcinoid syndrome. *Symptoms:* Dyspnoea; fatigue; oedema; ascites. *Signs:* Dysmorphic facies (congenital causes); prominent *a* wave in JVP; RV heave. In mild stenosis, there is an ejection click, ejection systolic murmur (which radiates to the left shoulder); widely split S_2. In severe stenosis, the murmur becomes longer and obscures A_2. P_2 becomes softer and may be inaudible. *Tests:* ECG: RAD, P-pulmonale, RVH, RBBB; echo/TOE (p110); CXR: prominent pulmonary arteries caused by post-stenotic dilatation. Cardiac catheterization is diagnostic. *Treatment:* Pulmonary valvuloplasty or valvotomy.

Pulmonary regurgitation *Causes:* Any cause of pulmonary hypertension (p194). *Signs:* Decrescendo murmur in early diastole at the left sternal edge (the Graham Steell murmur if associated with mitral stenosis and pulmonary hypertension).

Cardiac surgery

Cardiac surgery has come on a long way since 1923 when Dr Henry Souttar[58,59] used his finger to open a stenosed mitral valve in a beating heart.[6] Cardiac bypass allows prolonged access to the open, static heart, during which complex and high-precision repair and replacement of valves and aortic roots can occur. Transcatheter procedures are playing an increasing role in the management of cardiovascular disease. Key open heart procedures include:

Valve replacements *Mechanical valves* may be of the ball-cage (Starr-Edwards), tilting disc (Bjork-Shiley), or double tilting disc (St Jude) type. These valves are very durable but the risk of thromboembolism is high; patients require lifelong anticoagulation. *Xenografts* are made from porcine valves or pericardium. These valves are less durable and may require replacement at 8-10yrs but have the advantage of not necessitating anticoagulation. *Homografts* are cadaveric valves. They are particularly useful in young patients and in the replacement of infected valves. *Complications of prosthetic valves:* systemic embolism, infective endocarditis, haemolysis, structural valve failure, arrhythmias.

CABG See p123.

Cardiac transplantation Consider this when cardiac disease is *severely* curtailing quality of life, and survival is not expected beyond 6-12 months.

Surgery for congenital heart defects See p156.

Aortic root surgery Replacement/repair if dissection or aneurysmal.

5 Remember that it is the tricuspid valve which is the valve most vulnerable to events arriving by vein, eg pathogens from IV drug abusers or hormones (particularly 5-HT) from carcinoid tumours.
6 Souttar's own description of this landmark case is available online: H S Souttar. The surgical treatment of mitral stenosis. *BMJ* 1925: 2(3379): 603–606.

The heart in various, mostly rare, systemic diseases

This list reminds us to look at the heart *and* the whole patient, not just in exams (where those with odd syndromes congregate), but always.

Acromegaly: (p238) ↑BP; LVH; hypertrophic cardiomyopathy; high-output cardiac failure; coronary artery disease.

Amyloidosis: (p370) Restrictive cardiomyopathy. Bright myocardium on echo.

Ankylosing spondylitis: (p550) Conduction defects; AV block; AR.

Behçet's disease: (p694) Aortic regurgitation; arterial ± venous thrombi.

Beta thalassaemia: (p342) Dilated and restrictive cardiomyopathies.

Carcinoid syndrome: (p271) Tricuspid regurgitation and pulmonary stenosis.

Cushing's syndrome: (p224) Hypertension.

Down's syndrome: (*OHCS* p152) ASD; VSD; mitral regurgitation.

Ehlers-Danlos syndrome: (*OHCS* p642) Mitral valve prolapse; aortic aneurysm and dissection; hyperelastic skin; GI bleeds. Joints are loose and hypermobile; mutations exist, eg in genes for procollagen (COL3A1); there are six types.

Friedreich's ataxia: (p698) Hypertrophic cardiomyopathy, dilatation over time.

Haemochromatosis: (p288) AF; cardiomyopathy.

Holt-Oram syndrome: ASD or VSD with upper limb defects (eg polydactyly and triphalangeal thumb).[60]

Human immunodeficiency virus: (p398) Myocarditis; dilated cardiomyopathy; effusion; ventricular arrhythmias; SBE/IE; non-infective thrombotic (marantic) endocarditis; RVF (pulmonary hypertension); metastatic Kaposi's sarcoma.

Hypothyroidism: (p220) Sinus bradycardia; low pulse pressure; pericardial effusion; coronary artery disease; low-voltage ECG.

Kawasaki disease: (*OHCS* p646) Coronary arteritis similar to PAN; commoner than rheumatic fever (p142) as a cause of acquired heart disease.

Klinefelter's syndrome ♂: (*OHCS* p646) ASD. Psychopathy; learning difficulties; ↓libido; gynaecomastia; sparse facial hair and small firm testes. XXY.

Marfan's syndrome: (p706) Mitral valve prolapse; AR; aortic dissection. Look for long fingers and a high-arched palate.

Myotonic dystrophy (p510) Progressive conduction system disease; arrhythmias; LV dysfunction.

Noonan syndrome: (*OHCS* p650) ASD; pulmonary stenosis ± low-set ears.

Polyarteritis nodosa (PAN): (p556) Small and medium vessel vasculitis + angina; MI; arrhythmias; CCF; pericarditis and conduction defects.

Rheumatoid arthritis: Conduction defects; pericarditis; LV dysfunction; aortic regurgitation; coronary arteritis. Look for arthritis signs, p546.

Sarcoidosis: (p196) Infiltrating granulomas may cause complete AV block; ventricular or supraventricular tachycardia; myocarditis; CCF; restrictive cardiomyopathy. ECG may show Q waves.

Syphilis: (p412) Myocarditis; ascending aortic aneurysm.

Systemic lupus erythematosus: (p554) Pericarditis/effusion; myocarditis; Libman-Sacks endocarditis; mitral valve prolapse; coronary arteritis.

Systemic sclerosis: (p552) Pericarditis; pericardial effusion; myocardial fibrosis; myocardial ischaemia; conduction defects; cardiomyopathy.

Thyrotoxicosis: (p218) Pulse↑; AF ± emboli; wide pulse pressure; hyperdynamic apex; loud heart sounds; ejection systolic murmur; pleuropericardial rub; angina; high-output cardiac failure.

Turner syndrome ♀: Coarctation of aorta. Look for webbed neck. XO.

Williams syndrome: Supravalvular aortic stenosis (↓visuospatial IQ).

Infective endocarditis (IE)

►Fever + new murmur = endocarditis until proven otherwise. Any fever lasting >1wk in those known to be at risk[7] must prompt blood cultures.[61] *Acute* infective endocarditis (IE) tends to occur on 'normal' valves and may present with acute heart failure ± emboli; the commonest organism is *Staph. aureus*. Risk factors: skin breaches (dermatitis, IV lines, wounds); renal failure; immunosuppression; DM. Mortality: 5-50% (related to age and embolic events). Endocarditis on *abnormal valves* tends to run a *subacute course*. Risk factors: aortic or mitral valve disease; tricuspid valves in IV drug users; coarctation; patent ductus arteriosus; VSD; prosthetic valves. Endocarditis on prosthetic valves may be 'early' (within 60d of surgery, usually *Staph. epidermidis*, poor prognosis) or 'late'.

Causes *Bacteria:* Bacteraemia occurs all the time, eg when we chew (not just during dentistry or medical interventions—which is why routine prophylaxis for such procedures does not make sense).[61] *Strep. viridans* is the commonest (usually subacute) followed by *Staph. aureus*, *Strep. bovis* (need colonoscopy ?tumour), Enterococci and *Coxiella burnetii*. Rarely: **HACEK** Gram −ve bacteria (***H**aemophilus-**A**ctinobacillus-**C**ardiobacterium-**E**ikenella-**K**ingella*); diphtheroids; *Chlamydia*. *Fungi: Candida; Aspergillus; Histoplasma*. Usually in IV drug abusers, immunocompromised patients or those with prosthetic valves. High mortality, need surgical management. *Other:* SLE (Libman-Sacks endocarditis); malignancy.

Signs *Septic signs:* Fever, rigors, night sweats, malaise, weight loss, anaemia, splenomegaly, and clubbing (fig 3.46). *Cardiac lesions:* Any new murmur, or a change in pre-existing murmur, should raise the suspicion of endocarditis. Vegetations may cause valve destruction and severe regurgitation, or valve obstruction. An aortic root abscess causes prolongation of the PR interval, and may lead to complete AV block. LVF is a common cause of death. *Immune complex deposition:* Vasculitis (p556) may affect any vessel. Microscopic haematuria is common; glomerulonephritis and acute kidney injury may occur. Roth spots (boat-shaped retinal haemorrhage with pale centre); splinter haemorrhages (fig 3.47); Osler's nodes (painful pulp infarcts in fingers or toes). *Embolic phenomena:* Emboli may cause abscesses in the relevant organ, eg brain, heart, kidney, spleen, gut (or lung if right-sided IE) or skin: termed Janeway lesions (fig 3.48; painless palmar or plantar macules), which, together with Osler's nodes, are pathognomonic.

Diagnosis Use the Modified Duke criteria (BOX 'Modified Duke criteria').[62,63] *Blood cultures:* Do three sets at different times from different sites at peak of fever. 85-90% are diagnosed from the 1st two sets; 10% are culture-negative. *Blood tests:* Normochromic, normocytic anaemia, neutrophilia, high ESR/CRP. Rheumatoid factor positive (an immunological phenomenon). Also check U&E, Mg^{2+}, LFT. *Urinalysis:* For microscopic haematuria. *CXR:* Cardiomegaly, pulmonary oedema. *Regular ECGs:* To look for heart block. *Echocardiogram:* TTE (p110) may show vegetations, but only if >2mm. TOE (p110) is more sensitive, and better for visualizing mitral lesions and possible development of aortic root abscess. *CT:* To look for emboli (spleen, brain, etc.).

Treatment Liaise early with microbiologists and cardiologists.[62] Antibiotics: see BOX 'Antibiotic therapy for infective endocarditis'. *Surgery if:* Heart failure, valvular obstruction; repeated emboli; fungal IE; persistent bacteraemia; myocardial abscess; unstable infected prosthetic valve.[64]

Prognosis 50% require surgery. 20% inhospital mortality (Staphs 30%; bowel bacteria 14%; Streps 6%). 15% recurrence at 2yrs.

Prevention Antibiotic prophylaxis is no longer recommended for those at risk of IE undergoing invasive procedures. However, if they are given antibiotics for other reasons during a procedure, the antibiotic should cover the common IE organisms.

Recommendations Give clear information about prevention, including:
- The importance of maintaining good oral health.
- Symptoms that may indicate IE and when to seek expert advice.
- The risks of invasive procedures, including non-medical procedures such as body piercing or tattooing.[65]

7 Past IE or rheumatic fever; IV drug abuser; damaged or replaced valve; PPM or ICD; structural congenital heart disease (but not simple ASD, fully repaired VSD, or patent ductus); hypertrophic cardiomyopathy.

Modified Duke criteria for infective endocarditis

Major criteria:
- Positive blood culture:
  - Typical organism in 2 separate cultures *or*
  - Persistently +ve blood cultures, eg 3 >12h apart (or majority if >3) *or*
  - Single positive blood culture for *Coxiella burnetii*.
- Endocardium involved:
  - Positive echocardiogram (vegetation, abscess, pseudoaneurysm, dehiscence of prosthetic valve) *or*
  - Abnormal activity around prosthetic valve on PET/CT or SPECT/CT *or*
  - Paravalvular lesions on cardiac CT.

Minor criteria:
- Predisposition (cardiac lesion; IV drug abuse).
- Fever >38°C.
- Vascular phenomena (emboli, Janeway's lesions, etc.).
- Immunological phenomena (glomerulonephritis, Osler's nodes, etc.).
- Positive blood culture that does not meet major criteria.

How to diagnose: Definite infective endocarditis: 2 major *or* 1 major and 3 minor *or* all 5 minor criteria.

Antibiotic therapy for infective endocarditis

Prescribe antibiotics for infective endocarditis as follows.[66] For more information on individual antibiotics, see tables 9.4–9.9, pp386–7.
- Blind therapy—native valve or prosthetic valve implanted >1y ago: ampicillin, flucloxacillin and gentamicin. Vancomycin + gentamicin if penicillin-allergic. If thought to be Gram –ve: meropenem + vancomycin.
- Blind therapy—prosthetic valve: vancomycin + gentamicin + rifampicin.
- Staphs—native valve: flucloxacillin for >4wks. If allergic or MRSA: vancomycin .
- Staphs—prosthetic valves: flucloxacillin + rifampicin + gentamicin for 6wks (review need for gentamicin after 2wks). If penicillin-allergic or MRSA: vancomycin + rifampicin + gentamicin.
- Streps—fully sensitive to penicillin: benzylpenicillin 1.2g/4h IV for 4–6wks.[8]
- Streps—less sensitive: benzylpenicillin + gentamicin; if penicillin allergic or highly penicillin resistant: vancomycin + gentamicin.
- Enterococci: amoxicillin + gentamicin. If pen-allergic: vancomycin + gentamicin—for 4wks (6wks if prosthetic valve); review need for gentamicin after 2wks.
- HACEK organisms (*Haemophilus*, *Actinobacillus*, *Cardiobacterium*, *Eikenella*, *Kingella*): ceftriaxone for 4wks with native valve or 6wks with prosthetic.
- Fungal: *Candida*—amphotericin. *Aspergillus*—voriconazole.

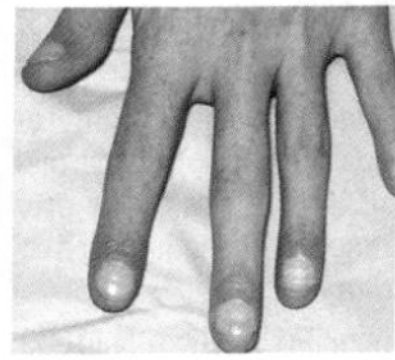

Fig 3.46 Clubbing with endocarditis.

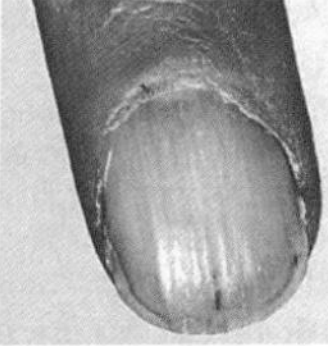

Fig 3.47 Splinter haemorrhages are normally seen under the fingernails or toenails. They are usually red-brown in colour.

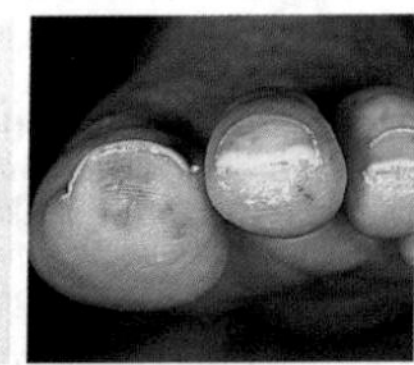

Fig 3.48 Janeway's lesions are non-tender erythematous, haemorrhagic, or pustular spots, eg on the palms or soles.

8 If *Strep bovis* is cultured, do colonoscopy, as a colon neoplasm is the likely portal of entry (table 6.3, p249).

Diseases of heart muscle

Acute myocarditis This is inflammation of myocardium, often associated with pericardial inflammation (myopericarditis).[67] *Causes:* See table 3.3. *Symptoms and signs:* ACS-like symptoms, heart failure symptoms, palpitations, tachycardia, soft S_1, S_4 gallop (p44). *Tests:* ECG: ST changes and T-wave inversion, atrial arrhythmias, transient AV block, QT prolongation. Bloods: CRP, ESR, & troponin may be raised; viral serology and tests for other likely causes. Echo: diastolic dysfunction, regional wall abnormalities. Cardiac MR if clinically stable. Endomyocardial biopsy is gold standard. ℞: Supportive. Treat the underlying cause. Treat arrhythmias and heart failure (p136). NSAID use is controversial. Avoid exercise as this can precipitate arrhythmias. *Prognosis:* 50% will recover within 4wks. 12–25% will develop DCM and severe heart failure. DCM can occur years after apparent recovery.

Dilated cardiomyopathy (DCM) A dilated, flabby heart of unknown cause. Associations: alcohol, ↑BP, chemotherapeutics, haemochromatosis, viral infection, autoimmune, peri- or postpartum, thyrotoxicosis, congenital (X-linked). *Prevalence:* 0.2%. *Presentation:* Fatigue, dyspnoea, pulmonary oedema, RVF, emboli, AF, VT. *Signs:* ↑Pulse, ↓BP, ↑JVP, displaced and diffuse apex, S_3 gallop, mitral or tricuspid regurgitation (MR/TR), pleural effusion, oedema, jaundice, hepatomegaly, ascites. *Tests: Blood:* BNP (p137), ↓Na^+ indicates a poor prognosis. *CXR:* cardiomegaly, pulmonary oedema. *ECG:* tachycardia, non-specific T-wave changes, poor R-wave progression. *Echo:* globally dilated hypokinetic heart and low ejection fraction. Look for MR, TR, LV mural thrombus. ℞: Bed rest, diuretics, β-blockers, ACE-i, anticoagulation, biventricular pacing, ICDs, LVADs, transplantation. *Mortality:* Variable, eg 40% in 2yrs.

Hypertrophic cardiomyopathy (HCM) LV outflow tract (LVOT) obstruction from asymmetric septal hypertrophy. HCM is the leading cause of sudden cardiac death in the young. *Prevalence:* 0.2%. Autosomal dominant inheritance, but 50% are sporadic. 70% have mutations in genes encoding β-myosin, α-tropomyosin, and troponin T. May present at any age. Ask about family history of sudden death. *Symptoms and signs:* Sudden death may be the first manifestation of HCM in many patients (VF is amenable to implantable defibrillators), angina, dyspnoea, palpitation, syncope, CCF. Jerky pulse; *a* wave in JVP; double-apex beat; systolic thrill at lower left sternal edge; harsh ejection systolic murmur. *Tests:* • *ECG:* LVH; progressive T-wave inversion; deep Q waves (inferior + lateral leads); AF; WPW syndrome (p133); ventricular ectopics; VT. • *Echo:* asymmetrical septal hypertrophy; small LV cavity with hypercontractile posterior wall; midsystolic closure of aortic valve; systolic anterior movement of mitral valve. • MRI: see fig 3.16. • *Cardiac catheterization* helps assess: severity of gradient; coronary artery disease or mitral regurgitation, but may provoke VT. • Electrophysiological studies may be needed (eg if WPW, p133). • Exercise test ± Holter monitor (p125) to risk stratify. ℞: β-blockers or verapamil for symptoms (the aim is reducing ventricular contractility). Amiodarone (p130) for arrhythmias (AF, VT). Anticoagulate for paroxysmal AF or systemic emboli. Septal myomectomy (surgical or chemical (with alcohol) to ↓LV outflow tract gradient) is reserved for those with severe symptoms. Consider implantable defibrillator—use http://www.doc2do.com/hcm/webHCM.html to assess risk of sudden cardiac death. *Mortality:* 5.9%/yr if <14yrs; 2.5%/yr if >14yrs. *Poor prognostic factors:* age <14yrs or syncope at presentation; family history of HCM/sudden death.

Restrictive cardiomyopathy *Causes:* Idiopathic; amyloidosis; haemochromatosis; sarcoidosis; scleroderma; Löffler's eosinophilic endocarditis; endomyocardial fibrosis. *Presentation:* Is like constrictive pericarditis (p154). Features of RVF predominate: ↑JVP, with prominent *x* and *y* descents; hepatomegaly; oedema; ascites. *Diagnosis:* Echo, MRI, cardiac catheterization. ℞: Treat the cause.

Cardiac myxoma (figs 3.49, 3.50) Rare benign cardiac tumour. Prevalence ≤5/10 000, ♀:♂≈2:1. Usually sporadic, but may be familial (Carney complex: cardiac and cutaneous myxomas, skin pigmentation, endocrinopathy, etc., p223). It may mimic infective endocarditis (fever, weight loss, clubbing, ↑ESR, systemic emboli), or mitral stenosis (left atrial obstruction, AF). A 'tumour plop' may be heard, and signs may vary according to posture. *Tests:* Echo. ℞: Excision.

How to inflame the heart

Table 3.3 Causes of myocarditis

Idiopathic	50% of cases
Viral	Enteroviruses, adenoviruses, HHV6, EBV, CMV, influenza, hepatitis, mumps, rubeola, Coxsackie, polio, HIV, HSV
Bacterial	*Staph*, *Strep*, *Clostridia*, diphtheria, TB, meningococcus, *Mycoplasma*, brucellosis, psittacosis
Spirochaetes	Leptospirosis, syphilis, Lyme disease
Protozoa	Chagas' (p423), *Leishmania*, toxoplasmosis
Drugs	Cyclophosphamide, trastuzumab, penicillin, chloramphenicol, sulfonamides, methyldopa, spironolactone, phenytoin, carbamazepine
Toxins	Cocaine, lithium, alcohol, lead, arsenic
Immunological	SLE, sarcoid, Kawasaki, scleroderma, heart transplant rejection

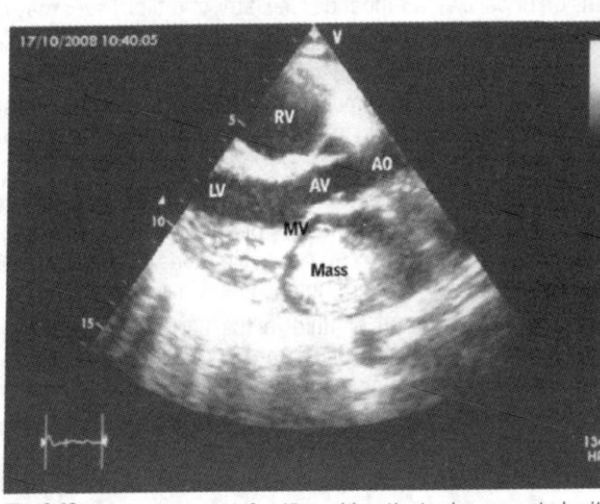

Fig 3.49 Echocardiogram of a 35-yr-old patient who presented with severe exertional dyspnoea and several episodes of syncope. Look at the large mass (cardiac myxoma) in left atrium. **Abbreviations:** RV: right ventricle; LV: left ventricle; AV: aortic valve; AO: aorta; MV: mitral valve.

Reproduced with permission from Hamid Reza Taghipour.

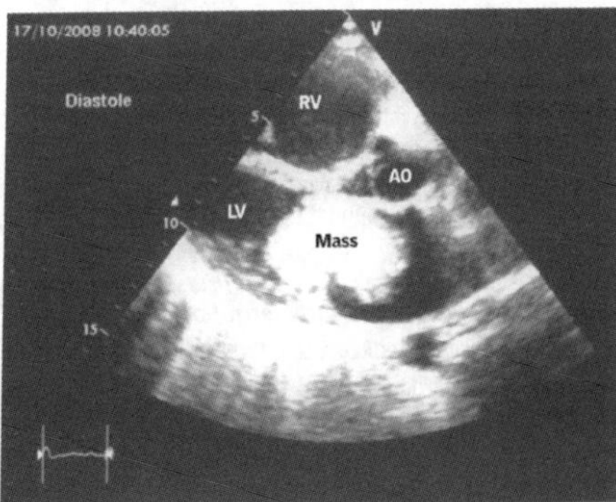

Fig 3.50 Echocardiogram of the same patient as fig 3.49 during diastole. Notice how the large mass of myxoma protrudes into the left ventricle during diastole, and obstructs the mitral valve almost completely. **Abbreviations:** RV: right ventricle; LV: left ventricle; AO: aorta.

Reproduced with permission from Hamid Reza Taghipour.

Pericardial diseases

Acute pericarditis This is inflammation of the pericardium.[68]
Causes: Idiopathic or secondary to:
- Viruses: eg coxsackie, echovirus, EBV, CMV, adenovirus, mumps, varicella, HIV.
- Bacteria: eg TB—commonest cause worldwide, Lyme disease, Q fever, pneumonia, rheumatic fever, Staphs, Streps, mycoplasma, legionella, MAI in HIV.
- Fungi and parasitic: v rare, usually in immunocompromised.
- Autoimmune: systemic autoimmune diseases eg SLE, RA; vasculitides eg Behçet, Takayasu; IBD; sarcoid; amyloid; Dressler's (p698).
- Drugs: eg procainamide, hydralazine, penicillin, isoniazid, chemotherapy.
- Metabolic: uraemia, hypothyroidism, anorexia nervosa.
- Others: trauma, surgery, malignancy, radiotherapy, MI, chronic heart failure.

Clinical features: Central chest pain worse on inspiration or lying flat ± relief by sitting forward. A pericardial friction rub (p46) may be heard. Look for evidence of a pericardial effusion or cardiac tamponade (see later in topic). Fever may occur.

Tests: *ECG* classically shows concave (saddle-shaped) ST segment elevation and PR depression, but may be normal or non-specific (10%); see fig 3.51. *Blood tests:* FBC, ESR, U&E, cardiac enzymes (NB: troponin may be raised); tests relating to possible aetiologies. Cardiomegaly on *CXR* may indicate a pericardial effusion. *Echo* (if suspected pericardial effusion). *CMR* and *CT* may show localized inflammation.

Treatment: NSAIDs or aspirin with gastric protection for 1-2weeks. Add colchicine 500mcg OD or BD for 3 months to reduce the risk of recurrence. Rest until symptoms resolve. Treat the cause. If not improving or autoimmune, consider steroids (may increase the risk of recurrence) or other immunosuppressive therapies.

Pericardial effusion Accumulation of fluid in the pericardial sac (normally 10-50mL).[68] *Causes:* Pericarditis, myocardial rupture (haemopericardium—surgical, stab wound, post-MI); aortic dissection; pericardium filling with pus; malignancy.

Clinical features: Dyspnoea, chest pain, signs of local structures being compressed—hiccoughs (phrenic N), nausea (diaphragm), bronchial breathing at left base (Ewart's sign: compressed left lower lobe). Muffled heart sounds. Look for signs of cardiac tamponade (below).

Diagnosis: *CXR* shows an enlarged, globular heart if effusion >300mL; fig 3.14. *ECG* shows low-voltage QRS complexes and may have alternating QRS morphologies (electrical alternans). *Echocardiography* shows an echo-free zone surrounding the heart.

Management: Treat the cause. Pericardiocentesis may be *diagnostic* (suspected bacterial pericarditis) or *therapeutic* (cardiac tamponade). See p773. Send pericardial fluid for culture, ZN stain/TB culture, and cytology.

Constrictive pericarditis The heart is encased in a rigid pericardium.[68]
Causes: Often unknown (UK); elsewhere TB, or after *any* pericarditis.

Clinical features: These are mainly of right heart failure with ↑JVP (with prominent *x* and *y* descents, p43); Kussmaul's sign (JVP rising paradoxically with inspiration); soft, diffuse apex beat; quiet heart sounds; S_3; diastolic pericardial knock, hepatosplenomegaly, ascites, and oedema.

Tests: *CXR:* small heart ± pericardial calcification. *CT/MRI*—helps distinguish from restrictive cardiomyopathy. *Echo. Cardiac catheterization.*

Management: Surgical excision. Medical ℞ to address the cause and symptoms.

Cardiac tamponade A pericardial effusion that raises intrapericardial pressure, reducing ventricular filling and thus dropping cardiac output.[68] ΔΔ Can lead rapidly to cardiac arrest.

Signs: ↑Pulse, ↓BP, pulsus paradoxus, ↑JVP, Kussmaul's sign, muffled S_1 and S_2.

Diagnosis: Beck's triad: falling BP; rising JVP; muffled heart sounds. *ECG:* low-voltage QRS ± electrical alternans. *Echo* is diagnostic: echo-free zone (>2cm, or >1cm if acute) around the heart ± diastolic collapse of right atrium and right ventricle.

Management: Seek expert help. The pericardial effusion needs urgent drainage (p773). Send fluid for culture, ZN stain/TB culture, and cytology.

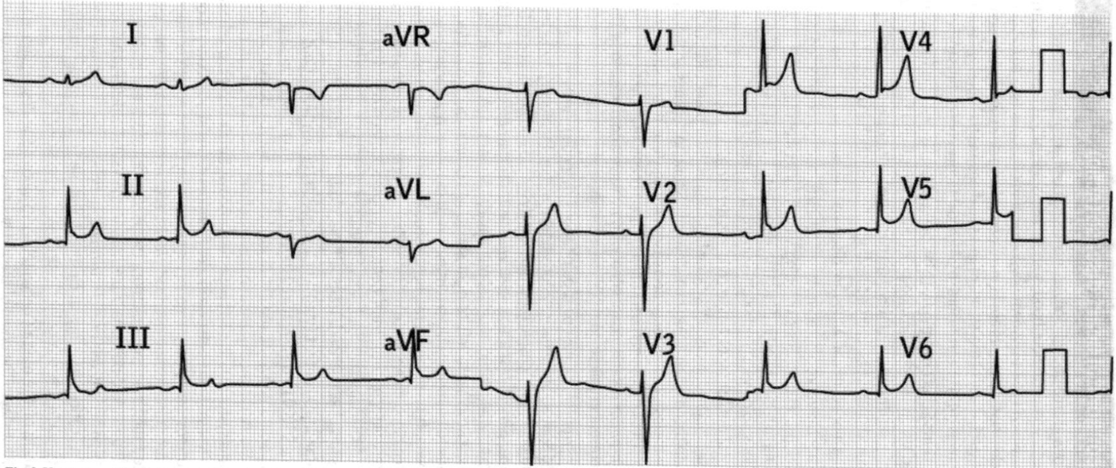

Fig 3.51 Pericarditis. Note the widespread 'saddle-shaped' ST elevation—particularly clear in V_5 and V_6.

Adult congenital heart disease (ACHD)

This is a growing area of cardiology as increasing numbers of children with congenital heart defects survive to adulthood, sometimes as a result of complex restructuring procedures which have their own physiological implications (see BOX 'Patients with one ventricle'). ACHD[69] patients are at increased risk of many conditions described elsewhere, for which many of the 'standard' investigations and therapies will apply: including arrhythmias (p124), heart failure (p134), and infective endocarditis (p150).

Investigations Echocardiography (± bubble contrast) is first line. Increasingly, cardiac CT and MR are used to provide precise anatomical and functional information. Cardiac catheterization generates data on oxygen saturation and pressure in different vessels and chambers. Exercise testing assesses functional capacity.

A few of the more common ACHDs are discussed below:

Bicuspid aortic valve These work well at birth and go undetected. Many eventually develop aortic stenosis (needing valve replacement) ± aortic regurgitation predisposing to IE/SBE ± aortic dilatation/dissection. Intense exercise may accelerate complications, so do yearly echocardiograms on affected athletes.[70]

Atrial septal defect (ASD) A hole connects the atria.

- *Ostium secundum* defects: 80% cases; hole high in the septum; often asymptomatic until adulthood when a L→R shunt develops. Shunting depends on the compliance of the ventricles. LV compliance decreases with age (esp. if ↑BP), so augmenting L→R shunting; hence dyspnoea/heart failure, typically aged 40–60yrs.
- *Ostium primum* defects: associated with AV valve anomalies, eg in Down's syndrome; present in childhood.

Signs and symptoms: Chest pain, palpitations, dyspnoea. Arrhythmias incl. AF; ↑JVP; wide, fixed split S_2; pulmonary systolic flow murmur. Pulmonary hypertension may cause pulmonary or tricuspid regurgitation, dyspnoea and haemoptysis. ↑Frequency of migraine. *Simple tests:* ECG: RBBB with LAD (primum defect) or RAD (secundum defect). CXR: small aortic knuckle, pulmonary plethora, atrial enlargement. *Complications:* • Reversal of left-to-right shunt, ie *Eisenmenger's complex*: initial L→R shunt leads to pulmonary hypertension which increases right heart pressures until they exceed left heart pressures, hence shunt reversal. This causes cyanosis as deoxygenated blood enters systemic circulation. • Paradoxical emboli eg causing CVAs (vein→artery via ASD; rare). *Treatment:* May close spontaenously. If not, primum defects are usually closed in childhood. Secundum defects should be closed if symptomatic or signs of RV overload. Transcatheter closure is more common than surgical.

Ventricular septal defect (VSD) A hole connects the ventricles. *Causes:* Congenital (prevalence 2:1000 births); acquired (post-MI). *Symptoms:* May present with severe heart failure in infancy, or remain asymptomatic and be detected incidentally in later life. *Signs:* Classically, a harsh pansystolic murmur is heard at the left sternal edge, with a systolic thrill, ± left parasternal heave. Smaller holes, which are haemodynamically less significant, give louder murmurs. Signs of pulmonary hypertension. *Complications:* AR, IE/SBE, pulmonary hypertension, Eisenmenger's complex (above), heart failure from volume overload. *Tests:* ECG: normal, LAD, LVH, RVH. CXR: normal heart size ± mild pulmonary plethora (small VSD) or cardiomegaly, large pulmonary arteries and marked pulmonary plethora (large VSD). Cardiac catheter: step up in O_2 saturation in right ventricle. *Treatment:* Initially medical as many close spontaneously. Indications for surgical closure: failed medical therapy, symptomatic VSD, shunt >3:1, SBE/IE. Endovascular closure may be possible.[71]

Coarctation of the aorta Congenital narrowing of the descending aorta; usually occurs just distal to the origin of the left subclavian artery. More common in boys. *Associations:* Bicuspid aortic valve; Turner's syndrome. *Signs:* Radiofemoral delay; weak femoral pulse; ↑BP; scapular bruit; systolic murmur (best heard over the left scapula); cold feet. *Complications:* Heart failure from high afterload; IE; intracerebral haemorrhage. *Tests:* CT or MRI-aortogram; CXR may show rib notching as blood diverts down intercostal arteries to reach the lower body, causing these vessels to dilate and erode local rib bone. *Treatment:* Surgery, or balloon dilatation ± stenting.

Tetralogy of Fallot See p157.

Fallot's tetralogy: what the non-specialist needs to know

Tetralogy of Fallot (TOF) is the most common cyanotic congenital heart disorder (prevalence: 3–6 per 10 000). It is also the most common cyanotic heart defect that survives to adulthood, accounting for 10% of all ACHD.[72] It is believed to be due to abnormalities in separation of the truncus arteriosus into the aorta and pulmonary arteries early in gestation (fig 3.52).

The 'tetralogy' of features are:

1. Ventricular septal defect (VSD).
2. Pulmonary stenosis.
3. Right ventricular hypertrophy.
4. The aorta overrides the VSD, accepting right heart blood.

A few patients also have an ASD, which makes up the pentad of Fallot.

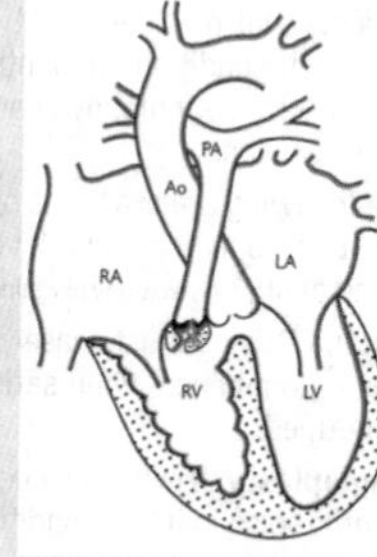

Fig 3.52 Tetralogy of Fallot.
Reproduced from Thorne *et al.*, *Adult Congenital Heart Disease*, 2009, with permission from Oxford University Press.

Presentation: Severity of illness depends greatly on the degree of pulmonary stenosis. Infants may be acyanotic at birth, with a pulmonary stenosis murmur as the only initial finding. Gradually (especially after closure of the ductus arteriosus) they become cyanotic due to decreasing flow of blood to the lungs and increasing right-to-left flow across the VSD. During a hypoxic spell, the child becomes restless and agitated. Toddlers may squat, which is typical of TOF, as it increases peripheral vascular resistance, thereby decreasing the degree of right to left shunt. Adult patients are often asymptomatic. In the unoperated adult patient, cyanosis is common, although extreme cyanosis or squatting is uncommon. In repaired patients, late symptoms include exertional dyspnoea, palpitations, clubbing, RV failure, syncope, and even sudden death. *Investigations: ECG* shows RV hypertrophy with a right bundle-branch block. *CXR* may be normal, or show the hallmark of TOF, which is the classic boot-shaped heart (fig 3.53). *Echocardiography* can show the anatomy as well as the degree of stenosis. *Cardiac CT* and *cardiac MRI* can give valuable information for planning the surgery.[73]

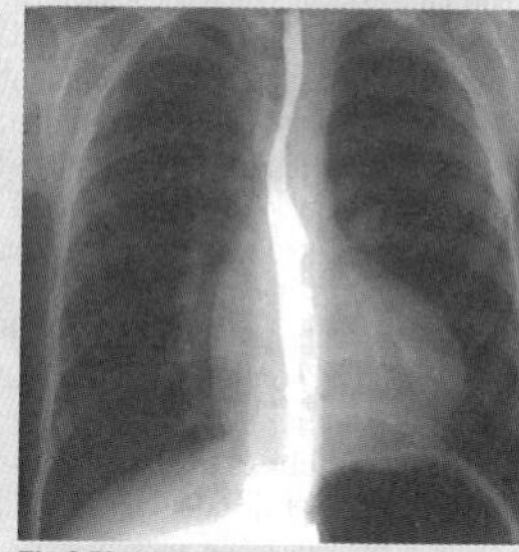

Fig 3.53 Boot-shaped heart.
Courtesy of Dr Edward Singleton.

Management: Surgery is usually done before 1yr of age, with closure of the VSD and correction of pulmonary stenosis.

Prognosis: Without surgery, mortality rate is ~95% by age 20. After repair, 85% of patients survive to 35yrs. Common problems in adulthood include pulmonary regurgitation, causing RV dilatation and failure; RV outflow tract obstruction; AR; LV dysfunction; and arrhythmias.

Patients with one ventricle

Many patients born with single-ventricle hearts (eg hypoplastic left heart syndrome) will undergo a Fontan procedure. This results in systemic venous blood flowing directly into the pulmonary arteries and the single ventricle being used to pump oxygenated blood into the aorta. The lack of a right heart results in many of the signs and symptoms of right heart failure and puts the patient at risk of rapid cardiac decompensation. ►►When looking after these patients, seek advice from specialist ACHD centres.

Driving and the heart

UK licences are inscribed 'You are required by law to inform Drivers Medical Branch, DVLA, Swansea SA99 1AT at once if you have any disability (physical or medical), which is, or may become likely to affect your fitness as a driver, unless you do not expect it to last more than 3 months'. It is the responsibility of drivers to inform the DVLA (the UK Driving and Vehicle Licensing Authority), and that of their doctors to advise patients that medical conditions[74] (and drugs) may affect their ability to drive and for which conditions patients should inform the DVLA. Drivers should also inform their insurance company of any condition disclosed to the DVLA. If in doubt, ask your defence union.

The following are examples of the guidance for holders of *standard* licences; different rules apply for group 2 vehicle licence-holders (eg lorries, buses). More can be found at https://www.gov.uk/guidance/cardiovascular-disorders-assessing-fitness-to-drive.

Angina Driving must cease when symptoms occur at rest or with emotion. Driving may recommence when satisfactory symptom control is achieved. DVLA need not be notified.

Angioplasty Driving must cease for 1wk, and may recommence thereafter provided no other disqualifying condition. DVLA need not be notified.

MI If successfully treated with angioplasty, cease driving for 1 week provided urgent intervention not planned and LVEF (left ventricular ejection fraction) >40%, and no other disqualifying condition. Otherwise, driving must cease for 1 month. DVLA need not be notified.

Dysrhythmias Including sinoatrial disease, AF/flutter, atrioventricular conduction defects, and narrow or broad complex tachycardias. Driving must cease if the dysrhythmia has caused or is likely to cause incapacity. Driving may recommence 4wks after successful control provided there is no other disqualifying condition.

Pacemaker implant Stop driving for 1wk, the patient must notify the DVLA.

Implanted cardioverter/defibrillator The licence is subject to annual review. Driving may occur when these criteria can be met:

- 6 months have passed since ICD implanted for secondary prevention.
- 1 month has passed since ICD implanted for primary prophylaxis.
- The device has not administered therapy (shock and/or symptomatic antitachycardia pacing) within the last 6 months (except during testing).
- No therapy (shock) in the last 2 years has been accompanied by *incapacity* (whether caused by the device or arrhythmia)—unless this was a result of device malfunction which has been corrected for at least 1 month or steps have been taken to avoid recurrence (eg ablation) which have been successful for at least 6 months.
- A period of 1 month off driving must occur following any revision of the device (generator and/or electrode) or alteration of antiarrhythmics.
- The device is subject to regular review with interrogation.
- There is no other disqualifying condition.

Syncope *Simple faint:* No restriction. *Unexplained syncope:* With probable cardiac aetiology—4wks off driving if cause identified and treated; otherwise 6 months off. Loss of consciousness or altered awareness associated with signs of seizure requires 6 months off driving. If the patient is known to be epileptic or has had another such episode in the preceeding 5yrs, they must abstain from driving for 1yr. See driving and epilepsy (BOX). Patients who have had a single episode of loss of consciousness with no cause found despite neurological and cardiac investigations, must abstain from driving for 6 months.

Hypertension Driving may continue unless treatment causes unacceptable side-effects. DVLA need not be notified.

Other conditions: UK DVLA states it must be informed if a driver suffers from medical conditions including:

- Epilepsy (the patient must have had at least two seizures in the last 5yrs). An epileptic patient who has suffered an epileptic attack while awake must not drive for 1yr from the date of the attack. Patients who have seizures that do not affect their consciousness (eg simple partial seizures) or seizures only during sleep may be allowed to drive. Being allowed to drive is conditional on the patient following medical advice and there not being reason to believe they are at high risk of further seizures.
- TIA or stroke. These patients should not drive for at least 1 month. There is no need to inform the DVLA unless there is residual neurological defect after 1 month, eg visual field defect. If TIAs have been recurrent and frequent, a 3-month period free of attacks may be required.
- Sudden attacks or disabling giddiness, fainting, or blackouts.
- Chronic neurological conditions including multiple sclerosis, Parkinson's (any 'freezing' or on-off effects), and motor neuron diseases.
- Severe mental disorders; including serious memory problems and severe psychiatric illness. Those with dementia should only drive if the condition is mild (do not rely on armchair judgements: on-the-road trials are better). Encourage relatives to contact DVLA if a dementing relative should not be driving. GPs may desire to breach confidentiality (the GMC approves) and inform DVLA of demented or psychotic patients (tel. 01792 783686). Many elderly drivers (~1 in 3) who die in accidents are found to have Alzheimer's.
- A pacemaker, defibrillator, or antiventricular tachycardia device fitted.
- Diabetes controlled by insulin or tablets. The main issues which may result in driving bans are impaired awareness of hypoglycaemia and impaired vision.
- Angina while driving.
- Any type of brain surgery, brain tumour. Severe head injury involving inpatient treatment at hospital.
- Continuing/permanent difficulty in the use of arms or legs which affects ability to control a vehicle.
- Dependence on or misuse of alcohol, illicit drugs, or chemical substances in the past 3yrs (do not include drink/driving offences).
- Any visual disability which affects *both* eyes (do not declare short/long sight or colour blindness).

Vision (new drivers) should be 6/9 on Snellen's scale in the better eye and 6/12 on the Snellen scale in the other eye, wearing glasses or contact lenses if needed, and 3/60 in each eye without glasses or contact lenses.

The above-listed rules apply to standard licences only, for group 2 entitlement (eg HGV drivers) see www.dvla.gov.uk/medical/ataglance.aspx.

4 Chest medicine

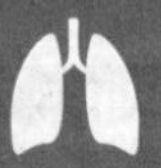

Contents

BRITISH MEDICAL JOURNAL

LONDON SATURDAY OCTOBER 30 1948

STREPTOMYCIN TREATMENT OF PULMONARY TUBERCULOSIS

A MEDICAL RESEARCH COUNCIL INVESTIGATION

The following gives the short-term results of a controlled investigation into the effects of streptomycin on one type of pulmonary tuberculosis. The inquiry was planned and directed by the Streptomycin in Tuberculosis Trials Committee, composed of the following members: Dr. Geoffrey Marshall (chairman), Professor J. W. S. Blacklock, Professor C. Cameron, Professor N. B. Capon, Dr. R. Cruickshank, Professor J. H. Gaddum, Dr. F. R. G. Heaf, Professor A. Bradford Hill, Dr. L. E. Houghton, Dr. J. Clifford Hoyle, Professor H. Raistrick, Dr. J. G. Scadding, Professor W. H. Tytler, Professor G. S. Wilson, and Dr. P. D'Arcy Hart (secretary). The centres at which the work was carried out and the specialists in charge of patients and pathological work were as follows:

Fig 4.1 In 1948, the Medical Research Council published a landmark paper in the *BMJ* about streptomycin as a treatment for pulmonary TB. The paper was regarded as a milestone in the history of clinical trials and set a precedent for the use of randomization in controlled trials. Before this, bed rest alone had been standard treatment for patients with pulmonary TB. After the successes of penicillin, there was excitement in the discovery that streptomycin proved effective against the tubercle bacilli. Patients aged 15 to 30 with 'acute progressive bilateral pulmonary tuberculosis of presumably recent origin, bacteriologically proved and unsuitable for collapse therapy' were entered into the trial. The streptomycin and bed rest group did better initially but the development of resistance was soon recognized. This was a new phenomenon which had not then been seen with penicillin. This led to the notion that combination therapies were needed to overcome TB drug resistance. The 'Edinburgh Method', described in 1957, advocated the use of triple therapy.

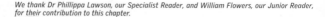

We thank Dr Phillippa Lawson, our Specialist Reader, and William Flowers, our Junior Reader, for their contribution to this chapter.

Respiratory health

The lungs provide a vital physiological function in allowing gas exchange, but are also at the vanguard of a constant battle between host, pathogens, and pollutants. Respiratory medicine exemplifies how careful epidemiology, science, and randomized controlled trials have revolutionized our understanding of common diseases, leading to preventative measures and effective treatments. However, the importance of poverty and general improvements in public health cannot be underestimated. Rates of TB in the UK declined well before the introduction of BCG vaccination and streptomycin, largely due to improvements in sanitation and less dense living conditions. Public health campaigns and taxation have helped lower smoking rates, although reductions in lung cancer will lag behind for many years.

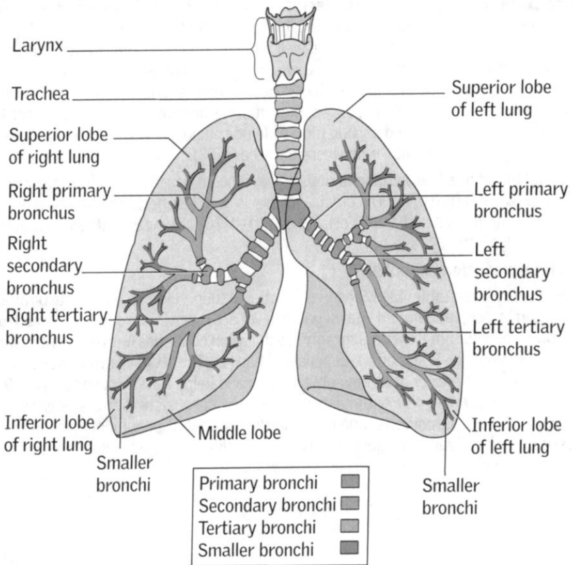

Fig 4.2 Segmental anatomy of the lungs and main bronchi. The left lung has two lobes and the right has three.

Bedside tests in chest medicine

There is no substitute for careful history taking and examination in making the 'correct' diagnosis. Tests should help clarify and assess severity. When examining the chest think about the anatomy, and the location of pathology (fig 4.2).

Sputum examination Collect a good sample; if necessary ask a physiotherapist to help. Note the appearance: clear and colourless (chronic bronchitis), yellow-green or brown (pulmonary infection), red (haemoptysis), black (smoke, coal dust), or frothy white-pink (pulmonary oedema). Send the sample to the laboratory for microscopy, culture/sensitivity. If indicated, ask for ZN stain, and PCR.

Peak expiratory flow (PEF) Measured by a maximal forced expiration through a peak flow meter. It correlates well with the forced expiratory volume in 1 second (FEV_1) & is used as an estimate of airway calibre in asthma, but is effort-dependent.

Pulse oximetry Allows non-invasive assessment of peripheral O_2 saturation (SpO_2). Useful for monitoring those who are acutely ill or at risk of deterioration. Target oxygen saturations are usually 94–98% in a well patient or 88–92% in those with certain pre-exisiting lung pathology (eg COPD). Oxygen saturation of <92% in a normally well person is a serious sign and arterial blood gases (ABGs) should be checked. Causes of erroneous readings: poor perfusion, movement, skin pigmentation, nail varnish, dyshaemoglobinaemias, and carbon monoxide poisoning. As with any bedside test, be sceptical, and check ABGs, whenever indicated (p188).

Arterial blood gas (ABG) analysis Heparinized blood is usually taken from the radial or femoral artery (see p771). The brachial artery is used less because of median nerve proximity and it is an end artery. pH, P_aO_2, P_aCO_2, HCO_3 are measured using an automated analyser.

ABG interpretation See pp188–9.

Spirometry (See table 4.1) Measures functional lung volumes. Forced expiratory volume in 1s (FEV_1) and forced vital capacity (FVC) are measured from a full forced expiration into a spirometer (Vitalograph®); exhalation continues until no more breath can be exhaled. FEV_1 is less effort-dependent than PEF. The FEV_1/FVC ratio gives a good estimate of the severity of airflow obstruction; and helps classify COPD severity. *Obstructive defect:* (fig 4.3) Asthma, bronchiectasis, COPD, cystic fibrosis. *Restrictive defect:* Fibrosis, sarcoidosis, pneumoconiosis, interstitial pneumonias, connective tissue diseases, pleural effusion, obesity, kyphoscoliosis, neuromuscular problems.

Table 4.1 Spirometry results (data source NICE COPD 2010 guidelines)

	FEV_1	FVC	FEV_1/FVC ratio
Normal	>80% predicted	>80% predicted	75-80%
Restrictive	<80% predicted	<80% predicted	>70% normal
Obstructive	<80% predicted	Normal or low	<70% predicted

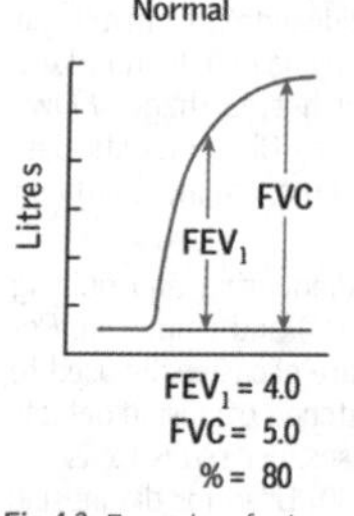

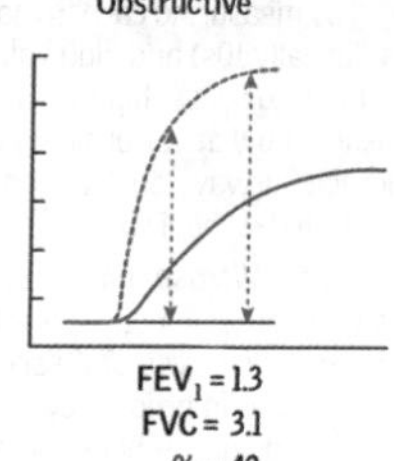

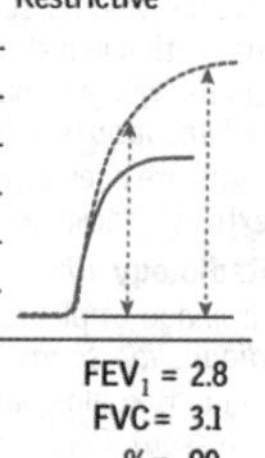

Fig 4.3 Examples of spirograms.

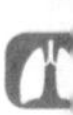

Further investigations in chest medicine

Lung function tests PEF, FEV_1, FVC (see p162). *Total lung capacity* (TLC) and *residual volume* (RV) are useful in distinguishing obstructive and restrictive diseases (see fig 4.4). TLC and RV are increased in obstructive airways disease and reduced in restrictive lung diseases and musculoskeletal abnormalities. The *gas transfer* coefficient (KCO) represents the carbon monoxide diffusing capacity (DLCO) corrected for alveolar volume. It is calculated by measuring carbon monoxide uptake from a single inspiration in a standard time (usually 10s) and lung volume by helium dilution. Low in emphysema and interstitial lung disease, high in alveolar haemorrhage.[1] *Flow-volume loop* (see fig 4.5) measures flow at various lung volumes. Characteristic patterns are seen with intra-thoracic airways obstruction (asthma, emphysema) and extra-thoracic airways obstruction (tracheal stenosis).

Radiology *Chest x-ray:* See p722. *Ultrasound:* Used in diagnosing and guiding drainage of pleural effusions (particularly loculated effusions) and empyema. *Radionuclide scans: Ventilation/perfusion* (V/Q, p738) *scans* are occasionally used to diagnose pulmonary embolism (PE), eg in pregnancy (unmatched perfusion defects are seen). *Bone scans* are used to diagnose bone metastases. *PET scans* to assess cancer and inflammation. *Computed tomography:* (CT, p730) Used for diagnosing and staging lung cancer, imaging the hila, mediastinum, and pleura, and guiding biopsies. Thin (1–1.5mm) section high-resolution CT (HRCT) is used in the diagnosis of interstitial lung disease, emphysema, and bronchiectasis. CT pulmonary angiography (CTPA) is used in the diagnosis of PE. *Pulmonary angiography:* Now rarely used for diagnosing pulmonary hypertension.

Fibreoptic bronchoscopy Performed under local anaesthetic via the nose or mouth. *Diagnostic indications:* Suspected lung carcinoma, slowly resolving pneumonia, pneumonia in the immunosuppressed, interstitial lung disease. Bronchoalveolar lavage fluid may be sent to the lab for microscopy, culture, and cytology. Mucosal abnormalities may be brushed (cytology) and biopsied (histopathology). *Therapeutic indications:* Aspiration of mucus plugs causing lobar collapse, removal of foreign bodies, stenting or treating tumours, eg laser. *Pre-procedure investigations:* FBC, coagulation, CXR, CT, spirometry, pulse oximetry, and ABG (if indicated). *Complications:* Hypoxia, bleeding, pneumothorax (fig 16.43, p749). *Diagnostic sensitivity* for cancer 50–90%, depends on tumour location; gene profiling of cell sample may improve this.[2] May also be used to deliver an ultrasound probe (endobronchial ultrasound), and treatments—eg stents, or cryotherapy.

Bronchoalveolar lavage (BAL) is performed at the time of bronchoscopy by instilling and aspirating a known volume of warmed, buffered 0.9% saline into the distal airway. *Diagnostic indications:* Suspected malignancy, pneumonia, in the immunosuppressed (especially HIV), bronchiectasis, suspected TB (if sputum negative), interstitial lung diseases (eg sarcoidosis, extrinsic allergic alveolitis, histiocytosis X). *Therapeutic indications:* alveolar proteinosis.[1] *Complications:* Hypoxia (give supplemental O_2), transient fever, transient CXR shadow, infection (rare).

Lung biopsy May be performed in several ways. *Percutaneous needle biopsy* is performed under radiological guidance and is useful for peripheral lung and pleural lesions. *Transbronchial biopsy* performed at bronchoscopy may help in diagnosing interstitial lung diseases, eg sarcoidosis, idiopathic pulmonary fibrosis. *Alternatives*: If unsuccessful, consider open lung biopsy or video-assisted thoracoscopy.

Surgical procedures are performed under general anaesthetic. *Rigid bronchoscopy* provides a wide lumen, enables larger mucosal biopsies, control of bleeding, and removal of foreign bodies. *Mediastinoscopy* and *mediastinotomy* enable examination and biopsy of the mediastinal lymph nodes/lesions. *Thoracoscopy* allows examination and biopsy of pleural lesions, drainage of pleural effusions, and talc pleurodesis and pleurectomy.

1 Pulmonary alveolar proteinosis causes cough, dyspnoea, and restrictive spirometry. It is caused by accumulation of surfactant-derived acidophilic phospholipid/protein compounds which fill alveoli and distal bronchioles. Diagnosis may require lung biopsy. Cause: primary genetic or antibody problem, or secondary to inflammation caused by inhaling silica, aluminium, or titanium.[3]

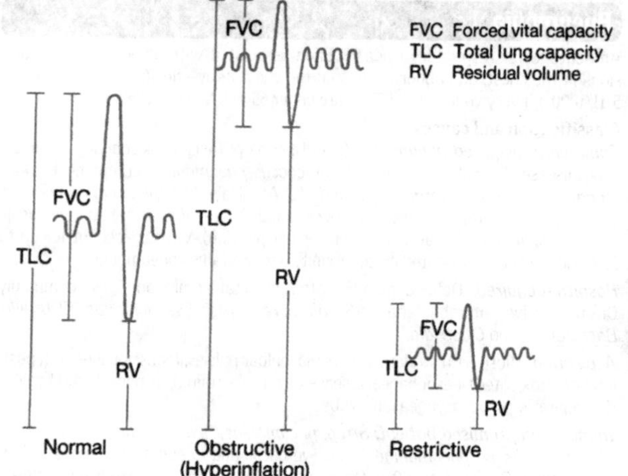

Fig 4.4 Lung volumes: physiological and pathological.

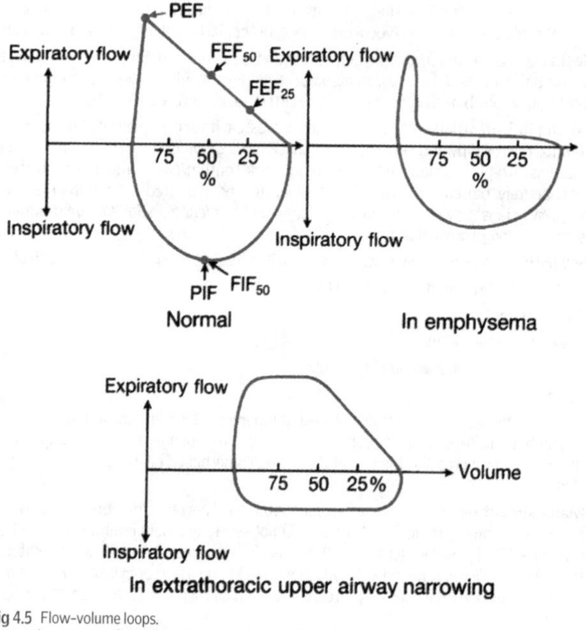

Fig 4.5 Flow-volume loops.
PEF=peak expiratory flow; FEF_{50}=forced expiratory flow at 50% TLC; FEF_{25}=forced expiratory flow at 25% TLC; PIF=peak inspiratory flow; FIF_{50}=forced inspiratory flow at 50% TLC.

Pneumonia

An acute lower respiratory tract infection associated with fever, symptoms and signs in the chest, and abnormalities on the chest x-ray—fig 16.2, p723. Incidence: 5-11/1000, ↑ if very young or old (30% are under 65yrs). Mortality: ~21% in hospital.

Classification and causes

Community-acquired pneumonia: (CAP) May be primary or secondary to underlying disease. Typical organisms: *Streptococcus pneumoniae* (commonest), *Haemophilus influenzae, Moraxella catarrhalis.* Atypicals: *Mycoplasma pneumoniae, Staphylococcus aureus, Legionella* species, and *Chlamydia*. Gram-negative bacilli, *Coxiella burnetii* and anaerobes are rarer (?aspiration). Viruses account for up to 15%. Flu may be complicated by community-acquired MRSA pneumonia.

Hospital-acquired: Defined as >48h after hospital admission. Most commonly Gram-negative enterobacteria or *Staph. aureus*. Also *Pseudomonas, Klebsiella, Bacteroides*, and *Clostridia*.

Aspiration: Those with stroke, myasthenia, bulbar palsies, ↓consciousness (eg postictal or intoxicated), oesophageal disease (achalasia, reflux), or poor dental hygiene risk aspirating oropharyngeal anaerobes.

Immunocompromised patient: Strep. pneumoniae, H. influenzae, Staph. aureus, M. catarrhalis, M. pneumoniae, Gram −ve bacilli and *Pneumocystis jirovecii* (formerly named *P. carinii*, pp400–1). Other fungi, viruses (CMV, HSV), and mycobacteria.

Clinical features *Symptoms:* Fever, rigors, malaise, anorexia, dyspnoea, cough, purulent sputum, haemoptysis, and pleuritic pain. *Signs:* Pyrexia, cyanosis, confusion (can be the only sign in the elderly—may also be hypothermic), tachypnoea, tachycardia, hypotension, signs of consolidation (reduced expansion, dull percussion, ↑tactile vocal fremitus/vocal resonance, bronchial breathing), and a pleural rub.

Tests *Assess oxygenation:* oxygen saturation, p162 (ABGs if S_aO_2 <92% or severe pneumonia) and BP. *Blood tests:* FBC, U&E, LFT, CRP (GPs should consider a point of care CRP to guide antibiotic prescribing where LRTI is suspected, NICE 2014[4]).

CXR (fig 16.2, p723): lobar or multilobar infiltrates, cavitation, or pleural effusion. *Sputum* for microscopy and culture. *Urine:* check for *Legionella/Pneumococcal* urinary antigens. Atypical organism/viral serology (PCR sputum/BAL, complement fixation tests acutely, paired serology). *Pleural fluid* may be aspirated for culture. Respiratory physicians may consider *bronchoscopy* and *bronchoalveolar lavage* if patient is immunocompromised or on ITU.

Severity 'CURB-65' is a simple, validated severity scoring system.[5,6] 1 point for each of:

Confusion (abbreviated mental test ≤8)

Urea >7mmol/L

Respiratory rate ≥30/min

BP <90 systolic and/or 60mmHg diastolic)

Age ≥65.

0–1, PO antibiotic/home treatment; 2, hospital therapy; ≥3, severe pneumonia indicates mortality 15–40%—consider ITU. It may 'underscore' the young—use clinical judgement. Other features increasing the risk of death are: comorbidity; bilateral/multilobar; P_aO_2 <8kPa.

Management ➤➤p816. *Antibiotics*—refer to your local hospital antibiotic policy. When none exists, consult table 4.2. If pneumonia not severe and not vomiting (CURB-65 1–2) give PO antibiotic; severe (CURB-65 >2) give IV. *Oxygen:* keep P_aO_2 >8.0 and/or saturation ≥94%. IV *fluids* (anorexia, dehydration, shock) and VTE prophylaxis. *Analgesia* if pleurisy. Consider ITU if shock, hypercapnia, or remains hypoxic. *Follow-up:* at 6 weeks (±CXR).

Complications (See p170.) Pleural effusion, empyema, lung abscess, respiratory failure, septicaemia, brain abscess, pericarditis, myocarditis, cholestatic jaundice. Repeat CRP and CXR in patients not improving to look for progression/complications.

Table 4.2 Empirical treatment of pneumonia (check local policy)

Clinical setting	Organisms	Antibiotic (further dosage details: pp386–7)
Community-acquired		
Mild not previously ℞ *CURB 0–1*	*Streptococcus pneumoniae* *Haemophilus influenzae*	Oral amoxicillin 500mg-1g/8h or clarithromycin 500mg/12h or doxycycline 200mg loading then 100mg/day (initially 5-day course)
Moderate *CURB 2*	*Streptococcus pneumoniae* *Haemophilus influenzae* *Mycoplasma pneumoniae*	Oral amoxicillin 500mg-1g/8h + clarithromycin 500mg/12h or doxycycline 200mg loading then 100mg/12h If IV required: amoxicillin 500mg/8h + clarithromycin 500mg/12h (7-day course)
Severe *CURB >3*	As above	Co-amoxiclav 1.2g/8h IV or cephalosporin IV (eg cefuroxime 1.5g/8h IV) AND clarithromycin 500mg/12h IV (7 days)
		Add flucloxacillin ± rifampicin if *Staph* suspected; vancomycin (or teicoplanin) if MRSA suspected. Treat for 10d (14-21d if *Staph*, *Legionella*, or Gram −ve enteric bacteria suspected)
	Panton-Valentine Leukocidin-producing *Staph. aureus* (PVL-SA)	Seek urgent help. Consider adding IV linezolid, clindamycin, and rifampicin
Atypical	*Legionella pneumophilia*	Fluoroquinolone combined with clarithromycin, or rifampicin, if severe. See p168
	Chlamydophila species	Tetracycline
	Pneumocystis jirovecii	High-dose co-trimoxazole (pp400–1)
Hospital-acquired		
	Gram-negative bacilli *Pseudomonas* Anaerobes	Aminoglycoside IV + antipseudomonal penicillin IV or 3rd-generation cephalosporin IV (p387)
Aspiration		
	Streptococcus pneumoniae Anaerobes	Cephalosporin IV + metronidazole IV
Neutropenic patients		
	Gram-positive cocci Gram-negative bacilli	Aminoglycoside IV + antipseudomonal penicillin IV or 3rd-generation cephalosporin IV
	Fungi (p177)	Consider antifungals after 48h

Pneumococcal vaccine

At-risk groups:

- All adults ≥65yrs old.
- Chronic heart, liver, renal, or lung conditions.
- Diabetes mellitus not controlled by diet.
- Immunosuppression, eg ↓spleen function, AIDS, or on chemotherapy or prednisolone >20mg/d, cochlear implant, occupation risk (eg welders), CSF fluid leaks. Vaccinate every 5yrs.

CI: Pregnancy, lactation, ↑T°, previous anaphylaxis to vaccine or one of its components.

Specific pneumonias

Pneumococcal pneumonia The commonest bacterial pneumonia. Affects all ages, but is commoner in the elderly, alcoholics, post-splenectomy, immunosuppressed, and patients with chronic heart failure or pre-existing lung disease. *Clinical features:* Fever, pleurisy, herpes labialis. CXR shows lobar consolidation. If mod/severe check for urinary antigen. *Treatment:* amoxicillin, benzylpenicillin, or cephalosporin.

Staphylococcal pneumonia May complicate influenza infection or occur in the young, elderly, intravenous drug users, or patients with underlying disease, eg leukaemia, lymphoma, cystic fibrosis (CF). It causes a bilateral cavitating bronchopneumonia. *Treatment:* flucloxacillin ± rifampicin, MRSA: contact lab; consider vancomycin.

***Klebsiella* pneumonia** Rare. Occurs in elderly, diabetics, and alcoholics. Causes a cavitating pneumonia, particularly of the upper lobes, often drug resistant. *Treatment:* cefotaxime or imipenem.

Pseudomonas A common pathogen in bronchiectasis and CF. It also causes hospital-acquired infections, particularly on ITU or after surgery. *Treatment:* anti-pseudomonal penicillin, ceftazidime, meropenem, or ciprofloxacin + aminoglycoside. Consider dual therapy to minimize resistance.

Mycoplasma pneumoniae Occurs in epidemics about every 4yrs. It presents insidiously with flu-like symptoms (headache, myalgia, arthralgia) followed by a dry cough. CXR: reticular-nodular shadowing or patchy consolidation often of one lower lobe, and worse than signs suggest. *Diagnosis:* PCR sputum or serology. Cold agglutinins may cause an autoimmune haemolytic anaemia. *Complications:* Skin rash (erythema multiforme, fig 12.22, p563), Stevens-Johnson syndrome, meningoencephalitis or myelitis; Guillain-Barré syndrome. *Treatment:* Clarithromycin (500mg/12h) or doxycycline (200mg loading then 100mg OD) or a fluroquinolone (eg ciprofloxacin or norfloxacin).

Legionella pneumophila Colonizes water tanks kept at <60°C (eg hotel air-conditioning and hot water systems) causing outbreaks. Flu-like symptoms (fever, malaise, myalgia) precede a dry cough and dyspnoea. Extra-pulmonary features include anorexia, D&V, hepatitis, renal failure, confusion, and coma. CXR shows bi-basal consolidation. Blood tests may show lymphopenia, hyponatraemia, and deranged LFTs. Urinalysis may show haematuria. *Diagnosis:* Urine antigen/culture. *Treatment:* fluoroquinolone for 2-3wks or clarithromycin (p387). 10% mortality.

Chlamydophila pneumoniae The commonest chlamydial infection. Person-to-person spread, biphasic illness: pharyngitis, hoarseness, otitis, followed by pneumonia. *Diagnosis: Chlamydophila* complement fixation test, PCR invasive samples.[7] *Treatment:* Doxycycline or clarithromycin. ***Chlamydophila psittaci*** Causes psittacosis, an ornithosis acquired from infected birds (typically parrots). Symptoms include headache, fever, dry cough, lethargy, arthralgia, anorexia, and D&V. Extra-pulmonary features are legion but rare, eg meningo-encephalitis, infective endocarditis, hepatitis, nephritis, rash, splenomegaly. CXR shows patchy consolidation. *Diagnosis: Chlamydophila* serology. *Treatment:* doxycycline or clarithromycin.

Viral pneumonia Influenza commonest (p396 and BOX), but 'swine flu' (H1N1) is now considered seasonal and covered by the annual 'flu vaccine. Others: measles, CMV, varicella zoster.

***Pneumocystis* pneumonia** Causes pneumonia in the immunosuppressed (eg HIV). The organism responsible was previously called *Pneumocystis carinii*, and now called *Pneumocystis jirovecii*.[8] It presents with a dry cough, exertional dyspnoea, ↓P_aO_2, fever, bilateral crepitations. CXR may be normal or show bilateral perihilar interstitial shadowing. *Diagnosis:* Visualization of the organism in induced sputum, bronchoalveolar lavage, or in a lung biopsy specimen. *Drugs:* High-dose co-trimoxazole (pp400–1), or pentamidine by slow IVI for 2-3 weeks (p401). Steroids are beneficial if severe hypoxaemia. Prophylaxis is indicated if the CD4 count is <200×10⁶/L or after the 1st attack.[9]

Avian influenza

Avian influenza A viruses rarely infect humans and most follow direct or close contact with infected poultry. The issue remains a public health priority because of the ability of the virus to mutate. Symptoms range from conjunctivitis to influenza-like illness (low pathogenic forms) to severe respiratory illness and multi-organ failure (highly pathogenic forms). H7N9 and H5N1 have been responsible for most human illnesses worldwide. ►Suspect avian flu if fever (>38°C), chest signs or consolidation on CXR, or life-threatening infection, and contact with poultry or others with similar symptoms.[10] NB: D&V, abdominal pain, pleuritic pain, and bleeding from the nose and gums are reported to be an early feature in some patients.[11]
Diagnosis: Viral culture ± reverse transcriptase-PCR with H5 & N1 specific primers.[12]
Management: ►Get help. Contain the outbreak,[2] p397, in the UK, via your consultant in communicable disease control.[13] Ventilatory support + O_2 and antivirals may be needed. Most viruses are susceptible to oseltamivir, peramivir, and zanamivir. Nebulizers and high-air flow O_2 masks are implicated in nosocomial spread.[11,14]
Precautions for close contacts of infected patients:
Hand hygiene, avoid shared utensils and face-to-face contact, wear high-efficiency masks and eye protection. Start empirical antiviral treatment (oseltamivir within 48 hours of exposure and zanamivir within 36 hours). Monitor for fever, cough, shortness of breath, diarrhoea, or other systemic symptoms developing.

Coronaviruses: SARS and MERS

Severe acute respiratory syndrome (SARS[15]) is caused by SARS-CoV virus—a coronavirus. Major features are persistent fever (>38°C), chills, rigors, myalgia, dry cough, headache, diarrhoea, and dyspnoea—with an abnormal CXR and ↓WCC. Respiratory failure is a complicating feature: ~20% progress to acute respiratory distress syndrome requiring invasive ventilation.[16] Mortality is 1-50%, depending on age, but no cases since 2004. Close contacts, or travel to an area with known cases should raise suspicion. The mechanism of transmission of SARS-COV is human-human. *Management:* seek expert help. Largely supportive with good infection control measures.

Middle East respiratory syndrome (MERS) is a viral respiratory disease caused by novel coronavirus (MERS COV) and was first identified in 2012 in Saudi Arabia. Symptoms include fever, cough, shortness of breath, and gastrointestinal upset. Incubation period 14 days. Human-to-human transmission has been reported in most cases, but camels play a pivotal host role in animal-to-human transmission. Large outbreaks linked to healthcare facilities have been reported in the Middle East and South Korea. The World Health Organization has reported mortality as high as 36% in known cases.[13]

2 Therapeutic or prophylactic antivirals are said to be the most effective single intervention followed by vaccine and basic public health measures.[17] But oseltamivir resistance and unavailability of a suitable vaccine during the early stages of a pandemic make non-drug interventions all the more important.

Complications of pneumonia

Respiratory failure (See p188.) Type I respiratory failure (P_aO_2 <8kPa) is relatively common. Treatment is with high-flow (60%) oxygen. *Transfer the patient to ITU if hypoxia does not improve with O_2 therapy or P_aCO_2 rises to >6kPa.* Be careful with O_2 in COPD patients; check ABGs frequently, and consider elective ventilation if rising P_aCO_2 or worsening acidosis. Aim to keep SaO_2 at 94–98%, P_aO_2 ≥8kPa.

Hypotension May be due to a combination of dehydration and vasodilation due to sepsis. If systolic BP is <90mmHg, give an intravenous fluid challenge of 250mL colloid/crystalloid over 15min. If BP does not rise, consider a central line and give IV fluids to maintain the systolic BP >90mmHg. If systolic BP remains <90mmHg despite fluid therapy, request ITU assessment for inotropic support.

Atrial fibrillation (p130.) Common in the elderly. It usually resolves with treatment of the pneumonia. β-blocker or digoxin may be required to slow the ventricular response rate in the short term.

Pleural effusion Inflammation of the pleura by adjacent pneumonia may cause fluid exudation into the pleural space. If this accumulates faster than it is reabsorbed, a pleural effusion develops. If small, it may be of no consequence. If larger and patient symptomatic, or infected (empyema), drainage is required (p192, p766).

Empyema Pus in the pleural space. It should be suspected if a patient with a resolving pneumonia develops a recurrent fever. Clinical features: CXR indicates a pleural effusion. The aspirated pleural fluid is typically yellow and turbid with a pH <7.2, ↓glucose, and ↑LDH. The empyema should be drained using a chest drain, inserted under radiological guidance. Adhesions and loculation can make this difficult.

Lung abscess A cavitating area of localized, suppurative infection within the lung (see fig 4.6).

Causes: •Inadequately treated pneumonia. •Aspiration (eg alcoholism, oesophageal obstruction, bulbar palsy). •Bronchial obstruction (tumour, foreign body). •Pulmonary infarction. •Septic emboli (septicaemia, right heart endocarditis, IV drug use). •Subphrenic or hepatic abscess.

Clinical features: Swinging fever; cough; purulent, foul-smelling sputum; pleuritic chest pain; haemoptysis; malaise; weight loss. Look for: finger clubbing; anaemia; crepitations. Empyema develops in 20–30%.

Tests: Blood: FBC (anaemia, neutrophilia), ESR, CRP, blood cultures. Sputum microscopy, culture, and cytology. *CXR:* walled cavity, often with a fluid level. Consider CT scan to exclude obstruction, and bronchoscopy to obtain diagnostic specimens.

Treatment: Antibiotics as indicated by sensitivities; continue until healed (4–6 wks). Postural drainage. Repeated aspiration, antibiotic instillation, or surgical excision may be required.

Septicaemia May occur as a result of bacterial spread from the lung parenchyma into the bloodstream. This may cause metastatic infection, eg infective endocarditis, meningitis. Treat with IV antibiotic according to sensitivities.

Pericarditis and myocarditis May also complicate pneumonia.

Jaundice This is usually cholestatic, and may be due to sepsis or secondary to antibiotic therapy (particularly flucloxacillin and co-amoxiclav).

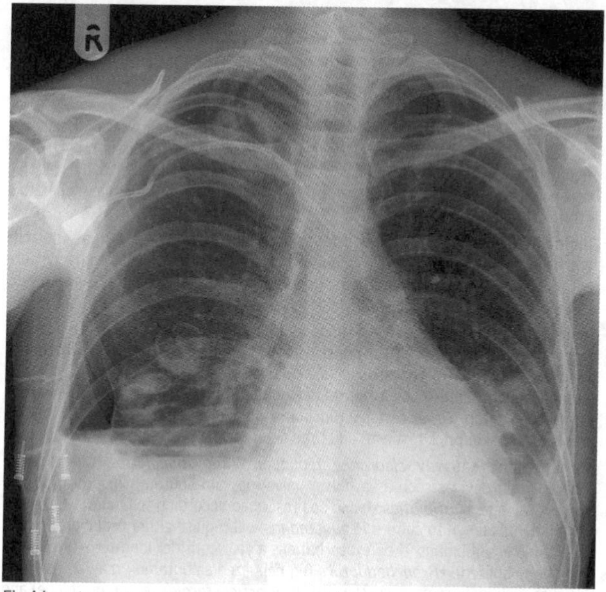

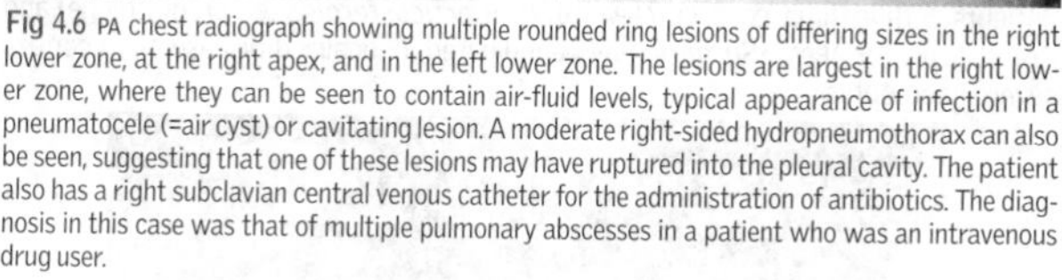

Fig 4.6 PA chest radiograph showing multiple rounded ring lesions of differing sizes in the right lower zone, at the right apex, and in the left lower zone. The lesions are largest in the right lower zone, where they can be seen to contain air-fluid levels, typical appearance of infection in a pneumatocele (=air cyst) or cavitating lesion. A moderate right-sided hydropneumothorax can also be seen, suggesting that one of these lesions may have ruptured into the pleural cavity. The patient also has a right subclavian central venous catheter for the administration of antibiotics. The diagnosis in this case was that of multiple pulmonary abscesses in a patient who was an intravenous drug user.

Image courtesy of Derby Hospitals NHS Foundation Trust Radiology Department.

Bronchiectasis

Pathology Chronic inflammation of the bronchi and bronchioles leading to permanent dilatation and thinning of these airways.[18] Main organisms: *H. influenzae*; *Strep. pneumoniae*; *Staph. aureus*; *Pseudomonas aeruginosa*.

Causes *Congenital:* Cystic fibrosis (CF); Young's syndrome; primary ciliary dyskinesia; Kartagener's syndrome (*OHCS* p646). *Post-infection:* Measles; pertussis; bronchiolitis; pneumonia; TB; HIV. *Other:* Bronchial obstruction (tumour, foreign body); allergic bronchopulmonary aspergillosis (ABPA, p177); hypogammaglobulinaemia; rheumatoid arthritis; ulcerative colitis; idiopathic.

Clinical features *Symptoms:* Persistent cough; copious purulent sputum; intermittent haemoptysis. *Signs:* Finger clubbing; coarse inspiratory crepitations; wheeze (asthma, COPD, ABPA). *Complications:* Pneumonia, pleural effusion; pneumothorax; haemoptysis; cerebral abscess; amyloidosis.

Tests *Sputum* culture. *CXR:* Cystic shadows, thickened bronchial walls (tramline and ring shadows); see fig 4.7. *HRCT chest* (p164) to assess extent and distribution of disease. *Spirometry* often shows an obstructive pattern; reversibility should be assessed. *Bronchoscopy* to locate site of haemoptysis, exclude obstruction and obtain samples for culture. *Other tests:* Serum immunoglobulins; CF sweat test; *Aspergillus* precipitins or skin-prick test RAST and total IgE.

Management •*Airway clearance techniques and mucolytics.* Chest physiotherapy and devices such as a flutter valve may aid sputum expectoration and mucus drainage. •*Antibiotics* should be prescribed according to bacterial sensitivities. Patients known to culture *Pseudomonas* will require either oral ciprofloxacin or suitable IV antibiotics. If ≥3 exacerbations a year consider long-term antibiotics (may be nebulized). •*Bronchodilators* (eg nebulized salbutamol) may be useful in patients with asthma, COPD, CF, ABPA (p177). •*Corticosteroids* (eg prednisolone) and itraconazole for ABPA. •*Surgery* may be indicated in localized disease or to control severe haemoptysis.

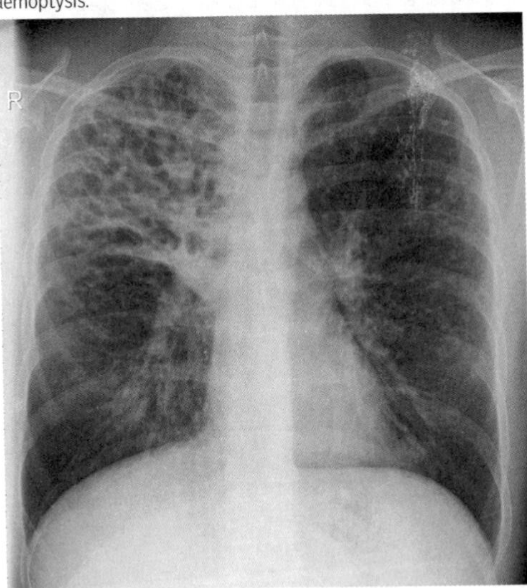

Fig 4.7 PA chest radiograph showing marked abnormal dilatation of the airways throughout the right upper lobe, subtle similar changes throughout the rest of the lung (particulalry periphery of the left upper zone). The fine background reticular pattern in the lungs suggests that there may also be some interstitial lung disease present.

Image courtesy of Nottingham University Hospitals NHS Trust Radiology Department.

Cystic fibrosis (CF)

One of the commonest life-threatening autosomal recessive conditions (1:2000 live births) affecting Caucasians. 1:25 people carry a copy of the faulty gene. All UK babies are screened at birth. Caused by mutations in the CF transmembrane conductance regulator (CFTR) gene on chromosome 7 (>1500 mutations have been identified). This is a Cl^- channel, and the defect leads to a combination of defective chloride secretion and increased sodium absorption across airway epithelium. The changes in the composition of airway surface liquid predispose the lung to chronic pulmonary infections and bronchiectasis. See OHCS ('Paediatrics', p162) for more detail.

Clinical features *Neonate:* Failure to thrive; meconium ileus; rectal prolapse. *Children and young adults: Respiratory:* cough; wheeze; recurrent infections; bronchiectasis; pneumothorax; haemoptysis; respiratory failure; cor pulmonale. *Gastrointestinal:* pancreatic insufficiency (diabetes mellitus, steatorrhoea); distal intestinal obstruction syndrome (meconium ileus equivalent); gallstones; cirrhosis. *Other:* male infertility; osteoporosis; arthritis; vasculitis (p556); nasal polyps; sinusitis; and hypertrophic pulmonary osteoarthropathy (HPOA). *Signs:* cyanosis; finger clubbing; bilateral coarse crackles.

Diagnosis *Sweat test:* Sweat sodium and chloride >60mmol/L; chloride usually > sodium. *Genetics:* Screening for known common CF mutations should be considered. *Faecal elastase* is a simple and useful screening test for exocrine pancreatic dysfunction.

Tests *Blood:* FBC, U&E, LFT; clotting; vitamin A, D, E levels; annual glucose tolerance test (p206). *Bacteriology:* Cough swab, sputum culture. *Radiology:* CXR; hyperinflation; bronchiectasis. *Abdominal ultrasound:* Fatty liver; cirrhosis; chronic pancreatitis; *Spirometry:* Obstructive defect. *Aspergillus serology/skin test* (20% develop ABPA, p177). *Biochemistry:* Faecal fat analysis.

Management Management should be multidisciplinary, eg physician, GP, physiotherapist, specialist nurse, and dietician, with attention to psychosocial as well as physical wellbeing. *Chest:* Physiotherapy (postural drainage, airway clearance techniques). Antibiotics are given for acute infective exacerbations and prophylactically. Chronic *Pseudomonas* infection is an important predictor of survival. Mucolytics may be useful (eg DNase, ie Dornase alfa, 2.5mg daily nebulized, or nebulized hypertonic saline). Bronchodilators. Annual CXR surveillance is recommended. *Gastrointestinal:* Malabsorption, GORD, distal obstruction syndrome. Pancreatic enzyme replacement; fat-soluble vitamin supplements (A, D, E, K); ursodeoxycholic acid for impaired liver function; cirrhosis may require liver transplantation. *Other:* Treatment of CF-related diabetes (screen annually with OGTT from 12yrs); screening/treatment of osteoporosis (DEXA bone scanning); arthritis, sinusitis, and vasculitis; fertility and genetic counselling. *Advanced lung disease:* Oxygen, diuretics (cor pulmonale); non-invasive ventilation; lung or heart/lung transplantation (post-transplant survival 5 years). *Prognosis:* Median survival is now ~41yrs in the UK, although a baby born today would expect to live longer.

Mutation-specific therapies for cystic fibrosis

Ivacaftor and lumacaftor target the CFTR protein. Ivacaftor, a CFTR potentiator, targets gating defects in disease causing CFTR mutations including G551D. Ivacaftor increases the open probability of CFTR channels and has been shown to improve clinical outcomes (lung function, weight, lung disease stability) in CF patients >6 years old.[19] Lumacaftor is a CFTR corrector, and has been shown to correct F508 del CFTR misprocessing and increase the amount of cell surface-localized protein. Ivacaftor and lumacaftor combination therapy, for patients with F508 del, have shown improved lung function and reduced pulmonary exacerbations.[20]

Gene therapy (transfer of CFTR gene using liposome or adenovirus vectors): phase 2b studies show modest but significant improvement in FEV_1 in those receiving gene therapy.[21] Further work into vectors for gene transfer is ongoing.

Lung tumours

Carcinoma of the bronchus Second most common cancer in the UK, accounting for 13% of all new cancer cases and 27% of cancer deaths (40 000 cases/yr in UK).[22] Incidence is increasing in women. Only 5% 'cured'. *Risk factors:* Cigarette smoking (causes 90% of lung ca). Others: passive smoking, asbestos, chromium, arsenic, iron oxides, and radiation (radon gas).

Histology: Clinically the most important division is between small cell (SCLC) and non-small cell (NSCLC). *NSCLC:* Squamous (35%); adenocarcinoma (27%), large cell (10%); adenocarcinoma *in situ* (rare, <1%). *Small cell (oat cell) (20%):* Arise from endocrine cells (Kulchitsky cells), often secreting polypeptide hormones resulting in paraneoplastic syndromes (eg production of ACTH, Cushing's syndrome). Most (70%) SCLC are disseminated at presentation.

Symptoms: Cough (80%); haemoptysis (70%); dyspnoea (60%); chest pain (40%); recurrent or slowly resolving pneumonia; lethargy, anorexia; weight loss.

Signs: Cachexia; anaemia; clubbing; HPOA (hypertrophic pulmonary osteoarthropathy, causing wrist pain); supraclavicular or axillary nodes. *Chest signs:* none, or consolidation; collapse; pleural effusion. *Metastases:* bone tenderness; hepatomegaly; confusion; fits; focal CNS signs; cerebellar syndrome; proximal myopathy; peripheral neuropathy.

Complications: Local: recurrent laryngeal nerve palsy; phrenic nerve palsy; SVC obstruction; Horner's syndrome (Pancoast's tumour); rib erosion; pericarditis; AF. *Metastatic:* brain; bone (bone pain, anaemia, ↑Ca^{2+}); liver; adrenals (Addison's). *Non-metastatic neurological:* confusion; fits; cerebellar syndrome; proximal myopathy; neuropathy; polymyositis; Lambert-Eaton syndrome (p512). See table 4.3.

Tests: CXR: peripheral nodule (fig 4.8); hilar enlargement; consolidation; lung collapse; pleural effusion; bony secondaries. *Cytology:* sputum and pleural fluid (send at least 20mL). *Fine needle aspiration* or *biopsy* (peripheral lesions/lymph nodes). *CT* to stage the tumour (p176) and guide bronchoscopy. *Bronchoscopy:* to give histology and assess operability, ± endobronchial ultrasound for assessment and biopsy. *^{18}F-deoxyglucose PET* or *PET/CT EBUS scan* to help in staging. *Radionuclide bone scan:* if suspected metastases. *Lung function tests:* help assess suitability for lobectomy.

Other lung tumours *Bronchial adenoma:* Rare, slow-growing. 90% are carcinoid tumours; 10% cylindromas. ℞: surgery. *Hamartoma:* Rare, benign; CT: lobulated mass ± flecks of calcification; ?excise to exclude malignancy.

Malignant mesothelioma A tumour of mesothelial cells that usually occurs in the pleura, and rarely in the peritoneum or other organs. It is associated with occupational exposure to asbestos but the relationship is complex.[23] 90% report previous exposure to asbestos, but only 20% of patients have pulmonary asbestosis. The latent period between exposure and development of the tumour may be up to 45yrs. Compensation is often available.

Clinical features: Chest pain, dyspnoea, weight loss, finger clubbing, recurrent pleural effusions. Signs of metastases: lymphadenopathy, hepatomegaly, bone pain/tenderness, abdominal pain/obstruction (peritoneal malignant mesothelioma).

Tests: CXR/CT: pleural thickening/effusion. Bloody pleural fluid.

Diagnosis: Made on histology, usually following a thoracoscopy. Often the diagnosis is only made post-mortem.

Management: Pemetrexed + cisplatin chemotherapy can improve survival.[24] Surgery is hard to evaluate (few randomized trials). Radiotherapy is controversial. Pleurodesis and indwelling intra-pleural drain may help.

Prognosis: Poor (especially without pemetrexed, eg <2yrs). >650 deaths/yr in UK.

Differential diagnosis of nodule in the lung on a CXR

- Malignancy (1° or 2°)
- Abscesses (p170)
- Granuloma
- Carcinoid tumour
- Pulmonary hamartoma
- Arterio-venous malformation
- Encysted effusion (fluid, blood, pus)
- Cyst
- Foreign body
- Skin tumour (eg seborrhoeic wart).

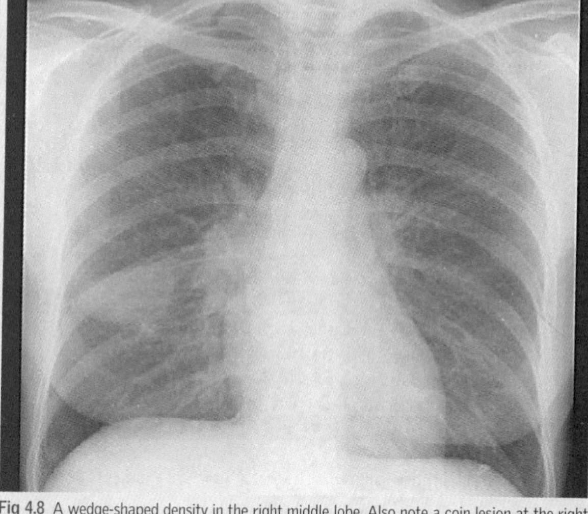

Fig 4.8 A wedge-shaped density in the right middle lobe. Also note a coin lesion at the right costophrenic angle. Right hilar lymphadenopathy.

Courtesy of Janet E. Jeddry, Yale Medical School.

Table 4.3 Non-metastatic extrapulmonary manifestations of bronchial cancer

System	Manifestations
Endocrine	Ectopic secretion; ACTH (Cushing's), ADH (dilutional hyponatraemia), PTH (hypercalcaemia), HCG (gynaecomastia)
Neurological	Cerebellar degeneration, myopathy, polyneuropathy, myasthenic syndrome
Vascular	Thrombophlebitis migrans (p562), anaemia, DIC
Cutaneous	Dermatomyositis, herpes zoster, acanthosis nigricans
Skeletal	Clubbing, HPOA

Lung tumours: staging and treatment

Assessing the extent of tumour spread (staging) is vital to determining the best course of treatment and also prognosis. All patients who may be suitable for surgery with curative intent should be offered PET-CT before treatment.[25] Some patients may undergo endobronchial ultrasound-guided transbronchial needle aspirations for mediastinal masses. TNM staging classification for non-small cell lung cancer is shown in table 4.4. You do not need to memorize this!

Table 4.4 TNM staging for non-small cell lung cancer

Primary tumour (T)	
TX	Malignant cells in bronchial secretions, no other evidence of tumour
TIS	Carcinoma *in situ*
T0	None evident
T1	≤3cm, in lobar or more distal airway
T2	>3cm and >2cm distal to carina or any size if pleural involvement or obstructive pneumonitis extending to hilum, but not all the lung
T3	Involves the chest wall, diaphragm, mediastinal pleura, pericardium, or <2cm from, but not at, carina. T >7cm diameter and nodules in same lobe
T4	Involves mediastinum, heart, great vessels, trachea, oesophagus, vertebral body, carina, malignant effusion, or nodules in another lobe
Regional nodes (N)	
N0	None involved (after mediastinoscopy)
N1	Peribronchial and/or ipsilateral hilum
N2	Ipsilateral mediastinum or subcarinal
N3	Contralateral mediastinum or hilum, scalene, or supraclavicular
Distant metastasis (M)	
M0	None
M1	a) Nodule in other lung, pleural lesions, or malignant effusion; b) distant metastases present

Stages					
Occult	I	II	IIIa	IIIb	IV
TX N0 M0	TIS/T1/T2 N0 M0	T1/T2 N1 M0	T3 N1 M0	T1–4 N3 M0	T1–4 N0–3 M1
		or T3 N0 M0	*or* T1–3 N2 M0	*or* T4 N0–2 M0	

Reproduced with permission from Edge, SB *et al.* (Eds.), *AJCC Cancer Staging Manual*, 7th Edition. New York: Springer; 2010.

Treatment ***NSCLC:*** *Lobectomy* (open or thoracoscopic) is the treatment of choice if medically fit and aim is curative intent or parenchymal sparing operation for patients with borderline fitness and smaller tumours ((T1a-b, N0, M0). *Radical radiotherapy* for patient with stage I, II, III NSCLC. *Chemotherapy ± radiotherapy* for more advanced disease. Regimens may be platinum based, eg with monoclonal antibodies targeting the epidermal growth factor receptor (cetuximab). ***SCLC:*** *consider surgery* with limited stage disease. *Chemotherapy ± radiotherapy* if well enough. *Palliation: Radiotherapy* is used for bronchial obstruction, SVC obstruction, haemoptysis, bone pain, and cerebral metastases. *SVC stent* + radiotherapy and dexamethasone for SVC obstruction. *Endobronchial therapy:* tracheal stenting, cryotherapy, laser, brachytherapy (radioactive source is placed close to the tumour). *Pleural drainage/ pleurodesis* for symptomatic pleural effusions. *Drugs:* analgesia; steroids; anti-emetics; cough linctus; bronchodilators; antidepressants.

Prognosis *Non-small cell:* 50% 2yr survival without spread; 10% with spread. *Small cell:* median survival is 3 months if untreated; 1-1½yrs if treated.

Prevention Stop smoking (p93). Prevent occupational exposure to carcinogens.

Aspergillus This group of fungi affects the lung in five ways:

1 *Asthma:* Type I hypersensitivity reaction to fungal spores (p178).

2 *Allergic bronchopulmonary aspergillosis (ABPA):* Results from type I and III hypersensitivity reactions to *Aspergillus fumigatus*. Affects 1-5% of asthmatics, 2-25% of CF patients.[26] Initially bronchoconstriction, then permanent damage occurs causing bronchiectasis (fig 4.9). *Symptoms:* wheeze, cough, sputum (plugs of mucus containing fungal hyphae, see p408), dyspnoea, and 'recurrent pneumonia'. *Investigations:* CXR (transient segmental collapse or consolidation, bronchiectasis); *Aspergillus* in sputum; positive *Aspergillus* skin test and/or *Aspergillus*-specific IgE RAST (radioallergosorbent test); positive serum precipitins; eosinophilia; raised serum IgE. *Treatment:* prednisolone 30-40mg/24h PO for acute attacks; maintenance dose 5-10mg/d. Itraconazole can be used in combination with corticosteroids. Bronchodilators for asthma. Sometimes bronchoscopic aspiration of mucus plugs is needed.

3 *Aspergilloma (mycetoma):* A fungus ball within a pre-existing cavity (often caused by TB or sarcoidosis). It is usually asymptomatic but may cause cough, haemoptysis (may be torrential), lethargy ± weight loss. *Investigations:* CXR (round opacity within a cavity, usually apical); sputum culture; strongly positive serum precipitins; *Aspergillus* skin test (30% +ve). *Treatment* (only if symptomatic): consider surgical excision for solitary symptomatic lesions or severe haemoptysis. Oral itraconazole and other antifungals have been tried with limited success. Local instillation of amphotericin paste under CT guidance yields partial success in carefully selected patients, eg in massive haemoptysis.

4 *Invasive aspergillosis: Risk factors:*[27] immunocompromise, eg HIV, leukaemia, burns, Wegener's (p714), and SLE, or after broad-spectrum antibiotic therapy. *Investigations:* sputum culture; BAL; biopsy; serum precipitins; CXR (consolidation, abscess). Early chest CT and serial serum measurements of galactomannan (an *Aspergillus* antigen) may be helpful. Diagnosis may only be made at lung biopsy or autopsy. *Treatment:* voriconazole is superior to IV amphotericin.[28] Alternatives: IV miconazole or ketoconazole (less effective). *Prognosis:* 30% mortality.

5 *Extrinsic allergic alveolitis (EAA):* See p198.

Other fungal infections *Candida* and *Cryptococcus* may cause pneumonia in the immunosuppressed (see p408).

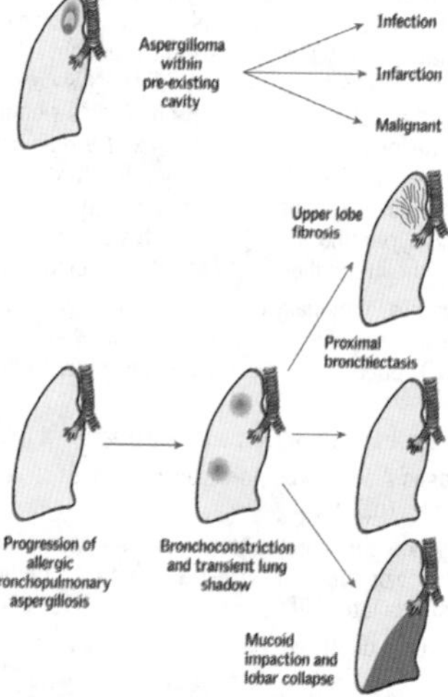

Fig 4.9 Aspergillosis.

Asthma

Asthma affects 5-8% of the population. It is characterized by recurrent episodes of dyspnoea, cough, and wheeze caused by reversible airways obstruction. Three factors contribute to airway narrowing: *bronchial muscle contraction*, triggered by a variety of stimuli; *mucosal swelling/inflammation*, caused by mast cell and basophil degranulation resulting in the release of inflammatory mediators; and *increased mucus production*.

Symptoms Intermittent dyspnoea, wheeze, cough (often nocturnal), and sputum (see table 4.5).

Precipitants: Cold air, exercise, emotion, allergens (house dust mite, pollen, fur), infection, smoking and passive smoking,[29] pollution, NSAIDs, β-blockers.

Diurnal variation Symptoms or peak flow may vary over the day. Marked morning dipping of peak flow is common and can tip the balance into a serious attack, despite having normal peak flow (fig 4.12) at other times.

Exercise: Quantify the exercise tolerance.

Disturbed sleep: Quantify as nights per week (a sign of severe asthma).

Acid reflux: 40-60% of those with asthma have reflux; treating it improves spirometry, but not necessarily symptoms.[30]

Other atopic disease: Eczema, hay fever, allergy, or family history?

The home (especially the bedroom): Pets? Carpet? Feather pillows or duvet? Floor cushions and other 'soft furnishings'?

Job: If symptoms remit at weekends or holidays, work may provide the trigger (15% of cases are work-related—more for paint sprayers, food processors, welders, and animal handlers).[31] Ask the patient to measure their peak flow at intervals at work and at home (at the same time of day) to confirm this (see fig 4.13).

Days per week off work or school.

Signs Tachypnoea; audible wheeze; hyperinflated chest; hyper-resonant percussion note; ↓air entry; widespread, polyphonic wheeze. ***Severe attack:*** Inability to complete sentences; pulse >110bpm; respiratory rate >25/min; PEF 33-50% predicted. ***Life-threatening attack:*** Silent chest; confusion; exhaustion; cyanosis (P_aO_2 <8kPa but P_aCO_2 4.6-6.0, SpO_2 <92%); bradycardia; PEF <33% predicted. *Near fatal:* ↑P_aCO_2.

Tests *Initial diagnosis:* See figs 4.10, 4.11. ***Acute attack:*** PEF, sputum culture, FBC, U&E, CRP, blood cultures. ABG analysis usually shows a normal or slightly ↓P_aO_2 but ↓P_aCO_2 (hyperventilation). If P_aO_2 is normal but the patient is hyperventilating, watch carefully and repeat the ABG a little later. ►*If P_aCO_2 is normal or raised,* transfer to high-dependency unit or ITU for ventilation, as this signifies failing respiratory effort. CXR (to exclude infection or pneumothorax). ***Chronic asthma:*** PEF monitoring (p162): a diurnal variation of >20% on ≥3d a wk for 2wks. *Spirometry:* obstructive defect (↓FEV_1/FVC, ↑RV p162); usually ≥15% improvement in FEV_1 following β_2 agonists or steroid trial. CXR: hyperinflation. Skin-prick tests may help to identify allergens. Histamine or methacholine challenge. *Aspergillus* serology.

Differential diagnosis Pulmonary oedema ('cardiac asthma'); COPD (may co-exist); large airway obstruction (eg foreign body, tumour); SVC obstruction (wheeze/dyspnoea not episodic); pneumothorax; PE; bronchiectasis; obliterative bronchiolitis (suspect in elderly).

Treatment Chronic asthma (p182). Emergency treatment (p810).

Associated diseases Acid reflux; polyarteritis nodosa (PAN, p556); Churg-Strauss syndrome (p696); ABPA (p177).

Natural history Most childhood asthmatics (see *OHCS* p164) either grow out of asthma in adolescence or suffer much less as adults. A significant number of people develop chronic asthma late in life.

Mortality ~900 asthma deaths in the UK in 2012, 50% were >65yrs old.

Table 4.5 Clinical features which increase or decrease probability of asthma in adults.

Increase probability of asthma	Lower probability of asthma
Wheeze, SOB, chest tightness	Prominent dizziness, lightheadedness, tingling
Diurnal variation	Chronic productive cough with no wheeze
Response to exercise, allergen, cold air	Normal examination when symptomatic
Symptoms after aspirin or β-blocker	Change in voice
History of atopy	Symptoms with colds only
Family history atopy/asthma	Significant smoking history (>20 pack year)
Widespread wheeze heard on auscultation	Cardiac disease
Unexplained low FEV_1 or PEF	Normal PEF when symptomatic
Unexplained peripheral blood eosinophilia	

(Data from https://www.brit-thoracic.org.uk/document-library/clinical-information/asthma/btsign-asthma-guideline-quick-reference-guide-2014)

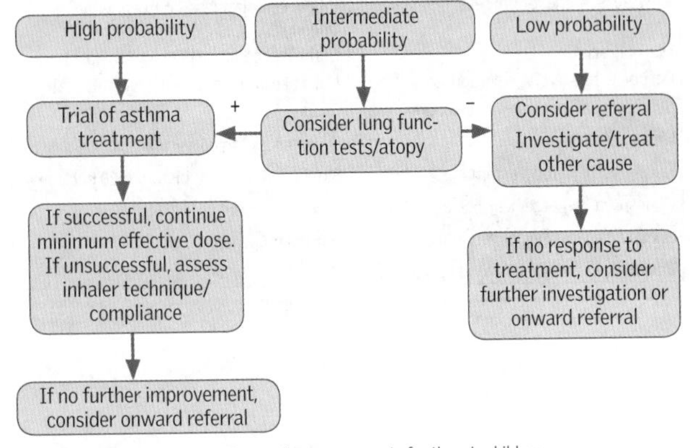

Fig 4.10 BTS/SIGN British guideline on the management of asthma in children.
Data from Fig 1, p21: https://www.brit-thoracic.org.uk/document-library/clinical-information/asthma/btssign-asthma-guideline-2014/

Suspected asthma in adults

Clinical investigation (spirometry or peak expiratory flow if spirometry not available)

High probability

Intermediate probability

Low probability

Trial of asthma treatment

FEV_1/FVC <0.7

FEV_1/FVC >0.7

Investigate or treat other cause

If successful, continue minimum effective dose. If unsuccessful, assess inhaler technique/ compliance

Consider referral/ treat other cause

If no response to treatment, consider further investigation or onward referral

If no further improvement, consider onward referral

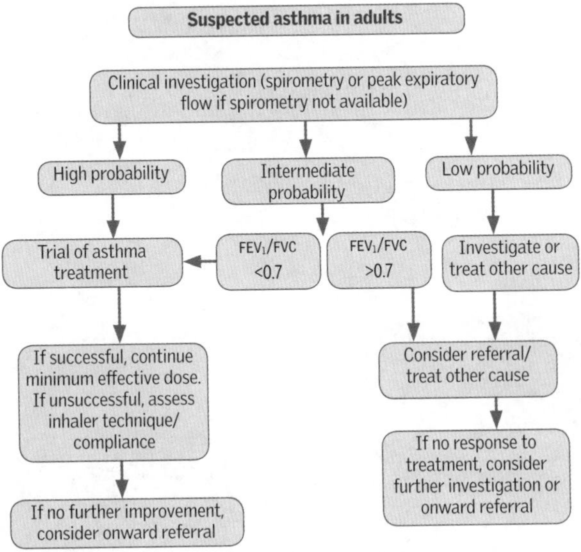

Fig 4.11 BTS/SIGN British guideline on the management of asthma in adults.
Data from Fig 2, p25: https://www.brit-thoracic.org.uk/document-library/clinical-information/asthma/btssign-asthma-guideline-2014/

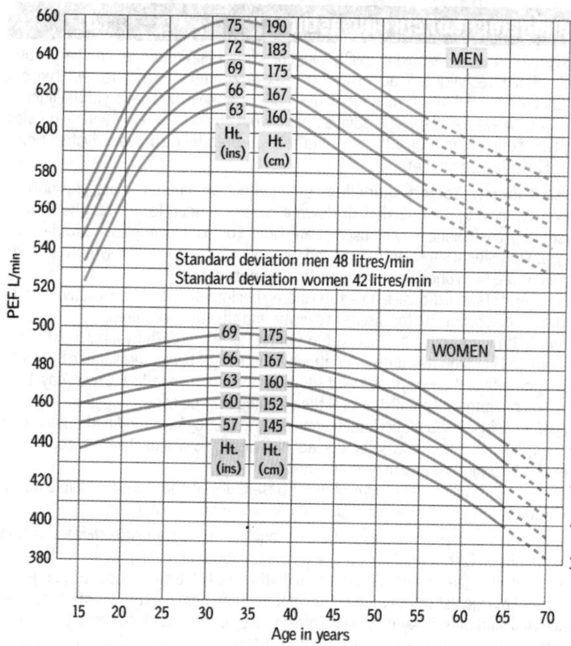

MEN
75 190
72 183
69 175
66 167
63 160
Ht. (ins) Ht. (cm)

Standard deviation men 48 litres/min
Standard deviation women 42 litres/min

WOMEN
69 175
66 167
63 160
60 152
57 145
Ht. (ins) Ht. (cm)

PEF L/min
Age in years

Fig 4.12 Normal peak expiratory flow (PEF).

Data from Nunn, AJ, Gregg, I. New regression equations for predicting peak expiratory flow in adults. *BMJ* 1989;298:1068–70.

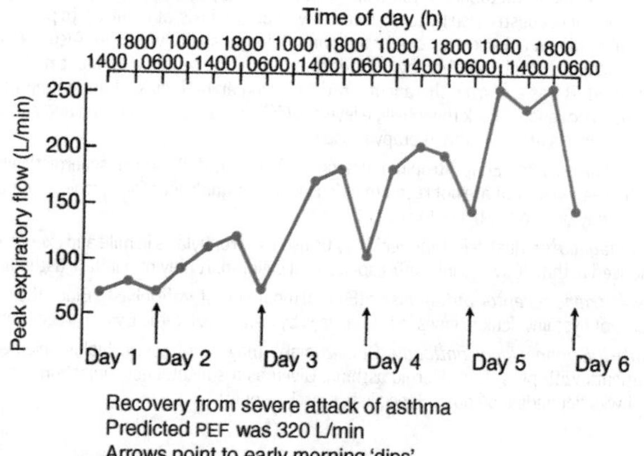

Fig 4.13 Examples of serial peak flow charts.

Management of chronic asthma

Lifestyle Help to quit smoking (p93). Avoid precipitants. Weight loss if overweight. Check inhaler technique. Teach use of a peak flow meter to monitor PEF twice a day. Educate to enable self-management by altering their medication in the light of symptoms or PEF. Give specific advice about what to do in an emergency; provide a written action plan. Consider teaching relaxed breathing to avoid dysfunctional breathing[32] (Papworth method).[3]

British Thoracic Society guidelines (BTS[33]) Start at the step most appropriate to severity; moving up if needed, or down if control is good for >3 months. Rescue courses of prednisolone may be used at any time. For drug examples see table 4.6.

- *Step 1:* Occasional short-acting inhaled β_2-agonist as required for symptom relief. If used more than once daily, or night-time symptoms, go to Step 2.
- *Step 2:* Add standard-dose inhaled steroid, eg beclometasone 200mcg/day, or start at the dose appropriate for disease severity, and titrate as required.
- *Step 3:* Add long-acting β_2-agonist (eg salmeterol 50mcg/12h by inhaler). If benefit—but still inadequate control—continue and ↑dose of beclometasone to 800mcg/day. If no effect then stop LABA and ↑dose of beclometasone to 800mcg/day. Leukotriene receptor antagonist or oral theophylline may be tried.
- *Step 4:* Consider trials of: beclometasone up to 2000mcg/day; modified-release oral theophylline; modified-release oral β_2-agonist tablets; oral leukotriene receptor antagonist, in conjunction with previous therapy.
- *Step 5:* Add regular oral prednisolone (1 dose daily, at the lowest possible dose). Continue with high-dose inhaled steroids. Refer for specialist input.

Drugs *β_2-adrenoceptor agonists:* Relax bronchial smooth muscle (↑cAMP), acting within minutes. Salbutamol is best given by inhalation (aerosol, powder, nebulizer), but may also be given PO or IV. SE: tachyarrhythmias, ↓K^+, tremor, anxiety. Long-acting inhaled β_2-agonist (eg salmeterol, formoterol) can help nocturnal symptoms and reduce morning dips. They may be an alternative to ↑steroid dose when symptoms are uncontrolled; doubts remain over whether they are associated with an increase in adverse events.[34] SE: as salbutamol, paradoxical bronchospasm.[35]

Corticosteroids: Best inhaled to minimize systemic effects, eg beclometasone via spacer (or powder), but may be given PO or IV. They act over days to ↓bronchial mucosal inflammation. Rinse mouth after inhaled steroids to prevent oral candidiasis. Oral steroids are used acutely (high-dose, short courses, eg prednisolone 40mg/24h PO for 7d) and longer term in lower dose (eg 5-10mg/24h) if control is not optimal on inhalers. Warn about SEs: p377.

Aminophylline: (Metabolized to theophylline) acts by inhibiting phosphodiesterase, thus ↓bronchoconstriction by ↑cAMP levels. Try as prophylaxis, at night, PO, to prevent morning dipping. Stick with one brand name (bioavailability variable). Also useful as an adjunct if inhaled therapy is inadequate. In acute severe asthma, it may be given IVI. It has a narrow therapeutic ratio, causing arrhythmias, GI upset, and fits in the toxic range. Check theophylline levels (p756), and do ECG monitoring and check plasma levels after 24h if IV therapy is used.

Anticholinergics: (Eg ipratropium, tiotropium.) May ↓muscle spasm synergistically with β_2-agonists but are not recommended in current guidelines for *chronic* asthma. They may be of more benefit in COPD.

Cromoglicate (Mast cell stabilizer.) May be used as prophylaxis in mild and exercise-induced asthma (always inhaled), especially in children. It may precipitate asthma.

Leukotriene receptor antagonists: (Eg oral montelukast, zafirlukast.) Block the effects of cysteinyl leukotrienes in the airways by antagonizing the $CystLT_1$ receptor.

Anti-IgE monoclonal antibody: Omalizumab[36] may be of use in highly selected patients with persistent allergic asthma. Given as a subcutaneous injection every 2-4 wks depending on dose. Specialists prescribe only.

3 Integrated breathing and relaxation training (Papworth method) is psychological *and* physical: patients learn to drop their shoulders, relax their abdomen, and breathe calmly and appropriately.

Table 4.6 Adult doses of common inhaled drugs used in bronchoconstriction

	Inhaled aerosol	Inhaled powder	Nebulized (supervised)
Salbutamol			
Dose example:	100–200mcg/6h	200–400mcg/6h	2.5–5mg/6h
Airomir® is a CFC-free example of a breath-actuated inhaler			
Terbutaline			
Single dose		500mcg	2.5mg/mL
Recommended regimen		500mcg/6h	5–10mg/6–12h
Salmeterol			
Dose/puff	25mcg	50mcg	—
Recommended regimen	50–100mcg/12h	50–100mcg/12h	—
Tiotropium bromide (COPD)			
Dose/puff	2.5mcg	9mcg	—
Recommended regimen	25mcg daily	18mcg daily	—
Steroids			
(Clenil Modulite®=beclometasone; Pulmicort®=budesonide;* Flixotide®=fluticasone)			
Fluticasone (Flixotide®)			
Doses available/puff	50, 100, 250, & 500mcg	As for aerosol	250mcg/mL
Recommended regimen	100–250mcg/12h	100–250mcg/12h max 1mg/12h	0.5–2mg/12h
Clenil Modulite®			
Doses available/puff	50 & 100mcg	—	—
	250mcg		
Recommended regimen	200mcg/12h then 400mcg/12h then 1000mcg/12h		

*Available as a Turbohaler®; Autohalers® are an alternative (breath-actuated) and don't need breathing coordination, eg Airomir® (salbutamol) and Qvar® (beclometasone). Accuhalers® deliver dry powders (eg Flixotide®, Serevent®).
Systemic absorption (via the throat) is less if inhalation is through a large-volume device, eg Volumatic® or AeroChamber Plus® devices. The latter is more compact. Static charge on some devices reduces dose delivery, so wash in water before dose; leave to dry (don't rub). It's pointless to squirt many puffs into a device: it is best to repeat single doses, and be sure to inhale *as soon as the drug is in the spacer*. SE: local (oral) candidiasis (p377); ↑rate of cataract if lifetime dose ≥2g beclometasone.[37]

►Prescribe beclometasone by brand name, and state that a CFC-free inhaler should be dispensed. This is because, dose for dose, Qvar® is twice as potent as the other available CFC-free brand (Clenil Modulite®).
Any dose ≥250mcg ≈ significant steroid absorption: carry a steroid card; this recommendation is being widened, and lower doses (beclometasone) are now said to merit a steroid card (manufacturer's information).

Chronic obstructive pulmonary disease (COPD)

Definitions COPD is a common progressive disorder characterized by airway obstruction (FEV_1 <80% predicted; FEV_1/FVC <0.7; see p162 and table 4.5) with little or no reversibility. It includes chronic bronchitis and emphysema. Usually patients have *either* COPD *or* asthma, not both: COPD is favoured by: •age of onset >35yrs •smoking (passive or active) or pollution related[38] •chronic dyspnoea •sputum production •minimal diurnal or day-to-day FEV_1 variation. *Chronic bronchitis* is defined *clinically* as cough, sputum production on most days for 3 months of 2 successive yrs. Symptoms improve if they stop smoking. There is no excess mortality if lung function is normal. *Emphysema* is defined *histologically* as enlarged air spaces distal to terminal bronchioles, with destruction of alveolar walls but often visualized on CT.

Prevalence 10–20% of the over-40s; 2.5×10^6 deaths/yr worldwide.[39]

Pink puffers and blue bloaters A traditional division but likely ends of a spectrum. *Pink puffers:* Have ↑alveolar ventilation, a near normal P_aO_2 and a normal or low P_aCO_2. They are breathless but are not cyanosed. They may progress to type I respiratory failure (p188). *Blue bloaters:* Have ↓alveolar ventilation, with a low P_aO_2 and a high P_aCO_2. They are cyanosed but not breathless and may go on to develop cor pulmonale. Their respiratory centres are relatively insensitive to CO_2 and they rely on hypoxic drive to maintain respiratory effort (p188)—►*supplemental oxygen should be given with care.*

Symptoms Cough; sputum; dyspnoea; wheeze. **Signs** Tachypnoea; use of accessory muscles of respiration; hyperinflation; ↓cricosternal distance (<3cm); ↓expansion; resonant or hyperresonant percussion note; quiet breath sounds (eg over bullae); wheeze; cyanosis; cor pulmonale.

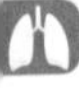

Complications Acute exacerbations ± infection; polycythaemia; respiratory failure; cor pulmonale (oedema; ↑JVP); pneumothorax (ruptured bullae); lung carcinoma.

Tests *FBC:* ↑*PCV*. *CXR:* Hyperinflation; flat hemidiaphragms; large central pulmonary arteries; ↓peripheral vascular markings; bullae. *CT:* Bronchial wall thickening; scarring; air space enlargement. *ECG:* Right atrial and ventricular hypertrophy (cor pulmonale). *ABG:* ↓P_aO_2 ± hypercapnia. *Spirometry* (p162, p165): obstructive + air trapping (FEV_1 <80% of predicted, FEV_1:FVC ratio <70%, ↑TLC, ↑RV, ↓DLCO in emphysema—see p160). Learn how to do spirometry from an experienced person: ensure *maximal* expiration of the full breath (it takes >4s; it's *not* a quick puff out).

Treatment *Chronic stable:* see BOX and fig 4.14; ►►*Emergency* ℞: p812. *Smoking cessation advice* with cordial vigour (p93). *Encourage exercise:* BMI is often low; *diet advice ± supplements*[40] may help (p584). *Mucolytics* (*BNF* 3.7) may help chronic productive cough (NICE).[41] Disabilities may cause serious, treatable *depression;* screen for this (p15). *Respiratory failure:* p188. *Oedema:* diuretics. *Flu and pneumococcal vaccinations:* p167 and p396.

Long-term O_2 therapy (LTOT): An MRC trial showed that if P_aO_2 was maintained ≥8.0kPa for 15h a day, 3yr survival improved by 50%. UK NICE guidelines suggest LTOT should be given for: **1** Clinically stable non-smokers with P_aO_2 <7.3kPa—despite maximal ℞. These values should be stable on two occasions >3wks apart. **2** If P_aO_2 7.3–8.0 *and* pulmonary hypertension (eg RVH; loud S_2), or polycythaemia, or peripheral oedema, or nocturnal hypoxia. **3** O_2 can also be prescribed for terminally ill patients.

Severity assessment in COPD

Severity assessment has implications for therapy and prognosis. The BODE index (Body mass index, airflow Obstruction, Dyspnoea and Exercise capacity) helps predict outcome and number and severity of exacerbations. The Global Initiative for COPD (GOLD) categorizes severity of COPD into four stages (mild, moderate, severe, and very severe) based on post-bronchodilator FEV_1% predicted, but it is not useful for predicting total mortality for 3 years of follow-up and onwards.[42]

British Thoracic Society (BTS)/NICE COPD guidelines

More advanced COPD

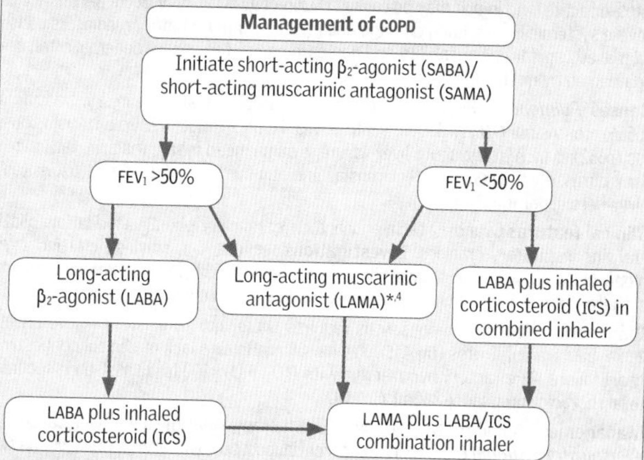

Management of COPD

Initiate short-acting β_2-agonist (SABA)/ short-acting muscarinic antagonist (SAMA)

- FEV_1 >50% → Long-acting β_2-agonist (LABA) or Long-acting muscarinic antagonist (LAMA)*[4]
- FEV_1 <50% → Long-acting muscarinic antagonist (LAMA)*[4] or LABA plus inhaled corticosteroid (ICS) in combined inhaler
- Long-acting β_2-agonist (LABA) → LABA plus inhaled corticosteroid (ICS) → LAMA plus LABA/ICS combination inhaler
- Long-acting muscarinic antagonist (LAMA) → LAMA plus LABA/ICS combination inhaler
- LABA plus inhaled corticosteroid (ICS) in combined inhaler → LAMA plus LABA/ICS combination inhaler

Fig 4.14 Management of COPD in primary and secondary care.
*Tiotropium (LAMA) is more effective than salmeterol in preventing exacerbations for patients with moderate-to-very-severe COPD.[43]

►Pulmonary rehabilitation is *greatly* valued by patients.

- Consider LTOT if P_aO_2 <7.3kPa (see 'Long-term O_2 therapy', earlier in topic OPPOSITE).
- Surgery may be appropriate in selected patients, eg recurrent pneumothoraces; isolated bullous disease. Lung volume reduction/endobronchial valve/transplant.
- NIV may be appropriate if hypercapnic on LTOT.
- NB: air travel is risky if FEV_1 <50% or P_aO_2 <6.7kPa on air.
- Consider palliative care input.

Indications for specialist referral

- Uncertain diagnosis, or suspected severe COPD, or a rapid decline in FEV_1.
- Onset of cor pulmonale.
- Bullous lung disease (to assess for surgery).
- Assessment for oral corticosteroids, nebulizer therapy, or LTOT.
- <10 pack-years smoking (= the number of packs/day × years of smoking) or COPD in patient <40yrs (eg is the cause α_1-antitrypsin deficiency? p290).
- Symptoms disproportionate to lung function tests.
- Frequent infections (to exclude bronchiectasis).

4 Cochrane meta-analyses (2007) of trials (including TORCH) favour steroids + LABA (long-acting β-agonist) vs either alone. LABA alone may ↑exacerbation rates, but no excess hospitalizations or mortality; steroid inhalers alone are associated with ↑mortality (by 33%) compared with steroids + LABA.[44] Steroid inhalers may ↑risk of pneumonia, but when combined with LABA, advantages outweigh disadvantages.

Acute respiratory distress syndrome (ARDS)

ARDS, or acute lung injury, may be caused by direct lung injury or occur secondary to severe systemic illness. Lung damage and release of inflammatory mediators cause increased capillary permeability and non-cardiogenic pulmonary oedema, often accompanied by multiorgan failure.

Causes *Pulmonary:* Pneumonia; gastric aspiration; inhalation; injury; vasculitis (p556); contusion. *Other:* Shock; septicaemia; haemorrhage; multiple transfusions; DIC (p352); pancreatitis; acute liver failure; trauma; head injury; malaria; fat embolism; burns; obstetric events (eclampsia; amniotic fluid embolus); drugs/toxins (aspirin, heroin, paraquat).

Clinical features Cyanosis; tachypnoea; tachycardia; peripheral vasodilation; bilateral fine inspiratory crackles. **Investigations** FBC, U&E, LFT, amylase, clotting, CRP, blood cultures, ABG. CXR shows bilateral pulmonary infiltrates. Pulmonary artery catheter to measure pulmonary capillary wedge pressure (PCWP).

Diagnostic criteria One consensus requires these four to exist:[45] **1** Acute onset. **2** CXR: bilateral infiltrates (**fig 4.15**). **3** PCWP <19mmHg or a lack of clinical congestive heart failure. **4** Refractory hypoxaemia with P_aO_2: FiO_2 <200 for ARDS. Others include total thoracic compliance <30mL/cmH_2O.

Chest medicine

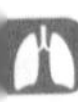

Management Admit to ITU; give supportive therapy; treat the underlying cause.

- *Respiratory support:* In early ARDS, continuous positive airway pressure (CPAP) with 40–60% oxygen may be adequate to maintain oxygenation. But most patients need mechanical ventilation. Indications for ventilation: P_aO_2: <8.3kPa despite 60% O_2; P_aCO_2: >6kPa. The large tidal volumes (10–15mL/kg) produced by conventional ventilation plus reduced lung compliance in ARDS may lead to high peak airway pressures ± pneumothorax. A low-tidal-volume, pressure-limited approach, with either low or moderate high positive end-expiratory pressure (PEEP), improves outcome.
- *Circulatory support:* Invasive haemodynamic monitoring with an arterial line and Swan–Ganz catheter aids the diagnosis and may be helpful in monitoring PCWP and cardiac output. A conservative fluid management approach improves outcome. Maintain cardiac output and O_2 delivery with inotropes (eg dobutamine 2.5–10mcg/kg/min IVI), vasodilators, and blood transfusion. Consider treating pulmonary hypertension with low-dose (20–120 parts per million) nitric oxide, a pulmonary vasodilator. Haemofiltration may be needed in renal failure and to achieve a negative fluid balance.[46,49]
- *Sepsis:* Identify organism(s) and treat. If septic, but no organisms cultured, use empirical broad-spectrum antibiotics (p167). Avoid nephrotoxic antibiotics.
- *Other:* Nutritional support: enteral is best: p584 & p586, with high-fat, antioxidant formulations. Steroids protect those at risk of fat embolization and with pneumocystosis and may improve outcome in subacute ARDS. Their role in established ARDS is controversial.[50,51]

Prognosis Overall mortality is 50–75%. Prognosis varies with age of patient, cause (pneumonia 86%, trauma 38%), and number of organs involved (three organs involved for >1wk is 'invariably' fatal).

Risk factors for ARDS

- Sepsis
- Hypovolaemic shock
- Trauma
- Pneumonia
- Diabetic ketoacidosis
- Gastric aspiration
- Pregnancy
- Eclampsia
- Amniotic fluid embolus
- Drugs/toxins
- Paraquat, heroin, aspirin
- Pulmonary contusion
- Massive transfusion
- Burns (p846)
- Smoke inhalation (p847)
- Near drowning
- Acute pancreatitis
- DIC (p352)
- Head injury
- ↑ICP
- Fat embolus
- Heart/lung bypass
- Tumour lysis syndrome (p529)
- Malaria.

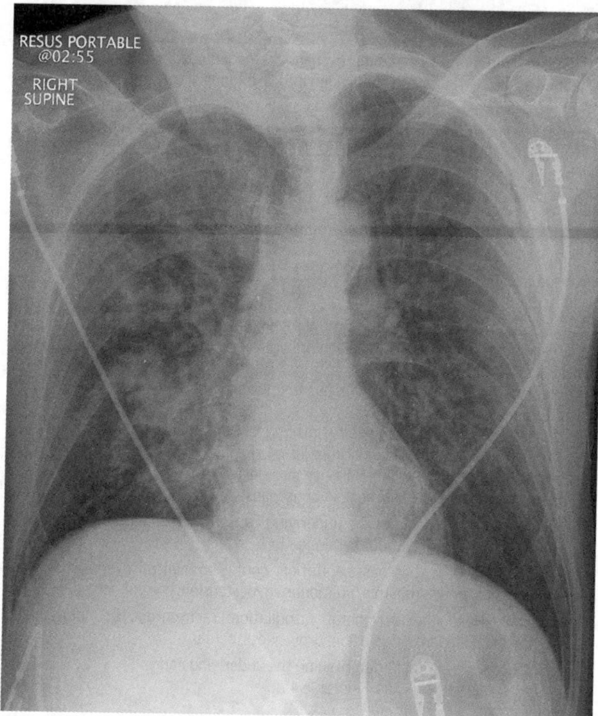

Fig 4.15 Supine chest radiograph showing air-space shadowing in a perihilar distribution spreading into the peripheries. This appearance can also be seen with infection and cardiogenic pulmonary oedema, but clues from the history, the heart size, and lack of pleural effusions can suggest ARDS over the latter. Remember though that this is a supine projection—the patient is lying flat with the X-ray beam AP—causing the cardiac shadow to be artificially enlarged and pleural effusions to level out on the posterior chest wall so they will not obscure the costophrenic angles unless very large.

Image courtesy of Nottingham University Hospitals NHS Trust Radiology Department.

Respiratory failure

Respiratory failure occurs when gas exchange is inadequate, resulting in hypoxia. It is defined as a P_aO_2 <8kPa and subdivided into two types according to P_aCO_2 level.

Type I respiratory failure Defined as hypoxia (P_aO_2 <8kPa) with a normal or low P_aCO_2. It is caused primarily by ventilation/perfusion (V/Q) mismatch, hypoventilation, abnormal diffusion, right to left cardiac shunts. Examples of V/Q mismatch:
- Pneumonia.
- Pulmonary oedema.
- PE.
- Asthma.
- Emphysema.
- Pulmonary fibrosis.
- ARDS (p186).

Type II respiratory failure Defined as hypoxia (P_aO_2 <8kPa) with hypercapnia (P_aCO_2 >6.0kPa). This is caused by alveolar hypoventilation, with or without V/Q mismatch. Causes include:
- *Pulmonary disease:* Asthma, COPD, pneumonia, end-stage pulmonary fibrosis, obstructive sleep apnoea (OSA, p194).
- *Reduced respiratory drive:* Sedative drugs, CNS tumour or trauma.
- *Neuromuscular disease:* Cervical cord lesion, diaphragmatic paralysis, poliomyelitis, myasthenia gravis, Guillain-Barré syndrome.
- *Thoracic wall disease:* Flail chest, kyphoscoliosis.

Clinical features are those of the underlying cause together with symptoms and signs of hypoxia, with or without hypercapnia.

Hypoxia: Dyspnoea; restlessness; agitation; confusion; central cyanosis. If long-standing hypoxia: polycythaemia; pulmonary hypertension; cor pulmonale.

Hypercapnia: Headache; peripheral vasodilation; tachycardia; bounding pulse; tremor/flap; papilloedema; confusion; drowsiness; coma.

Investigations are aimed at determining the underlying cause:
- Blood tests: FBC, U&E, CRP, ABG. See table 4.7.
- Radiology: CXR.
- Microbiology: sputum and blood cultures (if febrile).
- Spirometry (COPD, neuromuscular disease, Guillain-Barré syndrome).

Management Depends on the cause:

Type I respiratory failure:
- Treat underlying cause.
- Give oxygen (24–60%) by facemask.
- Assisted ventilation if P_aO_2 <8kPa despite 60% O_2.

Type II respiratory failure: The respiratory centre may be relatively insensitive to CO_2 and respiration could be driven by hypoxia.
- Treat underlying cause.
- Controlled oxygen therapy: start at 24% O_2. ►*Oxygen therapy should be given with care.* Nevertheless, don't leave the hypoxia untreated.
- Recheck ABG after 20min. If P_aCO_2 is steady or lower, increase O_2 concentration to 28%. If P_aCO_2 has risen >1.5kPa and the patient is still hypoxic, consider assisted ventilation (eg NIPPV, p813, ie non-invasive positive pressure ventilation).
- If this fails, consider intubation and ventilation, if appropriate.

When to consider ABG (arterial blood gas) measurement

- Any unexpected deterioration in an ill patient. (Technique: see p771.)
- Anyone with an acute exacerbation of a chronic chest condition.
- Anyone with impaired consciousness or impaired respiratory effort.
- Signs of CO_2 retention, eg bounding pulse, drowsy, tremor (flapping), headache.
- Cyanosis, confusion, visual hallucinations (signs of ↓P_aO_2; S_AO_2 is an alternative).
- To validate measurements from transcutaneous pulse oximetry (p162).

ABG interpretation

Normal pH is 7.35–7.45. pH <7.35 indicates acidosis and >7.45 indicates alkalosis. If the pCO_2 is in keeping with the pH, the problem is likely to be a respiratory problem (eg high pCO_2 and pH <7.35 = likely a respiratory acidosis). If the HCO_3^- is in keeping with the pH, this is suggestive of a metabolic problem (eg high HCO_3^- and pH > 7.45 = metabolic alkalosis).

Table 4.7 Interpreting blood gas analysis

	pH	$PaCO_2$	HCO_3^-
Metabolic acidosis	Low	Normal/low	Low
Respiratory acidosis	Low	High	Normal/high
Metabolic alkalosis	High	Normal/high	High
Respiratory alkalosis	High	Low	Normal/low

Steps to ABG interpretation:

1. pH: acidosis or alkalosis?
2. pCO_2: high/low? Does this fit with the pH? (if yes, think respiratory problem)
3. HCO_3^-: high/low? Does this fit with pH? (if yes, think metabolic problem)
4. PO_2: is this normal given the FiO_2 (fraction of inspired oxygen)?
5. Is there any compensation? (i.e. changes in PCO_2/HCO_3^- to try and correct an underlying imbalance). Is this partial (pH abnormal) or complete (pH normalized)?
6. Calculate the anion gap. Helpful in working out aetiology of metabolic acidosis.

Anion gap: $(Na^+ + K^+) - (Cl^- + HCO_3^-)$

See p670 for causes of raised anion gap (normal 10-18mmol/L).

Administering oxygen

Oxygen should be prescribed. Titrate the amount guided by the patient's S_aO_2 and clinical condition. Humidification is only required for longer-term delivery of O_2 at high flow rates and tracheostomies, but may ↑ expectoration in bronchiectasis.

Nasal cannulae: Preferred by patients, but O_2 delivery is relatively imprecise and may cause nasal soreness. The flow rate (1–4L/min) roughly defines the concentration of O_2 (24–40%). May be used to maintain S_aO_2 when nebulizers need to be run using air, eg COPD.

Simple face mask: Delivers a variable amount of O_2 depending on the rate of inflow. Less precise than venturi masks—so don't use if hypercapnia or type II respiratory failure. Risk of CO_2 accumulation (within the mask and so in inspired gas) if flow rate <5L/min. ►Be careful in those with COPD (p812).

Venturi mask: Provides a precise percentage or fraction of O_2 (FiO_2) at high flow rates. Start at 24-28% in COPD. Colours of masks:

BLUE = 24%, WHITE = 28%, YELLOW = 35%, RED = 40%, GREEN = 60%.

Non-rebreathing mask: These have a reservoir bag and deliver high concentrations of O_2 (60–90%), determined by the inflow (10-15L/min) and the presence of flap valves on the side. They are commonly used in emergencies, but are imprecise and should be avoided in those requiring controlled O_2 therapy.

Promoting oxygenation: Other ways to ↑ oxygenation to reach the target S_aO_2 (this should be given as a number on the drug chart):

- Treat anaemia (transfuse if essential).
- Improve cardiac output (treat heart failure).
- Chest physio to improve ventilation/perfusion mismatch.

Pulmonary embolism (PE)

Causes PEs usually arise from a venous thrombosis in the pelvis or legs. Clots break off and pass through the veins and the right side of the heart before lodging in the pulmonary circulation. Rare causes: RV thrombus (post-MI); septic emboli (right-sided endocarditis); fat, air, or amniotic fluid embolism; neoplastic cells; parasites.

Risk factors

- Recent surgery, especially abdominal/pelvic or hip/knee replacement.
- Thrombophilia, eg antiphospholipid syndrome (p374).
- Leg fracture.
- Prolonged bed rest/reduced mobility.
- Malignancy.
- Pregnancy/postpartum; combined contraceptive pill; HRT (lower risk).
- Previous PE.

Clinical features Small emboli may be asymptomatic, whereas large emboli are often fatal. *Symptoms:* Acute breathlessness, pleuritic chest pain, haemoptysis; dizziness; syncope. Ask about risk factors, past history or family history of thromboembolism. *Signs:* Pyrexia; cyanosis; tachypnoea; tachycardia; hypotension; raised JVP; pleural rub; pleural effusion. Look for signs of a cause, eg deep vein thrombosis.

Tests

- FBC, U&E, baseline clotting, D-dimers (BOX).
- ABG may show $\downarrow P_aO_2$ and $\downarrow P_aCO_2$.
- Imaging: CXR may be normal, or show oligaemia of affected segment, dilated pulmonary artery, linear atelectasis, small pleural effusion, wedge-shaped opacities or cavitation (rare). CTPA—see fig 4.16.
- ECG may be normal, or show tachycardia, right bundle branch block, right ventricular strain (inverted T in V_1 to V_4). The classical SI QIII TIII pattern (p98) is rare.

►Further investigations are shown on p818.

Treatment ►►See p818. If haemodynamically unstable, thrombolyse for massive PE (alteplase 10mg IV over 1min, then 90mg IVI over 2h; max 1.5mg/kg if <65kg). Haemodynamically stable: start LMWH or unfractionated heparin if underlying renal impairment and treat for 5 days. Then, start DOAC (direct oral anticoagulant) or warfarin (p350). For warfarin, stop heparin when INR is 2-3, due to intial prothrombotic effect of warfarin (target INR of 2-3). Consider placement of a *vena caval filter* if contra-indication to anticoagulation.

Unprovoked PE In patients with no known provoking risk factors, consider investigation for possible underlying malignany. Undertake full history, examination (including breast), CXR, FBC, calcium, LFTs, urinalysis. Patients >40yrs consider abdo-pelvic CT and mammography in women. Consider antiphospholipid and thrombophilia testing if family history positive (p374).

Prevention Give heparin to all immobile patients. Stop HRT and the combined contraceptive pill pre-op (if reliable with another form of contraception).

Pneumothorax

Causes Often spontaneous (especially in young, thin men) due to rupture of a subpleural bulla. Other causes: asthma; COPD; TB; pneumonia; lung abscess; carcinoma; cystic fibrosis; lung fibrosis; sarcoidosis; connective tissue disorders (Marfan's syn., Ehlers-Danlos syn.), trauma; iatrogenic (subclavian CVP line insertion, pleural aspiration/biopsy, transbronchial biopsy, liver biopsy, +ve pressure ventilation).

Clinical features *Symptoms:* May be asymptomatic (fit, young, and small pneumothorax) or there may be sudden onset of dyspnoea and/or pleuritic chest pain. Patients with asthma or COPD may present with a sudden deterioration. Mechanically ventilated patients may present with hypoxia or an increase in ventilation pressures. *Signs:* Reduced expansion, hyper-resonance to percussion, and diminished breath sounds on the affected side. With a *tension pneumothorax*, the trachea will be deviated away from the affected side, p749, p815. *Management:* See p815.

Investigating suspected PE

Diagnosis of PE is improved by adopting a stepwise approach, combining an objective probability score, with subsequent investigations, as follows.
Assess the clinical probability of a PE: Many systems exist and one of the most frequently used is the modified Wells Criteria (table 4.8).

Table 4.8 Modified two-level PE Wells score

Feature	Score
Clinical signs and symptoms of DVT (leg pain and pain on deep palpation of veins)	3
Heart rate >100 beats per minute	1.5
Recently bed-ridden (>3 days) or major surgery (<4 weeks)	1.5
Previous DVT or PE	1.5
Haemoptysis	1
Cancer receiving active treatment , treated in last 6/12, palliative	1
An alternative diagnosis is less likely than PE	3
Score <4 = PE unlikely; score >4 = PE likely	

Wells PS, Anderson DR, Rodger M, *et al.* 'Derivation of a Simple Clinical Model to Categorize Patients Probability of Pulmonary Embolism: Increasing the Models Utility with the SimpliRED D-dimer'. *Thromb Haemost* 2000; 83: 416–20.

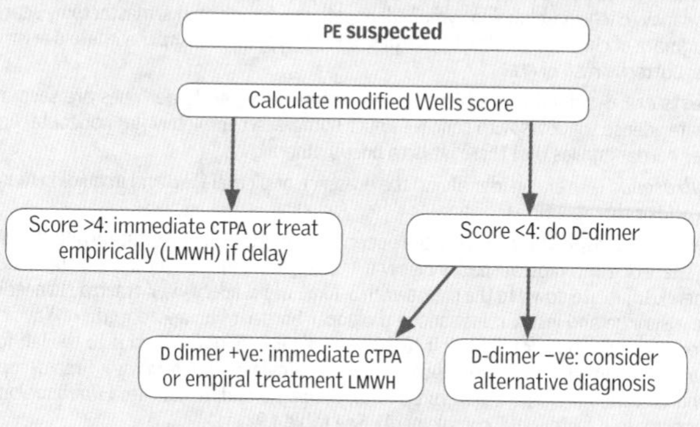

Length of treatment

- Provoked: 3 months and then reassess risk to benefit profile (depends on whether risk factor persists)
- Unprovoked: treatment is usually continued for >3 months (people with no identifiable risk factor)
- Malignancy: continue treatment with LMWH for 6 months or until cure of cancer
- Pregnancy: LMWH is continued until delivery/end of pregnancy

Fig 4.16 Investigation and management of PE.

Direct oral anticoagulants (DOACs)

Oral alternatives to warfarin (dabigatran, rivaroxaban, apixaban, edoxaban) have been available for treatment of PE since NICE approval in 2012. They have a rapid onset of action (without the need for LMWH overlap) and can be administered in fixed doses without the need for continuous monitoring. Monitoring is required to assess compliance, side effects (eg bleeding), and presence of VTE. Antidotes for DOACs are becoming available and in the USA idarucizumab is already licensed.

Pleural effusion

Definitions A pleural effusion is fluid in the pleural space. Effusions can be divided by their protein concentration into *transudates* (<25g/L) and *exudates* (>35g/L), see BOX. Blood in the pleural space is a *haemothorax*, pus in the pleural space is an *empyema*, and chyle (lymph with fat) is a *chylothorax*. Both blood and air in the pleural space is called a *haemopneumothorax*.

Causes *Transudates* may be due to ↑venous pressure (cardiac failure, constrictive pericarditis, fluid overload), or hypoproteinaemia (cirrhosis, nephrotic syndrome, malabsorption). Also occur in hypothyroidism and Meigs' syndrome (right pleural effusion and ovarian fibroma). *Exudates* are mostly due to increased leakiness of pleural capillaries secondary to infection, inflammation, or malignancy. Causes: pneumonia; TB; pulmonary infarction; rheumatoid arthritis; SLE; bronchogenic carcinoma; malignant metastases; lymphoma; mesothelioma; lymphangitis carcinomatosis.

Symptoms Asymptomatic—or dyspnoea, pleuritic chest pain.

Signs *Decreased expansion; stony dull percussion note; diminished breath sounds* occur on the affected side. Tactile vocal fremitus and vocal resonance are ↓ (inconstant and unreliable). Above the effusion, where lung is compressed, there may be *bronchial breathing*. With large effusions there may be *tracheal deviation* away from the effusion. Look for aspiration marks and signs of associated disease: malignancy (cachexia, clubbing, lymphadenopathy, radiation marks, mastectomy scar); stigmata of chronic liver disease; cardiac failure; hypothyroidism; rheumatoid arthritis; butterfly rash of SLE.

Tests *CXR:* Small effusions blunt the costophrenic angles, larger ones are seen as water-dense shadows with concave upper borders. A completely flat horizontal upper border implies that there is also a pneumothorax.

Ultrasound is useful in identifying the presence of pleural fluid and in guiding diagnostic or therapeutic aspiration.

Diagnostic aspiration: Percuss the upper border of the pleural effusion and choose a site 1 or 2 intercostal spaces below it (don't go too low or you'll be in the abdomen!). Infiltrate down to the pleura with 5-10mL of 1% lidocaine. Attach a 21G needle to a syringe and insert it just above the upper border of an appropriate rib (avoids neurovascular bundle). Draw off 10-30mL of pleural fluid and send it to the lab for *clinical chemistry* (protein, glucose, pH, LDH, amylase), *bacteriology* (microscopy and culture, auramine stain, TB culture), *cytology*, and, if indicated, *immunology* (rheumatoid factor, ANA, complement). See table 4.9.

Pleural biopsy: If pleural fluid analysis is inconclusive, consider parietal pleural biopsy. Thoracoscopic or CT-guided pleural biopsy increases diagnostic yield (by enabling direct visualization of the pleural cavity and biopsy of suspicious areas).

Management is of the underlying cause.

- *Drainage:* If the effusion is symptomatic, drain it, repeatedly if necessary. Fluid is best removed slowly (0.5-1.5L/24h). It may be aspirated in the same way as a diagnostic tap, or using an intercostal drain (see p766).
- *Pleurodesis* with talc may be helpful for recurrent effusions. Thorascopic mechanical pleurodesis is most effective for malignant effusions. Empyemas (p170) are best drained using a chest drain, inserted under ultrasound or CT guidance.
- *Intra-pleural alteplase and dornase alfa* may help with empyema.
- *Surgery:* Persistent collections and increasing pleural thickness (on ultrasound) requires surgery.[50]

Table 4.9 Pleural fluid analysis

Gross appearance	Cause
Clear, straw-coloured	Transudate, exudate
Turbid, yellow	Empyema, parapneumonic effusion[5]
Haemorrhagic	Trauma, malignancy, pulmonary infarction
Cytology	
Neutrophils ++	Parapneumonic effusion, PE
Lymphocytes ++	Malignancy, TB, RA, SLE, sarcoidosis
Mesothelial cells ++	Pulmonary infarction
Abnormal mesothelial cells	Mesothelioma
Multinucleated giant cells	RA
Lupus erythematosus cells	SLE
Malignant cells	Malignancy
Clinical chemistry	
*Protein <25g/L	Transudate
>35g/L	Exudate
25–35g/L	If pleural fluid protein/serum protein >0.5, effusion is an exudate (85% specific and sensitive)
Glucose <3.3mmol/L	Empyema, malignancy, TB, RA, SLE
pH <7.2	Empyema, malignancy, TB, RA, SLE
*↑LDH (pleural:serum >0.6)	Empyema, malignancy, TB, RA, SLE
↑Amylase	Pancreatitis, carcinoma, bacterial pneumonia, oesophageal rupture
Immunology	
Rheumatoid factor	RA
Antinuclear antibody	SLE
↓Complement levels	RA, SLE, malignancy, infection

* Light's criteria for defining an exudate: effusion protein/serum protein >0.5; effusion LDH/serum LDH >0.6; effusion LDH > ⅔ upper reference range. 98% sensitive and 83% specific.

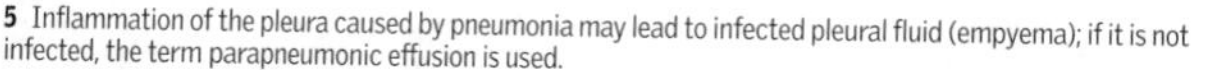
5 Inflammation of the pleura caused by pneumonia may lead to infected pleural fluid (empyema); if it is not infected, the term parapneumonic effusion is used.

Obstructive sleep apnoea syndrome

This disorder is characterized by intermittent closure/collapse of the pharyngeal airway causing apnoeic episodes during sleep. These are terminated by partial arousal.

Clinical features The typical patient is an obese, middle-aged man who presents because of snoring or daytime somnolence. His partner often describes apnoeic episodes during sleep.

- Loud snoring.
- Daytime somnolence.
- Poor sleep quality.
- Morning headache.
- Decreased libido.
- Nocturia.
- ↓Cognitive performance.

Complications Pulmonary hypertension; type II respiratory failure (p188). Sleep apnoea is also reported as an independent risk factor for hypertension.[51]

Investigations Simple studies (eg pulse oximetry, video recordings) may be all that are required for diagnosis. Polysomnography (which monitors oxygen saturation, airflow at the nose and mouth, ECG, EMG chest, and abdominal wall movement during sleep) is diagnostic. The occurrence of 15 or more episodes of apnoea or hypopnoea during 1h of sleep, on average, indicates significant sleep apnoea.

Management

- Weight reduction.
- Avoidance of tobacco and alcohol.
- Mandibular advancement device.
- CPAP via a nasal mask during sleep is effective and recommended by NICE for those with moderate to severe disease.[52]
- Surgery to relieve pharyngeal or nasal obstruction, eg tonsillectomy or polypectomy, is occasionally needed.

Cor pulmonale

Cor pulmonale is right heart failure caused by chronic pulmonary arterial hypertension. Causes include chronic lung disease, pulmonary vascular disorders, and neuromuscular and skeletal diseases (see BOX).

Clinical features Symptoms include dyspnoea, fatigue, and syncope. Signs: cyanosis; tachycardia; raised JVP with prominent a and v waves; RV heave; loud P_2, pansystolic murmur (tricuspid regurgitation); early diastolic Graham Steell murmur; hepatomegaly and oedema.

Investigations *FBC:* Hb and haematocrit↑ (secondary polycythaemia). *ABG:* hypoxia, with or without hypercapnia. *CXR:* enlarged right atrium and ventricle, prominent pulmonary arteries (see fig 4.17). *ECG:* P pulmonale; right axis deviation; right ventricular hypertrophy/strain.

Management

- *Treat underlying cause*—eg COPD and pulmonary infections.
- *Treat respiratory failure*—in the acute situation give 24% oxygen if P_aO_2 <8kPa. Monitor ABG and gradually increase oxygen concentration if P_aCO_2 is stable (p188). In COPD patients, long-term oxygen therapy (LTOT) for 16h/d increases survival (p184). Patients with chronic hypoxia when clinically stable should be assessed for LTOT.
- *Treat cardiac failure* with diuretics such as furosemide, eg 40–160mg/24h PO. Monitor U&E and give amiloride or potassium supplements if necessary. Alternative: spironolactone.
- Consider *venesection* if haematocrit >55%.
- Consider *heart-lung transplantation* in young patients.

Prognosis Poor. 50% die within 5yrs.

Causes of cor pulmonale

Lung disease
- COPD
- Bronchiectasis
- Pulmonary fibrosis
- Severe chronic asthma
- Lung resection.

Pulmonary vascular disease
- Pulmonary emboli
- Pulmonary vasculitis
- Primary pulmonary hypertension
- ARDS (p186)
- Sickle-cell disease
- Parasite infestation.

Thoracic cage abnormality
- Kyphosis
- Scoliosis
- Thoracoplasty.

Neuromuscular disease
- Myasthenia gravis
- Poliomyelitis
- Motor neuron disease.

Hypoventilation
- Sleep apnoea
- Enlarged adenoids in children.

Cerebrovascular disease

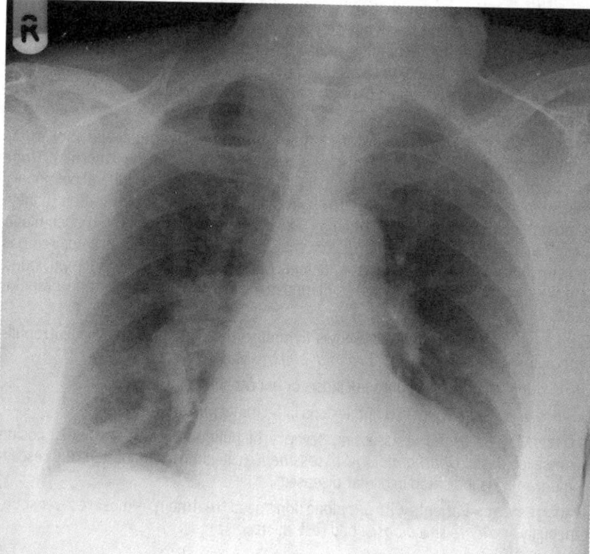

Fig 4.17 PA chest radiograph showing enlarged pulmonary arteries from pulmonary artery hypertension. When caused by interstitial lung disease and leading to right heart failure, this would be termed cor pulmonale. No signs of interstitial lung disease are identifiable in this image.

Image courtesy of Derby Hospitals NHS Foundation Trust Radiology Department.

Sarcoidosis

A multisystem granulomatous disorder of unknown cause. Prevalence highest in Northern Europe, eg UK: 10–20/10^5 population. Usually affects adults aged 20–40yrs, more common in women. African-Caribbeans are affected more frequently and more severely than Caucasians, particularly by extra-thoracic disease. Associated with HLA-DRB1 and DQB1 alleles. For other causes of granuloma see table 4.10.

Clinical features In 20–40%, the disease is discovered incidentally, after a routine CXR, and is thus asymptomatic. *Acute sarcoidosis* often presents with fever, erythema nodosum (fig 12.21, p563),[6] polyarthralgia, and bilateral hilar lymphodenopathy (BHL), also called Löfgren syndrome, which usually resolves spontaneously.

Pulmonary disease: 90% have abnormal CXRs with BHL (fig 4.18) ± pulmonary infiltrates or fibrosis; see later in topic for staging. *Symptoms:* Dry cough, progressive dyspnoea, ↓exercise tolerance, and chest pain. In 10–20%, symptoms progress, with concurrent deterioration in lung function.

Non-pulmonary signs: These are legion: lymphadenopathy; hepatomegaly; splenomegaly; uveitis; conjunctivitis; keratoconjunctivitis sicca; glaucoma; terminal phalangeal bone cysts; enlargement of lacrimal & parotid glands (fig 8.49, p355); Bell's palsy; neuropathy; meningitis; brainstem and spinal syndromes; space-occupying lesion; erythema nodosum (fig 12.21, p563); lupus pernio; subcutaneous nodules; cardiomyopathy; arrhythmias; hypercalcaemia; hypercalciuria; renal stones; pituitary dysfunction.

Tests *Blood:* ↑ESR, lymphopenia, ↑LFT, ↑serum ACE in ~60% (non-specific), ↑Ca^{2+}, ↑immunoglobulins. *24h urine:* ↑Ca^{2+}. *CXR* is abnormal in 90%: *Stage 0:* normal. *Stage 1:* BHL. *Stage 2:* BHL + peripheral pulmonary infiltrates. *Stage 3:* peripheral pulmonary infiltrates alone. Stage 4: progressive pulmonary fibrosis; bulla formation (honeycombing); pleural involvement. *ECG* may show arrhythmias or bundle branch block. *Lung function tests* may be normal or show reduced lung volumes, impaired gas transfer, and a restrictive ventilatory defect. *Tissue biopsy* (lung, liver, lymph nodes, skin nodules, or lacrimal glands) is diagnostic and shows non-caseating granulomata.

Bronchoalveolar lavage (BAL): Shows ↑lymphocytes in active disease; ↑neutrophils with pulmonary fibrosis. *Transbrochial biopsy:* May be diagnostic.

Ultrasound: May show nephrocalcinosis or hepatosplenomegaly.

Bone X-rays: Show 'punched out' lesions in terminal phalanges.

CT/MRI: May be useful in assessing severity of pulmonary disease or diagnosing neurosarcoidosis. *Ophthalmology assessment* (slit lamp examination, fluorescein angiography) is indicated in ocular disease.

Management ►Patients with *BHL* alone don't need treatment as most recover spontaneously.[53,54] *Acute sarcoidosis:* bed rest, NSAIDs.

Indications for corticosteroids:

- Parenchymal lung disease (symptomatic, static, or progressive).
- Uveitis.
- Hypercalcaemia.
- Neurological or cardiac involvement.

Prednisolone (40mg/24h) PO for 4–6 wks, then ↓dose over 1yr according to clinical status. A few patients relapse and may need a further course or long-term therapy.

Other therapy: In severe illness, IV methylprednisolone or immunosuppressants (methotrexate, hydroxychloroquine, ciclosporin, cyclophosphamide) may be needed. Anti-TNFα therapy may be tried in refractory cases, or lung transplantation.

Prognosis 60% of patients with thoracic sarcoidosis resolve over 2yrs. 20% respond to steroid therapy; in the rest, improvement is unlikely despite therapy.[7]

6 A detailed history and exam (including for synovitis) + CXR, 2 ASO (antistreptolysin-O) titres and a tuberculin skin test are usually enough to diagnose erythema nodosum.

7 ACE is also ↑ in: hyperthyroidism, Gaucher's, silicosis, TB, hypersensitivity pneumonitis, asbestosis, pneumocystosis.[55] ↑ACE levels in CSF help diagnose CNS sarcoidosis (when serum ACE may be normal).[56] ACE is *lower* in: Caucasians; and anorexia.[57]

Table 4.10 Differential diagnosis of granulomatous diseases

Infections	Bacteria	TB, leprosy, syphilis, cat scratch fever
	Fungi	*Cryptococcus neoformans* *Coccidioides immitis*
	Protozoa	*Schistosomiasis*
Autoimmune	Primary biliary cholangitis Granulomatous orchitis	
Vasculitis (p556)	Giant cell arteritis Polyarteritis nodosa Takayasu's arteritis Wegener's granulomatosis	
Organic dust disease	Silicosis, berylliosis	
Idiopathic	Crohn's disease De Quervain's thyroiditis Sarcoidosis	
Extrinsic allergic alveolitis		
Histiocytosis X		

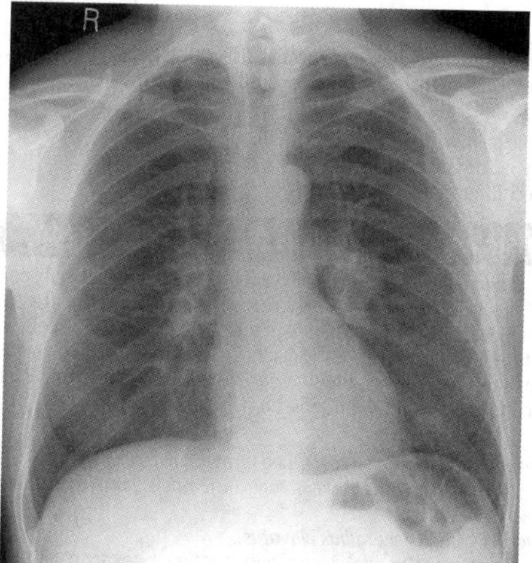

Fig 4.18 PA chest radiograph showing bilateral hilar lymphadenopathy. The important differentials for this appearance are: sarcoidosis, TB, lymphoma, pneumoconioses, and metastatic disease. This patient has sarcoidosis but there are no other stigmata (such as the presence of infiltrates, fibrosis, and honeycombing) on this image.

Image courtesy of Norfolk and Norwich University Hospitals NHS Trust Radiology Department.

Causes of BHL (bilateral hilar lymphadenopathy)

- Sarcoidosis
- Infection, eg TB, mycoplasma
- Malignancy, eg lymphoma, carcinoma, mediastinal tumours
- Organic dust disease, eg silicosis, berylliosis
- Hypersensitivity pneumonitis
- Histocytosis X (Langerhan's cell histiocytosis).

Interstitial lung disease (ILD)

This is the generic term used to describe a number of conditions that primarily affect the lung parenchyma in a diffuse manner.[58] They are characterized by chronic inflammation and/or progressive interstitial fibrosis (table 4.11), and share a number of clinical and pathological features. See table 4.11 and fig 4.19.

Clinical features Dyspnoea on exertion; non-productive paroxysmal cough; abnormal breath sounds; abnormal CXR or high-resolution CT; restrictive pulmonary spirometry with ↓DLCO (p164).

Pathological features Fibrosis and remodelling of the interstitium; chronic inflammation; hyperplasia of type II epithelial cells or type II pneumocytes.

Classification The ILDs can be broadly grouped into three categories:

Those with known cause, eg:

- Occupational/environmental, eg asbestosis, berylliosis, silicosis, cotton worker's lung (byssinosis).
- Drugs, eg nitrofurantoin, bleomycin, amiodarone, sulfasalazine, busulfan.
- Hypersensitivity reactions, eg hypersensitivity pneumonitis.
- Infections, eg TB, fungi, viral.
- Gastro-oesophageal reflux.

Those associated with systemic disorders, eg:

- Sarcoidosis.
- Rheumatoid arthritis.
- SLE, systemic sclerosis, mixed connective tissue disease, Sjögren's syndrome.
- Ulcerative colitis, renal tubular acidosis, autoimmune thyroid disease.

Idiopathic, eg:

- Idiopathic pulmonary fibrosis (IPF, p200).
- Cryptogenic organizing pneumonia.
- Non-specific interstitial pneumonitis.

Extrinsic allergic alveolitis (EAA)

In sensitized individuals, repetitive inhalation of allergens (fungal spores or avian proteins) provokes a hypersensitivity reaction which varies in intensity and clinical course depending on the antigen. In the acute phase, the alveoli are infiltrated with acute inflammatory cells. Early diagnosis and prompt allergen removal can halt and reverse disease progression, so prognosis can be good. With chronic exposure, granuloma formation and obliterative bronchiolitis occur.

Causes

- Bird-fancier's and pigeon-fancier's lung (proteins in bird droppings).
- Farmer's and mushroom worker's lung (*Micropolyspora faeni*, *Thermoactinomyces vulgaris*).
- Malt worker's lung (*Aspergillus clavatus*).
- Bagassosis or sugar worker's lung (*Thermoactinomyces sacchari*).

Clinical features *4–6h post-exposure:* Fever, rigors, myalgia, dry cough, dyspnoea, fine bibasal crackles. *Chronic:* Finger clubbing (50%), increasing dyspnoea, ↓weight, exertional dyspnoea, type I respiratory failure, cor pulmonale.

Tests *Acute: Blood:* FBC (neutrophilia); ↑ESR; ABGs; serum antibodies (may indicate exposure/previous sensitization rather than disease). *CXR:* upper-zone mottling/consolidation; hilar lymphadenopathy (rare). *Lung function tests:* Reversible restrictive defect; reduced gas transfer during acute attacks. *Chronic:* Blood tests: serum antibodies. *CXR:* upper-zone fibrosis; honeycomb lung. *CT chest:* nodules, ground glass appearance, extensive fibrosis. *Lung function tests:* restrictive defect. Bronchoalveolar lavage (BAL) fluid shows ↑lymphocytes and ↑mast cells.

Management *Acute:* Remove allergen and give O_2 (35–60%), PO prednisolone (40mg/24h PO), reducing course. *Chronic:* Allergen avoidance, or wear a facemask or +ve pressure helmet. Long-term steroids often achieve CXR and physiological improvement. Compensation (UK Industrial Injuries Act) may be payable.

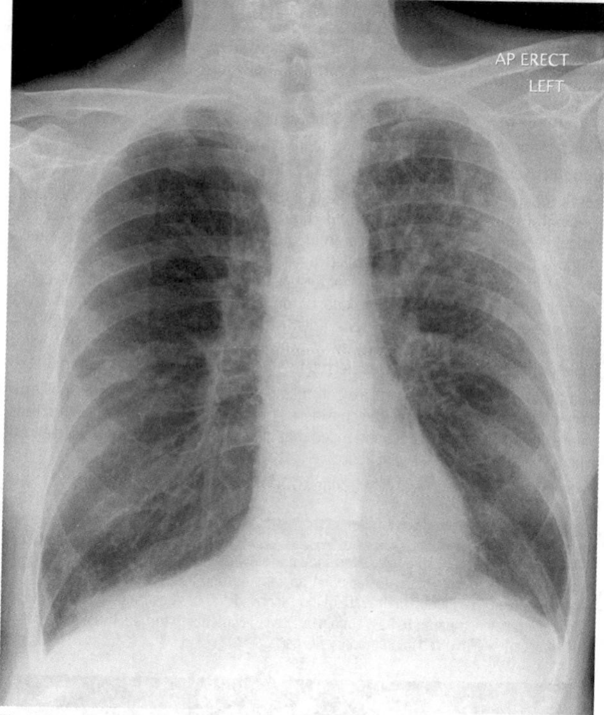

Fig 4.19 AP chest radiograph showing air-space shadowing in the left upper zone. Although this appearance often represents infection, it is non-specific. Differential diagnosis for this distribution of shadowing include lymphoma, alveolar cell carcinoma (both to be considered if not resolving in appearance on follow-up imaging), and haemorrhage.

Image courtesy of Nottingham University Hospitals NHS Trust Radiology Department.

Table 4.11 Causes of fibrotic shadowing on a CXR

Upper zone	Mid zone	Lower zone
TB Hypersensitivity pneumonitis	Sarcoidosis, histoplasmosis	Idiopathic pulmonary fibrosis
Ankylosing spondylitis		Asbestosis
Radiotherapy		
Progressive massive fibrosis (PMF)		

Idiopathic pulmonary fibrosis (IPF)

This is a type of idiopathic interstitial pneumonia. Inflammatory cell infiltrate and pulmonary fibrosis of unknown cause. It is the commonest cause of interstitial lung disease.

Symptoms Dry cough; exertional dyspnoea; malaise; ↓weight; arthralgia.

Signs Cyanosis; finger clubbing; fine end-inspiratory crepitations.

Complications Respiratory failure; ↑risk of lung cancer.

Tests *Blood:* ABG (↓P_aO_2; if severe, ↑P_aCO_2); ↑CRP; ↑immunoglobulins; ANA (30% +ve), rheumatoid factor (10% +ve). *Imaging:* (fig 4.20) ↓Lung volume; bilateral lower zone reticulo-nodular shadows; honeycomb lung (advanced disease). *CT:* Shows similar changes to the CXR but is more sensitive and is an essential for diagnosis. *Spirometry:* Restrictive (p162); ↓transfer factor. *BAL:* May indicate activity of alveolitis: ↑lymphocytes (good response/prognosis) or ↑neutrophils and ↑eosinophils (poor response/prognosis). *$^{99}TC^{m}$-DTPA scan:* (diethylene-triamine-penta-acetic acid) May reflect disease activity.[59] *Lung biopsy:* May be needed for diagnosis.The histological changes observed on biopsy are referred to as *usual interstitial pneumonia* (UIP).

Management Supportive care: oxygen, pulmonary rehabilitation, opiates, palliative care input. All patients should be considered for current clinical trials or lung transplantation.[60] It is strongly recommended that high-dose steroids are not used except where the diagnosis of IPF is in doubt.

Prognosis 50% 5yr survival rate (range 1–20yrs).

A new treatment emerges for sufferers of IPF

Nintedanib and pirfenidone have been shown to slow disease progression and offer some hope to sufferers of IPF. Pirfenidone, an immunosuppressant and antifibrotic agent, showed a reduction in the rate of lung scarring and has been shown to improve life expectancy compared to best supportive care.[61] Nintedanib targets three growth factor receptors involved in pulmonary fibrosis.

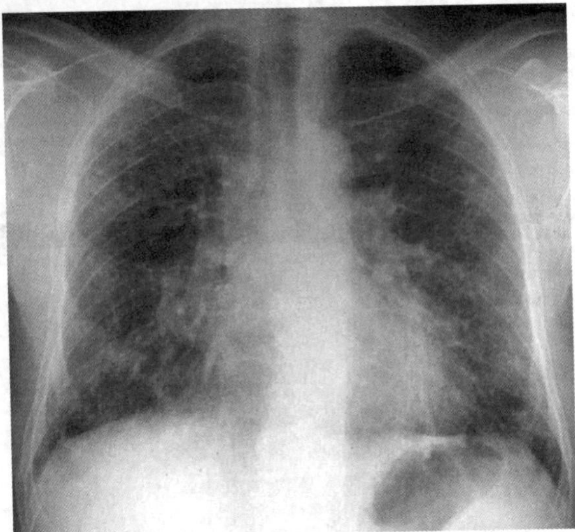

Fig 4.20 Interstitial lung disease due to idiopathic pulmonary fibrosis (a similar appearance to the interstitial oedema of moderate left heart failure, but without a big heart).

Courtesy of Prof P Scally.

Industrial dust diseases

Coal worker's pneumoconiosis (CWP) A common dust disease in countries that have or have had underground coal-mines. It results from inhalation of coal dust particles (1–3μm in diameter) over 15–20yrs. These are ingested by macrophages which die, releasing their enzymes and causing fibrosis.

Clinical features: Asymptomatic, but coexisting chronic bronchitis is common. CXR: many round opacities (1–10mm), especially in upper zone.

Management: Avoid exposure to coal dust; treat co-existing chronic bronchitis; claim compensation (in the UK, via the Industrial Injuries Act).

Progressive massive fibrosis (PMF) Due to progression of CWP, which causes progressive dyspnoea, fibrosis, and, eventually, cor pulmonale. CXR: usually bilateral, upper-mid zone fibrotic masses (1–10cm), develop from periphery towards hilum.

Management: Avoid exposure to coal dust; claim compensation (as for CWP).

Caplan's syndrome The association between rheumatoid arthritis, pneumoconiosis, and pulmonary rheumatoid nodules.

Silicosis (See fig 4.21.) Caused by inhalation of silica particles, which are very fibrogenic. A number of jobs may be associated with exposure, eg metal mining, stone quarrying, sandblasting, and pottery/ceramic manufacture.

Clinical features: Progressive dyspnoea, ↑incidence of TB, CXR shows diffuse miliary or nodular pattern in upper and mid-zones and egg-shell calcification of hilar nodes. Spirometry: restrictive ventilatory defect.

Management: Avoid exposure to silica; claim compensation (as for CWP).

Asbestosis Caused by inhalation of asbestos fibres. Asbestos was commonly used in the building trade for fire proofing, pipe lagging, electrical wire insulation, and roofing felt. Degree of asbestos exposure is related to degree of pulmonary fibrosis.

Clinical features: Similar to other fibrotic lung diseases with progressive dyspnoea, clubbing, and fine end-inspiratory crackles. Also causes pleural plaques, ↑risk of bronchial adenocarcinoma and mesothelioma.

Management: Symptomatic. Patients are often eligible for compensation through the UK Industrial Injuries Act.

Mesothelioma See p174.

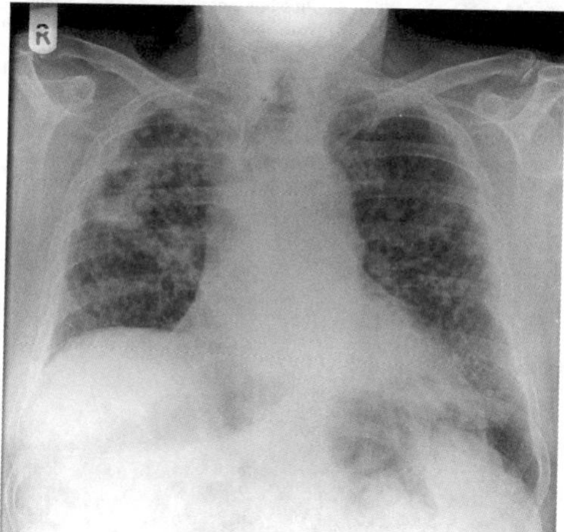

Fig 4.21 PA chest radiograph showing diffuse nodular opacities with a focal area of irregular soft tissue shadowing in the right upper zone, consistent with silicosis and developing progressive massive fibrosis (PMF). Image courtesy of Derby Hospitals NHS Foundation Trust Radiology Department.

5 Endocrinology

Contents

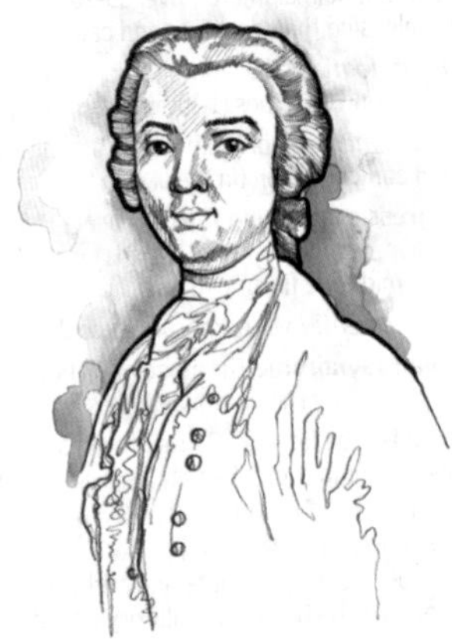

Fig 5.1 Our understanding of hormones, while still evolving, originated from a mix of random experiments, coincidental findings, and extraordinary sounding characters! One of these was the 'castrati' that featured in opera throughout the 16th, 17th, and 18th centuries. These were boys who were castrated before puberty. The voice of a castrato was pure and forceful, due to their enormous lung capacity and resulting breath control. They also experienced no temporal recession, and their arms and legs were long. One of the most well renowned was Farinelli, the stage name of Carlo Maria Michelangelo Nicola Broschi. It was said he had a well-modulated soprano voice with extraordinary breath control. His picture hangs in Handel's house in London. The practice was stopped in the early 20th century when it was acknowledged how inhumane the operation was.

We thank Dr Stephen Gilbey, our Specialist Reader for this chapter.

The essence of endocrinology

For scientists

- Define a syndrome, and match it to a gland malfunction.
- Measure the gland's output in the peripheral blood. Define clinical syndromes associated with too much or too little secretion (*hyper-* and *hypo-*syndromes, respectively; *eu-* means normal, neither ↑ nor ↓, as in *euthyroid*). Note factors that may make measurement variable, eg diurnal release of cortisol.
- If suspecting hormone deficiency, test by stimulating the gland that produces it (eg short ACTH stimulation test or *Synacthen*® test in Addison's). If the gland is not functioning normally, there will be a blunted response to stimulation.
- If suspecting hormone excess, test by inhibiting the gland that produces it (eg dexamethasone suppression test in Cushing's). If there is a hormone-secreting tumour then this will fail to suppress via normal feedback mechanisms.
- Find a way to image the gland. NB: non-functioning tumours or 'incidentalomas' may be found in health, see p224. Imaging alone does not make the diagnosis.
- Aim to halt disease progression; diet and exercise can stop progression of impaired fasting glucose to frank diabetes.[1,2] For other glands, halting progression will depend on understanding autoimmunity, and the interaction of genes and environment. In thyroid autoimmunity (an archetypal autoimmune disease), it is possible to track interactions between genes and environment (eg smoking and stress) via expression of immunologically active molecules (HLA class I and II, adhesion molecules, cytokines, CD40, and complement regulatory proteins).[3]

Endocrinologists love this reductionist approach, but have been less successful at understanding *emergent phenomena*—those properties and performances of ours that cannot be predicted from full knowledge of our perturbed parts. We understand the diurnal nature of cortisol secretion, for example, but the science of relating this to dreams, the consolidation of memory, and the psychopathology of families and other groups (such as the endocrinology ward round you may be about to join) is in its infancy. But as doctors we are steeped in the hormonal lives of patients (as they are in ours)—and we may as well start by recognizing this now.

For those doing exams

'What's wrong with *him*?' your examiner asks, boldly. While you apologize to the patient for this rudeness by asking, 'Is it alright if we speak about you as if you weren't here?', think to yourself that if you were a betting man or woman you would wager that the diagnosis will be endocrinological. In no other discipline are gestalt impressions so characteristic. To get good at recognizing these conditions, spend time in endocrinology outpatients and looking at collections of clinical photographs. Also, specific cutaneous signs are important, as follows.

Thyrotoxicosis: Hair loss; pretibial myxoedema (confusing term, p218); onycholysis (nail separation from the nailbed); bulging eyes (exophthalmos/proptosis).

Hypothyroidism: Hair loss; eyebrow loss; cold, pale skin; characteristic face. You might, perhaps should, fail your exam if you blurt out 'Toad-like face'.

Cushing's syndrome: Central obesity and wasted limbs (='lemon on sticks' see fig 5.2); moon face; buffalo hump; supraclavicular fat pads; striae.

Addison's disease: Hyperpigmentation (face, neck, palmar creases).

Acromegaly: Acral (distal) + soft tissue overgrowth; big jaws (macrognathia), hands and feet; the skin is thick; facial features are coarse.

Hyperandrogenism (♀): Hirsutism; temporal balding; acne.

Hypopituitarism: Pale or yellow tinged thinned skin, resulting in fine wrinkling around the eyes and mouth, making the patient look older.

Hypoparathyroidism: Dry, scaly, puffy skin; brittle nails; coarse hair.

Pseudohypoparathyroidism: Short stature, short neck, and short 4th and 5th metacarpals.

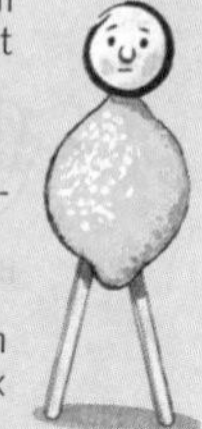

Fig 5.2 'Lemon on sticks.'

Endocrine physiology

Hormones are chemical messengers which act directly on nearby cells (paracrine effect), on the cell of origin (autocrine effect), at a distant site (endocrine effect), or as neurotransmitters (brain and gastrointestinal tract). Thirst, thermal regulation, appetite, sleep cycles, menstrual cycle, and stress/mood are all controlled by the hypothalamus. Releasing factors produced by the hypothalamus reach the pituitary via the portal system (pituitary stalk), see fig 5.3. The releasing factors stimulate or inhibit the production of hormones from the anterior pituitary, fig 5.4. Vasopressin and oxytocin are produced in the hypothalamus and stored and released from the posterior pituitary.

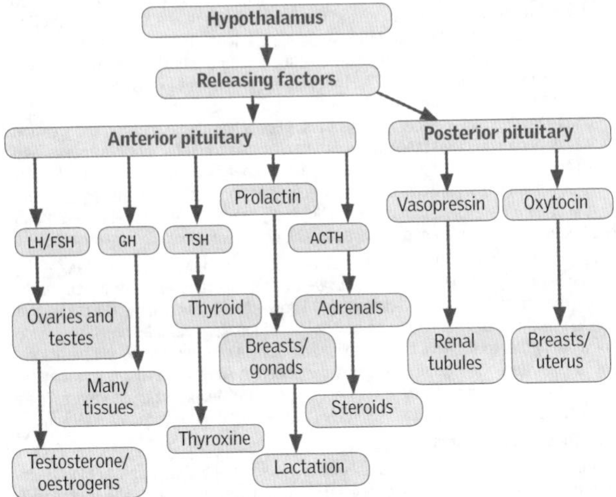

Fig 5.3 Hypothalamic-pituitary axis.

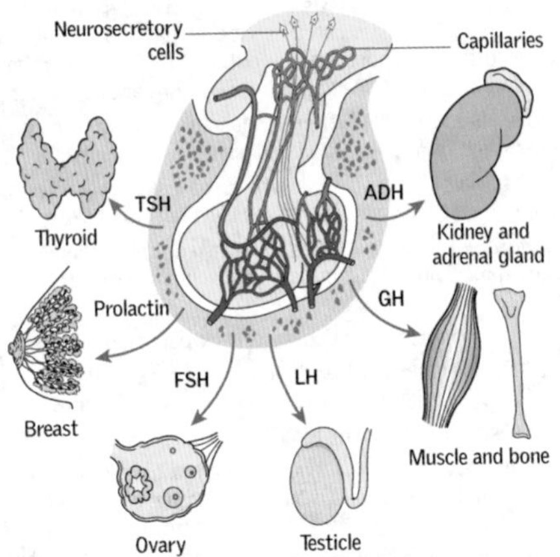

Fig 5.4 Neuroregulation and integration of endocrine axes makes us who we are—and who we are and what we do feeds back into our hormonal milieu. Multifactorial disruptions within the growth hormone (GH), luteinizing hormone (LH)-testosterone, adrenocorticotropin (ACTH)-cortisol and insulin axes play a major role in healthy maturation and ageing.

This page intentionally blank

Diabetes mellitus (DM): classification and diagnosis

DM results from lack, or reduced effectiveness, of endogenous insulin. Hyperglycaemia is one aspect of a far-reaching metabolic derangement, which causes serious microvascular (retinopathy, nephropathy, neuropathy) or macrovascular problems: stroke, MI, renovascular disease, limb ischaemia. *So think of DM as a vascular disease*:[1] adopt a holistic approach and consider other cardiovascular risk factors too.

Categories of diabetes and dyslipidaemia

Type 1 DM: Usually adolescent onset but may occur at *any* age. *Cause:* insulin deficiency from autoimmune destruction of insulin-secreting pancreatic β cells. Patients must have insulin, and are prone to ketoacidosis and weight loss. Associated with other autoimmune diseases (>90% HLA DR3 ± DR4). Concordance is only ~30% in identical twins, indicating environmental influence. Four genes are important: one (6q) determines islet sensitivity to damage (eg from viruses or cross-reactivity from cows' milk-induced antibodies). Latent autoimmune diabetes of adults (LADA) is a form of type 1 DM, with slower progression to insulin dependence in later life.

Type 2 DM: (Formerly non-insulin-dependent DM, NIDDM) is at 'epidemic' levels in many places, mainly due to changes in lifestyle, but also because of better diagnosis and improved longevity.[4] Higher prevalence in Asians, men, and the elderly (up to 18%). Most are over 40yrs, but teenagers are now getting type 2 DM (*OHCS* p156). *Cause:* ↓insulin secretion ± ↑insulin resistance. It is associated with obesity, lack of exercise, calorie and alcohol excess. ≥80% concordance in identical twins, indicating stronger genetic influence than in type 1 DM. Typically progresses from a preliminary phase of impaired glucose tolerance (IGT) or impaired fasting glucose (IFG). (►This is a unique window for lifestyle intervention.) Maturity onset diabetes of the young (MODY) is a rare autosomal dominant form of type 2 DM affecting young people.

Impaired glucose tolerance (IGT): Fasting plasma glucose <7mmol/L and OGTT (oral glucose tolerance) 2h glucose ≥7.8mmol/L but <11.1mmol/L.

Impaired fasting glucose (IFG): Fasting plasma glucose ≥ 6.1mmol/L but <7mmol/L (WHO criteria). Do an OGTT to exclude DM. The cut-off point is somewhat arbitrary. IGT and IFG denote different abnormalities of glucose regulation (post-prandial and fasting). There may be lower risk of progression to DM in IFG than IGT. Manage both with lifestyle advice (p93) + annual review. Incidence of DM if IFG and HbA1C at high end of normal (37–46mmol/mol) is ~25%.[5]

Other causes of DM ►Steroids; anti-HIV drugs; newer antipsychotics.

- Pancreatic: pancreatitis; surgery (where >90% pancreas is removed); trauma; pancreatic destruction (haemochromatosis, cystic fibrosis); pancreatic cancer.
- Cushing's disease; acromegaly; phaeochromocytoma; hyperthyroidism; pregnancy.
- Others: congenital lipodystrophy; glycogen storage diseases.

Metabolic syndrome (syndrome x) Definition from International Diabetes Federation: central obesity (BMI >30, or ↑waist circ, ethnic-specific values), plus two of BP ≥130/85, triglycerides ≥1.7mmol/L, HDL ≤1.03♂/1.29♀mmol/L, fasting glucose ≥5.6mmol/L or type 2 DM. ~20% are affected; weight, genetics, and insulin resistance important in aetiology. Vascular events—but probably not beyond the combined effect of individual risk factors. ℞: Exercise; ↓weight; treat individual components.

1 Chicken or egg? Most type 2 diabetes-associated genes have a function in the vasculature, and stress in β-cells can result from vascular defects in the pancreas, so maybe vascular events trigger DM.[6]

Diagnosis of diabetes mellitus: WHO criteria (rather arbitrary!)

- Symptoms of hyperglycaemia (eg polyuria, polydipsia, unexplained weight loss, visual blurring, genital thrush, lethargy) AND raised venous glucose detected once—fasting ≥7mmol/L or random ≥11.1mmol/L OR
- Raised venous glucose on two separate occasions—fasting ≥7mmol/L, random ≥11.1mmol/L *or* oral glucose tolerance test (*OGTT*)—2h value ≥11.1mmol/L
- HbA1c ≥48mmol/mol. Avoid in pregnancy, children, type 1 DM, and haemoglobinopathies.

►Whenever you have a needle in a vein, do a blood glucose (unless recently done); note if fasting or not. Non-systematic, but better than urine tests (false −ves).

Differentiating type 1 and 2 diabetes

Occasionally it may be difficult to differentiate whether a patient has type 1 or 2 DM, although they can present differently (see table 5.1). Features of type 1 include weight loss; persistent hyperglycaemia despite diet and medications; presence of autoantibodies: islet cell antibodies (ICA) and anti-glutamic acid decarboxylase (GAD) antibodies; ketonuria.

Table 5.1 Differences between type 1 and type 2 diabetes

	Type 1 DM	Type 2 DM
Epidemiology	Often starts before puberty	Older patients (usually)
Genetics	HLA D3 and D4 linked	No HLA association
Cause	Autoimmune β-cell destruction	Insulin resistance/β-cell dysfunction
Presentation	Polydipsia, polyuria, ↓weight, ketosis	Asymptomatic/complications, eg MI

►Not all new-onset DM in older people is type 2: if ketotic ± a poor response to oral hypoglycaemics (and patient is slim or has a family or personal history of autoimmunity), think of latent autoimmune diabetes in adults (LADA) and measure islet cell antibodies.

What is the best diet for obese patients with type 2 diabetes?

Dietary carbohydrate is a big determinant of postprandial glucose levels, and low-carbohydrate diets improve glycaemic control. How do low-carbohydrate, ketogenic diets (<20g of carbohydrate daily; LCKD) compare with low-glycaemic index, reduced-calorie diet (eg 500kcal/day deficit from weight maintenance diet)? In one randomized study over 24 weeks, LCKD had greater improvements in HbA1c (−15 vs −5mmol/L), weight (−11kg vs −7kg), and HDL. Diabetes drugs were reduced or eliminated in 95% of LCKD vs 62% of LGID participants.[6] NB: effects on renal function and mortality are unknown so these diets remain controversial.

Monitoring glucose control

1. Fingerprick glucose if on insulin (type 1/2). NB: *before* a meal informs about long-acting insulin doses; *after* meals inform about the dose of short-acting insulin.
2. Glycated haemoglobin (HbA1c) relates to mean glucose level over previous 8wks (RBC t½). Targets are negotiable, eg 48-57mmol/mol (depends on patient's wish and arterial risk, eg past MI or stroke). If at risk from the effects of hypoglycaemia, eg elderly patients prone to falls, consider less tight control. Tight control may not alter all-cause mortality.[7] Complications rise with rising HbA1c, so any improvement helps.
3. Be sure to ask about hypoglycaemic attacks (and whether symptomatic). Hypoglycaemic awareness may diminish if control is too tight, or with time in type 1 DM, due to ↓glucagon secretion. It may return if control is loosened.

Treating diabetes mellitus

General ►*Focus on education and lifestyle advice* (eg exercise to ↑insulin sensitivity), healthy eating: p244—↓saturated fats, ↓sugar, ↑starch-carbohydrate, moderate protein. Foods made just for diabetics are not needed. One could regard bariatric surgery as a cure for DM in selected patients. Be prepared to negotiate HbA1c target and review every 3–6 months. Assess *global* vascular risk; start a high-intensity statin (p115), eg atorvastatin as tolerated, control BP (p211). Give foot-care (p212). (Pre-) pregnancy care should be in a multidisciplinary clinic (*OHCS* p23). Advise informing DVLA and not to drive if hypoglycaemic spells (p159; loss of hypoglycaemia awareness may lead to loss of licence; permanent if HGV).

Type 1 DM Insulin (see BOX 'Using insulin').

Type 2 DM See fig 5.5.

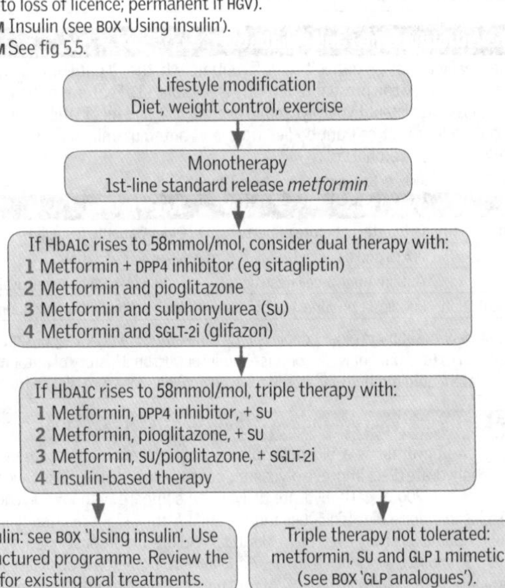

Fig 5.5 Management of type 2 diabetes. Aim for HbA1c 48mmol/mol or 53 if two or more agents.

Data from Algorithm for blood glucose lowering therapy in adults with type 2 diabetes, http://www.nice.org.uk/guidance/ng28/chapter/1-Recommendations#drug-treatment-2

Oral hypoglycaemic agents

Metformin: A biguanide. ↑ insulin sensitivity and helps weight. SE: nausea; diarrhoea (try modified-release version); abdominal pain; not hypoglycaemia. Avoid if eGFR ≤36mL/min (due to risk lactic acidosis).

DPP4 inhibitors/gliptins: (Eg sitagliptin.) Block the action of DPP-4, an enzyme which destroys the hormone incretin.

Glitazone: ↑ insulin sensitivity; SE: hypoglycaemia, fractures, fluid retention, ↑LFT (do LFT every 8wks for 1yr, stop if ALT up >3-fold). CI: past or present CCF; osteoporosis; monitor weight, and stop if ↑ or oedema.

Sulfonylurea: ↑ insulin secretion; eg gliclazide 40mg/d. SE: hypoglycaemia (monitor glucose); it ↑ weight.

SGLTI: Selective sodium-glucose co-transporter-2 inhibitor. Blocks the reabsorption of glucose in the kidneys and promotes excretion of excess glucose in the urine (eg empagliflozin, shown to reduce mortality from cardiovascular disease in patients with type 2 DM, when compared to placebo).[8]

Using insulin

Vital to educate to self-adjust doses in the light of exercise, fingerprick glucose, calorie intake, and carbohydrate counting. •Phone support (trained nurse 7/24). •Can modify diet wisely and avoid binge drinking (danger of delayed hypoglycaemia). •Partner can abort hypoglycaemia: sugary drinks; GlucoGel® PO if coma (no risk of aspiration). •Dose titration to target—eg by 2–4 UNIT steps.

►►It is vital to write UNITS in full when prescribing insulin to avoid misinterpretation of U for zero!

Subcutaneous insulins Short-, medium-, or long-acting. Strength: 100U/mL.

1 Ultra-fast acting (Humalog®; Novorapid®); inject at start of meal, or just after (unless sugar-laden)—helps match what is actually eaten (vs what is planned).
2 Isophane insulin (variable peak at 4–12h): favoured by NICE (it's cheap!).
3 Pre-mixed insulins (eg NovoMix® 30 = 30% short-acting and 70% long-acting).
4 Long-acting recombinant human insulin analogues (*insulin glargine*) are used at bedtime in type 1 or 2 DM. There is no awkward peak, so good if nocturnal hypoglycaemia is an issue. Caution if considering pregnancy. *Insulin detemir* is similar and has a role in intensive insulin regimens for overweight type 2 DM.

Common insulin regimens ►*Plan the regimen to suit the lifestyle, not vice versa.* Disposable pens: dial dose; insert needle 90° to skin. Vary injection site (outer thigh/abdomen); change needle daily.

- 'BD biphasic regimen': twice daily premixed insulins by pen (eg NovoMix 30®)—useful in type 2 DM or type 1 with regular lifestyle.
- 'QDS regimen': before meals ultra-fast insulin + bedtime long-acting analogue: useful in type 1 DM for achieving a flexible lifestyle (eg for adjusting doses with size of meals, or exercise).
- Once-daily before-bed long-acting insulin: a good initial insulin regimen when switching from tablets in type 2 DM. Typical dose to work up to (slowly!): ≥1U/24h for every unit of BMI in adults. Consider retaining metformin (±pioglitazone) if needed for tight control and patient is unable to use BD regimen.

Dose adjustment for normal eating (DAFNE): Multidisciplinary teams promoting autonomy can save lives. DAFNE found that training in flexible, intensive insulin dosing improved glycaemic control as well as well-being.[9] It is resource intensive.

Subcutaneous insulin dosing during intercurrent illnesses (eg influenza)

►► Advise patients to avoid stopping insulin during acute illness.

- Illness often increases insulin requirements despite reduced food intake.
- Maintain calorie intake, eg using milk.
- Check blood glucose ≥ 4 times a day and look for ketonuria. Increase insulin doses if glucose rising. Advise to get help from a specialist diabetes nurse or GP if concerned (esp. if glucose levels are rising or ketonuria). One option is 2-hourly ultra fast-acting insulin (eg 6–8U) preceded by a fingerprick glucose check.
- Admit if vomiting, dehydrated, ketotic (►►p832), a child, or pregnant.

Insulin pumps (continous subcutaneous insulin) Consider when attempts to reach HbA1c with multiple daily injections have resulted in disabling hypoglycaemia or person has been unable to achieve target HbA1c despite careful management.

Glucagon-like peptide (GLP) analogues (exenatide, liraglutide)

Work as incretin mimetics. Incretins are gut peptides that work by augmenting insulin release. Given by subcutaneous injection. Patients must have BMI >35 and specific psychological or other medical problems associated with obesity, or have a BMI lower than 35 kg/m², and for whom insulin therapy would have significant occupational implications, or weight loss would benefit other significant obesity-related comorbidities. To continue a GLP 1 mimetic, a person should have a beneficial metabolic response (a reduction of HbA1c by at least 11mmol/mol) and a weight loss of at least 3% of initial body weight in 6 months.

Complications of established diabetes

Prospective studies show that good control of hyperglycaemia is key to preventing microvascular complications in type 1 and 2 DM.[10] ►*Find out what problems are being experienced* (eg glycaemic control, morale, erectile dysfunction—p230).

Assess vascular risk BP control (see BOX 'Controlling blood pressure in diabetes') is crucial for preventing macrovascular disease and ↓mortality. Refer to *smoking* cessation services. Check *plasma lipids*.

Look for complications •Check injection sites for infection or lipohypertrophy (fatty change): advise on rotating sites of injection if present.

- *Vascular disease:* Chief cause of death. MI is 4-fold commoner in DM and is more likely to be 'silent'. Stroke is twice as common. Women are at high risk—DM removes the vascular advantage conferred by the female sex. Address other risk factors—diet, smoking, hypertension (p93). Suggest a statin (eg atorvastatin 20mg nocte) for all, even if no overt IHD, vascular disease, or microalbuminuria. Aspirin 75mg reduces vascular events (in context of secondary prevention). Safe to use in diabetic retinopathy.[11]
- *Nephropathy:* (p314.) Microalbuminuria is when urine dipstick is −ve for protein but the urine albumin:creatinine ratio (UA:CR) is ≳3mg/mmol (units vary, check lab) reflecting early renal disease and ↑vascular risk. If UA:CR >3, inhibiting the renin-angiotensin system with an ACE-i or sartan, even if BP is normal, protects the kidneys. Spironolactone may also help.[12] Refer if UA:CR >7 ± GFR falling by >5mL/min/1.73m²/yr.[13]
- *Diabetic retinopathy:* Blindness is *preventable*. ►*Annual retinal screening mandatory for all patients.* Refer to an ophthalmologist if pre-proliferative changes or if any uncertainty at or near the macula (the only place capable of 6/6 vision). ►Pre-symptomatic screening enables laser photocoagulation to be used, aimed to stop production of angiogenic factors from the ischaemic retina. Indications: maculopathy or proliferative retinopathy. See figs 5.6–5.9.
  - *Background retinopathy:* Microaneurysms (dots), haemorrhages (blots), and hard exudates (lipid deposits). Refer if near the macula, eg for intravitreal triamcinolone.
  - *Pre-proliferative retinopathy:* Cotton-wool spots (eg infarcts), haemorrhages, venous beading. These are signs of retinal ischaemia. Refer to a specialist.
  - *Proliferative retinopathy:* New vessels form. Needs urgent referral.
  - *Maculopathy:* (Hard to see in early stages.) Suspect if ↓acuity. Prompt laser, intravitreal steroids, or anti-angiogenic agents may be needed in macular oedema. *Pathogenesis:* Capillary endothelial change → vascular leak → microaneurysms → capillary occlusion → local hypoxia + ischaemia → new vessel formation. High retinal blood flow caused by hyperglycaemia (and ↑BP and pregnancy) triggers this, causing capillary pericyte damage. Microvascular occlusion causes *cotton-wool spots* (± *blot haemorrhages* at interfaces with perfused retina). *New vessels* form on the disc or ischaemic areas, proliferate, bleed, fibrose, and can detach the retina. Aspirin[2] (2mg/kg/d) may be recommended by ophthalmologists; there is no evidence that it ↑ bleeding.
- *Cataracts:* May be juvenile 'snowflake' form, or 'senile'—which occur earlier in diabetic subjects. Osmotic changes in the lens induced in acute hyperglycaemia reverse with normoglycaemia (so wait before buying glasses).
- *Rubeosis iridis:* New vessels on iris: occurs late and may lead to glaucoma.
- *Metabolic complications:* p832.
- *Diabetic feet:* p212.
- *Neuropathy:* p212.

2 As DM has so many vascular events, particularly encourage statin use (p690), esp. if LDL >3mmol/L **or** systolic BP >140. Even consider a statin *whatever* the pre-treatment cholesterol; discuss with your patient.

Controlling blood pressure in diabetes

Type 1 DM: Treat BP if >135/85mmHg, unless albuminuria or two or more features of metabolic syndrome, in which case it should be 130/80mmHg (NICE 2015). Use an ACE-i 1st line or angiotension receptor antagonist if intolerant. If hypertensive and underlying renal involvement, see local guidance, p304.

Type 2 DM: Target BP <140/80mmHg or <130/80mmHg if kidney, eye, or cerebrovascular damage. 1st-line drug treatment should be an ACE-i, except in those of African or Caribbean origin, where ACE-i plus diuretic or a calcium-channel antagonist (CCA) should be started. For pregnant women offer CCA. Do not offer aspirin for the primary prevention of cardiovascular disease to adults with type 1 DM (NICE 2015). Don't combine an ACE-i with an angiotension receptor antagonist.

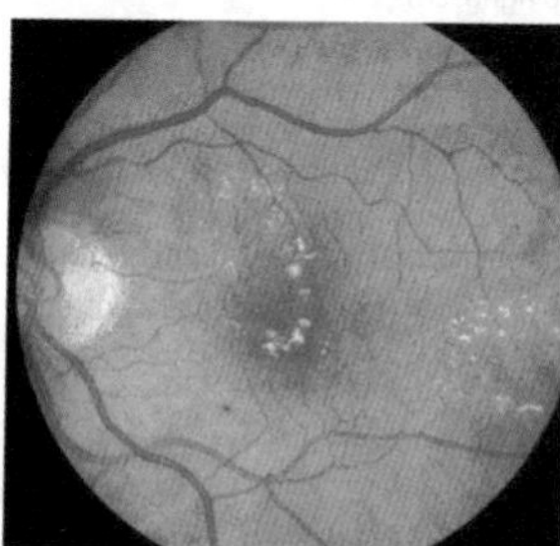

Fig 5.6 Background retinopathy, with microaneurysms and hard exudates.

Courtesy of Prof J Trobe.

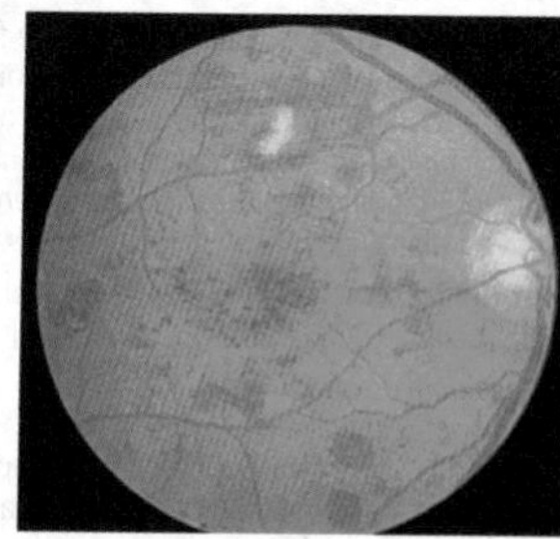

Fig 5.7 Pre-proliferative retinopathy, with haemorrhages and a cotton-wool spot.

Reproduced from Warrell *et al*, *Oxford Textbook of Medicine*, 2010, with permission from Oxford University Press.

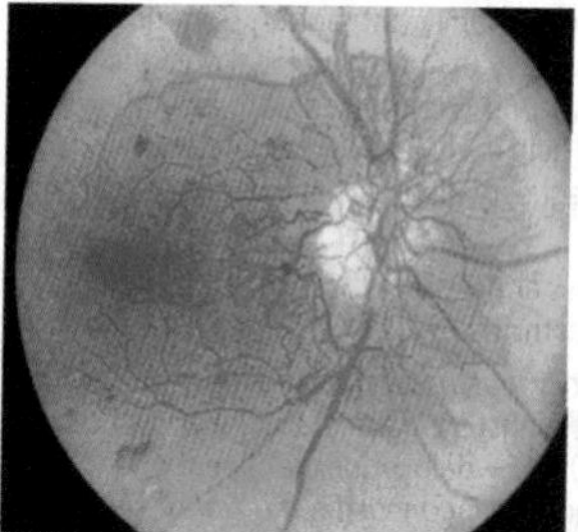

Fig 5.8 Proliferative retinopathy, with new vessel formation and haemorrhages.

Courtesy of Prof J Trobe.

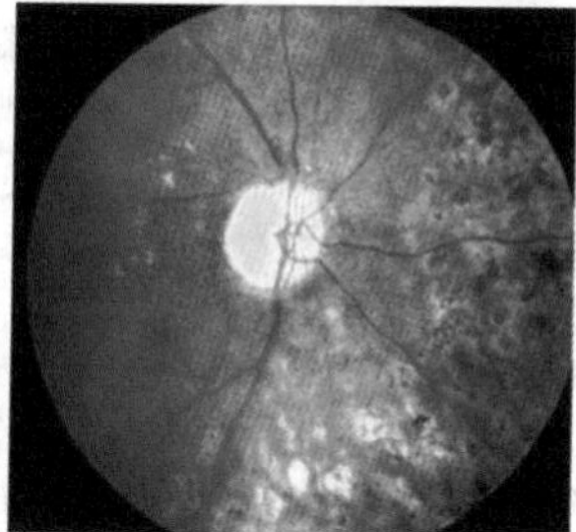

Fig 5.9 Scars from previous laser photocoagulation.

Courtesy of Prof J Trobe.

Improving quality of life: going beyond the pleasures of the flesh

'I cannot eat what I want because of your pitiful diet. Sex is out because diabetes has made me impotent. Smoking is banned, so what's left? I'd shoot myself if only I could see straight.' Start by acknowledging your patient's distress. Don't shrug it off—but don't take it at face value either. Life may be transformed by cataract surgery, sildenafil (unless contraindicated, p230), dietary negotiation, and sport (it needn't be shooting). Take steps to simplify care. Stop blood glucose self-monitoring if it's achieving nothing (known to ↓ quality of life). Even if all these interventions fail, you have one trump card up your sleeve: 'Let's both try to find one new thing of value before we next meet—and compare notes'. This opens the way to vicarious pleasure: a whole new world.

Diabetic neuropathy and diabetic foot care

►Refer *early* to foot services (podiatry, imaging, vascular surgery).
Amputations are common (135/week)—and preventable: *good care saves legs*. Examine feet regularly. Distinguish between ischaemia (critical toes ± absent foot pulses and worse outcome) and peripheral neuropathy (injury or infection over pressure points, eg the metatarsal heads). In practice, many have both.

Neuropathy ↓Sensation in 'stocking' distribution: test sensation with a 10g monofilament fibre (sensory loss is patchy so examine all areas), absent ankle jerks, neuropathic deformity (Charcot joint, fig 5.11): pes cavus, claw toes, loss of transverse arch, rocker-bottom sole. Caused by loss of pain sensation, leading to ↑mechanical stress and repeated joint injury. Swelling, instability, and deformity. ►Early recognition is vital (cellulitis or osteomyelitis are often misdiagnosed).

Ischaemia If the foot pulses cannot be felt, do Doppler pressure measurements. Any evidence of neuropathy or vascular disease raises risk of foot ulceration. *Educate* (daily foot inspection—eg with a mirror for the sole; comfortable shoes). *Regular chiropody* to remove callus, as haemorrhage and tissue necrosis may occur below, leading to ulceration. *Treat fungal infections* (p408). *Surgery* (including endovascular angioplasty balloons, stents, and subintimal recanalization) has a role.

Foot ulceration Typically painless, punched-out ulcer (fig 5.10) in an area of thick callus ± superadded infection. Causes cellulitis, abscess ± osteomyelitis.

Assess degree of:
1 Neuropathy (clinically).
2 Ischaemia (clinically + Doppler ± angiography).
3 Bony deformity, eg Charcot joint (clinically + x-ray). See fig 5.11.
4 Infection (swabs, blood culture, x-ray for osteomyelitis, probe ulcer to reveal depth).

Management: Regular chiropody. Bed rest ± therapeutic shoes. For Charcot joints: bed rest/crutches/total contact cast until oedema and local warmth reduce and bony repair is complete (≥8wks). Bisphosphonates may help. Charcot joints are also seen in tabes dorsalis, spina bifida, syringomyelia, and leprosy. Metatarsal head surgery may be needed. If there is cellulitis, admit for IV antibiotics. Common organisms: staphs, streps, anaerobes. Start empirically (as per your local guidance) with benzylpenicillin 1.2g/6h IV and flucloxacillin 1g/6h IV ± metronidazole 500mg/8h IV. IV insulin may improve healing. Get surgical help early. The degree of peripheral vascular disease, general health, and patient request will determine degree of vascular reconstruction/surgery.

►*Absolute indications for surgery:* Abscess or deep infection; spreading anaerobic infection; gangrene/rest pain; suppurative arthritis.

Diabetic neuropathies *Symmetric sensory polyneuropathy:* ('glove & stocking' numbness, tingling, and pain, eg worse at night). ℞: paracetamol → tricyclic (amitriptyline 10–25mg nocte; gradually ↑ to 150mg) → duloxetine, gabapentin, or pregabalin → opiates. Avoiding weight-bearing helps. *Mononeuritis multiplex:* (eg III & VI cranial nerves). Treatment: hard! If sudden or severe, immunosuppression may help (corticosteroids, IV immunoglobulin, ciclosporin). *Amyotrophy:* Painful wasting of quadriceps and other pelvifemoral muscles. Use electrophysiology to show, eg lumbosacral radiculopathy, plexopathy, or proximal crural neuropathy. Natural course: variable with gradual but often incomplete improvement. IV immunoglobulins have been used. *Autonomic neuropathy:* (p505) Postural BP drop; ↓cerebrovascular autoregulation; loss of respiratory sinus arrhythmia (vagal neuropathy); gastroparesis; urine retention; erectile dysfunction; gustatory sweating; diarrhoea (may respond to codeine phosphate). Gastroparesis (early satiety, post-prandial bloating, nausea/vomiting) is diagnosed by gastric scintigraphy with a ^{99}technetium-labelled meal; anti-emetics, erythromycin, or gastric pacing. Postural hypotension may respond to fludrocortisone (SE: oedema, ↑BP)/midodrine (α-agonist; SE: ↑BP).

Preventing loss of limbs: primary or secondary prevention?

Traditionally prevention involves foot care advice in diabetic clinics (eg 'Don't go bare-foot'), promoting euglycaemia and normotension. But despite this, the sight of a diabetic patient minus one limb is not rare, and must prompt us to redouble our commitment to primary prevention, ie stopping those at risk from ever getting diabetes. The sequelae of diabetic neuropathy can lead to gangrene, amputation, and the impact on quality of life can be profound. As one patient post amputation said, 'I begin again to walk, on crutches. What nuisance, what fatigue, what sadness, when I think about all my ancient travels, and how active I was just 5 months ago! Where are the runnings across mountains, the walks, the deserts, the rivers, and the seas? And now, the life of a legless cripple. For I begin to understand that crutches, wooden and articulated legs, are a pack of jokes...Goodbye to family, goodbye to future! My life is gone, I'm no more than an immobile trunk' (Arthur Rimbaud. Letter to his sister Isabelle, 10 July 1891).

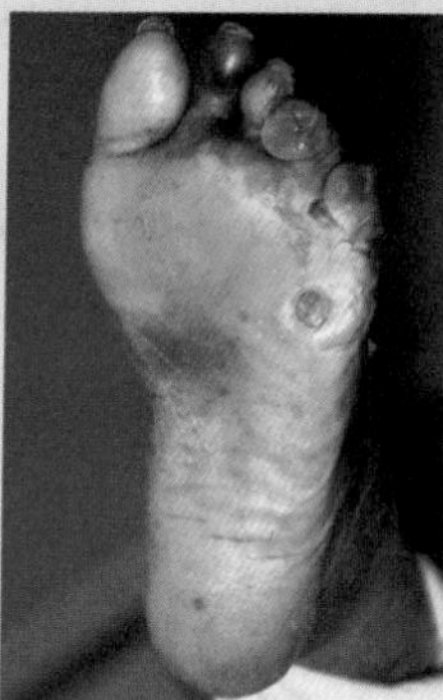

Fig 5.10 Gangrene (toes 2, 4, and 5). Reproduced from Warrell *et al*, *Oxford Textbook of Medicine*, 2010, with permission from Oxford University Press.

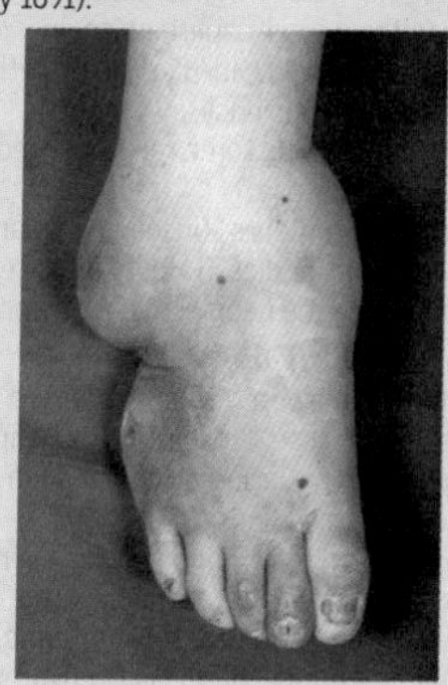

Fig 5.11 Charcot (neuropathic) joint. Reproduced from Warrell *et al*, *Oxford Textbook of Medicine*, 2010, with permission from Oxford University Press.

Special situations in diabetes

Pregnancy: (OHCS p23) 4% are complicated by DM: either pre-existing (<0.5%), or new-onset gestational diabetes (GDM) (>3.5%).

- All forms carry an increased risk to mother and fetus: miscarriage, pre-term labour, pre-eclampsia, congenital malformations, macrosomia, and a worsening of diabetic complications, eg retinopathy, nephropathy.
- Risk of GDM ↑ if: aged over 25; family history; +ve; ↑weight; non-Caucasian; HIV+ve; previous gestational DM.
- Pre-conception: offer general advice, and discuss risks. Control/reduce weight, aim for good glucose control, offer folic acid 5mg/d until 12 weeks.
- Screen for GDM with OGTT if risk factors at booking (16–18 weeks if previous GDM).
- Oral hypoglycaemics other than metformin should be discontinued. Metformin may be used as an adjunct or alternative to insulin in type 2 DM or GDM.

6wks postpartum, do a fasting glucose. Even if −ve, 50% go on to develop DM.

Surgery: Optimal blood sugar control pre, peri, and post operatively is important to minimize risk of infection and balance catabolic response to surgery. Type 1 diabetics should ideally be first on the list and BMs should have been stabilized 1–2 days pre major surgery. Consult local policy for how to manage insulin-treated/non-insulin-treated patients on morning of surgery (eg setting up glucose/insulin infusion).

Acute illness: Diabetics are prone to hyperglycaemia during periods of illness, in spite of reduced oral intake. Avoid stopping insulin in periods of acute illness.

Hypoglycaemia

▸▸**Hypoglycaemia** Commonest endocrine emergency—see p834. Prompt diagnosis and treatment essential—brain damage & death can occur if severe or prolonged. **Definition** Plasma glucose ≤3mmol/L. Threshold for symptoms varies. See BOX. **Symptoms** *Autonomic:* Sweating, anxiety, hunger, tremor, palpitations, dizziness. *Neuroglycopenic:* Confusion, drowsiness, visual trouble, seizures, coma. Rarely focal symptoms, eg transient hemiplegia. Mutism, personality change, restlessness, and incoherence may lead to misdiagnosis of alcohol intoxication or even psychosis.

Fasting hypoglycaemia *Causes:* The chief cause is insulin or sulfonylurea treatment in a diabetic, eg ↑activity, missed meal, accidental or non-accidental overdose (check for ciculating oral hypoglycaemics). In *non-diabetic*s you must **EXPLAIN** mechanism: **Ex**ogenous drugs, eg insulin, oral hypoglycaemics (p208)? access through diabetic in the family? Body-builders may misuse insulin to help stamina. Also: alcohol, eg a binge with no food; aspirin poisoning; ACE-i; β-blockers; pentamidine; quinine sulfate; aminoglutethamide; insulin-like growth factor.[14]

Pituitary insufficiency.

Liver failure, plus some rare inherited enzyme defects.

Addison's disease.

Islet cell tumours (insulinoma) and immune hypoglycaemia (eg anti-insulin receptor antibodies in Hodgkin's disease).

Non-pancreatic neoplasms, eg fibrosarcomas and haemangiopericytomas.

When to investigate:

- Whipple answered this (*Whipple's triad*): symptoms or signs of hypoglycemia + ↓plasma glucose + resolution of symptoms or signs post glucose rise.
- Document BM during attack and lab glucose if in hospital (monitors often not reliable at low readings).
- Take a drug history and exclude liver failure.
- 72h fasting may be needed (monitor closely). Bloods: glucose, insulin, C-peptide, and plasma ketones if symptomatic. If endogenous hyperinsulinism suspected, do insulin, C-peptide, proinsulin, β-hydroxybutyrate.

Interpreting results:

- Hypoglycaemic hyperinsulinaemia (HH): *Causes:* insulinoma, sulfonylureas, insulin injection (no detectable C-peptide—only released with endogenous insulin); non-insulinoma pancreatogenous hypoglycaemia syndrome, mutation in the insulin-receptor gene. Congenital HH follows mutations in genes involved in insulin secretion (ABCC8, KCNJ11, GLUD1, CGK, HADH, SLC16A1, HNF4A, ABCC8, & KCNJ11).[15]
- Insulin low or undetectable, no excess ketones. *Causes:* non-pancreatic neoplasm; anti-insulin receptor antibodies.
- ↓Insulin, ↑ketones. *Causes:* alcohol, pituitary insufficiency, Addison's disease.

Post-prandial hypoglycaemia May occur after gastric/bariatric surgery ('dumping', p623), and in type 2 DM. *Investigation:* Prolonged OGTT (5h, p206).

Treatment ▸▸See p834. If episodes are often, advise many small high-starch meals. If post-prandial ↓glucose, give slowly absorbed carbohydrate (high fibre). In diabetics, rationalize insulin therapy (p209).

The definition of hypoglycaemia is context-dependent

The brain stops working if plasma glucose levels get too low, so we are nervous of levels ≤3mmol/L. But some are asymptomatic at this level. So what is definitely abnormal? The answer may be 4mmol/L, allowing for inaccuracies in fingerprick BMs (NB: whole blood glucose is 10–15% < plasma glucose.) Think: '***In this ill patient when can I be sure that a low glucose is not contributing to their illness?***' If <4mmol/L, you may be wise to treat (p834)—just in case. Consider, is the patient on hypoglycaemics, have they binged on alcohol 24hrs pre test? Skipped meals? Is there an underlying illness, eg insulinoma? Unlikely, but possible. Keep an open mind; let the GP know. Counsel patient and relative about warning signs of hypoglycaemia. Be more inclined to investigate if the effects of even mild hypoglycaemia might be disastrous (eg in pilots) or if there are unexplained symptoms.

Insulinoma

This often benign (90–95%) pancreatic islet cell tumour is sporadic or seen with MEN-1 (p223). It presents as fasting hypoglycaemia, with Whipple's triad:

1. Symptoms associated with fasting or exercise.
2. Recorded hypoglycaemia with symptoms.
3. Symptoms relieved with glucose.

Screening test Hypoglycaemia + ↑plasma insulin during a long fast.

Suppressive tests Give IV insulin and measure C-peptide. Normally exogenous insulin suppresses C-peptide production, but this does not occur in insulinoma.

Imaging CT/MRI ± endoscopic pancreatic US ± IACS (see BOX; all fallible, so don't waste too much time before proceeding to intra-operative visualization ± intra-operative ultrasound). ^{18}F-L-3,4-dihydroxyphenylalanine PET-CT can help guide laparoscopic surgery.

Treatment Excision.

Nesidioblastosis See BOX. If this doesn't work, options are: ↑diet, diazoxide, dextrose IVI, enteral feeding, everolimus.

▸▸ **Diabetic ketoacidosis** Results from insulin deficiency (eg unknown diagnosis, intercurrent illness, interuption of insulin therapy). See p832.

Pursuing a voyage to the islets of Langerhans to the bitter end

A 50-year-old had episodic early-morning sweats and tremors and was found to have hyperinsulinaemic hypoglycaemia (= Nesidioblastosis). Selective intra-arterial calcium infusions (IACS) showed a 2-fold increase in insulin secretion after infusion of the splenic and superior mesenteric arteries, so setting the stage for 'hunt the insulinoma'.

But cross-sectional imaging and endoscopic ultrasound were normal. At laparotomy, no lesion was found despite mobilization of the pancreas, or during intra-operative ultrasound. 'Time to sew up and go home?' 'No!' said the surgeon, 'I'm going to do a distal pancreatectomy'. Histology showed no discrete insulinoma, but diffuse islet cell hyperplasia (*nesidioblastosis*). How much pancreas to resect? Too little and nothing is gained: too much spells pancreatic endocrine disaster. Luckily the surgeon guessed right, and the patient was cured by the procedure.[16]

Physiology

Thyroid-stimulating hormone (TSH=thyrotropin), a glycoprotein, is produced from the anterior pituitary (fig 5.12). The thyroid produces mainly T_4, which is 5-fold less active than T_3. 85% of T_3 is formed from peripheral conversion of T_4. Most T_3 and T_4 in plasma is protein bound, eg to thyroxine-binding globulin (TBG). The unbound portion is the active part. T_3 and T_4 ↑cell metabolism, via nuclear receptors, and are thus vital for growth and mental development. They also ↑catecholamine effects. Thyroid hormone abnormalities are usually due to problems in the thyroid gland itself, and rarely caused by the hypothalamus or the anterior pituitary.

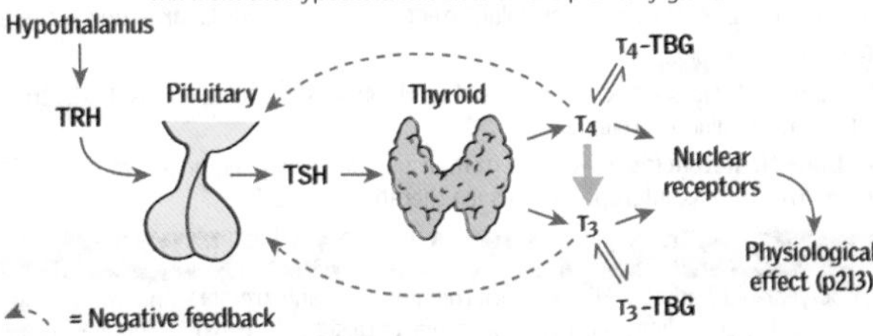

Fig 5.12 Pathways involved in thyroid function.

Basic tests See table 5.2. Free T_4 and T_3 are more useful than total T_4 and T_3 as the latter are affected by TBG. Total T_4 and T_3 are ↑ when TBG is ↑ and *vice versa*. TBG is ↑ in pregnancy, oestrogen therapy (HRT, oral contraceptives), and hepatitis. TBG is ↓ in nephrotic syndrome and malnutrition (both from protein loss), drugs (androgens, corticosteroids, phenytoin), chronic liver disease, and acromegaly. TSH is very useful:

- *Hyperthyroidism suspected:* Ask for T_3, T_4, and TSH. All will have ↓TSH (except the rare TSH-secreting pituitary adenoma). Most have ↑T_4, but ~1% have only raised T_3.
- *Hypothyroidism suspected or monitoring replacement ℞:* Ask for only T_4 and TSH. T_3 does not add any extra information. TSH varies through the day: trough at 2PM; 30% higher during darkness, so during monitoring, try to do at the same time.

Sick euthyroidism: In any systemic illness, TFTs may become deranged. The typical pattern is for 'everything to be low'. The test should be repeated after recovery.

Assay interference is caused by antibodies in the serum, interfering with the test.

Other tests

- *Thyroid autoantibodies:* Antithyroid peroxidase (TPO; formerly called microsomal) antibodies or antithyroglobulin antibodies may be increased in autoimmune thyroid disease: Hashimoto's or Graves' disease. If +ve in Graves', there is an increased risk of developing hypothyroidism at a later stage.
- *TSH receptor antibody:* May be ↑ in Graves' disease (useful in pregnancy).
- *Serum thyroglobulin:* Useful in monitoring the treatment of carcinoma (p600), and in detection of factitious (self-medicated) hyperthyroidism, where it is low.
- *Ultrasound:* This distinguishes cystic (usually, but not always, benign) from solid (possibly malignant) nodules. If a solitary (or dominant) large nodule, in a multinodular goitre, do a fine-needle aspiration to look for thyroid cancer; see fig 13.23, p601.
- *Isotope scan:* (^{123}Iodine, ^{99}technetium pertechnetate, etc; see fig 13.22, p601.) Useful for determining the cause of hyperthyroidism and to detect retrosternal goitre, ectopic thyroid tissue or thyroid metastases (+ whole body CT). If there are suspicious nodules, the question is: does the area have increased (hot), decreased (cold), or the same (neutral) uptake of isotope as the remaining thyroid (see fig 5.13). Few neutral and almost no hot nodules are malignant. 20% of 'cold' nodules are malignant. Surgery is most likely to be needed if: •rapid growth •compression signs •dominant nodule on scintigraphy •nodule ≥3cm •hypo-echogenicity. See also p738.

Screen the following for abnormalities in thyroid function

- Patients with atrial fibrillation.
- Patients with hyperlipidaemia (4–14% have hypothyroidism).
- Diabetes mellitus—on annual review.
- Women with type 1 DM during 1st trimester and post delivery (3-fold rise in incidence of postpartum thyroid dysfunction).
- Patients on amiodarone or lithium (6 monthly).
- Patients with Down's or Turner's syndrome, or Addison's disease (yearly).

Table 5.2 Interpreting TFTs

Hormone profile	Diagnosis
↑TSH, ↓T_4	Hypothyroidism
↑TSH, normal T_4	Treated hypothyroidism or subclinical hypothyroidism (p221)
↑TSH, ↑T_4	TSH-secreting tumour or thyroid hormone resistance
↑TSH, ↑T_4 and ↓T_3	Slow conversion of T_4 to T_3 (deiodinase deficiency; euthyroid hyperthyroxinaemia*) or thyroid hormone antibody artefact
↓TSH, ↑T_4 or ↑T_3	Hyperthyroidism
↓TSH, normal T_4 and T_3	Subclinical hyperthyroidism
↓TSH, ↓T_4	Central hypothyroidism (hypothalamic or pituitary disorder)
↓TSH, ↓T_4 and ↓T_3	Sick euthyroidism or pituitary disease
Normal **TSH**, abnormal T_4	Consider changes in thyroid-binding globulin, assay interference, amiodarone, or pituitary TSH tumour

*In 'consumptive hypothyroidism' deiodinase activity is ↑↑; suspect if thyroxine doses have to be ↑↑.

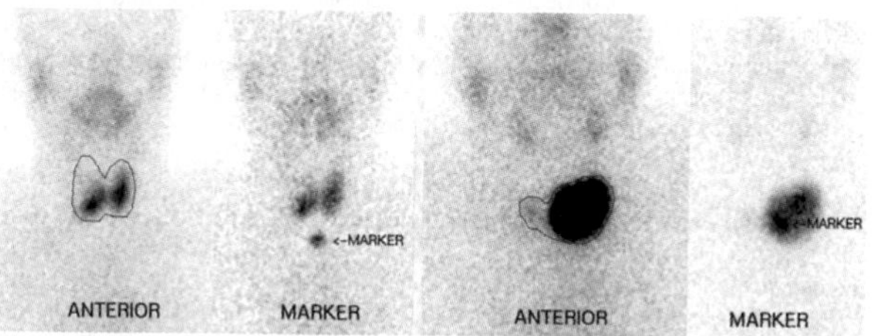

Fig 5.13 The images are from an isotope scan, with and without markers placed over the sternal notch. We can see on the left that the nodule is metabolically inactive ('cold'). The hot nodule (right pair) is a very avid nodule causing background thyroid suppression.

Image courtesy of Dr Y. T. Huang.

Thyrotoxicosis

The clinical effect of excess thyroid hormone, usually from gland hyperfunction.

Symptoms Diarrhoea; ↓weight; ↑appetite (if ↑↑, paradoxical weight *gain* in 10%); over-active; sweats; heat intolerance; palpitations; tremor; irritability; labile emotions; oligomenorrhoea ±infertility. Rarely psychosis; chorea; panic; itch; alopecia; urticaria.

Signs Pulse fast/irregular (AF or SVT; VT rare); warm moist skin; fine tremor; palmar erythema; thin hair; lid lag; lid retraction (exposure of sclera above iris; causing 'stare', (fig 5.14; eyelid lags behind eye's descent as patient watches your finger descend slowly). There may be goitre (fig 5.15); thyroid nodules; or bruit depending on the cause. *Signs of Graves' disease:* 1 *Eye disease* (BOX 'Thyroid eye disease'): exophthalmos, ophthalmoplegia. 2 *Pretibial myxoedema:* oedematous swellings above lateral malleoli: the term *myxoedema* is confusing here. 3 *Thyroid acropachy:* extreme manifestation, with clubbing, painful finger and toe swelling, and periosteal reaction in limb bones.

Tests ↓TSH (suppressed), T_4, and ↑T_3. There may be mild normocytic anaemia, mild neutropenia (in Graves'), ↑ESR, ↑Ca^{2+}, ↑LFT. *Also:* Check thyroid autoantibodies. Isotope scan if the cause is unclear, to detect nodular disease or subacute thyroiditis. If ophthalmopathy, test visual fields, acuity, and eye movements (see BOX 'Thyroid eye disease').

Causes

Graves' disease: Prevalence: 0.5% (⅔ of cases of hyperthyroidism). ♀:♂≈9:1. Typical age: 40–60yrs (younger if maternal family history). Cause: circulating IgG autoantibodies binding to and activating G-protein-coupled thyrotropin receptors, which cause smooth thyroid enlargement and ↑hormone production (esp. T_3), and react with orbital autoantigens. Triggers: stress; infection; childbirth. Patients are often hyperthyroid but may be, or become, hypo- or euthyroid. It is associated with other autoimmune diseases: vitiligo, type 1 DM, Addison's (table 5.3).

Toxic multinodular goitre: Seen in the elderly and in iodine-deficient areas. There are nodules that secrete thyroid hormones. Surgery is indicated for compressive symptoms from the enlarged thyroid (dysphagia or dyspnoea).

Toxic adenoma: There is a solitary nodule producing T_3 and T_4. On isotope scan, the nodule is 'hot' (p216), and the rest of the gland is suppressed.

Ectopic thyroid tissue: Metastatic follicular thyroid cancer, or struma ovarii: ovarian teratoma with thyroid tissue.

Exogenous: Iodine excess, eg food contamination, contrast media (▸▸thyroid storm, p834, if already hyperthyroid). Levothyroxine excess causes ↑T_4, ↓T_3, ↓thyroglobulin.

Others: 1 *Subacute de Quervain's thyroiditis:* self-limiting post-viral with painful goitre, ↑T° ± ↑ESR. Low isotope uptake on scan. ℞: NSAIDs. 2 *Drugs:* amiodarone (p220), lithium (hypothyroidism more common). 3 *Postpartum.* 4 TB (rare).

Treatment

1 *Drugs:* β-blockers (eg propranolol 40mg/6h) for rapid control of symptoms. *Antithyroid medication:* two strategies (equally effective):[17] **A** *Titration*, eg carbimazole 20–40mg/24h PO for 4wks, reduce according to TFTs every 1–2 months. **B** Block-replace: Give carbimazole + levothyroxine simultaneously (less risk of iatrogenic hypothyroidism). In Graves', maintain on either regimen for 12–18 months then withdraw. ~50% will relapse, requiring radioiodine or surgery. Carbimazole SE: agranulocytosis (↓↓neutrophils, can lead to dangerous sepsis; rare (0.03%)); warn to stop and get an urgent FBC if signs of infection, eg T°↑, sore throat/mouth ulcers.

2 *Radioiodine (^{131}I):* Most become hypothyroid post-treatment. There is no evidence for ↑cancer, birth defects, or infertility in women. CI: pregnancy, lactation. Caution in active hyperthyroidism as risk of thyroid storm (p835).

3 *Thyroidectomy (usually total):* Carries a risk of damage to recurrent laryngeal nerve (hoarse voice) and hypoparathyroidism. Patients will become hypothyroid, so thyroid replacement needed.

4 *In pregnancy and infancy:* Get expert help. See *OHCS* p24 & *OHCS* p182.

Complications Heart failure (thyrotoxic cardiomyopathy, ↑ in elderly), angina, AF (seen in 10–25%: control hyperthyroidism and warfarinize if no contraindication), osteoporosis, ophthalmopathy, gynaecomastia. ▸▸Thyroid storm (p835).

Thyroid eye disease

Seen in 25–50% of people with Graves' disease. The main known risk factor is smoking. The eye disease may not correlate with thyroid disease and the patient can be euthyroid, hypothyroid, or hyperthyroid at presentation. Eye disease may be the first presenting sign of Graves' disease, and can also be worsened by treatment, typically with radioiodine (usually a transient effect). Retro-orbital inflammation and lymphocyte infiltration results in swelling of the orbit.

Symptoms Eye discomfort, grittiness, ↑tear production, photophobia, diplopia, ↓acuity, afferent pupillary defect (p72) may mean optic nerve compression: ►*Seek expert advice at once as decompression may be needed.* Nerve damage does not necessarily go hand-in-hand with protrusion. Indeed, if the eye cannot protrude for anatomical reasons, optic nerve compression is more likely—a paradox!

Signs Exophthalmos—appearance of protruding eye; proptosis—eyes protrude beyond the orbit (look from above in the same plane as the forehead); conjunctival oedema; corneal ulceration; papilloedema; loss of colour vision. Ophthalmoplegia (especially of upward gaze) occurs due to muscle swelling and fibrosis.

Tests Diagnosis is clinical. CT/MRI of the orbits may reveal enlarged eye muscles.

Management Get specialist help. Treat hyper- or hypothyroidism. Advise to stop smoking (worse prognosis). Most have mild disease that can be treated symptomatically (artificial tears, sunglasses, avoid dust, elevate bed when sleeping to ↓periorbital oedema). Diplopia may be managed with a Fresnel prism stuck to one lens of a spectacle (aids easy changing as the exophthalmos changes). In more severe disease, try high-dose steroids (IV methylprednisolone is better than prednisolone 100mg/day PO)[18]—decreasing according to symptoms. Surgical decompression is used for severe sight-threatening disease, or for cosmetic reasons once the activity of eye disease has reduced (via an inferior orbital approach, using space in the ethmoidal, sphenoidal, and maxillary sinuses). Eyelid surgery may improve cosmesis and function. Orbital radiotherapy can be used to treat ophthalmoplegia but has little effect on proptosis. *Future options:* Anti-TNFα antibodies (eg infliximab).

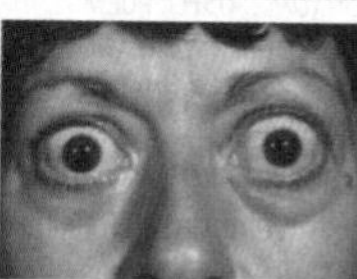

Fig 5.14 Thyroid eye disease: lid retraction causing a 'staring' appearance.

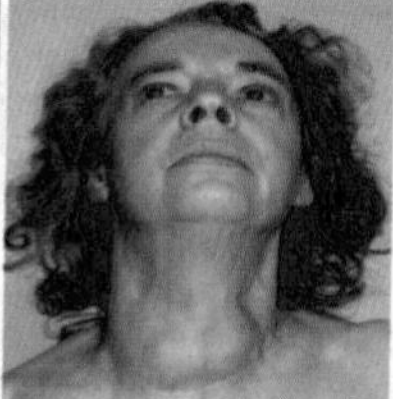

Fig 5.15 Goitre.

Causes of goitre

Diffuse
- Physiological
- Graves' disease
- Hashimoto's thyroiditis
- Subacute (de Quervain's) thyroiditis (painful).

Nodular
- Multinodular goitre
- Adenoma
- Carcinoma.

Table 5.3 Manifestations of Graves' disease—and pathophysiology

Pituitary	Suppressed TSH	↓Expression of thyrotropin β subunit
Heart	↑Rate; ↑contractility	↑Serum atrial natriuretic peptide
Liver	↑Peripheral T_3; LDL↓ (p690)	↑Type 1 5'-deiodinase; LDL receptors
Bone	↑Bone turnover; osteoporosis	↑Osteocalcin; ↑ALP; ↑urinary N-telopeptide
Genital ♂	↓Libido; erectile dysfunction	↑Sex hormone globulin; ↓testosterone
Genital ♀	Irregular menses	Oestrogen antagonism
Metabolic	↑Thermogenesis; ↑O_2 use	↑Fatty acid oxidation; ↑Na-K ATPase
White fat	↓Fat mass	↑Adrenergic-mediated lipolysis
CNS	Stiff person syndrome (rare)*	Antibodies to glutamic acid decarboxylase
Muscle	Proximal myopathy	↑Sarcoplasmic reticulum Ca^{2+}-activated ATPase
Thyroid	↑Secretion of T_3 and T_4	↑Type 2 5'-deiodinase activity in thyroid

*Emotional or tactile stimuli cause spasms; seen in any autoimmune state (eg type 1 DM); ℞: baclofen± IV Ig.

Hypothyroidism (myxoedema)

The clinical effect of lack of thyroid hormone. It is common (4/1000/yr). If treated, prognosis is excellent; untreated it is disastrous (eg heart disease, dementia). ►*As it is insidious, both you and your patient may not realize anything is wrong*, so be alert to subtle, non-specific symptoms, esp. in women ≳40yrs old (♀:♂≈6:1).

Symptoms Tiredness; sleepy, lethargic; ↓mood; cold-disliking; ↑weight; constipation; menorrhagia; hoarse voice; ↓memory/cognition; dementia; myalgia; cramps; weakness.

Signs BRADYCARDIC; reflexes relax slowly; ataxia (cerebellar); dry thin hair/skin; yawning/drowsy/coma (p834); cold hands ± ↓T°; ascites ± non-pitting oedema (lids; hands; feet) ± pericardial or pleural effusion; round puffy face/double chin/obese; defeated demeanour; immobile ± ileus; CCF. Also: neuropathy; myopathy; goitre (fig 5.16).

Diagnosis (p216) ►Have a low threshold for doing TFTs! ↑TSH (eg ≥4mU/L);[3] ↓T_4 (in rare secondary hypothyroidism: ↓T_4 and ↓TSH or ↔ due to lack from the pituitary, p232). Cholesterol and triglyceride↑; macrocytosis (less often normochromic anaemia too).

Causes of primary autoimmune hypothyroidism

- *Primary atrophic hypothyroidism:* ♀:♂≈6:1. Common. Diffuse lymphocytic infiltration of the thyroid, leading to atrophy, hence no goitre.
- *Hashimoto's thyroiditis:* Goitre due to lymphocytic and plasma cell infiltration. Commoner in women aged 60–70yrs. May be hypothyroid or euthyroid; rarely initial period of hyperthyroid ('Hashitoxicosis'). Autoantibody titres are very high.

Other causes of primary hypothyrodism

- ►World-wide the chief cause is *iodine deficiency*.
- *Post-thyroidectomy or radioiodine treatment*.
- *Drug-induced:* Antithyroid drugs, amiodarone, lithium, iodine.
- *Subacute thyroiditis:* Temporary hypothyroidism after hyperthyroid phase.

Secondary hypothyroidism Not enough TSH (due to hypopituitarism); very rare.

Hypothyroidism's associations Autoimmune is seen with other autoimmune diseases (type 1 DM, Addison's, and PA, p334). Turner's and Down's syndromes, cystic fibrosis, primary biliary cholangitis, ovarian hyperstimulation (*OHCS* p311); POEMS syndrome—polyneuropathy, organomegaly, endocrinopathy, m-protein band (plasmacytoma) + skin pigmentation/tethering. *Genetic:* Dyshormonogenesis: genetic (often autosomal recessive) defect in hormone synthesis, eg Pendred's syndrome (with deafness): there is ↑uptake on isotope scan, which is displaced by potassium perchlorate.

Pregnancy problems Eclampsia, anaemia, prematurity, ↓birthweight, stillbirth, PPH.

Treatment

- *Healthy and young:* Levothyroxine (T_4), 0–100mcg/24h PO; review at 12wks. Adjust 6-weekly by clinical state and to normalize but not suppress TSH (keep TSH >0.5mU/L). Thyroxine's *t½* is ~7d, so wait ~4wks before checking TSH to see if a dose change is right. NB: small changes in serum free T_4 have a logarithmic effect on TSH. Once normal, check TSH yearly. Enzyme inducers (p689) ↑metabolism of levothyroxine.
- *Elderly or ischaemic heart disease:* Start with 25mcg/24h; ↑dose by 25mcg/4wks according to TSH (►cautiously, as levothyroxine may precipitate angina or MI).
- *If diagnosis is in question and T_4 already given:* Stop T_4; recheck TSH in 6 weeks.

Amiodarone An iodine-rich drug structurally like T_4; 2% of users will get significant thyroid problems from it. Hypothyroidism can be caused by toxicity from iodine excess (T_4 release is inhibited). Thyrotoxicosis may be caused by a destructive thyroiditis causing hormone release. Here, radioiodine uptake can be undetectable and if this is the case, glucocorticoids may help. Get expert help. Thyroidectomy may be needed if amiodarone cannot be discontinued. *T½* of amiodarone ≈80d, so problems persist after withdrawal. If on amiodarone, check TFTs 6-monthly.

►►**Myxoedema coma** The ultimate hypothyroid state before death. See p834.

3 ►*Treat the patient not the blood level!* No exact cut-off in TSH can be given partly because risk of death from heart disease mirrors TSH even when in the normal range in women. Risk ≈ 1.4 if TSH 1.5–2.4 vs 1.7 if TSH 2.5–3.5. If TSH >3.65 and possibly symptomatic, a low dose of levothyroxine may be tried. Monitor symptoms, TSH and T_4 carefully. Over-exposure to thyroxine may cause osteoporosis ± AF.

Why are symptoms of thyroid disease so various, and so subtle?

Almost all our cell nuclei have receptors showing a high affinity for T_3: that known as TRα-1 is abundant in muscle and fat; TRα-2 is abundant in brain; and TRβ-1 is abundant in brain, liver, and kidney. These receptors, via their influence on various enzymes, affect the following processes:

- The metabolism of substrates, vitamins, and minerals.
- Modulation of all other hormones and their target-tissue responses.
- Stimulation of O_2 consumption and generation of metabolic heat.
- Regulation of protein synthesis, and carbohydrate and lipid metabolism.
- Stimulation of demand for co-enzymes and related vitamins.

Subclinical thyroid disease

Subclinical hypothyroidism Suspect if TSH >4mU/L with normal T_4 and T_3, and no symptoms. It is common: ~10% of those >55yrs have ↑TSH. Risk of progression to frank hypothyroidism is ~2%, and increases as ↑TSH; risk doubles if thyroid peroxidase antibodies are present, and is also increased in men. *Management:*

- Confirm that raised TSH is persistent (recheck in 2-4 months).
- Recheck the history: if any non-specific features (eg depression), discuss benefits of treating (p220) with the patient—maybe they will function better.
- Have a low threshold for carefully supervised treatment as your patient may not be so asymptomatic after all, and cardiac deaths *may* be prevented. Treat if: **1** TSH ≥10mu/L. **2** +ve thyroid autoantibodies. **3** Past (treated) Graves'. **4** Other organ-specific autoimmunity (type 1 DM, myasthenia, pernicious anaemia, vitiligo), as they are more likely to progress to clinical hypothyroidism. *If TSH 4-10, and vague symptoms*, treat for 6 months—only continue if symptoms improve (or the patient is trying to conceive). If the patient does not fall into any of these categories, monitor TSH yearly.
- Risks from well-monitored treatment of subclinical hypothyroidism are small (but there is an ↑risk of atrial fibrillation and osteoporosis if over-treated).

Subclinical hyperthyroidism occurs when ↓TSH, with normal T_4 and T_3. There is a 41% increase in relative mortality from all causes versus euthyroid control subjects—eg from AF and osteoporosis. *Management:*

- Confirm that suppressed TSH is persistent (recheck in 2-4 months).
- Check for a non-thyroidal cause: illness, pregnancy, pituitary or hypothalamic insufficiency (suspect if T_4 or T_3 are at the lower end of the reference range), use of TSH-suppressing medication, eg thyroxine, steroids.
- If TSH <0.1, treat on an individual basis, eg with symptoms of hyperthyroidism, AF, unexplained weight loss, osteoporosis, goitre.
- Options are carbimazole or propylthiouracil—or radioiodine therapy.
- If no symptoms, recheck 6-monthly.

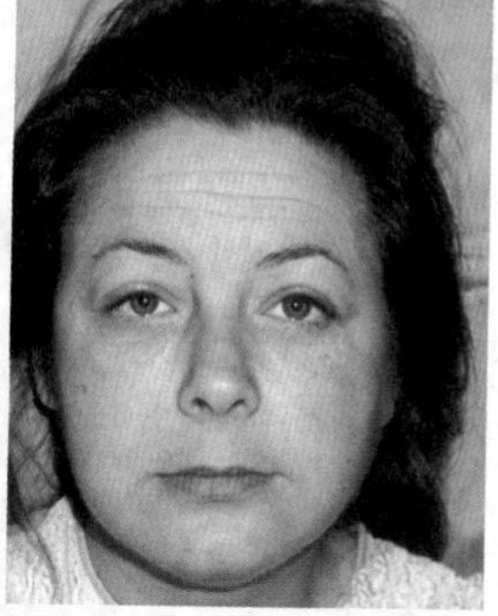

Fig 5.16 Facial appearance in hypothyroidism. Look for: pallor; coarse, brittle, diminished hair (scalp, axillary, and pubic); dull or blank expression lacking sparkle; coarse features; puffy lids. These signs are subtle: ►have a low threshold for measuring TSH.

Endocrinology

Parathyroid hormone and hyperparathyroidism

Parathyroid hormone (PTH) is normally secreted in response to low ionized Ca^{2+} levels, by four parathyroid glands situated posterior to the thyroid (p601). The glands are controlled by −ve feedback via Ca^{2+} levels. PTH acts by: •↑osteoclast activity releasing Ca^{2+} and PO_4^{3-} from bones •↑Ca^{2+} and ↓PO_4^{3-} reabsorption in the kidney •active 1,25 dihydroxy-vitamin D_3 production is ↑. Overall effect is ↑Ca^{2+} and ↓PO_4^{3-}.

Primary hyperparathyroidism *Causes:* ~80% solitary adenoma, ~20% hyperplasia of all glands, <0.5% parathyroid cancer. *Presentation:* Often 'asymptomatic' (►*not in retrospect!*), with ↑Ca^{2+} on routine tests. Signs relate to: **1** ↑Ca^{2+} (p676): weak, tired, depressed, thirsty, dehydrated-but-polyuric; also renal stones, abdominal pain, pancreatitis, and ulcers (duodenal:gastric≈7:1). **2** Bone resorption effects of PTH can cause pain, fractures, and osteopenia/osteoporosis. **3** ↑BP: ►so check Ca^{2+} in *everyone* with hypertension. *Association: MEN-1* (BOX 'Multiple endocrine neoplasia'). *Tests:* ↑Ca^{2+} & ↑PTH or inappropriately normal (other causes of this: thiazides, lithium, familial hypocalciuric hypercalcaemia, tertiary hyperparathyroidism). Also ↓PO_4^{3-} (unless in renal failure), ↑ALP from bone activity, 24h urinary ↑Ca^{2+}. *Imaging: osteitis fibrosa cystica* (due to severe resorption; rare) may show up as subperiosteal erosions, cysts, or brown tumours of phalanges ± acro-osteolysis (fig 5.17) ± 'pepper-pot' skull. *DEXA* (p683; for osteoporosis, p682). ℞: If mild: advise ↑fluid intake to prevent stones; avoid thiazides + high Ca^{2+} & vit D intake; see 6-monthly. Excision of the adenoma or of all four hyperplastic glands prevents fractures and peptic ulcers. *Indications:* high serum or urinary Ca^{2+}, bone disease, osteoporosis, renal calculi, ↓renal function, age ≤50yrs. *Complications:* Hypoparathyroidism, recurrent laryngeal nerve damage (∴hoarse), symptomatic Ca^{2+}↓ (hungry bones syndrome; check Ca^{2+} daily for ≥14d post-op). Pre-op US and MIBI scan may localize an adenoma; intra-operative PTH sampling is used to confirm removal. *Recurrence:* ~8% over 10yrs.[19] Cinacalcet (a 'calcimimetic') ↑sensitivity of parathyroid cells to Ca^{2+} (∴↓PTH secretion); monitor Ca^{2+} within 1 week of dose changes; SE: myalgia; ↓testosterone.

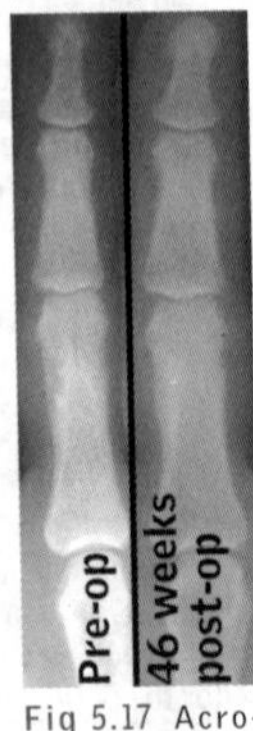

Fig 5.17 Acro-osteolysis.

©Dr I Maddison myweb.lsbu.ac.uk.

Secondary hyperparathyroidism ↓Ca^{2+}, ↑PTH (appropriately). *Causes:* ↓vit D intake, chronic renal failure. ℞: Correct causes. Phosphate binders; vit D; cinacalcet if PTH ≥85pmol/L and parathyroidectomy tricky.

Tertiary hyperparathyroidism ↑Ca^{2+}, ↑↑PTH (inappropriately). Occurs after prolonged secondary hyperparathyroidism, causing glands to act autonomously having undergone hyperplastic or adenomatous change. This causes ↑Ca^{2+} from ↑↑secretion of PTH unlimited by feedback control. Seen in chronic renal failure.

Malignant hyperparathyroidism Parathyroid-related protein (PTHrP) is produced by some squamous cell lung cancers, breast and renal cell carcinomas. This mimics PTH resulting in ↑Ca^{2+} (PTH is ↓, as PTHrP is not detected in the assay).

Hypoparathyroidism

Primary hypoparathyroidism PTH secretion is ↓ due to gland failure. *Tests:* ↓Ca^{2+}, ↑PO_4^{3-} or ↔, ↔ALP. *Signs:* Those of hypocalcaemia, p678 ± autoimmune comorbidities (BOX 'Autoimmune polyendocrine syndromes'). *Causes:* Autoimmune; congenital (Di George syn., *OHCS* p642). ℞: Ca^{2+} supplements + calcitriol (or synthetic PTH /12h SC: it prevents hypercalciuria).

Secondary hypoparathyroidism Radiation, surgery (thyroidectomy, parathyroidectomy), hypomagnesaemia (magnesium is required for PTH secretion).

Pseudohypoparathyroidism Failure of target cell response to PTH. *Signs:* Short metacarpals (esp. 4th and 5th, fig 5.18), round face, short stature, calcified basal ganglia (fig 5.19), ↓IQ. *Tests:* ↓Ca^{2+}, ↑PTH, ↔ or ↑ALP. ℞: As for 1° hypoparathyroidism.

Pseudopseudohypoparathyroidism The morphological features of pseudohypoparathyroidism, but with normal biochemistry. The cause for both is genetic.

Multiple endocrine neoplasia (MEN types 1, 2a, and 2b)

In MEN syndromes there are functioning hormone-producing tumours in multiple organs (they are inherited as autosomal dominants).[20] They comprise: •MEN-1 and 2 •Neurofibromatosis (p514) •Von Hippel-Lindau and Peutz-Jeghers syndromes (p712 & p708) •Carney complex (spotty skin pigmentation, schwannomas, myxoma of skin, mucosa, or heart, especially atrial myxoma), and endocrine tumours: eg pituitary adenoma, adrenal hyperplasia, and testicular tumour.

MEN-1:
- Parathyroid hyperplasia/adenoma (~95%; most ↑Ca^{2+}).
- Pancreas endocrine tumours (70%)—gastrinoma (p716) or insulinoma (p215), or, rarely, somatostatinoma (DM + steatorrhoea + gallstones/cholangitis), VIPoma (p258), or glucagonomas (±glucagon syndrome: migrating rash; glossitis; cheilitis, fig 8.5 p327; anaemia; ↓weight; ↑plasma glucagon; ↑glucose).
- Pituitary prolactinoma (~50%) or GH secreting tumour (acromegaly:[21] p239); also, adrenal and carcinoid tumours are associated.

The MEN-1 gene is a tumour suppressor gene. Menin, its protein, alters transcription activation. Many are sporadic, presenting in the 3rd–5th decades.

MEN-2a:
- Thyroid: medullary thyroid carcinoma (seen in ~100%, p600).
- Adrenal: phaeochromocytoma (~50%, usually benign and bilateral).
- Parathyroid hyperplasia (~80%, but less than 20% have ↑Ca^{2+}).

MEN-2b: Has similar features to MEN-2a plus mucosal neuromas and Marfanoid appearance (p706), but no hyperparathyroidism. Mucosal neuromas consist of 'bumps' on: lips, cheeks, tongue, glottis, eyelids, and visible corneal nerves.

The gene involved in MEN-2a and b is the ret proto-oncogene, a receptor tyrosine kinase. Tests for ret mutations are revolutionizing MEN-2 treatment by enabling a prophylactic thyroidectomy to be done before neoplasia occurs, usually before 3yrs of age. NB: ret mutations rarely contribute to sporadic parathyroid tumours.

Autoimmune polyendocrine syndromes

Autoimmune disorders cluster into two defined syndromes:

Type 1 Autosomal recessive, rare.
Cause: Mutations of **AIRE** (**A**uto **I**mmune**RE**gulator) gene on chromosome 21.
Features: •Addison's disease. •Chronic mucocutaneous candidiasis. •Hypoparathyroidism. Also associated with hypogonadism, pernicious anaemia, autoimmune primary hypothyroidism, chronic active hepatitis, vitiligo, alopecia.

Type 2 HLA D3 and D4 linked, common. *Cause:* Polygenic.
Features: •Addison's disease. •Type 1 diabetes mellitus (in 20%).
• Autoimmune thyroid disease—hypothyroidism or Graves' disease.
Also associated with primary hypogonadism, vitiligo, alopecia, pernicious anaemia, chronic atrophic gastritis, coeliac disease, dermatitis herpetiformis.

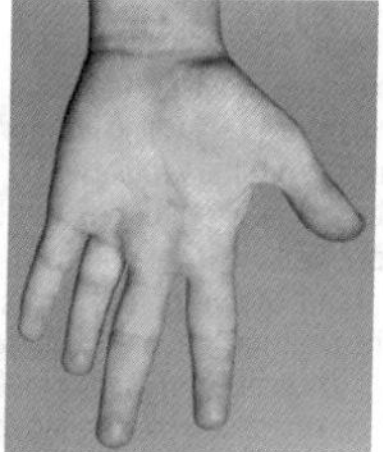

Fig 5.18 Pseudohypoparathyroidism: short 4th and 5th metacarpals.

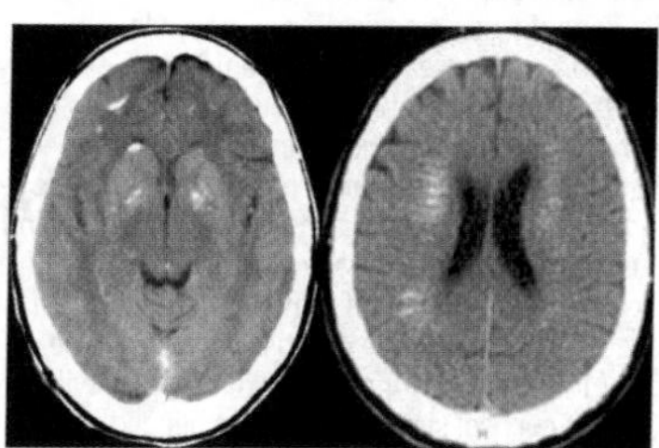

Fig 5.19 Cerebral calcification in pseudohypoparathyroidism: periventricular (left) and basal ganglia (right).
Courtesy of Professor Peter Scally.

Physiology The adrenal cortex produces steroids: 1 *Glucocorticoids* (eg cortisol), which affect carbohydrate, lipid, and protein metabolism. 2 *Mineralocorticoids*, which control sodium and potassium balance (eg aldosterone, p668). 3 *Androgens*, sex hormones which have weak effect until peripheral conversion to testosterone and dihydrotestosterone. Corticotropin-releasing factor (CRF) from the hypothalamus stimulates ACTH secretion from the pituitary, which in turn stimulates cortisol and androgen production by the adrenal cortex. Cortisol is excreted as urinary free cortisol and various 17-oxogenic steroids.

Cushing's syndrome This is the clinical state produced by chronic glucocorticoid excess + loss of the normal feedback mechanisms of the hypothalamo-pituitary-adrenal axis and loss of circadian rhythm of cortisol secretion (normally highest on waking). The chief cause is oral steroids. Endogenous causes are rare: 80% are due to ↑ACTH; of these a pituitary adenoma (Cushing's disease) is the commonest cause.

1 **ACTH-dependent causes (↑ACTH)**
- *Cushing's disease:* Bilateral adrenal hyperplasia from an ACTH-secreting pituitary adenoma (usually a microadenoma, p234). ♀:♂>1:1. Peak age: 30–50yrs. A low-dose dexamethasone test (BOX) leads to no change in plasma cortisol, but 8mg may be enough to more than halve morning cortisol (as occurs in normals).
- *Ectopic ACTH production:* Especially small cell lung cancer and carcinoid tumours, p271. Specific features: pigmentation (due to ↑↑ACTH), hypokalaemic metabolic alkalosis (↑↑cortisol leads to mineralocorticoid activity), weight loss, hyperglycaemia. Classical features of Cushing's are often absent. Dexamethasone even in high doses (8mg) fails to suppress cortisol production.
- *Rarely, ectopic CRF production:* Some thyroid (medullary) and prostate cancers.

2 **ACTH-independent causes (↓ACTH due to −ve feedback)**
- *Iatrogenic:* Pharmacological doses of steroids (common).
- *Adrenal adenoma/cancer:* (May cause abdo pain ± virilization in ♀, p230.) Because the tumour is autonomous, dexamethasone in any dose won't suppress cortisol.
- *Adrenal nodular hyperplasia:* (As for adrenal adenoma, no dexamethasone suppression.)
- *Rarely: Carney complex*, p223. *McCune-Albright syndrome*, see *OHCS* p650.

Symptoms ↑Weight; mood change (depression, lethargy, irritability, psychosis); proximal weakness; gonadal dysfunction (irregular menses; hirsutism; erectile dysfunction); acne; recurrent Achilles tendon rupture; occasionally virilization if ♀.

Signs Central obesity; plethoric, moon face; buffalo hump; supraclavicular fat distribution; skin & muscle atrophy; bruises; purple abdominal striae (fig 5.20); osteoporosis; ↑BP; ↑glucose; infection-prone; poor healing. Signs of the cause (eg abdo mass).

Tests Random plasma cortisols may mislead, as illness, time of day, and stress (eg venepuncture) influence results. Also, don't rely on imaging to localize the cause: non-functioning 'incidentalomas' occur in ~5% on adrenal CT and ~10% on pituitary MRI. MRI detects only ~70% of pituitary tumours causing Cushing's (many are too small).

Treatment Depends on the cause.
- *Iatrogenic:* Stop medications if possible.
- *Cushing's disease:* Selective removal of pituitary adenoma (trans-sphenoidally). Bilateral adrenalectomy if source unlocatable, or recurrence post-op (complication: *Nelson's syndrome:* ↑skin pigmentation due to ↑↑ACTH from an enlarging pituitary tumour, as adrenalectomy removes −ve feedback; responds to pituitary radiation).
- *Adrenal adenoma or carcinoma:* Adrenalectomy: 'cures' adenomas but rarely cures cancer. Radiotherapy & adrenolytic drugs (mitotane) follow if carcinoma.
- *Ectopic ACTH:* Surgery if tumour is located and hasn't spread. Metyrapone, ketoconazole, and fluconazole ↓cortisol secretion pre-op or if awaiting effects of radiation. Intubation + mifepristone (competes with cortisol at receptors) + etomidate (blocks cortisol synthesis) may be needed, eg in severe ACTH-associated psychosis.

Prognosis Untreated Cushing's has ↑vascular mortality.[22] Treated, prognosis is good (but myopathy, obesity, menstrual irregularity, ↑BP, osteoporosis, subtle mood changes and DM often remain—so follow up carefully, and manage individually).

Investigating suspected Cushing's syndrome

First, confirm the diagnosis (a raised plasma cortisol), then localize the source on the basis of laboratory testing. Use imaging studies to confirm the likely source.

1st-line tests *Overnight dexamethasone suppression test* is a good outpatient test. Dexamethasone 1mg PO at midnight; do serum cortisol at 8AM. Normally, cortisol suppresses to <50nmol/L; no suppression in Cushing's syndrome. False −ve rate: <2%; false +ves: 2% normal, 13% obese, and 23% of inpatients. *NB:* false +ves (*pseudo-Cushing's*) are seen in depression, obesity, alcohol excess, and inducers of liver enzymes (↑rate of dexamethasone metabolism, eg phenytoin, phenobarbital, rifampicin, p689). *24h urinary free cortisol* (normal: <280nmol/24h) is an alternative.

2nd-line tests If 1st-line tests abnormal: *48h dexamethasone suppression test:* Give dexamethasone 0.5mg/6h PO for 2d. Measure cortisol at 0 and 48h (last test at 6h after last dose). Again, in Cushing's syndrome, there is a failure to suppress cortisol. *48h high-dose dexamethasone suppression test:* (2mg/6h.) May distinguish pituitary (suppression) from others causes (no/part suppression). *Midnight cortisol:* Admit (unless salivary cortisol used). Often inaccurate due to measurement issues. Normal circadian rhythm (cortisol *lowest* at midnight, *highest* early morning) is lost in Cushing's syndrome. Midnight blood, via a cannula during sleep, shows cortisol ↑ in Cushing's.

Localization tests (Where is the lesion?) If the 1st- and 2nd-line tests are +ve—*Plasma ACTH. If ACTH is undetectable*, an adrenal tumour is likely → CT/MRI adrenal glands. If no mass, proceed to *adrenal vein sampling. If ACTH is detectable*, distinguish a pituitary cause from ectopic ACTH production by high-dose suppression test or *corticotropin-releasing hormone (CRH) test:* 100mcg ovine or human CRH IV. Measure cortisol at 120min. Cortisol rises with pituitary disease but not with ectopic ACTH production.

If tests indicate that cortisol responds to manipulation, Cushing's disease is likely. Image the pituitary (MRI) and consider *bilateral inferior petrosal sinus blood sampling.*

If tests indicate that cortisol does not respond to manipulation, hunt for the source of ectopic ACTH—eg IV contrast CT of chest, abdomen, and pelvis ± MRI of neck, thorax, and abdomen, eg for small ACTH secreting carcinoid tumours.

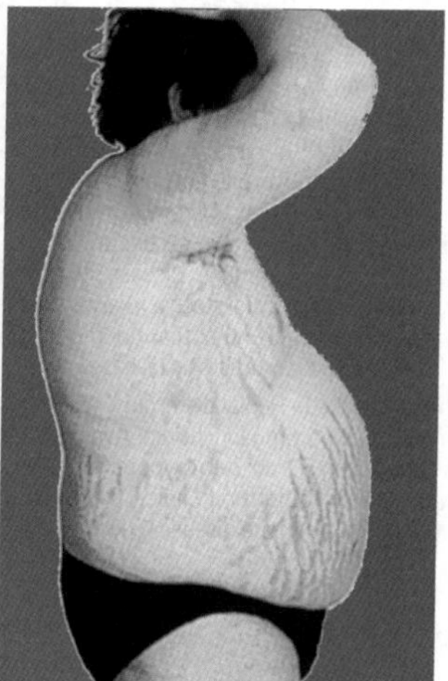

Fig 5.20 Hypercortisolism weakens skin; even normal stretching (or the pressure of obesity, as here) can make its elastin break—on healing we see these depressed purple scars (striae). Cortisone or rapid growth contributes to striae in other contexts: pregnancy, adolescence, weight lifting, sudden-onset obesity, or from strong steroid creams. Striae mature into silvery crescents looking like the underside of willow leaves. Unsightly immature striae may be improved by YAG lasers.

Addison's disease (adrenal insufficiency)

Primary adrenocortical insufficiency (Addison's disease) is rare (~0.8/100 000), but can be fatal. Destruction of the adrenal cortex leads to glucocorticoid (cortisol) and mineralocorticoid (aldosterone) deficiency (see fig 5.21). Signs are capricious: it is '*the unforgiving master of non-specificity and disguise*'.[23] You may diagnose a viral infection or anorexia nervosa in error (K^+ is ↓ in the latter but ↑ in Addison's).

Physiology:

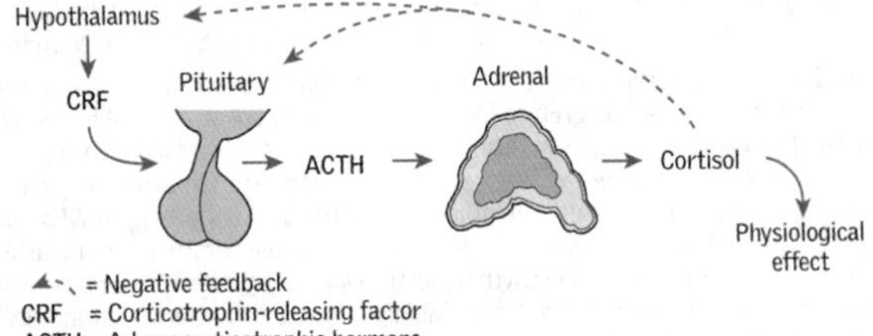

Fig 5.21 Pathways involved in adrenal function.

Causes: 80% are due to autoimmunity in the UK. *Other causes:* TB (commonest cause worldwide), adrenal metastases (eg from lung, breast, renal cancer), lymphoma, opportunistic infections in HIV (eg CMV, *Mycobacterium avium*, p400); adrenal haemorrhage (►►Waterhouse-Friderichsen syndrome p714; antiphospholipid syndrome; SLE), congenital (late-onset congenital adrenal hyperplasia).

Secondary adrenal insufficiency The commonest cause is iatrogenic, due to long-term steroid therapy leading to suppression of the pituitary-adrenal axis. This only becomes apparent on withdrawal of the steroids. Other causes are rare and include hypothalamic-pituitary disease leading to ↓ACTH production. Mineralocorticoid production remains intact, and there is no hyperpigmentation as ↓ACTH.

Symptoms Often diagnosed late: lean, tanned, tired, tearful ± weakness, anorexia, dizzy, faints, flu-like myalgias/arthralgias. *Mood:* depression, psychosis. *GI:* nausea/vomiting, abdominal pain, diarrhoea/constipation. *Think of Addison's in all with unexplained abdominal pain or vomiting*. Pigmented palmar creases & buccal mucosa (↑ACTH; cross-reacts with melanin receptors). Postural hypotension. Vitiligo. ►►*Signs of critical deterioration* (p836): Shock (↓BP, tachycardia), T°↑, coma.

Tests ↓Na^+ & ↑K^+ (due to ↓mineralocorticoid), ↓glucose (due to ↓cortisol). Also: uraemia, ↑Ca^{2+}, eosinophilia, anaemia. Δ: *Short ACTH stimulation test (Synacthen® test):* Do plasma cortisol before and ½h after tetracosactide (Synacthen®) 250mcg IM. Addison's is excluded if 30min cortisol >550nmol/L. Steroid drugs may interfere with assays: ask lab. NB: in pregnancy and contraceptive pill, cortisol levels may be reassuring but falsely ↑, due to ↑cortisol-binding globulin. *Also:* •*ACTH:* In Addison's, 9AM ACTH is ↑ (>300ng/L: inappropriately high). It is low in secondary causes •*21-Hydroxylase adrenal autoantibodies:* +ve in autoimmune disease in >80% •*Plasma renin & aldosterone:* to assess mineralocortocoid status. *AXR/CXR:* Any past TB, eg upper zone fibrosis or adrenal calcification? If no autoantibodies, consider further tests (eg adrenal CT) for TB, histoplasma, or metastatic disease.

Treatment ►►See p836 for Addisonian crisis (shocked). Replace steroids: ~15–25mg hydrocortisone daily, in 2–3 doses, eg 10mg on waking, 5mg lunchtime. Avoid giving late (may cause insomnia). Mineralocorticoids to correct postural hypotension, ↓Na^+, ↑K^+: fludrocortisone PO from 50–200mcg daily. Adjust both on clinical grounds. If there is a poor response, suspect an associated autoimmune disease (check thyroid, do coeliac serology: p266).

Steroid use Advise wearing a bracelet declaring steroid use. Add 5–10mg hydrocortisone to daily intake before strenuous activity/exercise. Double steroids in febrile illness, injury, or stress. Give out syringes and in-date IM hydrocortisone, and show how to inject 100mg IM if vomiting prevents oral intake (seek medical help; admit for IV fluids if dehydrated).

Follow-up Yearly (BP, U&E); watch for autoimmune diseases (pernicious anaemia).[4]

Prognosis (treated) Adrenal crises and infections do cause excess deaths: mean age at death for men is ~65yrs (11yrs <estimated life expectancy; women lose ~3yrs).

⚠ Exogenous steroid use

Replacement steroids are vital in those taking long-term steroids when acutely unwell. Adrenal insufficiency may develop with deadly hypovolaemic shock, if additional steroid is not given. ▸▸See p836.

Steroid use: Warn against abruptly stopping steroids. Emphasize that prescribing doctors/dentists/surgeons *must* know of steroid use: give *steroid card*.

Excerpt from the notes of Miss E.L.R., 92 days before her death from undiagnosed Addison's disease. From the Coroner's Court...

'Typical day—wakes up at 11.30, still feels tired, then will have some breakfast and usually fall asleep on the couch. The most energy req. activity in last 1 month is—cooking herself a pasta meal. Then, totally exhausted will sleep more in pm, then eat some dinner. Goes to bed at 11pm—latest. Not able to concentrate...Used to weigh 45kg. Now weighs 42kg.'[24]

Placed on a page about Addison's disease, we might think there are sufficient clues to raise the suspicion of Addison's (even though her electrolytes were not particularly awry, and her pigmentation was barely perceptible). But change the context to our last busy clinic. We are a little distracted. The memory of Addison's is fading. Who among us will hear the alarm bell ring?

4 Autoimmune polyglandular syndromes types 1-4: 1 Monogenic syndrome (AIRE gene on chromosome 21); signs: candidiasis, hypoparathyroidism + Addison's. 2 (Schmidt syndrome.) Adrenal insufficiency + auto immune thyroid disease ± DM ± pleuritis/pericarditis. 3 Autoimmune thyroid disease + other autoimmune conditions but *not* Addison's. 4 Autoimmune combinations not included in 1-3.

Hyperaldosteronism

Primary hyperaldosteronism Excess production of aldosterone, independent of the renin-angiotensin system, causing ↑sodium and water retention, and ↓renin release. Consider if: hypertension, hypokalaemia, or alkalosis in someone not on diuretics. Sodium tends to be mildly raised or normal.

Symptoms: Often asymptomatic or signs of hypokalaemia (p674): weakness (even quadriparesis), cramps, paraesthesiae, polyuria, polydipsia. ↑BP but not always.

Causes: ~⅔ due to a solitary aldosterone-producing adenoma (linked to mutations in K^+ channels)[5]—*Conn's syndrome*. ~⅓ due to bilateral adrenocortical hyperplasia. Rare causes: adrenal carcinoma; or glucocorticoid-remediable aldosteronism (GRA)—the ACTH regulatory element of the 11β-hydroxylase gene fuses to the aldosterone synthase gene, ↑aldosterone production, & bringing it under the control of ACTH.

Tests: U&E, renin and aldosterone, and adrenal vein sampling. Do not rely on a low K^+, as >20% are normokalaemic. For GRA (suspect if there is a family history of early hypertension), genetic testing is available. *Treatment:* •*Conn's*: laparoscopic adrenalectomy. Spironolactone (25–100mg/24h PO) for 4wks pre-op controls BP and K^+. •*Hyperplasia:* treated medically: spironolactone or amiloride. •*GRA:* dexamethasone 1mg/24h PO for 4wks, normalizes biochemistry but not always BP. If BP is still ↑, use spironolactone as an alternative. •*Adrenal carcinoma:* surgery ± post-operative adrenolytic therapy with mitotane—prognosis is poor.

Secondary hyperaldosteronism Due to a high renin from ↓renal perfusion, eg in renal artery stenosis, accelerated hypertension, diuretics, CCF, or hepatic failure.

Bartter's syndrome This is a major cause of congenital (autosomal recessive) salt wasting—via a sodium and chloride leak in the loop of Henle via mutations in channels and transporters. Presents in childhood with failure to thrive, polyuria, and polydipsia. BP is *normal*. Sodium loss leads to volume depletion, causing ↑renin and aldosterone production, leading to hypokalaemia and metabolic alkalosis, ↑urinary K^+ and Cl^-. *Treatment:* K^+ replacement, NSAIDs (to inhibit prostaglandins), and ACE-i.

Phaeochromocytoma

Rare catecholamine-producing tumours. They arise from sympathetic paraganglia cells (=phaeochrome bodies), which are collections of chromaffin cells. They are usually found within the adrenal medulla. Extra-adrenal tumours (paragangliomas) are rarer, and often found by the aortic bifurcation (the organs of Zuckerkandl). Phaeochromocytomas *roughly* follow the 10% rule: 10% are malignant, 10% are extra-adrenal, 10% are bilateral, and 10% are familial. Recent data suggest higher preponderance in patients with genetic mutations affecting several genes including SDH (succinyl dehydrogenase). Thus, family history is crucial and referral for genetic screening (particularly <50 years old). A dangerous but treatable cause of hypertension (in <0.1%). *Associations* ~90% are sporadic; 10% are part of hereditary cancer syndromes (p215), eg thyroid, MEN-2A and 2B, neurofibromatosis, von Hippel–Lindau syndrome (SDH mutations). *Classic triad* Episodic headache, sweating, and tachycardia (± ↑, ↓, or ↔BP, see BOX 'Features of phaeochromocytoma').

Tests •*Biochemical:* 24h urine for metanephrines/metadrenaline (better than catecholamines and vanillylmandelic acid[25]), ↑WCC. •*Localization:* Abdominal CT/MRI, or meta-iodobenzylguanidine (chromaffin-seeking isotope) scan (can find extra-adrenal tumours, p738). **Treatment** *Surgery:* α-blockade pre-op: phenoxybenzamine (α-blocker) is used before β-blocker to avoid crisis from unopposed α-adrenergic stimulation, β-block too if heart disease or tachycardic. *Consult the anaesthetist. Post-op:* Do 24h urine metanephrine 2wks post-op, monitor BP (risk of ↓↓BP). ►►*Emergency* ℞: p837. If malignant, chemotherapy or therapeutic radiolabelled MIBG may be used. *Follow-up:* Lifelong: malignant recurrence may present late, genetic screening.

5 Tumours from the zona glomerulosa, zona fasciculata, or zona reticularis associate with syndromes of ↑ mineralocorticoids, glucocorticoids, or androgens respectively, usually; remember 'GFR≈miner GA'.

Hypertension: a common context for hyperaldosteronism tests

Think of Conn's in these contexts:

- Hypertension associated with hypokalaemia.
- Refractory hypertension, eg despite ≥3 antihypertensive drugs.
- Hypertension occurring before 40yrs of age (especially in women).

The approach to investigation remains controversial, but the simplest is to look for a suppressed renin and ↑aldosterone (may be normal if there is severe hypokalaemia). CT or MRI of the adrenals is done to localize the cause. This should be done after hyperaldosteronism is proven, due to the high number of adrenal incidentalomas. If imaging shows a unilateral adenoma, *adrenal vein sampling* may be done (venous blood is sampled from both adrenals). If one side reveals increased aldosterone:cortisol ratio compared with the other (>3-fold difference), an adenoma is likely, and surgical excision is indicated. If no nodules or bilateral nodules are seen, think about adrenal hyperplasia or GRA.

►NB: renal artery stenosis is a more common cause of refractory ↑BP and ↓K^+ (p315).

Features of phaeochromocytoma (often episodic and often vague)

Try to diagnose before death: suspect if BP hard to control, accelerating, or episodic.

- *Heart:* ↑Pulse; palpitations/VT; dyspnoea; faints; angina; MI/LVF; cardiomyopathy.[6]
- *CNS:* Headache; visual disorder; dizziness; tremor; numbness; fits; encephalopathy; Horner's syndrome (paraganglioma); subarachnoid/CNS haemorrhage.
- *Psychological:* Anxiety; panic; hyperactivity; confusion; episodic psychosis.
- *Gut:* D&V; abdominal pain over tumour site; mass; mesenteric vasoconstriction.
- *Others:* Sweats/flushes; heat intolerance; pallor; ↑T°; backache; haemoptysis.

Symptoms may be precipitated by straining, exercise, stress, abdominal pressure, surgery, or by agents such as β-blockers, IV contrast agents, or the tricyclics. The site of the tumour may determine precipitants, eg if pelvic, precipitants include sexual intercourse, parturition, defecation, and micturition. Adrenergic crises may last minutes to days. Suddenly patients feel 'as if about to die'—and then get better, or go on to develop a stroke or cardiogenic shock. On examination, there may be no signs, or hypertension ± signs of heart failure/cardiomyopathy (± paradoxical shock, similar to Takotsubo's[6]), episodic thyroid swelling, glycosuria during attacks, or terminal haematuria from a bladder phaeochromocytoma.

6 *Takotsubo cardiomyopathy* (=stress- or catecholamine-induced cardiomyopathy/broken heart syndrome) may cause sudden chest pain mimicking MI, with ↑ST segments, and its signature apical ballooning on echo (also ↓ejection fraction) occurring during catecholamine surges. It is a cause of MI in the presence of normal arteries. The stress may be medical (SAH, p478) or psychological.

Hirsutism, virilism, gynaecomastia, and impotence

Hirsutism is common (10% of women) and usually benign. It implies male pattern hair growth in women. Causes are familial, idiopathic, or are due to ↑androgen secretion by the *ovary* (eg polycystic ovarian syndrome, ovarian cancer, *OHCS* p281), the *adrenal gland* (eg late-onset congenital adrenal hyperplasia, *OHCS* p251, Cushing's syndrome, adrenal cancer), or *drugs* (eg steroids). *Polycystic ovarian syndrome (PCOS)* causes secondary oligo- or amenorrhoea, infertility, obesity, acne, and hirsutism (*OHCS* p252). Ultrasound: bilateral polycystic ovaries. Blood tests: ↑testosterone (if ≥6nmol/L, look for an androgen-producing adrenal or ovarian tumour), ↓sex-hormone binding globulin, ↑LH:FSH ratio (not consistent), TSH, lipids. Address any feelings of lack of conformity to society's perceived norms of feminine beauty.
Management: Healthy eating, optimize weight, shaving; laser photoepilation; wax; creams, eg eflornithine, or electrolysis (expensive/time-consuming, but effective); bleach (1:10 hydrogen peroxide).
- Oestrogens: combined contraceptive pill (*OHCS* p302)—Yasmin® is one choice as its progestogen, drospirenone, is an antimineralocorticoid. Alternatively, co-cyprindiol provided there are no contraindications, such as uncontrolled hypertension and current breast cancer. Stop co-cyprindiol 3–4 months after hirsutism has completely resolved because of increased VTE risk. If COCs are contraindicated or have not worked (after 6/12), refer the woman to secondary care for specialist treatment:
- Metformin (helps with insulin resistance) and spironolactone are sometimes tried.
- Clomifene is used for infertility (a fertility expert should prescribe).

Virilism Onset of amenorrhoea, clitoromegaly, deep voice, temporal hair recession + hirsutism. Look for an androgen-secreting adrenal or ovarian tumour.

Gynaecomastia (ie abnormal amount of breast tissue in men; may occur in normal puberty.) Oestrogen/androgen ratio↑ (vs galactorrhoea in which prolactin is↑). *Causes:* Hypogonadism (see BOX 'Male hypogonadism'), liver cirrhosis (↑oestrogens), hyperthyroidism, tumours (oestrogen-producing, eg testicular, adrenal; HCG-producing, eg testicular, bronchial); drugs: oestrogens, spironolactone, digoxin, testosterone, marijuana; if stopping is impossible, consider testosterone if hypogonadism ± anti-oestrogen (tamoxifen).

Impotence *(= erectile dysfunction)* Erections result from neuronal release of nitric oxide (NO) which, via cGMP and Ca^{2+}, hyperpolarizes and thus relaxes vascular and trabecular smooth muscle cells, allowing engorgement. Common after 50yrs, and often multifactorial. A psychological facet is common (esp. if erectile dysfunction occurs only in some situations, if onset coincides with stress, and if early morning erections still occur: these also persist in early organic disease).
Organic causes: The big three: smoking, alcohol, and diabetes (reduce NO +autonomic neuropathy). Also *endocrine:* hypogonadism, hyperthyroidism, ↑prolactin; *neurological:* cord lesions, MS, autonomic neuropathy; *pelvic surgery*, eg bladder-neck, prostate; *radiotherapy*; *atheroma*; *renal* or *hepatic failure*; *prostatic hyperplasia*; *penile anomalies*, eg post-priapism, or Peyronie's (p708); *drugs:* digoxin, β-blockers, diuretics, antipsychotics, antidepressants, oestrogens, finasteride, narcotics.
Workup: After a full sexual and psychological history do: U&E, LFT, glucose, TFT, LH, FSH, lipids, testosterone, prolactin ± Doppler. Is penile arterial pressure enough for inflow? Is penile sensation OK (if not, ?CNS problem)? Is the veno-occlusive mechanism OK?
℞: •Treat causes. •Counselling. •Oral phosphodiesterase (PDE5) inhibitors ↑cGMP. Erection isn't automatic (depends on erotic stimuli). Sildenafil 25-100mg ½–1h pre-sex (food and alcohol upset absorption). *SE:* Headache (16%); flushing (10%); dyspepsia (7%); stuffy nose (4%); transient blue-green tingeing of vision (inhibition of retinal PDE6). *CI:* See BOX 'Contraindications and cautions to PD5 Inhibitors'. Tadalafil (long $t_{½}$) 10–20mg ½–36h pre-sex. Don't use >once daily. Vardenafil (5–20mg). •Vacuum aids (ideal for penile rehabilitation after radical prostatectomy), intracavernosal injections, transurethral pellets, and prostheses (inflatable or malleable; partners may receive unnatural sensations). •Corpus cavernosum tissue engineering (eg on acellular collagen scaffolds) is in its infancy.

Contraindications and cautions to PD5 inhibitors

►►**Contraindications**

- Concurrent use of nitrates.
- BP high or systolic <90mmHg/arrhythmia.
- Degenerative retinal disorders, eg retinitis pigmentosa.
- Unstable angina/stroke <6 months ago.
- Myocardial infarction <90 days ago.

Cautions ►Angina (especially if during intercourse).

- Bleeding; peptic ulcer (sildenafil).
- Marked hepatic or renal impairment.
- Peyronie's disease or cavernosal fibrosis.
- Risk of priapism (sickle-cell anaemia, myeloma, leukaemia).
- Concurrent complex antihypertensive regimens.
- Dyspnoea on minimal effort (sexual activity may be unsupportable).

Use in coronary artery disease has been a question, but is probably OK.[26]

Interactions: Nitrates (contraindication); cytochrome p450 (CYP3A) inducers: macrolides, protease inhibitors, theophyllines, azole antifungals, rifampicin, phenytoin, carbamazepine, phenobarbital, grapefruit juice (↑bioavailability). Caution if α-blocker use; avoid vardenafil with type 1A (eg quinidine; procainamide) and type 3 anti-arrhythmics (sotalol; amiodarone)—as well as nitrates as above-mentioned.

Male hypogonadism

Hypogonadism is failure of testes to produce testosterone, sperm, or both. Features: small testes, ↓libido, erectile dysfunction, loss of pubic hair, ↓muscle bulk, ↑fat, gynaecomastia, osteoporosis, ↓mood. If prepubertal: ↓virilization; incomplete puberty; eunuchoid body; reduced secondary sex characteristics. Causes include:

Primary hypogonadism is due to testicular failure, eg from •local trauma, torsion, chemotherapy/irradiation •post-orchitis, eg mumps, HIV, brucellosis, leprosy •renal failure, liver cirrhosis, or alcohol excess (toxic to Leydig cells) •chromosomal abnormalities, eg Klinefelter's syndrome (47XXY)—delayed sexual development, small testes, and gynaecomastia. Anorchia is rare.

Secondary hypogonadism ↓Gonadotropins (LH & FSH), eg from •hypopituitarism •prolactinoma •Kallman's syndrome—isolated gonadotropin-releasing hormone deficiency, often with anosmia and colour blindness •systemic illness (eg COPD; HIV; DM) •Laurence-Moon-Biedl and Prader-Willi syndromes (*OHCS* p648 & p652) •Age.

Ʀ: (p232) If total testosterone ≤8nmol/L, on 2 mornings (or <15 if ↑LH too) and ↓muscle bulk, testosterone may help, eg 1% dermal gel (Testogel®). Heart, bladder, and sexual function may perk up in age-related hypogonadism. Beware medicalizing ageing! CI ↑Ca^{2+}; nephrosis; polycythaemia; prostate, breast♂ or liver ca. Monitor PSA.

Hypopituitarism

Hypopituitarism entails ↓secretion of anterior pituitary hormones (figs 5.3, 5.22). They are affected in this order: growth hormone (GH), gonadotropins: follicle-stimulating hormone (FSH) and luteinizing hormone (LH), thyroid-stimulating hormone (TSH), and adrenocorticotrophic hormone (ACTH), prolactin (PRL). Panhypopituitarism is deficiency of all anterior hormones, usually caused by irradiation, surgery, or pituitary tumour.

Causes are at three levels. 1 *Hypothalamus:* Kallman's syndrome (p231), tumour, inflammation, infection (meningitis, TB), ischaemia. 2 *Pituitary stalk:* Trauma, surgery, mass lesion (craniopharyngioma, p234), meningioma, carotid artery aneurysm. 3 *Pituitary:* Tumour, irradiation, inflammation, autoimmunity,[7] infiltration (haemochromatosis, amyloid, metastases), ischaemia (pituitary apoplexy, p234; DIC[8]; Sheehan's syndrome[9]).

Features are due to:

1 *Hormone lack:* •*GH:* central obesity, atherosclerosis, dry wrinkly skin, ↓strength, ↓balance, ↓well-being, ↓exercise ability, ↓cardiac output, osteoporosis, ↓glucose. •*Gonadotropin (FSH; LH):* ♀ oligomenorrhoea or amenorrhoea, ↓fertility, ↓libido, osteoporosis, breast atrophy, dyspareunia. ♂ Erectile dysfunction, ↓libido, ↓muscle bulk, hypogonadism (↓hair, all over; small testes; ↓ejaculate volume; ↓spermatogenesis). •*Thyroid:* as for hypothyroidism (p220). •*Corticotropin:* as for adrenal insufficiency (p226). NB: no ↑skin pigmentation as ↓ACTH. •*Prolactin:* rare: absent lactation.

2 *Causes:* Eg pituitary tumour (p234), causing mass effect, or hormone secretion with ↓secretion of other hormones—eg prolactinoma, acromegaly, rarely Cushing's.

Tests (The triple stimulation test is now rarely done.)

- *Basal tests:* LH and FSH (↓ or ↔), testosterone or oestradiol (↓); TSH (↓ or ↔), T_4 (↓); prolactin (may be ↑, from loss of hypothalamic dopamine that normally inhibits its release), insulin-like growth factor-1 (IGF-1; ↓—used as a measure of GH axis, p238), cortisol (↓). Also do U&E (↓Na^+ from dilution), ↓Hb (normochromic, normocytic).
- *Dynamic tests:* 1 Short Synacthen® test: (p226) to assess the adrenal axis.
  2 Insulin tolerance test (ITT): done in specialist centres to assess the adrenal and GH axes. CI: epilepsy, heart disease, adrenal failure. Consult lab first. It involves IV insulin to induce hypoglycaemia, causing stress to ↑cortisol and GH secretion. It is done in the morning (water only taken from 22:00h the night before). Have 50% glucose and hydrocortisone to hand and IV access. Glucose must fall below 2.2mmol/L and the patient should become symptomatic when cortisol and GH are taken. Normal: GH >20mu/L, and peak cortisol >550nmol/L.
  3 Arginine + growth hormone-releasing hormone test.
  4 Glucagon stimulation test is alternative when ITT is contraindicated.
- *Investigate cause:* MRI scan to look for a hypothalamic or pituitary lesion.

Treatment Refer to an endocrinologist for assessment of pituitary fuction and to oversee hormone replacement and treatment of underlying cause.

- *Hydrocortisone* for 2° adrenal failure (p226) ►before other hormones are given.
- Thyroxine if hypothyroid (p220, but TSH is useless for monitoring).
- Hypogonadism (for symptoms and to prevent osteoporosis). ♂: options include *testosterone enanthate* 250mg IM every 3 weeks, daily topical gels or buccal mucoadhesive tablets. Patches (eg Testogel®) are also used. ♀: (premenopausal). *Oestrogen:* transdermal oestradiol patches, or contraceptive pill (exceeds replacement needs) ± testosterone or dehydroepiandrosterone (DHEA, in hypoandrogenic women; a small amount may improve well-being and sexual function, and help bone mineral density and lean body mass).
- *Gonadotropin* therapy is needed to induce fertility in both men and women.
- Growth hormone (GH). Somatotrophin mimics human GH. It addresses problems of ↑fat mass, ↓bone mass, ↓lean body mass (muscle bulk), ↓exercise capacity, and problems with heat intolerance.

7 Autoimmune hypophysitis (=inflamed pituitary) mimics pituitary adenoma. It may be triggered by pregnancy or immunotherapy blocking CTLA-4. No pituitary auto-antigen is yet used diagnostically.
8 Snake bite is a common cause in India (eg when associated with acute kidney injury).
9 Sheehan's syndrome is pituitary necrosis after postpartum haemorrhage.

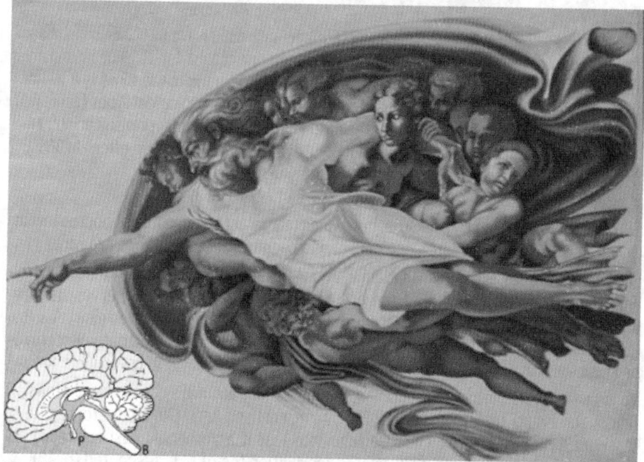

Fig 5.22 Neuroendocrinology: emotions ⇄ thoughts ⇄ actions. As Michelangelo foretold (in his *Creation of Adam*) 'all gods and demons that have ever existed are within us as possibilities, desires, and ways of escape'. Within the dark red vault of our skull we see human and god-like forms reaching out, as thoughts escape into actions—with legs extending into our brainstem (B) and a fist is pushing from our hypothalamus into the pituitary stalk (P). Above the pituitary we have thoughts, ideas, impulses, and neurotransmitters. Below we have hormones. Between is the realm of neuroendocrinology—the neurosecretory cells which turn emotions into the releasing factors for the pituitary hormones (fig 5.4).

Image courtesy of Gary Bevans; quote from Frank Lynn Meshberger. *Michelangelo, Renaissance Man of the Brain, Too?*

Pituitary tumours

Pituitary tumours (almost always benign adenomas) account for 10% of intracranial tumours (see figs 5.23, 5.24). They may be divided by size: a microadenoma is a tumour <1cm across, and a macroadenoma is >1cm. There are three histological types (table 5.4):

1 *Chromophobe* 70%. Many are non-secretory,[10] some cause hypopituitarism. Half produce prolactin (PRL); a few produce ACTH or GH. Local pressure effect in 30%.
2 *Acidophil* 15%. Secrete GH or PRL. Local pressure effect in 10%.
3 *Basophil* 15%. Secrete ACTH. Local pressure effect rare.

Symptoms are caused by pressure, hormones (eg galactorrhoea), or hypopituitarism (p232). FSH-secreting tumours can cause macro-orchidism in men, but are rare.

Features of local pressure Headache, visual field defects (bilateral temporal hemianopia, due to compression of the optic chiasm), palsy of cranial nerves III, IV, VI (pressure or invasion of the cavernous sinus; fig 5.25). Also, diabetes insipidus (DI) (p240; more likely from hypothalamic disease); disturbance of hypothalamic centres of T°, sleep, and appetite; erosion through floor of sella leading to CSF rhinorrhoea.

Tests MRI defines intra- and supra-sellar extension; accurate assessment of visual fields; screening tests: PRL, IGF-1 (p238), ACTH, cortisol, TFTs, LH/FSH, testosterone in ♂, short Synacthen® test. Glucose tolerance test if acromegaly suspected (p238). If Cushing's suspected, see p225. Water deprivation test if DI is suspected (p240).

Treatment Start hormone replacement as needed (p232). Ensure steroids are given before levothyroxine, as thyroxine may precipitate an adrenal crisis. For Cushing's disease see p225, prolactinoma p236, acromegaly p238.

- *Surgery:* (fig 5.26) Most pituitary surgery is trans-sphenoidal, but if there is supra-sellar extension, a trans-frontal approach may be used. For prolactinoma, 1st-line treatment is medical with a dopamine agonist, p236. *Pre-op:* ensure hydrocortisone 100mg IV/IM. Subsequent cortisol replacement and reassessment varies with local protocols: get advice. *Post-op:* retest pituitary function (p232) to assess replacement needs. Repeating dynamic tests for adrenal function ≥6 weeks post-op.
- *Radiotherapy:* (Eg stereotactic.) Good for residual or recurrent adenomas (good rates of tumour control and normalization of excess hormone secretion).[27]

Post-op Recurrence may occur late after surgery, so life-long follow-up is required. Fertility should be discussed: this may be reduced post-op due to ↓gonadotropins.

Pituitary apoplexy Rapid pituitary enlargement from a bleed into a tumour may cause mass effects, cardiovascular collapse due to acute hypopituitarism, and death. Suspect if acute onset of headache, meningism, ↓GCS, ophthalmoplegia/visual field defect, especially if there is a known tumour (may present like subarachnoid haemorrhage). *℞:* Urgent steroids (hydrocortisone 100mg IV) and meticulous fluid balance ± cabergoline (dopamine agonist, if prolactinoma) ± surgery; find the cause, eg a predisposition to thrombosis, from antiphospholipid syndrome.

Craniopharyngioma Not strictly a pituitary tumour: it originates from Rathke's pouch so is situated between the pituitary and 3rd ventricle floor. They are rare, but are the commonest childhood intracranial tumour. Over 50% present in childhood with growth failure; adults may present with amenorrhoea, ↓libido, hypothalamic symptoms (eg DI, hyperphagia, sleep disturbance) or tumour mass effect. *Tests:* CT/MRI (calcification in 50%, may also be seen on skull x-ray). *Treatment:* Surgery ± post-op radiation; test pituitary function post-op.

Table 5.4 Frequency of hormones secreted by pituitary adenomas based on immunohistochemistry

Hormone	%	Hormone	%
PRL only (→prolactinoma)	35%	ACTH (→Cushing's disease)	7%
GH only (→acromegaly)	20%	LH/FSH/TSH	≥1%*
PRL and GH	7%	No obvious hormone	30%

*Sensitive methods of TSH measurement have improved recognition of TSH-secreting tumours. These are now more frequently found at microadenoma stage, medially located, and *without* associated hormone hypersecretion. In these tumours, somatostatin analogues (p238) are very helpful. See also Socin *et al. Eur J Endocrinol.* 2003;148:433–42.

10 If <1cm, usually 'incidentaloma'; most non-functioning macroadenomas are revealed by mass effect and/or hypopituitarism. Here, recurrence after surgery is common, so follow carefully with MRIs.

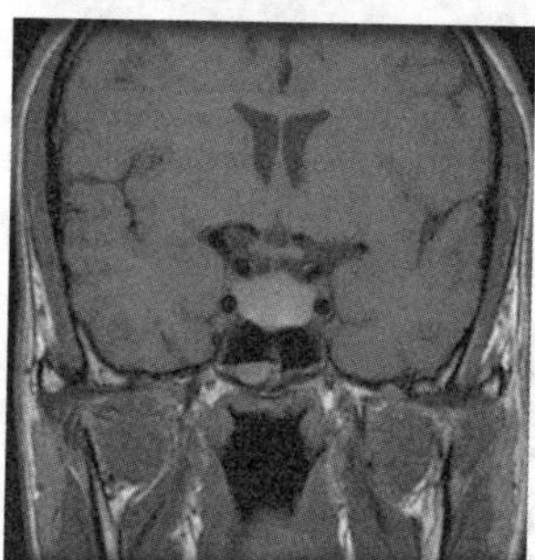

Fig 5.23 Sagittal T1-weighted MRI of the brain (no gadolinium contrast) showing a lesion in the pituitary fossa, most likely a haemorrhagic pituitary adenoma. Differential diagnosis includes a Rathke's cleft cyst.

Courtesy of Norwich Radiology Dept.

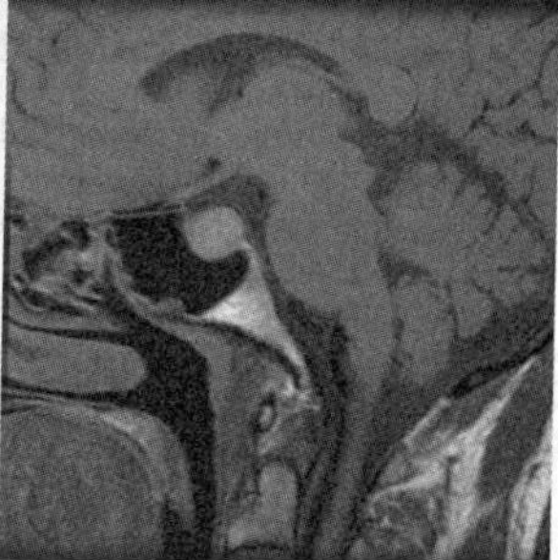

Fig 5.24 Coronal T1-weighted MRI of the brain (no gadolinium contrast) showing a lesion in the pituitary fossa (see fig 5.23).

Courtesy of Norwich Radiology Dept.

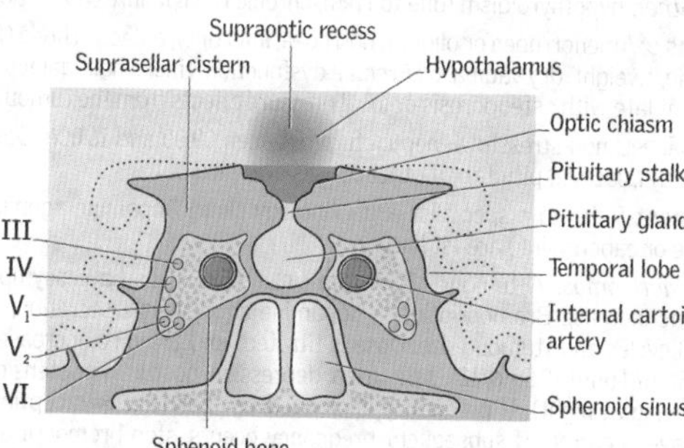

Fig 5.25 The pituitary gland's relationships to cranial nerves III, IV, V, and VI.
Reproduced from Turner and Wass, *Oxford Handbook of Endocrinology and Diabetes*, 2009, with permission from Oxford University Press.

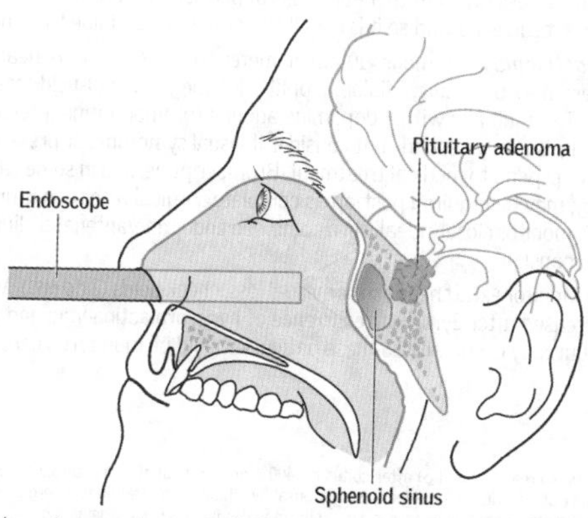

Fig 5.26 Endoscopic surgery is now possible for pituitary surgery.

Hyperprolactinaemia

This is the commonest hormonal disturbance of the pituitary. It presents earlier in women (menstrual disturbance) but later in men (eg with erectile dysfunction and/or mass effects). Prolactin stimulates lactation.[11,12] Raised levels lead to hypogonadism, infertility, and osteoporosis, by inhibiting secretion of gonadotropin-releasing hormone (hence ↓LH/FSH and ↓testosterone or oestrogen).

Causes of raised plasma prolactin (PRL; >390mU/L) PRL is secreted from the anterior pituitary and release is inhibited by dopamine produced in the hypothalamus. Hyperprolactinaemia may result from **1** Excess production from the pituitary, eg prolactinoma. **2** Disinhibition, by compression of the pituitary stalk, reducing local dopamine levels. **3** Use of a dopamine antagonist. A PRL of 1000–5000mU/L may result from any, but >5000 is likely to be due to a prolactinoma, with macroadenomas (>10mm) having the highest levels, eg 10 000–100 000.

- *Physiological:* Pregnancy; breastfeeding; stress. Acute rises occur post-orgasm.[11]
- *Drugs (most common cause):* Metoclopramide; haloperidol; methyldopa; oestrogens; ecstasy/MDMA;[12] antipsychotics (a reason for 'non-compliance': sustained hyperprolactinaemia may cause ↓libido, anorgasmia, and erectile dysfunction).
- *Diseases: Prolactinoma:* micro- or macroadenoma; *Stalk damage:* pituitary adenomas, surgery, trauma; *Hypothalamic disease:* craniopharyngioma, other tumours; *Other:* hypothyroidism (due to ↑TRH), chronic renal failure (↓excretion).

Symptoms ♀: Amenorrhoea or oligomenorrhoea; infertility; galactorrhoea (fig 5.27). Also: ↓libido, ↑weight, dry vagina. ♂: Erectile dysfunction, ↓facial hair, galactorrhoea. May present late with osteoporosis or local pressure effects from the tumour (p234).

Tests Basal PRL: non-stressful venepuncture between 09.00 and 16.00h. Do a pregnancy test, TFT, U&E. MRI pituitary if other causes are ruled out.

Management Refer to a specialist endocrinology clinic. Dopamine agonists (bromocriptine or cabergoline) are 1st line.

Microprolactinomas: A tumour <10mm on MRI (~25% of us have asymptomatic microprolactinomas). Bromocriptine, a dopamine agonist, ↓PRL secretion, restores menstrual cycles and ↓tumour size. Dose is titrated up: 1.25mg PO; increase weekly by 1.25–2.5mg/d until ~2.5mg/12h. SE: nausea, depression, postural hypotension (minimize by giving at night). If pregnancy is planned, use barrier contraception until 2 periods have occurred. If subsequent pregnancy occurs, stop bromocriptine after the 1st missed period. An alternative dopamine agonist is cabergoline: more effective and fewer SE, but there are fewer data on safety in pregnancy. NB: ergot alkaloids (bromocriptine and cabergoline) can cause fibrosis (eg echocardiograms are needed). Trans-sphenoidal surgery may be considered if intolerant of dopamine agonists. It has a high success rate, but there are risks of permanent hormone deficiency and prolactinoma recurrence, and so it is usually reserved as a 2nd-line treatment.

Macroprolactinomas: A tumour >10mm diameter on MRI. As they are near the optic chiasm, there may be ↓acuity, diplopia, ophthalmoplegia, visual-field loss, and optic atrophy. Treat initially with a dopamine agonist (bromocriptine if fertility is the goal). Surgery is rarely needed , but consider if visual symptoms or pressure effects which fail to respond to medical treatment. Bromocriptine, and in some cases radiation therapy, may be required post-op as complete surgical resection is uncommon. If pregnant, monitor closely ideally in a combined endocrine/antenatal clinic as there is ↑risk of expansion.

Follow-up Monitor PRL. If headache or visual loss, check fields (? do MRI). Medication can be decreased after 2yrs, but recurrence of hyperprolactinaemia and expansion of the tumour may occur, and so these patients should be monitored carefully.

11 The prolactin increase (♂ and ♀) after coitus is ~400% greater than after masturbation; post-orgasmic prolactin is part of a feedback loop decreasing arousal by inhibiting central dopaminergic processes. The size of post-orgasmic prolactin increase is a neurohormonal index of sexual satisfaction.

12 MDMA also ↑oxytocin; prolactin + oxytocin are thought to mediate post-orgasmic well-being.

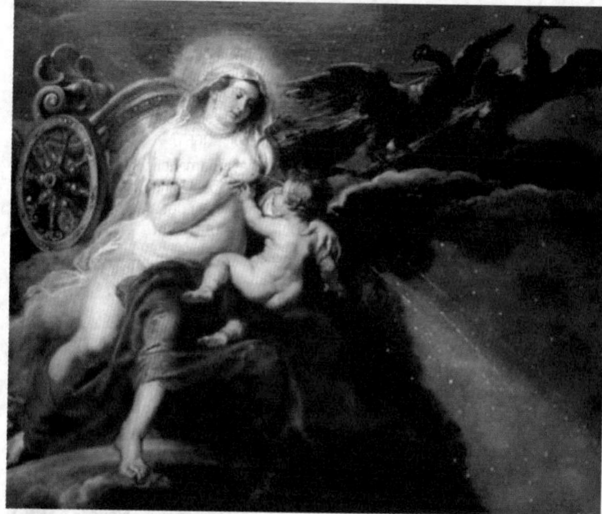

Fig 5.27 Galactorrhoea can be prolific enough to create medium-sized galaxies (bottom right). In the *Birth of the Milky Way* Hera is depicted by Rubens in her chariot, being drawn through the night sky by ominous black peacocks. Between journeys, she enjoyed discussing difficult endocrinological topics with her husband Zeus (who was also her brother), such as whether women or men find sexual intercourse more enjoyable. Hera inclined to the latter—and it is on this flimsy evidence, and her gorgeous galactorrhoea, that we diagnose her hyperprolactinaemia (which is known to decrease desire, lubrication, orgasm, and satisfaction). In the end, this issue was settled, in favour of Zeus's view, by Tiresias, who had unique insight into this intriguing question: every time this soothsayer saw two snakes entwined, (s)he changed sex, so coming to know a thing or two about gender and pleasure. This is a primordial example of an 'N of 1' trial, where the subject is his or her own control. Generalizability can be a problem with this methodology.

Acromegaly

This is due to ↑secretion of GH (growth hormone) from a pituitary tumour (99%) or hyperplasia, eg via ectopic GH-releasing hormone from a carcinoid tumour. ♀:♂≈1:1. Incidence: UK 3/million/yr. ~5% are associated with MEN-1 (p223). GH stimulates bone and soft tissue growth through ↑secretion of insulin-like growth factor-1 (IGF-1).

Symptoms Acroparaesthesia (*akron*=extremities); amenorrhoea; ↓libido; headache; ↑sweating; snoring; arthralgia; backache; fig 5.28: 'My rings don't fit, nor my old shoes, and now I've got a wonky bite (malocclusion) and curly hair. I put on lots of weight, all muscle and looked good for a while; now I look so haggard'.

Signs (BOX 'Signs of acromegaly'.) Often predate diagnosis by >4yrs. If acromegaly occurs before bony epiphyses fuse (rare), gigantism occurs.

Complications (May present with CCF or ketoacidosis.)
- Impaired glucose tolerance (~40%), DM (~15%).
- Vascular: ↑BP, left ventricular hypertrophy (±dilatation/CCF), cardiomyopathy, arrhythmias. There is ↑risk of ischaemic heart disease and stroke (?due to ↑BP ± insulin resistance and GH-induced increase in fibrinogen and decrease in protein S).
- Neoplasia: ↑colon cancer risk; colonoscopy may be needed.[21]

Acromegaly in pregnancy (Subfertility is common.) Pregnancy may be normal; signs and chemistry may remit. Monitor glucose.

Tests ↑Glucose, ↑Ca^{2+}, and ↑PO_4^{3-}. *GH:* Don't rely on random GH as secretion is pulsatile and during peaks acromegalic and normal levels overlap. GH also ↑ in: stress, sleep, puberty, and pregnancy. Normally GH secretion is inhibited by high glucose, and GH hardly detectable. In acromegaly GH release fails to suppress.
- If basal serum GH is >0.4mcg/L (1.2mIU/L) and/or if ↑IGF-I (p232), an oral glucose tolerance test (OGTT) is needed. If the lowest GH value during OGTT is above 1mcg/L (3mIU/L), acromegaly is confirmed. With general use of very sensitive assays, it has been said that this cut-off be decreased to 0.3mcg/L (0.9mIU/L).[28] *Method:* Collect samples for GH glucose at: 0, 30, 60, 90, 120, 150min. Possible false +ves: puberty, pregnancy, hepatic and renal disease, anorexia nervosa, and DM.
- MRI scan of pituitary fossa. • Look for hypopituitarism (p232).
- Visual fields and acuity. • ECG, echo. Old photos if possible.

Treatment Aim to correct (or prevent) tumour compression by excising the lesion, and to reduce GH and IGF-I levels to at least a 'safe' GH level of <2mcg/L (<6mIU/L). A 3-part strategy: **1** Trans-sphenoidal surgery is often 1st line. **2** If surgery fails to correct GH/IGF-I hypersecretion, try somatostatin analogues (SSA) and/or radiotherapy, SSA being generally preferred. Example: octreotide (Sandostatin LAR®, given monthly IM), or lanreotide (Somatuline LA®). SE: pain at the injection site; gastrointestinal: abdominal cramps, flatulence, loose stools, ↑gallstones; impaired glucose tolerance. **3** The GH antagonist pegvisomant (recombinant GH analogue) is used if resistant or intolerant to SSA. It suppresses IGF-1 to normal in 90%, but GH levels may rise; rarely tumour size increases, so monitor closely. *Radiotherapy:* If unsuited to surgery or as adjuvant; may take years to work. *Follow-up:* Yearly GH, IGF-1 ± OGTT; visual fields; vascular assessment. BMI; photos (fig 5.29).

Prognosis May return to normal (any excess mortality is mostly vascular). 16% get diabetes with SSAs vs ~13% after surgery.

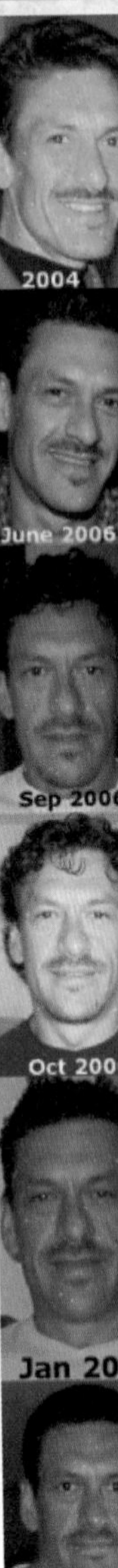

Fig 5.28 Acromegaly. Courtesy of Omar Rio. *My life with acromegaly*. (http://odelrio.blogspot.com)

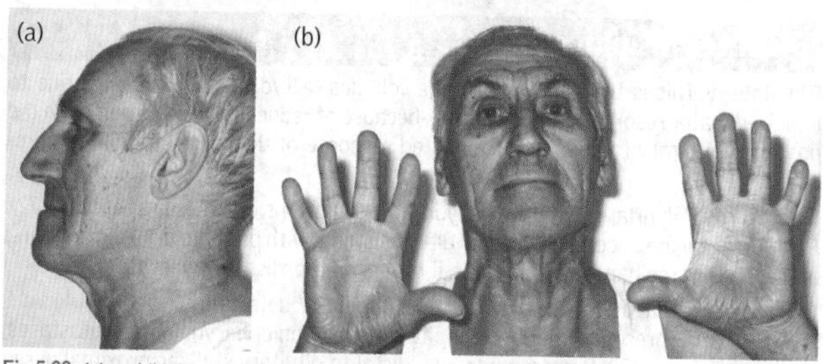

Fig 5.29 (a) and (b) Coarsening of the face and ↑growth of hands and mandible (prognathism).

Signs of acromegaly

- ↑Growth of hands (fig 5.29b; may be spade-like), jaw (fig 5.29a) and feet (sole may encroach on the dorsum).
- Coarsening face; wide nose.
- Big supraorbital ridges.
- Macroglossia (big tongue).
- Widely spaced teeth.
- Puffy lips, eyelids, and skin (oily and large-pored); also skin tags.
- Scalp folds (*cutis verticis gyrata*; due to expanding but tethered skin).
- Skin darkening (fig 5.29).
- Acanthosis nigricans (fig 12.28, p563).
- Laryngeal dyspnoea (fixed cords).
- Obstructive sleep apnoea.
- Goitre (↑thyroid vascularity).
- Proximal weakness + arthropathy.
- Carpal tunnel signs in 50%, p503.
- Signs from any pituitary mass: hypopituitarism ± local mass effect (p232; ↓vision; hemianopia); fits.

Dysmorphia, personal identity, and acromegaly

We might have devoted this box to a grotesque homunculus depicting the signs of acromegaly: all disconnected lips, hands, feet, brows, and noses. But our integrative ethics disallow this, and ask us instead to see if acromegaly can reveal something universal about our patients and ourselves. What is it like to feel in the grip of some 'alien puberty' or 'empty pregnancy'? These analogies are physiological as well as metaphorical.[14,15] The changes of acromegaly are not so insidious that the patient thinks all is fine: there is often partial knowledge and a few dark thoughts on looking into the mirror. Even when we lay our lives end-to-end for inspection (fig 5.28), changes are subtle. It can take the observations of others to force us to come face-to-face with the truth of our new unfolding self. In one patient the comment was 'So are you pregnant again?' 'Why do you ask?' 'Because your nose is as big as it was when you were last pregnant'. So here we have the well-known 'physiological acromegaly of pregnancy'[14] predating the pathological, as the carnival of personal identity moves from helter-skelter to roller-coaster.

14 GH variants made by the placenta rise exponentially until 37wks' gestation; pituitary GH gradually drops to near-undetectable levels. 'Gestational acromegaly' probably develops to foster fetoplacental growth; its side-effects include facial oedema, carpal tunnel symptoms, and nose enlargement.
15 Puberty sees GH- and gonad-mediated rises in bone and muscle mass + other 'acromegalic' effects.

Diabetes insipidus (DI)

Physiology This is the passage of large volumes (>3L/day) of dilute urine due to impaired water resorption by the kidney, because of reduced ADH secretion from the posterior pituitary (cranial DI) or impaired response of the kidney to ADH (nephrogenic DI).

Symptoms Polyuria; polydipsia; dehydration; symptoms of hypernatraemia (p672). *Polydipsia* can be uncontrollable and all-consuming, with patients drinking anything and everything to hand: in such cases, if beer is on tap, disaster will ensue!

Causes of cranial DI •*Idiopathic* (≤50%). •*Congenital:* defects in ADH gene, DIDMOAD.[16] •*Tumour* (may present with DI + hypopituitarism): craniopharyngioma, metastases, pituitary tumour. •*Trauma:* temporary if distal to pituitary stalk as proximal nerve endings grow out to find capillaries in scar tissue and begin direct secretion again. •Hypophysectomy. •Autoimmune hypophysitis (p232). •*Infiltration:* histiocytosis, sarcoidosis.[17] •*Vascular:* haemorrhage.[18] •*Infection:* meningoencephalitis.

Causes of nephrogenic DI •Inherited. •*Metabolic:* low potassium, high calcium. •*Drugs:* lithium, demeclocycline. •Chronic renal disease. •Post-obstructive uropathy.

Tests U&E, Ca^{2+}, glucose (exclude DM), serum and urine osmolalities. Serum osmolality estimate $\approx 2\times(Na^+ + K^+)$ + urea + glucose (all in mmol/L). Normal plasma osmolality is 285–295mOsmol/kg, and urine can be concentrated to more than twice this concentration. Significant DI is excluded if urine to plasma (U:P) osmolality ratio is more than 2:1, provided plasma osmolality is no greater than 295mOsmol/kg. In DI, despite raised plasma osmolality, urine is dilute with a U:P ratio <2. In primary polydipsia there may be dilutional hyponatraemia—and as hyponatraemia may itself cause mania, be cautious of saying 'It's water intoxication from psychogenic polydipsia'.

Diagnosis *Water deprivation test:* See BOX 'The 8-hour water deprivation test'. NB: it is often difficult to differentiate primary polydipsia from partial DI. ΔΔ: DM; diuretics or lithium use; *primary polydipsia* causes symptoms of polydipsia and polyuria with dilute urine. Its cause is poorly understood;[19] it may be associated with schizophrenia or mania (±Li^+ therapy), or, rarely, hypothalamic disease (neurosarcoid; tumour; encephalitis; brain injury; HIV encephalopathy). As part of this syndrome, the kidneys may lose their ability to fully concentrate urine, due to a wash-out of the normal concentrating gradient in the renal medulla.

Treatment *Cranial DI:* MRI (head); test anterior pituitary function (p232). Give desmopressin, a synthetic analogue of ADH (eg Desmomelt® tablets).

Nephrogenic: Treat the cause. If it persists, try bendroflumethiazide 5mg PO/24h. NSAIDs lower urine volume and plasma Na^+ by inhibiting prostaglandin synthase: prostaglandins locally inhibit the action of ADH.

►►Emergency management

- Do urgent plasma U&E, and serum and urine osmolalities. Monitor urine output carefully and check U&E twice a day initially.
- IVI to keep up with urine output. If severe hypernatraemia, do not lower Na^+ rapidly as this may cause cerebral oedema and brain injury. If Na^+ is ≥170, use 0.9% saline initially—this contains 150mmol/L of sodium. Aim to reduce Na^+ at a rate of less than 12mmol/L per day. Use of 0.45% saline can be dangerous.
- Desmopressin 2mcg IM (lasts 12–24h) may be used as a therapeutic trial.

16 DIDMOAD is a rare autosomal recessive disorder: Diabetes Insipidus, Diabetes Mellitus, Optic Atrophy and Deafness (also known as Wolfram's syndrome).
17 Suspect neurosarcoidosis if ↑CSF protein (seen in 34%), facial nerve palsy (25%), CSF pleocytosis (23%), diabetes insipidus (21%), hemiparesis (17%), psychosis (17%), papilloedema (15%), ataxia (13%), seizures (12%), optic atrophy (12%), hearing loss (12%), or nystagmus (9%).
18 Sheehan's syndrome is pituitary infarction from shock, eg postpartum haemorrhage. It is rare.
19 Most of us could drink 20L/d and not be hyponatraemic; some get hyponatraemic drinking 5L/d; they may have Psychosis, Intermittent hyponatraemia, and Polydipsia (PIP syndrome), ?from ↑intravascular volume leading to ↑atrial natriuretic peptide, p137, hence natriuresis and hyponatraemia.

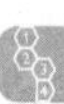

The 8-hour water deprivation test

Tests the ability of kidneys to concentrate urine for diagnosis of DI (dilute urine in spite of dehydration), and then to localize the cause (table 5.5). Do not do the test before establishing that urine volume is >3L/d (output less than this with normal plasma Na^+ and osmolality excludes significant disturbance of water balance).

- Stop test if *urine* osmolality >600mOsmol/kg in Stage 1 (DI is excluded).
- Free fluids until 07.30. Light breakfast at 06.30, no tea, no coffee, no smoking.

Stage 1 Fluid deprivation (0–8h): for diagnosis of DI. Start at 08.00.

- Empty bladder, then no drinks and only dry food.
- Weigh hourly. If >3% weight lost during test, order urgent serum osmolality. If >300mOsmol/kg, proceed to Stage 2. If <300, continue test.
- Collect urine every 2h; measure its volume and osmolality.
- Venous sample for osmolality every 4h.
- Stop test after 8h (16.00) if urine osmolality >600mOsmol/kg (ie normal).

Stage 2 Differentiate cranial from nephrogenic DI.

- Proceed if urine still dilute—ie urine osmolality <600mOsmol/kg.
- Give desmopressin 2mcg IM. Water can be drunk now.
- Measure urine osmolality hourly for the next 4h.

Table 5.5 Interpreting the water deprivation test

Diagnosis	Urine osmolality
Normal	Urine osmolality >600mOsmol/kg in Stage 1 U:P ratio >2 (normal concentrating ability)
Primary polydipsia	Urine concentrates, but less than normal, eg >400–600mOsmol/kg
Cranial DI	Urine osmolality increases to >600mOsmol/kg *after* desmopressin (if equivocal an extended water deprivation test may be tried (no drinking from 18:00 the night before))
Nephrogenic DI	No increase in urine osmolality after desmopressin

Syndrome of inappropriate ADH secretion (SIADH)

In SIADH, ADH continues to be secreted in spite of low plasma osmolality or large plasma volume. Diagnosis requires concentrated urine (Na^+ >20mmol/L and osmolality >100mOsmol/kg) in the presence of hyponatraemia and low plasma osmolality. Causes are numerous. See p673.

6 Gastroenterology

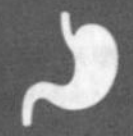

Contents

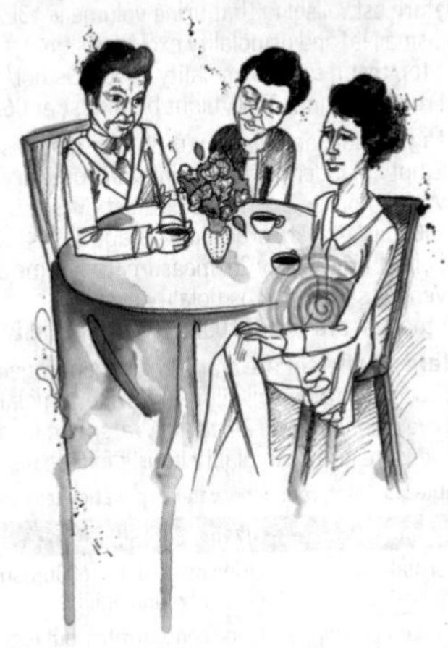

Fig 6.1 Families are rarely what they seem: Otto, Aurelia, and Sylvia seem to be having a nice cup of tea, but Warren (the son and brother) is absent, Otto's leg is missing, Aurelia is beside herself with anxiety, and neither is fully aware of the turmoil spiralling out of control in their unstable daughter, Sylvia. How the gut weaves in and out of our patients' stories is one of gastroenterology's perpetually fascinating and significant riddles. So whenever you are presented with an image in gastroenterology, ask what is missing, and try to work out the forces which are perpetuating or relieving symptoms. This is all very helpful, but it can never be relied on to tame or predict what happens next. So what *did* happen next? See BOX to find out.

We thank Dr Simon Campbell, our Specialist Reader for this chapter.

Lumen

We learn about gastroenterological diseases as if they were separate entities, independent species collected by naturalists, each kept in its own dark matchbox—collectors' items collecting dust in a desiccated world on a library shelf. But this is not how illness works. Otto had diabetes, but refused to see a doctor until it was far advanced, and an amputation was needed. He needed looking after by his wife Aurelia. But she had her children Warren and Sylvia to look after too. And when Otto was no longer the bread-winner, she forced herself to work as a teacher, an accountant, and at any other job she could get. Otto's illness manifested in Aurelia's duodenum—as an ulcer. The gut often bears the brunt of other people's worries. Inside every piece of a gut is a lumen[1]—the world is in the gut, and the gut is in the world. But the light does not always shine. So when the lumen filled with Aurelia's blood, we can expect the illness to impact on the whole family. Her daughter knows where blood comes from ('straight from the heart ... pink fizz'). After Otto died, Sylvia needed long-term psychiatric care, and Aurelia moved to be near her daughter. The bleeding duodenal ulcer got worse when Sylvia needed electroconvulsive therapy. The therapy worked and now, briefly, Sylvia, before her own premature death, is able to look after Aurelia, as she prepares for a gastrectomy.

The story of each illness told separately misses something; but even taken in its social context, this story is missing something vital—the poetry, in most of our patients lived rather than written—tragic, comic, human, and usually obscure—but in the case of this family not so obscure. Welling up, as unstoppable as the bleeding from her mother's ulcer came the poetry of Sylvia Plath.

1 *Lumen* is Latin for light (hence its medical meaning of a tubular cavity open to the world at both ends), as well as being the SI unit of light flux falling on an object—ie the power to illuminate. All doctors have this power, whether by insightfully interpreting patients' lives and illnesses to them, or by acts of kindness—even something so simple as bringing a cup of tea.

Healthy, enjoyable eating

'There's a lot of people in this world who spend so much time watching their health that they haven't the time to enjoy it.' Josh Billings (1818–85).

Updates to guidelines on healthy eating perhaps provide fodder for journalists who have been served a diet both rich and varied in apparently contradictory advice. Nonetheless, for many of our increasingly overweight population, simply eating less (eg 2500 calories/d for men and 2000 for women) and balancing intake across food groups seems a sensible start. Diet is of course not independent of lifestyle, and we should continue to promote a balanced diet in the context of the full range of public health messages. Unravelling these confounding threads in population-level data will always pose a challenge—while some studies show vegetarians may be less likely to die from ischaemic heart disease, is this effect because vegetarians in the UK are more likely to be non-smokers? Overly proscriptive application of such population-level data in advice given to individuals (as journalists may be prone to do) will always be flawed and risks drowning important fundamental concepts in a sea of cynicism.

Current recommendations must take into account three facts
- Obesity costs health services as much as smoking—1 in 4 UK adults is obese.
- Diabetes mellitus is burgeoning: in some places prevalence is >7% (p206).
- Past advice has not changed eating habits in large sections of the population.

Advice is likely to focus on the following

Body mass index: (BMI; table 6.1.) Aim for 18.5–25. Controlling quantity may be more important than quality. In hypertension, eating the 'right' things lowers BP only marginally, but controlling weight causes a more significant reduction.

Base meals on starch: (Bread, rice, potatoes, pasta.) These provide a slower release form of carbohydrate compared to diets containing refined sugar, and beware of the high sugar contents of, eg soft drinks.

Eat enough fruit and vegetables: Aiming for 5 portions a day.

Eat foods high in fat, salt, or sugar infrequently.

Eat some meat, fish, eggs, and beans: Aim for 2 portions of fish a week, including oily fish (those rich in omega-3 fatty acid, such as mackerel, herring, pilchards, salmon). Non-dairy sources of protein include beans and nuts. Aim to reduce intake of red or processed meat to <70g/day.

Eat some milk and dairy products: Select those options with lower fat, sugar and salt where possible.

Moderate alcohol use (adults <65yrs): ≤14U/wk for both men and women, spread over 3 or more days. There is no 'safe' level.

Supplements: There is scant evidence for most nutritional supplements in those able to follow a balanced diet. Women attempting to conceive should take 400mcg/day folic acid from (pre-)conception until at least 12wks. Vitamin D supplements (10mcg/day) may benefit breast-feeding mothers, those ≥65yrs old, those whose skin is not typically exposed to sun, or those with very dark skin. Lower doses may be recommended for infants and young children.

►*This diet is not appropriate for all:* • <5yrs old. • Need for low residue (eg Crohn's, UC, p264) or special diet (coeliac disease, p266). *Emphasis may be different in:* Dyslipidaemia (p690); DM (p206); obesity; constipation (p260); liver failure (p274); chronic pancreatitis (p270); renal failure (less protein)(p304); ↑BP (see p140).

Difficulties It is an imposition to ask us to change our diet (children often refuse point-blank); a more subtle approach is to take a food we enjoy (crisps) and make it healthier (eg low-salt crisps made from jacket potatoes and fried in sunflower oil).

Losing weight—why and how?

The risks of too much sugar Excess sugar causes caries, diabetes, obesity—which itself contributes to osteoarthritis, cancer, hypertension, and increased oxidative stress—so raising cardiovascular mortality and much more.

Losing weight Motivational therapy. Consider referral to a dietician—a needs-specific diet may be best. In conjunction with exercise and diet strategies, targeted weight-loss can also be achieved successfully with psychotherapy.

Drugs or surgery for obesity? The most desirable treatment for obesity is still primary prevention, but pharmacotherapy does work. *Orlistat* lowers fat absorption (hence SE of oily faecal incontinence)—see *OHCS* p514. *Surgery:* Carries potential for significant weight loss in appropriately selected patients but also significant morbidity (see p626).

Calculating body mass index

Table 6.1 BMI=(weight in kg)/(height in m)^2

BMI	State	Some implications within the categories
<18.5	Underweight	Consider pathology (inc. eating disorder)
18.5–25	On target	
25–30	Overweight	Weight loss should be considered
30–40	Obesity	>32 is unsuitable for day-case general surgery
>40	Extreme/morbid obesity	>40 is an indication for bariatric surgery

Caveats: BMI does not take into account the distribution of body fat, and is harder to interpret for children and adolescents. ►*Waist circumference* >94cm in men and >80cm in women reflects omental fat and correlates better with risk than does BMI. BMI is still a valid way of comparing populations: average BMI in the USA is 28.8; in Japan, 22. A nation can be lean without being poor. As nations continue to adopt the lifestyle trends of the USA, this impacts sustainability.

The mouth

The diagnosis will often come out of your patient's mouth, so open it! So many GI investigations are indirect...now is your chance for direct observation.

Leucoplakia (fig 6.2) Is an oral mucosal white patch that will not rub off and is not attributable to any other known disease. It is a premalignant lesion, with a transformation rate, which ranges from 0.6% to 18%. Oral hairy leucoplakia is a shaggy white patch on the side of the tongue seen in HIV, caused by EBV. ►When in doubt, refer all intra-oral white lesions (see BOX).

Aphthous ulcers (fig 6.3) 20% of us get these shallow, painful ulcers on the tongue or oral mucosa that heal without scarring. *Causes of severe ulcers:* Crohn's and coeliac disease; Behçet's (p694); trauma; erythema multiforme; lichen planus; pemphigus; pemphigoid; infections (herpes simplex, syphilis, Vincent's angina, p712). ℞: *Minor ulcers:* avoid oral trauma (eg hard toothbrushes or foods such as toast) and acidic foods or drinks. *Tetracycline* or antimicrobial mouthwashes (eg chlorhexidine) with topical steroids (eg triamcinolone gel) and topical analgesia. *Severe ulcers:* possible therapies include systemic corticosteroids (eg oral *prednisolone* 30-60mg/d PO for a week) or thalidomide (absolutely contraindicated in pregnancy).►Biopsy any ulcer not healing after 3 weeks to exclude malignancy; refer to an oral surgeon if uncertain.

Candidiasis (thrush) (fig 6.4) Causes white patches or erythema of the buccal mucosa. Patches may be hard to remove and bleed if scraped. *Risk factors:* Extremes of age; DM; antibiotics; immunosuppression (long-term corticosteroids, including inhalers; cytotoxics; malignancy; HIV). ℞: *Nystatin* suspension 400000U (4mL swill and swallow/6h). *Fluconazole* for oropharyngeal thrush.

Cheilitis (angular stomatitis) Fissuring of the mouth's corners is caused by denture problems, candidiasis, or deficiency of iron or riboflavin (vitamin B_2). (fig 8.5, p327.)

Gingivitis Gum inflammation ± hypertrophy occurs with poor oral hygiene, drugs (phenytoin, ciclosporin, nifedipine), pregnancy, vitamin C deficiency (scurvy, p268), acute myeloid leukaemia (p356), or Vincent's angina (p712).

Microstomia (fig 6.5) The mouth is too small, eg from thickening and tightening of the perioral skin after burns or in epidermolysis bullosa (destructive skin and mucous membrane blisters ± ankyloglossia) or systemic sclerosis (p552).

Oral pigmentation Perioral brown spots characterize Peutz-Jeghers' (p708). Pigmentation anywhere in the mouth suggests Addison's disease (p226) or drugs (eg antimalarials). Consider malignant melanoma. *Telangiectasia:* Systemic sclerosis; Osler-Weber-Rendu syndrome (p708). *Fordyce glands:* (Creamy yellow spots at the border of the oral mucosa and the lip vermilion.) Sebaceous cysts, common and benign. *Aspergillus niger* colonization may cause a black tongue.

Teeth (fig 6.6) A blue line at the gum-tooth margin suggests lead poisoning. Prenatal or childhood tetracycline exposure causes a yellow-brown discolouration.

Tongue This may be furred or dry (xerostomia) in dehydration, drug therapy,[3] after radiotherapy, in Crohn's disease, Sjögren's (p710), and Mikulicz's syndrome (p706).

Glossitis: Means a smooth, red, sore tongue, eg caused by iron, folate, or B_{12} deficiency (fig 8.27, p335). If local loss of papillae leads to ulcer-like lesions that change in colour and size, use the term *geographic tongue* (harmless migratory glossitis).

Macroglossia: The tongue is too big. Causes: myxoedema; acromegaly; amyloid (p370). A *ranula* is a bluish salivary retention cyst to one side of the frenulum, named after the bulging vocal pouch of frogs' throats (genus *Rana*).

Tongue cancer: Appears as a raised ulcer with firm edges. Risk factors: smoking, alcohol.[4] Spread: anterior ⅓ of tongue drains to submental nodes; middle ⅓ to submandibular nodes; posterior ⅓ to deep cervical nodes (see BOX, p599). *Treatment:* Radiotherapy or surgery. 5yr survival (early disease): 80%. ►When in doubt, refer.

3 Drugs causing xerostomia: ACE-i; antidepressants; antihistamines; antipsychotics; antimuscarinics/anticholinergics; bromocriptine; diuretics; loperamide; nifedipine; opiates; prazosin; prochlorperazine, etc.
4 Betel nut (*Areca catechu*) chewing, common in South Asia, may be an independent risk factor.

White intra-oral lesions

- Idiopathic keratosis
- Leucoplakia
- Lichen planus
- Poor dental hygiene
- Candidiasis
- Squamous papilloma
- Carcinoma
- Hairy oral leucoplakia
- Lupus erythematosus
- Smoking
- Aphthous stomatitis
- Secondary syphilis.

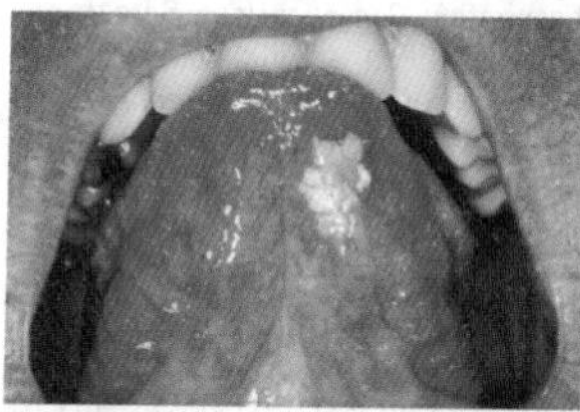

Fig 6.2 Leucoplakia on the underside of the tongue. It is important to refer leucoplakia because it is premalignant.

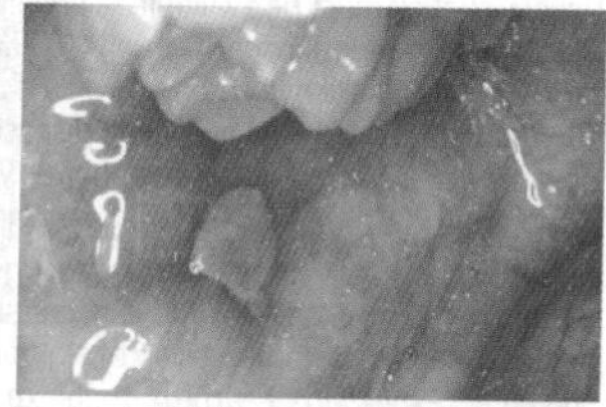

Fig 6.3 An aphthous ulcer inside the cheek. The name is tautological: *aphtha* in Greek means ulceration.

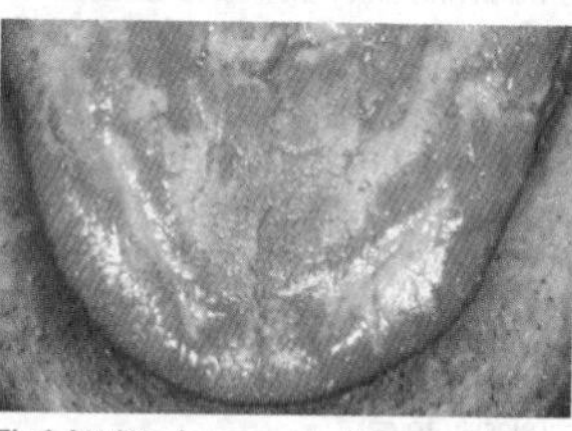

Fig 6.4 White fur on an erythematous tongue caused by oral candidiasis. Oropharyngeal candidiasis in an apparently fit patient may suggest underlying HIV infection.

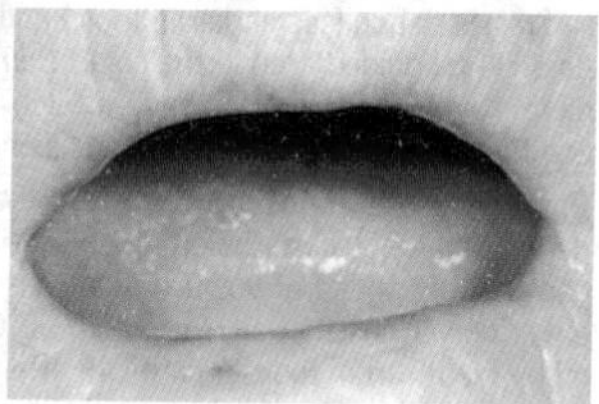

Fig 6.5 Microstomia (small, narrow mouth), eg from hardening of the skin in scleroderma which narrows the mouth. It is cosmetically and functionally disabling.[1]

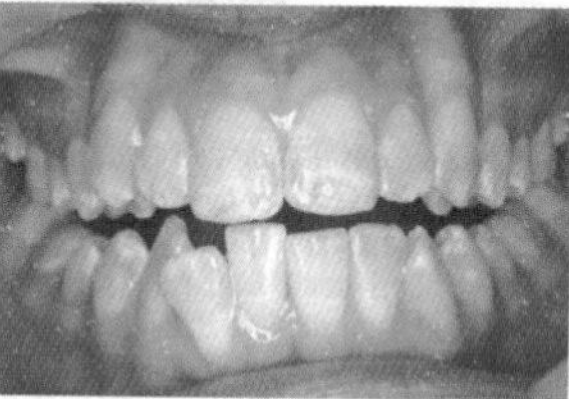

Fig 6.6 White bands on the teeth can be caused by excessive fluoride intake.

Endoscopy and biopsy

►Consent is needed for all these procedures; see p568.

Upper GI endoscopy *Indications:* See table 6.2. *Pre-procedure:* Stop PPIs 2wks pre-op if possible (∵ pathology-masking). Nil by mouth for 6h before. Don't drive for 24h if sedation is used. *Procedure:* Sedation optional, eg midazolam 1-5mg slowly IV (to remain conscious; if deeper sedation is needed, propofol via an anaesthetist (narrow therapeutic range)); nasal prong O_2 (eg 2L/min; monitor respirations & oximetry). The pharynx may be sprayed with local anaesthetic before the endoscope is passed. Continuous suction must be available to prevent aspiration. *Complications:* Sore throat; amnesia from sedation; perforation (<0.1%); bleeding (if on aspirin, clopidogrel, warfarin, or DOACs these need stopping only if therapeutic procedure). *Duodenal biopsy:* The gold standard test for coeliac disease (p266); also useful in unusual causes of malabsorption, eg giardiasis, lymphoma, Whipple's disease.

Sigmoidoscopy Views the rectum + distal colon (to ~splenic flexure). Flexible sigmoidoscopy has largely displaced rigid sigmoidoscopy for diagnosis of distal colonic pathology, but ~25% of cancers are still out of reach. It can be used therapeutically, eg for decompression of sigmoid volvulus (p611). *Preparation:* Phosphate enema PR. *Procedure:* Learn from an expert; do PR exam first. Do biopsies—macroscopic appearances may be normal, eg IBD, amyloidosis, microscopic colitis.

Colonoscopy *Indications:* See table 6.3. *Preparation:* Stop iron 1wk prior; discuss with local endoscopy unit bowel preparation and diet required. *Procedure:* Do PR first. Sedation (see earlier in topic) and analgesia are given before colonoscope is passed and guided around the colon. *Complications:* Abdominal discomfort; incomplete examination; haemorrhage after biopsy or polypectomy; perforation (<0.1%). See figs 6.7–6.11. Post-procedure: no alcohol, and no operating machinery for 24h.

Video capsule endoscopy (VCE) To evaluate obscure GI bleeding (p326) and to detect small bowel pathology. Use small bowel imaging (eg contrast) or patency capsule test ahead of VCE if patient has abdominal pain or symptoms suggesting small bowel obstruction. *Preparation:* Clear fluids only the evening before then nil by mouth from morning until 4h after capsule swallowed. *Procedure:* Capsule is swallowed (fig 6.12)—this transmits video wirelessly to capture device worn by patient. Normal activity can take place for the day. *Complications:* Capsule retention in 1% (endoscopic or surgical removal is needed)—avoid MRI for 2 wks after unless AXR confirms capsule has cleared; obstruction, incomplete exam (eg slow transit, achalasia). *Problems:* No therapeutic options; poor localization of lesions; may miss more subtle lesions.

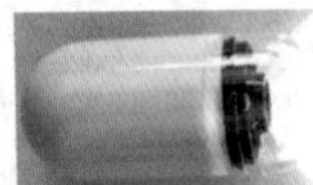

Fig 6.12 PillCam®.

Liver biopsy *Route: Percutaneous* if INR in range else *transjugular* with FFP. *Indications:* ↑LFT of unknown aetiology; assessment of fibrosis in chronic liver disease (this indication being replaced by ultrasound-based elastography); suspected cirrhosis or suspected hepatic lesions/cancer. *Pre-op:* Nil by mouth for 8h. Are INR <1.5 and platelets $>50\times10^9$/L? Give analgesia. *Procedure:* Sedation may be given. Do under US/CT guidance; the liver borders are percussed and where there is dullness in the mid-axillary line in expiration, lidocaine 2% is infiltrated down to the liver capsule. Breathing is rehearsed and a needle biopsy is taken with the breath held in expiration. Afterwards lie on the right side for 2h, then in bed for 4h; check pulse and BP every 15 mins for 1h, every 30 mins for 2h, then hourly until discharge 4h post-biopsy. *Complications:* Local pain; pneumothorax; bleeding (<0.5%); death (<0.1%).

Table 6.2 Indications for upper GI endoscopy

Diagnostic indications	Therapeutic indications
Haematemesis/melaena	Treatment of bleeding lesions
Dysphagia	Variceal banding and sclerotherapy
Dyspepsia (≥55yrs old + alarm symptoms or treatment refractory, p252)	Argon plasma coagulation for suspected vascular abnormality
Duodenal biopsy (?coeliac)	Stent insertion, laser therapy
Persistent vomiting	Stricture dilatation, polyp resection
Iron deficiency (cancer)	

Table 6.3 Indications for colonoscopy

Diagnostic indications	Therapeutic indications
Rectal bleeding—when settled, if acute	Haemostasis (eg by clipping vessel)
Iron-deficiency anaemia (bleeding cancer)	Bleeding angiodysplasia lesion (argon beamer photocoagulation)
Persistent diarrhoea	
Positive faecal occult blood test	Colonic stent deployment (cancer)
Assessment or suspicion of IBD	Volvulus decompression (flexi sig)
Colon cancer surveillance	Pseudo-obstruction Polypectomy

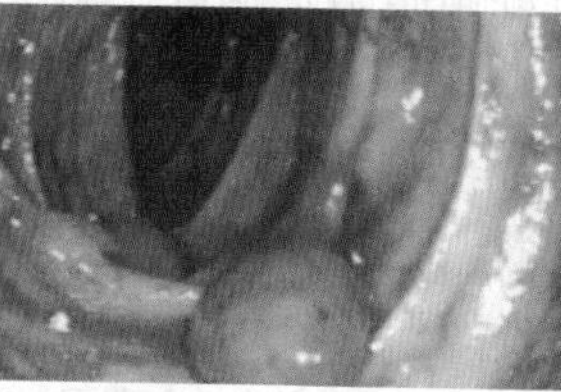

Fig 6.7 A big polyp seen on colonoscopy. An advantage of colonoscopy over barium enema is the ability to biopsy or intervene at the same time—in this case, polypectomy.

Image courtesy of Dr Anthony Mee.

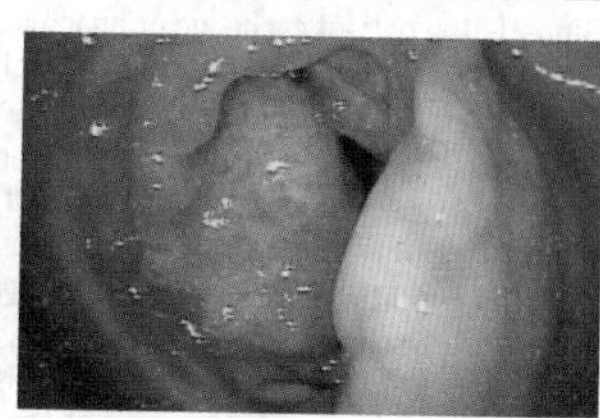

Fig 6.8 Colonoscopic image of an adenocarcinoma—p616. Compared with a colonic polyp (fig 6.7), the carcinoma is irregular in shape and colour, larger and more aggressive.

Image courtesy of Dr J Simmons.

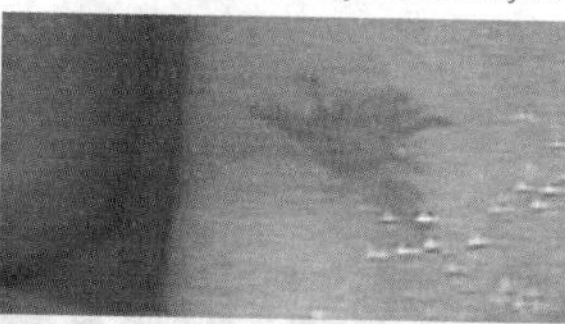

Fig 6.9 Angiodysplasia lesion seen at colonoscopy. Bleeding may be brisk. ℞: endoscopic obliteration. It is associated with aortic stenosis (Heyde's syndrome).[2]

Image courtesy of Dr Anthony Mee.

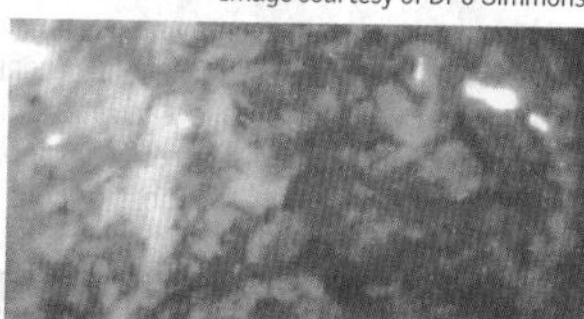

Fig 6.10 Colonic mucosa in active UC (p262); it is red, inflamed, and friable (bleeds on touching). Signs of severity: mucopurulent exudate, mucosal ulceration ± spontaneous bleeding. If quiescent, there may only be a distorted or absent mucosal vascular pattern.

Image courtesy of Dr J Simmons.

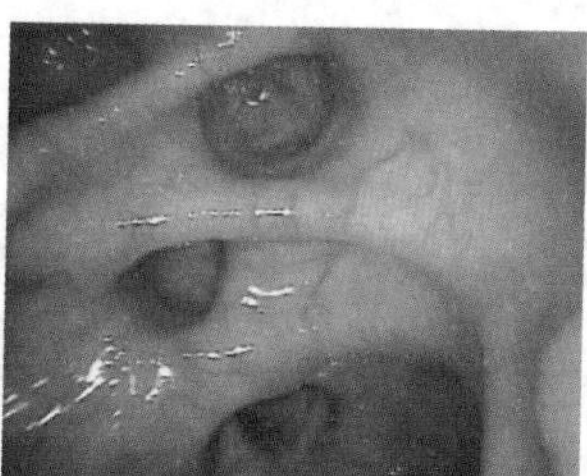

Fig 6.11 Colonoscopic image showing diverticulosis (p628). Navigating safely through the colon, avoiding the false lumina of the diverticula, can be a challenge. Don't go there if diverticula are inflamed (diverticulitis): perforation is a big risk. *Other CI to colonoscoy:* MI in last month; ischaemic colitis (*Oxford Handbook of Gastroenterology and Hepatology*, Second Edition (Bloom *et al.*), p165).

Image courtesy of Dr J Simmons.

Dysphagia

Dysphagia is difficulty in swallowing and should prompt urgent investigation to exclude malignancy (unless of short duration, and associated with a sore throat).

Causes Oral, pharyngeal, or oesophageal? Mechanical or motility related? (See BOX 'Causes of dysphagia'.)

Five key questions to ask

1 Was there difficulty swallowing solids *and* liquids from the start?
Yes: motility disorder (eg achalasia, CNS, or pharyngeal causes).
No: Solids *then* liquids: suspect a stricture (benign or malignant).

2 Is it difficult to initiate a swallowing movement?
Yes: Suspect bulbar palsy, especially if patient coughs on swallowing.

3 Is swallowing painful (odynophagia)?
Yes: Suspect ulceration (malignancy, oesophagitis, viral infection or *Candida* in immunocompromised, or poor steroid inhaler technique) or spasm.

4 Is the dysphagia intermittent or is it constant and getting worse?
Intermittent: suspect oesophageal spasm.
Constant and worsening: suspect malignant stricture.

5 Does the neck bulge or gurgle on drinking?
Yes: Suspect a pharyngeal pouch (see *OHCS* p570).

Signs Is the patient cachectic or anaemic? Examine the mouth; feel for supraclavicular nodes (left supraclavicular node = Virchow's node—suggests intra-abdominal malignancy); look for signs of systemic disease, eg systemic sclerosis (p552), CNS disease.

Tests FBC (anaemia); U&E (dehydration). Upper GI endoscopy ± biopsy (fig 6.13). If suspicion of pharyngeal pouch consider contrast swallow (± ENT opinion). Video fluoroscopy may help identify neurogenic causes. Oesophageal manometry for dysmotility.

Specific conditions *Oesophagitis:* See p254. *Diffuse oesophageal spasm:* Causes intermittent dysphagia ± chest pain. Contrast swallow/manometry: abnormal contractions.[5] *Achalasia:* Coordinated peristalsis is lost and the lower oesophageal sphincter fails to relax (due to degeneration of the myenteric plexus), causing dysphagia, regurgitation, and ↓weight. Characteristic findings on manometry or contrast swallow showing dilated tapering oesophagus. Treatment: endoscopic balloon dilatation, or Heller's cardiomyotomy—then proton pump inhibitors (PPIs, p254). Botulinum toxin injection if a non-invasive procedure is needed (repeat every few months). Calcium channel blockers and nitrates may also relax the sphincter. *Benign oesophageal stricture:* Caused by gastro-oesophageal reflux (GORD, p254), corrosives, surgery, or radiotherapy. Treatment: endoscopic balloon dilatation. *Oesophageal cancer:* (p618.) Associations: ♂, GORD, tobacco, alcohol, Barrett's oesophagus (p695), tylosis (palmar hyperkeratosis), Plummer-Vinson syndrome (post-cricoid dysphagia, upper oesophageal web + iron-deficiency). *CNS causes:* Ask for help from a speech and language therapist.

Nausea and vomiting

Consider pregnancy where appropriate! Other causes, p56.

What's in the vomit? Reports of 'coffee grounds' *may* indicate upper GI bleeding but represent one of the most over-called signs in clinical medicine — always verify yourself and look for other evidence of GI bleeding; recognizable food ≈ gastric stasis; feculent ≈ small bowel obstruction.

Timing Morning ≈ pregnancy or ↑ICP; 1h post food ≈ gastric stasis/gastroparesis (DM); vomiting that relieves pain ≈ peptic ulcer; preceded by loud gurgling ≈ GI obstruction.

Tests *Bloods:* FBC, U&E, LFT, Ca^{2+}, glucose, amylase. *ABG:* A metabolic (hypochloraemic) alkalosis from loss of gastric contents (pH >7.45, ↑HCO_3^-) indicates severe vomiting. *Plain AXR:* If suspected bowel obstruction (p728). *Upper GI endoscopy:* (See p248.) If suspicion of bleed or persistent vomiting. Consider head CT in case ↑ICP.

Treatment Identify and *treat underlying causes*. Symptomatic relief: table 6.4. Be pre-emptive, eg pre-op for post-op symptoms. Try oral route first. 30% need a 2nd-line anti-emetic, so be prepared to prescribe more than one. Give IV fluids with K^+ replacement if severely dehydrated or nil-by-mouth, and monitor electrolytes and fluid balance.

Causes of dysphagia

Mechanical block

Malignant stricture (fig 6.13)
- Pharyngeal cancer
- Oesophageal cancer
- Gastric cancer

Benign strictures
- Oesophageal web or ring (p250)
- Peptic stricture

Extrinsic pressure
- Lung cancer
- Mediastinal lymph nodes
- Retrosternal goitre
- Aortic aneurysm
- Left atrial enlargement

Pharyngeal pouch

Motility disorders

Achalasia (see p250)
Diffuse oesophageal spasm
Systemic sclerosis (p552)
Neurological bulbar palsy (p507)
- Pseudobulbar palsy (p507)
- Wilson's or Parkinson's disease
- Syringobulbia (p516)
- Bulbar poliomyelitis (p436)
- Chagas' disease (p423)
- Myasthenia gravis (p512)

Others

Oesophagitis (p254; reflux or *Candida*/HSV)
Globus (='I've got a lump in my throat': try to distinguish from true dysphagia)

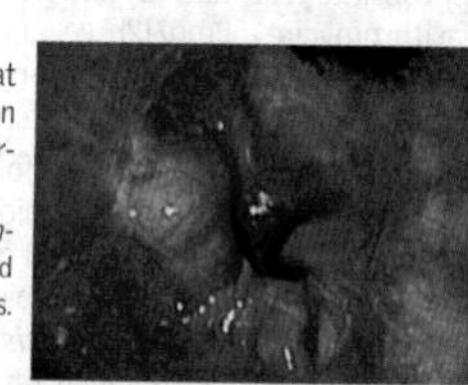

Fig 6.13 A malignant lower oesophageal stricture seen at endoscopy. Note the asymmetry and heaped edges. Benign strictures have a smoother appearance and tend to be circumferential.

Reproduced from Bloom *et al.*, *Oxford Handbook of Gastroenterology and Hepatology*, 2012, with permission from Oxford University Press.

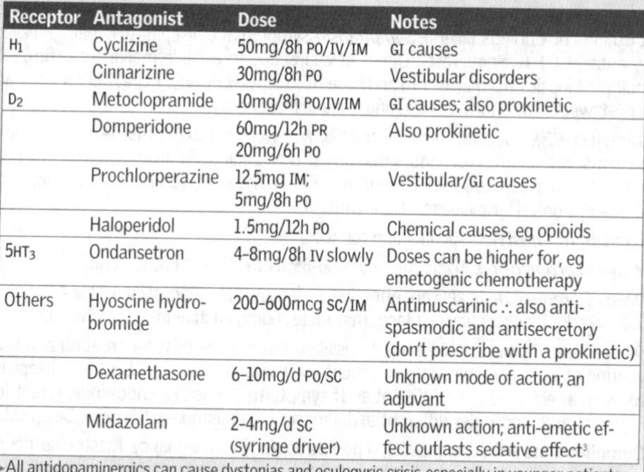

Remembering your anti-emetics

One way of recalling anti-emetics involves using (simplified) pharmacology.

Table 6.4 Pharmacology of common anti-emetics

Receptor	Antagonist	Dose	Notes
H_1	Cyclizine	50mg/8h PO/IV/IM	GI causes
	Cinnarizine	30mg/8h PO	Vestibular disorders
D_2	Metoclopramide	10mg/8h PO/IV/IM	GI causes; also prokinetic
	Domperidone	60mg/12h PR 20mg/6h PO	Also prokinetic
	Prochlorperazine	12.5mg IM; 5mg/8h PO	Vestibular/GI causes
	Haloperidol	1.5mg/12h PO	Chemical causes, eg opioids
$5HT_3$	Ondansetron	4–8mg/8h IV slowly	Doses can be higher for, eg emetogenic chemotherapy
Others	Hyoscine hydrobromide	200–600mcg SC/IM	Antimuscarinic ∴ also antispasmodic and antisecretory (don't prescribe with a prokinetic)
	Dexamethasone	6–10mg/d PO/SC	Unknown mode of action; an adjuvant
	Midazolam	2–4mg/d SC (syringe driver)	Unknown action; anti-emetic effect outlasts sedative effect[3]

►All antidopaminergics can cause dystonias and oculogyric crisis, especially in younger patients.

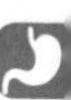

5 Non-propulsive contractions manifest as tertiary contractions or 'corkscrew oesophagus' (fig 16.34, p743) and suggest a motility disorder and may lead to ↓acid clearance. Symptoms and radiology may not match. Nutcracker oesophagus denotes distal peristaltic contractions >180mmHg. It may cause pain, relieved by nitrates or sublingual nifedipine.

Dyspepsia and peptic ulcer disease

War The stomach is a battle ground between the forces of attack (acid, pepsin, *Helicobacter pylori*, bile salts) and defence (mucin secretion, cellular mucus, bicarbonate secretion, mucosal blood flow, cell turnover). Gastric antisecretory agents, eg H_2receptor antagonists (H2RAs), and proton pump inhibitors (PPIs) may only work if you have optimized cytoprotection (antacids and sucralfate work this way). Success may depend on you being not just a brilliant general, but also a tactician, politician, and diplomat. Plan your strategy carefully[4] (fig 6.14). As in any war, neglecting psychological factors can prove disastrous. The aim is not outright victory but *maintaining the balance of power* so all may prosper.

Symptoms Epigastric pain often related to hunger, specific foods, or time of day, fullness after meals, heartburn (retrosternal pain); tender epigastrium. Beware **Alarm** symptoms: **A**naemia (iron deficiency); **l**oss of weight; **a**norexia; **r**ecent onset/progressive symptoms; **m**elaena/haematemesis; **s**wallowing difficulty.

H. pylori (See table 6.5.) *If ≲55yrs old:* 'Test and treat' for *H. pylori*;[6] if +ve give appropriate PPI and 2 antibiotic combination, eg lansoprazole 30mg/12h PO, clarithromycin 250mg/12h PO, and amoxicillin 1g/12h PO for 1wk. If −ve give acid suppression alone. ►Refer for urgent endoscopy (p248) *all* with dysphagia, as well as those ≳55 with *alarm symptoms* or with treatment-refractory dyspepsia.

Duodenal ulcer (DU, fig 6.15.) 4-fold commoner than GU. *Major risk factors: H. pylori* (90%); drugs (NSAIDs; steroids; SSRI). *Minor:* ↑Gastric acid secretion; ↑gastric emptying (↓duodenal pH); blood group O; smoking.
Symptoms: Asymptomatic or epigastric pain (relieved by antacids) ± ↓weight. *Signs:* Epigastric tenderness. *Diagnosis:* Upper GI endoscopy. Test for *H. pylori*. Measure gastrin concentrations when off PPIs if Zollinger-Ellison syndrome (p716) is suspected. *ΔΔ:* Non-ulcer dyspepsia; duodenal Crohn's; TB; lymphoma; pancreatic cancer (p270). *Follow-up:* None; if good response to ℞ (eg PPI).

Gastric ulcers (GU.) Occur mainly in the elderly, on the lesser curve. Ulcers elsewhere are more often malignant. *Risk factors: H. pylori* (~80%); smoking; NSAIDs; reflux of duodenal contents; delayed gastric emptying; stress, eg neurosurgery or burns (Cushing's or Curling's ulcers). *Symptoms:* Asymptomatic or epigastric pain (relieved by antacids) ± ↓weight. *Tests:* Upper GI endoscopy to exclude malignancy (fig 6.14); multiple biopsies from ulcer rim and base (histology, *H. pylori*). Repeat endoscopy after 6–8 weeks to confirm healing and exclude malignancy.

Gastritis *Risk factors:* Alcohol, NSAIDS, *H. pylori*, reflux/hiatus hernia, atrophic gastritis, granulomas (Crohn's; sarcoidosis), CMV, Zollinger-Ellison syndrome & Ménétrier's disease (p716 & 706). *Symptoms:* Epigastric pain, vomiting; *Tests:* Upper GI endoscopy only if suspicious features (fig 6.14).

Treatment *Lifestyle:* ↓Alcohol and tobacco.

H. pylori eradication: Triple therapy is 80–85% effective at eradication.[7]

Drugs to reduce acid: PPIs are effective, eg lansoprazole 30mg/24h PO for 4 (DU) or 8 (GU) wks. H_2 blockers have a place (ranitidine 300mg each night PO for 8wks).

Drug-induced ulcers: Stop drug if possible. PPIs may be best for treating and preventing GI ulcers and bleeding in patients on NSAID or antiplatelet drugs. Misoprostol is an alternative with different SE. If symptoms persist, re-endoscope, retest for *H. pylori*, and reconsider differential diagnoses (eg gallstones). *Surgery:* See p622.

Complications ►►Bleeding (p256), ►►perforation (p606), malignancy, ↓gastric outflow.

Functional (non-ulcer) dyspepsia Common. *H. pylori* eradication (only after a +ve result) *may* help. Some evidence favours PPIs and psychotherapy. Low-dose amitriptyline (10–20mg each night PO) may help. Antacids, antispasmodics, H_2 blockers, misoprostol, prokinetic agents, bismuth, or sucralfate all have less evidence.

6 *H. pylori* is the commonest bacterial pathogen found worldwide (>50% of the world population over 40yrs has it). It's a class I carcinogen causing gastritis (p252), duodenal/gastric ulcers & gastric cancer/lymphoma (MALT, p362), also associated with coronary artery disease, B_{12} and iron deficiency.
7 1 week of therapy sufficient; 2 weeks increases erradication rates by ~5% but also increases SE. For resistant infections switch to a 2nd-line antibiotic combination (see *BNF*).

Table 6.5 Tests (other than serology) should be performed after >2 wks off ppi

		Sensitivity	Specificity
Invasive tests	CLO test	95%	95%
	Histology	95%	95%
	Culture	90%	100%
Non-invasive	^{13}C breath test*	95%	95%
	Stool antigen	95%	94%
	Serology	92%	83%

* The ^{13}C breath test is the most accurate non-invasive *Helicobacter* test.

Differential diagnosis of dyspepsia

- Non-ulcer dyspepsia
- Duodenal/gastric ulcer
- Duodenitis
- Oesophagitis/GORD
- Gastric malignancy
- Gastritis (p257)

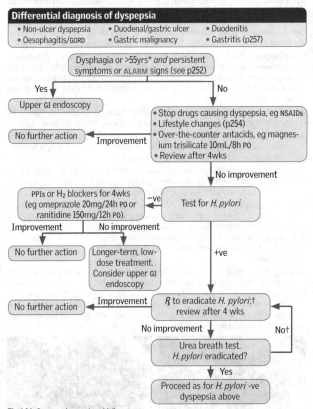

Dysphagia or >55yrs* *and* persistent symptoms or ALARM signs (see p252)

- Yes → Upper GI endoscopy
- No →
  - Stop drugs causing dyspepsia, eg NSAIDs
  - Lifestyle changes (p254)
  - Over-the-counter antacids, eg magnesium trisilicate 10mL/8h PO
  - Review after 4wks
  - Improvement → No further action
  - No improvement → Test for *H. pylori*

Test for *H. pylori*:

- −ve → PPIs or H_2 blockers for 4wks (eg omeprazole 20mg/24h PO or ranitidine 150mg/12h PO).
  - Improvement → No further action
  - No improvement → Longer-term, low-dose treatment. Consider upper GI endoscopy
- +ve → ℞ to eradicate *H. pylori*;† review after 4 wks
  - Improvement → No further action
  - No improvement → Urea breath test. *H. pylori* eradicated?
    - No† → ℞ to eradicate *H. pylori*;† review after 4 wks
    - Yes → Proceed as for *H. pylori* -ve dyspepsia above

Fig 6.14 See NICE dyspepsia guidelines.[4]
*Nothing magical happens on the 55th birthday—this is simply an inflection point in population risk data. We should not be overly rigid in applying these rules to the patient in front of us—though those who hold the purse strings may at time seek to reduce costs by strict enforcement of such guidelines.
†Don't treat +ve cases of *H. pylori* more than twice. If still +ve refer for specialist opinion.

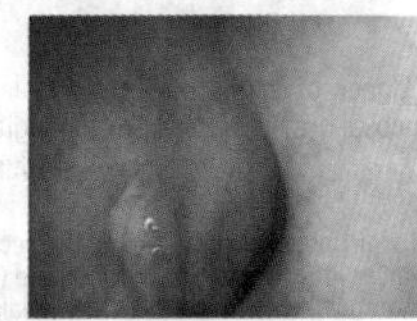

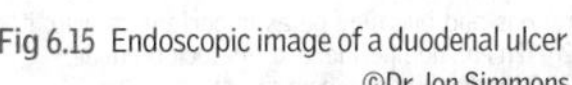

Fig 6.15 Endoscopic image of a duodenal ulcer
©Dr Jon Simmons.

Gastro-oesophageal reflux disease (GORD)

GORD is common, and caused by reflux of stomach contents (acid ± bile)[8] causing troublesome symptoms and/or complications. If reflux is prolonged, it may cause oesophagitis (fig 6.16), benign oesophageal stricture, or Barrett's oesophagus (fig 6.17 and p695; it is pre-malignant). **Causes** Lower oesophageal sphincter hypotension, hiatus hernia (see BOX), oesophageal dysmotility (eg systemic sclerosis), obesity, gastric acid hypersecretion, delayed gastric emptying, smoking, alcohol, pregnancy, drugs (tricyclics, anticholinergics, nitrates), *Helicobacter pylori*?[9]

Symptoms *Oesophageal:* Heartburn (burning, retrosternal discomfort after meals, lying, stooping, or straining, relieved by antacids); belching; acid brash (acid or bile regurgitation); waterbrash (↑↑salivation: 'My mouth fills with saliva'); odynophagia (painful swallowing, eg from oesophagitis or ulceration). *Extra-oesophageal:* Nocturnal asthma, chronic cough, laryngitis (hoarseness, throat clearing), sinusitis.

Complications Oesophagitis, ulcers, benign stricture, iron-deficiency. *Metaplasia →dysplasia→neoplasia:* GORD may lead to Barrett's oesophagus (p695; distal oesophageal epithelium undergoes metaplasia from squamous to columnar, fig 6.17). 0.1–0.4%/yr of those with Barrett's progress to oesophageal cancer (higher if dysplasia is present).

ΔΔ Oesophagitis from corrosives, NSAIDs, herpes, *Candida*; duodenal or gastric ulcers or cancers; non-ulcer dyspepsia; oesophageal spasm; cardiac disease.

Tests Endoscopy if dysphagia, or if ≥55yrs old with *alarm symptoms* (p252) or with treatment-refractory dyspepsia. 24h oesophageal pH monitoring ± manometry help diagnose GORD when endoscopy is normal.

Treatment *Lifestyle:* Weight loss; smoking cessation; small, regular meals; reduce hot drinks, alcohol, citrus fruits, tomatoes, onions, fizzy drinks, spicy foods, caffeine, chocolate; avoid eating <3h before bed. Raise the bed head.

Drugs: Antacids, eg magnesium trisilicate mixture (10mL/8h), or alginates, eg Gaviscon® (10–20mL/8h PO) relieve symptoms. Add a PPI, eg lansoprazole 30mg/24h PO. For refractory symptoms, add an H_2 blocker and/or try twice-daily PPI. Avoid drugs affecting oesophageal motility (nitrates, anticholinergics, Ca^{2+} channel blockers—relax the lower oesophageal sphincter) or that damage mucosa (NSAIDs, K^+ salts, bisphosphonates).

Surgery: (Eg laparoscopic Nissen fundoplication, or novel options including laparoscopic insertion of a magnetic bead band or radiofrequency-induced hypertrophy.) These all aim to ↑resting lower oesophageal sphincter pressure. Consider in severe GORD (confirm by pH-monitoring/manometry) if drugs are not working. Atypical symptoms (cough, laryngitis) are less likely to improve with surgery compared to patients with typical symptoms.

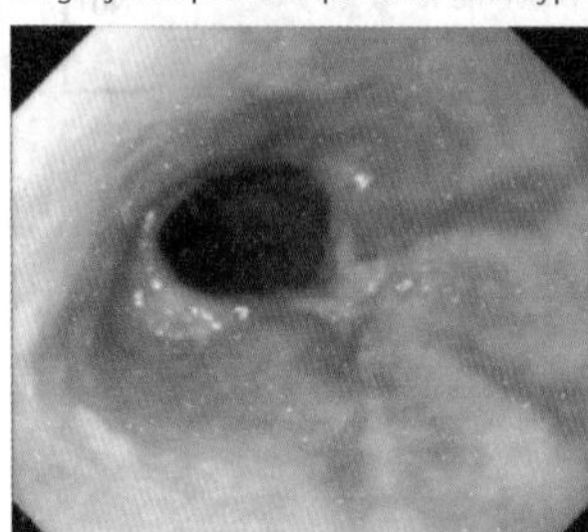

Fig 6.16 Upper GI endoscopy showing longitudinal mucosal breaks in severe oesophagitis.
©Dr A Mee.

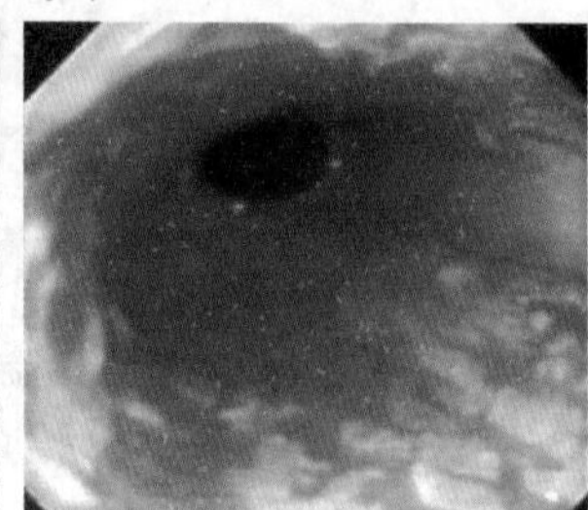

Fig 6.17 Barrett's oesophagus.
©Dr A Mee.

8 The reflux of duodenal fluid, pancreatic secretions and bile may be as important as acid; it may respond to similar lifestyle measures, sucralfate (2g/12h PO), domperidone, or metoclopramide.
9 *H. pylori* association with GORD controversial, but eradication may help symptoms.

Hiatus hernia

Sliding hiatus hernia (80%) The gastro-oesophageal junction slides up into the chest—see fig 6.18. Acid reflux often happens as the lower oesophageal sphincter becomes less competent in many cases.

Paraoesophageal hernia (rolling hiatus hernia) (20%) The gastro-oesophageal junction remains in the abdomen but a bulge of stomach herniates up into the chest alongside the oesophagus—see figs 6.18, 6.19. As the gastro-oesophageal junction remains intact, GORD is less common.

Clinical features Common: 30% of patients >50yrs, especially obese women. Although most small hernias are asymptomatic, patients with large hernias may develop GORD.

Imaging Upper GI endoscopy visualizes the mucosa (?oesophagitis) but cannot reliably exclude a hiatus hernia.

Treatment Lose weight. Treat GORD. Surgery indications: intractable symptoms despite aggressive medical therapy, complications (see p254). Although paraoesophageal hernias may strangulate the risk of this drops dramatically after 65 yrs. Prophylactic repair is only undertaken in those considered at high risk, due to operative mortality (≈1-2%).

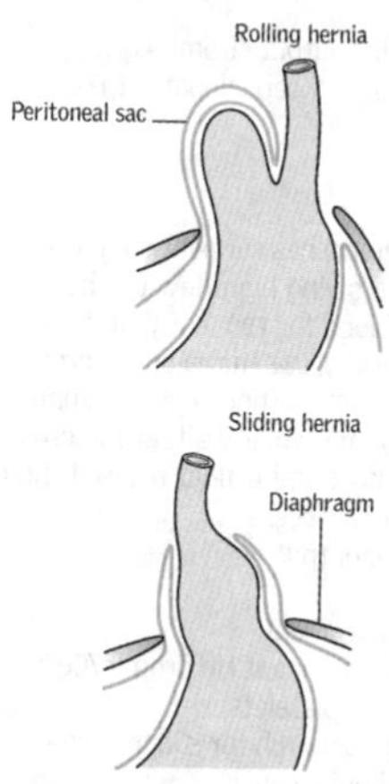

Fig 6.18 Hiatus hernia—sliding and rolling.

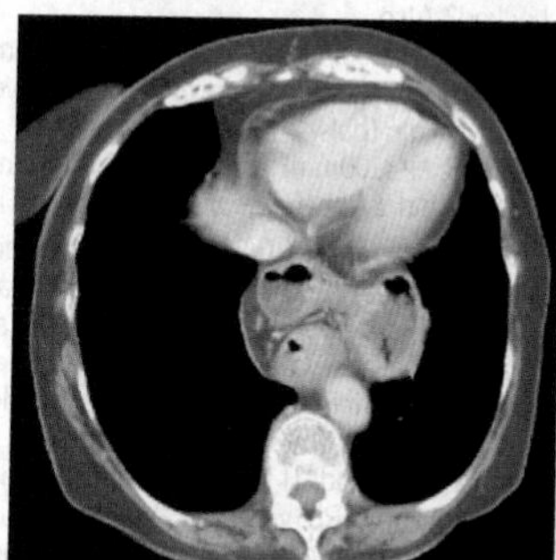

Fig 6.19 CT chest (IV contrast) showing the rolling components of a hiatus hernia anterior to the oesophagus. Between the oesophagus and the vertebral column on the left-hand side is the aorta.

©Dr S Golding.

Upper gastrointestinal bleeding

Haematemesis is vomiting of blood. It may be bright red or look like coffee grounds. *Melaena* (Greek *melas* = black) means black motions, often like tar, and has a characteristic smell of altered blood. Both indicate upper GI bleeding.

Common causes	Rare causes
• Peptic ulcers • Mallory-Weiss tear • Oesophageal varices • Gastritis/gastric erosions • Drugs (NSAIDs, aspirin, steroids, thrombolytics, anticoagulants) • Oesophagitis • Duodenitis • Malignancy • No obvious cause	• Bleeding disorders • Portal hypertensive gastropathy • Aorto-enteric fistula[10] • Angiodysplasia • Haemobilia • Dieulafoy lesion[11] • Meckel's diverticulum • Peutz-Jeghers' syndrome • Osler-Weber-Rendu syndrome.

Take a brief history and examine to assess severity. *Ask about* past GI bleeds; dyspepsia/known ulcers; known liver disease or oesophageal varices (p257); dysphagia; vomiting; weight loss. Check drugs (see BOX on common and rare causes) and alcohol use. Is there serious co-morbidity (bad prognosis), eg cardiovascular disease, respiratory disease, hepatic or renal impairment, or malignancy? *Look for* signs of chronic liver disease (p276) and do a PR to check for melaena. Is the patient shocked? Also:

- Peripherally cool/clammy; capillary refill time >2s; urine output <0.5mL/kg/h.
- ↓GCS (tricky to assess in decompensated liver disease) or encephalopathy (p275).
- Tachycardic (pulse >100bpm).
- Systolic BP <100mmHg; postural drop >20mmHg.
- Calculate the *Rockall score* (tables 6.6, 6.7).

Acute management (p820.) Skill in resuscitation determines survival, so get good at this! Summary:[5] start by protecting the airway and giving high-flow O_2, then:

- ►► Insert 2 large-bore (14–16G) IV cannulae and take blood for FBC (early Hb may be normal because haemodilution has not yet taken place), U&E (↑urea out of proportion to creatinine indicative of massive blood meal), LFT, clotting, and crossmatch.
- ►► Give IV fluids (p821) to restore intravascular volume while waiting for crossmatched blood. If haemodynamically deteriorating despite fluid resuscitation, give group O Rh−ve blood. Avoid saline if cirrhotic/varices.
- ►► Insert a urinary catheter and monitor hourly urine output.
- ►► Organize a CXR, ECG, and check ABG.
- ►► Consider a CVP line to monitor and guide fluid replacement.
- ►► Transfuse (with crossmatched blood if needed) if significant Hb drop (<70g/L).
- ►► Correct clotting abnormalities (vitamin K (p274), FFP, platelets).
- ►► If suspicion of varices then give terlipressin IV eg 1-2mg/6h for ≤3d; relative risk of death ↓ by 34%. Initiate broad-spectrum IV antibiotic cover.
- ►► Monitor pulse, BP, and CVP (keep >5cmH_2O) at least hourly until stable.
- ►► Arrange an urgent *endoscopy* (p248).
- ►► If endoscopic control fails, surgery or emergency mesenteric angiography/embolization may be needed. For uncontrolled oesophageal variceal bleeding, a Sengstaken-Blakemore tube may compress the varices, but should only be placed by someone with experience.

Further management ►Anatomy is important in assessing risk of rebleeding. Posterior DUs are highest risk as they are nearest to the gastroduodenal artery.

- Re-examine after 4h and consider the need for FFP if >4 units transfused.
- Hourly pulse, BP, CVP, urine output (4hrly if haemodynamically stable may be OK).
- Transfuse to keep Hb >70g/L; ensure a current valid group & save sample.
- Check FBC, U&E, LFT, and clotting daily.
- Keep nil by mouth if at high rebleed risk (see BOX 'Management of peptic ulcer bleeds' and p256)—ask the endoscopist.

10 A patient with an aortic graft repair and upper GI bleeding is considered to have an aorto-enteric fistula until proven otherwise: CT abdomen is usually required as well as endoscopy.
11 A Dieulafoy lesion is the rupture of an unusually big arteriole, eg in the fundus of the stomach.

Rockall risk-scoring for upper GI bleeds

Table 6.6 Rockall score calculation

Pre-endoscopy	0 pts	1 pt	2 pts	3 pts
Age	<60yrs	60–79yrs	≥80yrs	
Shock: systolic BP & pulse rate	BP >100mmHg Pulse <100/min	BP >100mmHg Pulse >100/min	BP <100mmHg	
Comorbidity	Nil major	Heart failure; ischaemic heart disease	Renal failure Liver failure	Metastases
Post-endoscopy Diagnosis	Mallory–Weiss tear; no lesion; no sign of recent bleeding	All other diagnoses	Upper GI malignancy	
Signs of recent haemorrhage on endoscopy	None, or dark red spot		Blood in upper GI tract; adherent clot; visible vessel	

Initial Rockall score is based on pre-endoscopy criteria; these are added to post-endoscopy criteria for final score which predicts risk of rebleeding and death (table 6.7). The *Glasgow Blatchford score (GBS)* is used pre-endoscopy to identify patients at low risk of requiring intervention. If GBS≈0, admission can be avoided—ie Hb ≳130g/L (or ≳120g/L if ♀); systolic BP ≳110mmHg; pulse <100/min; urea <6.5mmol/L; no melaena or syncope + no past/present liver disease or heart failure.

Table 6.7 GI bleed mortality by Rockall score

Score	Mortality with initial scoring	Mortality after endoscopy
0	0.2%	0%
1	2.4%	0%
2	5.6%	0.2%
3	11.0%	2.9%
4	24.6%	5.3%
5	39.6%	10.8%
6	48.9%	17.3%
7	50.0%	27.0%
8+	-	41.1%

Management of peptic ulcer bleeds based on endoscopic findings

High-risk *Active bleeding, adherent clot, or non-bleeding visible vessel.* Achieve endoscopic haemostasis (2 of: clips, cautery, adrenaline). Admit to monitored bed; start PPI (eg omeprazole 40mg/12h IV/PO; meta-analyses show 72h IVI eg omeprazole 80mg bolus then 8mg/h *not* superior). If haemodynamically stable start oral intake of clear liquids 6h after endoscopy. Treat if positive for *H. pylori* (p253).

Low-risk *Flat, pigmented spot or clean base.* No need for endoscopic haemostasis. Consider early discharge if patient otherwise low risk. Give oral PPI (p252). Regular diet 6h after endoscopy if stable. Treat if positive for *H. pylori* (p253).

Gastro-oesophageal varices

Submucosal venous dilatation 2° to ↑portal pressures (►may not have documented liver disease—suspect varices if alcohol history); bleeding can be brisk, particularly if underlying coagulopathy 2° to loss of hepatic synthesis of clotting factors.

Causes of portal hypertension *Pre-hepatic:* Thrombosis (portal or splenic vein). *Intra-hepatic:* Cirrhosis (80% in UK); schistosomiasis (commonest worldwide); sarcoid; myeloproliferative diseases; congenital hepatic fibrosis. *Post-hepatic:* Budd-Chiari syndrome (p696); right heart failure; constrictive pericarditis; veno-occlusive disease. *Risk factors for variceal bleeds:* ↑Portal pressure, variceal size, endoscopic features of the variceal wall and advanced liver disease.

Management Endoscopic banding (oesophageal) or sclerotherapy (gastric). *Prophylaxis: 1°:* ~30% of cirrhotics with varices bleed vs ~15% with non-selective β-blockade (propranolol 20–40mg/12h PO) or repeat endoscopic banding. *2°:* after a 1st variceal bleed, 60% rebleed within 1yr. Use banding and non-selective β-blockade; transjugular intrahepatic porto-systemic shunt (TIPS) for resistant varices.

Diarrhoea

Diarrhoea is characterized by increased stool frequency and volume and decreased consistency—though patients' perspectives of these may vary wildly.

History As ever, a careful history will help narrow myriad causes to just a few. *Acute or chronic?* If acute (<2wks) suspect gastroenteritis—any risk factors: Travel? Diet change? Contact with D&V? Any fever/pain? HIV; achlorhydria, eg PA, p334, or on acid suppressants, eg PPI? Chronic diarrhoea alternating with constipation suggests irritable bowel (p266). ↓Weight, nocturnal diarrhoea, or anaemia mandate close follow-up (coeliac/UC/Crohn's?).
Bloody diarrhoea: Campylobacter, Shigella/Salmonella (p431), *E. coli*, amoebiasis (p432), UC, Crohn's, colorectal cancer (p616), colonic polyps, pseudomembranous colitis, ischaemic colitis (p620). *Fresh PR bleeding:* p629.
Mucus: Occurs in IBS (p266), colorectal cancer, and polyps.
Frank pus: Suggests IBD, diverticulitis, or a fistula/abscess.
Explosive: Eg cholera; *Giardia*; *Yersinia* (p425); *Rotavirus*.
Steatorrhoea: Characterized by ↑gas, offensive smell, and floating, hard-to-flush stools—consider pancreatic insufficiency (p267) or biliary obstruction.

Look for Dehydration—dry mucous membranes, ↓skin turgor; capillary refill >2s; shock. Any fever, ↓weight, clubbing, anaemia, oral ulcers (p246), rashes or abdominal mass or scars? Any goitre/hyperthyroid signs? Do rectal exam for masses (eg rectal cancer) or impacted faeces:

- *Blood: FBC:* ↓MCV/Fe deficiency, eg coeliac or colon ca; ↑MCV if alcohol abuse or ↓B_{12} absorption, eg in coeliac or Crohn's; eosinophilia if parasites. ↑*ESR/CRP:* infection, Crohn's/UC, cancer. *U&E:* ↓K^+ ≈ severe D&V. ↓*TSH:* thyrotoxicosis. *Coeliac serology:* p266.
- *Stool: MC&S:* bacterial pathogens, ova cysts, parasites, *C. diff* toxin (CDT, see BOX 'Causes of diarrhoea'), viral PCR. *Faecal elastase:* if suspect chronic pancreatitis (malabsorption, steatorrhoea).
- *Lower GI endoscopy:* (Malignancy? colitis?) ►If acutely unwell, limited flexible sigmoidoscopy with biopsies. Full colonoscopy (including terminal ileum) can assess for more proximal disease If normal, consider small bowel radiology or video capsule.

Management Treat cause. Food handlers: no work until stool samples are -ve. If a hospital outbreak, wards may need closing. *Oral rehydration* is better than IV, but ►if sustained diarrhoea or vomiting, IV fluids with appropriate electrolyte replacement may be needed. Codeine phosphate 30mg/8h PO or loperamide 2mg PO after each loose stool (max 16mg/day) ↓stool frequency (avoid in colitis; both may precipitate toxic megacolon). Avoid antibiotics unless infective diarrhoea is causing systemic upset (fig 6.20). *Antibiotic-associated diarrhoea*[12] may respond to probiotics (eg lactobacilli).

Causes of diarrhoea

Common
- Gastroenteritis (p428)
- Traveller's diarrhoea (p429)
- *C. difficile* (BOX '*Clostridium difficile*')
- IBS (p266)
- Colorectal cancer
- Crohn's; UC; coeliac.

Less common causes (Esp. if painful)
- Microscopic colitis[13]
- Chronic pancreatitis
- Bile salt malabsorption
- Laxative abuse
- Lactose intolerance
- Ileal/gastric resection
- Overflow diarrhoea
- Bacterial overgrowth.

Non-GI or rare causes
- Thyrotoxicosis
- Autonomic neuropathy
- Addison's disease
- Ischaemic colitis
- Tropical sprue
- Gastrinoma
- Carcinoid
- Pellagra
- VIPoma[14]
- Amyloid.

Drugs
(Many, see *BNF*.)
- Antibiotics[12]
- Propranolol
- Cytotoxics
- Laxatives
- PPI
- NSAIDs
- Digoxin
- Alcohol.

12 Erythromycin is prokinetic, others cause overgrowth of bowel organisms, or alter bile acids.
13 Think of this in any chronic watery diarrhoea; diagnosis by biopsy. Associated with a range of drugs including NSAIDs and PPIs. Stop the offending drug where possible. Treat with budesonide.
14 Vasoactive intestinal polypeptide-secreting tumour; suspect if ↓K^+ and acidosis; ↑Ca^{2+}; ↓Mg^{2+}.

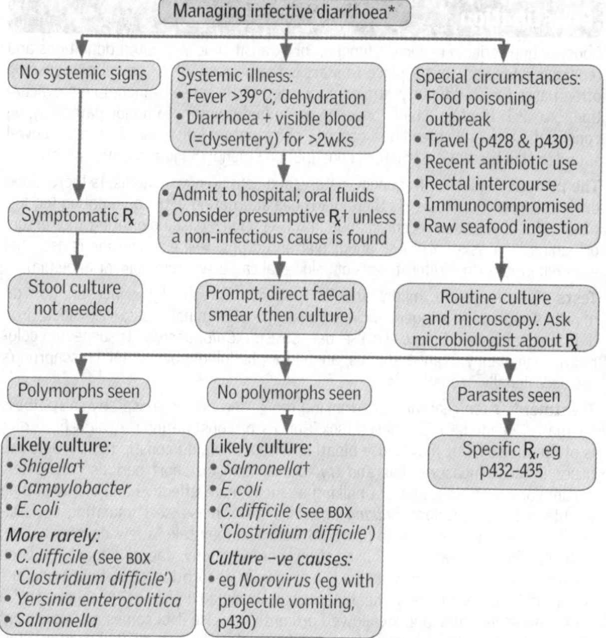

Fig 6.20 Managing infective diarrhoea.

*Be aware of local pathogens, and be prepared to close wards and hospitals if contagion is afoot.

†Prompt specific ℞: eg ciprofloxacin 500mg/12h PO for 6d may be needed before sensitivities are known. Metronidazole is also tried, as *Giardia* is a common cause of watery diarrhoea in travellers.

Clostridium difficile: the cause of pseudomembranous colitis

First isolated from stools of healthy neonates, *C. difficile* was named owing to difficulties in culture. Today, '*difficile*' might better refer to challenges of containment.

Signs: ↑T°; colic; diarrhoea with systemic upset—↑↑CRP, ↑WCC, ↓albumin, and colitis (with yellow adherent plaques on inflamed non-ulcerated mucosa—the pseudomembrane) progressing to toxic megacolon and multi-organ failure.

Asymptomatic carriage: 2–5% of all adults. Only problematic with gut ecology disrupted by, eg antibiotics, leading to rapid proliferation and toxin expression.

Predictors of fulminant C. diff colitis: >70yrs, past *C. diff* infection; use of anti-peristaltic drugs; severe leucocytosis; haemodynamic instability.

Detection: Urgent testing of suspicious stool (characteristic smell—ask the nurses). Two-stage process with rapid screening test for *C. diff* protein (or PCR) followed by specific ELISA for toxins. AXR for toxic megacolon.

℞: Stop causative antibiotic if possible. Mild disease: metronidazole 400mg/8h PO for 10–14d (vancomycin 125mg/6h PO is better in severe disease). Intensive regimens of vancomycin 500mg/6h with IV and PR vancomycin may be needed for non-responders. ►Urgent colectomy may be needed if toxic megacolon, ↑LDH, or if deteriorating.

Recurrent disease: Common (≈25%). Fidaxomicin, a minimally absorbed oral antibiotic, is associated with lower relapse rates. Faecal transplantation (introduction of a suspension prepared from the faeces of a screened donor via endoscopy or via NG/NJ tube) is a highly effective, if aesthetically unappealing, method of treatment.

Preventing spread: Meticulous cleaning and appropriate bed management policies, use of disposable gloves and aprons, hand-washing (not just gel—kill the spores).

Constipation

Constipation reflects pelvic dysfunction or ↑transit time. Accepted definitions and reported rates vary, but a place to start is the passage of ≤2 bowel motions/wk, often passed with difficulty, straining, or pain, and a sense of incomplete evacuation. ♀:♂≈2:1. Doctors' chief concerns are to find pointers to major pathology, eg constipation+rectal bleeding≈cancer; constipation+distension+active bowel sounds≈stricture/GI obstruction; constipation+menorrhagia≈hypothyroidism.

The patient Ask about frequency, nature, and consistency of stools. Is there blood or mucus in/on the stools? Is there diarrhoea alternating with constipation (eg IBS, p266)? Has there been recent change in bowel habit? Is she digitating the rectum or vagina to pass stool?[15] Ask about diet and drugs. ►PR examination is essential even when referring (refer if signs of colorectal ca, eg ↓weight, pain, or anaemia).

Tests None in young, mildly affected patients. Threshold for investigation diminishes with age; triggers include:[6] ↓weight, abdominal mass, +PR blood, iron deficiency anaemia. *Blood:* FBC, ESR, U&E, Ca^{2+}, TFT. *Colonoscopy:* If suspected colorectal malignancy. Transit studies; anorectal physiology; biopsy for Hirschprung's are occasionally needed.

Treatment Often reassurance, drinking more, and diet/exercise advice (p245) is all that is needed. Treat causes (BOX 'Causes of constipation'). A high-fibre diet is often advised, but may cause bloating without helping constipation. ►Only use drugs if these measures fail, and try to use them for short periods only. Often, a stimulant such as senna ± a bulking agent is more effective and cheaper than agents such as lactulose. *Bulking agents:* ↑Faecal mass, so stimulating peristalsis. They must be taken with plenty of fluid and may take a few days to act. CI: difficulty in swallowing; GI obstruction; colonic atony; faecal impaction. Bran powder 3.5g 2-3 times/d with food (may hinder absorption of dietary trace elements if taken with every meal). Ispaghula husk, eg 1 Fybogel® sachet after a meal, mixed in water and swallowed promptly (or else it becomes an unpleasant sludge). Methylcellulose, eg Celevac® 3-6 tablets/12h with ≥300mL water. Sterculia, eg Normacol® granules, 10mL sprinkled on food daily. *Stimulant laxatives:* Increase intestinal motility, so do not use in intestinal obstruction or acute colitis. Avoid prolonged use as it *may* cause colonic atony. Abdominal cramps are an important SE. Pure stimulant laxatives are bisacodyl tablets (5-10mg at night) or suppositories (10mg in the mornings) and senna (2-4 tablets at night). Docusate sodium and dantron[16] have stimulant and softening actions. Glycerol suppositories act as a rectal stimulant. Sodium picosulfate (5-10mg at night) is a potent stimulant. *Stool softeners:* Particularly useful when managing painful anal conditions, eg fissure. Arachis oil enemas lubricate and soften impacted faeces. Liquid paraffin should not be used for a prolonged period (SE: anal seepage, lipoid pneumonia, malabsorption of fat-soluble vitamins). *Osmotic laxatives:* Retain fluid in the bowel. Lactulose, a semisynthetic disaccharide, produces osmotic diarrhoea of low faecal pH that discourages growth of ammonia-producing organisms. It is useful in hepatic encephalopathy (initial dose: 30-50mL/12h). SE: bloating, so its role in treating constipation is limited. Macrogol (eg Movicol®) is another example. Magnesium salts (eg magnesium hydroxide; magnesium sulfate) are useful when rapid bowel evacuation is required. Sodium salts (eg Microlette® and Micralax® enemas) should be avoided as they may cause sodium and water retention. Phosphate enemas are useful for rapid bowel evacuation prior to procedures.

If these don't help Prucalopride is an elective $5HT_4$ agonist with prokinetic properties; Lubiprostone is a chloride-channel activator that increases intestinal fluid secretion; Linaclotide is a guanylate cyclase-C agonist that also increases fluid secretion and decreases visceral pain. A multidisciplinary approach with behaviour therapy, habit training ± sphincter biofeedback may help.

15 *Rectocele:* front wall of the rectum bulges into the back wall of the vagina.
16 Dantron causes colon & liver tumours in animals, so reserve use for the very elderly or terminally ill.

Causes of constipation

General
- Poor diet ± lack of exercise
- Poor fluid intake/dehydration
- Irritable bowel syndrome
- Old age
- Post-operative pain
- Hospital environment (↓privacy; having to use a bed pan).

Anorectal disease (Esp. if painful.)
- ►► Anal or colorectal cancer
- Fissures (p630), strictures, herpes
- Rectal prolapse
- Proctalgia fugax (p630)
- Mucosal ulceration/neoplasia
- Pelvic muscle dysfunction/levator ani syndrome.

Intestinal obstruction
- ►► Colorectal carcinoma (p616)
- Strictures (eg Crohn's disease)
- Pelvic mass (eg fetus, fibroids)
- Diverticulosis (rectal bleeding is a commoner presentation)
- Pseudo-obstruction (p611).

Metabolic/endocrine
- Hypercalcaemia (p676)
- Hypothyroidism (rarely *presents* with constipation)
- Hypokalaemia (p674)
- Porphyria
- Lead poisoning.

Drugs (Pre-empt by diet advice.)
- Opiates (eg morphine, codeine)
- Anticholinergics (eg tricyclics)
- Iron
- Some antacids, eg with aluminium
- Diuretics, eg furosemide
- Calcium channel blockers.

Neuromuscular (Slow transit from decreased propulsive activity.)
- Spinal or pelvic nerve injury (eg trauma, surgery)
- Aganglionosis (Chagas' disease, Hirschsprung's disease)
- Systemic sclerosis
- Diabetic neuropathy.

Other causes
- Chronic laxative abuse (rare—diarrhoea is commoner)
- Idiopathic slow transit
- Idiopathic megarectum/colon.

Defining gastrointestinal dysfunction—the Rome criteria

'Here was history in the stones of the street and the atoms of the sunshine... she went about in a kind of repressed ecstasy of contemplation, seeing often... a great deal more than was there.'

Henry James, *The Portrait of a Lady.*

While the tools of contemporary gastroenterology are well placed to explore the comparatively simple domains of structural lesions and inflammation, for those patients troubled by 'functional' disorders of motility and pain, we lack methods to understand nervous activity in their guts. Instead, unlike James' heroine Isabel Archer, as she explored late 19th-century Rome, we are left seeing a greal deal less than perhaps is there. The failure to see, then becomes a failure to comprehend (the endoscopy and CT were normal, so there must be nothing wrong?)—then a failure to believe and ultimately to treat an illness.

Before we subject any intervention to the rigors of medical trials, we should first agree a classification of the disease process we are aiming to treat. Some of medicine's darkest alcoves reflect less a lack of potential treatments and more a lack of any agreement on where classification boundaries lie. Failure to define and distinguish pathologies then leads to a literature studded with small conflicting studies on heterogeneous patients which feeds a perception of a condition as 'untreatable'.

There is nothing romantic about constipation, and gastrointestinal dysfunction in general, other than the association of the definitions of these disorders with Rome. By the late 1980s, these confused areas exemplified the above-described challenges. Recognition of the need for order and classification to support studies led to an international collaboration, born out of the University of Rome. A process of expert debate and discussion reached consensus definitions that could support scientific studies. The experts then periodically reconvene in the eternal city to revisit and evaluate these 'Rome consensus' definitions. Rather more prosaically, the Rome foundation itself is now headquartered in Raleigh, North Carolina, USA.

Ulcerative colitis (UC)

UC is a relapsing and remitting inflammatory disorder of the colonic mucosa. It may affect just the rectum (proctitis, as in ~30%) or extend to involve part of the colon (left-sided colitis, in ~40%) or the entire colon (pancolitis, in ~30%). It 'never' spreads proximal to the ileocaecal valve (except for backwash ileitis). **Cause** Inappropriate immune response against (?abnormal) colonic flora in genetically susceptibile individuals. **Pathology** Hyperaemic/haemorrhagic colonic mucosa ± pseudopolyps formed by inflammation. Punctate ulcers may extend deep into the lamina propria—inflammation is normally not transmural. Continuous inflammation limited to the mucosa differentiates it from Crohn's disease. **Prevalence** 100–200/100 000. **Incidence** 10–20/100 000/yr; typically presents ~20–40yrs. UC is 3-fold as common in non-smokers (the opposite is true for Crohn's disease)—symptoms may relapse on stopping smoking.

Symptoms Episodic or chronic diarrhoea (± blood & mucus); crampy abdominal discomfort; bowel frequency relates to severity (see table 6.8); urgency/tenesmus≈proctitis. Systemic symptoms in attacks: fever, malaise, anorexia, ↓weight.

Signs May be none. In acute, severe UC there may be fever, tachycardia, and a tender, distended abdomen. *Extraintestinal signs:* Clubbing; aphthous oral ulcers; erythema nodosum (p265); pyoderma gangrenosum; conjunctivitis; episcleritis; iritis; large joint arthritis; sacroiliitis; ankylosing spondylitis; PSC (p282); nutritional deficits.

Tests *Blood:* FBC, ESR, CRP, U&E, LFT, blood culture. *Stool MC&S/CDT:* (See p258.) To exclude *Campylobacter, C. difficile, Salmonella, Shigella, E. coli,* amoebae. *Faecal calprotectin:* A simple, non-invasive test for GI inflammation with high sensitivity. *AXR:* No faecal shadows; mucosal thickening/islands (fig 16.9, p729); colonic dilatation (see 'Complications'). *Lower GI endoscopy:* Limited flexible sigmoidoscopy if acute to assess and biopsy; full colonoscopy once controlled to define disease extent (see p249, fig 6.10).

Table 6.8 Assessing severity in UC (Truelove & Witts criteria modified to include CRP)

Variable	Mild UC	Moderate UC	Severe UC
Motions/day	≤4	5	≥6
Rectal bleeding	Small	Moderate	Large
T°C	Apyrexial	37.1–37.8°C	>37.8°C
Resting pulse	<70 beats/min	70–90 beats/min	>90 beats/min
Haemoglobin	>110g/L	105–110g/L	<105g/L
ESR (do CRP too)	<30		>30 (or CRP >45mg/L)

Data from Truelove *et al.*, 'Cortisone in ulcerative colitis', *BMJ*; 2(4947): 1041–8.

Complications *Acute:* Toxic dilatation of colon (mucosal islands, colonic diameter >6cm) with risk of perforation; venous thromboembolism: give prophylaxis to all inpatients regardless of rectal bleeding (p350); ↓K^+ *Chronic:* Colonic cancer: risk related to disease extent and activity≈5–10% with pancolitis for 20yrs. Neoplasms may occur in flat, normal-looking mucosa. To spot precursor areas of dysplasia, surveillance colonoscopy eg 1–5yrs (depending on risk), with multiple random biopsies or biopsies guided by differential uptake by abnormal mucosa of dye sprayed endoscopically.

Treatment Goals are to induce, then maintain disease remission.[7]
Mild UC: • 5-ASA,[17] eg mesalazine (=mesalamine) is the mainstay for remission-induction/maintenance. Given PR (suppositories or enemas) for distal disease (eg Pentasa® 1g daily); or PO for more extensive disease (eg Pentasa® 2g daily; once-daily dosing as effective as split dose; combine PR+PO if flare). • Topical steroid foams PR (eg hydrocortisone as Colifoam®), or prednisolone 20mg retention enemas (Predsol®) less effective than PR 5-ASA but may be added in addition.

Moderate UC: If 4–6 motions/day, but otherwise well, induce remission with oral *prednisolone* 40mg/d for 1wk, then taper by 5mg/week over following 7wks. Then maintain on 5-ASA (SEs: rash, haemolysis, hepatitis, pancreatitis, paradoxical worsening of colitis ►monitor FBC and U&E at start, then at 3 months, then annually).

17 5-aminosalicylic acid (5-ASA or mesalazine) must be stabilized in oral preparations to survive gastric pH. Alternatively, olsalazine is a dimer of 5-ASA or balsalazide is a prodrug, both of which are cleaved in the colon. Rare hypersensitivity reactions: worsening colitis, pancreatitis, pericarditis, nephritis.

Severe UC: If unwell and ≥6 motions/d, admit for: IV hydration/electrolyte replacement; IV steroids, eg hydrocortisone 100mg/6h or methylprednisolone 40mg/12h; rectal steroids, eg hydrocortisone 100mg in 100mL 0.9% saline/12h PR; thromboembolism prophylaxis (p350); ensure multiple stool MC&S/CDT to exclude infection.

- Monitor T°, pulse, and BP—and record stool frequency/character on a stool chart.
- Twice-daily exam: document distension, bowel sounds, and tenderness.
- Daily FBC, ESR, CRP, U&E ± AXR. Consider blood transfusion (eg if Hb <80g/L).
- If on day 3-5 CRP >45 or >6 stools/d, ►►action is needed.[18] *Rescue therapy* with ciclosporin or infliximab, can avoid colectomy, but involve surgeons early in shared care.
- If improving, transfer to prednisolone PO (40mg/24h). Schedule maintenance infliximab if used for rescue, or azathioprine if ciclosporin rescue.
- If fails to improve then urgent colectomy by d7-10—the challenge is not to delay surgery so long as to accumulate significant steroid exposure and debilitation that will delay post-surgical recovery.

It's time for immunomodulation if... Patients flare on steroid tapering or require ≥2 courses of steroids/year eg azathioprine (2-2.5mg/kg/d PO). 30% of patients will develop SEs requiring treatment cessation including abdominal pain, nausea, pancreatitis, leucopenia, abnormal LFTs. Monitor FBC, U+E, LFT weekly for 4 wks, then every 4 wks for 3 months, then at least 3-monthly.

Biologic therapy For patients intolerant of immunomodulation, or developing symptoms despite an immunomodulator, *monoclonal antibodies to TNFα* (infliximab, adalimumab, golimumab) or to adhesion molecules involved in gut lymphocyte trafficking (vedolizumab) play an important role (see BOX 'Therapies in Crohn's disease' p265).

Surgery This is needed at some stage in ~20%, eg *subtotal colectomy + terminal ileostomy* for failure of medical therapy or fulminant colitis with toxic dilatation/ perforation. Subsequently *completion proctectomy* (permanent stoma) vs *ileo-anal pouch*. Pouches mean stoma reversal and the possibility of long-term continence but pouch opening frequency may still be around 6×/day and recurrent pouchitis can be troublesome (give antibiotics, eg metronidazole + ciprofloxacin for 2wks).

Diagnosing IBD-unclassified (IBD-U)

After full investigation, IBD may not obviously be Crohn's or UC. IBD-U refers to isolated colonic IBD where the diagnosis remains unknown (small bowel involvement=Crohn's). This situation is rare in adults but commoner in children. Over time the phenotype tends to become clearer (generally UC>Crohn's). Colectomy ± pouch formation may be needed, though pouch failure rate is higher than in UC.

18 Day 3 stool frequency >8×/day *or* frequency 3-8×/day & CRP >45 =85% chance of colectomy *this admission*.

Crohn's disease

A chronic inflammatory disease characterized by transmural granulomatous inflammation affecting any part of the gut from mouth to anus (esp. terminal ileum in ~70%). Unlike UC, there is unaffected bowel between areas of active disease (skip lesions). **Cause** As with UC an inappropriate immune response against the (?abnormal) gut flora in a genetically susceptible individual.[19] **Prevalence** 100-200/100 000. **Incidence** 10-20/100 000/yr; typically presents ~20-40yrs. **Associations** Smoking ↑risk ×3-4; NSAIDs may exacerbate disease.

Symptoms Diarrhoea, abdominal pain, weight loss/failure to thrive. Systemic symptoms: fatigue, fever, malaise, anorexia.

Signs Bowel ulceration (fig 6.22); abdominal tenderness/mass; perianal abscess/fistulae/skin tags; anal strictures. *Beyond the gut:* (fig 6.21) Clubbing, skin, joint, & eye problems.

Complications Small bowel obstruction; toxic dilatation (colonic diameter >6cm, toxic dilatation is rarer than in UC); abscess formation (abdominal, pelvic, or perianal); fistulae (present in ~10%), eg entero-enteric, colovesical (bladder), colovaginal, perianal, enterocutaneous; perforation; colon cancer; PSC (p282), malnutrition.

Tests *Blood:* FBC, ESR, CRP, U&E, LFT, INR, ferritin, TIBC, B_{12}, folate. *Stool:* MC&S and CDT (p258) to exclude eg *C. difficile*, *Campylobacter*, *E. coli;* faecal calprotectin is a simple, non-invasive test for GI inflammation with high sensitivity. *Colonoscopy + biopsy:* Even if mucosa looks normal. *Small bowel:* To detect isolated proximal disease by eg *capsule endoscopy* (p248, use dummy patency capsule 1st that disintegrates if it gets stuck); *MRI* increasingly used to assess pelvic disease and fistulae, small bowel disease activity and strictures; *US* in skilled hands can provide small bowel imaging.

Treatment (See BOX.[8]) Find out how your patient deals with what may be a brutal disease (no intimacy...no sex...no hope...'I live with this alone and will die alone'). With a collaborative approach, courage, attention to detail, and a dose of humour, this can change. Help quit smoking. ►*Optimize nutrition.* Assess severity: ↑T°, ↑pulse, ↑ESR, ↑WCC, ↑CRP, + ↓albumin may merit admission for IV steroids.

Mild-moderate: Symptomatic but systemically well. Prednisolone 40mg/d PO for 1wk, then taper by 5mg every wk for next 7wks. An alternative dietary approach based upon 'elemental' or 'polymeric' diets is effective in children but less used for adults. Plan maintenance therapy (see BOX).

Severe: Admit for IV hydration/electrolyte replacement; IV steroids, eg hydrocortisone 100mg/6h or methylprednisolone 40mg/12h; thromboembolism prophylaxis (p350); ensure multiple stool MC&S/CDT to exclude infection.

- Monitor T°, pulse, BP, and record stool frequency/character on a stool chart.
- Physical examination daily. Daily FBC, ESR, CRP, U&E, and plain AXR.
- Consider need for blood transfusion (if Hb <80g/L) and nutritional support.
- If improving switch to oral prednisolone (40mg/d). If not, *biologics* have a role.
- Consider abdominal sepsis complicating Crohn's disease especially if abdominal pain (ultrasound, CT, & MRI are often required to assess this). Seek surgical advice.

Perianal disease: Occurs in about 50%. MRI and examination under anaesthetic (EUA) are an important part of assessment. Treatment includes oral antibiotics, immunosuppressant therapy ± anti-TNFα, and local surgery ± seton insertion.

19 Much of the genetic risk is shared with UC—small differences in genetics combined with environmental modifiers may explain the very different phenotypes.

Therapies in Crohn's disease

Azathioprine (AZA) (2-2.5mg/kg/d PO) used if refractory to steroids, relapsing on steroid taper, or requiring ≥2 steroid courses/yr. Takes 6-10wks to work. 30% will develop SEs requiring treatment cessation including abdominal pain, nausea, pancreatitis, leucopenia, abnormal LFTs. Monitor FBC, U&E, LFT weekly for 4wks, then every 4wks for 3 months, then at least 3-monthly. Alternative immunomodulators include 6-mercaptopurine and methotrexate (CI: ♀ of reproductive age).

5-ASA Unlike in UC, have no role in the management of Crohn's.

Biologics *Anti-TNFα:* TNFα plays an important role in pathogenesis of Crohn's disease, therefore monoclonal antibodies to TNFα, eg infliximab and adalimumab, can ↓disease activity. They counter neutrophil accumulation and granuloma formation and cause cytotoxicity to CD4+ T cells, thus clearing cells driving the immune response. These drugs play a vital role in both induction and maintenance therapy. CI: sepsis, active/latent TB, ↑LFT >3-fold above top end of normal. SE: rash. Avoid in people with known underlying malignancy. TB may reactivate when on infliximab, so screen patients before starting the treatment (CXR, PPD, interferon gamma release assay (IGRA)). Combined AZA and infliximab can ↑ efficacy of ℞ at 12 months, but there are long-term safety issues (eg increased lymphoma risk). *Anti-integrin:* Monoclonal antibodies targeting adhesion molecules involved in gut lymphocyte trafficking, eg vedolizumab, reduce disease activity and have a more gut-specific mechanism of activiy. *Anti-IL12/23:* Represents a new cytokine target with an emerging role in treatment, eg ustekinumab.

Nutrition Enteral is preferred (eg polymeric diet); consider TPN as a last resort. *Elemental diets:* (Eg E028®.) Contain amino acids and can give remission. *Low residue diets:* Help symptoms in those with active disease or strictures.

Surgery 50-80% need ≥1 operation in their life. It never cures. Indications: drug failure (most common); GI obstruction from stricture; perforation; fistulae; abscess. Surgical aims are: **1** resection of affected areas—but beware short bowel syndrome (p580) **2** to control perianal or fistulizing disease **3** defunction (rest) distal disease eg with a temporary ileostomy. Pouch surgery is avoided in Crohn's (∵ ↑ risk of recurrence).

Poor prognosis Age <40yrs; steroids needed at 1st presentation; perianal disease; isolated terminal ileitis; smoking.

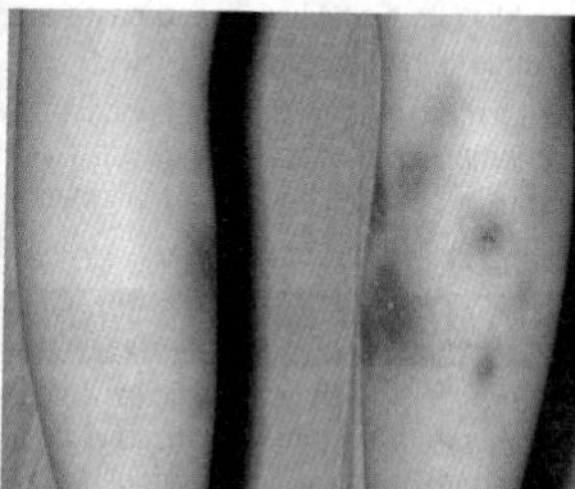

Fig 6.21 Beyond the gut... 'I hate how this stupid illness is crippling me...' As well as erythema nodosum on the shins (above; also caused by sarcoid, drugs, streptococci, and TB), Crohn's can associate with sero −ve arthritis of large or small joints, spondyloarthropathy, ankylosing spondylitis, sacroiliitis, pyoderma gangrenosum, conjunctivitis, episcleritis, and iritis.

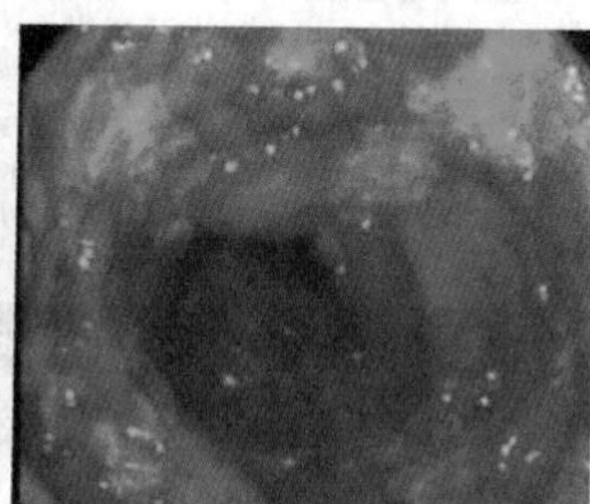

Fig 6.22 Deep fissured ulcers seen at colonoscopy. The end result? 'My family does not or will not even talk to me about the disease ... I don't know when urgency to race for the bathroom will happen so I don't go out and have been living a hermit life...'

Gastrointestinal malabsorption

Causes See BOX 'Causes of gastrointestinal malabsorption'.

Symptoms Diarrhoea; ↓weight; lethargy; steatorrhoea; bloating.

Deficiency signs Anaemia (↓Fe, B_{12}, folate); bleeding disorders (↓vit K); oedema (↓protein); metabolic bone disease (↓vit D); neurological features, eg neuropathy.

Tests FBC (↓ or ↑MCV); ↓Ca^{2+}; ↓Fe; ↓B_{12} + folate; ↑INR; lipid profile; coeliac tests (see 'Coeliac disease'). *Stool:* Sudan stain for fat globules; stool microscopy (infestation); elastase. *Breath hydrogen analysis:* For bacterial overgrowth.[20] Take samples of end-expired air; give glucose; take more samples at ½h intervals; early ↑exhaled hydrogen = overgrowth. *Endoscopy + small bowel biopsy.*

Infectious malabsorption *Giardia*, *Cryptosporidium*, *Isospora belli*, *Cyclospora cayetanensis*, microsporidia. *Tropical sprue:* Villous atrophy + malabsorption occurring in the Far and Middle East and Caribbean—the cause is unknown. Tetracycline 250mg/6h PO + folic acid 5mg/d PO for 3-6mnths may help.

Coeliac disease

►Suspect this if diarrhoea + weight loss or anaemia (esp. if iron or B_{12} ↓). T-cell-responses to gluten (alcohol-soluble proteins in wheat, barley, rye ± oats) in the small bowel causes villous atrophy and malabsorption. **Associations** HLA DQ2 in 95%; the rest are DQ8; autoimmune disease; dermatitis herpetiformis. **Prevalence** 1 in 100-300 (commoner if Irish). Any age (peaks in childhood and 50-60yrs). ♀:♂ >1:1. Relative risk in 1st-degree relatives is 6×.

Presentation Stinking stools/steatorrhoea; diarrhoea; abdominal pain; bloating; nausea + vomiting; aphthous ulcers; angular stomatitis (p327, fig 8.5); ↓weight; fatigue; weakness; osteomalacia; failure to thrive (children). ~30% less severe: may mimic IBS.

Diagnosis ↓Hb; ↑RCDW (p325); ↓B_{12}, ↓ferritin. Antibodies: anti-transglutaminase is single preferred test (but is an IgA antibody—check IgA levels to exclude subclass deficiency). Where serology positive or high index of suspicion proceed to duodenal biopsy while on a gluten-containing diet: expect subtotal villous atrophy, ↑intra-epithelial WBCs + crypt hyperplasia. Where doubt persists, HLA DQ2 and DQ8 genotyping may help.

Treatment *Lifelong gluten-free diet*—patients become experts. Rice, maize, soya, potatoes, and sugar are OK. Limited consumption of oats (≤50g/d) may be tolerated in patients with mild disease. Gluten-free biscuits, flour, bread, and pasta are prescribable. Monitor response by symptoms and repeat serology.[9]

Complications Anaemia; dermatitis herpetiformis (*OHCS* p588); osteopenia/osteoporosis; hyposplenism (offer 'flu and pneumococcal vaccinations); GI T-cell lymphoma (rare; suspect if refractory symptoms or ↓weight); ↑risk of malignancy (lymphoma, gastric, oesophageal, colorectal); neuropathies.

Irritable bowel syndrome (IBS)

IBS denotes a mixed group of abdominal symptoms for which no organic cause can be found. Most are probably due to disorders of intestinal motility, enhanced visceral perception (the 'brain-gut' axis: see BOX 'Managing IBS'), or microbial dysbiosis. Several diagnostic criteria exist (see BOX 'Defining gastrointestinal dysfunction' p261). **Prevalence** 10-20%; age at onset: ≤40yrs; ♀:♂ ≥2:1.

Diagnosis Only diagnose IBS if recurrent abdominal pain (or discomfort) associated with at least 2 of: • relief by defecation • altered stool form • altered bowel frequency (constipation and diarrhoea may alternate). Other features: urgency; incomplete evacuation; abdominal bloating/distension; mucus PR; worsening of symptoms after food. Symptoms are chronic (>6 months), and often exacerbated by stress, menstruation, or gastroenteritis (post-infectious IBS). *Signs:* Examination may be normal, but general abdominal tenderness is common. Insufflation of air during lower GI endoscopy (*not* usually needed) may reproduce the pain. *Think of other diagnoses if:* Age >60yrs; history <6 months; anorexia; ↓weight; waking at night with pain/diarrhoea; mouth ulcers; abnormal CRP, ESR.

Causes of gastrointestinal malabsorption

Common in the UK: Coeliac disease; chronic pancreatitis; Crohn's disease.

Rarer:

- ↓*Bile:* primary biliary cholangitis; ileal resection; biliary obstruction; colestyramine.
- *Pancreatic insufficiency:* pancreatic cancer; cystic fibrosis.
- *Small bowel mucosa:* Whipple's disease (p716); radiation enteritis; tropical sprue; small bowel resection; brush border enzyme deficiencies (eg lactase insufficiency); drugs (metformin, neomycin, alcohol); amyloid (p370).
- *Bacterial overgrowth:*[20] spontaneous (esp. in elderly); in jejunal diverticula; post-op blind loops. DM & PPI use are also risk factors. Try metronidazole 400mg/8h PO. Don't confuse with afferent loop syndrome (p622).
- *Infection:* giardiasis; diphyllobothriasis (B_{12} malabsorption); strongyloidiasis.
- *Intestinal hurry:* post-gastrectomy dumping; post-vagotomy; gastrojejunostomy.

Managing IBS

Make a *positive* diagnosis (p266) and other diagnoses, so:

- If the history is classic, FBC, ESR, CRP & coeliac serology (p266) are sufficient.
- If ≥60yrs or *any* marker or organic disease (↑T°, blood PR, ↓weight): colonoscopy.
- Have a low threshold for referring if family history of ovarian or bowel cancer.
- ♀: excluding ovarian cancer requires serum CA-125 (*OHCS* p281); endometriosis (*OHCS* p288) often mimics IBS: consider if pain cyclical.
- If IBS criteria not met, consider clinical context and decide upon: stool culture; B_{12}/folate; TSH; faecal calprotectin (p262).

Refer if: **1** Diagnostic uncertainty (you or the patient!). **2** If changing symptoms in 'known IBS'. **3** Refractory to management: stress or depression (seen in ≥50%) or refractory symptoms (here, NICE favours cognitive therapy, *OHCS* p390), *chronic pain overlap syndromes* (fibromyalgia + chronic fatigue + chronic pelvic pain) or detrusor problems.

Treatment: Should focus on controlling symptoms, initially using lifestyle/dietary measures, then cognitive therapy (*OHCS* p390) or pharmacotherapy if required:

- *Constipation:* ensure adequate water and fibre intake and promote physical activity; (↑fibre intake can worsen flatulence/bloating so avoid insoluble fibre, such as bran; oats are better). Simple laxatives (p260, but beware lactulose which ferments and can aggravate bloating).If 2 of these fail, try prucalopride, linaclotide, or lubiprostone; or self-administered anal irrigation.
- *Diarrhoea:* avoid sorbitol sweeteners, alcohol, and caffeine; reduce dietary fibre content; encourage patients to identify their own 'trigger' foods; try a bulking agent ± loperamide 2mg after each loose stool.
- *Colic/bloating:* oral antispasmodics: mebeverine 135mg/8h or hyoscine butylbromide 10mg/8h (over the counter). Combination probiotics in sufficient doses (eg VSL#3®) may help flatulence or bloating. Diets low in fermentable, poorly absorbed saccharides and alcohols may provide benefit (the low FODMAP diet).
- *Psychological symptoms/visceral hypersensitivity:* emphasize the positive! You have excluded sinister pathology and over time, symptoms tend to improve. Consider cognitive behavioural therapy (*OHCS* p390), hypnosis, and tricyclics, eg amitriptyline 10–20mg at night (SE: drowsiness, dry mouth); explain that this is at a low dose for visceral pain (ie you are not prescribing the higher licensed dose for depression).

20 Bacterial overgrowth proximal to the colon causes diarrhoea, abdominal pain, and vitamin malabsorption. Causes: old age, autonomic neuropathy (eg diabetic), ileocaecal valve resection; PPI usage; amyloidosis.

Nutritional disorders

►Always consider that more than one nutritional disorder is likely to be present (table 6.9).

Scurvy is due to lack of vitamin C.[21] Is the patient poor, pregnant, or on an odd diet? *Signs:* **1** Listlessness, anorexia, cachexia (p35). **2** Gingivitis, loose teeth, and foul breath (halitosis). **3** Bleeding from gums, nose, hair follicles, or into joints, bladder, gut. **4** Muscle pain/weakness. **5** Oedema. *Diagnosis:* No test is completely satisfactory. WBC ↓ascorbic acid. ℞: Dietary education; ascorbic acid ≥250mg/24h PO.

Beriberi There is heart failure with general oedema (wet beriberi) or neuropathy (dry beriberi) due to lack of vitamin B_1 (thiamine). For treatment and diagnostic tests, see Wernicke's encephalopathy (p714).

Pellagra = lack of nicotinic acid. Classical triad: **d**iarrhoea, **d**ementia, **d**ermatitis (Casal's necklace) ± neuropathy, depression, insomnia, tremor, rigidity, ataxia, fits. It may occur in carcinoid syndrome and anti-TB drugs (isoniazid). It is endemic in China and Africa. ℞: Education, electrolyte replacement, nicotinamide 100mg/4h.

Xerophthalmia This vitamin A deficiency syndrome is a big cause of blindness in the Tropics. Conjunctivae become dry and develop oval/triangular spots (Bitôt's spots). Corneas become cloudy and soft. Give vitamin A (*OHCS* p460). ►Get special help if pregnant: vitamin A embryopathy must be avoided. Re-educate and monitor diet.

Table 6.9 Deficiency syndromes and the sites of nutrient absorption

Vitamin/nutrient	Site of absorption	Deficiency syndrome
A[F]	Small intestine	Xerophthalmia
B_1 (thiamine)	Small intestine	Beriberi; Wernicke's encephalopathy (p714)
B_2 (riboflavin)	Proximal small intestine	Angular stomatis; cheilitis (p246)
B_6 (pyridoxine)	Small intestine	Polyneuropathy
B_{12}	Terminal ileum	Macrocytic anaemia (p332); neuropathy; glossitis
C	Proximal ileum	Scurvy
D[F]	Jejunum as free vitamin	Rickets (p684); osteomalacia (p684)
E[F]	Small intestine	Haemolysis; neurological deficit
K[F]	Small intestine	Bleeding disorders (p344)
Folic acid	Jejunum	Macrocytic anaemia (p332)
Nicotinamide	Jejunum	Pellagra
Mineral		
Calcium	Duodenum + jejunum	p676
Copper	Stomach + jejunum	Menkes' kinky hair syndrome
Fluoride	Stomach	Dental caries
Iodide	Small intestine	Goitre; cretinism
Iron	Duodenum + jejunum	Microcytic anaemia (p326)
Magnesium	Small intestine	p679
Phosphate	Small intestine	Osteoporosis; anorexia; weakness
Selenium	Small intestine	Cardiomyopathy (p679)
Zinc	Jejunum	Acrodermatitis enteropathica; poor wound healing (p679)

F = fat-soluble vitamin, thus deficiency is likely if there is fat malabsorption.

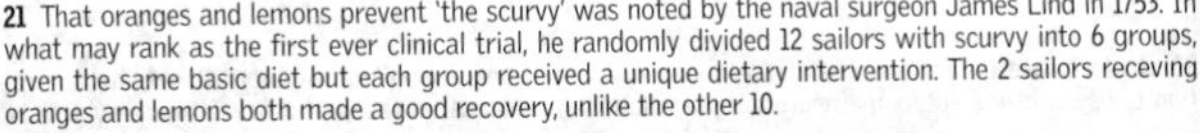

21 That oranges and lemons prevent 'the scurvy' was noted by the naval surgeon James Lind in 1753. In what may rank as the first ever clinical trial, he randomly divided 12 sailors with scurvy into 6 groups, given the same basic diet but each group received a unique dietary intervention. The 2 sailors receving oranges and lemons both made a good recovery, unlike the other 10.

Food mountains, the pellagra paradox, and the sorrow that weeping cannot symbolize

'The sweet smell is a great sorrow on the land. Men who can graft the trees and make the seed fertile and big can find no way to let the hungry people eat their produce ... The works of the roots of the vines, of the trees, must be destroyed to keep up the price ...

There is a crime here that goes beyond denunciation. There is a sorrow here that weeping cannot symbolize. There is a failure here that topples all our success. The fertile earth, the straight tree rows, the sturdy trunks, and the ripe fruit. And children dying of pellagra must die because a profit cannot be taken from an orange. And coroners must fill in the certificates—died of malnutrition—because the food must rot, must be forced to rot.

The people come with nets to fish for potatoes in the river, and the guards hold them back; they come in rattling cars to get the dumped oranges, but the kerosene is sprayed. And they stand still and watch the potatoes float by, listen to the screaming pigs being killed in a ditch and covered with quicklime, watch the mountains of oranges slop down to a putrefying ooze; and in the eyes of the people there is a failure; and in the eyes of the hungry there is a growing wrath. In the souls of the people the grapes of wrath are filling and growing heavy, growing heavy for the vintage.' (J Steinbeck *The Grapes of Wrath*)

How do John Steinbeck's grapes grow in our 21st-century soil? Too well; a double harvest, it turns out, as not only is much of the world starving, amid plenty (for those who can pay) but also there is a new 'sorrow in our land that weeping cannot symbolize': pathological 'voluntary' *self-starvation*, again amid plenty, in pursuit of the body-beautiful according to images laid down by media gods. If gastroenterologists had one wish it might not be the ending of all their diseases, but that humankind stand in a right relationship with Steinbeck's fertile earth, his straight trees, his sturdy trunks, and his ripe fruit.

Chronic pancreatitis

Epigastric pain 'bores' through to the back, eg relieved by sitting forward or hot water bottles on epigastrium/back (look for *erythema ab igne*'s mottled dusky greyness); bloating; steatorrhoea; ↓weight; brittle diabetes. Symptoms relapse and worsen.

Causes Alcohol; smoking; autoimmune; rarely: familial; cystic fibrosis; haemochromatosis; pancreatic duct obstruction (stones/tumour); congenital (*pancreas divisum*).

Tests *Ultrasound* ± *CT:* pancreatic calcifications confirm the diagnosis, *MRCP*; *AXR*. Speckled calcification; faecal elastase.

Treatment *Drugs:* Give analgesia (coeliac-plexus block may give brief relief); lipase, eg Creon®; fat-soluble vitamins. Insulin needs may be high or variable (beware hypoglycaemia). *Diet:* No alcohol; low fat may help. Medium-chain triglycerides (MCT oil) may be tried (no lipase needed for absorption, but diarrhoea may be worsened). *Surgery:* For unremitting pain; narcotic abuse (beware of this); ↓weight: eg pancreatectomy or pancreaticojejunostomy (a duct drainage procedure).

Complications Pseudocyst; diabetes; biliary obstruction; local arterial aneurysm; splenic vein thrombosis; gastric varices; pancreatic carcinoma.

Carcinoma of the pancreas

Epidemiology ≈3% of all malignancy; ~9000 deaths/yr (UK). UK incidence is rising. **Typical patient** ♂ >70yrs old. **Risk factors** Smoking, alcohol, carcinogens, DM, chronic pancreatitis, ↑waist circumference (ie adiposity), and possibly a high-fat and red or processed meat diet. **Pathology** Mostly ductal adenocarcinoma (metastasize early; present late). 60% arise in the pancreas head, 25% in the body, 15% tail. A few arise in the ampulla of Vater (ampullary tumour) or pancreatic islet cells (insulinoma, gastrinoma, glucagonomas, somatostatinomas (p223), VIPomas); both have a better prognosis. **Genetics** ~95% have mutations in the KRAS2 gene.

The patient Tumours in the head of the pancreas present with *painless obstructive jaundice*. 75% of tumours in the body and tail present with epigastric pain (radiates to back and relieved by sitting forward). Either may cause anorexia, weight loss, diabetes, or acute pancreatitis. *Rarer features:* Thrombophlebitis migrans (eg an arm vein becomes swollen and red, then a leg vein); ↑Ca^{2+}; marantic endocarditis; portal hypertension (splenic vein thrombosis); nephrosis (renal vein metastases). *Signs:* Jaundice + palpable gallbladder (Courvoisier's 'law', p272); epigastric mass; hepatomegaly; splenomegaly; lymphadenopathy; ascites.

Tests *Blood:* Cholestatic jaundice. ↑CA 19-9 (p531) is non-specific, but helps assess prognosis. *Imaging:* US or CT can show a pancreatic mass ± dilated biliary tree ± hepatic metastases. They can guide biopsy and help staging prior to surgery/stent insertion. ERCP/MRCP (p742) show biliary tree anatomy and may localize the site of obstruction. EUS (endoscopic sonography) is an emerging adjunct for diagnosis and staging. *℞:* Most ductal cancers present with metastatic disease; <20% are suitable for radical surgery. *Surgery:* Resection (pancreatoduodenectomy: Whipple's, p271, fig 6.23) is a major undertaking best considered only where no distant metastases and where vascular invasion is still at a minimum. Post-op morbidity is high (mortality <5%); non-curative resection confers no survival benefit. *Laparoscopic excision:* Tail lesions are easiest. *Post-op chemotherapy:* Delays disease progression. *Palliation of jaundice:* Endoscopic or percutaneous stent insertion may help jaundice and anorexia. Rarely, palliative bypass surgery is done for duodenal obstruction or unsuccessful ERCP. *Pain:* Disabling pain may need big doses of opiates (p575), or radiotherapy. Coeliac plexus infiltration with alcohol may be done at the time of surgery, or percutaneously. Referral to a palliative care team is essential.

Prognosis Often dismal. Mean survival <6 months. 5yr survival: 3%. Overall 5yr survival after Whipple's procedure 5–14%. Prognosis is better if: tumour <3cm; no nodes involved; −ve resection margins at surgery; ampullary or islet cell tumours.

Carcinoid tumours

This is a specialized area! A diverse group of tumours of enterochromaffin cell (neural crest) origin, by definition capable of producing 5HT. Common sites: appendix (45%), ileum (30%), or rectum (20%).[22] They also occur elsewhere in the GI tract, ovary, testis, and bronchi. 80% of tumours >2cm across will metastasize (ie consider all as malignant). **Symptoms and signs** Initially few. GI tumours can cause appendicitis, intussusception, or obstruction. Hepatic metastases may cause RUQ pain. Tumours may secrete bradykinin, tachykinin, substance P, VIP, gastrin, insulin, glucagon, ACTH (∴ Cushing's syndrome), parathyroid, and thyroid hormones. 10% are part of MEN-1 syndrome (p223); 10% occur with other neuroendocrine tumours.

Carcinoid syndrome Occurs in ~5% and implies hepatic involvement.

Symptoms and signs: Bronchoconstriction; paroxysmal flushing especially in upper body (± migrating weals); diarrhoea; CCF (tricuspid incompetence and pulmonary stenosis from 5HT-induced fibrosis). ►*Carcinoid crisis:* See BOX 'Carcinoid crisis'.

Tests ↑24h urine 5-hydroxyindoleacetic acid (5HIAA, a 5HT metabolite; levels change with drugs and diet: discuss with lab). CXR + chest/pelvis MRI/CT help locate primary tumours. Plasma chromogranin A (reflects tumour mass); ^{111}Indium octreotide scintigraphy (octreoscan) and positron emission tomography (p739) also have a role. Echocardiography and BNP (p137) can be used to investigate carcinoid heart disease.

Treatment *Carcinoid syndrome:* Octreotide (somatostatin analogue) blocks release of tumour mediators and counters peripheral effects. Long-acting alternative: lanreotide. Loperamide for diarrhoea. *Tumour therapy:* Resection is the only cure for carcinoid tumours so it is vital to find the primary site. At surgery, tumours are an intense yellow. Procedures depend on site, eg rectal carcinoid tumours <1cm can be resected endoscopically. Debulking (eg enucleating), embolization, or radiofrequency ablation of hepatic metastases can ↓ symptoms. Give octreotide cover to avoid precipitating a massive carcinoid crisis.

Median survival 5–8yrs (~3yrs if metastases are present, but may be up to 20yrs; so beware of giving up too easily, even in metastatic disease).

►►Carcinoid crisis

When a tumour outgrows its blood supply or is handled too much during surgery, mediators flood out. There is life-threatening vasodilation, hypotension, tachycardia, bronchoconstriction, and hyperglycaemia. It is treated with high-dose octreotide, supportive measures, and careful management of fluid balance (ie a central line is needed—see p775 for insertion technique).

Whipple's procedure

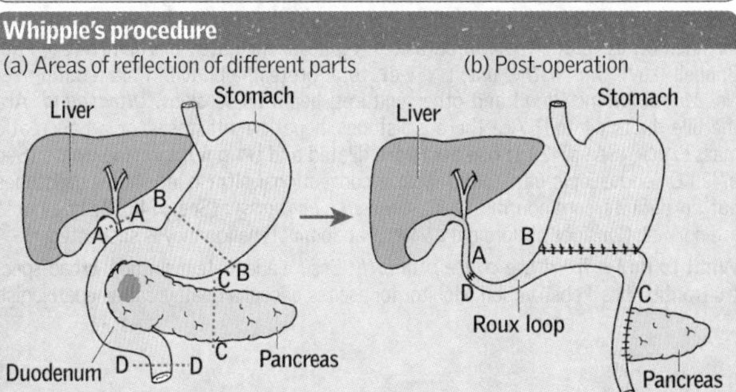

Fig 6.23 Whipple's procedure may be used for removing masses in the head of the pancreas—typically from pancreatic carcinoma or, rarely, a carcinoid tumour.[10]

22 Some are never clinically detected: 1 in 300 autopsies have a small bowel carcinoid tumour.

Jaundice

Jaundice refers to yellowing of skin, sclerae, and mucosae from ↑plasma bilirubin (visible at ≳60μmol/L fig 6.24). Jaundice is classified by the site of the problem (pre-hepatic, hepatocellular, or cholestatic/obstructive) or by the type of circulating bilirubin (conjugated or unconjugated, fig 6.25).

Unconjugated hyperbilirubinaemia As unconjugated bilirubin is water-insoluble, it does not enter urine, resulting in unconjugated hyperbilirubinaemia.

Overproduction: Haemolysis (p338, eg malaria/DIC, etc); ineffective erythropoiesis.
Impaired hepatic uptake: Drugs (paracetamol, rifampicin), ischaemic hepatitis.
Impaired conjugation: Eponymous syndromes: Gilbert's, p700; Crigler–Najjar, p696.
Physiological neonatal jaundice: Caused by a combination of the above, *OHCS* p115.

Conjugated hyperbilirubinaemia As conjugated bilirubin is water-soluble, it is excreted in urine, making it dark. Less conjugated bilirubin enters the gut and the faeces become pale. When severe, it can be associated with an intractable pruritus which is best treated by relief of the obstruction.

Hepatocellular dysfunction: There is hepatocyte damage, usually with some cholestasis. *Causes:* Viruses: hepatitis (p278), CMV (p405), EBV (p405); drugs (see table 6.10); alcohol; cirrhosis (see BOX 'Causes of jaundice'); liver metastases/abscess; haemochromatosis; autoimmune hepatitis (AIH); septicaemia; leptospirosis; syphilis; α_1-antitrypsin deficiency (p290); Budd–Chiari (p696); Wilson's disease (p285); failure to excrete conjugated bilirubin (Dubin–Johnson & Rotor syndromes, p698, p710); right heart failure; toxins, eg carbon tetrachloride; fungi (fig 6.26).

Impaired hepatic excretion (cholestasis): Primary biliary cholangitis; primary sclerosing cholangitis; drugs (see table 6.10); common bile duct gallstones; pancreatic cancer; compression of the bile duct, eg lymph nodes at the porta hepatis; cholangiocarcinoma; choledochal cyst; Caroli's disease;[23] Mirrizi's syndrome (obstructive jaundice from common bile duct compression by a gallstone impacted in the cystic duct, often associated with cholangitis).

The patient *Ask:* About blood transfusions, IV drug use, body piercing, tattoos, sexual activity, travel abroad, jaundiced contacts, family history, alcohol use, and *all* medications (eg old drug charts; GP records). *Examine:* For signs of chronic liver disease (p276), hepatic encephalopathy (p275), lymphadenopathy, hepatomegaly, splenomegaly, ascites, and a palpable gallbladder (if seen with painless jaundice the cause is not gallstones—Courvoisier's 'law').[24] Pale stools + dark urine ≈ cholestatic jaundice.

Tests See p276 for screening tests in suspected liver disease. *Urine:* Bilirubin is absent in pre-hepatic causes; in obstructive jaundice, urobilinogen is absent. *Haematology:* FBC, clotting, film, reticulocyte count, Coombs' test and haptoglobins for haemolysis (p336), malaria parasites (eg if unconjugated bilirubin/fever); Paul Bunnell (EBV). *Chemistry:* U&E, LFT, γ-GT, total protein, albumin.[25] Paracetamol levels. *Microbiology:* Blood and other cultures; hepatitis serology. *Ultrasound:* Are the bile ducts dilated? Are there gallstones, hepatic metastases, or a pancreatic mass? *ERCP:* (See p742.) If bile ducts are dilated and LFT not improving. *MRCP:* (See p742.) Or endoscopic ultrasound (EUS) if conventional ultrasound shows gallstones but no definite common bile duct stones. *Liver biopsy:* (See p248.) If bile ducts are normal. Consider abdominal *CT/MRI* if abdominal malignancy is suspected.

What to do? ►►*Treat the cause promptly.* Ensure adequate hydration; broad-spectrum antibiotics if obstruction. Monitor for ascites, encephalopathy; call a hepatologist.

23 Multiple segmental cystic or saccular dilatations of intrahepatic bile ducts with congenital hepatic fibrosis. It may present in 20yr-olds, with portal hypertension ± recurrent cholangitis/cholelithiasis.
24 Pancreatic or gallbladder cancer is more likely, as stones lead to a fibrotic, unexpandable gallbladder.
25 Albumin & INR are the best indicators of hepatic synthetic function. ↑Transaminases (ALT, AST) indicate hepatocyte damage. ↑ALP suggests obstructive jaundice, but also occurs in hepatocellular jaundice, malignant infiltration, pregnancy (placental isoenzyme), Paget's disease, and childhood (bone isoenzyme).

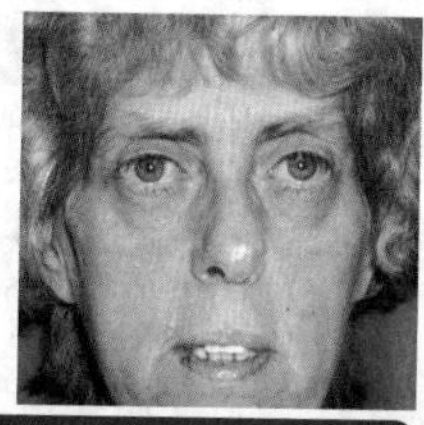

Fig 6.24 It's easy to miss mild jaundice, especially under fluorescent light, so take your patient to the window, and as you both gaze at the sky, use the opportunity to broaden the horizons of your enquiries... where have you been... where are you going...who are you with... what are you taking...? In the gaps, your patient may tell you the diagnosis—alcohol or drug abuse, sexual infections/hepatitis, or worries about the side-effects of their TB or HIV medication or a spreading cancer 'from this lump here which I haven't told anyone about yet'. Reproduced from Roper, *Clinical Skills*, 2014, with permission from Oxford University Press.

The pathway of bilirubin metabolism

In the liver, bilirubin is conjugated with glucuronic acid by hepatocytes, making it water-soluble. Conjugated bilirubin is secreted in bile and passes into the gut. Some is taken up again by the liver (via the enterohepatic circulation) and the rest is converted to urobilinogen by gut bacteria. Urobilinogen is either reabsorbed and excreted by the kidneys, or converted to stercobilin, which colours faeces brown.

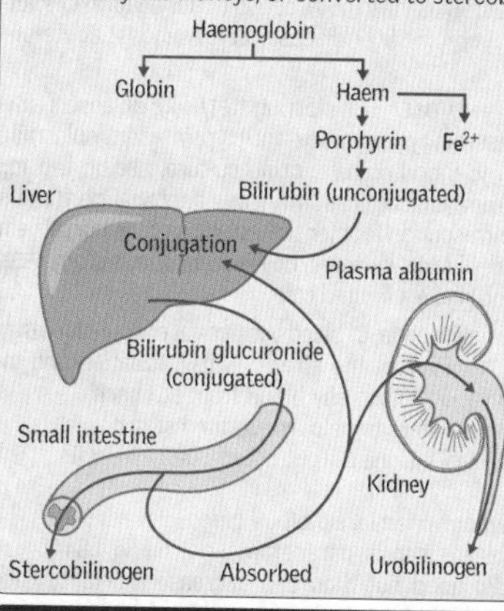

Fig 6.25 Bilirubin is formed by the breakdown of haemoglobin in a 3-step process: hepatic uptake, conjugation, and excretion.

Causes of jaundice in a previously stable patient with cirrhosis

- Sepsis (esp. UTI, pneumonia, or peritonitis)
- Malignancy: eg hepatocellular carcinoma
- Alcohol; drugs (table 6.10)
- GI bleeding.

Signs of decompensation: Jaundice; ascites; UGI bleed; encephalopathy.

Table 6.10 Examples of drug-induced jaundice

Haemolysis	• Antimalarials (eg dapsone)	
Hepatitis	• Paracetamol overdose (p844)	• Sodium valproate
	• Isoniazid, rifampicin, pyrazinamide	• Halothane
	• Monoamine oxidase inhibitors	• Statins
	• Flucloxacillin (may be weeks after Rx)	• Sulfonylureas
Cholestasis	• Fusidic acid, co-amoxiclav, nitrofurantoin	• Prochlorperazine
	• Steroids (anabolic; the Pill)	• Chlorpromazine

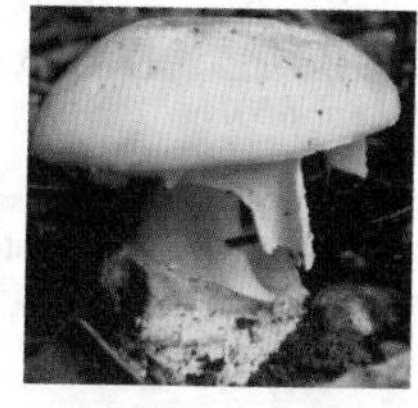

Fig 6.26 *Amanita phalloides* (Latin for 'phallic toadstool'; also known as the 'death cap') is a lethal cause of jaundice. It is the most toxic mushroom known. After ingestion (its benign appearance is confusing), amatoxins induce hepatic necrosis leaving few options other than transplantation.

©Ian Herriott. NB: don't use this image for identification!

Liver failure

Definitions Liver failure may be recognized by the development of coagulopathy (INR>1.5) and encephalopathy. This may occur suddenly in the previously healthy liver = *acute liver failure* (hyperacute = onset ≤7d; acute = 8–21d; subacute = 4–26wks.) More often it occurs on a background of cirrhosis = *chronic liver failure*. *Fulminant hepatic failure* is a clinical syndrome resulting from massive necrosis of liver cells leading to severe impairment of liver function.

Causes *Infections:* Viral hepatitis (esp. B, C, CMV), yellow fever, leptospirosis. *Drugs:* Paracetamol overdose, halothane, isoniazid. *Toxins: Amanita phalloides* mushroom (fig 6.26), carbon tetrachloride. *Vascular:* Budd-Chiari syn. (p696), veno-occlusive disease. *Others:* Alcohol, fatty liver disease, primary biliary cholangitis, primary sclerosing cholangitis, haemochromatosis, autoimmune hepatitis, α_1-antitrypsin deficiency, Wilson's disease, fatty liver of pregnancy (*OHCS* p25), malignancy.

Signs Jaundice, hepatic encephalopathy (see BOX 'Hepatic encephalopathy'), *fetor hepaticus* (smells like pear drops), asterixis/flap (p50), constructional apraxia (cannot copy a 5-pointed star?). Signs of chronic liver disease (p276) suggest acute-on-chronic hepatic failure.

Tests *Blood:* FBC (?infection,[26] ?GI bleed), U&E,[27] LFT, clotting (↑PT/INR), glucose, paracetamol level, hepatitis, CMV and EBV serology, ferritin, α_1-antitrypsin, caeruloplasmin, autoantibodies (p284). *Microbiology:* Blood culture; urine culture; ascitic tap for MC&S of ascites—neutrophils >250/mm^3 indicates spontaneous bacterial peritonitis (p276). *Radiology:* CXR; abdominal ultrasound; Doppler flow studies of the portal vein (and hepatic vein in suspected Budd-Chiari syndrome, p696). *Neurophysiology:* EEG, evoked potentials (and neuroimaging) have a limited role.

Management ►►Beware sepsis, hypoglycaemia, GI bleeds/varices, & encephalopathy:
- Nurse with a 20° head-up tilt in ITU. Protect the airway with intubation and insert an NG tube to avoid aspiration and remove any blood from stomach.
- Insert urinary and central venous catheters to help assess fluid status.
- Monitor T°, respirations, pulse, BP, pupils, urine output hourly. Daily weights.
- Check FBC, U&E, LFT, and INR daily.
- 10% glucose IV, 1L/12h to avoid hypoglycaemia. Do blood glucose every 1–4h.
- Treat the cause, if known (eg GI bleeds, sepsis, paracetamol poisoning, p844).
- If malnourished, get dietary help: good nutrition can decrease mortality. Give thiamine and folate supplements (p714).
- Treat seizures with phenytoin (p826).[11]
- Haemofiltration or haemodialysis, if renal failure develops (BOX 'What is hepatorenal syndrome?').
- Try to avoid sedatives and other drugs with hepatic metabolism (BOX 'Prescribing in liver failure' and *BNF*).
- Consider PPI as prophylaxis against stress ulceration, eg omeprazole 40mg/d IV/PO.
- Liaise early with nearest transplant centre regarding appropriateness.

Treat complications *Cerebral oedema:* On ITU: 20% mannitol IV; hyperventilate.

Ascites: Restrict fluid, low-salt diet, weigh daily, diuretics (p276).

Bleeding: Vitamin K 10mg/d IV for 3d, platelets, FFP + blood as needed ± endoscopy.

Blind ℞ of infection: Ceftriaxone 1–2g/24h IV, *not* gentamicin (↑risk of renal failure).

↓Blood glucose: If ≤2mmol/L or symptomatic, ℞ 50mL of 50% glucose IV; check often.

Encephalopathy: Avoid sedatives; 20° head-up tilt in ITU; correct electrolytes; lactulose 30–50mL/8h (aim for 2–4 soft stools/d) is catabolized by bacterial flora to short-chain fatty acids which ↓colonic pH and trap NH_3 in the colon as NH_4^+; Rifaximin 550mg/12h is a non-absorbable oral antibiotic that ↓ numbers of nitrogen-forming gut bacteria.

Worse prognosis if Grade III–IV encephalopathy, age >40yrs, albumin <30g/L, ↑INR, drug-induced liver failure, late-onset hepatic failure worse than fulminant failure.

26 Neutrophilic leucocytosis need not mean a secondary infection: alcoholic hepatitis may be the cause.
27 Urea is synthesized in the liver, so is a poor test of renal function in liver failure; use creatinine instead

Prescribing in liver failure

Avoid drugs that constipate (↑risk of encephalopathy), oral hypoglycaemics, and saline-containing IVIs. *Warfarin* effects are enhanced. *Hepatotoxic drugs include* paracetamol, methotrexate, isoniazid, azathioprine, phenothiazines, oestrogen, 6-mercaptopurine, salicylates, tetracycline, mitomycin.

Hepatic encephalopathy: letting loose some false neurotransmitters

As the liver fails, nitrogenous waste (as ammonia) builds up in the circulation and passes to the brain, where astrocytes clear it (by processes involving the conversion of glutamate to glutamine). This excess glutamine causes an osmotic imbalance and a shift of fluid into these cells—hence cerebral oedema. Grading:

I Altered mood/behaviour; sleep disturbance (eg reversed sleep pattern); dyspraxia ('Please copy this 5-pointed star'); poor arithmetic. No liver flap.
II Increasing drowsiness, confusion, slurred speech ± liver flap, inappropriate behaviour/personality change (ask the family—don't be too tactful).
III Incoherent; restless; liver flap; stupor.
IV Coma.

►What else could be clouding consciousness? Hypoglycaemia; sepsis; trauma; postictal.

What is hepatorenal syndrome (HRS)?

Cirrhosis + ascites + renal failure ≈ HRS—*if other causes of renal impairment have been excluded*. Abnormal haemodynamics causes splanchnic and systemic vasodilation, but renal *vasoconstriction*. Bacterial translocation, cytokines, and mesenteric angiogenesis cause splanchnic vasodilation, and altered renal autoregulation is involved in the renal vasoconstriction.

Types of HRS: HRS 1 is a rapidly progressive deterioration in circulatory and renal function (median survival <2wks), often triggered by other deteriorating pathologies. Terlipressin resists hypovolaemia. Haemodialysis may be needed. *HRS 2* is a more steady deterioration (survival ~6 months). Transjugular intrahepatic portosystemic stent shunting may be required (TIPS, p257).

Other factors in cirrhosis may contribute to poor renal function (p277).

Transplants: Liver transplant may be required. After >8–12wks of pre-transplant dialysis, some may be considered for combined liver-kidney transplantation.

King's College Hospital criteria in acute liver failure

Paracetamol-induced liver failure

- Arterial pH <7.3 24h after ingestion.

Or all of the following:

- Prothrombin time (PT) >100s
- Creatinine >300μmol/L
- Grade III or IV encephalopathy.

Non-paracetamol liver failure

- PT >100s.

Or 3 out of 5 of the following:

1. Drug-induced liver failure
2. Age <10 or >40yrs old
3. >1wk from 1st jaundice to encephalopathy
4. PT >50s
5. Bilirubin ≥300μmol/L.

Fulfilling these criteria predicts poor outcome in acute liver failure and should prompt consideration for transplantation (p277).

Cirrhosis

Cirrhosis (Greek *kirrhos* = yellow) implies irreversible liver damage. Histologically, there is loss of normal hepatic architecture with bridging fibrosis and nodular regeneration.

Causes Most often chronic alcohol abuse, HBV, or HCV infection. Others: see BOX 'Causes of cirrhosis'.

Signs Leuconychia: white nails with lunulae undemarcated, from hypoalbuminaemia; Terry's nails—white proximally but distal ⅓ reddened by telangiectasias; clubbing; palmar erythema; hyperdynamic circulation; Dupuytren's contracture; spider naevi (fig 6.27); xanthelasma; gynaecomastia; atrophic testes; loss of body hair; parotid enlargement (alcohol); hepatomegaly, or small liver in late disease; ascites; splenomegaly.

Complications *Hepatic failure:* Coagulopathy (failure of hepatic synthesis of clotting factors); encephalopathy (p259); hypoalbuminaemia (oedema); sepsis (pneumonia; septicaemia); spontaneous bacterial peritonitis (SBP); hypoglycaemia. *Portal hypertension:* Ascites (fig 6.28); splenomegaly; portosystemic shunt including oesophageal varices (± life-threatening upper GI bleed) and *caput medusae* (enlarged superficial periumbilical veins). *HCC:* ↑risk.

Tests *Blood:* LFT: ↔ or ↑bilirubin, ↑AST, ↑ALT, ↑ALP, ↑γGT. Later, with loss of synthetic function, look for ↓albumin ± ↑PT/INR. ↓WCC & ↓platelets indicate hypersplenism. *Find the cause:* ferritin, iron/total iron-binding capacity (p288); hepatitis serology (p278); immunoglobulins (p290); autoantibodies (ANA, AMA, SMA, p553); α-feto protein (p286); caeruloplasmin in patients <40yrs old (p285); α_1-antitrypsin (p290). *Liver ultrasound + duplex:* May show a small liver or hepatomegaly, splenomegaly, focal liver lesion(s), hepatic vein thrombus, reversed flow in the portal vein, or ascites. *MRI:* ↑Caudate lobe size, smaller islands of regenerating nodules, and the presence of the right posterior hepatic notch are more frequent in alcoholic cirrhosis than in virus-induced cirrhosis. *Ascitic tap:* Should be performed and fluid sent for urgent MC&S—neutrophils >250/mm^3 indicates spontaneous bacterial peritonitis (see later in topic for treatment). *Liver biopsy:* (See p248.) Confirms the clinical diagnosis.

Management *General:* Good nutrition is vital. Alcohol abstinence (p280). Avoid NSAIDs, sedatives, and opiates. Colestyramine helps pruritus (4g/12h PO, 1h after other drugs). Consider ultrasound ± α-fetoprotein every 6 months to screen for HCC (p286) in those where this information will change management. *Specific:* For hepatitis-induced cirrhosis see p278. High-dose ursodeoxycholic acid in PBC (p282) may improve LFT and improve transplant-free survival. Penicillamine for Wilson's disease (p285). *Ascites:* Fluid restriction (<1.5L/d), low-salt diet (40–100mmol/d). Give *spironolactone* 100mg/24h PO; ↑dose as tolerated (max 400mg/24h)—it counters deranged renin-angiotensin-aldosterone (RAA) axis. Chart daily weight and aim for weight loss of ≤½kg/d. If response is poor, add furosemide ≤120mg/24h PO; do U&E (watch Na$^+$) often. Therapeutic paracentesis with concomitant albumin infusion (6–8g/L fluid removed) may be required. *Spontaneous bacterial peritonitis (SBP):* ►Must be considered in any patient with ascites who deteriorates suddenly (may be asymptomatic). Common organisms are *E. coli*, *Klebsiella*, and streptococci. ℞: eg piperacillin with tazobactam 4.5g/8h for 5d or until sensitivities known. Give prophylaxis for high-risk patients (↓albumin, ↑PT/INR, low ascitic albumin) or those who have had a previous episode: eg ciprofloxacin 500mg PO daily. *Encephalopathy:* Recurrent episodes may be reduced in frequency with prophylactic lactulose and rifaximin (p274). *Renal failure:* ↓hepatic clearance of immune complexes leads to trapping in kidneys (∴ IgA nephropathy ± hepatic glomerulosclerosis). See also p275 for hepatorenal syndrome.

Prognosis Overall 5yr survival is ~50%. Poor prognostic indicators: encephalopathy; serum Na$^+$<110mmol/L; serum albumin <25g/L; ↑INR.

Liver transplantation is the only definitive treatment for cirrhosis (p277). *Acute indications:* Acute liver failure meeting King's College criteria (see BOX 'King's College Hospital criteria in acute liver failure' p275) *Chronic indications:* Advanced cirrhosis of any cause; hepatocellular cancer (1 nodule <5cm or ≤5 nodules <3cm).

Fig 6.27 Spider naevi: a central arteriole, from which numerous vessels radiate (like the legs of a spider). These fill from the centre unlike telangiectasias that fill from the edge. They occur most commonly in skin drained by the superior vena cava. ≤5 are normal (especially in ♀). Causes include liver disease, OCP, and pregnancy (ie changes in oestrogen metabolism).

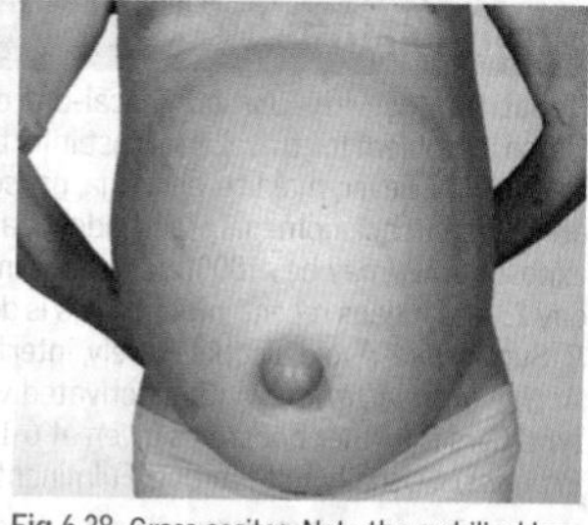

Fig 6.28 Gross ascites. Note the umbilical hernia (p613), gynaecomastia, and veins visible on the anterior abdominal wall.

Causes of cirrhosis

- Chronic alcohol use
- Chronic HBV or HCV infection[28]
- Genetic disorders: haemochromatosis (p288); α_1-antitrypsin deficiency (p290); Wilson's disease (p285)
- Hepatic vein events (Budd–Chiari, p696)
- Non-alcoholic steatohepatitis (NASH)
- Autoimmunity: primary biliary cholangitis (p282); primary sclerosing cholangitis (p282); autoimmune hepatitis (p284)
- Drugs: eg amiodarone, methyldopa, methotrexate.

Is cirrhosis becoming decompensated? ►►Prepare to make an arrest...

Cirrhosis may lie in wait for years before committing one of its three great crimes against the person: jaundice, ascites, or encephalopathy. There are almost always accomplices who, if arrested *now*, may stop a killing from unfolding. These usual suspects are: ►dehydration ►constipation ►covert alcohol use ►infection (eg spontaneous peritonitis, see earlier in topic) ►opiate over-use—or ►an occult GI bleed. If all have alibis, think of portal vein thrombosis, and call in the Chief Inspector.

Liver transplantation

The first liver transplant was in Denver, USA, in 1963. Now 800–1000 are performed each year in the UK (indications see p284). The limiting step for the procedure is often the waiting-list for a donor organ, which may be *cadaveric* (heart-beating or non-heart-beating) or from *live donors* (right lobe). *Contraindications* include extrahepatic malignancy; severe cardiorespiratory disease; systemic sepsis; expected non-compliance with drug therapy; ongoing alcohol consumption (in those with alcohol-related liver disease). Refer earlier rather than later, eg when ascites is refractory or after a 1st episode of bacterial peritonitis. Prioritization in the UK is based upon the UKELD (UK end-stage liver disease) score, calculated from serum Na^+, creatinine, bilirubin, and INR.[29]

Post-op: 12–48h on ITU, with enteral feeding starting as soon as possible and close monitoring of LFT. Immunosuppression examples: tacrolimus ± mycophenolate mofetil (or azathioprine) + prednisolone. Hyperacute rejection is a result of ABO incompatibility. Acute rejection (T-cell mediated, at 5–10d): the patient feels unwell with pyrexia and tender hepatomegaly—often managed by altering the immunosuppressives. Other complications: sepsis (esp. Gram –ve and CMV), hepatic artery thrombosis, chronic rejection (at 6–9 months), disease recurrence, and, rarely, graft-versus-host disease. Average patient survival at 1yr is ~80% (5yr survival 60–90%; depends on the pre-op disease).

28 Clues as to which patients with chronic HCV will get cirrhosis: platelet count ≤140 × 10^9/L, globulin/albumin ratio ≥1, and AST/ALT ratio ≥1—100% +ve predictive value but lower sensitivity (~30%).
29 Online calculators available, eg at www.odt.nhs.uk

Viral hepatitis

Hepatitis A RNA virus. *Spread:* Faecal-oral or shellfish. Endemic in Africa and S America, so a problem for travellers. Most infections are in childhood. *Incubation:* 2–6wks. *Symptoms:* Fever, malaise, anorexia, nausea, arthralgia—then: jaundice (rare in children), hepatosplenomegaly, and adenopathy. *Tests:* AST and ALT rise 22-40d after exposure (ALT may be >1000IU/L), returning to normal over 5–20wks. IgM rises from day 25 and means recent infection. IgG is detectable for life.
℞: Supportive. Avoid alcohol. Rarely, interferon alfa for fulminant hepatitis.
Active immunization: With inactivated viral protein. 1 IM dose gives immunity for 1yr (20yrs if further booster is given at 6–12 months).
Prognosis: Usually self-limiting. Fulminant hepatitis is rare. Chronicity doesn't occur.

Hepatitis B virus (HBV, a DNA virus.) *Spread:* Blood products, IV drug abusers (IVDU), sexual, direct contact. *Deaths:* 1 million/yr. *Risk groups:* IV drug users and their sexual partners/carers; health workers; haemophiliacs; men who have sex with men; haemodialysis (and chronic renal failure); sexually promiscuous; foster carers; close family members of a carrier or case; staff or residents of institutions/prisons; babies of HBsAg +ve mothers; adopted child from endemic area.
Endemic in: Far East, Africa, Mediterranean. *Incubation:* 1–6 months.
Signs: Resemble hepatitis A but arthralgia and urticaria are commoner.
Tests: HBsAg (surface antigen) is present 1–6 months after exposure. HBeAg (e antigen) is present for 1½–3 months after acute illness and implies high infectivity. HBsAg persisting for >6 months defines carrier status and occurs in 5–10% of infections; biopsy may be indicated unless ALT↔ and HBV DNA <2000iu/mL. Antibodies to HBcAg (anti-HBc) imply past infection; antibodies to HBsAg (anti-HBs) alone imply vaccination. HBV PCR allows monitoring of response to therapy. See fig 6.29 and table 6.11. *Vaccination:* See p287. Passive immunization (specific anti-HBV immunoglobulin) may be given to non-immune contacts after high-risk exposure.
Complications: Fulminant hepatic failure, cirrhosis, HCC, cholangiocarcinoma, cryoglobulinaemia, membranous nephropathy, polyarteritis nodosa (p556).
℞: Avoid alcohol. Immunize sexual contacts. Refer all with chronic liver inflammation (eg ALT ≳30IU/L), cirrhosis, or HBV DNA >2000IU/mL for antivirals (choice is 48 wks pegylated (PEG) interferon alfa-2a vs long-term but better tolerated nucleos(t)ide analogues, eg tenofovir, entecavir). The aim is to clear HBsAg and ►prevent cirrhosis and HCC (risk is ↑↑ if HBsAg and HBeAg +ve).

Hepatitis C virus (HCV) RNA flavivirus. *Spread:* Blood: transfusion, IV drug abuse, sexual contact. UK prevalence: >200 000. Early infection is often mild/asymptomatic. ~85% develop silent chronic infection; ~25% get cirrhosis in 20yrs—of these, ≤4% get hepatocellular cancer (HCC)/yr. *Risk factors for progression:* Male, older, higher viral load, use of alcohol, HIV, HBV. *Tests:* LFT (AST:ALT <1:1 until cirrhosis develops, p276), anti-HCV antibodies confirms exposure; HCV-PCR confirms ongoing infection/chronicity; liver biopsy or non-invasive elastography if HCV-PCR +ve to assess liver damage and need for treatment. Determine HCV genotype (1–6).
℞: BOX; quit alcohol. *Other complications:* Glomerulonephritis; cryoglobulinaemia; thyroiditis; autoimmune hepatitis; PAN; polymyositis; porphyria cutanea tarda.

Hepatitis D virus (HDV) Incomplete RNA virus (needs HBV for its assembly). HBV vaccination prevents HDV infection. 5% of HBV carriers have HDV co-infection. It may cause acute liver failure/cirrhosis. *Tests:* Anti-HDV antibody (only ask for it if HBsAg +ve). ℞: As interferon alfa has limited success, liver transplantation may be needed.

Hepatitis E virus (HEV) RNA virus. Similar to HAV; common in Indochina (commoner in older men and also commoner than hepatitis A in UK); mortality is high in pregnancy. It is associated with pigs. Epidemics occur (eg Africa). Vaccine is available in China (not Europe). *Δ:* Serology. ℞: Nil specific.

Other infective causes of hepatitis EBV; CMV; leptospirosis; malaria; Q fever; syphilis; yellow fever.

Table 6.11 Serological markers of HBV infection

	Incubation	Acute	Carrier	Recovery	Vaccinated
LFT		↑↑↑	↑	Normal	Normal
HBsAg	+	+	+		
HBeAg	+	+	+/−		
Anti-HBs				+	+
Anti-HBe			+/−		
Anti-HBc IgM		+	+/−		
Anti-HBc IgG		+	+	+	

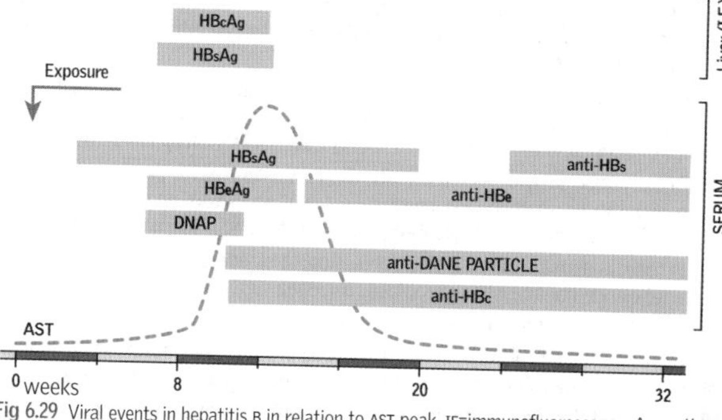

Fig 6.29 Viral events in hepatitis B in relation to AST peak. IF=immunofluorescence; Ag=antigen; HBs=hep. B surface; HBc=hep. B core; HBe=hep. B e antigen; DNAP=DNA polymerase.

The virologists' triumph: curing HCV

Since the original isolation of HCV in the late 1980s, riding the wave of the AIDS scare, less than three decades have elapsed. In this time, the comparatively simple genome of HCV has proven far easier than HIV to combat and the treatment of HCV has undergone nothing less than a revolution to the point where many common genotypes are considered curable.

All patients with sustained detectable HCV should be considered for treatment. Options are evolving rapidly, but centre on the use of inhibitors of non-structural viral proteins (eg ledipasvir+sofosbuvir) which are much better tolerated than the previous mainstay of treatment, pegylated interferon. Interferon-free regimens therefore eliminate major barriers to compliance including treatment duration and SEs, as well as achieving superior results: contemporary antiviral regimens can now realistically achieve the complete absence of PCR detectable virus in the blood 6 months post-treatment in almost 100% of genotype 1 patients, including patients with established cirrhosis. Ribavirin, a nucleoside analogue, can also increasingly be avoided in genotype 1, though it remains a useful treatment for the harder to treat genotypes 2 and 3. Here, reported rates of sustained undetectable viral levels now routinely exceed 90%. The costs of treatment are staggering, but cost-effectiveness analysis is favourable given the high cure rates and the significant public health burden of HCV. Genotypes 4, 5, or 6 are prevalent in lower-income countries and have received less attention but limited data where resources do exist suggest similarly good response rates.

Meanwhile, the threat of HIV remains. HCV prevalence is ~7% for sexually transmitted HIV and >90% for IV transmission. Untreated HIV may accelerate progress of HCV-induced liver fibrosis. All HIV/HCV co-infected patients should be assessed for combination antiviral therapy. Given the potential for toxicities and viral resistance mutation, such therapies should be planned and delivered through expert services.

Alcoholism

An alcoholic is one whose problematic pattern of alcohol use leads to clinically significant impairment or distress, manifested by multiple psychosocial, behavioural, or physiological features. Other addictions may coexist. Lifetime prevalence: ♂~10% (♀≈4%). ►Denial is a leading feature, so be sure to question relatives.

Organs affected ►Don't forget the risk of trauma while intoxicated.
The liver: Normal in 50%; ↑ or ↑↑γGT[30]—but may be ↑↑ in *any* type of liver inflammation, eg fatty liver, AIH (p284), HBV. *Fatty liver:* Acute/reversible, but may progress to cirrhosis if drinking continues (also seen in obesity, DM, and with amiodarone). *Alcoholic hepatitis:* See BOX 'Managing alcoholic hepatitis'. 80% progress to cirrhosis (hepatic failure in 10%). *Cirrhosis:* (See p276.) 5yr survival is 48% if drinking continues (if not, 77%). Biopsy: Mallory bodies ± neutrophil infiltrate (can be indistinguishable from NASH, p277).

CNS: Self neglect; ↓memory/cognition: high-potency vitamins IM may reverse it (p714; don't delay!); cortical atrophy; retrobulbar neuropathy; fits; falls; wide-based gait; neuropathy; confabulation/Korsakoff's (p704) ± Wernicke's encephalopathy (p714).

Gut: Obesity; D&V; gastric erosions; peptic ulcers; varices (p257); pancreatitis (acute or chronic); cancer (many types); oesophageal rupture (∵ vomiting against a closed glottis; suspect if shock and surgical emphysema in the neck: Boerhaave's syndrome).

Blood: ↑MCV; anaemia from: marrow depression, GI bleeding, alcoholism-associated folate deficiency, haemolysis; sideroblastic anaemia. See p326.

Heart: Arrhythmias; ↑BP; cardiomyopathy; sudden death in binge drinkers.

Reproduction: Testicular atrophy; ↓testosterone/progesterone; ↑oestrogen; fetal alcohol syndrome—↓IQ, short palpebral fissure, absent philtrum, and small eyes.

Withdrawal starts 10–72h after last drink. *Signs:* ↑Pulse; ↓BP; tremor; confusion; fits; hallucinations (*delirium tremens*)—may be visual or tactile, eg animals crawling all over skin. Consider it in any new (≲3d) ward patient with acute confusion.

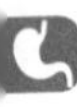

Management *Alcohol withdrawal:* There is almost no role for hospital inpatient 'detox' as a sole indication for admission however attractive the idea of a 'quick fix' may be—community-based services are much better placed to support cessation. Admit only if complicating or coexisting medical problems require inpatient treatment. Check BP + TPR/4h. Beware ↓BP. For the 1st 3d give generous chlordiazepoxide, eg 10–50mg/6h PO with additional doses PRN, then sum total dose and plan weaning regimen over 5–7d. Vitamins may be needed (p714). *Prevention:* (*OHCS* p512.) Alcohol-free beers; price may help promote lower-risk drinking. NB: there are no absolutes: risk is a continuum. *Suggest:* 1 Graceful ways of declining a drink, eg 'I'm seeing what it's like to go without for a bit'. 2 Not buying him- or herself a drink when it is his/her turn. 3 'Don't lift your glass to your lips until after the slowest drinker in your group takes a drink.' 4 'Sip, don't gulp.' Give follow-up and encouragement. *Treating established alcoholics:* May be rewarding, particularly if they really want to change. If so, group therapy or self-help (eg Alcoholics Anonymous) may be useful—especially if self-initiated and determined. Encourage the will to change.

Relapse 50% will relapse soon after starting treatment. Acamprosate (p449)may help intense anxiety, insomnia, and craving. CI: pregnancy, severe liver failure, creatinine >120μmol/L. SE: D&V, ↑ or ↓libido; dose example: 666mg/8h PO if >60kg and <65yrs old.It should be started as soon as acute withdrawal is complete and continued for ~1yr. Disulfiram can be used to treat chronic alcohol dependence. It causes acetaldehyde build-up (like metronidazole) with extremely unpleasant effects to *any* alcohol ingestion—eg flushing, throbbing headache, palpitations. Care must be taken to avoid alcohol (eg toiletries, food, medicines) since severe reactions can occur. ►Confer with experts if drugs are to be used.

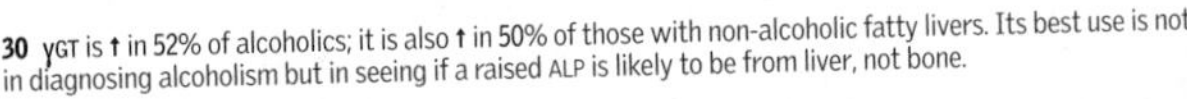

30 γGT is ↑ in 52% of alcoholics; it is also ↑ in 50% of those with non-alcoholic fatty livers. Its best use is not in diagnosing alcoholism but in seeing if a raised ALP is likely to be from liver, not bone.

Screening for unhealthy alcohol use

Several screening tools have been validated (eg AUDIT) but these typically require detailed questioning and careful scoring. For simplicity, a single-item question has much to recommend it, such as 'How many times in the past year have you had five (four for ♀) or more drinks in a day?' (+ve if >0; 82% sensitive, 79% specific). This can be followed up with the easily remembered **CAGE** questions: Ever felt you ought to **c**ut down on your drinking? Have people **a**nnoyed you by criticizing your drinking? Ever felt **g**uilty about your drinking? Ever had an **e**ye-opener in the morning? Those answering 'yes' to ≥2 may be exhibiting dependency (sensitivity 43–94%; specificity 70–97%), but accuracy does change according to background population. Those who refuse, or give unconvincing answers may have more to tell in their biochemistry: look for ↑γGT, ↑ALT, ↑MCV, AST:ALT>2, ↓urea, ↓platelets.

Managing alcoholic hepatitis

The patient: Malaise; ↑TPR; anorexia; D&V; tender hepatomegaly ± jaundice; bleeding; ascites. *Blood:* ↑WCC; ↓platelets (toxic effect or ∵ hypersplenism); ↑INR; ↑AST; ↑MCV; ↑urea. ►Jaundice, encephalopathy or coagulopathy ≈ *severe* hepatitis.

- Most need hospitalizing; urinary catheter and CVP monitoring may be needed.
- Screen for infections ± ascitic fluid tap and treat for SBP (p276).
- Stop alcohol consumption: for withdrawal symptoms, if chlordiazepoxide by the oral route is impossible, try lorazepam IM.
- Vitamins: vit K: 10mg/d IV for 3d. Thiamine 100mg/d PO (high-dose B vitamins can also be given IV as Pabrinex®—1 pair of ampoules in 50mL 0.9% saline IVI over ½h).
- Optimize nutrition (35–40kcal/kg/d non-protein energy). Use ideal body weight for calculations, eg if malnourished.
- Don't use low-protein diets even if severe encephalopathy is present. Give >1.2g/kg/d of protein; this prevents encephalopathy, sepsis, and some deaths.
- Daily weight; LFT; U&E; INR. If creatinine ↑, get help with this—HRS (p275). ↓Na^+ is common, but water restriction may make matters worse.
- Steroids may confer benefit in those with severe disease. The Maddrey Discriminant Factor (DF) = (4.6 × patient's prothrombin time in sec − control time) + bilirubin (μmol/L) roughly reflects mortality. If Maddrey score >31 and encephalopathy then consider prednisolone 40mg/d for 5d tapered over 3wks. ►CI: sepsis; variceal bleeding. The largest study to date (STOPAH) showed only a non-significant trend towards benefit with this regimen.

Prognosis: Mild episodes hardly affect mortality; if severe, mortality × 50% at 30d. 1yr after admission for alcoholic hepatitis, 40% are dead...a sobering thought.

Primary biliary cholangitis (PBC)

Interlobular bile ducts are damaged by chronic autoimmune granulomatous[31] inflammation causing cholestasis which may lead to fibrosis, cirrhosis, and portal hypertension. **Cause** Unknown environmental triggers (?pollutants, xenobiotics, non-pathogenic bacteria) + genetic predisposition (eg IL12A locus) leading to loss of immune tolerance to self-mitochondrial proteins. **Antimitochondrial antibodies (AMA)** are the hallmark of PBC. **Prevalence** ≤4/100 000. ♀:♂ ≈ 9:1. **Risk ↑ if** +ve family history (seen in 1–6%); many UTIs; smoking; past pregnancy; other autoimmune diseases; ↑use of nail polish/hair dye. **Typical age at presentation** ~50yrs.

The patient Often asymptomatic and diagnosed after incidental finding ↑ALP. Lethargy, sleepiness, and pruritus may precede jaundice by years. *Signs:* Jaundice; skin pigmentation; xanthelasma (p691); xanthomata; hepatosplenomegaly. *Complications:* Those of cirrhosis (p276); osteoporosis is common. Malabsorption of fat-soluble vitamins (A, D, E, K) due to cholestasis and ↓bilirubin in the gut lumen results in osteomalacia and coagulopathy; HCC (p286).

Tests *Blood:* ↑ALP, ↑γGT, and mildly ↑AST & ALT; late disease: ↑bilirubin, ↓albumin, ↑prothrombin time. 98% are AMA M2 subtype +ve, eg in a titre of 1:40 (see earlier in topic). Other autoantibodies (p553) may occur in low titres. Immunoglobulins are ↑ (esp. IgM). TSH & cholesterol ↑ or ↔. *Ultrasound:* Excludes extrahepatic cholestasis. *Biopsy:* Not usually needed (unless drug-induced cholestasis or hepatic sarcoidosis need excluding); look for granulomas around bile ducts ± cirrhosis.[31]

Treatment *Symptomatic:* Pruritus: try colestyramine 4–8g/24h PO; naltrexone and rifampicin may also help. Diarrhoea: codeine phosphate, eg 30mg/8h PO. Osteoporosis prevention: p682. *Specific: Fat-soluble vitamin prophylaxis:* vitamin A, D, and K. Consider high-dose ursodeoxycholic acid (UDCA)—it may improve survival and delay transplantation. SE: ↑weight. *Monitoring:* Regular LFT; ultrasound ± AFP twice-yearly if cirrhotic. *Liver transplantation:* (See p277.) For end-stage disease or intractable pruritus. Histological recurrence in the graft: ~17% after 5yrs; although graft failure can occur as a result of recurrence, it is rare and unpredictable.

Prognosis Highly variable. The Mayo survival model is a validated predictor of survival that combines age, bilirubin, albumin, PT time, oedema, and need for diuretics.

Primary sclerosing cholangitis (PSC)

Progressive cholestasis with bile duct inflammation and strictures (figs 6.30, 6.31).

Symptoms/signs Pruritus ± fatigue; if advanced: ascending cholangitis, cirrhosis, and hepatic failure. *Associations:* •♂ sex. •HLA-A1; B8; DR3. •AIH (p284); >80% of Northern European patients also have IBD, usually UC; this combination is associated with ↑↑risk of colorectal malignancy.

Cancers Bile duct, gallbladder, liver, and colon cancers are more common, so do yearly colonoscopy + ultrasound; consider cholecystectomy for gallbladder polyps.[32]

Tests ↑ALP, then ↑bilirubin; hypergammaglobulinaemia and/or ↑IgM; AMA −ve, but ANA, SMA, and ANCA may be +ve; see BOX and p553. *ERCP* (fig 6.30) or *MRCP* (fig 6.31) reveal duct anatomy and damage. *Liver biopsy* shows a fibrous, obliterative cholangitis.

Treatment *Liver transplant* is the mainstay for end-stage disease; recurrence occurs in up to 30%; 5yr graft survival is >60%. Prognosis is worse for those with IBD, as 5–10% develop colorectal cancer post-transplant. *Ursodeoxycholic acid* may improve LFT but has not shown evidence of survival benefit. High doses, eg 25–30mg/kg/d, may be harmful. Colestyramine 4–8g/24h PO for pruritus (naltrexone and rifampicin may also help). Antibiotics for bacterial cholangitis.

31 Other causes of liver granulomas: TB, sarcoid, infections with HIV (eg toxoplasmosis, CMV, mycobacteria), PAN, SLE, granulomatosis with polyangiitis, lymphoma, syphilis, isoniazid, quinidine, carbamazepine, allopurinol. Signs: PUO; ↑LFT.

32 Usually gallbladder polyps are an incidental finding on ultrasound, and they can often be left if <1cm diameter, but in PSC they are much more likely to become malignant.

Testing for autoantibodies—the anguish of partial understanding

The diagnostic approach to several inflammatory conditions includes the measurement of autoantibodies. Consequently and all too often, attempts to acquire (and test) medical knowledge may promote these antibody panels to a position as the final arbiter of disease diagnosis which, with their varying sensitivities and specificities, they are quite unfit to assume. Indeed, often just such a work-up shows strange overlap conditions between apparently different diseases: strange until we realize that these markers are just surrogates for processes that we lack a complete aetiological explanation for and in which the antibodies themselves may just be bystanders. Process that we lack the tools to visualize, as cells of the immune system continue their onslaught against their perceived enemies, driven by reasons that none present seem willing to reveal to our crude probing with blood tests, X-rays and biopsies. While the body knows no diseases, only pain and death, our minds attempt to impose a unitary disease on unsuspecting and sometimes innocent cells.

For example, clinically we observe that autoimmune hepatitis (AIH) frequently overlaps with PSC and IBD. A battery of antibody tests may sometimes help understand the dominant process, but equally may mystify matters still further if we attempt to apply our inadequate classifiers ('*But why is the ANCA not positive*?' cries the student, enraged at the failure of the miserable patient's B lymphocytes to do the honourable thing). As ever, management should be individualized dependent on liver and bowel histology, serum immunoglobulin levels, the degree of biochemical cholestasis, cholangiography, and, yes, autoantibodies.

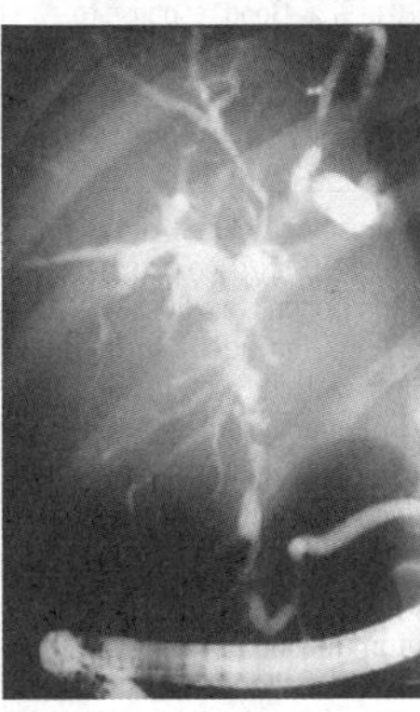

Fig 6.30 ERCP showing many strictures in the biliary tree with a characteristic 'beaded' appearance.

© Dr Anthony Mee.

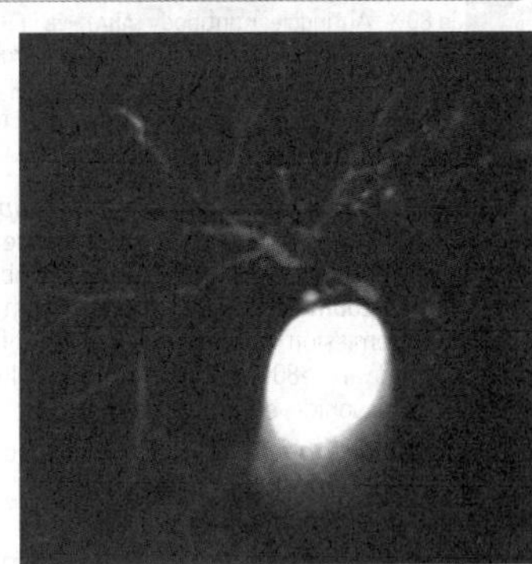

Fig 6.31 MRCP showing features of PSC. The intrahepatic ducts show multifocal strictures. Strictures can be hard to differentiate from cholangiocarcinoma (coexistence of UC may promote this development). Stenting may be needed.

©Norwich Radiology Department.

Autoimmune hepatitis (AIH)

An inflammatory liver disease of unknown cause[33] characterized by abnormal T-cell function and autoantibodies directed against hepatocyte surface antigens. Classification is by autoantibodies (see table 6.12). AIH predominantly affects young or middle-aged women (bimodal, ie 10-30yrs—or >40yrs old). Up to 40% present with acute hepatitis and signs of autoimmune disease, eg fever, malaise, urticarial rash, polyarthritis, pleurisy, pulmonary infiltration, or glomerulonephritis. The remainder present with gradual jaundice or are asymptomatic and diagnosed incidentally with signs of chronic liver disease. Amenorrhoea is common and disease tends to attenuate during pregnancy. **Complications** Those associated with cirrhosis (p276) and drug therapy.

Tests Serum bilirubin, AST, ALT, and ALP all usually ↑, hypergammaglobulinaemia (esp. IgG), +ve autoantibodies (see table 6.12). Anaemia, ↓WCC, and ↓platelets indicate hypersplenism. *Liver biopsy:* (See p248.) Mononuclear infiltrate of portal and periportal areas and piecemeal necrosis ± fibrosis; cirrhosis≈worse prognosis. *MRCP:* (See p742.) Helps exclude PSC if ALP ↑ disproportionately.

Diagnosis Depends on excluding other diseases (no lab test is pathognomonic). Diagnostic criteria based on IgG levels, autoantibodies, and histology in the absence of viral disease are helpful. Sometimes diagnosis is a challenge—there is overlap with other chronic liver disease: eg PBC (p282), PSC (p282) and chronic viral hepatitis.

Table 6.12 Classifying autoimmune hepatitis: types I-II

I	Seen in 80%. Typical patient: ♀<40yrs. Antismooth muscle antibodies (ASMA) +ve in 80%. Antinuclear antibody (ANA) +ve in 10%. ↑IgG in 97%. Good response to immunosuppression in 80%. 25% have cirrhosis at presentation.
II	Commoner in Europe than USA. More often seen in children, and more commonly progresses to cirrhosis and less treatable. Typically anti-liver/kidney microsomal type 1 (LKM1) antibodies +ve. ASMA and ANA −ve.

Management *Immunosuppressant therapy:* Prednisolone 30mg/d PO for 1 month; ↓ by 5mg a month to a maintenance dose of 5-10mg/d PO. Corticosteroids can sometimes be stopped after 2yrs but relapse occurs in 50-86%. Azathioprine (50-100mg/d PO) may be used as a steroid-sparing agent to maintain remission. Remission is achievable in 80% of patients within 3yrs. 10- and 20yr survival rates are >80%. SEs are a big problem (p376)—partly ameliorated by a switch to budesonide, eg in non-cirrhotic AIH.

Liver transplantation: (See p277.) Indicated for decompensated cirrhosis or if there is failure to respond to medical therapy, but recurrence may occur. It is effective (actuarial 10yr survival is 75%).

Prognosis Appears not to matter whether symptomatic or asymptomatic at presentation (10yr survival ~80% for both). The presence of cirrhosis at presentation reduces 10yr survival from 94% to 62%. Overlap syndromes: AIH-PBC (primary biliary cholangitis) overlap is worse than AIH-AIC (autoimmune cholangitis).

Associations of autoimmune hepatitis

- Pernicious anaemia
- Ulcerative colitis
- Glomerulonephritis
- Autoimmune thyroiditis
- Autoimmune haemolysis
- Diabetes mellitus
- PSC (p282)
- HLA A1, B8, and DR3 haplotype.

33 Hepatotropic viruses (eg measles, herpes viruses) and some drugs appear to trigger AIH in genetically predisposed individuals exposed to a hepatotoxic *milieu intérieur*. Viral interferon can inactivate cytochrome P450 enzymes (∴ ↓ metabolism of ex- or endogenous hepatotoxins). Resulting modifications to proteins may generate autoantigens driving CD4 T-helper cell activation.

Non-alcoholic fatty liver disease (NAFLD)

The commonest liver disorder in Western industrialized countries (prevalence≈20%), NAFLD[12] represents ↑fat in hepatocytes (steatosis) visualized, eg on ultrasound *that cannot be attributed to other causes* (most commonly alcohol so consider NAFLD if drink ♂<18U/wk, ♀<9U). If inflammation is also present (↑LFT, typically ↑ALT) = non-alcoholic steatohepatitis (NASH). Rule out other causes of liver disease (p284) and check for associated metabolic disorders (obesity, dyslipidaemia, diabetes, hypertension). Progression to cirrhosis may occur—biopsy or elastography may be needed (p248). **Risk factors for progression** Older age; obesity; DM; NASH. **Treatment** Control risk factors, including obesity (bariatic surgery helps). Address cardiovascular risk (commonest cause of death, see p93). Avoid alcohol consumption. No drug is of proven benefit, though vitamin E may improve histology in fibrosis (eg 400IU/d—higher doses associated with excess mortality). **Follow-up** Monitor for complications (NASH, cirrhosis, DM). If cirrhotic, screen for HCC with ultrasound ± AFP twice-yearly.

Wilson's disease/hepatolenticular degeneration

Wilson's disease is a rare (3/100 000) inherited disorder of copper excretion with excess deposition in liver and CNS (eg basal ganglia). It is treatable, so screen all with cirrhosis.

Genetics An autosomal recessive disorder of a copper transporting ATPase, ATP7B.

Physiology Total body copper content is ~125mg. Intake≈3mg/day (absorbed in proximal small intestine). In the liver, copper is incorporated into caeruloplasmin. In Wilson's disease, copper incorporation into caeruloplasmin in hepatocytes and excretion into bile are impaired. Copper accumulates in liver, and later in other organs.

Signs Children present with *liver disease* (hepatitis, cirrhosis, fulminant liver failure); young adults often start with *CNS signs:* tremor; dysarthria, dysphagia; dyskinesias; dystonias; dementia; Parkinsonism; ataxia/clumsiness.
Mood: Depression/mania; labile emotions; ↑↓libido; personality change. ►Ignoring these may cause years of needless misery: often the doctor who is good at combining the analytical and integrative aspects will be the first to make the diagnosis.
Cognition: ↓Memory; slow to solve problems; ↓IQ; delusions; mutism.
Kayser-Fleischer (KF) rings: Copper in iris (see 6 in following list); they are not invariable.
Also: Haemolysis; blue lunulae (nails); arthritis; hypermobile joints; grey skin.

Tests ►Equivocal copper studies need expert interpretation.

1. *Urine:* 24h copper excretion is *high*, eg >100mcg/24h (normal <40mcg).
2. ↑*LFT:* non-specific (but ALT >1500 is *not* part of the picture).
3. *Serum copper:* typically <11μmol/L.
4. ↓*Serum caeruloplasmin:* <200mg/L (<140mg/L is pathognomonic)—beware incidental low values in protein-deficiency states (eg nephrotic syndrome, malabsorption).
5. *Molecular genetic testing* can confirm the diagnosis.
6. *Slit lamp exam: KF rings:* in iris/Descemet's membrane (fig 5.42 *OHCS* p452).
7. *Liver biopsy:* ↑Hepatic copper (copper >250mcg/g dry weight); hepatitis; cirrhosis.
8. *MRI:* degeneration in basal ganglia, fronto-temporal, cerebellar, and brainstem.

Management *Diet:* Avoid foods with high copper content (eg liver, chocolate, nuts, mushrooms, legumes, and shellfish). Check water sources (eg wells, pipes) for copper. *Drugs:* Lifelong penicillamine (500mg/6–8h PO for 1yr, maintenance 0.75–1g/d). SEs: nausea, rash, ↓WCC, ↓Hb, ↓platelets, haematuria, nephrosis, lupus. Monitor FBC and urinary copper and protein excretion. *Liver transplantation:* (See p277.) If severe liver disease. *Screen siblings:* Asymptomatic homozygotes need treating.

Prognosis Pre-cirrhotic liver disease is reversible; CNS damage less so. There are no clear clinical prognostic indicators. Fatal events: liver failure, bleeding, infection.

Liver tumours

The commonest (90%) liver tumours are metastases (see fig 6.32), eg from breast, bronchus, or the gastrointestinal tract (see table 6.14). Primary hepatic tumours are much less common and may be benign or malignant (see table 6.13).

Symptoms Fever, malaise, anorexia, ↓weight, RUQ pain (∵ liver capsule stretch). Jaundice is late, except with cholangiocarcinoma. Benign tumours are often asymptomatic. Tumours may rupture causing intraperitoneal haemorrhage.

Signs Hepatomegaly (smooth, or hard and irregular, eg metastases, cirrhosis, HCC). Look for signs of chronic liver disease (p276) and evidence of decompensation (jaundice, ascites). Feel for an abdominal mass. Listen for a bruit over the liver (HCC).

Tests *Blood:* FBC, clotting, LFT, hepatitis serology, α-fetoprotein (↑ in 50–80% of HCC, though levels do not correlate with size, stage, or prognosis). *Imaging:* US or CT to identify lesions and guide biopsy. MRI is better at distinguishing benign from malignant lesions. Do ERCP (p742) and biopsy if cholangiocarcinoma is suspected. *Liver biopsy:* (See p248.) May achieve a histological diagnosis; ►careful multidisciplinary discussion is required if potentially resectable, as bleeding or seeding along the biopsy tract can occur. If the lesion could be a metastasis, find the primary, eg by CXR, mammography, colonoscopy, CT, MRI, or marrow biopsy.

Liver metastases Signify advanced disease. Treatment and prognosis vary with the type and extent of primary tumour. Chemotherapy may be effective (eg lymphomas, germ cell tumours). Small, solitary metastases may be amenable to resection (eg colorectal cancer). In most, treatment is palliative. *Prognosis:* Often <6 months.

Hepatocellular carcinoma (HCC) Primary hepatocyte neoplasia accounts for 90% of primary liver cancers; it is common in China & Africa (40% of cancers vs 2% in UK). *The patient:* Fatigue, ↓appetite, RUQ pain, ↓weight, jaundice, ascites, haemobilia.[34] ♂:♀≈3. *Causes:* HBV is the leading cause worldwide (esp. if high viral load; p278). HCV;[35] AIH (p284); cirrhosis (alcohol, haemochromatosis, PBC); non-alcoholic fatty liver; aflatoxin; *Clonorchis sinensis*; anabolic steroids.
Δ: 3-phase CT (delayed wash-out of contrast in a suspect mass); MRI; biopsy.
Treatment: Resecting solitary tumours <3cm across ↑ 3yr survival from 13% to 59%; but ~50% have recurrence by 3yrs.[36] Liver transplant gives a 5yr survival rate of 70%.[37] Percutaneous ablation, tumour embolization (TACE[38]), and sorafenib are options. *Prevention:* ►HBV vaccination (BOX and table 6.15). ►Don't reuse needles. ►Screen blood. ►↓Aflatoxin exposure (sun-dry maize). *AFP ± ultrasound (eg 6-monthly screen):* Consider if at ↑ risk: eg all with cirrhosis; or chronic HBV in Africans or older Asians.

Cholangiocarcinoma (Biliary tree cancer.) ~10% of liver primaries. *Causes:* Flukes (*Clonorchis*, p435); PSC (screening by CA19-9 may be helpful, p282); biliary cysts; Caroli's disease, p272; HBV; HCV; DM; N-nitroso toxins.
The patient: Fever, abdominal pain (±ascites), malaise, ↑bilirubin; ↑↑ALP.
Pathology: Usually slow-growing. Most are distal extrahepatic or perihilar.
Management: 70% inoperable at presentation. Of those that are, 76% recur. *Surgery:* eg major hepatectomy + extrahepatic bile duct excision + caudate lobe resection. 5yr survival ~30%. Post-op complications include liver failure, bile leak, and GI bleeding. *Stenting* of obstructed extrahepatic biliary tree, percutaneously or via ERCP (p742), improves quality of life. *Liver transplantation* rarely possible. *Prognosis:* ~5 months.

Benign tumours *Haemangiomas:* The commonest benign liver tumours. They are often an incidental finding on ultrasound or CT and don't require treatment. Avoid biopsy! *Adenomas:* Common. Causes: anabolic steroids, oral contraceptive pill; pregnancy. Only treat if symptomatic, or >5cm.

34 Haemobilia is late in HCC. Think of bleeding into the biliary tree whenever Quincke's triad obtains: RUQ pain, upper GI haemorrhage, and jaundice. It may be life-threatening.
35 5yr cumulative risk if cirrhosis is present is 30% in Japan and 17% in USA.
36 Operative mortality: 1.6%. Recurrence is more likely if histology showed neoplastic emboli in small vessels. Get early warning of recurrence by arranging imaging, eg if AFP >5.45mcg/L (esp. if trend is rising). Fibrolamellar HCC, which occurs in children and young adults, has a better prognosis.
37 Milan criteria for liver transplantation in HCC: 1 nodule <5cm or 2-3 nodules <3cm.
38 TACE=transarterial chemoembolization, eg with drug-eluting beads; it causes fever and abdo pain in 50%.

Table 6.13 Primary liver tumours

Malignant (prognosis—regardless of type—is poor)	Benign
HCC	Cysts
Cholangiocarcinoma	Haemangioma;* common, ♀:♂≈5:1
Angiosarcoma	Adenoma
Hepatoblastoma	Focal nodular hyperplasia
Fibrosarcoma & hepatic gastrointestinal stromal tumour (GIST†, formerly leiomyosarcoma)	Fibroma Benign GIST (=leiomyoma)

* Haemangiomas are hyperechoic on ultrasound; may be part of von Hippel-Lindau syndrome; may need surgery if diagnosis is uncertain (may be confused with HCC) or they are enlarging on 6-monthly US.

† GISTs are mesenchymal tumours that are more likely to be found in the gut as a spherical mass arising from the muscularis propria, eg with GI bleeding. If unresectable, imatinib ↑ 2yr survival from 26% to 76%.

Table 6.14 Origins of secondary liver tumours

Common in men	Common in women	Less common (either sex)
Stomach	Breast	Pancreas
Lung	Colon	Leukaemia
Colon	Stomach	Lymphoma
	Uterus	Carcinoid tumours

Vaccinating to prevent hepatitis B (and associated complications)

Use hepatitis B vaccine 1mL into deltoid; repeat at 1 & 6 months (child: 0.5mL × 3 into the anterolateral thigh). *Indications:* Everyone (WHO advice, even in areas of 'low' endemicity—in 2014 this meant that 82% of the world's children received protection against HBV). This contrasts with the approach in eg the UK and USA of targeting at-risk groups (p278). The immunocompromised and others may need further doses. Serology helps time boosters and finds non-responders (correlates with older age, smoking, and ♂ sex). ►*Know your own antibody level!*

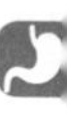

Table 6.15 Post-immunization anti-HBs titres and actions

Anti-HBs (IU/L)	Actions and comments (advice differs in some areas)
>1000	Good level of immunity; retest in ~4yrs.
100–1000	Good level of immunity; if level approaches 100, retest in 1yr.
<100	Inadequate; give booster and retest.
<10	Non-responder; give another set of 3 vaccinations. Retest; if <10 get consent to check hepatitis B status: HBsAg +ve means chronic infection; anti-HB core +ve represents past infection and immunity. If a non-responder is deemed susceptible to HBV, and has recently come in contact with risky bodily fluids, offer 2 doses of anti-hep B immunoglobulin.

NB: protection begins some weeks after dose 1, so it won't work if exposure is recent; here, specific antihepatitis B immunoglobulin is best if not already immunized.

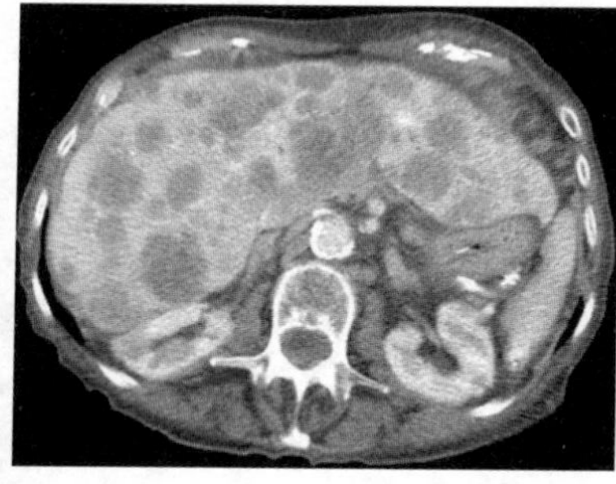

Fig 6.32 Axial CT of the liver after IV contrast showing multiple round lesions of varying size, highly suggestive of hepatic metastases.
Courtesy of Norwich Radiology Dept.

Hereditary haemochromatosis (HH)

An inherited disorder of iron metabolism in which ↑intestinal iron absorption leads to iron deposition in joints, liver, heart, pancreas, pituitary, adrenals, and skin. Middle-aged men are more frequently and severely affected than women, in whom the disease tends to present ~10yrs later (menstrual blood loss is protective).

Genetics HH is one of the commonest inherited conditions in those of Northern European (especially Celtic) ancestry (carrier rate of ~1 in 10 and a frequency of homozygosity of ~1 in 200–400). The gene responsible for most HH is HFE: the 2 commonest mutations are termed C282Y and H63D. C282Y accounts for 60–90% of HH, and H63D accounts for 1–3%, with compound heterozygotes accounting for 4–7%. Penetrance is variable—a significant fraction of C282Y homozygotes will not develop signs of iron overload during follow-up, complicating screening decisions.

The patient *Early on:* Nil—or tiredness; arthralgia (2nd+3rd MCP joints + knee pseudogout); ↓libido. *Later:* Slate-grey skin pigmentation; signs of chronic liver disease (p276); hepatomegaly; cirrhosis (esp. if drinks alcohol); dilated cardiomyopathy. *Endocrinopathies:* DM ('bronze diabetes' from iron deposition in pancreas); hypogonadism (p232) from ↓pituitary dysfunction.

Tests *Blood:* ↑LFT, ↑ferritin (♂>200/♀>150ng/mL; but inflammation will also ↑ferritin); ↑transferrin saturation[39] should all trigger suspicion. Confirm by HFE genotyping.

Images: Chondrocalcinosis (fig 6.33). Liver & cardiac MRI: Fe overload.

Liver biopsy: Perl's stain quantifies iron loading[40] and assesses disease severity.

Management *Venesect:* ~0.5–2 units/1–2wks, until ferritin ≤50mcg/L (may take 2yrs). Iron will continue to accumulate, so maintenance venesection is needed for life (1u every 2–3 months to maintain haematocrit <0.5, ferritin <100mcg/L, and transferrin saturation <40%). Consider desferrioxamine (p342) if intolerant of this. *Monitor:* LFT and glucose/diabetes (p206). HbA1c levels may be falsely low as venesection ↓the time available for Hb glycosylation. If cirrhotic, screen for HCC with ultrasound ± AFP twice-yearly.

Over-the-counter drugs: Ensure vitamin preparations contain no iron.

Diet: A well-balanced diet should be encouraged—there is no need to avoid iron-rich foods. Avoid alcohol. Avoid uncooked seafood (may contain bacteria that thrive on increased plasma iron concentrations, eg *Listeria monocytogenes*, *Vibrio vulnificus*).

Screening: Serum ferritin, transferrin saturation, and HFE genotype. ►Screen 1st-degree relatives by genetic testing even if they are asymptomatic and have normal LFT ideally prior to age where significant iron deposition likely to have occurred (eg 18–30yrs). Since C282Y homozygotes may never develop iron overload, population screening should not be performed.

Prognosis Venesection returns life expectancy to normal if non-diabetic and non-cirrhotic (and liver histology *can* improve). Arthropathy may improve or worsen. Gonadal failure may reverse in younger men. ►If cirrhosis, 22–30% get hepatocellular cancer, especially if: age >50yrs (risk ↑×13), HBsAg +ve (risk ↑×5), or alcohol abuse (risk ↑×2).

39 Transferrin saturation >45% is a sensitive threshold for further screening but will lead to some false +ves.
40 Although generally not required, biopsy quantifies hepatic iron loading and fibrosis. This helps determine the severity of liver disease, particularly in those with other underlying causes of chronic liver disease.

A bit about iron metabolism

60% of body iron is in haemoglobin, and erythropoiesis requires ~5-30mg iron/day—provided by macrophages (recycling of haeme iron after phagocytosis of old RBCs). Intestinal iron absorption (1-2mg/day) compensates for daily iron losses.

Red meats, liver, seafoods, enriched breakfast cereals and pulses, and some spices (eg paprika) are iron-rich. Most dietary iron is Fe^{3+}, which is reduced by low gastric pH and ascorbic acid (vitamin C) to better-absorbed Fe^{2+}. Absorption occurs mainly in the duodenum and jejunum, though very small amounts are absorbed in the stomach and ileum. Iron requirements are greater for women (menstrual loss), when growing, in pregnancy, and in chronic infection.

Hepcidin, a peptide synthesized in hepatocytes, secreted in plasma, is a negative regulator of gut iron absorption and haeme iron recycling by macrophages. Hepcidin synthesis is stimulated by iron and repressed by iron deficiency and by ↑marrow erythropoiesis (eg in anaemia, bleeding, haemolysis, dyserythropoiesis, or erythropoietin injections). Defects in the normal triggering of hepcidin by iron excess is a rare cause of haemochromatosis unrelated to HFE mutations, whereas a defect in hepcidin repression is responsible for an iron refractory iron deficiency anaemia.

In HH, the total body iron is up to 10-fold that of a normal person, with loading found particularly in the liver and pancreas (×100). Hepatic disease classically starts with fibrosis, progressing to cirrhosis as a late feature.

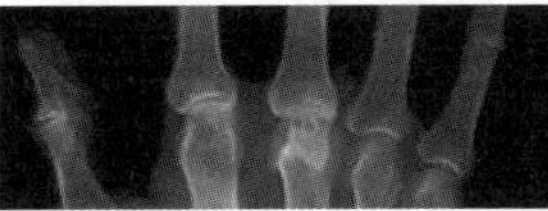

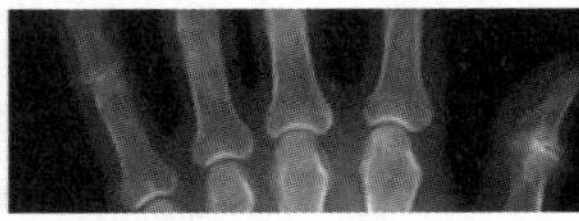

Fig 6.33 Haemochromatosis causes stressed joints to deteriorate faster than resting joints: the 2nd and 3rd MCP joints have osteophytes and narrowed joint spaces compared to the normal hand (right image) in this man who only used his dominant hand for his production line job.

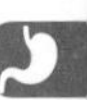

α_1-antitrypsin (A1AT) deficiency

A1AT deficiency is an inherited disorder affecting lung (emphysema) and liver (cirrhosis and HCC). A1AT is a glycoprotein and one of a family of serine protease inhibitors made in the liver that control inflammatory cascades. Deficiency is called a serpinopathy. It makes up 90% of serum α_1-globulin on electrophoresis (p687). A1AT deficiency is the chief genetic cause of liver disease in children. In adults, its lack is more likely to cause emphysema. Lung A1AT protects against tissue damage from neutrophil elastase—a process that is also induced by cigarette smoking (p184). **Prevalence** ~1:4000 (higher in Caucasians).

Genetics Genetic variants of A1AT are typed by electrophoretic mobility as *medium* (M), *slow* (S), or *very slow* (Z). S and Z types are due to single amino acid substitutions at positions 264 and 342, respectively. These result in ↓production of α_1-antitrypsin (S=60%, Z=15%). The normal genotype is PiMM, the high risk homozygote is PiZZ; heterozygotes are PiMZ and PiSZ (at low risk of developing liver disease).

The patient Symptomatic patients usually have the PiZZ genotype: dyspnoea from emphysema; cirrhosis; cholestatic jaundice. Cholestasis often remits in adolescence.

Tests *Serum α_1-antitrypsin* (α_1AT) levels ↓, usually (eg <11μmol/L or <75% of lower limit of normal, which is ~0.9g/L; labs vary). Note the 'usually'. Because A1AT is part of the acute-phase response, inflammation may hide a low level. Unless you do genotyping, you will inevitably mis-label some cirrhosis as cryptogenic. *Lung function testing:* Shows reductions in FEV_1 with obstructive pattern (p162). There may be some bronchdilator reversibility. *Liver biopsy:* (See p248.) Periodic acid Schiff (PAS) +ve; diastase-resistant globules. *Phenotyping:* By isoelectric focusing requires expertise to distinguish SZ and ZZ phenotypes. Phenotyping can miss null phenotypes. *Prenatal diagnosis:* Possible by DNA analysis of chorionic villus samples obtained at 11-13wks' gestation.

Management Smoking cessation. Prompt treatment/preventative vaccination for lung infections. Giving IV A1AT pooled from human plasma is expensive but COPD exacerbations *may* be prevented (no good randomized trials). *Liver transplantation:* Needed in decompensated cirrhosis. *Lung transplantation:* Improves survival and has a comparable survival to transplantation in non-A1AT-deficient COPD. *Inhaled A1AT:* Has been tried in lung disease.

Prognosis Some patients have life-threatening symptoms in childhood, whereas others remain asymptomatic and healthy into old age. Worse prognosis if male, a smoker, or obese. Emphysema is the cause of death in most, liver disease in ~5%. In adults, cirrhosis ± HCC affect 25% of A1AT-deficient adults >50yrs.

Approaches to abnormal liver function tests (LFTs)

Abnormal LFTs can be found in ~17% of the asymptomatic general population. Also, remember that a normal LFT does not exclude liver disease.

Tests of hepatocellular injury or cholestasis

Aminotransferases: (AST, ALT) Released in the bloodstream after hepatocellular injury. ALT is more specific for hepatocellular injury (but also expressed in kidney and muscle). AST is also expressed in the heart, skeletal muscle, and RBCs.

Alkaline phosphatase: May originate from liver, bone (so raised in growing children) or placenta.

Gamma-glutamyltransferase (GGT; γGT): Present in liver, pancreas, renal tubules, and intestine—but not bone, so it helps tell if a raised ALP is from bone (GGT↔) or liver (GGT↑). NB: it is not specific to alcohol damage to the liver.

Tests of hepatic function Serum albumin, serum bilirubin, PT (INR).

Hepatocellular predominant liver injury ↑AST & ↑ALT. Evaluate promptly, consider medications, collateral history from family ('Could he be consuming ↑alcohol?'); ultrasound for fatty liver, metastases, viral serology (hepatitis A, B, C, E, EBV, CMV).

Alcoholic liver disease: AST/ALT ratio is typically 2:1 or more. When the history is not reliable, normal ALP, ↑GGT, and macrocytosis suggest this condition.

Acute viral hepatitis: ↑ALT; bilirubin may be ↔. NB: AST may be ↑↑, p278, p281.

Chronic viral hepatitis: ↑ALT; HBV & C are a leading cause worldwide.

Autoimmune hepatitis (AIH): Occurs mainly in young and middle-aged females.

Fatty infiltration of the liver: (See p285.) Probably the chief cause of mildly raised LFTs in the general population and may be recognized on ultrasound.

Ischaemic hepatitis: Can be seen in conditions when effective circulatory volume is low (eg MI, hypotension, haemorrhage). ↑↑↑ALT, as well as LDH.

Drug-induced hepatitis: As no specific serology identifies most culprits, a good history is vital. Paracetamol overdose causes most acute liver failure in the UK.

Cholestasis predominant liver injury ALP and GGT are ↑; AST and ALT mildly↑.

Management For each specific diagnosis, manage accordingly. If asymptomatic and other tests are −ve, try lifestyle modification. Help reduce weight and alcohol use (p280 & *OHCS* p512); control DM & dyslipidaemia; stop hepatotoxic drugs.

Follow-up Repeat tests after 1-2 months; if still ↑, do US (±abdominal CT). If diagnosis still unclear, get help: is biopsy needed? Consider (if you haven't already) α_1-antitrypsin levels, serum caeruloplasmin (Wilson's disease), coeliac serology, ANA and ASMA (AIH, p284).

7 Renal medicine

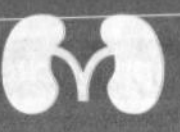

Contents

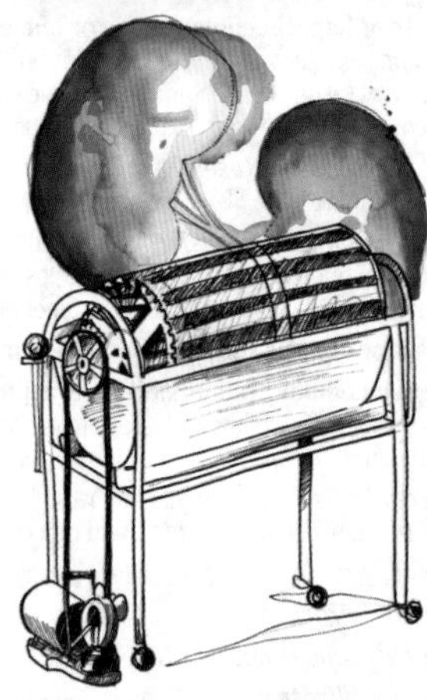

Fig 7.1 A 'rotating drum artificial kidney': one of the earliest dialysis machines built by Willem Kolff in 1943. Exiled to a remote Dutch hospital during the Nazi occupation of the Netherlands, the resourceful inventor assembled a junkyard construction using a water pump from a Ford model T, an aluminium drum from a downed warplane, washing machine parts, orange juice cans, and sausage skins. The first 16 patients to use the machine died. Then, in 1945, 67-year-old Sofia Maria Schafstadt ('Patient Number 17') was referred reluctantly to Kolff with 'poisoning'. Her blood was passed through his sausage-skin tube which was wrapped around the drum, rotating like a washing machine in a bath of salt water. A total of 80L of her blood was treated in this way, removing 60g of urea. After 11 hours she opened her eyes to declare, 'I'm going to divorce my husband'. This she duly achieved, as well as making medical history. Kolff chose not to patent his life-saving invention but donated copies to hospitals across the world.

We thank Dr Andrew Mooney, our Specialist Reader, for his contribution to this chapter.

Renal disease presents as:

1 Asymptomatic disease

- *Non-visible haematuria:* (NVH, microscopic haematuria.) Detected on urine dipstick on repeated testing. Most is not due to renal disease and urological investigation is first-line for all those aged >40 years. See p294.
- *Asymptomatic proteinuria:* Normal renal protein excretion is less than 150mg/24 hours (non-pregnant). Quantification by 24h urine collection is unreliable and rarely used in clinical practice. A spot urinary protein to creatinine ratio (P:CR) >15mg/mmol or urinary albumin to creatinine ratio (A:CR) >2.5(♂) or 3.5(♀)mg/mmol may signify either glomerular (common) or tubular (rare) pathology.
- *Abnormal renal function (GFR):* The glomerular filtration rate (GFR) is a measure of how much blood the kidneys are cleaning per minute. Direct measurement is invasive and time-consuming. Estimations derived from equations based on serum creatinine are widely used to give an eGFR (see p669). Errors in eGFR are caused by non-steady-state conditions, conditions which alter serum creatinine (diet, muscle mass), and eGFR is less accurate at higher levels of GFR. eGFR is therefore only part of the assessment of renal function.
- *High blood pressure:* A renal aetiology should be excluded if hypertension occurs with any indicators of renal disease: haematuria, proteinuria, ↓eGFR.
- *Electrolyte abnormalities:* Disorders of sodium, potassium, and acid-base balance (pp301 and 670–5) may be due to underlying renal disease.

2 With renal tract symptoms

- *Urinary symptoms: Dysuria* is a sensation of discomfort with micturition and may be accompanied by *urgency*, *frequency*, and *nocturia*. UTI is the primary differential. Consider prostatic aetiology if there is difficulty initiating voiding, poor stream and dribbling. *Oliguria* (<400mL/24 hours or <0.5mL/kg/hour) and *anuria* should trigger assessment and investigation for *acute kidney injury* (AKI) (see pp298–301). *Polyuria* is the voiding of abnormally high volumes of urine, usually from high fluid intake. Consider also DM, diabetes insipidus (p240), hypercalcaemia (p676), renal medullary disorders (causing impaired concentration of urine).
- *Loin pain:* Ureteric colic is severe and radiates anteriorly and to the groin. It is caused by a renal stone, clot, or a sloughed papilla. For pain confined to the loin consider pyelonephritis, renal cyst pathology, and renal infarct.
- *Visible haematuria:* (VH, macroscopic.) Urological investigation is required to exclude renal tract malignancy. Nephrological causes include polycystic kidney disease and glomerular disease (IgA p311, anti-glomerular basement membrane (anti-GBM) disease p311, Alport syndrome p320).
- *Nephrotic syndrome:* Proteinuria >3g/24 hours (=P:CR >300mg/mmol) with hypoalbuminaemia (<30g/L) and peripheral oedema. Renal biopsy is usually indicated in adults (p310).
- *Symptomatic chronic kidney disease:* Dyspnoea, anorexia, weight loss, pruritus, bone pain, sexual dysfunction, cognitive decline (pp302–5).

3 A systemic disorder with renal involvement

- *DM:* (p314.)
- *Metabolic*: Sickle cell disease (p315), tuberous sclerosis (p320), Fabry disease (p320), cystinosis (p321).
- *Auto-immune:* ANCA-associated vasculitis (p314, 556), SLE (p314), Henoch-Schonlein purpura (p311), systemic sclerosis (p315), sarcoid (p318), Sjögren's syndrome (p318, 710).
- *Infection*: Sepsis is a common cause of AKI. Specific renal involvement may occur with TB (p392), malaria, chronic hepatitis (p278), HIV (pp398–403).
- *Malignancy*: Obstruction, hypercalcaemia, direct toxicity, eg myeloma (p314).
- *Pregnancy:* Pre-eclampsia, obstruction.
- *Drugs used in systemic disorders:* NSAIDs, ACE-i, ARB, aminoglycosides, chemotherapy.

Urine

Perform dipstick urinalysis whenever you suspect renal disease. This is a crude way of checking whether the urine contains anything that it should not, eg protein, blood, glucose. Abnormalities can indicate intrinsic renal disease or renal tract abnormalities and usually require further investigation. However, a dipstick-positive catheter sample is difficult to interpret.

►Look for a urine dip result (before the catheter was inserted). A positive result indicates the need for specialist advice from nephrology/urology. A negative result *may* help to reassure you about the absence of intrinsic renal disease.

Proteinuria

Requires quantification. 24h collections are rarely used due to inaccuracy. Albumin:creatinine ratio (A:CR) or protein:creatinine ratio (P:CR) is performed on a random spot urine sample. Normal A:CR is <2.5(♂) or <3.5(♀). P:CR is <15. Approximate equivalent levels of proteinuria are given in table 7.1.

Table 7.1 Conversion factors

Protein excretion g/24h	A:CR mg/mmol	P:CR mg/mmol
0.15 (physiological)	2.5 ♂ or 3.5 ♀	15
0.5	30	50
1	70	100
3 (nephrotic range)	250	300

Causes of raised A:CR/P:CR: The higher the proteinuria, the more chance it is caused by glomerular disease, eg glomerulonephritis, DM, amyloidosis, myeloma (though dipsticks do not detect light chains). Proteinuria is associated with an ↑risk of cardiovascular disease and death. *False positive:* Postural (repeat using an early morning sample), post-exercise, fever, heart failure.

Microalbuminuria: Ultra-sensitive dipsticks are available to measure albuminuria (albumin excretion 30-300mg/24h). Suggests early glomerular disease, eg DM, ↑BP.

Haematuria

Blood in the urine may arise from anywhere in the renal tract. Transient causes should be excluded, eg UTI, menstruation. Classified as:

- visible (VH): previously known as macroscopic, frank
- non-visible (NVH): found on dipstick/microscopy, previously known as microscopic. NVH is subdivided according to the presence of urinary tract symptoms: symptomatic (sNVH) or asymptomatic (aNVH).

Causes: Malignancy (kidney, ureter, bladder), calculi, IgA nephropathy, Alport syndrome (p320), other glomerulonephritis (p310), polycystic kidney disease (p320), schistosomiasis. Do not attribute haematuria to anticoagulation without investigation. *False positive:* Myoglobin triggers same dipstick reaction—check microscopy.

Management: VH, sNVH, and aNVH >40yr should undergo urological assessment, imaging, and cystoscopy to exclude renal tract malignancy and calculi.
A renal aetiology should be considered, and renal referral made, for NVH with:

- eGFR <60
- coexistent proteinuria (A:CR >30 or P:CR >50)
- hypertension >140/90mmHg
- family history of renal disease.

A cause is not established in 19-68% of patients with NVH. These patients should be monitored via BP, eGFR, and repeat A:CR/P:CR every 6 months-1 year. Increasing proteinuria and deteriorating eGFR warrant repeat referral and investigation.

Others

Glucose: DM, pregnancy, sepsis, proximal renal tubular pathology (p316). *Ketones:* Starvation, ketoacidosis. *Leucocytes:* UTI (p296), vaginal discharge. *Nitrites:* UTI (enteric Gram−ve organism). *Bilirubin:* Haemolysis. *Urobilinogen:* Liver disease, haemolysis. *Specific gravity:* Normal range: 1.005-1.030, limited surrogate for urine osmolality, affected by proteinuria. *pH:* NR: 4.5-9, usually acidic with meat containing diet (acid-base balance: p670, renal tubular acidosis pp316-7).

Urine microscopy

Cells:

Red blood cells:

- >2 red cells/mm^3 is abnormal.
- Can come from anywhere in the urinary tract. Isomorphic red cells are similar to circulating red cells and may suggest bleeding from a genitourinary or external source. Dysmorphic red cells are abnormal in size/shape. Although they may indicate bleeding from the glomerulus (especially in exam questions!), assessment is subjective and dysmorphism also occurs due to changes in pH, osmolality, protein, and due to tubular passage.

White blood cells: (fig 7.2a)

- >10 white cells/mm^3 in an unspun specimen is abnormal.
- Causes include UTI, glomerulonephritis, tubulointerstitial nephritis, renal transplant rejection, and malignancy.

Squamous epithelial cells:

- Often seen, not pathological.

Casts:

Casts are cylindrical bodies formed in the lumen of distal tubules. They are formed of Tamm-Horsfall protein combined with cells.

- Hyaline cast (fig 7.2b)—seen in normal urine.
- Red cell cast (fig 7.2c)—signify an inflammatory process in the glomerulus, eg glomerulonephritis (p311).
- White cell cast (fig 7.2d)—pyelonephritis, interstitial nephritis (p318), glomerulonephritis (p311).
- Granular cast (fig 7.2e)—formed from degenerated tubular cells, seen in any chronic kidney disease.

Crystals:

Crystals are common in old or cold urine and may not signify pathology. They are important in stone formers.

- Uric acid (fig 7.2f)(p680)—uric acid stones, tumour lysis syndrome.
- Calcium oxalate (fig 7.2g)—stones (p638), high oxalate diet, ethylene glycol poisoning.
- Cystine (fig 7.2h)—seen in cystinuria (p321).

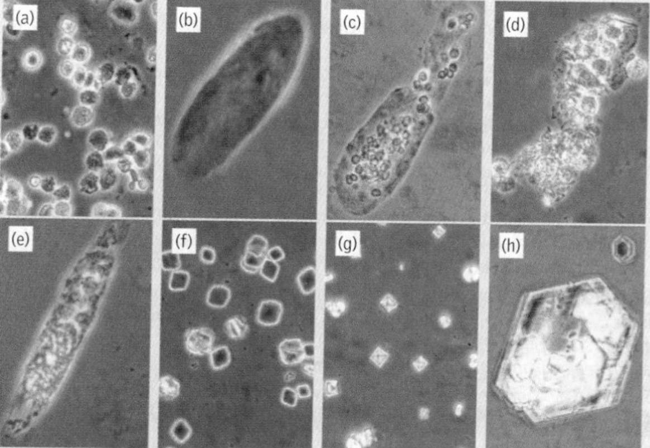

Fig 7.2 (a) White cells; (b) hyaline cast; (c) red cell cast; (d) white cell cast; (e) granular cast; (f) uric acid crystals; (g) calcium oxalate crystals; (h) cystine crystal.

Images (a) to (h) reproduced from Turner *et al.*, *Oxford Textbook of Clinical Nephrology*, 2005, with permission from Oxford University Press.

Urinary tract infection (UTI)

Definitions *Bacteriuria:* Bacteria in the urine; may be asymptomatic or symptomatic. Bacteriuria is not a disease. *UTI:*[1] A diagnosis based on symptoms and signs. Tests which prove bacteria in urine may provide additional information. There is no 'gold-standard' bacterial count. *Lower UTI:* Bladder (cystitis), prostate (prostatitis). *Upper UTI:* Pyelonephritis = infection of kidney/renal pelvis. *Abacterial cystitis/urethral syndrome:* A diagnosis of exclusion in patients with dysuria and frequency, without demonstrable infection. *Urethritis:* See pp412–3.

Incidence Annual incidence of UTI in women is 10–20%. 10% of men and 20% of women >65 years have asymptomatic bacteriuria (>65 years MSU is no longer diagnostic and clinical assessment is mandatory). Pyelonephritis = 3 per 1000 patient years.

Classification
- *Uncomplicated:* normal renal tract structure and function.
- *Complicated:* structural/functional abnormality of genitourinary tract, eg obstruction, catheter, stones, neurogenic bladder, renal transplant.

Risk factors
- ↑*Bacterial inoculation:* Sexual activity, urinary incontinence, faecal incontinence, constipation.
- ↑*Binding of uropathogenic bacteria:* Spermicide use, ↓oestrogen, menopause.
- ↓*Urine flow:* Dehydration, obstructed urinary tract (p640).
- ↑*Bacterial growth:* DM, immunosuppression, obstruction, stones, catheter, renal tract malformation, pregnancy.

Symptoms
- *Cystitis:* Frequency, dysuria, urgency, suprapubic pain, polyuria, haematuria.
- *Acute pyelonephritis:* Fever, rigor, vomiting, loin pain/tenderness, costovertebral pain, associated cystitis symptoms, septic shock.
- *Prostatitis:* Pain: perineum, rectum, scrotum, penis, bladder, lower back. Fever, malaise, nausea, urinary symptoms, swollen or tender prostate on PR. See p645.

Signs Fever, abdominal or loin tenderness. Check for a distended bladder, enlarged prostate. If *vaginal discharge*, consider PID, see p413.

►Do not rely on classical symptoms and signs in a catheterized patient.

Tests In non-pregnant women, if ≥3 (or one severe) symptoms of cystitis, and no vaginal discharge, treat empirically without further tests.
- *Dipstick:* Use in non-pregnant women <65 years with less than three symptoms. A negative dipstick reduces probability of UTI to <20%. Do not use in pregnant women. Limited data for men. No diagnostic value in catheterized sample.
- *MSU culture:* Conventional cut off >10^5 colony-forming units (cfu)/mL (but best diagnostic criterion may be >10^2–10^3cfu/mL). Use in pregnant women, men, children, and if fail to respond to empirical antibiotics. Catheterized sample only if septic.
- *Blood tests:* If systemically unwell: FBC, U&E, CRP, and blood culture (positive in only 10–25% of pyelonephritis). Consider fasting glucose.
- *Imaging:* Consider USS and referral to urology for assessment (cystoscopy, urodynamics, CT) in men with upper UTI; failure to respond to treatment; recurrent UTI (>2/year); pyelonephritis; unusual organism; persistent haematuria.

Organisms Usually anaerobes and Gram-negative bacteria from bowel and vaginal flora. *E. coli* is the main organism (75–95% in community but ↓ in hospital). *Staphylococcus saprophyticus* (a skin commensal) in 5–10%. Other enterobacteriaceae such as *Proteus mirabilis* and *Klebsiella pneumonia.* For sterile pyuria see table 7.2.

Table 7.2 Causes of sterile pyuria (↑ numbers of white cells but sterile on standard culture)

Infection related	Non-infection related	
►TB	Calculi	Polycystic kidney
Recently treated UTI	Renal tract tumour	Recent catheter
Inadequately treated UTI	Papillary necrosis	Pregnancy
Fastidious culture requirement	Tubulointerstitial nephritis	SLE
Appendicitis, prostatitis, chlamydia	Chemical cystitis	Drugs, eg steroids

Managing UTI

►Do not use antibiotics for the treatment of asymptomatic bacteriuria in non-pregnant women, men, and adults with catheters.

Non-pregnant women:

- If three or more symptoms (or one severe) of cystitis, and no vaginal discharge, treat empirically with 3-day course of trimethoprim, or nitrofurantoin (if eGFR >30).
- If first-line empirical treatment fails, culture urine and treat according to antibiotic sensitivity.
- In upper UTI, take a urine culture and treat initially with a broad-spectrum antibiotic according to local guidelines/sensitivities, eg co-amoxiclav. Hospitalization should be considered due to risk of antibiotic resistance. Avoid nitrofurantoin as it does not achieve effective concentrations in the blood.

Pregnant women:

Get expert help: UTI in pregnancy is associated with preterm delivery and intrauterine growth restriction. Asymptomatic bacteriuria should be confirmed on a second sample. Treat with an antibiotic. Refer to local guidance advice for antibiotic choice (avoid ciprofloxacin, trimethoprim in 1st trimester, nitrofurantoin in 3rd trimester). Confirm eradication.

Men:

- Treat lower UTI with a 7-day course of trimethoprim or nitrofurantoin (if eGFR >30).
- If symptoms suggest prostatitis (pain in pelvis, genitals, lower back, buttocks) consider a longer (4-week) course of a fluoroquinolone (eg ciprofloxacin) due to ability to penetrate prostatic fluid.
- If upper or recurrent UTI, refer for urological investigation.

Catheterized patients:

- All catheterized patients are bacteriuric. Send MSU only if symptomatic. Symptoms of UTI may be non-specific/atypical. Possible symptoms include fever, flank/suprapubic pain, change in voiding pattern, vomiting, confusion, sepsis.
- Change long-term catheter before starting an antibiotic.
- Refer to local guidelines for initial antibiotic choice. Where possible use a narrow-spectrum antibiotic according to culture sensitivity.

Urinary tract tuberculosis

- A cause of sterile pyuria: dysuria, frequency, suprapubic pain but negative standard culture. Ask about malaise, fever, night sweats, weight loss, back/flank pain, visible haematuria (p393).
- Can also cause an interstitial nephritis (p318) and renal amyloidosis (p315). Glomerulonephritis is rare.
- Diagnose by microscopy with acid-fast techniques and mycobacterial culture of an early morning MSU and/or urinary tract tissue.
- Treat with rifampicin and isoniazid for 6 months in conjunction with pyrazinamide and ethambutol for 2 months (see p394).

The 'Piss Prophets'

Beware the fallacies, deceit and juggling of the piss-pot science used by all those who pretend knowledge of diseases by the urine. Thomas Brian, 1655.

Medieval texts[1] give the following maxims regarding urinary change and disease:

- White or straw coloured urine = weak and cold liver and stomach
- Foamy urine = eructation (belching)
- Light coloured, turbid urine = mucus
- Lead circle on thin urine = pathological melancholy
- Bubbles on the surface = disease of the head
- Watery urine = love sickness
- Swampy, black, stinking urine = fatal
- Lead coloured urine = a disintegrating uterus
- Reddish, cloudy urine with bubbles = asthma or an irregular heart beat.

1 *Uroscopy in Early Modern Europe* by Michael Stolberg, Routledge, 2016, p53–6.

Acute kidney injury (AKI): a clinical approach

Definition

Acute kidney injury (AKI) is a syndrome of decreased renal function, measured by serum creatinine or urine output, occurring over hours-days. It includes different aetiologies and may be multifactorial.

Different definitions of AKI exist. In 2012, there was an attempt to amalgamate different diagnostic criteria into a single definition and staging system. The Kidney Diseases: Improving Global Outcomes (KDIGO) guidelines[2] define AKI as:

- rise in creatinine >26µmol/L within 48h.
- rise in creatinine >1.5 × baseline (ie before the AKI) within 7 days.
- urine output <0.5mL/kg/h for >6 consecutive hours.

The severity of AKI is then staged according to the highest creatinine rise or longest period/severity of oliguria (table 7.3).

Table 7.3 KDIGO staging system for AKI

Stage	Serum creatinine	Urine output
1	>26.5µmol/L (0.3mg/dL) or 1.5–1.9 × baseline	<0.5mL/kg/h for 6–12h
2	2.0–2.9 × baseline	<0.5mL/kg/h for >12h
3	>353.6µmol/L (4.0mg/dL) or >3.0 × baseline or renal replacement therapy	<0.3mL/kg/h for >24h or anuria for >12h

Although there are limitations to the use of serum creatinine, including the effects of muscle mass and dilution, no other biomarker has been able to supersede it (yet). The clinical approach to AKI is shown in fig 7.3.[3]

Epidemiology

AKI is common, occurring in up to 18% of hospital patients and ~50% of ICU patients. Risk factors for AKI include pre-existing CKD, age, male sex, and comorbidity (DM, cardiovascular disease, malignancy, chronic liver disease, complex surgery).

Causes

Commonest causes:

1. Sepsis.
2. Major surgery.
3. Cardiogenic shock.
4. Other hypovolaemia.
5. Drugs.
6. Hepatorenal syndrome.
7. Obstruction.

Aetiology can be divided according to site (table 7.4) as:

- pre-renal: ↓perfusion to the kidney.
- renal: intrinsic renal disease.
- post-renal: obstruction to urine.

Table 7.4 Aetiology of AKI

Where?	Pathology	Example
Pre-renal	↓Vascular volume	Haemorrhage, D&V, burns, pancreatitis
	↓Cardiac output	Cardiogenic shock, MI
	Systemic vasodilation	Sepsis, drugs
	Renal vasoconstriction	NSAIDS, ACE-i, ARB, hepatorenal syndrome
Renal	Glomerular (pp310–13)	Glomerulonephritis, ATN (prolonged renal hypoperfusion causing intrinsic renal damage)
	Interstitial (p318)	Drug reaction, infection, infiltration (eg sarcoid)
	Vessels (pp314–5)	Vasculitis, HUS, TTP, DIC
Post-renal	Within renal tract	Stone, renal tract malignancy, stricture, clot
	Extrinsic compression	Pelvic malignancy, prostatic hypertrophy, retroperitoneal fibrosis

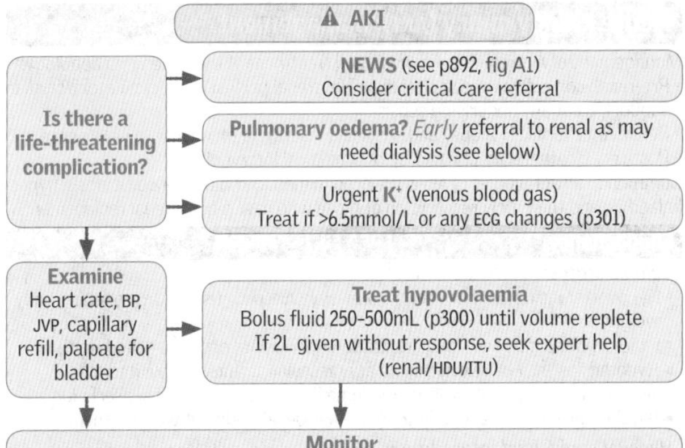

Monitor

- Fluid balance—consider urinary catheter and hourly urine output
- K^+—check response to treatment and at least daily until creatinine falls
- Observations—minimum every 4 hours
- Lactate if signs of sepsis
- Daily creatinine until ↓ (lags ~24 hours behind clinical response)

Investigate

- Urine dipstick (pre-catheter) and quantification of any proteinuria. Haematuria/proteinuria may suggest intrinsic renal disease
- USS within 24 hours (unless cause obvious or AKI improving). Small kidneys (<9cm) suggest CKD. Asymmetry may suggest renal vascular disease
- Check liver function (hepatorenal)
- Check platelets—if low need blood film to check for haemolysis (HUS/TTP)
- Investigate for intrinsic renal disease if indicated: immunoglobulins, paraprotein, complement, autoantibodies (ANA, ANCA, anti-GBM)

Support

- Treat sepsis (p792)
- Stop nephrotoxic medication—NSAIDs, ACE-i, ARB, aminoglycosides
- Stop drugs that may ↑complications: diuretics (especially K^+-sparing), metformin, antihypertensives
- Check all drug dosages are appropriate for renal impairment
- Consider gastroprotection (H2 antagonist, PPI) and nutritional support
- Avoid radiological contrast (or ↓risk: p319).

Fig 7.3 The clinical approach to AKI.[3]

Referring to the renal team

Request that advice/review is necessary due to:

- AKI not responding to treatment
- AKI with complications: ↑K^+, acidosis, fluid overload
- stage 3 AKI (table 7.3)
- AKI with difficult fluid balance (eg hypoalbuminaemia, heart failure, pregnancy)
- AKI due to possible intrinsic renal disease (table 7.4)
- AKI with hypertension.

Know: Creatinine trend and pre-morbid result if available, K^+, bicarbonate/lactate, Hb, platelet count (+film), urine dipstick (before catheter), clinical observations (NEWS) since admission, fluid input/output, examination findings (hypo/hypervolaemia), USS result, comorbidity (eg DM), drugs given (what? when? nephrotoxic?).

Acute kidney injury (AKI): management

Management of AKI requires diagnosis and treatment of the underlying aetiology:

- Pre-renal: correct volume depletion and/or ↑renal perfusion via circulatory/cardiac support, treat any underlying sepsis.
- Renal: refer for likely biopsy and specialist treatment of intrinsic renal disease.
- Post-renal: catheter, nephrostomy, or urological intervention.

Common to all aetiologies of AKI is the need to manage fluid balance, acidosis, hyperkalaemia, and the timely recognition of those who may require renal replacement.

Fluid balance

Volume status:

- Hypovolaemia: ↓BP, ↓urine volume, non-visible JVP, poor tissue turgor, ↑pulse, daily weight loss.
- Fluid overload: ↑BP, ↑JVP, lung crepitations, peripheral oedema, gallop rhythm.

►Hypotension may be relative in old age, vascular stiffness, untreated ↑BP.
►JVP does not reflect intravascular volume if right-sided heart disease/failure.
►↓BP, skin turgor, capillary refill changes may be late—do not wait for them.

Hypovolaemia, fluid resuscitation:

- If hypovolaemic, renal perfusion will improve with volume replacement.[4]
- Care in cardiac disease (↓renal perfusion despite adequate circulating volume) and sepsis/third-spacing (↑extravascular volume).
- *Dynamic assessment is essential:* examine before and after all fluid given to ensure an adequate response and to reduce the risk of fluid overload.
  1 Give 500mL crystalloid over 15 min.
  2 Reassess fluid state. Get expert help if unsure or if patient remains shocked.
  3 Further boluses of 250-500mL crystalloid with clinical review after each.
  4 Stop when euvolaemic or seek expert help when 2L given.

Which crystalloid? Any crystalloid can be used (follow local guidelines). 0.9% ('normal') saline is non-buffered, contains ↑chloride, and may cause hyperchloraemic acidosis. 'Balanced' or buffered crystalloids include Hartmann's, Ringer's lactate, and Plasma-Lyte®. Because they are 'balanced' they are often used preferentially. However, they contain 4-5mmol/L of K^+ so caution if ↑$K^+$and oligo/anuria.
What about colloid? Blood components should be used in resuscitation due to haemorrhage. Human albumin solutions may be given only under specialist advice in hepatorenal syndrome and as second line to crystalloids in septic shock.

Hypervolaemia, fluid overload:

Occurs due to aggressive fluid resuscitation, oliguria, and in sepsis due to ↑capillary permeability. Monitor weight daily in patients receiving IV fluids. Treat with:

- Oxygen supplementation if required.
- Fluid restriction. Consider oral and IV volumes. Give antibiotics in minimal fluid and consider concentrated nutritional support preparations.
- Diuretics. Only in symptomatic fluid overload. They are ineffective and potentially harmful if used to treat oliguria without fluid overload.
- Renal replacement therapy (p306). AKI with fluid overload and oligo/anuria needs urgent referral to renal/critical care.

Acidosis

- Mild = pH 7.30-7.36 (~bicarbonate >20mmol/L).
- Moderate = pH 7.20-7.29 (~bicarbonate 10-19mmol/L).
- Severe = pH <7.2 (~bicarbonate <10mmol/L): refer to renal/critical care.

Treatment is of the underlying disorder which will stop acid production. Where the effect of treatment may be delayed, acidosis will persist and renal replacement may be indicated (p306).

Medical management of acidosis is controversial. Giving sodium bicarbonate will generate CO_2. Adequate ventilation is therefore needed to prevent respiratory acidosis worsening the clinical picture. Sodium bicarbonate also represents a sodium and a volume load which can precipitate fluid overload in the vulnerable patient.

Hyperkalaemia

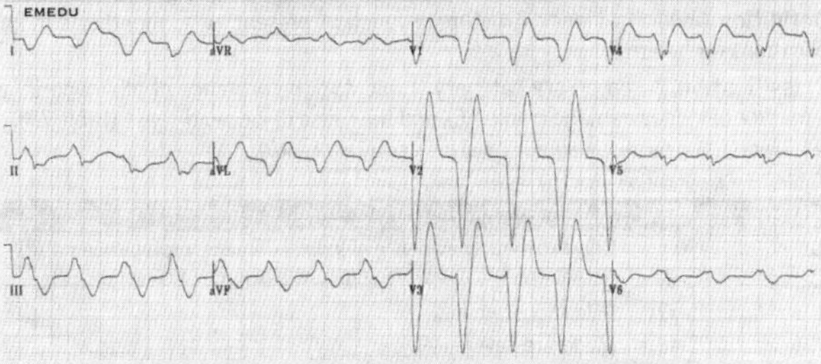

Fig 7.4 ECG showing severe hyperkalaemia; note broadening of QRS complexes.

ECG changes: In order: tall 'tented' T waves; increased PR interval; small or absent P wave; widened QRS complex (fig 7.4); 'sine wave' pattern; asystole. There is considerable inter-individual susceptibility.

►*Don't wait for a lab result: use the blood gas analyser.*

►►Treat[5] K^+ >6.5mmol/L or any with ECG changes (ECG for all K^+ >6.0mmol/L):

1. 10mL of 10% calcium chloride[2] (or 30mL of 10% calcium gluconate) IV via a big vein over 5-10min, repeated if necessary and if ECG changes persist. This is cardioprotective (for 30-60min) but does not treat K^+ level.
2. Intravenous insulin (10u soluble insulin) in 25g glucose (50mL of 50% or 125mL of 20% glucose). Insulin stimulates intracellular uptake of K^+, lowering serum K^+ by 0.65-1.0mmol/L over 30-60min. Monitor hourly for hypoglycaemia (in 11-75% of treated patients) which may be delayed in renal impairment (up to 6 hours after infusion).
3. Salbutamol also causes an intracellular K^+ shift but high doses are required (10-20mg via nebulizer) and tachycardia can limit use (10mg dose in IHD, avoid in tachyarrhythmias).
4. Definitive treatment requires K^+ removal. If the underlying pathology cannot be corrected renal replacement may be indicated. Safe transfer to an offsite renal unit requires K^+ <6.5mmol/L—discuss with renal team and critical care.

Use of intravenous sodium bicarbonate is controversial with insufficient evidence that it has any additional benefit over the treatment steps listed here. There is a risk of both sodium and fluid overload. Bolus doses of 8.4% sodium bicarbonate should not be used.

Renal replacement therapy (RRT) in AKI

RRT options in AKI include haemodialysis and haemofiltration (p306). Peritoneal dialysis is rare for AKI in adults and in high-income countries but can be used.

Possible indications for renal replacement therapy:

- Fluid overload unresponsive to medical treatment.
- Severe/prolonged acidosis.
- Recurrent/persistent hyperkalaemia despite medical treatment.
- Uraemia eg pericarditis, encephalopathy (more common in CKD).

The decision to start RRT should be individualized, aiming to provide organ support and prevent complications, rather than waiting for them to occur. The complexity of AKI and variation in thresholds for starting RRT prevent robust meta-analysis. Fluid overload is likely to be an important predictor of worse outcome.

Possible complications of RRT: Risks of dialysis catheter insertion and maintenance, procedural hypotension, bleeding due to the requirement for anticoagulation, altered nutrition and drug clearance.

2 Calcium chloride contains 3x calcium than the same volume of gluconate. Concern exists about the ↓bioavailability of calcium gluconate. Both salts carry a risk of tissue necrosis with extravasation.

Chronic kidney disease (CKD)

Definition Abnormal kidney structure or function, present for >3 months, with implications for health.[6]

Classification Based on GFR category (table 7.5), the presence of albuminuria as a marker of kidney damage (table 7.6), and the cause of kidney disease (table 7.7). (Problems using formula to grade renal disease by eGFR p669).

Table 7.5 Classification of CKD by GFR (mL/min/1.73m²)

Category	GFR	Notes
G1	>90	Only CKD if other evidence of kidney damage: protein/haematuria,
G2	60–89	pathology on biopsy/imaging, tubule disorder, transplant
G3a	45–59	Mild-moderate ↓GFR
G3b	30–44	Moderate-severe ↓GFR
G4	15–29	Severe ↓GFR
G5	<15	Kidney failure

Table 7.6 Classification of CKD by albuminuria

Category	Albumin excretion (mg/24h)	Albumin:creatinine ratio (A:CR) (mg/mmol)
A1	<30	<3
A2	30–300	3–30
A3	>300	>30

Table 7.7 Classification of CKD based on underlying disease

Renal pathology	Examples	
	Primary renal disease	Systemic disease
Glomerular	Minimal change, membranous	Diabetes, amyloid
Tubulointerstitial	UTI, pyelonephritis, stones	Drugs, toxins, sarcoid
Blood flow/vessels	Renal limited vasculitis	Heart failure, TTP
Cystic/congenital	Renal dysplasia	Alport syndrome, Fabry disease
Transplant	Recurrence of renal disease	Rejection, calcineurin toxicity

The most common causes of CKD in the UK are diabetes (24%), glomerulonephritis (13%), and ↑BP/renovascular disease (11%).[7]

Prognosis ↓GFR and albuminuria are independently associated with a higher risk of:
- all-cause mortality
- cardiovascular mortality
- progressive kidney disease and kidney failure
- AKI.

Patients with CKD are much more likely to die of CVD than to need renal replacement therapy. The risk of adverse outcome in CKD can be represented as a 'heat map' according to GFR and albuminuria categories (fig 7.5).

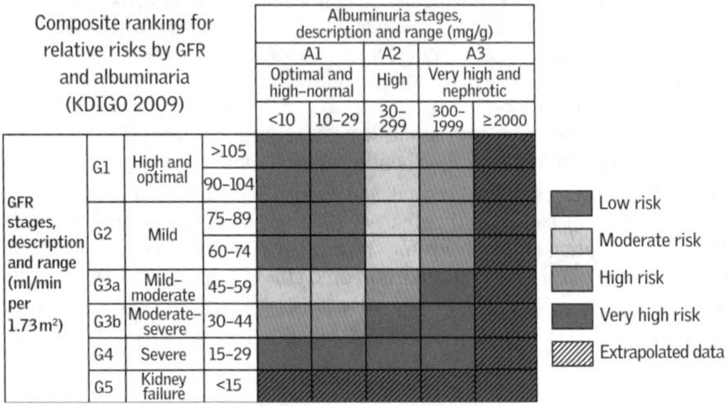

Fig 7.5 Composite risk of adverse outcome by GFR and albuminuria.

Reprinted from *Kidney International*, 80, AS Levey *et al*., Chronic kidney disease: definition, classification, and prognosis, 17–28, 2011, with permission from Elsevier.

The patient with CKD: a clinical approach

History

- *Does the patient really have CKD?* Does the eGFR reflect the true GFR (p669)? Is the eGFR corrected for ethnicity/drugs (eg trimethoprim alters creatinine concentration but not GFR)? Evidence of chronicity, ie >3 months—is there a previous creatinine on record?
- *Possible cause:* Ask about previous UTI, lower urinary tract symptoms, PMH of ↑BP, DM, IHD, systemic disorder, renal colic. Check drug history including when medications started. Family history including renal disease and subarachnoid haemorrhage. Systems review: look out for more than is immediately obvious, consider rare causes, ask about eyes, skin, joints, ask about symptoms suggestive of systemic disorder ('When did you last feel well?') and malignancy.
- *Current state:* Patients may have symptomatic CKD if GFR <30. Includes symptoms of fluid overload (SOB, peripheral oedema), anorexia, nausea, vomiting, restless legs, fatigue, weakness, pruritus, bone pain, amenorrhoea, impotence.

Examination

- *Periphery:* Peripheral oedema. Signs of peripheral vascular disease or neuropathy. A vasculitic rash. Gouty tophi. Joint disease. Arteriovenous fistula (thrill, bruit, recently needling?). Signs of immunosuppression: bruising from steroids, skin malignancy. Uraemic flap/encephalopathy if GFR <15.
- *Face:* Anaemia, xanthelasma, yellow tinge (uraemia), jaundice (hepatorenal), gum hypertrophy (ciclosporin), Cushingoid (steroids), periorbital oedema (nephrotic syndrome), taut skin/telangiectasia (scleroderma), facial lipodystrophy (glomerulonephritis).
- *Neck:* JVP for fluid state, tunnelled line (if removed, look for small scar over internal jugular, and a larger scar in 'breast pocket' area), scar from parathyroidectomy, lymphadenopathy.
- *Cardiovascular:* BP, sternotomy, cardiomegaly, stigmata of endocarditis. If right-sided heart failure/tricuspid regurgitation, JVP does not reflect fluid state.
- *Respiratory:* Pulmonary oedema or effusion.
- *Abdomen:* PD catheter or scars from previous catheter (small scars just below umbilicus and to side of midline), signs of previous transplant (scar, palpable graft), ballotable polycystic kidneys ± palpable liver.

Investigation

- *Blood:* U&E (compare with previous), Hb (normochromic, normocytic anaemia), glucose (DM), ↓Ca^{2+}, ↑PO_4^{3-}, ↑PTH (renal osteodystrophy). Directed investigation of intrinsic renal disease: ANA, ANCA, antiphospholipid antibodies, paraprotein, complement, cryoglobulin, anti-GBM, hepatitis serology, anti-PLA2R (membranous nephropathy). Note: ESR is not helpful as ↑ in CKD and proteinuric states.
- *Urine:* Dipstick, MC&S, A:CR or P:CR (p294), Bence Jones.
- *Imaging:* USS for size, symmetry, anatomy, corticomedullary differentiation, and to exclude obstruction. In CKD kidneys may be small (<9cm) except in infiltrative disorders (amyloid, myeloma), APKD, and DM. If asymmetrical consider renovascular disease. Scarring may be seen on USS but isotope scans are more sensitive.
- *Histology:* Consider renal biopsy (p310) in progressive disease, nephrotic syndrome, systemic disease, AKI without recovery. Biopsy is unlikely to change treatment if GFR stable and P:CR <150. DM with neuropathy/retinopathy may not need biopsy unless atypical, ie nephrotic, haematuria, other systemic symptoms.

Monitoring renal function in CKD

GFR and albuminuria should be monitored at least annually, according to risk. If high risk, monitor every 6 months (fig 7.5, orange), if very high risk, monitor at least every 3–4 months (fig 7.5, red). Small fluctuations are common but a drop in eGFR stage with ↓eGFR ≥25% is significant. Rapid progression is ↓eGFR >5/yr.

Risk factors for decline: ↑BP, DM, metabolic disturbance, volume depletion, infection, NSAIDs, smoking. All CKD has ↑risk of superimposed AKI and needs monitoring and prompt treatment during intercurrent illness.

Chronic kidney disease (CKD): management

CKD encompasses a range of disease from mild disease without progression to advanced, symptomatic disease requiring renal replacement.

Management of CKD[6,8] requires:

1. Appropriate referral to nephrology.
2. Treatment to slow renal disease progression.
3. Treatment of renal complications of CKD.
4. Treatment of other complications of CKD.
5. Preparation for renal replacement therapy (dialysis/transplantation) (p306).

Referral to nephrology

Consider referral for:

- stage G4 and G5 CKD (table 7.5)
- moderate proteinuria A:CR >70mg/mmol unless due to DM and already treated
- proteinuria A:CR >30mg/mmol with haematuria
- declining eGFR:
  - ↓eGFR by ≥25% + ↓GFR category (table 7.5)
  - sustained ↓eGFR ≥15% within 12 months
- ↑BP poorly controlled despite ≥4 antihypertensive drugs at therapeutic dose
- known or suspected rare or genetic cause of CKD.

Treatment to slow renal disease progression

BP: Target systolic BP is <140mmHg (range 120–139mmHg) and diastolic <90mmHg. If DM or A:CR >70 then systolic target is <130mmHg (range 120–129) and diastolic <80mmHg.

Renin-angiotensin system: Offer treatment with a renin-angiotensin system antagonist (ACE-i, ARB) to:

- DM and A:CR >3mg/mmol.
- Hypertension and A:CR >30mg/mmol.
- Any CKD with A:CR >70mg/mmol.

Do not combine renin-angiotensinsin antagonists due to risk of hyperkalaemia and hypotension. Check K^+ and renal function prior to, and 1–2 weeks after, starting treatment or changing dose. Stop if K^+ >6mmol/L, ↓eGFR >25%, or ↓creatinine >30%: exclude other possible causes and consider a lower dose.

Glycaemic control: Target HbA1c of ~53mmol/mol (7.0%) unless risk of hypoglycaemia, comorbidity or limited life expectancy.

Lifestyle: Offer advice about exercise, healthy weight, and smoking cessation. Salt intake should be reduced to <2g of sodium/day (=<5g sodium chloride/day).

Treatment of renal complications of CKD

Anaemia: Check Hb when eGFR <60. Investigate (especially if anaemic with eGFR >30) and treat other deficiencies: iron (hypochromic red cells >6%, transferrin saturation <20%, ferritin <100), B_{12}, and folate. Do not miss chronic blood loss. Iron therapy may need to be given IV. Consider treatment with an erythropoietic stimulating agent (ESA, 'Epo') if Hb <110g/L and likely to benefit in terms of function and quality of life. Pure red cell aplasia is a very rare, severe complication of ESA treatment due to anti-erythropoietin antibodies and usually causes Hb <60g/L: exclude more common causes of anaemia first.

Acidosis: Consider sodium bicarbonate supplements for patients with eGFR <30 and low serum bicarbonate (<20mmol/L). Caution in patients with hypertension and fluid overload due to sodium component.

Oedema: Restrict fluid and sodium intake. High doses of loop diuretics may be needed. Combination of a loop and thiazide diuretic can have a powerful effect: distal tubule sodium excretion (and its inhibition with a thiazide) is more significant when already treated with a loop diuretic (fig 7.13). Diuretic treatment should only be given with careful monitoring of fluid state and renal function.

CKD bone-mineral disorders: CKD causes ↑ in serum phosphate and reduced hydroxlyation of vitamin D by the kidney. Measure calcium, phosphate, ALP, PTH, and 25-OH vit D if eGFR <30.

- Treat if phosphate >1.5mmol/L (>1.7mmol/L if RRT) with dietary restriction ± phosphate binders. The use of binders which do not contain calcium may be beneficial in preventing vascular calcification.
- Give vitamin D supplements (colecalciferol, ergocalciferol) if deficient. If ↑PTH persists or is increasing, treat with an activated vit D analogue eg 1α-calcidol or calcitriol. Paricalcitol suppresses PTH with less effect on gut absorption of calcium and phosphate and is less likely to cause ↑calcium/phosphate.

Restless legs/cramps: Exclude iron deficiency as a possible exacerbating factor. Give sleep hygiene advice. Treatment for severe cases with gabapentin/pregabalin/dopamine agonists is off licence and may be complicated by side-effects (falls, cognitive impairment, impulse-control disorder).

Diet: Expert dietary advice should be available regarding protein intake, K^+ if hyperkalaemic, and phosphate restriction (eg dairy products).

Treatment of other complications of CKD

Cardiovascular disease: CKD confers ↑risk of cardiovascular disease due to ↑BP, vascular stiffness, inflammation, oxidative stress, and abnormal endothelial function (CV risk often higher than the risk of kidney failure).

- Antiplatelets (low-dose aspirin) for CKD at risk for atherosclerotic events unless bleeding risk outweighs benefit (mortality benefit unclear in CKD).
- Atorvastatin 20mg (and higher if GFR >30) for primary and secondary prevention of cardiovascular disease.
- CKD should not affect treatment for heart failure but ↑monitoring of GFR and K^+.
- GFR <60 may affect troponin and BNP values. Interpret results cautiously with consideration for the GFR.

Preparation for renal replacement therapy (RRT)

Planning for RRT should begin in progressive CKD when the risk of renal failure is 10–20% within a year. Referral to nephrology less than 1 year before RRT is required is considered a late referral.

All suitable patients should be listed for a deceased donor transplantation 6 months before the anticipated start of RRT. All suitable patients should be informed about the advantages of a pre-emptive living kidney transplant and efforts made to find a donor (p308).

Prescribing in CKD

►Never prescribe in renal failure before checking how administration should be altered due to a ↓GFR. This will be determined largely by the extent to which a drug is renally excreted. This is significant for aminoglycosides, penicillins, cephalosporins, heparin, lithium, opiates, and digoxin. Loading doses should not be changed.

If precision is required for dosing (eg chemotherapy) then GFR should not be estimated from creatinine: a cystatin C or direct measure of GFR should be used.

If the patient is receiving renal replacement (haemofiltration, peritoneal or haemodialysis), dose modification depends on the extent to which a drug is cleared from the circulation by dialysis/filtration.

The best prescribing guide to consult is the *Renal Drug Database/Handbook* (www.renaldrugdatabase.com), an invaluable resource detailing dose modification in renal failure and in renal replacement for almost any drug you could wish to use. All hospitals should have access: speak to your pharmacist.

Renal replacement therapy (RRT): dialysis and filtration

Long-term dialysis is started when it is necessary to manage one or more symptoms of renal failure including:

- inability to control volume status, including pulmonary oedema
- inability to control blood pressure
- serositis
- acid-base or electrolyte abnormalities
- pruritus
- nausea/vomiting/deterioration in nutritional status
- cognitive impairment.

►RRT is a misnomer for dialysis: renal function is not replaced, rather there is provision of just enough clearance to ameliorate the symptoms of kidney failure.

GFR at commencement of dialysis is usually ~5–10. When transplantation is awaited or not possible, there are two main options: haemodialysis and peritoneal dialysis.

Haemodialysis (HD) (fig 7.6) Blood is passed over a semi-permeable membrane against dialysis fluid flowing in the opposite direction. Diffusion of solutes occurs down the concentration gradient. A hydrostatic gradient is used to clear excess fluid as required (ultrafiltration). Access is preferentially via an arteriovenous fistula which provides ↑blood flow and longevity. This should be created prior to need for RRT to avoid the infection risk associated with central venous dialysis catheters. HD is needed 3 times/week or more. Daily HD increases the 'dose' and improves outcomes. Home HD should be offered to all suitable patients. *Problems:* Access (arteriovenous fistula: thrombosis, stenosis, steal syndrome; tunnelled venous line: infection, blockage, recirculation of blood), dialysis dysequilibrium (between cerebral and blood solutes leading to cerebral oedema ∴ start HD gradually), hypotension, time consuming.

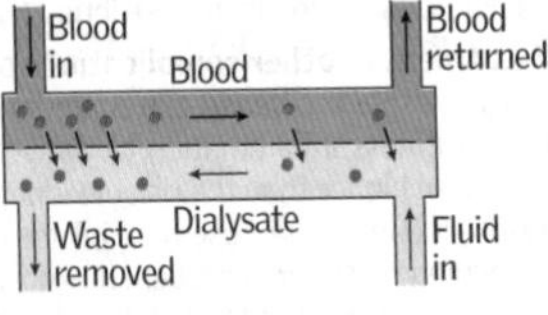

Fig 7.6 Haemodialysis.

Peritoneal dialysis (PD) Uses the peritoneum as a semi-permeable membrane. A catheter is inserted into the peritoneal cavity and fluid infused. Solutes diffuse slowly across. Ultrafiltration is achieved by adding osmotic agents (glucose, glucose polymers) to the fluid. It is a continuous process with intermittent drainage and refilling of the peritoneal cavity, performed at home. *Problems:* Catheter site infection, PD peritonitis, hernia, loss of membrane function over time.

Haemofiltration (fig 7.7) Water cleared by positive pressure, dragging solutes into the waste by convection. The ultrafiltrate (waste) is replaced with an appropriate volume of ('clean') fluid either before (predilution) or after (post-dilution) the membrane. ↓Haemodynamic instability so used in critical care when HD not possible due to ↓BP. Not used for chronic RRT unless in combination with HD (haemodiafiltration) for haemodynamic stability and ↑middle molecule clearance, eg β2-microglobulin.

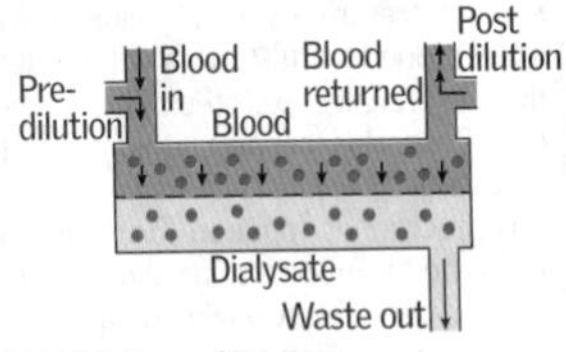

Fig 7.7 Haemofiltration.

Complications of RRT Annual mortality is significant, mostly due to *cardiovascular disease:* ↑BP, calcium/phosphate dysregulation, vascular stiffness, inflammation, oxidative stress, abnormal endothelial function. *Protein-calorie malnutrition:* Increases morbidity and mortality. *Renal bone disease:* High bone turnover, renal osteodystrophy, osteitis fibrosa. *Infection:* Uraemia causes granulocyte and T-cell dysfunction with ↑sepsis-related mortality. *Amyloid:* β2-microglobulin accumulates in long-term dialysis causing carpal tunnel syndrome, arthralgia, visceral effects.

Conservative management is for those who opt not to receive RRT due to lack of benefit on quality or quantity of life. Focus is on preserving residual renal function, symptom control, and advanced planning with patient and family for end-of-life care.

When a patient on dialysis presents...

1. Do they ***need dialysis*** now? Examine for fluid overload and check K^+. If on PD are they well enough to perform it themselves? Refer urgently to renal on-call.
2. When will they need dialysis? When are they due to dialyse next? Weigh them. All patients on dialysis have a ***target weight*** at which they are considered euvolaemic. How much are they above it? Do they have any useful urine output (ie that may help them lose volume/K^+)? Refer to renal in a timely manner.
3. What is your diagnosis? History and examination as for any other patient. ***Do not measure BP on fistula arm***. Remember ↑risk for CVD but troponin has ↓specificity in ESRF.
4. Treat. Remember to ***dose adjust for renal failure***—includes antibiotics, opiates, insulin, and low-molecular-weight heparin (see www.renaldrugdatabase.com, p305). Care with fluid replacement in sepsis: be guided by clinical examination and target weight. If unsure get expert help. If volume depleted give a 250mL bolus of (non-K^+ containing) crystalloid over 15min with close observation. Avoid maintenance fluids in those who normally have a fluid restriction. ***Do not use a dialysis line or fistula for IV access***—if a cannula is necessary, preferentially use the back of the hand, save other vessels for future fistulas.
5. Surgery needs senior anaesthetic and renal input. Aim for pre-op K^+ <5.5mmol/L (<5.0mmol/L if major surgery with risk of tissue breakdown/haemolysis). ***Check K^+ urgently post-op*** (venous gas in recovery). In elective surgery, plan dialysis provision pre- and post-op.

Warning: there is no normal

Ten years is a long time. For those ten years, or just over 3,560 times, I attached myself to a peritoneal dialysis machine and underwent nine hours and fifty minutes of nightly therapy. I subsequently learned to do a lot of crosswords and read a ridiculous amount of books. In ten years I had just three incidents: an inguinal hernia due to thinking that I could move a sofa (I could not), a parathyroidectomy (my knees were much happier afterwards), and one unfortunate bout of peritonitis (once was enough). Statistically speaking, I am an anomaly: the 'average' life span of a peritoneal dialysis patient is four years.

Admittedly, I did not initially cope well with needing to be on dialysis. After having lived successfully with a transplant, a return to dialysis felt like failure. I did not want the hassle of treatment. I did not want piles of boxes cluttering up our home. Mostly, I did not want a PD catheter jutting out of my belly. But what I originally believed to be unacceptable, gradually became tolerable. This took time. It took care and support. It took experiencing relative health, and seeing that dialysis life, although different to existing with a transplant, could be lived well.

Natasha Boone , author and illustrator, www.normalnotnormal.com; www.natashaboone.com

The man in a red canoe who saved a million lives

Mostly we commute to work each day driven by motives we would rather not look at too deeply. But one renal physician used a red canoe to commute each day from his houseboat to the hospital. He could have been a very rich man but instead Belding Scribner gave his invention away, and continued his modest existence.

He invented the Scribner shunt—a U of teflon connecting an artery to a vein, allowing haemodialysis to be something that could be repeated as often as needed. Before Scribner, glass tubes had to be painfully inserted into blood vessels, which would be damaged by the procedure so that haemodialysis could be done for only a few cycles. Clyde Shields was his first patient in 1960, and said that his first treatment 'took so much of the waste I'd stored up out of me that it was just like turning on the light from darkness'. Scribner took something that was 100% fatal and turned it into a condition with a 90% survival.

On 19 June 2003, his canoe was found afloat but empty. And like those ancient Indian burial canoes found at Wiskam which have been polished to an unimaginable lustre by the action of the shifting sands around the Island of the Dead, so we polish and cherish the image of this man who gave everything away to help others.

Renal replacement therapy (RRT): transplantation

Transplantation (figs 7.8, 7.9) should be considered for every patient with, or progressing towards, stage G5 kidney disease (p302). It is the treatment of choice for kidney failure provided risks do not exceed benefits. Many will not make the transplant list due to comorbidity or frailty.

Contraindications

- Absolute: cancer with metastases.
- Temporary: active infection, HIV with viral replication, unstable CVD.
- Relative: congestive heart failure, CVD.

Types of graft

- *Living donor:* Best graft function and survival, especially if HLA matched.
- *Deceased donor:* (See organ donation p13.)
  1. Donor after brain death (DBD, heart-beating donor).
  2. Expanded criteria donor (ECD) is from an older kidney or from a patient with a history of CVA, BP, or CKD. This impacts on the long-term prognosis of the transplant but offers a better outcome than remaining on dialysis.
  3. Donor after cardiac death (DCD, non-heart-beating donor) with ↑risk of delayed graft function.

Immunosuppression

A combination of drugs are used. Aim is to use the minimal effective dose with the lowest drug-related toxicity. Protocol used depends upon the immunological risk of the recipient and type of donated kidney.

Monoclonal antibodies: Eg basiliximab, daclizumab (selectively block activated T cells via CD-25), alemtuzumab (T- and B-cell depletion). Used at the time of transplantation ('induction'). ↓Acute rejection and graft loss, ↑infection risk if non-selective.

Calcineurin inhibitors: Eg tacrolimus, ciclosporin. These drugs inhibit T-cell activation and proliferation. ↑Inter-individual variation and narrow therapeutic index mean drug level monitoring is required. Clearance is dependent on cytochrome p450 isoenzymes so beware of drug interactions including macrolide antibiotics and antifungal drugs. Side effects: nephrotoxicity in the graft, modification of CV risk factors: ↑BP, ↑cholesterol, NODAT (new-onset diabetes after transplantation).

Antimetabolites: Eg mycophenolic acid (MPA), azathioprine. MPA is now used preferentially due to better prevention of acute rejection and graft survival (not in pregnancy, MPA is teratogenic). Side effects: anaemia, leucopenia, and GI toxicity.

Glucorticosteroids: ↓Transcription of inflammatory cytokines. First-choice treatment for acute rejection. Significant side-effects (BP, hyperlipidaemia, DM, impaired wound healing, osteoporosis, cataracts, skin fragility) have led to protocols with early withdrawal of steroids and the use of steroid-free immunosuppression regimens.

Complications

Surgical: Bleed, thrombosis, infection, urinary leaks, lymphocele, hernia.

Delayed graft function: Affects up to 40% of grafts, more common in DCD.

Rejection: Acute or chronic. Acute is divided into antibody mediated (rare unless known pre-sensitized recipient) or cellular (most common). Causes ↓renal function, diagnosed on graft biopsy. Treatment with high-dose steroids and ↑immunosuppression. Chronic antibody-mediated rejection causes progressive dysfunction of the graft. Most graft loss is now thought to be due to an immune response by donor-specific antibodies causing damage to the kidney microcirculation. Complex pathology and lack of controlled studies mean treatment is not clear. The results of monoclonal antibody trials are awaited.

Infection: ↑Risk of all infections. Typically hospital acquired/donor derived in month 1, opportunistic in months 1–6 (therefore prophylactic treatment for CMV and *Pneumocystis jirovecii* given), usual spectrum of community-acquired infection after 6–12 months. Late viral infection should always be considered: eg CMV, HSV.

Malignancy: Up to 25× ↑risk of cancer with immunosuppression, particularly skin, post-transplant lymphoproliferative disorder (PTLD), and gynaecological.

CVD: 3–5× ↑risk of premature CVD compared to general population (but ~80% less than dialysis). BP, NODAT, rejection, and renal history (uraemic cardiomyopathy) contribute.

Prognosis

Acute rejection <15%, 1-year graft survival >90%. Longer-term graft loss ~4%/year. Factors contributing to graft loss:

- Donor factors: age, comorbidity, living/deceased, DBD/DCD.
- Rejection.
- Infection.
- BP/CVD.
- Recurrent renal disease in graft.

Most common outcome is death with a functioning transplant (ie transplant 'outlives' the patient).

When a patient with a renal transplant presents...

1. Discuss everything with the local renal transplant unit: they will be happy to advise, review, transfer, and follow-up any renal transplant recipient.
2. What is the eGFR/creatinine? How does that compare with previous results? If you do not have any, ask the transplant unit.
3. Examine for and treat any reversible cause of AKI. Fluid state assessment (p300) is important—if you are unsure, get expert help. Correction of volume depletion and treatment of any sepsis should be prompt.
4. Consider viral/opportunistic infections and atypical presentations due to immunosuppression, eg CMV, *Pneumocystis jirovecii*.
5. ***Do not stop any immunosuppressive medication.*** If the patient is unable to tolerate oral medication then immunosuppression must be given NG or converted to an IV dose (conversion depends on drug: check with your pharmacist).
6. Check for medication interactions: macrolide antibiotics (erythromycin, clarithromycin) can cause calcineurin inhibitor toxicity.
7. Dose all drugs according to renal function: penicillins, cephalosporins, aminoglycosides, insulin, opiates, and low-molecular-weight heparin.
8. Check with the transplant unit before you give low-molecular-weight heparin for VTE prophylaxis: they may want to do a transplant biopsy.

Thank you for life

It feels good to be able to put pen to paper at last and to thank you from the bottom of my heart for the gift of life your daughter has given me and for the kindness and compassion you have shown.... I want to say to you that it was a wonderful thing that you did as a mother that in your deep sadness showed a caring and giving heart. I have a much better quality of life now since coming off dialysis 5 years ago. My father died of kidney failure when I was 3 years old. He was someone I would have loved to have known. I often think about your daughter, who she was and what she was like. Despite not knowing her, I think about her with affection and much respect. These last years must have been extremely painful for you all. I really hope that you, your family and friends have found peace in your lives.

Love Deborah (renal transplant recipient, 1998)

Reproduced from: Royal College of Physicians, Department of Health, NHS Blood and Transplant. *Thank you for life: letters from transplant recipients to donors' families*. London: RCP, 2010.

for the first time in eleven YEARS I have NO tubes in me.

Fig 7.8 'Alive' by Natasha Boone. www.natashaboone.com

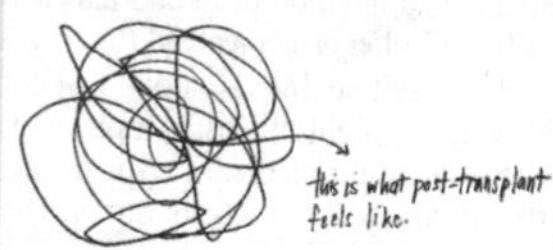

Fig 7.9 Post-transplant scribble by Natasha Boone. www.natashaboone.com

Glomerulonephritis

The term glomerulonephritis (GN) encompasses a number of conditions which:
- are caused by pathology in the glomerulus
- present with proteinuria, haematuria, or both
- are diagnosed on a renal biopsy
- cause CKD
- can progress to kidney failure (except minimal change disease).

The names of the diseases come from either the histological appearance (eg membranous glomerulonephritis), or the associated systemic condition (eg lupus nephritis).

Nephrotic or nephritic?
The glomerulonephritides classically present on a spectrum ranging from nephrosis (proteinuria due to podocyte pathology, p312), to nephritis (haematuria due to inflammatory damage, p311). This is illustrated in fig 7.10. However, if a GN causes scarring, then proteinuria can occur. Proteinuria can therefore complicate the longer-term clinical picture of any GN, including those that are classically 'nephritic'.

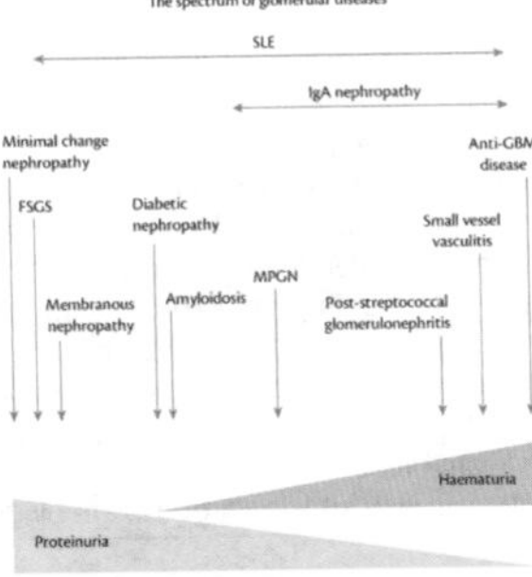

Fig 7.10 The spectrum of glomerular disease ranging from proteinuria (nephrosis) to haematuria (nephritis).

Figure adapted from Turner *et al.*, *Oxford Textbook of Clinical Nephrology*, 2015, with permission from Oxford University Press

Investigation Assess damage and potential cause. *Blood:* FBC, U&E, LFT, CRP; immunoglobulins, electrophoresis, complement (C3, C4); autoantibodies (p553): ANA, ANCA, anti-dsDNA, anti-GBM; blood culture, ASOT, hepatitis serology. *Urine:* MC&S, Bence Jones protein, A:CR/P:CR (p294), RBC casts (p295). *Imaging:* CXR (pulmonary haemorrhage), renal ultrasound (size and anatomy for biopsy). *Renal biopsy:* Required for diagnosis.

Renal biopsy

Pre-procedure: BP (<160/95 or according to local protocol), FBC (Hb>9, plt>100), clotting (PT and APTT <1.2), G&S. Written informed consent including possible complications: mild back/loin pain, visible haematuria (~5%, usually clears), bleeding, need for transfusion (~1%), angiographic intervention (~≤0.5%). Stop anticoagulants (aspirin 1 week, warfarin to PT <1.2, low-molecular-weight heparin 24h).
Post-procedure: Bed rest for a minimum of 4h. Monitor pulse, BP, symptoms, and urine colour. Do not discharge home until macroscopic haematuria settled. Aspirin or warfarin can be restarted the next day if procedure uncomplicated.
Result: Examination of glomerular lesions provides GN diagnosis. Includes: proportion of glomeruli involved (focal vs diffuse), how much of each glomerulus is involved (segmental vs global), hypercellularity, sclerosis. Immunohistology for deposits (Ig, light chains, complement). Electron microscopy for ultrastructure: precise location of deposits, podocyte appearance. Also examines tubulointerstitium (atrophy, fibrosis, inflammation) and any vessels.

Management General management as for CKD (pp304–5) including BP control and inhibition of renin-angiotensin axis. Specific treatment including immunosuppression depends on histological diagnosis, disease severity, disease progression, and comorbidity.

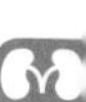

Nephritic glomerulonephritis

Nephritic glomerulonephritides[9] include:

IgA nephropathy

Commonest primary GN in high-income countries *Presentation:* Asymptomatic non-visible haematuria, or episodic visible haematuria which may be 'synpharyngitic': within 12–72h of infection. ↑BP. Proteinuria usually <1g. Slow, indolent disease: 20–50% progress to renal failure over 30yr. Worse prognosis in ♂, ↑BP, ↑creatinine, proteinuria. *Diagnosis:* Renal biopsy: IgA deposition in mesangium. *Treatment:* ACE-i/ARB reduce proteinuria and protect renal function. Corticosteroids and fish oil if persistent proteinuria >1g despite 3–6 months of ACE-i/ARB and GFR >50.

Henoch-Schönlein purpura (HSP)

Small vessel vasculitis and systemic variant of IgA nephropathy with IgA deposition in skin/joints/gut in addition to kidney. *Presentation:* Purpuric rash on extensor surfaces (typically on the legs, p702), flitting polyarthritis, abdominal pain (GI bleeding), and nephritis. *Diagnosis:* Usually clinical. Confirmed with positive IF for IgA and C3 in skin. Renal biopsy is identical to IgA nephropathy. *Treatment:* Renal disease is managed as IgA nephropathy. Steroids may be used for gut involvement.

Post-streptococcal GN

Occurs after a throat (~2 weeks) or skin (~3–6 weeks) infection. Streptococcal antigen deposits in the glomerulus leading to immune complex formation and inflammation. *Presentation:* Varies from haematuria to acute nephritis: haematuria, oedema, ↑BP and oliguria. *Diagnosis:* Evidence of streptococcal infection: ↑ASOT, ↑anti-DNAse B. Also ↓C3. *Treatment:* Supportive, antibiotics to clear the nephritogenic bacteria.

Anti-glomerular basement membrane (anti-GBM) disease

Previously known as Goodpasture's disease. Rare. Auto-antibodies to type IV collagen which is present in glomerular and alveolar basement membranes. *Presentation:* Renal disease (oliguria/anuria, haematuria, AKI, renal failure) and lung disease (pulmonary haemorrhage in 50–90% ∴ SOB, haemoptysis). Dialysis-dependence at presentation and ↑crescents on biopsy predict poor prognosis. *Diagnosis:* Anti-GBM in circulation/kidney (fig 7.11). *Treatment:* Plasma exchange, corticosteroids, and cyclophosphamide.

Rapidly progressive GN

Any aggressive GN, rapidly progressing to renal failure over days or weeks. Causes include small vessel/ANCA vasculitis (p314), lupus nephritis (p314), anti-GBM disease. Other GNs may 'transform' to become rapidly progressive including IgA, membranous. *Diagnosis:* Breaks in the GBM allow an influx of inflammatory cells so that crescents are seen on renal biopsy (may be referred to as crescentic GN) (fig 7.12). *Treatment:* Corticosteroids and cyclophosphamide. Other treatments depend on aetiology eg plasma exchange for anti-GBM/ANCA vasculitis, possible role for monoclonal antibodies in lupus nephritis.

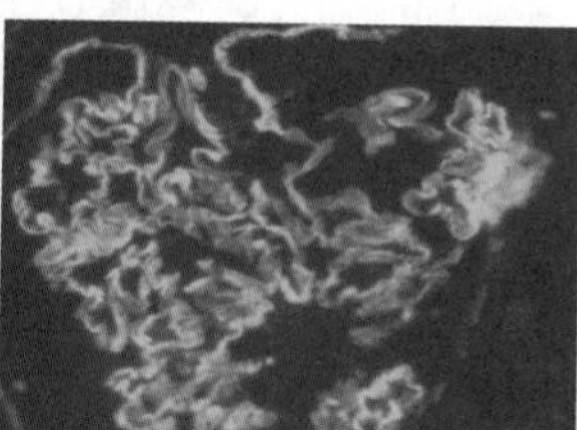

Fig 7.11 Immunofluorescence for IgG, showing linear staining characteristic of anti-GBM disease.

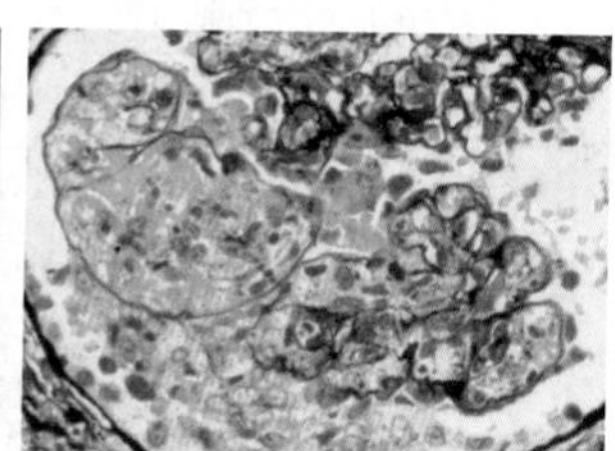

Fig 7.12 Crescentic GN: a proliferation of epithelial cells and macrophages with rupture of Bowman's capsule.

Nephrotic syndrome

►If there is oedema, dipstick the urine to avoid missing renal disease.

Definition The nephrotic syndrome is a triad of:
- proteinuria >3g/24h (P:CR >300mg/mmol, A:CR >250mg/mmol, p294)
- hypoalbuminaemia (usually <30g/L, can be <10g/L)
- oedema.

Aetiology Primary renal disease or secondary to a systemic disorder.
- *Primary renal disease:* Minimal change disease, membranous nephropathy (may be associated with underlying inflammation/malignancy), focal segmental glomerulosclerosis (FSGS), membranoproliferative GN.
- *Secondary causes:* DM, lupus nephritis, myeloma, amyloid, pre-eclampsia.

Pathophysiology The filtration barrier of the kidney is formed by podocytes, the glomerular basement membrane (GBM), and endothelial cells. Proteinuria results from podocyte pathology: abnormal function in minimal change disease, immune-mediated damage in membranous nephropathy, and podocyte injury/death in FSGS; or pathology in the GBM/endothelial cell: membranoproliferative GN.

Presentation Generalized, pitting oedema, which can be rapid and severe. Look in dependent areas (ankles if mobile, sacral pad/elbows if bed-bound) and areas of low tissue resistance, eg periorbitally. *History:* Ask about systemic symptoms, eg joint, skin. Consider malignancy and chronic infection. ΔΔ: CCF (↑JVP, pulmonary oedema), liver disease (↓albumin).

Management

1 *Reduce oedema*
Fluid (1L/day) and salt restriction. Diuresis with loop diuretics, eg furosemide. If gut oedema affects oral absorption of diuretics, give IV. Use daily weights to guide. Aim 0.5–1kg weight loss per day to avoid intravascular volume depletion and secondary AKI. Thiazide diuretics can be added if oedema remains resistant to high-dose loop diuretics. Albumin infusion increases proteinuria and remains controversial with no consistent evidence of benefit.

2 *Treat underlying cause*
Adults need a renal biopsy (p310). This is technically more difficult when there is gross oedema so diuresis may be required first. Treatment known to induce remission should be given, eg corticosteroids in minimal change disease. Look for and treat any underlying systemic disease, infection, or malignancy.
In children, minimal change disease is the commonest aetiology and steroids induce remission in the majority. Biopsy is therefore avoided in children unless there is no response to steroids, or if clinical features suggest another cause: age <1yr, family history, extrarenal disease (eg arthritis, rash, anaemia), renal failure, haematuria.

3 *Reduce proteinuria*
ACE-i/ARB reduce proteinuria (may not be needed in minimal change disease).

4 *Complications*
- *Thromboembolism.* Hypercoagulable due to ↑clotting factors, ↓anti-thrombin III, and platelet abnormalities. ↑Risk of VTE including DVT/PE (~10% adult patients) and renal vein thrombosis (loin pain, haematuria, ↑LDH, AKI if bilateral). Treat with heparin (may need to dose adjust low-molecular-weight heparin if ↓GFR) and warfarin. If low bleeding risk, consider prophylaxis when albumin <20g/L.
- *Infection.* Urine losses of immunoglobulins and immune mediators lead to ↑risk of urinary, respiratory, and CNS infection. Infection also seen in areas of fluid accumulation: cellulitis, peritonitis, empyema. Ensure pneumococcal vaccination given. ↑Risk of varicella with steroid treatment: post-exposure prophylaxis in non-immune, do not give live vaccine if immunosuppressed.
- *Hyperlipidaemia.* ↑Cholesterol (>10mmol/L), ↑LDL, ↑triglycerides, ↓HDL. Thought due to hepatic synthesis in response to ↓oncotic pressure and defective lipid breakdown. Abnormalities are proportional to proteinuria. The benefits of statins in CKD are extrapolated to nephrotic syndrome where there is ↓evidence.

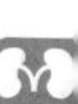

Nephrotic glomerulonephritis

Nephrotic glomerulonephritides[9] include:

Minimal change disease
~25% of adult nephrotic syndrome. Idiopathic (most) or in association with drugs (NSAIDs, lithium) or paraneoplastic (haematological malignancy, usually Hodgkin's lymphoma). Does not cause renal failure (if progressive CKD consider missed FSGS).
Diagnosis: Light microscopy is normal (hence the name). Electron microscopy shows effacement of podocyte foot processes.
Treatment: Prednisolone 1mg/kg for 4–16 weeks. 75% of adults will respond, >50% relapse. Frequent relapses are managed with ↑ or longer-term immune suppression (cyclophosphamide, calcineurin inhibitors).

Focal segmental glomerulosclerosis (FSGS)
Commonest glomerulonephritis seen on renal biopsy. Primary (idiopathic) or secondary (HIV, heroin, lithium, lymphoma, any cause of ↓kidney mass/nephrons, kidney scarring due to another glomerulonephritis). All at risk of progressive CKD and kidney failure: ↑proteinuria worsens prognosis. Disease will recur in 30–50% of kidney transplants.
Diagnosis: Glomeruli have scarring of certain segments (ie focal sclerosis). May miss early disease if <10 glomeruli in biopsy sample.
Treatment: ACE-i/ARB and blood pressure control in all. Corticosteroids only in primary (idiopathic) disease: remission in ~25%, partial remission in up to 50%. Calcineurin inhibitors may be considered second line. Plasma exchange and rituximab have been used for recurrence in transplants.

Membranous nephropathy
~25% of adult nephrotic syndrome. Primary (idiopathic) or secondary to:
- malignancy: lung, breast, GI, prostate, haematological
- infection: hepatitis B/C, *Streptococcus*, malaria, schistosomiasis
- immunological disease: SLE, rheumatoid arthritis, sarcoidosis, Sjögren's
- drugs: gold, penicillamine.

Indolent disease with spontaneous remission in ~25%.
Diagnosis: Anti-phospholipase A2 receptor antibody in 70–80% of idiopathic disease. Diffusely thickened GBM due to subepithelial deposits (IgG4 dominant in idiopathic, other IgGs in secondary disease). 'Spikes' on silver stain.
Treatment: ACE-i/ARB and blood pressure control in all. Immunosuppression ('Ponticelli' regimen: corticosteroids plus cyclophosphamide/chlorambucil) only in those at high risk of progression (proteinuria >4g without response to ACE-i/ARB for 6 months, ↑creatinine by 30% in 6–12 months but eGFR still >30). The role of targeted immunosuppression in those positive for anti-phospholipase A2 receptor antibodies remains unknown. In secondary disease proteinuria can remit with treatment of the underlying cause.

Membranoproliferative glomerulonephritis
~10% of adult nephrotic syndrome (higher in low- and middle-income countries due to infection). Divided into:
- *immune-complex associated:* driven by increased or abnormal immune complexes which deposit in the kidney and activate complement. An underlying cause can be found in most adult cases, eg infection, cryoglobulinaemia, monoclonal gammopathy, autoimmunity
- *C3 glomerulopathy:* due to a genetic or acquired defect in the alternative complement pathway, eg C3 nephritic factor. Progressive kidney dysfunction is common.

Diagnosis: A proliferative glomerulonephritis with electron dense deposits. Immunoglobulin deposition distinguishes immune-complex-associated disease from C3 glomerulopathy.
Treatment: ACE-i/ARB and blood pressure control in all. Underlying cause in immune-complex disease. Trial of immunosuppression if no underlying cause found and progressive decline in renal function. Treatments to block or modify C3 activation are awaited.

Diabetic nephropathy

DM nephropathy[10] is the commonest cause of end-stage renal failure: ~30–40% of patients requiring renal replacement. Predicted prevalence ↑ by 25–40% over next 20 years. Hyperglycaemia leads to ↑growth factors, renin-angiotensin-aldosterone activation, production of advanced glycosylation end-products, and oxidative stress. Causes ↑glomerular capillary pressure, podocyte damage, and endothelial dysfunction. Albuminuria is first clinical sign. Later scarring (glomerulosclerosis), nodule formation (Kimmelstiel-Wilson lesions), and fibrosis with progressive loss of renal function. Coexisting ↑BP accelerates the disease course.

Diagnosis: Microalbuminuria ('moderately increased albuminuria') = A:CR 3–30mg/mmol (p294, 302). Regression at this level of disease is possible. Not detected on standard dipstick ∴ must send A:CR. Screen annually.

Treatment:

- Intensive DM control prevents microalbuminuria and reduces risk of progression to macroalbuminuria ('severely increased albuminuria') = A:CR >30mg/mmol. HbA1c of 53mmol/mol (7%) reduces the development of all microvascular complications. However, less impact on CVD risk and hard renal outcomes including progression to kidney failure. Consider risk of hypoglycaemia.
- BP <130/80. Use ACE-i or ARB for CV and renal protection above BP control. Can prevent progression from normoalbuminuria to microalbuminuria to macroalbuminuria in hypertensive DM. (Less clear benefit in normotensive DM but recommended if A:CR >30mg/mmol.) No head-to-head studies of ACE-i/ARB in DM but equivalence outside DM. If cough with ACE-i switch to ARB. No benefit to dual therapy and ↑risk of ↑K^+. Data on direct renin inhibitors (eg aliskiren) awaited.
- Sodium restriction to <2g/day (=<5g sodium chloride/day).
- Statins to reduce CV risk (p305). Unclear benefit once on dialysis: do not initiate but do not need to discontinue if tolerated.

Lupus nephritis

SLE is a systemic autoimmune disease with antibodies against nuclear components, eg double-stranded (ds)DNA. Deposition of antibody complexes causes inflammation and tissue damage. *Presentation:* Rash, photosensitivity, ulcers, arthritis, serositis, CNS effects, cytopenias, and renal disease. Nephropathy is common (50% in first year, 75% overall). Can present as nephritis (p310) or nephrosis (p312). *Diagnosis:* Clinical. Antibody profile: ANA is sensitive but not specific. Anti-dsDNA has a specificity of 75–100% and titres correlate with disease activity. Consider biopsy if A:CR >30, P:CR >50. *Treatment:* Depends on histological class. Classes I and II show mild changes with little risk of renal disease progression: ACE-i/ARB for renal protection and hydroxychloroquine for extra-renal disease. Classes III-V require immunosuppression: mycophenolate, glucocorticoids, cyclophosphamide, rituximab.

Small vessel vasculitis

Multiple classification systems exist. Clinical phenotype and ANCA subtype are important. ANCA-associated vasculitis (AAV) occurs with or without specificity for proteinase 3 (PR3) and myeloperoxidase (MPO). AAV classically presents at an older age (>60yrs) and accounts for 20% of biopsy findings >80yrs. Ask about lethargy, fever, myalgia, anorexia ('When did you last feel well?'). Ask about respiratory symptoms and investigate for pulmonary haemorrhage. *Diagnosis:* Clinical + ANCA + biopsy: rapidly progressive GN (p311) without immune deposits ('pauci-immune'). *Treatment:* High-dose glucocorticoids plus cyclophosphamide or rituximab. Plasma exchange if presents with renal failure or pulmonary haemorrhage.

Myeloma (See p368.)

Associated renal disease in up to 40%: tubular obstruction due to light chain casts ('myeloma kidney'); deposition of Ig/light chains in glomerulus (causes proteinuria); hypercalcaemia; renal tract infection due to immunoparesis. *Treatment:* Adequate hydration, bisphosphonates for hypercalcaemia (care if GFR <30), anti-myeloma treatment including glucocorticoids. It remains unclear whether there is a benefit in removing light chains by either plasma exchange or large pore haemodialysis.

Amyloid

Pathological folding of proteins leads to extracellular accumulation and organ dysfunction including kidney disease. Classified according to protein: light chains in myeloma = AL amyloid; serum amyloid A in chronic inflammation = AA amyloid; also rare familial types. *Diagnosis:* Congo red staining on biopsy, SAP scan. *Treatment:* Underlying condition. New therapies target amyloid production, aggregation, and breakdown.

Haemolytic uraemic syndrome (HUS)

Presents with a microangiopathic haemolytic anaemia (Hb <100g/L, ↑LDH, ↓haptoglobin, fragments on blood film), ↓platelets and AKI due to thrombosis of the glomerular capillaries (microangiopathy). In children, primarily associated with haemorrhagic colitis due to Shiga toxin-producing *E. coli* (STEC) eg O157:H7. Atypical HUS caused by dysregulation/uncontrolled activation of complement = ~5% of HUS. Can be precipitated by pregnancy. *Diagnosis:* Triad of haemolytic anaemia, ↓platelets, and AKI with haematuria/proteinuria. ?Evidence of STEC. Look for abnormalities in the complement pathway: levels of C3, C4, factors H and I, complement mutation screen. *Treatment:* STEC-HUS: supportive. aHUS: plasma infusion/exchange, eculizumab (anti-C5) in England via the national aHUS centre, Newcastle-Upon-Tyne.

Thrombotic thrombocytopenic purpura (TTP)

Symptoms overlap with HUS (see previous paragraph). Pentad: microangiopathic haemolytic anaemia, ↓platelets, AKI, neurological symptoms (headache, palsies, seizure, confusion, coma), and fever. Due to a congenital deficiency of, or acquired antibodies to, the ADAMTS13 protease which normally cleaves multimers of von Willebrand factor (vWF). Large vWF multimers cause platelet aggregation and fibrin deposition in small vessels, leading to a multisystem thrombotic microangiopathy. *Diagnosis:* Clinical. ADAMTS13 activity. *Treatment:* ►*TTP is a haematological emergency: get expert help.* Plasma infusion/exchange removes antibodies/replaces ADAMTS13 and may be life-saving. Corticosteroids. Consider rituximab for non-responders/relapse.

Atherosclerotic renovascular disease

Part of a systemic atheromatous vascular disease including cardio-, cerebro-, and peripheral vascular disease (ask about claudication, check foot pulses), ↑BP, and ↑lipids. Leads to renin-angiotensin upregulation which causes treatment-resistant ↑BP and/or a deterioration in renal function on ACE-i/ARB. Acute decompensated heart failure (no LV impairment on echo) with flash pulmonary oedema in up to 10%. *Diagnosis:* >1.5cm asymmetry in renal size (but ↓sensitivity and ↓specificity). Doppler studies of native kidneys not consistently accurate for diagnosis. CT or MR (avoids contrast) angiography. *Treatment:* Modification of CV risk factors: statin, aspirin, antihypertensive treatment. Historically, ACE-i/ARB were considered contraindicated due to concern about renin-dependent renal perfusion and deterioration in function on ACE-i/ARB. However, ↓mortality seen with ACE-i/ARB. ↓eGFR by <25% 'sacrificed' for longer-term renal and cardiac outcome. Large RCTs of medical treatment vs revascularization have failed to show an advantage to revascularization ∴ only considered in flash pulmonary oedema, rapid/oligo-anuric renal failure.

Scleroderma renal crisis

Occurs in ~5% of systemic sclerosis. ↑Risk with: diffuse disease, anti-RNA polymerase III antibodies and <2yr from diagnosis. *Diagnosis:* Accelerated hypertension (new >150/85mmHg) and AKI (↓eGFR by >30%). Biopsy: collapsed glomeruli, onion-skin thickening of arterioles. *Treatment:* ACE-i/ARB. IV vasodilators to ↓vascular resistance and for digital ischaemia. Care with β-blockers as ↑HR compensating for ↓stroke volume. May recover renal function after many months.

Sickle cell nephropathy

Hbss is associated with hyperfiltration (lower than expected creatinine) and albuminuria. Although up to 75% of young patients will have some degree of CKD, progression to renal failure is usually associated with another trigger, eg papillary necrosis, infection. *Diagnosis:* Clinical. Biopsy only if looking for another diagnosis, eg AKI without clinical cause, nephrotic syndrome. *Treatment:* ACE-i/ARB. Inconsistent data re hydroxycarbamide and ↓hyperfiltration. ↑Mortality on dialysis: aim to transplant.

The renal tubule: disorders and diuretics

Tubular disorders and the action of diuretics can be considered according to the affected segment of the nephron (fig 7.13 and table 7.8).

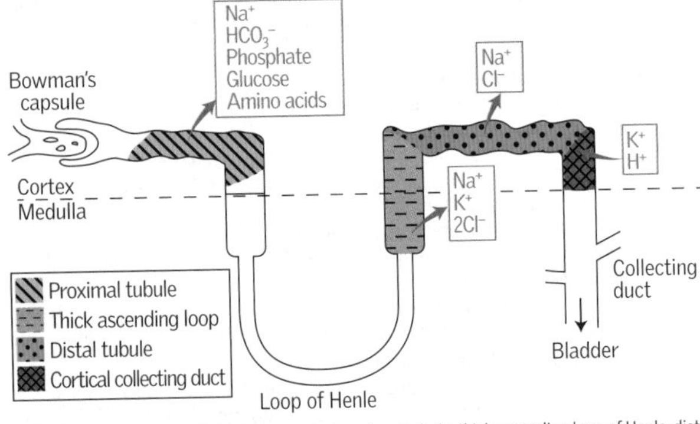

Fig 7.13 The nephron divided into segments (proximal tubule, thick ascending loop of Henle, distal tubule, collecting duct) with key solute movement (red).

Table 7.8 Summary table of tubular disorders and diuretic action (RTA = renal tubular acidosis)

Nephron segment	Solute movement	Tubular pathlogy	Diuretic
Proximal tubule	Reabsorption: Na^+, HCO_3^-, phosphate, sugars, amino acids	Fanconi syndrome Proximal (type 2) RTA	Mannitol Carbonic anhydrase inhibitor
Thick ascending loop	Reabsorption: Na^+, K^+, Cl^-	Bartter syndromes	Loop
Distal tubule	Reabsorption: Na^+, Cl^-	Gitelman syndrome	Thiazide
Cortical collecting duct	Excretion: K^+, H^+	Distal (type 1) RTA Type 4 RTA	K^+-sparing
Collecting duct	Excretion: water	Diabetes insipidus (p240)	V2 antagonists ('vaptan') (p320)

Proximal tubule

Physiology

Reabsorbs Na^+ (~70%), bicarbonate, phosphate, amino acids, sugars, uric acid.

Pathology

Fanconi syndrome: Generalized impairment of proximal tubular function leading to glycosuria (in a non-diabetic), phosphaturia, uricosuria, aminoaciduria, and tubular-proteinuria (negative dipstick but positive urine P:CR p294). Phosphaturia leads to phosphate loss from bone, demineralization, and growth impairment. *Treatment:* replace phosphate. *Proximal (type 2) renal tubular acidosis (RTA):* Failure of bicarbonate reabsorption. Distal reabsorption intact so serum bicarbonate usually ≥12mmol/L. Accompanied by Fanconi syndrome unless rare familial cause. *Aetiology:* light chain disease, drugs (eg tenofovir), heavy metals. *Diagnosis:* IV bicarbonate increases bicarbonate loss in urine and causes rapid rise in urine pH to ~7.5. *Treatment:* bicarbonate and potassium replacement.

Diuretics

Osmotic diuretic (eg mannitol): Used to ↓ICP and intra-ocular pressure. Freely filtered but poorly reabsorbed, holding water by osmosis. Na^+, K^+, Ca^{2+}, Cl^-, Mg^{2+}, HCO_3^- may be affected. Risk of pulmonary oedema if oligo/anuric. *Carbonic anhydrase inhibitor (eg acetazolamide):* Used in altitude sickness, glaucoma. Metabolic acidosis due to ↑bicarbonate excretion. Risk of nephrocalcinosis.

Thick ascending loop of Henle

Physiology

Reabsorbs Na^+ (~10–30%) and other electrolytes. Key transport via electroneutral $Na^+/K^+/2Cl^-$ co-transporter.

Pathology

Bartter syndromes: Due to impaired salt transport in the thick ascending loop. Sodium reabsorption increases further along the nephron in exchange for K^+ and H^+ ∴ all cause a hypokalaemic, hypochloraemic, metabolic alkalosis. Usually present in childhood. Divided into subtypes depending on transport molecule defect. Type 1 mimics a loop diuretic. Elevated prostaglandin levels are also a feature. Treatment is with salt replacement and the use of NSAIDs (after volume repletion).

Diuretics

Loop diuretics (eg furosemide, bumetanide): Block the $Na^+/K^+/2Cl^-$ co-transporter in the thick ascending loop of Henle, hence increase the solute load of the filtrate and reduce water resorption. Increase excretion of water, Na^+, Cl^-, phosphate, Mg^{2+}, Ca^{2+}, K^+, and H^+. They are readily absorbed from the GI tract (unless it is oedematous in which case IV may be needed) with peak concentration within 30–120min. Widely used in peripheral oedema (heart failure, ascites). They can also be used to treat hypercalcaemia. Side effects include hypokalaemic metabolic alkalosis, hypovolaemia, and ototoxicity.

Distal tubule

Physiology

Reabsorbs Na^+ (~5–10%) and other electrolytes. Key transport via NaCl co-transporter.

Pathology

Gitelman syndrome: Loss of function of the NaCl co-transporter. Milder than Bartter syndrome: usually presents in adolescence/adulthood with incidental finding of electrolyte abnormalities. Mimics thiazide diuretic administration. Treat with electrolyte supplementation.

Diuretics

Thiazide (eg bendroflumethiazide) and thiazide-like diuretics (eg indapamide, chlortalidone, metolazone): Inhibit the NaCl transporter ∴ decrease NaCl reabsorption and increase water loss. Used to treat ↑BP (p140). Side effects: hyponatraemia, hypokalaemia, and hypomagnesaemia. However, calcium excretion is reduced (in contrast to loop diuretics) ∴ can be used to treat recurrent kidney stones in patients with hypercalciuria. Excretion of uric acid is reduced (care in gout). Glucose intolerance can occur (mechanism may be related to hypokalaemia) so care in DM. Increase in LDL cholesterol is not significant with chronic use at low dose, especially in the context of beneficial BP reduction.

Cortical collecting duct

Physiology

Acid-base and K^+ homeostasis. Aldosterone acts to retain $Na^+$and excrete K^+.

Pathology

Distal (type 1) renal tubular acidosis (RTA): Failure of acid (H^+) excretion. Primary genetic disease or secondary to autoimmune disease (eg Sjögren's syndrome, SLE), toxins (eg lithium). Can cause, or be caused by, nephrocalcinosis (eg medullary sponge kidney, sarcoid). Leads to bone demineralization, renal calculi. Hypokalaemia can be severe. Diagnosis: urine fails to acidify (pH >5.3) despite metabolic acidosis. Treat with bicarbonate replacement and management of underlying disease. *Type 4 RTA*: Hyperkalaemia and acidosis due to (real or apparent) hypoaldosteronism, eg adrenal insufficiency, DM, ACE-i/ARB, K^+-sparing diuretics.

Diuretics

K^+-sparing: aldosterone antagonists, eg spironolactone, eplerenone, amiloride. Used in aldosteronism, heart failure, cirrhosis, K^+-wasting states. Decrease Na^+ and K^+ excretion. Can cause ↑K^+, acidosis. Oestrogenic effects with spironolactone.

Tubulointerstitial nephropathy and nephrotoxins

The renal tubules and the interstitium make up ~80% of the kidney. Damage to one is usually associated with damage to the other = tubulointerstitial nephropathy. Can be acute or chronic.

Acute tubulointerstitial nephritis (ATIN)

Presents with AKI. Eosinophilia in ~30%. An 'allergic triad' of fever, rash, and arthralgia occurs in ~10%. Should be considered in all cases of AKI for which there is no obvious pre-renal or post-renal precipitant (p298). Biopsy shows an inflammatory cell infiltrate in the interstitium ±tubule ('tubulitis'). Prognosis improves with early recognition although residual CKD in up to 40%. *Aetiology:*

- Drugs: antibiotics, NSAIDs, PPIs, diuretics, ranitidine, anticonvulsants, warfarin. ►Take a full drug history including over-the-counter and herbal preparations.
- Infection: *Streptococcus, Pneumococcus, Staphylococcus, Campylobacter, E. coli, Mycoplasma,* CMV, EBV, HSV, hepatitis A-C.
- Autoimmune disease: SLE, sarcoid, Sjögren's syndrome, ANCA.

Treatment: Stop causative agent or treat underlying cause. Steroids are used despite a paucity of RCT evidence.

Chronic tubulointerstitial nephritis (CTIN)

Insidious onset and slowly progressive renal impairment. Biopsy shows interstitial fibrosis and tubular atrophy. Most commonly due to drugs (>70%) or infection. Possible causes include:

- drugs: NSAIDs (p319), lithium, calcineurin inhibitors, aminosalicylates (eg mesalazine, sulfasalazine), chemotherapy (eg cisplatin)
- infection: TB, pyelonephritis, leptospirosis, HIV
- immune disease: sarcoid, Sjögren's syndrome
- specific nephrotoxins: lead, cadmium, mercury, aristolochic acid (p319)
- haematological disorders: myeloma
- genetic interstitial disease.

Treatment: Stop causative agent or treat underlying cause. Reduce risk of progression as per CKD management: ACE-i/ARB, BP control, glucose, lipids (pp304–5). Future: antifibrotic agents?

Nephrotoxins

Many agents may be toxic to the kidneys either by direct damage to the tubules, or by causing an interstitial nephritis (see earlier in topic). Examples (not an exhaustive list and idiosyncratic reactions are possible):

Analgesics: NSAIDs (p319).

Antimicrobials: Aminoglycosides (p319), sulfamethoxazole (in co-trimoxazole), penicillins, rifampicin, amphotericin, aciclovir.

Anticonvulsants: Lamotrigine, valproate, phenytoin.

Other drugs: PPIs, cimetidine, furosemide, thiazides, ACE-i/ARB, lithium, iron, calcineurin inhibitors, cisplatin.

Anaesthetic agents: Methoxyflurane, enflurane.

Radiocontrast material: (p319.)

Proteins: Igs in myeloma, light chain disease, Hb in haemolysis, myoglobin in rhabdomyolysis (p319).

Crystals: Urate (p319).

Bacteria: Streptococci, *Legionella, Brucella, Mycoplasma, Chlamydia,* TB, *Salmonella, Campylobacter,* leptospirosis, syphilis.

Viruses: EBV, CMV, HIV, polyomavirus, adenovirus, measles.

Parasites: Toxoplasma, Leishmania.

Other: Ethylene glycol, radiation (p319), aristolochic acid (p319).

Analgesic nephropathy
Caused by NSAIDs, aspirin, paracetamol. ↓Prevalence since phenacetin withdrawn. Risk determined by frequency and duration of use. *Presentation:* History of chronic pain (headache, musculoskeletal). Often silent until advanced CKD. *Diagnosis:* Urinalysis: normal or sterile pyuria, mild proteinuria. USS: small and irregular kidneys. IVU: classic 'cup and spill' appearance. Non-contrast CT: ↓renal mass, papillary calcification. Biopsy: CTIN secondary to papillary necrosis. ↑Risk of atherosclerosis. *Treatment:* Discontinue analgesia. Manage CKD (pp304–5). USS or CT urogram if sudden flank pain to exclude obstruction from sloughed papilla.

Aminoglycosides (gentamicin >tobramycin >amikacin >streptomycin)
Cause AKI due to tubular necrosis. Risk factors: ↑dose, prolonged use, CKD, volume depletion, other nephrotoxins. *Presentation:* Typically mild, non-oliguric AKI after 1–2 weeks of therapy. Recovery can be delayed/incomplete. *Treatment:* Prevention. Single daily dose may be less nephrotoxic ►Check levels (p756).

Radiocontrast nephropathy
AKI 48–72 hours after IV contrast. Risk factors: CKD, DM, ↑dose of contrast, volume depletion, other nephrotoxins. *Treatment:* None. ►Prevention is key: pre-hydrate with IV cystalloid (no consistent benefit shown for bicarbonate above 0.9% sodium chloride). Use local protocol or consider 3mL/kg/h 1 hour before, and 1mL/kg/h for 6h after. Acetylcysteine evidence is weak. Discontinue other nephrotoxic medication for 24h pre- and post-procedure. Tell the radiologist about risk factors so they can use the lowest dose of low/iso-osmolar contrast.

Rhabdomyolysis
Results from skeletal muscle breakdown, with release of intracellular contents (K^+, myoglobin) into the extracellular space. ↑Cytokines and ↓nitric oxide cause renal vasoconstriction. Myoglobin is filtered by the glomeruli causing obstruction and inflammation. *Presentation:* History of trauma, surgery, immobility, hyperthermia, seizures. Muscle pain, swelling, tenderness. AKI. Red-brown urine. *Diagnosis:* Serum myoglobin: short half-life, may be missed. Plasma CK ×5 upper limit. Myoglobinuria (tea- or cola-coloured urine) is falsely +ve for blood on dipstick with *no* RBC seen on microscopy. ↑K^+, ↑↑PO_4^{3-}, ↓Ca^{2+}. *Treatment:* Supportive. Urgent treatment for hyperkalaemia (p301). IV fluid rehydration: maintain urine output 300mL/h until myoglobinuria has ceased; up to 1.5L fluid/h may be needed. If oliguric, monitor CVP in HDU/ICU setting. Renal replacement may be needed. (Alkalinization of urine hypothesized to ↓crystallization and ↓toxic metabolites but no RCT evidence to support use over other crystalloids and beware ↓Ca^{2+}.)

Urate nephropathy
In acute crystal nephropathy, uric acid crystals precipitate within the tubulointerstitium causing ↓GFR and secondary inflammation. Seen in tumour lysis syndrome when a high tumour burden and sensitivity to chemotherapy cause ↑uric acid which precipitates in association with ↑phosphate. In addition, serum uric acid is a risk factor for CKD: hypothesized stimulus for arterial disease with pathological autoregulation of renal blood flow, renin, and ↑BP. *Treatment:* Tumour lysis: aggressive hydration, allopurinol/rasburicase to ↓synthesis of uric acid. Chronic disease: unclear whether diet/treatment to ↓uric acid (allopurinol, febuxostat) improves outcome.

Radiation nephritis
Renal impairment due to ionizing radiation. Presents 6 months–years after total body irradiation, local field radiotherapy, or targeted radionucleotide therapy. Presents with ↑BP, proteinuria/haematuria, progression to renal failure. Prognosis linked to ↑BP. *Treatment:* ↓Radiation dose with shielding. As CKD (pp304–5) with strict BP control.

Aristolochic acid nephropathy
Herbal remedies containing aristolochic acid can cause progressive CKD. Disproportionate anaemia, mild proteinuria, and renal dysfunction. Biopsy: extensive fibrosis and tubular atrophy. Risk of urothelial malignancy ×5, occurs in up to 40%. Aristolochic acid thought to be underlying cause of *Balkan endemic nephropathy:* cluster of CKD/renal failure in Balkan areas where aristolochic acid is detected in wheat. *Treatment:* Avoid exposure. Treat as CKD (pp304–5). Screen for malignancy. Consider therapeutic trial of steroids (limited data).

Autosomal dominant polycystic kidney disease (ADPKD)
1 in 400-1000 (~7 million worldwide). *De novo* mutation in ~10%. 2/3 will require renal replacement. 85% have mutations in PKD1 (chromosome 16) and reach ESRF by 50s. Mutation in PKD2 (chromosome 4) has a slower course, reaching ESRF by 70s. *Presentation:* May be clinically silent unless cysts become symptomatic due to size/haemorrhage (fig 7.14). Loin pain, visible haematuria, cyst infection, renal calculi, ↑BP, progressive renal failure. *Extrarenal:* liver cysts, intracranial aneurysm→SAH (p478), mitral valve prolapse, ovarian cyst, diverticular disease. *Diagnosis:* USS is modality of choice. Renal cysts are common and ↑prevalence with age so diagnostic criteria are age-specific: 15-39yrs ≥3 cysts, 40-59yrs >2 cysts in each kidney give a positive predictive value of 100% for both PKD1 and PKD2 mutations. Sensitivity is >93% for PKD1 but only 69% for diagnosis of PKD2 <30 years. Liver (90% by age 50) and pancreatic cysts (~10%) support the diagnosis. Genetic testing available but ~1500 different mutations are described so use limited to diagnostic uncertainty, potential donors, and pre-implantation diagnosis. (Non-contrast) CT for renal colic as cysts obscure view on USS. Screening for intracranial aneurysms (MRI) recommended for age <65yrs if personal/family history of aneurysm/SAH. *Treatment:* Water intake 3-4L/day (if eGFR >30) may suppress cyst growth. ↑BP should be treated to target <130/80mmHg: 1st-line ACE-i/ARB, 2nd-line thiazide-like, 3rd-line β-blocker (not calcium channel blocker as ↓Ca^{2+} entry is part of pathology although no specific outcome data). Treat infection. Haematuria usually managed conservatively. Persistent/severe pain may need cyst decompression. Plan for RRT including pre-emptive transplantation. Ongoing research evaluating drugs which inhibit cyst growth including vasopressin antagonists (tolvaptan: decrease in kidney volume seen), somatostatin analogues, metformin, and transcription inhibitors.

Autosomal recessive polycystic kidney disease
1 in 20 000, chromosome 6. Presents ante/perinatally with renal cysts ('salt and pepper' appearance on USS), congenital hepatic fibrosis→portal hypertension. Poor prognosis if neonatal respiratory distress. No specific therapy. (See *OHCS* p132.)

Renal phakomatoses
Tuberous sclerosis complex: 1 in 6000, autosomal dominant. Two genes: TSC1 (chromosome 9) and TSC2 (chromosome 16). Multisystem disorder with hamartoma formation in skin, brain (→epilepsy), eye, heart, and lung (see *OHCS* p638). In kidney: angiomyolipomata in 90% with risk of aneurysm and haemorrhage, cystic disease in 50%. Replacement of renal tissue leads to kidney failure. mTORC1 inhibitors (eg sirolimus, everolimus) block pathological cell signalling and reduce tumour volume.
Von Hippel-Lindau syndrome: 1 in 36 000, autosomal dominant (p712). Mutation in VHL gene (chromosome 3) leads to uncontrolled activation of growth factors. Phenotype is a familial, multisystem cancer syndrome including renal cysts and clear cell renal carcinoma at mean age 40s, ~70% risk by age 60 (VHL tumour-suppressor gene is inactivated in most sporadic renal cell cancers). Manage by screening for tumours. Possibility of future therapies which inhibit growth factor signalling.

Alport syndrome
1 in 5000. ~80-85% X-linked. Due to mutations in the COL4A5 gene, which encodes the α5 chain of type IV collagen. Haematuria, proteinuria, and progressive renal insufficiency. Average age of renal failure in men 30-40yrs. Female 'carriers' can exhibit the phenotype, renal failure in ~30% by 60yrs. High-tone sensorineural hearing loss. Anterior lenticonus: bulging of lens seen on slit-lamp examination (see *OHCS* p638). Type IV collagen is the antigen in anti-GBM disease (p311) so there is a risk of anti-GBM disease following transplantation as the graft type IV collagen is recognized as 'foreign'.

Fabry disease
1 in 40 000-120 000. X-linked. Lysosomal storage disorder due to a deficiency of the enzyme α-galactosidase-A. Causes proteinuria and progressive renal failure in most men and some female 'carriers'. Lipid deposits are seen in urine and on renal biopsy ('zebra body'). Treatment with IV enzyme replacement can stabilize kidney function if proteinuria controlled to <1g/24h.

Cystinuria

1 in 17 000. Autosomal recessive defect prevents reabsorption of cystine and dibasic amino acids in proximal tubule. Leads to cystinuria and cystine stone formation. Treatment: diet, ↑fluid intake, and urine alkalinization. Current drugs which increase cystine solubility have adverse side-effect profiles.

Cystinosis

1 in 100 000–200 000. Autosomal recessive. Lysosomal storage disorder with accumulation of cystine. In nephropathic forms causes proximal tubule dysfunction, Fanconi syndrome (p316), and progressive renal impairment. Also visual impairment, myopathy, hypothyroidism. Oral cysteamine ↓intralysosomal cystine, and delays ESRF, but is poorly tolerated (GI symptoms, skin deposits, fever, seizures).

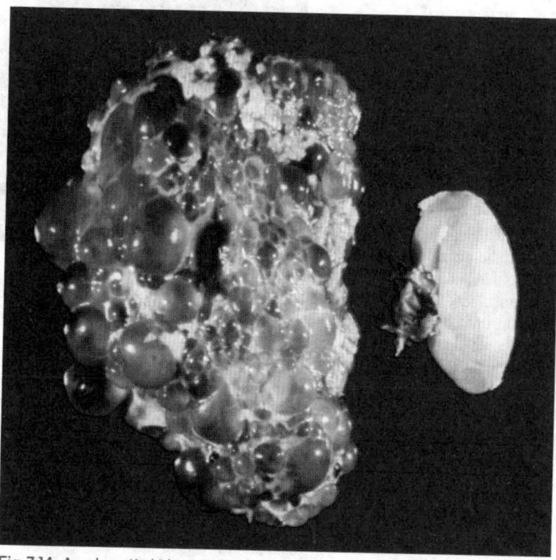

Fig 7.14 A polycystic kidney (left) compared with a normal-sized kidney (right). The progressive increase in size can lead to abdominal discomfort. There may be haemorrhage into a cyst causing haematuria, or infection.

Courtesy of the PKD Foundation.

8 Haematology

Contents

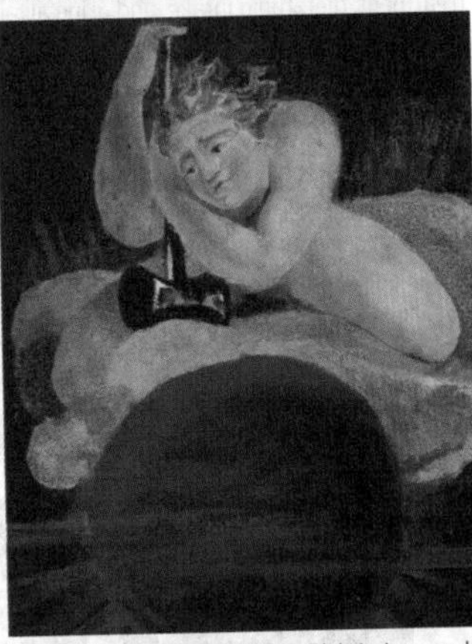

Fig 8.1 Here we see William Blake's Los working alone and at night, hammering a red cell into shape in the forge of the human heart. '*For every space larger than a red globule of Man's blood/ Is visionary, and is created by the Hammer of Los:/ And every Space smaller than a Globule of Man's blood opens/ Into Eternity of which this vegetable Earth is but a shadow./ The red Globule is the unwearied Sun by Los created./ To measure Time and Space to mortal Men ...*' (William Blake's *Milton* (1804–1810), lines 17–24.) When we ourselves are working alone and at night, hammering away at some difficult problem within the arteries of the hospital, we can lose sight of the context in which our own red globule sits. Unfortunately, as with Los' task, ours is one with an eternity of duties within and external to it. Rather than becoming overwhelmed by a seemingly endless job list, we must take our focus from the single red cell to the surrounding interconnected systems; by prioritizing our tasks and asking for help when we need it, we might not face such a solitary and interminable fate.

We thank our Specialist Reader, Dr Drew Provan, for his contribution to this chapter.

A sense of humourism

Whilst our understanding of blood has changed emphatically with the advent of medical research, its importance in health and disease is a common theme throughout human history and culture. Hippocrates (460–370BC) first described the four bodily fluids, or humours (Latin umor = body fluid): blood, phlegm, and yellow and black bile. This is not bile and phlegm as we know it; rather, it was postulated by Fahråeus (1921, the Swedish physician who pioneered the ESR, p372) that humourism arose from watching blood coagulate *in vitro*: distilling into layers of bilious yellow serum floating on a scurf of white cells, with the dark red-black clot of erythrocytes lurking in the depths of the sample.

These four humours were later elaborated by Roman physician, surgeon, and philosopher Claudius Galen (c.129–c.201AD) who attributed physical and behavioural traits to each humour: sanguine people are warm hearted and confident, the phlegmatic practical and rational, those with a choleric nature are fiery and passionate, while the melancholic (melas=black, khole=bile) are depressed yet creative.[1] It was thought that an imbalance of any of these elements was the source of disease, a belief which led to the wide-scale recommendation of the removal of the excess bodily fluid: expectoration, purging, and most popularly, blood-letting. William Harvey, Sydenham, and Dupytren are among the famous names who celebrated this cure, Harvey stating that 'daily experience satisfies us that blood-letting has a most salutary effect in many diseases, and is indeed the foremost among all the general remedial means'. Many tools were developed to aid this procedure, notably a collecting bowl with a convenient notch for the antecubital fossa or neck: the predecessor of the modern kidney dish.

Such was the conviction of the healing brought about by bloodletting that 'haematomania' reigned despite a suspicious degree of mortality. Indeed, it may have even killed inaugural US president George Washington in 1799: on developing laryngitis he was enthusiastically bled four times by his personal physician, and died 24 hours after symptom onset.

Eventually, the credibility of this practice waned, and by 1860 it had virtually disappeared. However, venesection still plays an important role in the management of haemachromatosis (see p288) and polycythaemia rubra vera (p366).

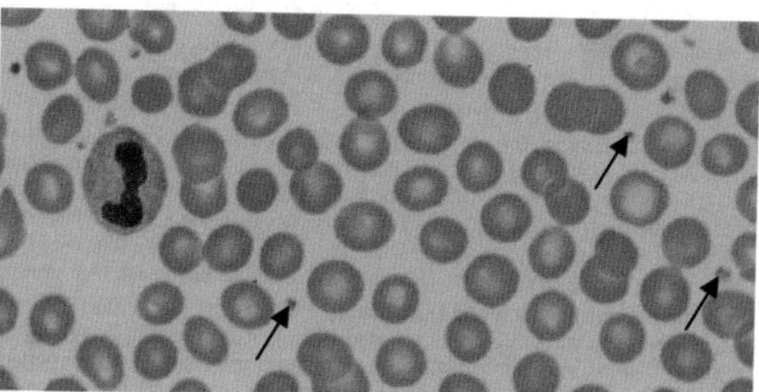

Fig 8.2 A normal blood film, with a neutrophil, red cells, and platelets (arrows).

1 Compare these personalities with those of the 2015 anthropomorphic Pixar film 'Inside Out'.

Anaemia

Anaemia is defined as a low haemoglobin (Hb) concentration, and may be due either to a low red cell mass or increased plasma volume (eg in pregnancy). A low Hb (at sea level) is <135g/L for men and <115g/L for women. Anaemia may be due to reduced production or increased loss of RBCs and has many causes. These will often be distinguishable by history, examination, and inspection of the blood film (fig 8.2, p323).

Symptoms Due to the underlying cause or to the anaemia itself: fatigue, dyspnoea, faintness, palpitations, headache, tinnitus, anorexia—and angina if there is pre-existing coronary artery disease.

Signs May be absent even in severe anaemia. There may be pallor (eg of the conjunctivae, see fig 8.3, although this is not a reliable sign). In severe anaemia (Hb <80g/L), there may be signs of a hyperdynamic circulation, eg tachycardia, flow murmurs (ejection-systolic loudest over apex), and cardiac enlargement; or retinal haemorrhages (rarely). Later, heart failure may occur: here, rapid blood transfusion can be fatal.

Types of anaemia The first step in diagnosis is to look at the mean cell volume (MCV). *Normal* MCV is 76–96 femtolitres (10^{15} fL = 1L).

Low MCV (microcytic anaemia):

1 Iron-deficiency anaemia (IDA), the most common cause: see p326.
2 Thalassaemia (suspect if the MCV is 'too low' for the Hb level and the red cell count is raised, though definitive diagnosis needs DNA analysis): see p342.
3 Sideroblastic anaemia (very rare): p326.

NB: there is iron accumulation in the last two conditions, and so tests will show increased serum iron and ferritin with a low total iron-binding capacity (TIBC).

Normal MCV (normocytic anaemia):

1 Acute blood loss.
2 Anaemia of chronic disease (or ↓MCV).
3 Bone marrow failure.
4 Renal failure.
5 Hypothyroidism (or ↑MCV).
6 Haemolysis (or ↑MCV).
7 Pregnancy.

NB: if ↓WCC or ↓platelet in normocytic anaemia, suspect marrow failure: see p364.

High MCV (macrocytic anaemia):

1 B_{12} or folate deficiency.
2 Alcohol excess—or liver disease.
3 Reticulocytosis (p328, eg with haemolysis).
4 Cytotoxics, eg hydroxycarbamide.
5 Myelodysplastic syndromes.
6 Marrow infiltration.
7 Hypothyroidism.
8 Antifolate drugs (eg phenytoin).

Haemolytic anaemias: These do not fit into the above-mentioned classification as the anaemia may be normocytic or, if there are many young (hence larger) RBCs and reticulocytes, macrocytic (p332). Suspect if there is a reticulocytosis (>2% of RBCs; or reticulocyte count >100×10^9/L), mild macrocytosis, ↓haptoglobin, ↑bilirubin, ↑LDH, or ↑urobilinogen. These patients will often be mildly jaundiced (but note that haemolysis causes pre-hepatic jaundice so there will be no bilirubin in their urine).

Does the patient need a blood transfusion? Probably not if Hb >70g/L. Chronic anaemia in particular can be well-tolerated (though it is crucial to ascertain the cause), and in IDA iron supplements will raise the Hb more safely and cost-effectively. In *acute* anaemia (eg haemorrhage with active peptic ulcer), transfusion for those with Hb <70g/L may be indicated. Other factors to consider include comorbidities (particularly IHD) and whether the patient is symptomatic.

In severe anaemia with heart failure, transfusion is vital to restore Hb to a safe level, eg 60–80g/L, but this must be done with great care. Give it *slowly* with 10–40mg furosemide IV/PO with alternate units (dose depends on previous exposure to diuretics; do not mix with blood). Check for signs of worsening overload: rising JVP and basal crackles: in this eventuality, stop and treat.

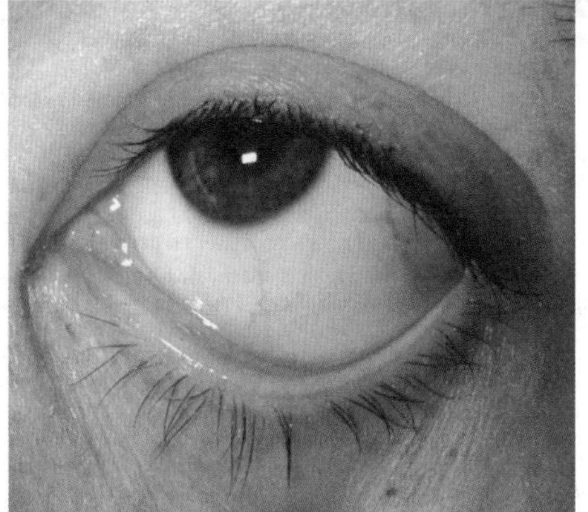

Fig 8.3 'Conjunctival pallor', *the* classic sign of anaemia, is a confusing term as the conjunctiva is translucent, transmitting the colour of structures under it. The 'pallor' refers to the vasculature on the inner surface of the lid which is lacking Hb. It is this colour but it should be:

Red cell distribution width (RCDW or RDW)

In health or in unifactorial anaemia, all the red cells in a sample are about the same size, and the graph of their volume distribution forms a narrow peak. In mixed anaemias, however, this peak broadens, reflecting an abnormally large RDW—this may be the first clue to dual pathology. In coeliac disease, for example, poor absorption of iron (↓MCV) *and* folate (↑MCV) may occur simultaneously, resulting in a combination of microcytes and macrocytes in the circulation. The visual analogue of this is anisocytosis (p328) on a blood film. The laboratory measure is a ↑RDW, where RDW = the standard deviation of MCV divided by the mean MCV, multiplied by 100. Reference interval: 11.5–14.6%. If the MCV is high and the RDW is *normal*, the cause is likely to be alcohol, liver disease, or a marrow problem (chemotherapy or aplastic anaemia).

Iron-deficiency anaemia (IDA)

This is common (seen in up to 14% of menstruating women).

Causes •Blood loss, eg menorrhagia or GI bleeding[2] (upper p256; lower p629).
• Poor diet or poverty may cause IDA in babies or children (but rarely in adults).
• Malabsorption (eg coeliac disease) is a cause of refractory IDA.
• In the tropics, hookworm (GI blood loss) is the most common cause.

Signs Chronic IDA (signs now rare): koilonychia (fig 8.4 and p76), atrophic glossitis, angular cheilosis (fig 8.5), and, rarely, post-cricoid webs (Plummer–Vinson syndrome).

Tests Blood film: microcytic, hypochromic anaemia with anisocytosis and poikilocytosis (figs 8.6, 8.7). ↓MCV, ↓MCH, and ↓MCHC. Confirmed by ↓ferritin (also ↓serum iron with ↑TIBC, but these are less reliable, see table 8.1). ►NB: ferritin is an acute phase protein and ↑ with inflammation, eg infection, malignancy. Transferrin is also ↑ in IDA but is less affected by inflammation. Check coeliac serology in all (p266): if negative then refer all males and females who are not menstruating for urgent gastroscopy *and* colonoscopy. Consider stool microscopy for ova if relevant travel history. Faecal occult blood is not recommended as sensitivity is poor. ►*IDA with no obvious source of bleeding mandates careful GI workup.*[2]

Treatment Treat the cause. Oral iron, eg ferrous sulfate 200mg/8h PO. SE: nausea, abdominal discomfort, diarrhoea or constipation, black stools. Hb should rise by 10g/L/week, with a modest reticulocytosis (young RBC, p328). Continue for at least 3 months after Hb normalizes to replenish stores. IV iron is only indicated if the oral route is impossible or ineffective, eg functional iron deficiency in chronic renal failure, where there is inadequate mobilization of iron stores in response to erythropoietin therapy.

The usual reason that IDA fails to respond to iron replacement is that the patient has rejected the pills—check compliance. Is the reason for the problem GI disturbance? Altering the dose of elemental iron with a different preparation may help. Alternatively, there may be continued blood loss, malabsorption, anaemia of chronic disease; or misdiagnosis, eg when thalassaemia is to blame.

Anaemia of chronic disease (secondary anaemia)

The commonest anaemia in hospital patients (and the 2nd commonest, after IDA, worldwide). It arises from three problems (in which the polypeptide, hepcidin, plays a key role): **1** Poor use of iron in erythropoiesis. **2** Cytokine-induced shortening of RBC survival. **3** ↓Production of and response to erythropoietin.

Causes Many, eg chronic infection, vasculitis, rheumatoid, malignancy, renal failure.

Tests Ferritin normal or ↑ in mild normocytic or microcytic anaemia (eg Hb >80g/L; see table 8.1). Check blood film, B_{12}, folate, TSH, and tests for haemolysis (p336).

Treatment Treating the underlying disease may help (eg in 60% of patients with RA), as may erythropoietin (SE: flu-like symptoms, hypertension, mild rise in the platelet count and thromboembolism). Also effective in improving quality of life in malignant disease. IV iron can safely overcome the functional iron deficiency. Hepcidin inhibitors and inflammatory modulators show promise.

Sideroblastic anaemia

Microcytic anaemia does not always mean iron deficiency! 20% of older people with an MCV <75fL are not iron deficient. ►*Think of sideroblastic anaemia whenever microcytic anaemia is not responding to iron.* This condition is characterized by ineffective erythropoiesis, leading to ↑iron absorption, iron loading in marrow ± haemosiderosis (endocrine, liver, and heart damage due to iron deposition).

Causes Congenital (rare, x-linked) or acquired, eg idiopathic as one of the myelodysplastic/myeloproliferative diseases, can also follow chemotherapy, anti-TB drugs irradiation, alcohol or lead excess. **Tests** Look for ↑ferritin, a hypochromic blood film and disease-defining sideroblasts in the marrow (figs 8.8, 8.9; table 8.1). **Treatment** Remove the cause. Pyridoxine ± repeated transfusions for severe anaemia.

2 In one study, 11% presenting to their GP with IDA had GI carcinoma. Plan both upper and lower GI investigation: there may be abnormalities on both.

Table 8.1 Interpreting plasma iron studies

	Iron	TIBC	Ferritin
Iron deficiency	↓	↑	↓
Anaemia of chronic disease	↓	↓	↑
Chronic haemolysis	↑	↓	↑
Haemochromatosis	↑	↓ (or ↔)	↑
Pregnancy	↑	↑	↔
Sideroblastic anaemia	↑	↔	↑

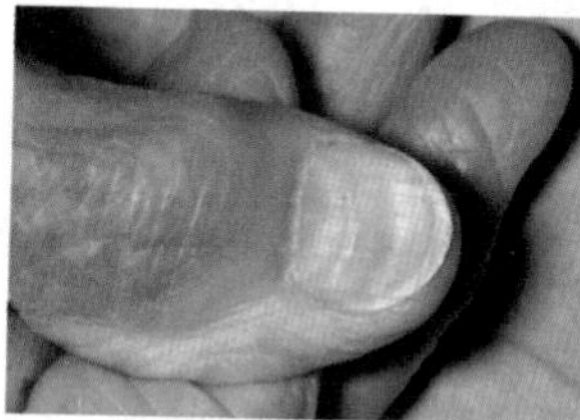

Fig 8.4 Koilonychia: spoon-shaped nails.

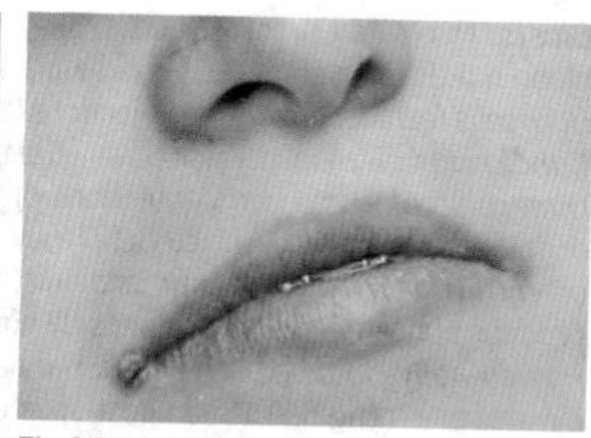

Fig 8.5 Angular cheilosis (also known as stomatitis): ulceration at the side of the mouth. Also a feature of vitamin B_{12} and B_2 (riboflavin) deficiency, and glucagonoma (p223).

Courtesy of Dr Joseph Thompson: AskAnOrthodontist.com.

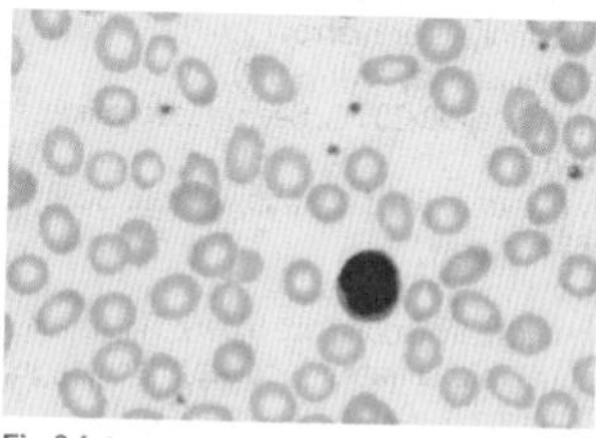

Fig 8.6 Microcytic hypochromic cells.

Courtesy of Prof. Krzysztof Lewandowski

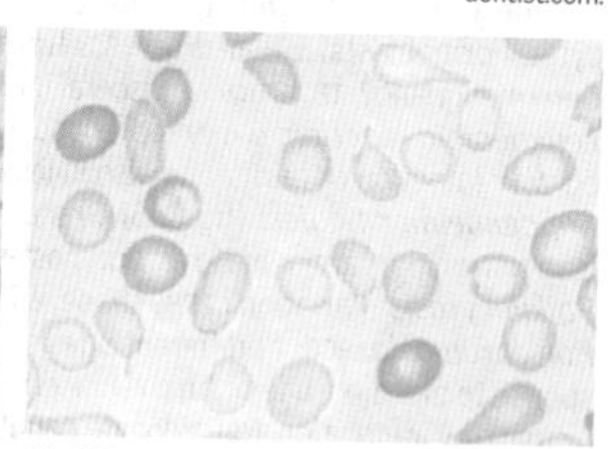

Fig 8.7 Poikilocytosis and anisocytosis.

Courtesy of Prof. Christine Lawrence.

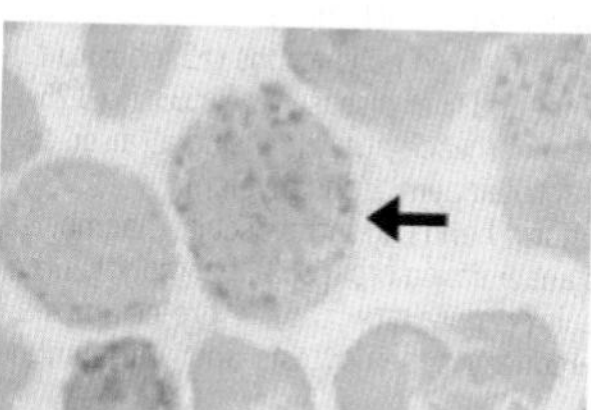

Fig 8.8 Ring sideroblasts in the marrow, with a perinuclear ring of iron granules, found in sideroblastic anaemia.

Courtesy of Prof. Christine Lawrence.

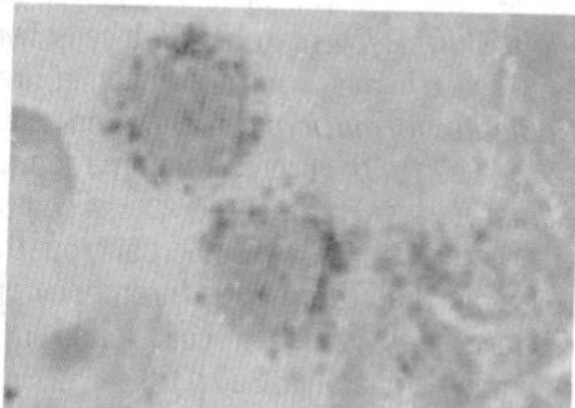

Fig 8.9 Two ringed sideroblasts showing how the distribution of perinuclear mitochondrial ferritin can vary. The problem in congenital sideroblastic anaemia is disordered mitochondrial haem synthesis.

Courtesy of Prof. Tangün and Dr Köroğlu.

The peripheral blood film

►Many haematological (and other) diagnoses are made by careful examination of the peripheral blood film. It is also necessary for interpretation of the FBC indices.

Features Include:

Acanthocytes: (fig 8.10) Spicules on RBCs (∵ unstable RBC membrane lipid structure); causes: splenectomy, alcoholic liver disease, abetalipoproteinaemia, spherocytosis.
Anisocytosis: Variation in RBC size, eg megaloblastic anaemia, thalassaemia, IDA.
Basophilic RBC stippling: (fig 8.11) Denatured RNA found in RBCs, indicating accelerated erythropoiesis or defective Hb synthesis. Seen in lead poisoning, megaloblastic anaemia, myelodysplasia, liver disease, haemoglobinopathy, eg thalassaemia.
Blasts: Nucleated precursor cells. They should not normally appear in peripheral blood but do in myelofibrosis, leukaemia, and malignant marrow infiltration.
Burr cells (echinocytes): RBC projections (less marked than in acanthocytes); fig 8.12.
Cabot rings: Seen in: pernicious anaemia; lead poisoning; bad infections (fig 8.13).[3]
Dimorphic picture: Two populations of red cells. Seen after treatment of Fe, B_{12}, or folate deficiency, in mixed deficiency (↓Fe with ↓B_{12} or folate), post-transfusion, or with primary sideroblastic anaemia, where a clone of abnormal erythroblasts produce abnormal red cells, alongside normal red cell production.
Howell-Jolly bodies: DNA nuclear remnants in RBCs, which are normally removed by the spleen (fig 8.14). Seen post-splenectomy and in hyposplenism (eg sickle-cell disease, coeliac disease, congenital, UC/Crohn's, myeloproliferative disease, amyloid). Also in dyserythropoietic states: myelodysplasia, megaloblastic anaemia.
Hypochromia: (p326.) Less dense staining of RBCs due to ↓Hb synthesis, seen in IDA, thalassaemia, and sideroblastic anaemia (iron stores unusable, p366).
Left shift: Immature neutrophils released from the marrow, eg in infection (fig 8.15).
Leukoerythroblastic film: Immature cells (myelocytes, promyelocytes, metamyelocytes, normoblasts) ± tear-drop RBCs from haemolysis or marrow infiltration/infection (malignancy; TB; brucella; visceral leishmaniasis; parvovirus B19).
Leukaemoid reaction: A marked leucocytosis (WCC >50×10^9/L). Seen in severe illness, eg with infection or burns, and also in leukaemia.
Pappenheimer bodies: (fig 8.16) Granules of siderocytes containing iron. Seen in lead poisoning, carcinomatosis, and post-splenectomy.
Poikilocytosis: Variation in RBC shape, eg in IDA, myelofibrosis, thalassaemia.
Polychromasia: RBCs of different ages stain unevenly (young are bluer). This is a response to bleeding, haematinic replacement (ferrous sulfate, B_{12}, folate), haemolysis, or marrow infiltration. Reticulocyte count is raised.
Reticulocytes: (Normal range: 0.8-2%; or <85×10^9/L.) (fig 8.17) Young, larger RBCs (contain RNA) signifying active erythropoiesis. Increased in haemolysis, haemorrhage, and if B_{12}, iron, or folate is given to marrow that lack these.
Right shift: Hypermature white cells: hypersegmented polymorphs (>5 lobes to nucleus) seen in megaloblastic anaemia, uraemia, and liver disease. See p333, fig 8.25.
Rouleaux formation: (fig 8.18) Red cells stack on each other (causing a raised ESR; p372). Seen with chronic inflammation, paraproteinaemia, and myeloma.
Schistocytes: Fragmented RBCs sliced by fibrin bands, in intravascular haemolysis (p339, fig 8.31). Look for microangiopathic anaemia, eg DIC (p352), haemolytic uraemic syndrome, thrombotic thrombocytopenic purpura (TTP: p315), or pre-eclampsia.
Spherocytes: Spherical cells found in hereditary spherocytosis and autoimmune haemolytic anaemia. See p338.
Target cells: (Also known as Mexican hat cells, fig 8.14 and fig 8.41, p343.) These are RBCs with central staining, a ring of pallor, and an outer rim of staining seen in liver disease, hyposplenism, thalassaemia—and, in small numbers, in IDA.
Tear-drop RBCs: Seen in extramedullary haematopoiesis; see leukoerythroblastic film.

3 Cabot 'figure-of-eight' rings may be microtubules from mitotic spindles. It is easy to confuse them with malaria parasites, p416 (especially if stippling gives a 'chromatin dot' artefact, as here). Richard Clarke Cabot (1868-1939) liked diagnostic challenges: he founded the notoriously hard but beautifully presented weekly clinicopathological exercises of the Massachusetts General Hospital which made the *New England Journal of Medicine* so famous. He also wisely recommended that: 'before you tell the truth to the patient, be sure you know the truth, and that the patient wants to hear it'.

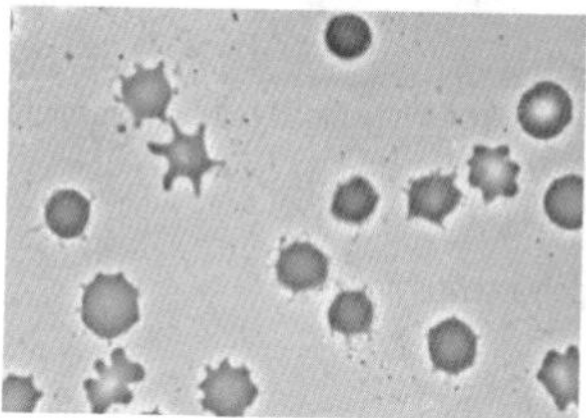

Fig 8.10 Acanthocytosis.

©Dr N Medeiros.

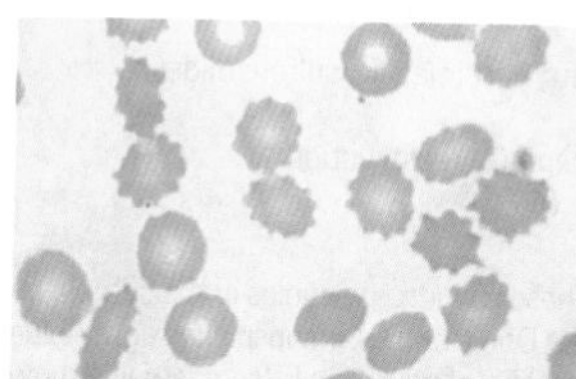

Fig 8.12 Burr cells: the cause may be renal or liver failure, or an EDTA storage artefact.

©Prof. Christine Lawrence.

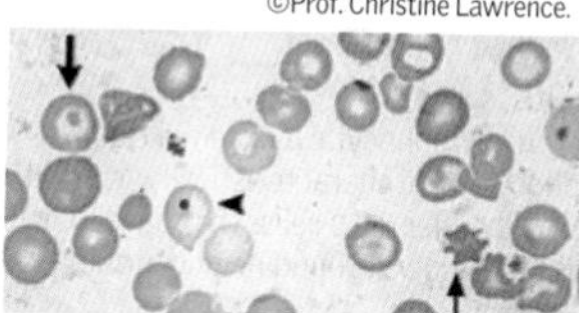

Fig 8.14 Film in hyposplenism: target cell (short arrow), acanthocyte (long arrow), and a Howell–Jolly body (arrow head).

From the *New England Journal of Medicine*, Bain, B, 'Diagnosis from the blood smear', 353(5), 498. Copyright © 2005 Massachusetts Medical Society. Reprinted with permission from Massachusetts Medical Society.

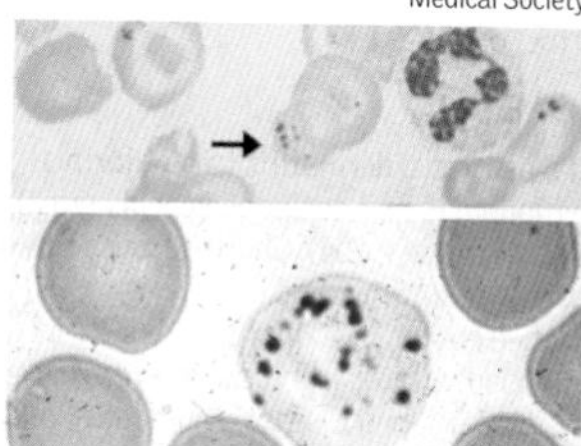

Fig 8.16 Pappenheimer bodies.

Top image ©Prof. Christine Lawrence, bottom image ©Crookston Collection.

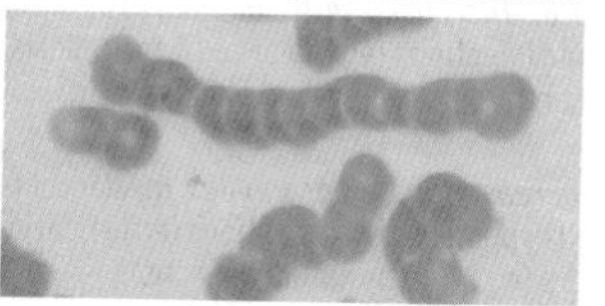

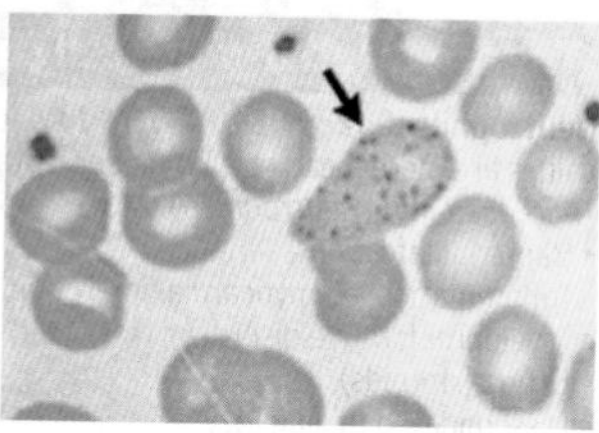

Fig 8.11 Basophilic stippling.

From the *New England Journal of Medicine*, Bain, B, 'Diagnosis from the blood smear', 353(5), 498. Copyright © 2005 Massachusetts Medical Society. Reprinted with permission from Massachusetts Medical Society.

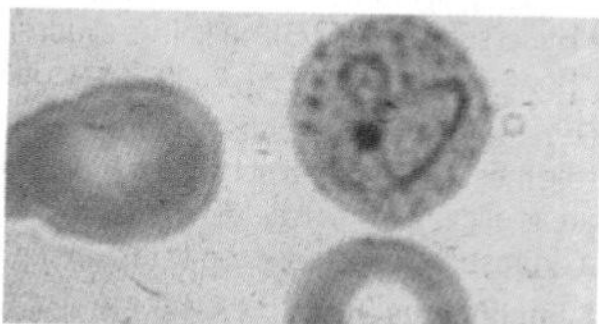

Fig 8.13 A Cabot ring.[3]

©Crookston Collection.

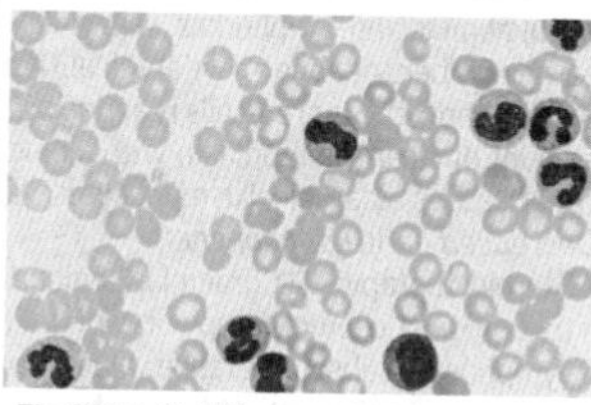

Fig 8.15 Left shift: presence of immature neutrophils in the blood. See p328.

©Prof. Krzysztof Lewandowski.

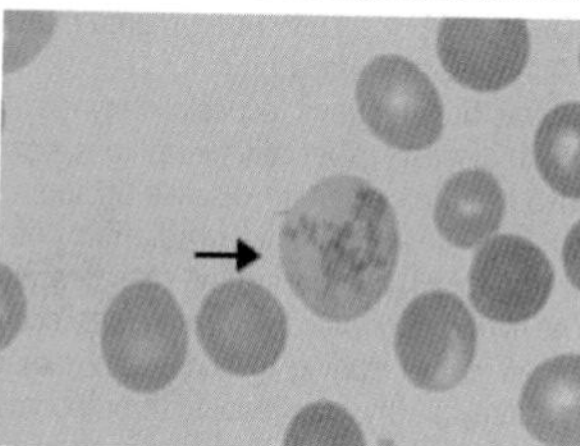

Fig 8.17 Reticulocytes. RNA in RBCs; supravital staining (azure B; cresyl blue) is needed.

©Dr N Medeiros.

Fig 8.18 Rouleaux formation.

©Dr N Medeiros.

The differential white cell count

Neutrophils (figs 8.19, 8.20) 2–7.5 × 10^9/L (40–75% of white blood cells: but absolute values are more meaningful than percentages).

Increased in (ie *neutrophilia*):
- Bacterial infections.
- Inflammation, eg myocardial infarction, polyarteritis nodosa.
- Myeloproliferative disorders.
- Drugs (steroids).
- Disseminated malignancy.
- Stress, eg trauma, surgery, burns, haemorrhage, seizure.

Decreased in (ie *neutropenia*—see p352):
- Viral infections.
- Drugs: post-chemotherapy, cytotoxic agents, carbimazole, sulfonamides.
- Severe sepsis.
- Neutrophil antibodies (SLE, haemolytic anaemia)—↑destruction.
- Hypersplenism (p373), eg Felty's syndrome (p698).
- Bone marrow failure—↓production (p364).

Other neutrophil responses to infection: These include: • vacuoles in the cytoplasm (the most specific sign of bacterial infection); • Döhle bodies: inconspicuous grey-blue areas of cytoplasm (residual ribosomes). Up to 17% of neutrophils from females show a drumstick-shaped Barr body (arrow, fig 8.20d). It is the inactivated X chromosome.

Lymphocytes (fig 8.21) 1.5–4.5 × 10^9/L (20–45%).

Increased in (ie *lymphocytosis*):
- Acute viral infections.
- Chronic infections, eg TB, brucellosis, hepatitis, syphilis.
- Leukaemias and lymphomas, especially chronic lymphocytic leukaemia (CLL).

Large numbers of abnormal ('atypical') lymphocytes are characteristically seen with EBV infection: these are T cells reacting against EBV-infected B cells. They have a large amount of clearish cytoplasm with a blue rim that flows around neighbouring RBCs. Other causes of 'atypical' lymphocytes: see p405.

Decreased in (ie *lymphopenia*):
- Steroid therapy; SLE; uraemia; Legionnaire's disease; HIV infection; marrow infiltration; post chemotherapy or radiotherapy.

T-lymphocyte subset reference values: CD4 count: 537–1571/mm^3 (low in HIV infection). CD8 count: 235–753/mm^3; CD4/CD8 ratio: 1.2–3.8.

Eosinophils (fig 8.22) 0.04–0.4 × 10^9/L (1–6%).

Increased in (ie *eosinophilia*):
- Drug reactions, eg with erythema multiforme, p562.
- Allergies: asthma, atopy.
- Parasitic infections (especially invasive helminths).
- Skin disease: especially pemphigus, eczema, psoriasis, dermatitis herpetiformis.

Also seen in malignant disease (including lymphomas and eosinophilic leukaemia), PAN, adrenal insufficiency, irradiation, Löffler's syndrome (p704), Churg–Strauss syndrome (p696) and during the convalescent phase of any infection.

The hypereosinophilic syndrome (HES) occurs when eosinophila >1.5 × 10^9/L is sustained for >6 weeks leading to end-organ damage (endomyocardial fibrosis and restrictive cardiomyopathy, skin lesions, thromboembolic disease, lung disease, neuropathy, and hepatosplenomegaly). The cause is often unknown, though if FIP1L1-PDFRA genotype, diagnose myeloproliferative HES or eosinophilic leukaemia. ℞: PO steroids ± mepolizumab (anti-interleukin-5 monoclonal antibody). Imatinib is 1st choice for myoproliferative HES.

Monocytes (fig 8.23) 0.2–0.8 × 10^9/L (2–10%). *Increased in* (ie *monocytosis*): the aftermath of chemo- or radiotherapy, chronic infections (eg malaria, TB, brucellosis, protozoa), malignant disease (including M4 and M5 acute myeloid leukaemia (p356), and Hodgkin's disease), myelodysplasia.

Basophils (fig 8.24) 0–0.1 × 10^9/L (0–1%). *Increased in* (ie *basophilia*): myeloproliferative disease, viral infections, IgE-mediated hypersensitivity reactions (eg urticaria, hypothyroidism), and inflammatory disorders (eg UC, rheumatoid arthritis).

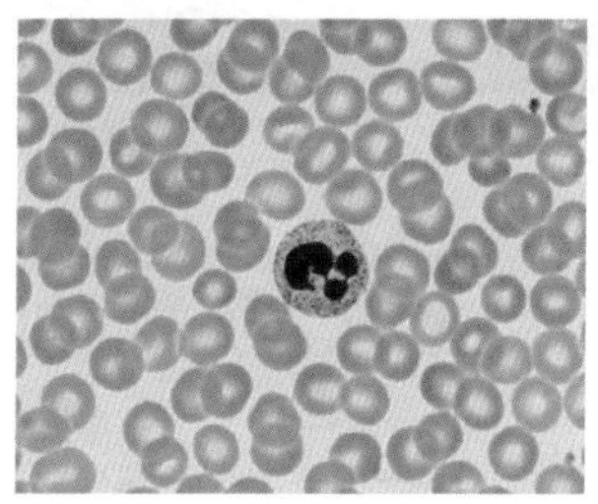

Fig 8.19 Neutrophil. These ingest and kill bacteria, fungi, and damaged cells.

Courtesy of Prof. Krzysztof Lewandowski.

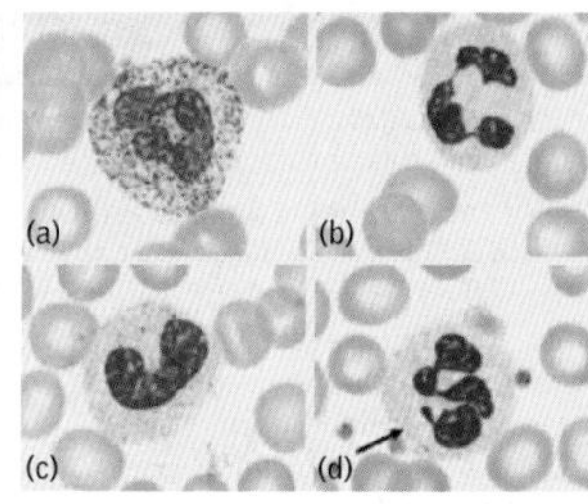

Fig 8.20 Neutrophils: (a) 'toxic granulation' seen in infection or pregnancy; (b) normal appearances; (c) 'left shift': immature forms are released with few lobes to their nuclei, seen in infection; (d) Barr body (arrow, see text).

Courtesy of Prof. Tangün and Dr Köroğlu.

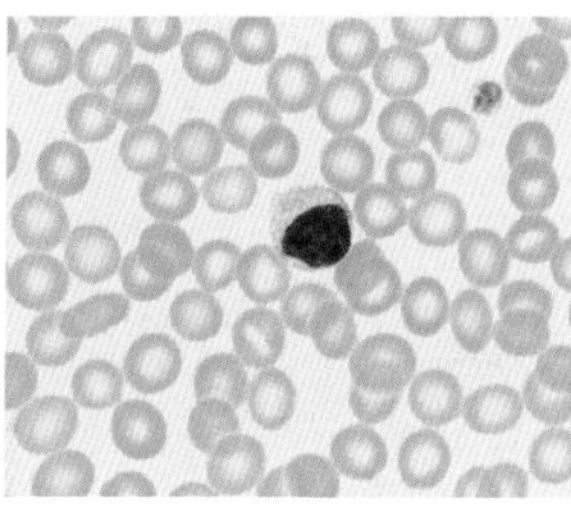

Fig 8.21 Lymphocyte: divided into T & B types, which have important roles in cell-mediated immunity and antibody production.

Courtesy of Prof. Krzysztof Lewandowski.

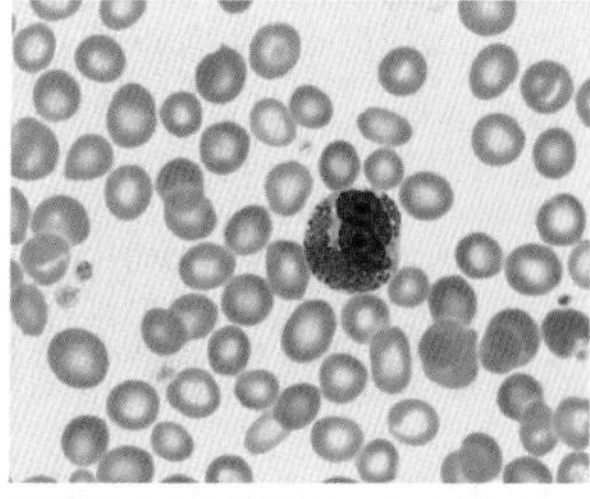

Fig 8.22 Eosinophil: these mediate allergic reactions and defend against parasites.

Courtesy of Prof. Krzysztof Lewandowski.

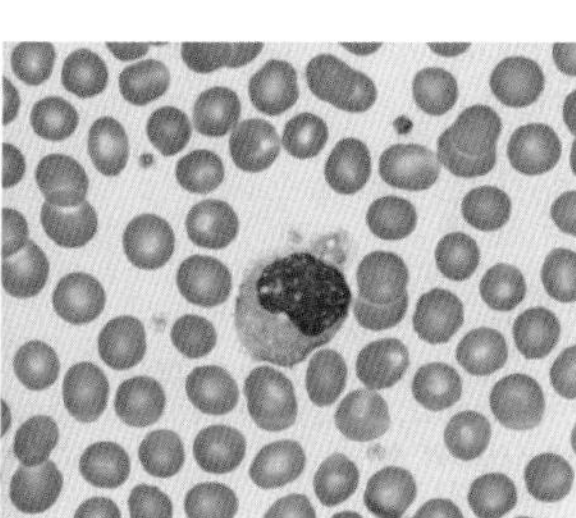

Fig 8.23 Monocyte: precursors of tissue macrophages.

Courtesy of Prof. Krzysztof Lewandowski.

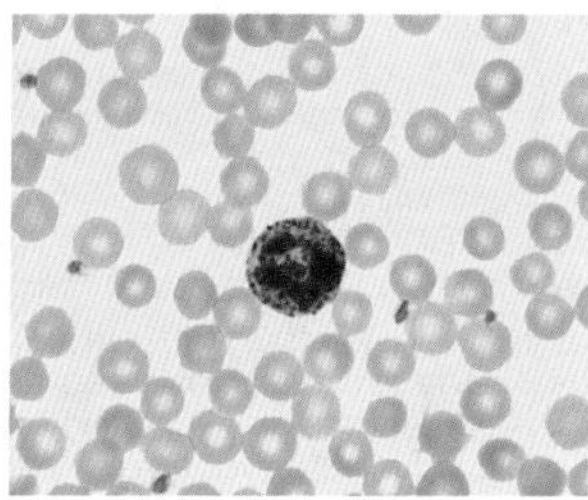

Fig 8.24 Basophil. The cytoplasm is filled with dark-staining granules, containing histamine, myeloperoxidase and other enzymes. On binding IgE, histamine is released from the basophil.

Courtesy of Prof. Krzysztof Lewandowski.

Macrocytic anaemia

Macrocytosis (MCV >96fL) is common, and may not always be accompanied by anaemia (eg in alcohol excess).

Causes of macrocytosis (MCV >96fL)

- *Megaloblastic:* (fig 8.25) a megaloblast is a cell in which nuclear maturation is delayed compared with the cytoplasm. This occurs with B_{12} (p334) and folate deficiency: both are required for DNA synthesis. Another cause is cytotoxic drugs.
- *Non-megaloblastic:* Alcohol excess, reticulocytosis (eg in haemolysis), liver disease, hypothyroidism, pregnancy.
- *Other haematological disease:* Myelodysplasia (fig 8.26), myeloma, myeloproliferative disorders, aplastic anaemia.

Tests B_{12} and folate deficiency result in similar blood film and bone marrow biopsy appearances.
Blood film: Hypersegmented neutrophils (fig 8.25) in B_{12} and folate deficiency. Target cells if liver disease; see fig 8.14, p329 and fig 8.41, p343.
Other tests: LFT (include γGT), TFT, serum B_{12}, and serum folate (or red cell folate—a more reliable indicator of folate status, as serum folate only reflects *recent* intake).
Bone marrow biopsy is indicated if the cause is not revealed by the above tests. It is likely to show one of the following four states:

1. Megaloblastic marrow.
2. Normoblastic marrow (eg in liver disease, hypothyroidism).
3. Abnormal erythropoiesis (eg sideroblastic anaemia, p326, leukaemia, aplasia).
4. Increased erythropoiesis (eg haemolysis).

Folate Found in green vegetables, nuts, yeast, and liver; it is synthesized by gut bacteria. Body stores can last for 4 months. Maternal folate deficiency causes fetal neural tube defects. It is absorbed by duodenum/proximal jejunum.

Causes of deficiency:

- Poor diet, eg poverty, alcoholics, elderly.
- Increased demand, eg pregnancy or ↑cell turnover (seen in haemolysis, malignancy, inflammatory disease, and renal dialysis).
- Malabsorption, eg coeliac disease, tropical sprue.
- Alcohol.
- Drugs: anti-epileptics (phenytoin, valproate), methotrexate, trimethoprim.

Treatment: Assess for an underlying cause, eg poor diet, malabsorption. Treat with folic acid 5mg/day PO for 4 months, ►never without B_{12} unless the patient is known to have a normal B_{12} level, as in low B_{12} states it may precipitate, or worsen, subacute combined degeneration of the cord (p334). In pregnancy, prophylactic doses of folate (400mcg/day) are given from conception until at least 12wks; this helps prevent spina bifida, as well as anaemia.

NB: in unwell patients (eg CCF) with megaloblastic anaemia, it may be necessary to treat before serum B_{12} and folate results are known. Do tests then treat with large doses of hydroxocobalamin, eg 1mg/48h IM—see *BNF*, with folic acid 5mg/24h PO. Blood transfusions are very rarely needed (see p324).

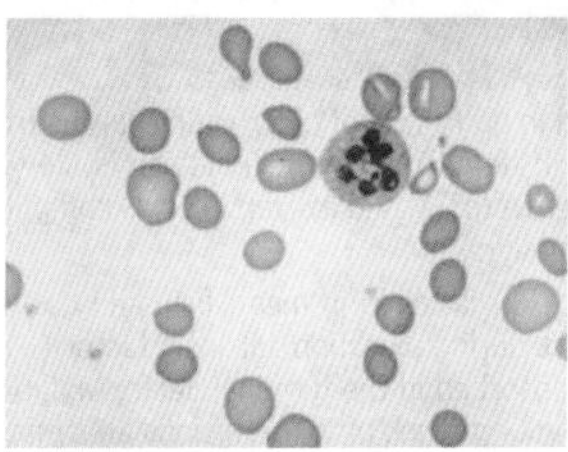

Fig 8.25 Megaloblastic anaemia: peripheral blood film showing many macrocytes and one hypersegmented neutrophil (normally there should be ≤5 segments).

From the *New England Journal of Medicine*, Bain, B, 'Diagnosis from the blood smear', 353(5), 498. Copyright © 2005 Massachusetts Medical Society. Reprinted with permission from Massachusetts Medical Society.

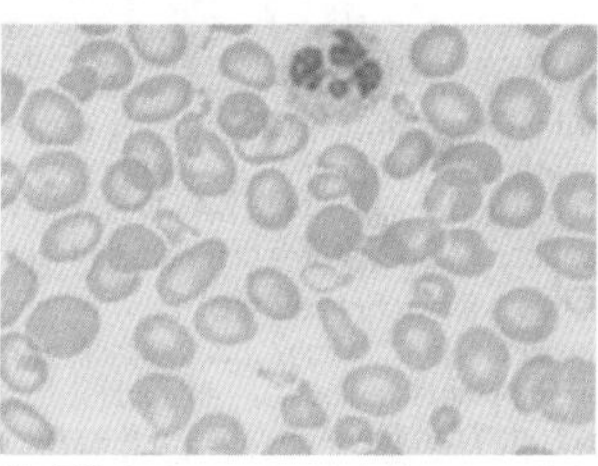

Fig 8.26 Oval macrocytes seen here in myelodysplastic syndromes. Note aniso- and poikilocytosis with small fragmented cells (schistocytes). NB: B_{12} and folate deficiencies also cause oval macrocytes, but macrocytes caused by alcohol and liver disease are usually round.

Courtesy of Prof. Tangün and Dr Köroğlu.

B_{12} deficiency and pernicious anaemia

Vitamin B_{12} deficiency is common, occurring in up to 15% of older people. B_{12} helps synthesize thymidine, and hence DNA, so in deficiency RBC production is slow. Untreated, it can lead to megaloblastic anaemia (p332) and irreversible CNS complications. ► Body stores of B_{12} are sufficient for 4yrs.

Causes of deficiency • Dietary (eg vegans: B_{12} is found in meat, fish, and dairy products, but not in plants). • Malabsorption: during digestion, intrinsic factor (IF) in the stomach binds B_{12}, enabling it to be absorbed in the terminal ileum. Malabsorption can therefore arise in the *stomach* due to lack of IF (pernicious anaemia, post gastrectomy) or the *terminal ileum* (ileal resection, Crohn's disease, bacterial overgrowth, tropical sprue, tapeworms). • Congenital metabolic errors.

Features *General:* Symptoms of anaemia (p324), 'lemon tinge' to skin due to combination of pallor (anaemia) and mild jaundice (due to haemolysis), glossitis (beefy-red sore tongue; fig 8.27), angular cheilosis (p326).

Neuropsychiatric: Irritability, depression, psychosis, dementia.

Neurological: Paraesthesiae, peripheral neuropathy. Also *subacute combined degeneration of the spinal cord,* a combination of peripheral sensory neuropathy with both upper *and* lower motor neuron signs due to ↓B_{12}. The patient may display the classical triad of: • extensor plantars (UMN) • absent knee jerks (LMN) • absent ankle jerks (LMN). The onset is insidious (*subacute*) and signs are symmetrical. There is a combination of posterior (dorsal) column loss, causing the sensory and LMN signs, and corticospinal tract loss, causing the motor and UMN signs (p446). The spinothalamic tracts are preserved so pain and temperature sensation may remain intact even in severe cases. Joint-position and vibration sense are often affected first leading to ataxia, followed by stiffness and weakness if untreated. ► The neurological signs of B_{12} deficiency can occur without anaemia.

Pernicious anaemia (PA) This is an autoimmune condition in which atrophic gastritis leads to a lack of IF secretion from the parietal cells of the stomach. Dietary B_{12} therefore remains unbound and conseqeuently cannot be absorbed by the terminal ileum.

Incidence: 1:1000; ♀:♂≈1.6:1; usually >40yrs; higher incidence if blood group A.

Associations: Other autoimmune diseases (p553): thyroid disease (~25%), vitiligo, Addison's disease, hypoparathyroidism. Carcinoma of stomach is ~3-fold more common in pernicious anaemia, so have a low threshold for upper GI endoscopy.

Tests: • ↓Hb. • ↑MCV. • WCC and ↓platelets if severe. • ↓Serum B_{12}[4]. • Reticulocytes may be ↓ as production impaired. • Hypersegmented neutrophils (p332). • Megaloblasts in the marrow. • Specific tests for PA: 1 Parietal cell antibodies: found in 90% with PA, but also in 3–10% without. 2 IF antibodies: specific for PA, but lower sensitivity.

Treatment: Treat the cause if possible. If due to malabsorption, give hydroxocobalamin (B_{12}) 1mg IM alternate days for 2wks (or, if CNS signs, until improvement stops), then 1mg IM every 3 months for life. If the cause is dietary, then oral B_{12} can be given after the initial IM course (50–150mcg/daily, between meals). Improvement is indicated by a transient marked reticulocytosis (↑MCV), after 4–5 days.

Practical hints: • Beware of diagnosing PA in those under 40yrs old: look for GI malabsorption (small bowel biopsy, p266).
- Watch for hypokalaemia due to uptake into new haematopoietic cells.
- Transfusion is best avoided, but PA with high-output CCF may require transfusion, after doing tests for FBC, folate, B_{12}, and marrow sampling.
- As haematopoiesis accelerates on treatment, additional iron may be needed.
- Hb rises ~10g/L per week; WCC and platelet count should normalize in 1wk.

Prognosis: Supplementation usually improves peripheral neuropathy within the first 3–6 months, but has little effect on cord signs. Patients do best if treated as soon as possible after the onset of symptoms: don't delay!

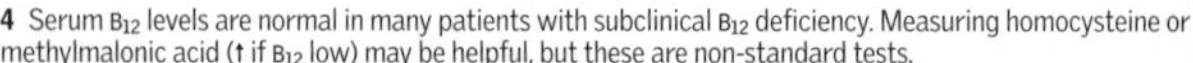

4 Serum B_{12} levels are normal in many patients with subclinical B_{12} deficiency. Measuring homocysteine or methylmalonic acid (↑ if B_{12} low) may be helpful, but these are non-standard tests.

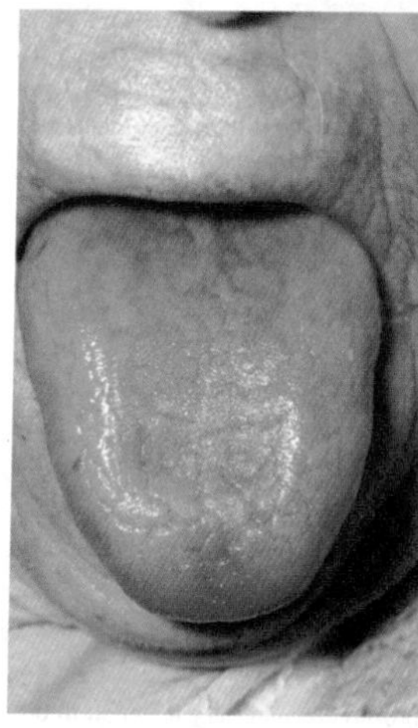

Fig 8.27 The big, beefy tongue of B_{12} deficiency glossitis. Other causes of glossitis: iron (or Zn) deficiency, pellagra, contact dermatitis/specific food intolerances, Crohn's disease, drugs (minocycline, clarithromycin, some ACE-i), TB of the tongue. Glossitis may be the presenting feature of coeliac disease or alcoholism.

An approach to haemolytic anaemia

Haemolysis is the premature breakdown of RBCs, before their normal lifespan of ~120d. It occurs in the circulation (*intravascular*) or in the reticuloendothelial system, ie macrophages of liver, spleen, and bone marrow (*extravascular*). In sickle-cell anaemia, lifespan may be as short as 5d. Haemolysis may be asymptomatic, but if the bone marrow does not compensate sufficiently, a haemolytic anaemia results.

An approach is first to confirm haemolysis and then find the cause—try to answer these four questions:

1 *Is there increased red cell breakdown?*
- Anaemia with normal or ↑MCV.
- ↑Bilirubin: unconjugated, from haem breakdown (pre-hepatic jaundice).
- ↑Urinary urobilinogen (no urinary conjugated bilirubin).
- ↑Serum LDH, as it is released from red cells.

2 *Is there increased red cell production?*
- ↑Reticulocytes, causing ↑MCV (reticulocytes are large immature RBCs) and polychromasia.

3 *Is the haemolysis mainly extra- or intravascular?*
Extravascular haemolysis may lead to splenic hypertrophy and splenomegaly. Features of intravascular haemolysis are:
- ↑Free plasma haemoglobin: released from RBCs.
- Methaemalbuminaemia: some free Hb is broken down in the circulation to produce haem and globin; haem combines with albumin to make methaemalbumin.
- ↓Plasma haptoglobin: mops up free plasma Hb, then removed by the liver.
- Haemoglobinuria: causes red-brown urine, in absence of red blood cells.
- Haemosiderinuria: occurs when haptoglobin-binding capacity is exceeded, causing free Hb to be filtered by the renal glomeruli, with absorption of free Hb via the renal tubules and storage in the tubular cells as haemosiderin. This is detected in the urine as sloughed tubular cells by Prussian blue staining ~1 week after onset (implying a chronic intravascular haemolysis).

4 *Why is there haemolysis?* Causes are on p338.

History Family history, race, jaundice, dark urine, drugs, previous anaemia, travel.

Examination Jaundice, hepatosplenomegaly, gallstones (pigmented, due to ↑bilirubin from haemolysis), leg ulcers (due to poor blood flow).

Tests FBC, reticulocytes, bilirubin, LDH, haptoglobin, urinary urobilinogen. Thick and thin films for malaria screen if history of travel. The blood film may show polychromasia and macrocytosis due to reticulocytes, or point to the diagnosis:
- Hypochromic microcytic anaemia (thalassaemia).
- Sickle cells (sickle-cell anaemia).
- Schistocytes (fig 8.30, p339; microangiopathic haemolytic anaemia).
- Abnormal cells in haematological malignancy.
- Spherocytes (hereditary spherocytosis or autoimmune haemolytic anaemia).
- Elliptocytes (fig 8.36, p339; hereditary elliptocytosis).
- Heinz bodies, 'bite' cells (fig 8.32, p339; glucose-6-phosphate dehydrogenase deficiency).

Further tests (if the cause is still not obvious)
- Osmotic fragility testing will confirm the presence of membrane abnormalities which have been identified on the film.
- Hb electrophoresis will detect haemoglobinopathies.
- The direct antiglobulin (Coombs) test (DAT, fig 8.28) identifies red cells coated with antibody or complement, the presence of which indicates an immune cause.
- Enzyme assays are reserved for when other causes have been excluded.

Direct Coombs test/Direct antiglobulin test

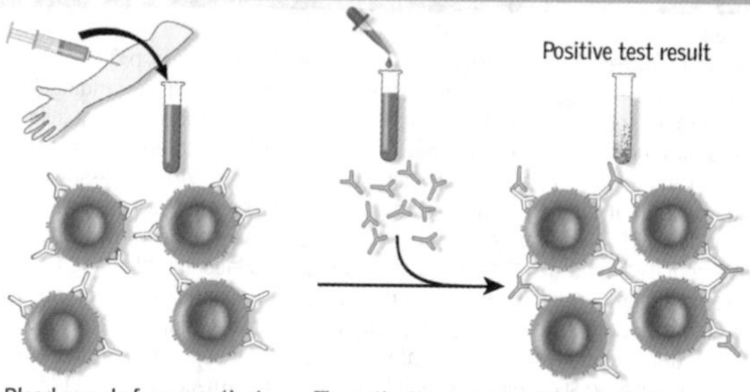

Positive test result
Anti-human Ig's (Coombs antibodies) are added to the solution.
Human anti-RBC antibody
Blood sample from a patient with immune mediated haemolytic anaemia: antibodies are shown attached to antigens on the RBC surface.
The patient's washed RBCs are incubated with antihuman antibodies (Coombs reagent).
RBCs agglutinate: antihuman antibodies form links between RBCs by binding to the human antibodies on the RBCs.

Indirect Coombs test/Indirect antiglobulin test

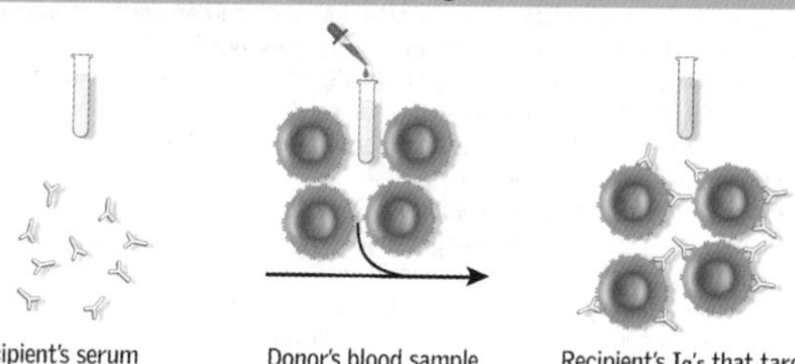

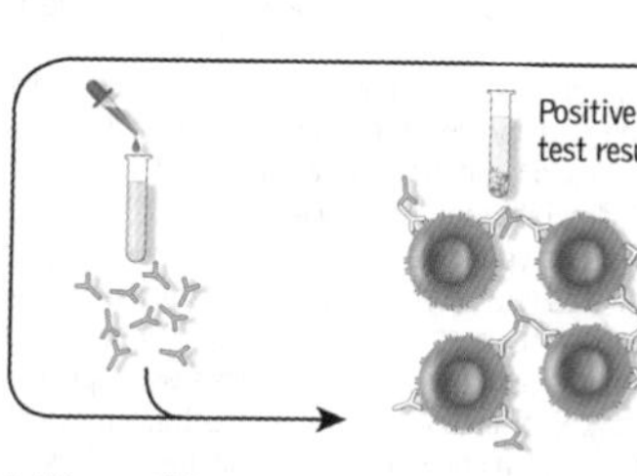

Recipient's serum is obtained, containing antibodies (Ig's).
Donor's blood sample is added to the tube with serum.
Recipient's Ig's that target the donor's red blood cells form antibody-antigen complexes.

Fig 8.28 The *direct* Coombs test detects antibodies on RBCs. The *indirect* Coombs test is used in pre-natal testing and before blood transfusion. It detects antibodies against RBCs that are free in serum: serum is incubated with RBCs of known antigenicity. If agglutination occurs, the indirect Coombs test is positive.

With kind permission of Aria Rad.

Causes of haemolytic anaemia

Acquired

1 *Immune-mediated/direct antiglobulin test +ve:* (Coombs test, p337.)

- *Drug-induced:* causing formation of RBC autoantibodies from binding to RBC membranes (eg penicillin) or production of immune complexes (eg quinine).
- *Autoimmune haemolytic anaemia (AIHA;* fig 8.29*):* mediated by autoantibodies causing mainly extravascular haemolysis and spherocytosis. Classify according to optimal binding temperature to RBCs: *Warm AIHA:* IgG-mediated, bind at body T° 37°C. ℞: Steroids/immunosuppressants (± splenectomy). *Cold AIHA:* IgM-mediated, bind at ↓T° (<4°C), activating cell-surface complement. Causes a chronic anaemia made worse by cold, often with Raynaud's or acrocyanosis. ℞: keep warm. Chlorambucil may help. *Causes:* most are idiopathic; 2° causes of warm AIHA include lymphoproliferative disease (CLL, lymphoma), drugs, autoimmune disease, eg SLE. Cold AIHA may follow infection (mycoplasma; EBV).
- *Paroxysmal cold haemoglobinuria:* seen with viruses/syphilis. It is caused by Donath-Landsteiner antibodies sticking to RBCs in the cold, causing self-limiting complement-mediated haemolysis on rewarming.
- *Isoimmune:* acute transfusion reaction (p349); haemolysis of the newborn.

2 *Direct antiglobulin/Coombs −ve AIHA:* (2% of all AIHA.) Autoimmune hepatitis; hepatitis B & C; post flu and other vaccinations; drugs (piperacillin, rituximab).

3 *Microangiopathic haemolytic anaemia (MAHA):* Mechanical damage to RBCs in circulation, causing intravascular haemolysis and schistocytes (figs 8.30, 8.31). Causes include haemolytic-uraemic syndrome (HUS), TTP (p315), DIC, pre-eclampsia, and eclampsia. Prosthetic heart valves can also cause mechanical damage.

4 *Infection:* Malaria (p416): RBC lysis and 'blackwater fever' (haemoglobinuria). ►All infections can exacerbate haemolysis.

5 *Paroxysmal nocturnal haemoglobinuria:* Rare acquired stem cell disorder, with haemolysis (esp. at night→haemoglobinuria, fig 15.8, p705), marrow failure + thrombophilia. *Tests:* urinary haemosiderin +ve; if suspect in Coombs -ve intravascular haemolysis, seek confirmation by flow cytometry. ℞: anticoagulation; monoclonal anticomplement antibodies (eg eculizumab); stem cell transplantation.

Hereditary

1 *Enzyme defects:*

- *Glucose-6-phosphate dehydrogenase (G6PD) deficiency (X-linked):* the chief RBC enzyme defect, affects 100 million (mainly ♂) in Mediterranean, Africa, Middle/Far East. Most are asymptomatic, but may get oxidative crises due to ↓glutathione production, precipitated by drugs (eg primaquine, sulfonamides, aspirin), exposure to *Vicia faba* (broad beans/favism), or illness. In attacks, there is rapid anaemia and jaundice. Film: bite- and blister-cells (figs 8.32, 8.33). *Tests:* Enzyme assay (>8wks after crisis as young RBCs may have enough enzyme so results normal). ℞: Avoid precipitants (eg, henna, fig 8.34); transfuse if severe.
- *Pyruvate kinase deficiency (AUTOSOMAL RECESSIVE):* ↓ATP production causes ↓RBC survival. Homozygotes have neonatal jaundice; later, haemolysis with splenomegaly ± jaundice. *Tests:* enzyme assay. ℞: often not needed; splenectomy may help.

2 *Membrane defects:* All are Coombs −ve; all need folate; splenectomy helps some.

- *Hereditary spherocytosis (AUTOSOMAL DOMINANT):* prevalence: 1:3000. Less deformable spherical RBCs, so trapped in spleen→extravascular haemolysis. *Signs:* Splenomegaly, jaundice. *Tests:* Mild if Hb >110g/L and reticulocytes <6%; film: fig 8.35. ↑Bilirubin (→gallstones).
- *Hereditary elliptocytosis (AUTOSOMAL DOMINANT):* film: fig 8.36. Mostly asymptomatic (somewhat protects from malaria). 10% display a more severe phenotype (±death *in utero*).
- *Hereditary ovalocytosis and stomatocytosis* are rarer. Refer to a haematologist.

3 *Haemoglobinopathy:* • *Sickle-cell disease* (p340). • *Thalassaemia* (p342).

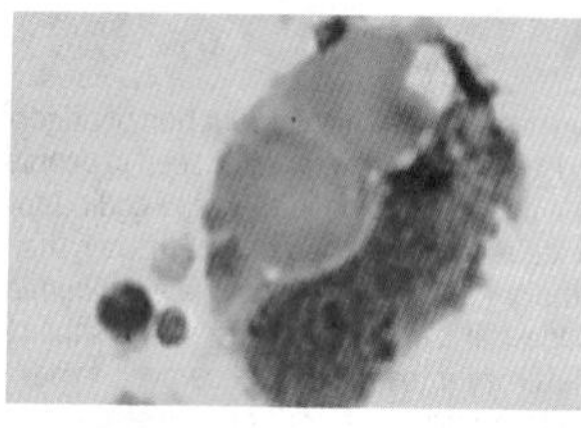

Fig 8.29 Autoimmune haemolytic anaemia: antibody-coated red cells undergoing phagocytosis by monocytes.

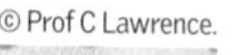

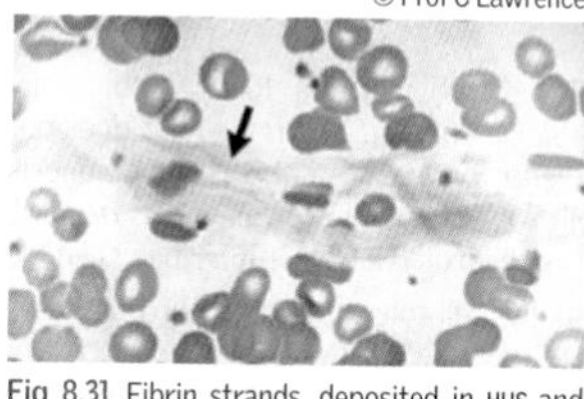

Fig 8.31 Fibrin strands, deposited in HUS and TTP (p315), slicing up RBCs (microangiopathy).

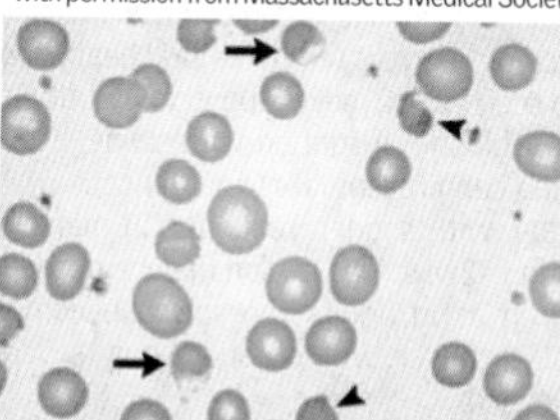

Fig 8.33 Blister-cells (arrows) in G6PD, following removal of Heinz bodies. Also contracted red cells (arrowheads).

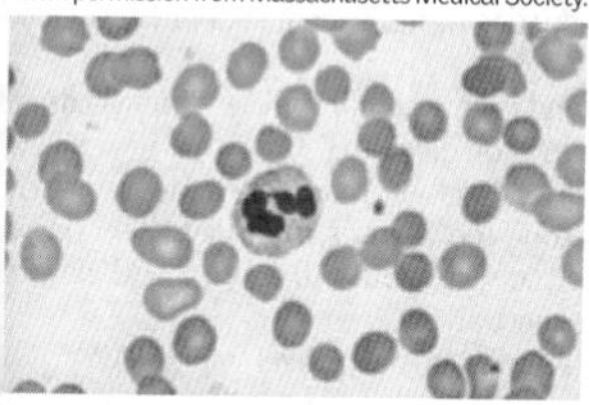

Fig 8.35 Hereditary spherocytosis. Osmotic fragility tests: RBCs show ↑fragility in hypotonic solutions.

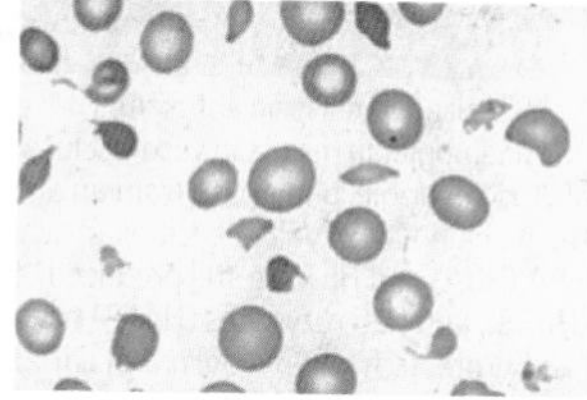

Fig 8.30 Microangiopathic anaemia, eg from DIC: numerous cell fragments (schistocytes) are present.

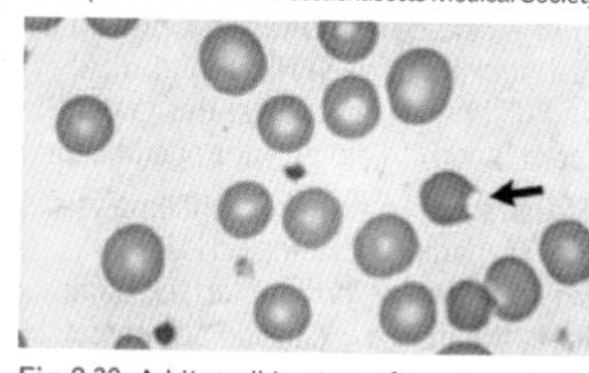

Fig 8.32 A bite-cell in G6PD, after removal of a Heinz body by the spleen; these are formed from denatured Hb during oxidative crises.

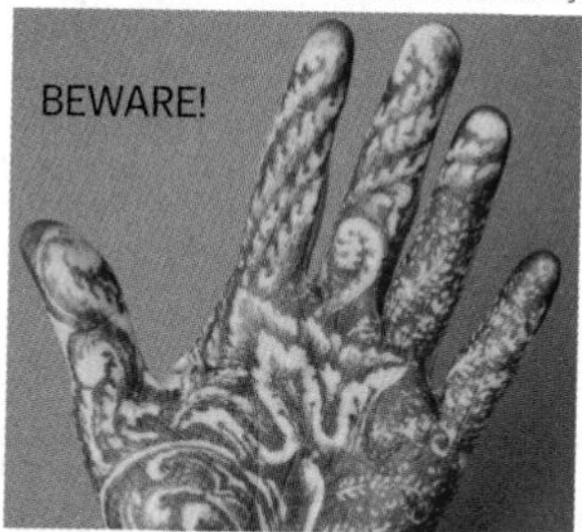

Fig 8.34 Avoid henna use in G6PD deficiency!

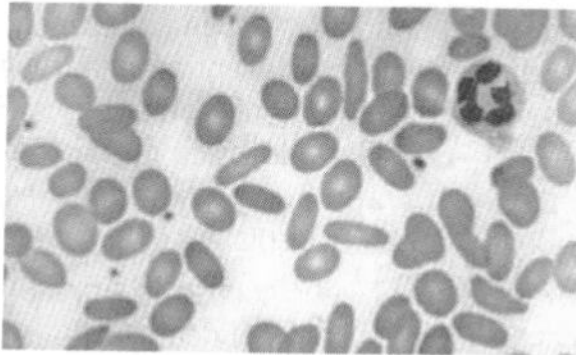

Fig 8.36 Hereditary elliptocytosis.

Sickle-cell anaemia

Sickle-cell anaemia is an autosomal recessive disorder in which production of abnormal haemoglobin results in vaso-occlusive crises. It is most commonly seen in people of African origin, and arises from an amino acid substitution in the gene coding for the β chain (Glu → Val at position 6) which leads to production of HbS rather than HbA (HbA_2 and HbF are still produced). Homozygotes (SS) have sickle-cell *anaemia* (HbSS), and heterozygotes (HbAS) have sickle-cell *trait*, which causes no disability (and protects from *falciparum* malaria). Heterozygotes may still, however, experience symptomatic sickling in hypoxia, eg in unpressurized aircraft or anaesthesia (so all those of African descent need a pre-op sickle-cell test).

Pathogenesis HbS polymerizes when deoxygenated, causing RBCs to deform, producing sickle cells, which are fragile and haemolyse, and also block small vessels.

Prevalence 1:700 people of African descent.

Tests Haemolysis is variable. Hb ≈ 60–90g/L, ↑reticulocytes 10–20%, ↑bilirubin. *Film:* sickle cells and target cells (fig 8.37). *Sickle solubility test:* +ve, but does not distinguish between HbSS and HbAS. *Hb electrophoresis:* Confirms the diagnosis and distinguishes SS, AS states, and other Hb variants. ►Aim for diagnosis *at birth* (cord blood) to aid prompt pneumococcal prophylaxis (vaccine, p167 ± penicillin V).

Signs/symptoms Chronic haemolysis is usually well tolerated (except in crises; see BOX 'Managing sickle-cell crises').

Vaso-occlusive 'painful' crisis: Common, due to microvascular occlusion. Often affects the marrow, causing severe pain, triggered by cold, dehydration, infection, or hypoxia. Hands and feet are affected if <3yrs old leading to *dactylitis*. Occlusion may cause *mesenteric ischaemia*, mimicking an acute abdomen. CNS infarction occurs in ~10% of children, leading to *stroke, seizures*, or *cognitive defects*. Transcranial Doppler ultrasonography indicates risk of impending stroke, and blood transfusions can prevent this by reducing HbS. Also *avascular necrosis* (eg of femoral head), *leg ulcers* (fig 8.38) and low-flow *priapism* (also seen in CML, may respond to hydration, α-agonists, eg phenylephrine, or aspiration of blood + irrigation with saline; if for >12h prompt cavernosus-spongiosum shunting can prevent later impotence).

Aplastic crisis: This is due to parvovirus B19, with sudden reduction in marrow production, especially RBCs. Usually self-limiting <2wks; transfusion may be needed.

Sequestration crisis: Mainly affects children as in adults the spleen becomes atrophic. There is pooling of blood in the spleen ± liver, with organomegaly, severe anaemia, and shock. Urgent transfusion is needed.

Complications • Splenic infarction occurs before 2yrs old, due to microvascular occlusion, leading to ↑susceptibility to infection (40% of childhood sickle deaths are caused this way). • Poor growth. • Chronic renal failure. • Gallstones. • Retinal disease. • Iron overload (see BOX 'A 7-year-old ...'). • Lung damage: hypoxia→fibrosis→pulmonary hypertension.

Management of chronic disease ►Get help from a haematologist.

- Hydroxycarbamide if frequent crises (↑production of fetal haemoglobin, HbF). Dose example: 20mg/kg/d if eGFR >60mL/min.
- Splenic infarction leads to hyposplenism and immunocompromise. Prophylaxis, in terms of antibiotics and immunization, should be given (p373).
- Febrile children risk septicaemia: repeated admission may be avoided by early rescue out-patient antibiotics, eg ceftriaxone (eg 2 doses, 50mg/kg IV on day 0 and 1). Consider admission if Hb <50g/L, WCC <5 or >30 × 10^9/L, T° >40°C, severe pain, dehydration, lung infiltration. Seek expert advice.
- Bone marrow transplant can be curative but remains controversial.

Prevention Genetic counselling; prenatal tests (*OHCS* pp154–5). Parental education can help prevent 90% of deaths from sequestration crises.

Managing sickle-cell crises

- Give *prompt*, generous analgesia, eg IV opiates (see p574). ►Most sickle patients will have a personalized analgesia plan—ask them! ►Seek expert help early.
- Crossmatch blood, check FBC and reticulocyte count.
- Do a septic screen: blood cultures, MSU ± CXR if T°↑ or chest signs.
- Rehydrate with IVI and keep warm. Give O_2 by mask if ↓P_aO_2 or O_2 sats <95%.
- Consider starting antibiotics empirically if T° >38°, unwell, or chest signs.
- Measure PCV, reticulocytes, liver, and spleen size twice daily.
- Give blood transfusion if Hb or reticulocytes fall sharply. This helps oxygenation, and is as good as exchange transfusion. Match blood for the blood group antigens Rh(C, D, E) and Kell, to prevent alloantibody formation.
- Exchange transfusion is reserved for those who are rapidly worsening: it is a process where blood is removed and donor blood is given in stages. Indications: severe chest crisis, suspected CNS event, or multiorgan failure—when the proportion of HbS should be reduced to <30%.
- Inform their haematologist of admission *early*.

The acute chest syndrome: Entails pulmonary infiltrates involving complete lung segments, causing pain, fever, tachypnoea, wheeze, and cough. It is serious. Incidence: ~0.1 episodes/patient/yr. 13% in the landmark Vichinsky study needed ventilation, 11% had CNS symptoms, and 9% of those over 20 years old died. Prodromal painful crisis occur ~2.5 days before any abnormalities on CXR in 50% of patients. The chief causes of the infiltrates are fat embolism from bone marrow or infection with *Chlamydia*, *Mycoplasma*, or viruses. ℞: O_2, analgesia, empirical antibiotics (cephalosporin + macrolide) until culture results known. Bronchodilators (eg salbutamol, p182) have proved to be effective in those with wheezing or obstructive pulmonary function at presentation. Blood transfusion (exchange if severe). *Take to ITU* if P_aO_2 cannot be kept above 9.2kPa (70mmHg) when breathing air.

Patient-controlled analgesia is a good option if supportive measures and oral analgesia do not control pain. Start with morphine 1mg/kg in 50mL 5% glucose (paediatric dose) and try a rate of 1mL/h, allowing the patient to deliver extra boluses of 1mL when needed. Check respiratory rate and GCS every ¼h + O_2 sats if chest/abdominal pain. Liaise with the local pain service.

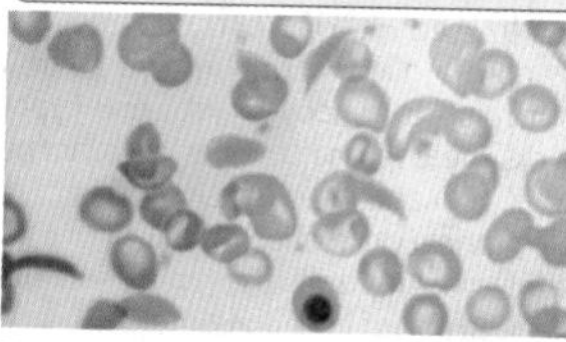

Fig 8.37 Sickle-cell film: there are sickle cells, target cells, and a nucleated red cell.

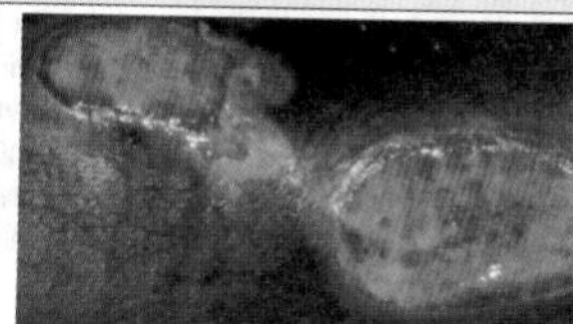

Fig 8.38 Leg ulcers in sickle-cell disease.

A 7-year-old tells us what it's like to have sickle-cell disease

'I have been hospitalized over 50 times for complications from this disease. To keep it controlled I started having monthly transfusions. After repeated transfusions my body began to get too much iron so I had to start getting infusions. I was taking the medication desferal[5] which my mummy had to insert a needle in my belly hooked up to a pump which I had to carry on my back in my neat Spiderman backpack. I was hooked up to the machine for 10 hours a day 5 days a week but it was okay I still got to play!!! I suffered from pain crisis which makes my legs and back hurt like someone is hitting me with a hammer.

You may notice that I may move slow or look tired when it is time for my blood transfusion. That is because the transfusions are like a heartbeat for my body, without it I can't survive. When I'm in pain the only thing that helps is morphine... I tell my mummy when she's crying I WILL BE OK!!'

5 This was necessary until a once-daily oral iron chelator came along: deferasirox.

Thalassaemia

The thalassaemias are genetic diseases of unbalanced Hb synthesis, with underproduction (or no production) of one globin chain (see table 8.2 and BOX). Unmatched globins precipitate, damaging RBC membranes, causing their haemolysis while still in the marrow. They are common in areas from the Mediterranean to the Far East.

The β thalassaemias Usually caused by point mutations in β-globin genes on chromosome 11, leading to ↓β chain production (β^+) or its absence (β^0). Various combinations of mutations are possible (eg β^0/β^0, β^+/β^+, or β^+/β^0).

Tests: FBC, MCV, film, iron, HbA_2, HbF, Hb electrophoresis. MRI where myocardial siderosis suspected (from iron overload).

β thalassaemia minor or trait (eg β/β^+; heterozygous state): this is a carrier state, and is usually asymptomatic. Mild, well-tolerated anaemia (Hb >90g/L) which may worsen in pregnancy. MCV <75fL, HbA_2 >3.5%, slight ↑HbF. Often confused with iron-deficiency anaemia.

β thalassaemia intermedia: describes an intermediate state with moderate anaemia but not requiring transfusions. There may be splenomegaly. There are a variety of causes including mild homozygous β thalassaemia mutations, eg β^+/β^+, or co-inheritance of β thalassaemia trait with another haemoglobinopathy, eg HbC thalassaemia (one parent has the HbC trait, and the other has β^+). Sickle-cell β^+ thalassaemia produces a picture similar to sickle-cell anaemia.

β thalassaemia major: denotes significant abnormalities in both β-globin genes, and presents in the 1st year, with severe anaemia and failure to thrive. Extramedullary haematopoiesis (RBCs made outside the marrow) occurs in response to anaemia, causing characteristic head shape, eg skull bossing (figs 8.39, 8.40) and hepatosplenomegaly (also due to haemolysis). There is osteopenia (may respond to zoledronic acid). Skull x-ray shows a 'hair on end' sign due to ↑marrow activity. Life-long blood transfusions are needed, with resulting iron overload/deposition seen after ~10yrs as endocrine failure (pituitary, thyroid, pancreas→diabetes mellitus), liver disease, and cardiac toxicity. The film shows very hypochromic, microcytic cells + target cells + nucleated RBCs. ↑↑HbF, HbA_2 variable, HbA absent.

Treatment: ►Promote fitness; healthy diet. Folate supplements help.

- Regular (~2–4 weekly) life-long transfusions to keep Hb >90g/L, to suppress the ineffective extramedullary haematopoiesis and to allow normal growth. ►Iron overload is a big problem causing hypothyroidism, hypocalcaemia, and hypogonadism. Can be mitigated by iron-chelators (deferiprone PO + desferrioxamine SC twice weekly. SE: pain, deafness, cataracts, retinal damage, ↑risk of *Yersinia*). Large doses of ascorbic acid can also help by ↑urinary excretion of iron.
- Splenectomy if hypersplenism persists with increasing transfusion requirements (p373)—this is best avoided until >5yrs old due to risk of infections.
- Hormonal replacement or treatment for endocrine complications, eg diabetes mellitus, hypothyroidism. Growth hormone treatment has had variable success.
- A histocompatible marrow transplant can offer the chance of a cure.

Prevention: Approaches include genetic counselling or antenatal diagnosis using fetal blood or DNA, then 'therapeutic' abortion.

The α thalassaemias (fig 8.41) There are two separate α-globin genes on each chromosome 16 ∴ there are four genes (termed αα/αα). The α thalassaemias are mainly caused by gene deletions. If all four α genes are deleted (--/--), death is *in utero* (*Bart's hydrops*). Here, HbBarts (γ_4) is present, which is physiologically useless. HbH disease occurs if three genes are deleted (--/-α); there may be moderate anaemia and features of haemolysis: hepatosplenomegaly, leg ulcers, and jaundice. In the blood film, there is formation of β_4 tetramers (=HbH) due to excess β chains, HbBarts, HbA, and HbA_2. If two genes are deleted (--/αα or -α/-α), there is an asymptomatic carrier state, with ↓MCV. With one gene deleted, the clinical state is normal.

Structure of haemoglobin

Table 8.2 The three main types of Hb in adult blood

Type	Peptide chains	% in adult blood	% in fetal blood
HbA	$\alpha_2\beta_2$	97	10–50
HbA_2	$\alpha_2\delta_2$	2.5	Trace
HbF	$\alpha_2\gamma_2$	0.5	50–90

Adult haemoglobin (HbA) is a tetramer of 2 α- and 2 β-globin chains each containing a haem group. In the first year of life, adult haemoglobin replaces fetal haemoglobin (HbF).

It might be thought that because the molecular details of the thalassaemias are so well worked out they represent a perfect example of the reductionist principle at work: find out *exactly* what is happening *within* molecules, and you will be able to explain all the manifestations of a disease. But this is not so. We have to recognize that two people with the identical mutation at their β loci may have quite different diseases. Co-inheritance of other genes and conditions (eg α thalassaemia) is part of the explanation, as is the efficiency of production of fetal haemoglobin. The reasons lie beyond simple co-segregation of genes promoting the formation of fetal Hb. The rate of proteolysis of excess α-globin chains may also be important—as may mechanisms that have little to do with genetic or molecular events.

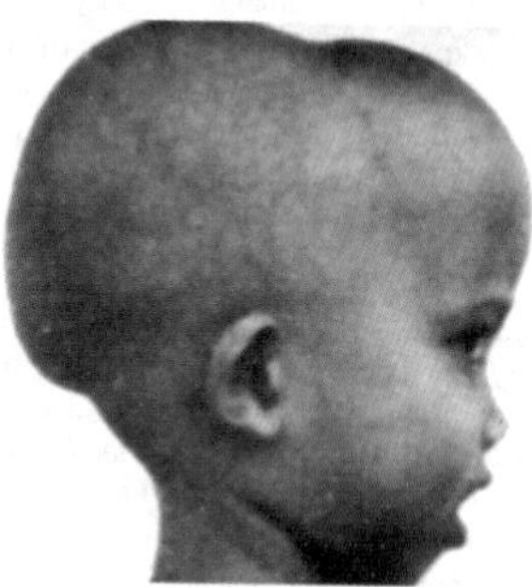

Fig 8.39 β thalassaemia major: bossing due to extramedullary haematopoiesis.

©Dr E van der Enden.

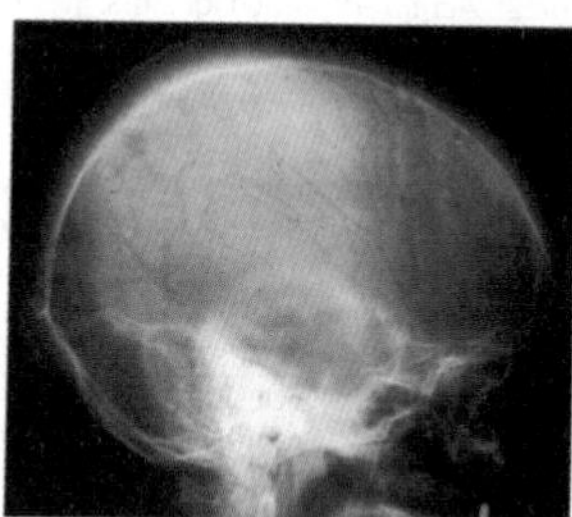

Fig 8.40 β thalassaemia major: skull x-ray.

©Crookston collection.

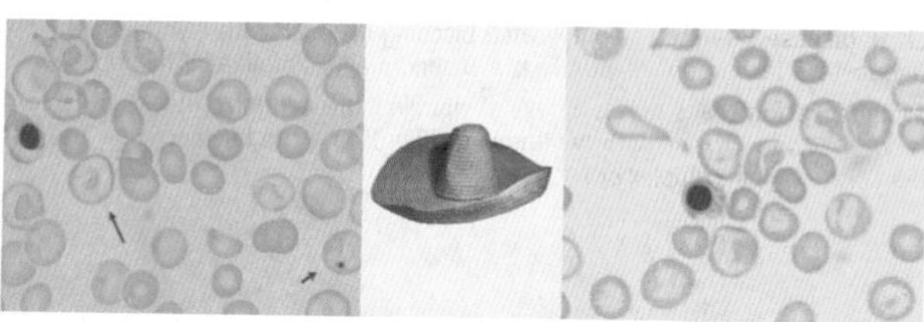

Fig 8.41 α thalassaemia showing Mexican hat cells (also called target cells)—one of which is arrowed on the left panel. Note also the tear-drop cell on the right panel, and the 2 normoblasts (nucleated red cells, one on each panel). The shorter arrow on the left panel points to a Howell-Jolly body. Note that the cells which are not Mexican hats are rather small (microcytic). There is also poikilocytosis (*poikilos* is Greek for varied—so this simply means that the red blood cells are of varied shape).

Courtesy of Prof. Tangün and Dr Köroğlu.

Bleeding disorders

After injury, three processes halt bleeding: vasoconstriction, gap-plugging by platelets, and the coagulation cascade (fig 8.42). Disorders of haemostasis fall into these three groups. The pattern of bleeding is important—vascular and platelet disorders lead to prolonged bleeding from cuts, bleeding into the skin (eg easy bruising and purpura), and bleeding from mucous membranes (eg epistaxis, bleeding from gums, menorrhagia). Coagulation disorders cause delayed bleeding into joints and muscle.

1 **Vascular defects** *Congenital:* Osler-Weber-Rendu syndrome (p708), connective tissue disease (eg Ehlers-Danlos syndrome, *OHCS* p642, pseudoxanthoma elasticum). *Acquired:* Senile purpura, infection (eg meningococcal, measles, dengue fever), steroids, scurvy (perifollicular haemorrhages), Henoch-Schönlein purpura (p702).

2 **Platelet disorders** *Decreased marrow production:* Aplastic anaemia (p364), megaloblastic anaemia, marrow infiltration (eg leukaemia, myeloma), marrow suppression (cytotoxic drugs, radiotherapy). *Excess destruction: Immune:* immune thrombocytopenia (ITP, see BOX 'Immune thrombocytopenia'), other autoimmune causes, eg SLE, CLL, drugs, eg heparin, viruses; *Non-immune:* DIC (p352), thrombotic thrombocytopenic purpura (TTP), or HUS (p315), sequestration (in hypersplenism). *Poorly functioning platelets:* Seen in myeloproliferative disease, NSAIDs, and ↑urea.

3 **Coagulation disorders** *Congenital:* Haemophilia, von Willebrand's disease (p712). *Acquired:* Anticoagulants, liver disease, DIC (p352), vitamin K deficiency.

Haemophilia A Factor VIII deficiency; inherited in an X-linked recessive pattern in 1:10000 male births—usually due to a 'flip tip' inversion in the factor VIII gene in the X chromosome. There is a high rate of new mutations (30% have no family history). *Presentation* depends on severity and is often early in life or after surgery/trauma—with bleeds into joints leading to crippling arthropathy, and into muscles causing haematomas (↑pressure can lead to nerve palsies and compartment syndrome). *Diagnose* by ↑APTT and ↓factor VIII assay. *Management:* Seek expert advice. Avoid NSAIDs and IM injections (fig 8.43). *Minor bleeding:* pressure and elevation of the part. Desmopressin (0.3mcg/kg/12h IVI over 20min) raises factor VIII levels, and may be sufficient. *Major bleeds* (eg haemarthrosis): ↑factor VIII levels to 50% of normal, eg with recombinant factor VIII. *Life-threatening bleeds* (eg obstructing airway) need levels of 100%. *Genetic counselling: OHCS* p154.

Haemophilia B (Christmas disease) Factor IX deficiency (inherited, X-linked recessive); behaves clinically like haemophilia A. *Treat* with recombinant factor IX.

Acquired haemophilia is a bleeding diathesis causing big mucosal bleeds in males and females caused by suddenly appearing autoantibodies that interfere with factor VIII. *Tests:* ↑APPT; ↑VIII autoantibody; factor VIII activity <50%. ℞: Steroids.

Liver disease Produces a complicated bleeding disorder with ↓synthesis of clotting factors, ↓absorption of vitamin K, and abnormalities of platelet function.

Malabsorption Leads to less uptake of vitamin K (needed for synthesis of factors II, VII, IX, and X). *Treat* with IV vitamin K (10mg). In acute haemorrhage, use human prothrombin complex or FFP.

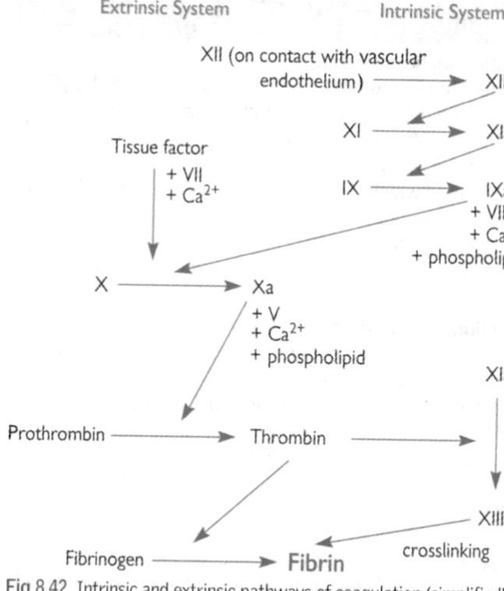

Fig 8.42 Intrinsic and extrinsic pathways of coagulation (simplified!).

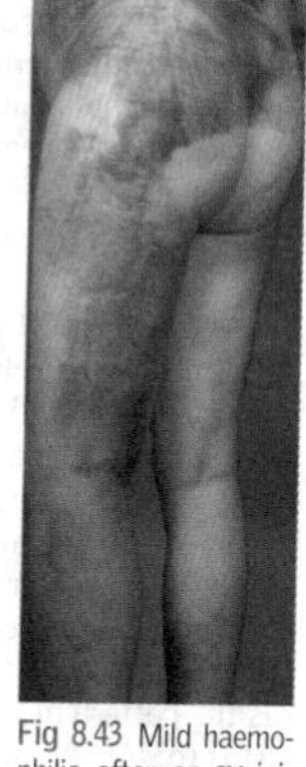

Fig 8.43 Mild haemophilia after an IM injection. ►Give vaccines etc SC!

Fibrinolysis

The fibrinolytic system works by generating plasmin, which causes fibrin dissolution. The process starts with the release of tissue plasminogen activator (t-PA) from endothelial cells, a process stimulated by fibrin formation. t-PA converts inactive plasminogen to plasmin which can then cleave fibrin, as well as several other factors. t-PA and plasminogen both bind fibrin thus localizing fibrinolysis to the area of the clot.

Fibrinolytic agents activate this system and can be utilized in order to break down pathological thrombi, eg in: acute MI, acute ischaemic stroke, DVT, PE, and central retinal venous or arterial thrombosis. In all cases the risk of adverse effects of thrombolysis (eg haemorrhage) must be outweighed by the potential benefits. Streptokinase, a streptococcal exotoxin that binds and activates plasminogen, was the first licensed agent but risks anaphylaxis on repeat dosing. Alteplase is recombinant t-PA. Newer agents include tenecteplase and reteplase.

Immune thrombocytopenia (ITP)

ITP is caused by antiplatelet autoantibodies. It is acute (usually in children, 2wks after infection with sudden self-limiting purpura: *OHCS* p197) or chronic (seen mainly in women). Chronic ITP runs a fluctuating course of bleeding, purpura (esp. dependent pressure areas), epistaxis, and menorrhagia. There is no splenomegaly. *Tests:* ↑Megakaryocytes in marrow, antiplatelet autoantibodies often present. ℞: None if mild. If symptomatic or platelets <20 × 10^9/L, prednisolone 1mg/kg/d, and reduce after remission; aim to keep platelets >30 × 10^9/L—takes a few days to work. Platelet transfusions are not used (except during splenectomy or life-threatening haemorrhage) as these are quickly destroyed by the autoantibodies. IV immunoglobulin may temporarily raise the platelet count, eg for surgery, pregnancy. If relapse, choices include splenectomy or B-cell depletion with rituximab. Eltrombopag (an oral thrombopoietin-receptor agonist) and romiplostim (an injectable thrombopoietin analogue) are alternative options for those with refractory disease.

An approach to bleeding

There are three sets of questions to be answered:

1 Is there an emergency needing immediate resuscitation or senior help?
- Is the patient about to exsanguinate (dizzy on sitting up, shock, coma)?
- Is there hypovolaemia (postural hypotension, oliguria)?
- Is there CNS bleeding (meningism, CNS and retinal signs)?
- Is there an underlying condition which escalates apparently minor bleeding into an evolving catastrophe? For example:
  - Bleeding in pregnancy or the puerperium.
  - GI bleeding in a jaundiced patient (ie coagulation factors already depleted).
  - Bleeding in someone who is already anaemic (esp if other comorbidities).

2 Why is the patient bleeding? Is bleeding normal, given the circumstances (eg surgery, trauma, parturition), or does the patient have a bleeding disorder (BOX 'Is this pre-op patient at risk of excessive bleeding?')?
- Is there a secondary cause, eg drugs (warfarin), alcohol, liver disease, sepsis?
- Is there unexplained bleeding, bruising, or purpura?
- Past or family history of excess bleeding, eg during trauma, dentistry, surgery?
- Is the pattern of bleeding indicative of vascular, platelet, or coagulation problems (p344)? Are old venepuncture or cannula sites bleeding (DIC, p352)? Look for associated conditions (eg with DIC).
- Is a clotting screen abnormal (table 8.3)? Check FBC, platelets, PT, APTT, and thrombin time. Consider D-dimers, bleeding time, and a factor VIII assay. ►If both PT and APTT are very raised, with low platelets and ↑D-dimers, consider DIC (p352).

3 In cases of bleeding disorders, what is the mechanism? Investigate with FBC, film, and coagulation screen (citrate tube; false results if under-filled):
- *Prothrombin time (PT):* Thromboplastin is added to test the *extrinsic system*. PT is expressed as a ratio compared to control (international normalized ratio (INR), normal range = 0.9–1.2). It tests for abnormalities in factors I, II, V, VII, X. Prolonged by: warfarin, vitamin K deficiency, liver disease, DIC.
- *Activated partial thromboplastin time (APTT):* Kaolin is added to test the *intrinsic system*. Tests for abnormalities in factor I, II, V, VIII, IX, X, XI, XII. Normal range 35–45s. Prolonged by: heparin treatment, haemophilia, DIC, liver disease.
- *Thrombin time:* Thrombin is added to plasma to convert fibrinogen to fibrin. Normal range: 10–15s. Prolonged by: heparin treatment, DIC, dysfibrinogenaemia.
- *D-dimers* are a fibrin degradation product, released from cross-linked fibrin during fibrinolysis (p345). This occurs during DIC, or in the presence of venous thromboembolism—deep vein thrombosis (DVT) or pulmonary embolism (PE). D-dimers may also be raised in inflammation, eg with infection or malignancy.

Management Depends on the degree of bleeding. If shocked, resuscitate (p790). If bleeding continues in the presence of a clotting disorder or a massive transfusion, discuss the need for FFP, cryoprecipitate, factor concentrates, or platelets with a haematologist. In ITP (p345), steroids ± IV immunoglobulin may be used. Especially in pregnancy (*OHCS* p88), consult an expert. Is there overdose with anticoagulants (p842)? In haemophiliac bleeds, *consult early* for coagulation factor replacement. *Never* give IM injections.

Table 8.3 Clotting screen abnormalities in coagulopathies

Disorder	INR	APTT	Thrombin time	Platelet count	Notes
Heparin	↑	↑↑	↑↑	↔	
DIC	↑↑	↑↑	↑↑	↓	↑D-dimer, p346
Liver disease	↑	↑	↔/↑	↔/↓	AST↑
Platelet defect	↔	↔	↔	↔	
Vit K deficiency	↑↑	↑	↔	↔	
Haemophilia	↔	↑↑	↔	↔	see p344
von Willebrand's	↔	↑↑	↔	↔	see p712

Special tests may be available (factor assays: ►consult a haematologist).

Towards a better assay for clotting function

Bleeding time, a barbaric and unreliable test (the clue is in the name), is no longer used. Amongst the range of techniques to replicate the clotting process *in vitro* is thromboelastography (TEG). TEG permits rapid and more precise assays of clotting function under massive transfusion situations (eg major surgery, especially trauma). In particular, advances in this field have been driven by recent military usage.

Is this pre-op patient at risk of excessive bleeding?

Take a bleeding history! The more structured this is the better. Enquire about factors which may indicate increased bleeding risk, such as:

- past history of excessive, prolonged, or unexplained bleeding
- comorbidities such as lupus or liver disease
- on agents known to affect haemostasis.

In such cases, or if bleeding would be disastrous, further tests may be indicated after discussion with a haematologist.

Blood transfusion and blood products

►Blood should only be given if strictly necessary *and there is no alternative*. Outcomes may be *worse* after an inappropriate transfusion.

- Know and use local procedures to ensure that the right blood gets to the right patient at the right time.
- Take blood for crossmatching from only one patient at a time. Label immediately. This minimizes risk of wrong labelling of samples.
- When giving blood, monitor TPR and BP every ½h.
- Use a dedicated line where practicable (or dedicated lumen of multilumen line).

Group-and-save (G&S) requests Know your local guidelines for elective surgery. Having crossmatched blood to hand may not be needed if a blood sample is already in the lab, with group determined, without any atypical antibodies (ie G&S).

Products[2] *Whole blood:* The only option for the first 250 years of transfusion history, but now rarely used. *Red cells:* (Packed to make haematocrit ~70%.) Use to correct anaemia or blood loss. 1U ↑Hb by 10-15g/L. In anaemia, transfuse until Hb ~80g/L. *Platelets:* (p364.) Usually only needed if bleeding or count is <20 × 10^9/L. 1U should ↑platelet count by >20 × 10^9/L. Failure to do so suggests refractory cause: discuss with haematologist. If surgery is planned, get advice if count is <100 × 10^9/L. *Fresh frozen plasma (FFP):* Use to correct clotting defects: eg DIC (p352); warfarin overdosage where vitamin K would be too slow; liver disease; thrombotic thrombocytopenic purpura (p315). It is expensive and carries all the risks of blood transfusion. Do not use as a simple volume expander. *Human albumin solution* is produced as 4.5% or 20% protein solution and is used to replace protein. 20% albumin can be used temporarily in the hypoproteinaemic patient (eg liver disease; nephrosis) who is fluid overloaded, without giving an excessive salt load. Also used as replacement in abdominal paracentesis (p765). *Others* Cryoprecipitate (a source of fibrinogen); coagulation concentrates (self-injected in haemophilia); immunoglobulins.

Complications of transfusion ►Management of acute reactions:[2] see BOX 'Transfusion reactions' and table 8.4.

- *Early (within 24h):* Acute haemolytic reactions (eg ABO or Rh incompatibility); anaphylaxis; bacterial contamination; febrile reactions (eg from HLA antibodies); allergic reactions (itch, urticaria, mild fever); fluid overload; transfusion-related acute lung injury (TRALI, ie ARDS due to antileucocyte antibodies in donor plasma).
- *Delayed (after 24h):* Infections (eg viruses: hepatitis B/C, HIV; bacteria; protozoa; prions); iron overload (treatment, p342); GVHD; post-transfusion purpura—potentially lethal fall in platelet count 5-7d post-transfusion requiring specialist treatment with IV immunoglobulin and platelet transfusions.

Massive blood transfusion This is defined as replacement of an individual's entire blood volume (>10U) within 24h. Complications: ↓platelets; ↓Ca^{2+}; ↓clotting factors; ↑K^+; hypothermia. ►Seek early and ongoing support from haematologist and blood bank who should advise on products and monitoring. In acute haemorrhage, use crossmatched blood if possible, but if not, use 'universal donor' group O Rh−ve blood, changing to crossmatched blood as soon as possible.

Transfusing patients with heart failure If Hb ≲50g/L with heart failure, transfusion with packed red cells is vital to restore Hb to a safe level, eg 60-80g/L, but must be done with care. Give each unit over 4h with furosemide (eg 40mg slow IV/PO; don't mix with blood) with alternate units. Check for ↑JVP and basal lung crackles; consider CVP line.

Autologous transfusion There is a role for patients having their own blood stored pre-op for later use. Erythropoietin (EPO, p304) can increase the yield of autologous blood in normal people. Intraoperative cell salvage with retransfusion is also being used more often, especially in cardiac, vascular, and emergency surgery, Cost-analysis shows that it may be worthwhile on an economic basis alone.

Transfusion reactions

All UK blood products are now leucocyte-depleted (white cells <5×10^6/L) so as to reduce the incidence of complications such as alloimmunization to HLA class I antigens and febrile transfusion reactions.

Table 8.4 Management of transfusion reactions

Acute haemolytic reaction (eg ABO incompatibility) Agitation, ↑T° (rapid onset), ↓BP, flushing, abdominal/chest pain, oozing venepuncture sites, DIC.	**STOP** transfusion. Check identity and name on unit; tell haematologist; send unit + FBC, U&E, clotting, cultures, & urine (haemoglobinuria) to lab. Keep IV line open with 0.9% saline. Treat DIC (p352).
Anaphylaxis Bronchospasm, cyanosis, ↓BP, soft tissue swelling.	**STOP** the transfusion. Maintain airway and give oxygen. Contact anaesthetist. ►►See p794.
Bacterial contamination ↑T° (rapid onset), ↓BP, and rigors.	**STOP** the transfusion. Check identity against name on unit; tell haematologist and send unit + FBC, U&E, clotting, cultures & urine to lab. Start broad-spectrum antibiotics.
TRALI (See p348) Dyspnoea, cough; CXR 'white out'.	**STOP** the transfusion. Give 100% O_2. ►►Treat as ARDS, p186. Donor should be removed from donor panel.
Non-haemolytic febrile transfusion reaction Shivering and fever usually ½–1h after starting transfusion.	**SLOW** or **STOP** the transfusion. Give an antipyretic, eg paracetamol 1g. Monitor closely. If recurrent, use WBC filter.
Allergic reactions Urticaria and itch.	**SLOW** or **STOP** the transfusion; chlorphenamine 10mg slow IV/IM. Monitor closely.
Fluid overload Dyspnoea, hypoxia, tachycardia, ↑JVP and basal crepitations.	**SLOW** or **STOP** the transfusion. Give oxygen and a diuretic, eg furosemide 40mg IV initially. Consider CVP line.

Blood transfusion and Jehovah's Witnesses

Adult human beings (with mental 'capacity' see p568) have an absolute right to refuse any medical treatment, even if to do so seems illogical or could result in their death. To treat patients despite such a refusal would amount to battery under common law, or could even amount to a degrading act or torture, against which the European Convention on Human Rights gives absolute, inalienable protection.

The biblical verse '*no soul of you shall eat blood*' (Leviticus 17:12) is one of several that have been interpreted by some religious groups to extend to acceptance of blood products in a medical context. Jehovah's Witnesses, for example, may refuse potentially vital blood transfusions on such grounds. These views must be respected, but complex issues arise if the patient is a child, or an adult who may not be able to give or withhold consent in an informed way. In an immediately life-threatening situation where further delay may cause harm, treatment such as blood products may be given in the child's best interest, but the team should always involve senior paediatricians and hospital ethicists where practical. If the requirement is less immediate, then the clinicians should seek further legal advice, which might involve approaching the Courts.

Main indications

- *Therapeutic:* Venous thromboembolic disease: DVT and PE.
- *Prophylactic:* Prevention of DVT/PE in high-risk patients (p375), eg post-op. Prevention of stroke, eg in chronic AF or prosthetic heart valves.

Heparin 1 *Low-molecular-weight heparin (LMWH):* Eg dalteparin, enoxaparin, tinzaparin. The preferred option in the prevention and initial treatment of venous thromboembolism. Inactivates factor Xa (but not thrombin). *t½* is 2- to 4-fold longer than standard heparin, and response is more predictable: only needs to be given once or twice daily SC, and laboratory monitoring is usually not required. See *BNF* for doses. It accumulates in renal failure: decrease dose for prophylaxis, use UFH for therapeutic treatment

2 *Unfractionated heparin (UFH):* IV or SC. Binds antithrombin (an endogenous inhibitor of coagulation), increasing its ability to inhibit thrombin, factor Xa, and IXa. Rapid onset and has a short *t½*. Monitor and adjust dose with APTT (p346).

SE for both: ↑Bleeding (eg at operative site, gastrointestinal, intracranial), heparin-induced thrombocytopenia (HIT), osteoporosis with long-term use. HIT and osteoporosis are less common with LMWH than UFH. Beware hyperkalaemia.

CI: Bleeding disorders, platelets $<60\times10^9$/L, previous HIT, peptic ulcer, cerebral haemorrhage, severe hypertension, neurosurgery.

Warfarin Used PO OD as long-term anticoagulation. The therapeutic range is narrow, varying with the condition being treated (see BOX 'Warfarin guidelines and target levels for INR')—and effects are reflected in the INR. Warfarin inhibits the reductase enzyme responsible for regenerating the active form of vitamin K, producing a state analogous to vitamin K deficiency. *CI:* Peptic ulcer, bleeding disorders, severe hypertension, pregnancy (teratogenic, see *OHCS* p640). Use with caution in elderly and those with past GI bleeds. In the UK, warfarin tablets are 0.5mg (white), 1mg (brown), 3mg (blue), or 5mg (pink). ►Interactions: p757.

DOACs (Direct oral anticoagulants.) Rivaroxaban, apixaban (factor Xa inhibitors) and dabigatran (a direct thrombin inhibitor) do not require regular monitoring and dose adjustment; just a quarterly assessment and annual blood test. They offer an attractive alternative to warfarin (particularly where monitoring and maintaining a therapeutic INR is difficult). *CI:* severe renal/liver impairment; active bleeding; lesion at risk of bleeding; ↓clotting factors. Interactions: heparin, clopidogrel.

Others Fondaparinux is a pentasaccharide Xa inhibitor and is used in acute coronary syndrome or in place of LMWH for prophylaxis.

Beginning therapeutic anticoagulation (Follow local guidelines, and see *BNF*.) For treatment of venous thromboembolism, LMWH or UFH are typically used initially. When transitioning to warfarin, give heparin in combination (as early as day 1) and continue until INR is in target therapeutic range on 2 consecutive days (see BOX 'Warfarin dosage'). Start warfarin at 5–10mg given at 18.00 on days 1 and 2, then check INR on day 3 (it takes 48–72h for anticoagulant effect to develop). Adjust subsequent doses according to the INR (see table 8.5), which needs to be measured on alternate days until stable, then weekly or less often. When transitioning to a DOAC switch from heparin (ie do not coadminister DOAC and heparin). DOACs and warfarin may both be initiated as monotherapy in chronic AF (DOACs also in less extensive thromboembolism).

Antidotes If UFH overdose: stop infusion. If there is bleeding, protamine sulphate counteracts UFH: discuss with a haematologist. Warfarin: see BOX 'Warfarin dosage' and table 8.6. DOACs: challenging and evolving area (including monoclonal anti-drug antibodies eg idarucizumab for dabigatran)—discuss with haematologist.

Warfarin guidelines and target levels for INR

- Pulmonary embolism and DVT. Aim for INR of 2-3; 3.5 if recurrent PE or DVT whilst anticoagulated.
- Atrial fibrillation: for stroke prevention (p130). Target INR 2-3.
- Prosthetic metallic heart valves: for stroke prevention. Target INR 2-3 if aortic valve or 2.5-3.5 if mitral valve.

Duration of anticoagulation in DVT/PE: First episodes of DVT or PE require at least 3 months of anticoagulation. Consider extending this to 6 months in patients with more extensive, life-threatening clot at presentation, for those with transient but persistent risk factors (eg prolonged immobility) or if evidence of persistent clot at 3 months. For those with recurrent unprovoked emboli or underlying thrombophilia (p374), consider bleeding risks against benefits of indefinite treatment.

Warfarin dosage and what to do when the INR is much too high

Below is a rough guide to warfarin dosing for target INR of 2-3.

Table 8.5 Suggested dosing for day 3 of warfarin loading

INR	<2	2	2.5	2.9	3.3	3.6	4.1
3rd dose	5mg	5mg	4mg	3mg	2mg	0.5mg	0mg
Maintenance	≥6mg	5.5mg	4.5mg	4mg	3.5mg	3mg	*

*Miss a dose; give 1-2mg the next day; if INR >4.5, miss 2 doses.

Table 8.6 When the INR is much too high (see also BNF)

INR 5-8, no bleed	Withold 1-2 doses. Restart warfarin at a lower maintanence dose once INR <5.
INR 5-8, minor bleed*	Stop warfarin and admit for urgent IV vitamin K (give slowly). Restart warfarin when INR <5.
INR >8, no bleed	Stop warfarin and seek haematology advice.
NR >8, minor bleed*	Stop warfarin and admit for urgent IV vitamin K. Check INR daily—repeat vitamin K if INR too high after 24h. Restart warfarin at a lower dose when INR <5.
Any major bleed (including intracranial haemorrhage)	Stop warfarin. Give prothrombin complex concentrate 50 units/kg (if unavailable, give FFP 15mL/kg≈1L for a 70kg man) and 5-10mg vitamin K IV. Discuss with haematologist.

*Minor bleeding includes epistaxis.

Vitamin K may take several hours to work and can cause prolonged resistance when restarting warfarin, so should be avoided if possible when long-term anticoagulation is needed. Prothrombin complex concentrate contains a concentrate of factors II, VII, IX, and X and provides a more complete and rapid reversal of warfarin than FFP.

Leukaemia and the on-call junior doctor

Leukaemia divides into four main types depending on the cell line involved (table 8.7).

Table 8.7 Principal subtypes of leukaemia

	Lymphoid	Myeloid
Acute	Acute lymphoblastic leukaemia (ALL)	Acute myeloid leukaemia (AML)
Chronic	Chronic lymphocytic leukaemia (CLL)	Chronic myeloid leukaemia (CML)

These patients (esp. AML) fall ill suddenly and deteriorate fast, eg with: ▸▸infection, ▸▸bleeding (℞: platelets ± FFP), and ▸▸hyperviscosity (p372). Take non-specific confusion/drowsiness or just 'I feel a bit ill today' *seriously*: do blood cultures, FBC, U&E, LFT, Ca^{2+}, glucose, and clotting. Consider CNS bleeding—CT if in doubt. With any new patient, find out the agreed aim of treatment: cure; prolonging disease-free survival; or palliation with minimal toxicity? Direct your efforts accordingly; get help if lack of clarity here.

Neutropenic regimen (For when neutrophil count $\le 0.5 \times 10^9$/L.)[3] ▸Close liaison with a microbiologist and haematologist is vital. Abide by infection control procedures! Use a *risk-assessment tool* (eg MASCC, see BOX).

- Full barrier nursing in a side room if possible. Hand-washing is vital.
- Avoid IM injections (danger of an infected haematoma).
- Look for infection (mouth, axillae, perineum, IVI site). Take swabs.
- Check: FBC, platelets, INR, U&E, LFT, LDH, CRP. Take cultures (blood ×3—peripherally ± Hickman line; urine, sputum, stool if diarrhoea); CXR if clinically indicated.
- Wash perineum after defecation. Swab moist skin with chlorhexidine. Avoid unnecessary rectal examinations. Oral hygiene (eg hydrogen peroxide mouth washes/2h) and *Candida* prophylaxis are important (p246).
- Check vital signs 4-hrly. High-calorie diet; avoid foods with high risk of microbial contamination. Vases containing cut flowers pose a *Pseudomonas* risk.

Use of antibiotics in neutropenia ▸Treat any known infection promptly.

- If T° >38°C or T° >37.5°C on two occasions, >1h apart, or the patient is septic, start blind combination therapy according to local guidelines—eg piperacillin-tazobactam—p386 (+vancomycin, p386, if Gram+ve organisms suspected or isolated, eg Hickman line sepsis). Continue until afebrile for 72h or 5d course, and until neutrophils $>0.5\times10^9$/L. If fever persists despite antibiotics, think of CMV, fungi (eg *Candida*; *Aspergillus*, p408) and central line infection.
- Consider treatment for *Pneumocystis* (p400, eg co-trimoxazole, though beware as this can worsen neutropenia). Remember TB.

Other dangers • *Tumour lysis syndrome:* Results in ↑K^+, ↑urate and AKI. See p529.

- *Hyperviscosity:* (p372). If WCC is $>100\times10^9$/L WBC thrombi may form in brain, lung, and heart (leukostasis). Avoid transfusing before lowering WCC, eg with hydroxycarbamide or leukapheresis, as viscosity rises (↑risk of leukostasis).
- *DIC:* The release of procoagulants into the circulation causes widespread activation of coagulation, consuming clotting factors and platelets and causing ↑risk of bleeding. Fibrin strands fill small vessels, haemolysing passing RBCs. Fibrinolysis is also activated. *Causes:* Malignancy, sepsis, trauma, obstetric events. *Signs:* (fig 8.44) Bruising, bleeding anywhere (eg venepuncture sites), renal failure. *Tests:* ↓Platelets; ↑PT; ↑APTT; ↓fibrinogen (correlates with severity); ↑↑fibrin degradation products (D-dimers). Film: broken RBCs (schistocytes). *℞:* Treat the cause. Replace platelets if $<50\times10^9$/L, cryoprecipitate to replace fibrinogen, FFP to replace coagulation factors. Heparin is controversial. The use of all-transretinoic acid (ATRA) has significantly reduced the risk of DIC in acute promyelocytic leukaemia (the commonest leukaemia associated with DIC).
- *Preventing sepsis:* Give fluoroquinolone (eg ciprofloxacin) before neutropenia gets serious. Granulocyte colony stimulators (G-CSF) can increase the production of WBCs (granulocytes) from bone marrow, but should not be given routinely in chemotherapy. Herpes, pneumocystis, and CMV prophylaxis has a role.

MASCC score

The Multinational Association for Supportive Care in Cancer (MASCC) assessment tool can be used to predict the risk of serious complications in febrile neutropaenia, and can inform management decisions: if the total score is ≳21, risk of septic complications is low and admission may be avoided.

- Solid tumour or lymphoma with no previous fungal infection 4
- Outpatient status at onset of fever (not needing admission) 3
- Age <60yrs 2
- Burden of illness:
  - Mild (or no) symptoms 5
  - Moderate symptoms 3
  - Severe symptoms 0
- No hypotension (systolic BP >90mmHg) 5
- No COPD 4
- No dehydration 3

Note the subjectivity of the 'burden of illness' and the omission of potentially vital variables such as CRP (which, should it fail to fall after starting antibiotics predicts treatment failure). As with all other scores, the MASCC score should therefore be interpreted within the context of the individual clinical picture.

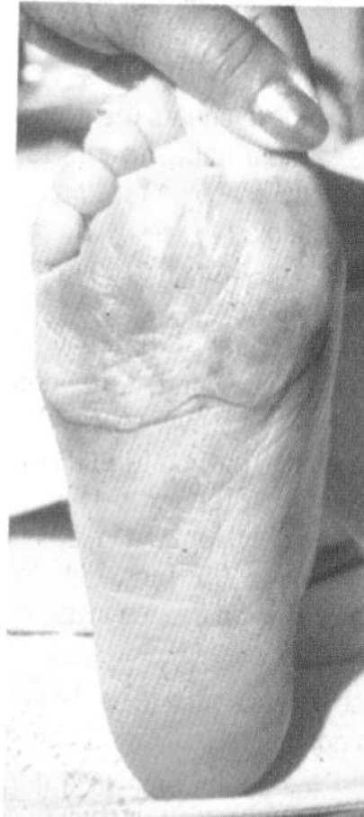

Fig 8.44 The appearance of disseminated intravascular coagulation (DIC) on the sole.
Courtesy of the Crookston Collection.

Acute lymphoblastic leukaemia (ALL)

A malignancy of lymphoid cells, affecting B- or T-lymphocyte cell lineages, arresting maturation and promoting uncontrolled proliferation of immature blast cells, with marrow failure and tissue infiltration. Ionizing radiation (eg X-rays) during pregnancy, and Down's syndrome are important associations.It is the commonest cancer of childhood, and is rare in adults. CNS involvement is common.

Classification Based on three systems:

1 *Morphological:* The FAB system (French, American, British) divides ALL into three types (L1, L2, L3) by microscopic appearance. Provides limited information (figs 8.45–8.48).

2 *Immunological:* Surface markers are used to classify ALL into:
• Precursor B-cell ALL • T-cell ALL • B-cell ALL.

3 *Cytogenetic:* Chromosomal analysis. Abnormalities are detected in up to 85%, which are often translocations.[6] Useful for predicting prognosis, eg poor with Philadelphia chromosome (p358), and for detecting disease recurrence.

Signs and symptoms (fig 8.49) Due to:
- Marrow failure: anaemia (↓Hb), infection (↓WCC), and bleeding (↓platelets).
- Infiltration: hepato- and splenomegaly, lymphadenopathy—superficial or mediastinal, orchidomegaly, CNS involvement—eg cranial nerve palsies, meningism.

Common infections: Especially chest, mouth, perianal, and skin. Bacterial septicaemia, zoster, CMV, measles, candidiasis, *Pneumocystis* pneumonia (p400).

Tests • Characteristic blast cells on blood film and bone marrow. WCC usually high.
- CXR and CT scan to look for mediastinal and abdominal lymphadenopathy.
- Lumbar puncture should be performed to look for CNS involvement.

Treatment ►Educate and motivate patient to promote engagement with therapy.
- *Support:* Blood/platelet transfusion, IV fluids, allopurinol (prevents tumour lysis syndrome). Insert a subcutaneous port system/Hickman line for IV access.
- *Infections:* These are dangerous, due to neutropenia caused by the disease and treatment: give immediate IV antibiotics. Start the neutropenic regimen (p352) and give prophylactic antivirals, antifungals, and antibiotics.
- *Chemotherapy:* Complex multi-drug, multi-phase regimens that may take years:
  - *Remission induction:* eg vincristine, prednisolone, L-asparaginase + daunorubicin.
  - *Consolidation:* high-medium-dose therapy in 'blocks' over several weeks.
  - *CNS prophylaxis:* intrathecal (or high-dose IV) methotrexate ± CNS irradiation.
  - *Maintenance:* prolonged chemotherapy, eg mercaptopurine (daily), methotrexate (weekly), and vincristine + prednisolone (monthly) for 2yrs. Relapse is common in blood, CNS, or testis (examine these sites at follow-up). More details: *OHCS* p194.
- *Matched related allogeneic marrow transplantations:* Once in 1st remission is the best option in standard-risk younger adults.

Haematological remission: Means no evidence of leukaemia in the blood, a normal or recovering blood count, and <5% blasts in a normal regenerating marrow.

Prognosis Cure rates for children are 70–90%; for adults only 40% (higher when imatinib/rituximab, p358, are used). Poor prognosis if: adult, male, Philadelphia chromosome (p358: BCR-ABL gene fusion due to translocation of chromosomes 9 and 22), presentation with CNS signs, ↓Hb, WCC >100×10^9/L, or B-cell ALL. PCR is used to detect minimal residual disease, undetectable by standard means. Prognosis in relapsed Ph-negative ALL is poor (but improvable by marrow transplant).

Personalized treatment ►*One size does not fit all!* Aim to tailor therapy to the exact gene defect, and according to individual metabolism. Monoclonal antibodies, gene-targeted retinoids, cytokines, vaccines, and T-cell infusions are relevant here. Biomarkers, eg thiopurine methyltransferase, can predict toxicity from thiopurines.

6 Eg t(12:21) ETV6-RUNX1, t(1;19) TCF3-PBX1, t(9;22) BCR-ABL1, and rearrangement of MLL.

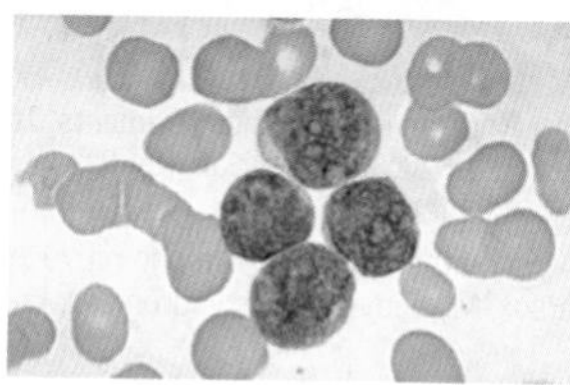

Fig 8.45 Blood film in ALL, L1 subtype. Small blasts with scanty cytoplasm.

Courtesy of Prof. Christine Lawrence.

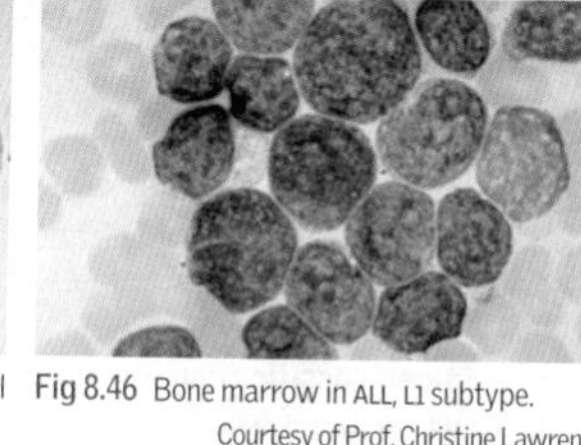

Fig 8.46 Bone marrow in ALL, L1 subtype.

Courtesy of Prof. Christine Lawrence.

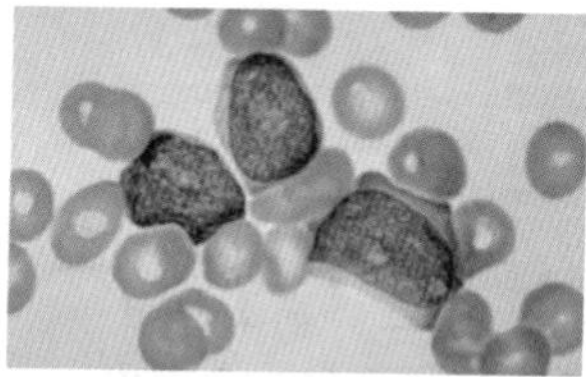

Fig 8.47 Blood film in ALL, L2 subtype. Larger blast cells with greater morphological variation and more abundant cytoplasm.

Courtesy of Prof. Christine Lawrence.

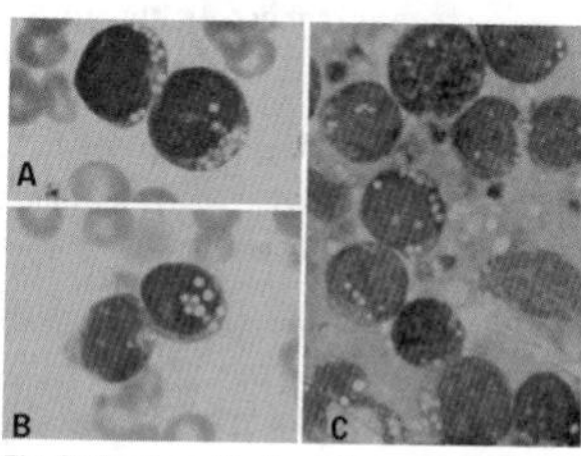

Fig 8.48 ALL L3. Blasts with vacuolated basophilic cytoplasm. A and B: blood films. C: lymph node.

Courtesy of Prof. Tangün and Dr Köroğlu.

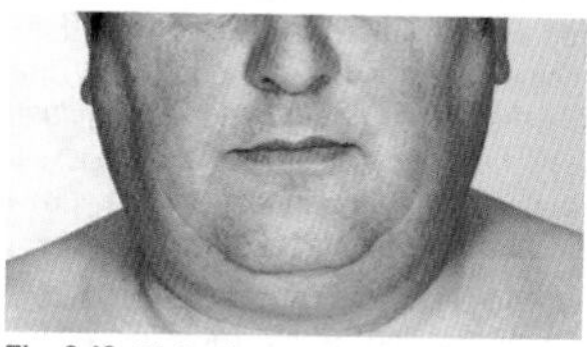

Fig 8.49 Bilateral parotid infiltration in ALL. (Enlarged salivary glands are also seen in mumps, HIV, bulimia, myxoedema, etc., p594.)

Acute myeloid leukaemia (AML)

Neoplastic proliferation of blast cells derived from marrow myeloid elements. It progresses rapidly (death in ~2 months if untreated; ~20% 3yr survival after ℞).

Incidence The commonest acute leukaemia of adults (1/10 000/yr; increases with age). AML can be a long-term complication of chemotherapy, eg for lymphoma. Also associated with myelodysplastic states (see BOX 'Myelodysplastic syndromes'), radiation, and syndromes, eg Down's.

Morphological classification There is much heterogeneity (see BOX 'Heterogeneity in AML'). Four types based on WHO histological classification, cytogenetics, and molecular genetics:

1 AML with recurrent genetic abnormalities.
2 AML multilineage dysplasia (eg 2° to pre-existing myelodysplastic syndrome).
3 AML, therapy related (in those previously treated with cytotoxic drugs).
4 AML, other (not fitting above-listed; further subclassified as M0–M7 by maturation).

Signs and symptoms • *Marrow failure:* Anaemia, infection, or bleeding. DIC occurs in acute promyelocytic leukaemia, a subtype of AML, where there is release of thromboplastin (p352). • *Infiltration:* Hepatomegaly, splenomegaly, gum hypertrophy (fig 8.50), skin involvement. CNS involvement at presentation is rare.

Diagnosis WCC is often ↑, but can be normal or even low. Blast cells may be few in the peripheral blood, so diagnosis depends on bone marrow biopsy, immunophenotyping, and molecular methods. On biopsy, AML is differentiated from ALL by Auer rods (figs 8.51–8.53). Cytogenetic analysis (eg type of mutation) guides treatment recommendations and prognosis.

Complications • Predisposition to infection by both the disease and the treatment; may be bacterial, fungal, or viral—prophylaxis is given for each during therapy. Be alert to septicaemia (p352): common organisms present oddly and rare organisms can infect commonly (particularly the fungi *Candida* and *Aspergillus*). Be aware that AML itself causes fever. • Chemotherapy causes ↑plasma urate levels (from tumour lysis)—so give allopurinol with chemotherapy, and keep well hydrated with IV fluids. • Leukostasis (p352) may occur if ↑↑WCC.

Treatment • *Supportive care:* As for ALL. Walking exercises can relieve fatigue.

- *Chemotherapy:* Very intensive, resulting in long periods of marrow suppression with neutropenia + platelets ↓. The main drugs used include daunorubicin and cytarabine, with ~5 cycles given in 1-week blocks to get a remission (RAS mutations occur in ~20% of patients with AML and enhance sensitivity to cytarabine).
- *Bone marrow transplant (BMT):* Pluripotent haematopoietic stem cells are collected from the marrow. *Allogeneic* transplants from HLA-matched donors (held on international databases) are indicated in refractory or relapsing disease. The idea is to destroy leukaemic cells and the immune system by, eg cyclophosphamide + total body irradiation, then repopulate the marrow with donor cells infused IV. Ciclosporin ± methotrexate are used to reduce the effect of the new marrow attacking the patient's body (GVHD).
  - *Complications:* GVHD (may help explain the curative effect of BMT); opportunistic infections; relapse of leukaemia; infertility.
  - *Prognosis:* Lower relapse rates ~60% long-term survivors, but significant mortality of ~10%. Autologous BMT (where stem cells are taken from the patient themselves) is used in intermediate prognosis disease, although some studies suggest better survival rates with intensive chemotherapy regimens.
  - *Autologous mobilized peripheral blood stem cell transplantation* may offer faster haemopoietic recovery and less morbidity.
- Supportive care, or lower-dose chemotherapy for disease control, may be more appropriate in elderly patients, where intensive therapies have poorer outcomes.

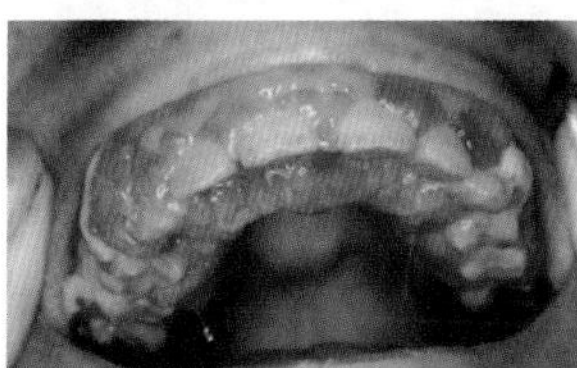
Fig 8.50 Gum hypertrophy in AML.
Courtesy of Prof. Christine Lawrence.

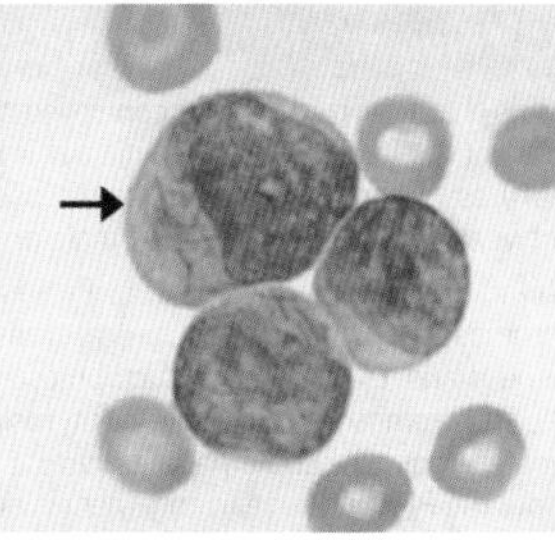
Fig 8.51 Auer rods (crystals of coalesced granules) found in AML myeloblast cells.
Courtesy of Prof. Christine Lawrence.

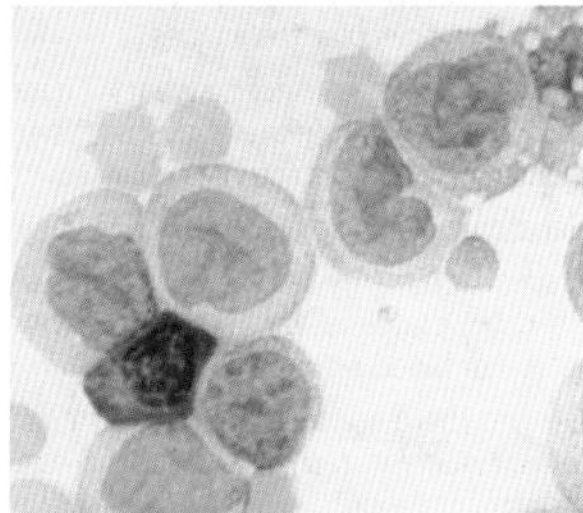
Fig 8.52 AML with monoblasts and myeloblasts on the peripheral blood film.
Courtesy of Prof. Christine Lawrence.

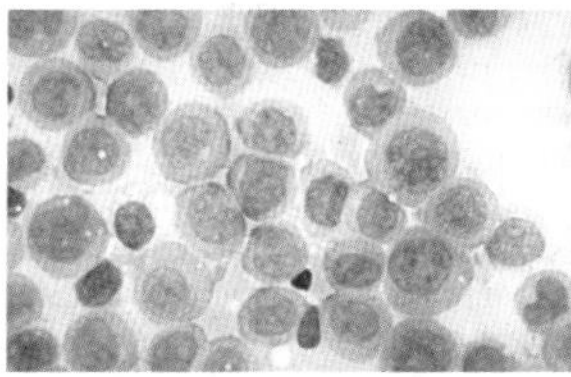
Fig 8.53 Marrow in AML: multiple monoblasts.
Courtesy of Prof. Christine Lawrence.

Myelodysplastic syndromes (MDS, myelodysplasia)

These are a heterogeneous group of disorders that manifest as marrow failure with risk of life-threatening infection and bleeding (median survival varies from 6 months to 6 years according to disease type). Mostly primary, but can develop secondary to chemotherapy or radiotherapy. 30% transform to acute leukaemia. *Tests:* Pancytopenia (p364), with ↓reticulocyte count. Marrow cellularity is usually increased due to ineffective haematopoiesis. Ring sideroblasts may also be seen in the marrow (fig 8.9, p327).

Treatment:
- Multiple transfusions of red cells or platelets as needed.
- Erythropoietin ± G-CSF (p352) may lower transfusion requirement.
- Allogeneic stem cell transplantation is one option (curative but often inappropriate owing to age-related comorbidities—most are >70yrs old).
- Low-intensity treatments that are not curative but may improve quality of life in symptomatic disease include thalidomide analogues (eg lenalidomide) or hypomethylating agents (eg azacitidine and decitabine).

Heterogeneity in AML

Consider four types of heterogeneity as we move through medical history: morphologic, immunophenotypic, cytogenetic, and molecular. Genomic technologies enable an ever more detailed molecular analysis of AML and this can be used to inform prognosis and guide risk stratification. Epigenetic and other profiling reveals more and more biomarkers, eg mutations in the genes encoding DNA (cytosine-5)-methyltransferase 3A (DNMT3A).

Chronic myeloid leukaemia (CML)

CML is characterized by an uncontrolled clonal proliferation of myeloid cells (fig 8.54). It accounts for 15% of leukaemias. It is a myeloproliferative disorder (p366) having features in common with these diseases, eg splenomegaly. It occurs most often between 40-60yrs, with a slight male predominance, and is rare in childhood.

Philadelphia chromosome (Ph) Present in >80% of those with CML. It is a hybrid chromosome comprising reciprocal translocation between the long arm of chromosome 9 and the long arm of chromosome 22—t(9;22)—forming a fusion gene BCR/ABL on chromosome 22, which has tyrosine kinase activity. Those without Ph have a worse prognosis. Some patients have a masked translocation—cytogenetics do not show the Ph, but the rearrangement is detectable by molecular techniques.

Symptoms Mostly chronic and insidious: ↓weight, tiredness, fever, sweats. There may be features of gout (due to purine breakdown), bleeding (platelet dysfunction), and abdominal discomfort (splenic enlargement). ~30% are detected by chance.

Signs Splenomegaly (>75%)—often massive. Hepatomegaly, anaemia, bruising (fig 8.55).

Tests ↑↑WBC (often $>100\times10^9$/L) with whole spectrum of myeloid cells, ie ↑neutrophils, monocytes, basophils, eosinophils. ↓Hb or ↔, platelets variable. ↑Urate, ↑B_{12}. Bone marrow hypercellular. Cytogenetic analysis of blood or bone marrow for Ph.

Natural history Variable, median survival 5-6yrs. There are three phases: *Chronic*, lasting months or years of few, if any, symptoms. • *Accelerated phase*, with increasing symptoms, spleen size, and difficulty in controlling counts. • *Blast transformation*, with features of acute leukaemia ± death. **Treatment** See BOX.

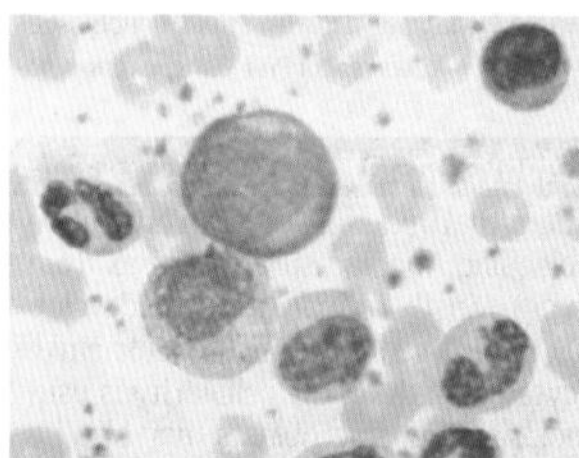

Fig 8.54 CML: numerous granulocytic cells at different stages of differentiation.

Courtesy of Prof. Christine Lawrence.

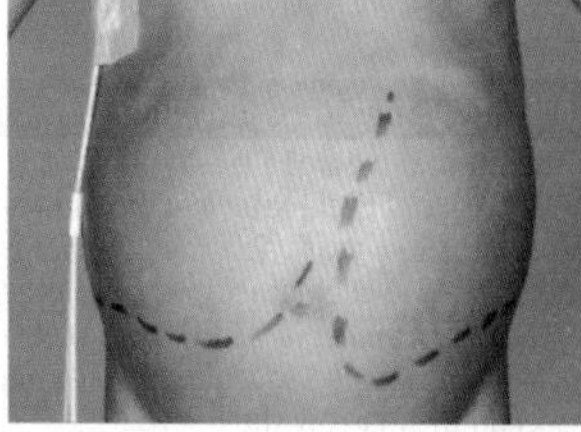

Fig 8.55 Hepatosplenomegaly in CML.

Treating CML

CML is the first example of a cancer where knowledge of the genotype has led to a specifically targeted drug—*imatinib*, a BCR-ABL tyrosine kinase inhibitor. This has transformed therapy over the last 10yrs. Side effects are usually mild: nausea, cramps, oedema, rash, headache, arthralgia. May cause myelosuppression.

More potent 2nd-generation BCR-ABL inhibitors: *dasatinib*, *nilotinib*, *bosutinib*, and *ponatinib*. Dasatinib and nilotinib allow more patients to achieve deeper, more rapid responses associated with improved outcomes, and dasatinib has been used in imatinib-resistant blast crises (though NICE says that it is often not cost-effective). *Hydroxycarbamide* is also used.

Those with lymphoblastic transformation may benefit from treatment as for ALL. Treatment of myeloblastic transformation with chemotherapy rarely achieves lasting remission, and allogeneic transplantation offers the best hope.

Stem cell transplantation. Allogeneic transplantation from an HLA-matched sibling or unrelated donor offers the only cure, but carries significant morbidity and mortality. Guidelines suggest that this approach should be only rarely used 1st line in young patients (where mortality rates are lower). Other patients should be offered a BCR-ABL inhibitor. Patients are then reviewed annually to decide whether to continue, to offer combination therapy or stem cell transplantation.

Chronic lymphocytic leukaemia (CLL)

CLL is the commonest leukaemia (>25%; incidence: ~5/100 000/yr). ♂:♀≈2:1. The hallmark is progressive accumulation of a malignant clone of functionally incompetent B cells. Mutations, trisomies, and deletions (eg del17p13) influence risk (table 8.8).

Table 8.8 Staging and survival in CLL

Rai stage:			
	0	Lymphocytosis alone	Median survival >13yrs
	I	Lymphocytosis + lymphadenopathy	8yrs
	II	Lymphocytosis + spleno- or hepatomegaly	5yrs
	III	Lymphocytosis + anaemia (Hb <110g/L)	2yrs
	IV	Lymphocytosis + platelets <100 × 10^9/L	1yr

Symptoms Often none, presenting as a surprise finding on a routine FBC. Patients may be anaemic or infection-prone, or have ↓weight, sweats, anorexia if severe.

Signs Enlarged, rubbery, non-tender nodes (fig 8.56). Splenomegaly, hepatomegaly.

Tests ↑Lymphocytes—may be marked (fig 8.57). Later: autoimmune haemolysis (p338), marrow infiltration: ↓Hb, ↓neutrophils, ↓platelets.

Complications 1 Autoimmune haemolysis. 2 ↑Infection due to hypogammaglobulinaemia (=↓IgG), bacterial, viral especially herpes zoster. 3 Marrow failure.

Treatment Consider drugs if symptomatic. Fludarabine + rituximab ± cyclophosphamide is 1st line (there is synergism). Ibrutinib, chlorambucil, bendamustine, and ofatumumab all have a role. Steroids help autoimmune haemolysis. *Radiotherapy* helps lymphadenopathy and splenomegaly. *Stem-cell transplantation* may have a role in carefully selected patients. *Supportive care:* Transfusions, IV human immunoglobulin if recurrent infection.

Natural history ⅓ never progress (or even *regress*), ⅓ progress slowly, and ⅓ progress actively. CD23 and β2 microglobulin correlate with bulk of disease and rates of progression. Death is often due to infection or transformation to aggressive lymphoma (Richter's syndrome).

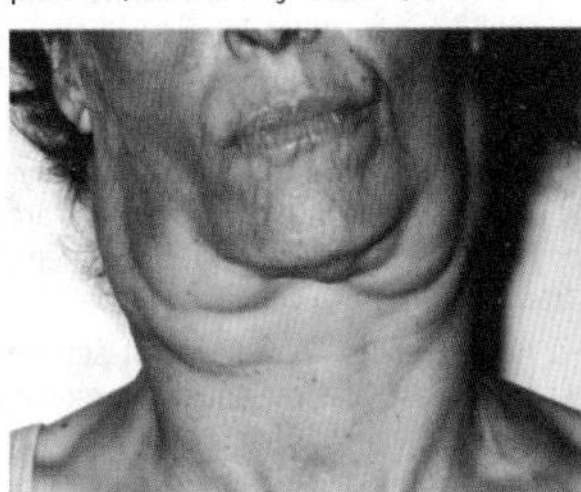

Fig 8.56 Bilateral cervical lymphadenopathy in CLL.

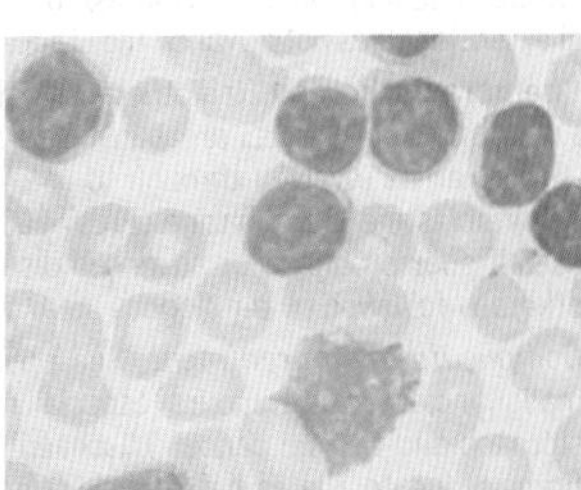

Fig 8.57 CLL: many lymphocytes and a 'smear' cell: a fragile cell damaged in preparation.

Courtesy of Prof. Christine Lawrence.

Haematology

Hodgkin's lymphoma (HL)

Lymphomas are disorders caused by malignant proliferations of lymphocytes. These accumulate in the lymph nodes causing lymphadenopathy, but may also be found in peripheral blood or infiltrate organs. Lymphomas are histologically divided into Hodgkin's and non-Hodgkin's types. In Hodgkin's lymphoma,[7] characteristic cells with mirror-image nuclei are found, called Reed–Sternberg cells (figs 8.58–8.60).

Incidence Two peaks: young adults (HL is the commonest malignancy in 15–24yr olds) and elderly. ♂:♀≈2:1. *Risk factors*: An affected sibling; EBV (p405); SLE; post-transplantation.

Symptoms Often presents with enlarged, non-tender, 'rubbery' superficial lymph nodes (60–70% cervical, fig 8.61, also axillary or inguinal). Node size may fluctuate, and they can become matted. 25% have constitutional upset, eg fever, weight loss, night sweats, pruritus, and lethargy. There may be alcohol-induced lymph node pain. Mediastinal lymph node involvement can cause mass effect, eg bronchial or SVC obstruction (p528), or direct extension, eg causing pleural effusions.

Signs Lymphadenopathy. Also, cachexia, anaemia, spleno- or hepatomegaly.

Tests *Tissue diagnosis:* Lymph node excision biopsy if possible. Image-guided needle biopsy, laparotomy, or mediastinoscopy may be needed. *Bloods:* FBC, film, ESR, LFT, LDH, urate, Ca^{2+}. ↑ESR or ↓Hb indicate a worse prognosis. LDH↑ as it is released during cell turnover. *Imaging:* CXR, CT/PET of thorax, abdo, and pelvis.

Staging (Ann Arbor system.) Influences treatment and prognosis. Done by imaging ±marrow biopsy if B symptoms, or stage III–IV disease.

- **I** Confined to single lymph node region.
- **II** Involvement of two or more nodal areas on the same side of the diaphragm.
- **III** Involvement of nodes on both sides of the diaphragm.
- **IV** Spread beyond the lymph nodes, eg liver or bone marrow.

Each stage is either 'A'—no systemic symptoms other than pruritus; or 'B'—presence of B symptoms: weight loss >10% in last 6 months, unexplained fever >38°C, or night sweats (needing change of clothes). 'B' indicates worse disease. Localized extra-nodal extension does not advance the stage, but is indicated by subscripted 'E', eg I-A_E.

Chemoradiotherapy Radiotherapy + short courses of chemotherapy for stages I-A and II-A (eg with ≤3 areas involved). Longer courses of chemotherapy for II-A with >3 areas involved through to IV-B. '**ABVD**': **A**driamycin (doxorubicin), **B**leomycin, **V**inblastine, **D**acarbazine cures ~80% of patients. More intensive regimens are used if poor prognosis or advanced disease.[8] In relapsed disease: high-dose chemotherapy followed by autologous stem cell transplantation.

Complications of treatment: See pp524–7. *Radiotherapy* may ↑ risk of second malignancies—solid tumours (especially lung and breast, also melanoma, sarcoma, stomach and thyroid cancers), ischaemic heart disease, hypothyroidism, and lung fibrosis due to the radiation field. *Chemotherapy* SE include myelosuppression, nausea, alopecia, infection. AML (p356), non-Hodgkin's lymphoma, and infertility may be due to both chemo- and radiotherapy—see p525.

5-year survival Depends on stage and grade (table 8.9): >95% in I-A lymphocyte-predominant disease; <40% with IV-B lymphocyte-depleted.

Emergency presentations Infection; SVC obstruction—↑JVP, sensation of fullness in the head, dyspnoea, blackouts, facial oedema (seek expert help; see p528).

7 Thomas Hodgkin (1798–1866); rediscovered by Samuel Wilks (1824–1911) who magnanimously gave the disease Hodgkin's name.
8 Eg BEACOPP (bleomycin/etoposide/doxorubicin/cyclophosphamide/vincristine/procarbazine/prednisone). In IIB, III, or IV, BEACOPP gives better initial control, but 7yr event-free survival is similar: 78% vs 71%.

Table 8.9 HL subtypes

Classification *(% of cases)*	Prognosis
Nodular sclerosing (70%)	Good
Mixed cellularity* (20–25%)	Good
Lymphocyte rich (5%)	Good
Lymphocyte depleted* (<1%)	Poor
NB: nodular lymphocyte predominant Hodgkin's is recognized as a separate entity, behaving as an indolent B-cell lymphoma. **Higher incidence and worse prognosis if HIV +ve.*	

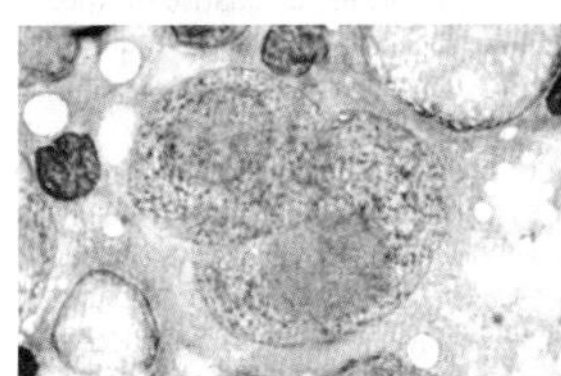

Fig 8.58 A Reed-Sternberg cell with two nuclei, characteristic of Hodgkin's lymphoma.

Courtesy of Prof. Christine Lawrence.

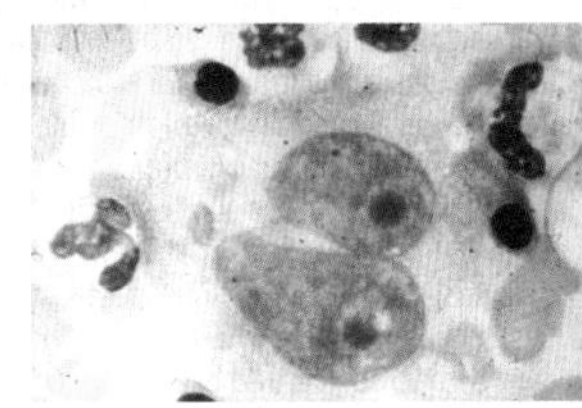

Fig 8.59 Another Reed-Sternberg cell.

Courtesy of the Crookston collection.

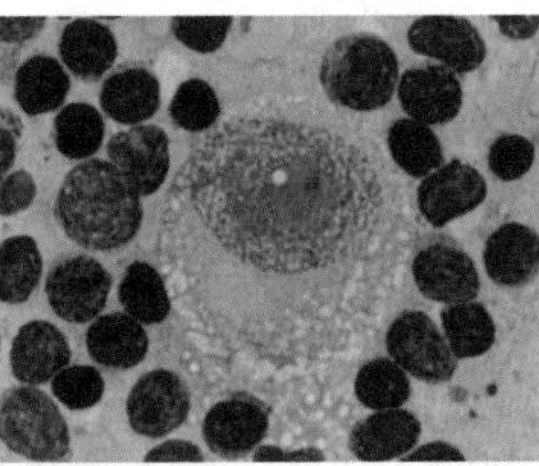

Fig 8.60 Mononuclear Reed-Sternberg cell in a lymph node.

©Prof. Tangün and Dr Köroğlu.

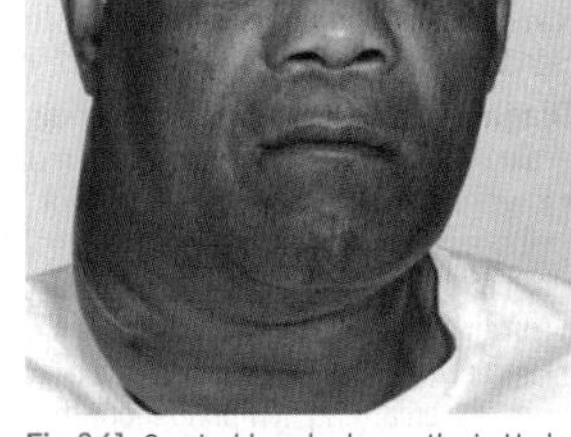

Fig 8.61 Cervical lymphadenopathy in Hodgkin's disease.

Quality of life, lymphoma, and the role of expressive writing

Being treated for Hodgkin's lymphoma is arduous. Our job is often to give encouragement—the more this is personalized for our individual patient the better.

One method is to encourage our patients to write about their experiences. In one study this gave clear-cut benefits in lymphoma patients. Participants report positive responses to writing, and half said that writing changed their thoughts about their illness in a positive way (this increased on subsequent follow-up). Textual analysis identifies themes related to experiences of positive change, transformation, and self-affirmation through reflection. These techniques are akin to those used in post-traumatic stress—and remind us that some of our treatments are as destabilizing to our patients as any shipwreck or earthquake. 'I can whine, I can complain, I can moan, and bitch, about all of the above, but I won't.... The true feat isn't escaping death, rather, learning how to live.'

Sometimes narrating lymphoma experiences reveals bitterness, loss of control, and a feeling that life has been rendered void. Here our role is to receive these negatives and to try to keep the channels of communication open, as dialogue is the only validated means of filling these voids. The need to enhance support networks and bolster social ties may trump all our pharmacological imperatives.

Non-Hodgkin's lymphoma

This includes all lymphomas without Reed-Sternberg cells (p360)—a diverse group. Most are derived from B-cell lines; diffuse large B-cell lymphoma (DLBCL) is commonest. Not all centre on nodes (extranodal tissues generating lymphoma include mucosa-associated lymphoid tissue, eg gastric MALT, later in topic). Incidence has doubled since 1970 (to 2:10 000). **Causes** Immunodeficiency—drugs; HIV (usually high-grade lymphoma from EBV transformed cells, p405); HTLV-1, p405; *H. pylori*; toxins; congenital.

Signs and symptoms • Superficial lymphadenopathy (75% at presentation).

- Extranodal disease (50%) *Gut* (commonest): **1** *Gastric MALT* is caused by *H. pylori*, and may regress with its eradication (p252). Symptoms: as for gastric Ca (p619), with systemic features (see below). MALT usually involves the antrum, is multifocal, and metastasizes late. **2** *Non-MALT gastric lymphomas* (60%) are usually diffuse large-cell B lymphomas—high-grade and not responding well to *H. pylori* eradication. **3** *Small-bowel lymphomas* eg IPSID (immunoproliferative small intestine disease p370), or EATCL (enteropathy/coeliac-associated intra-epithelial T-cell lymphoma)—presents with diarrhoea, vomiting, abdominal pain, and ↓weight. Poor prognosis. *Skin:* (2nd commonest—see fig 8.62) Eg clonal T cells in mycosis fungoides (accounts for ~50%—p596). *Oropharynx:* Waldeyer's ring lymphoma causes sore throat/obstructed breathing. *Other possible sites:* Bone, CNS, and lung.
- Systemic features—fever, night sweats, weight loss (less common than in Hodgkin's lymphoma, and indicates disseminated disease).
- Pancytopenia from marrow involvement—anaemia, infection, bleeding (↓platelets).

Tests *Blood:* FBC, U&E, LFT. ↑LDH≈worse prognosis, reflecting ↑cell turnover. *Marrow and node biopsy* for classification (complex, based on the WHO system of high- or low-grade). *Staging:* Ann Arbor system (p360)—CT ± PET of chest, abdomen, pelvis. Send *cytology* of any effusion; LP for CSF cytology if CNS signs.

Diagnosis/management is multidisciplinary, synthesizing details from clinical evaluation, histology, immunology, molecular genetics, and imaging. *Generally:*

- Low-grade lymphomas are indolent, often incurable and widely disseminated. Include: follicular lymphoma, marginal zone lymphoma/MALT, lymphocytic lymphoma (closely related to CLL and treated similarly), lymphoplasmacytoid lymphoma (produces IgM = Waldenström's macroglobulinaemia, p370). See fig 8.63.
- High-grade lymphomas are more aggressive, *but often curable*. There is often rapidly enlarging lymphadenopathy with systemic symptoms. Include: Burkitt's lymphoma (childhood disease with characteristic jaw lymphadenopathy; figs 8.64, 8.65), lymphoblastic lymphomas (like ALL), diffuse large B-cell lymphoma.

Treatment Huge range of options, depending on disease subtype. *Low grade:* If symptomless, none may be needed. Radiotherapy may be curative in localized disease. Chlorambucil is used in diffuse disease. Remission may be maintained by using interferon alfa or rituximab (see later in paragraph). Bendamustine is effective both with rituximab and as a monotherapy in rituximab-refractory patients. *High grade:* (eg large B-cell lymphoma, DLBCL), '**R-CHOP' regimen**: Rituximab, Cyclophosphamide, Hydroxydaunorubicin, vincristine (Oncovin®) and Prednisolone. Granulocyte colony-stimulating factors (G-CSFs) help neutropenia—eg filgrastim or lenograstim (at low doses it may be cost-effective).

Survival Histology is important. Prognosis is worse if, at presentation: • Age >60yrs. • Systemic symptoms. • Bulky disease (abdominal mass >10cm). • ↑LDH. • Disseminated disease. Typical 5yr survival for treated patients: ~30% for high-grade and >50% for low-grade lymphomas, but the picture is very variable.

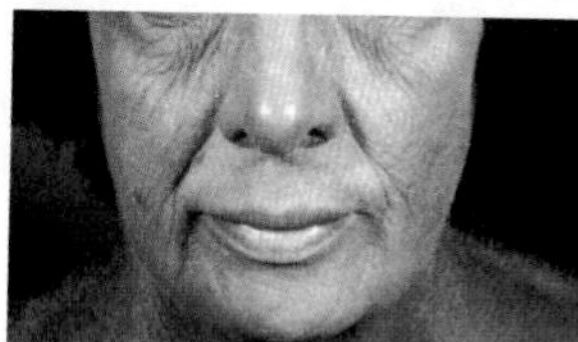

Fig 8.62 Cutaneous T-cell lymphoma, which has caused severe erythroderma (Sézary syndrome) in a Caucasian woman.

Courtesy of Prof. Christine Lawrence.

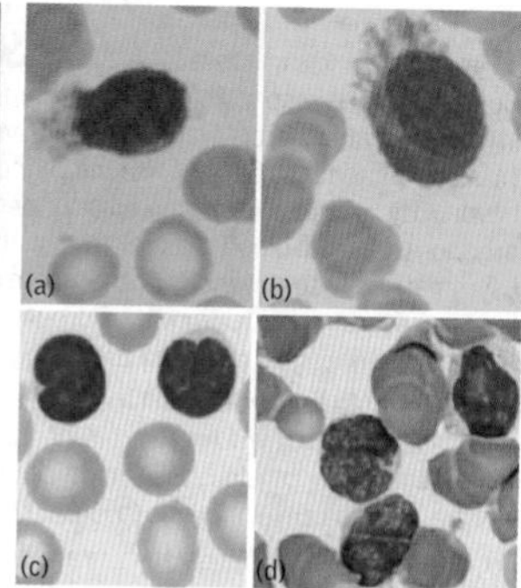

Fig 8.63 (a) and (b): villous lymphocytes (splenic marginal zone lymphoma). (c): 'buttock cells' with cleaved nuclei (follicular lymphoma). (d): Sézary cells with convoluted nuclei.

Courtesy of Prof. Tangün & Dr Köroğlu.

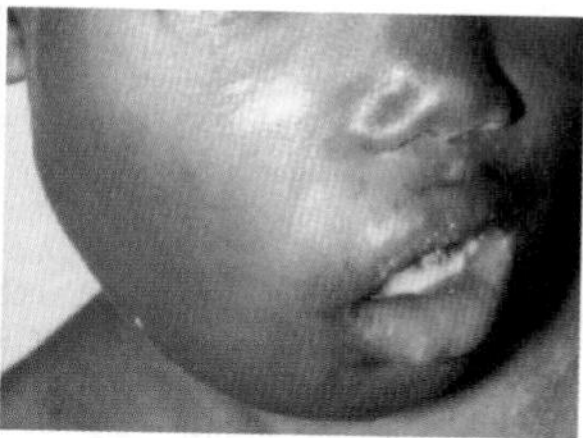

Fig 8.64 Burkitt's lymphoma, with characteristic jaw lymphadenopathy.

Courtesy of Dr Tom D Thacher.

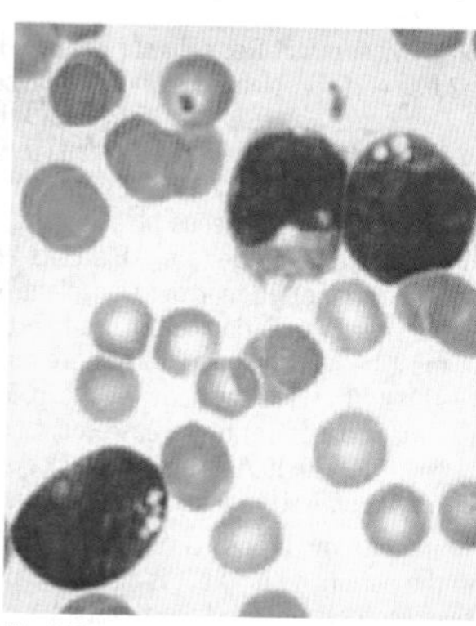

Fig 8.65 Burkitt's lymphoma, with three basophilic vacuolated lymphoma cells.

From the *New England Journal of Medicine*, Bain, B, 'Diagnosis from the blood smear', 353(5), 498. Copyright © 2005 Massachusetts Medical Society. Reprinted with permission from Massachusetts Medical Society.

The role of rituximab in untreated follicular lymphoma

Rituximab kills CD20+ve cells by antibody-directed cytotoxicity ± apoptosis induction. It also sensitizes cells to CHOP. It is cost-effective when used with:

- cyclophosphamide, vincristine, and prednisolone (CVP)
- cyclophosphamide, doxorubicin, vincristine, and prednisolone (CHOP)
- cyclophosphamide, doxorubicin, etoposide, prednisolone, and interferon alfa (CHVPi)
- mitoxantrone, chlorambucil, and prednisolone (MCP)
- chlorambucil.

It also has a role in maintaining remission, and in relapsed disease.

Pancytopenia and bone marrow failure

Bone marrow is responsible for haematopoiesis. In adults, this normally takes place in the central skeleton (vertebrae, sternum, ribs, skull) and proximal long bones. In some anaemias (eg thalassaemia), increased demand induces haematopoiesis beyond the marrow (extramedullary haematopoiesis), in liver and spleen, causing organomegaly. All blood cells arise from an early pluripotent stem cell, which divides asymmetrically to produce another stem cell and a progenitor cell committed to a lineage (see fig 8.66). Committed progenitors further differentiate into myeloid or lymphocyte lineages, releasing their progeny into the blood.

Pancytopenia Reduction in all the major cell lines: red cells, white cells, and platelets. Causes are due to: 1 ↓*Marrow production:* Aplastic anaemia (see BOX), infiltration (eg acute leukaemia, myelodysplasia, myeloma, lymphoma, solid tumours, TB), megaloblastic anaemia, myelofibrosis (p366). 2 ↑*Peripheral destruction:* Hypersplenism.

Agranulocytosis Implies that granulocytes (WBCs with neutrophil, basophil, or eosinophil granules) have stopped being made, leaving the patient at risk of fatal infections. Many drugs can be the culprit: eg carbimazole, procainamide, sulfonamides, gold, clozapine, dapsone. ►When starting drugs known to cause agranulocytosis, warn patients to report *any* fever. Neutropenia (WCC $\le 0.5 \times 10^9$/L) may declare itself initially as a sore throat. Stop the drug, commence neutropenic regimen and consider G-CSF if indicated (p352).

Marrow support Red cells survive for ~120d, platelets for ~8d, and neutrophils for 1-2d, so early problems are mainly from neutropenia and thrombocytopenia.

1 *Red cell transfusion:* Transfusing 1U should raise Hb by ~10-15g/L (p348). Transfusion may drop the platelet count (you may need to give platelets before or after).
2 *Platelets:* Traumatic bleeds, purpura, and easy bruising occur if platelets $<50 \times 10^9$/L. Spontaneous bleeding may occur if platelets $<20 \times 10^9$/L, with intracranial haemorrhage rarely. Platelets are stored at room temperature (22°C; not in the fridge). In marrow transplant or if severely immunosuppressed, platelets may need irradiation before use to prevent transfusion-associated GVHD. Platelets must be ABO compatible. They are not used in ITP (p345). Indications: • Platelets $<10 \times 10^9$/L. • Haemorrhage (eg DIC, p352). • Before invasive procedures (eg biopsy, lumbar puncture) to increase count to $>50 \times 10^9$/L. 4U of platelets should raise the count to $>40 \times 10^9$/L in adults; check dose needed with lab.
3 *Neutrophils:* Use neutropenic regimen if the count $<0.5 \times 10^9$/L (p352).

Bone marrow biopsy Gives diagnostic information where there are abnormalities in the peripheral blood; it is also an important staging test in the lymphoproliferative disorders. Ideally take an aspirate *and* trephine usually from the posterior iliac crest (aspirates can be taken from the anterior iliac crest or sternum). The aspirate provides a film which is examined by microscope. The trephine is a core of bone which allows assessment of bone marrow cellularity, architecture, and the presence of infiltrative disease (eg neoplasia). Coagulation disorders may need to be corrected pre-biopsy. Apply pressure afterwards (lie on that side for 1-2h if platelets are low).

Aplastic anaemia

This is a rare (~5 cases per million/year) stem cell disorder in which bone marrow stops making cells, leading to pancytopenia. Presents with features of anaemia (↓Hb), infection (↓WCC), or bleeding (↓platelets). *Causes:* Most cases are autoimmune, triggered by drugs, viruses (eg parvovirus, hepatitis), or irradiation. May also be inherited, eg Fanconi anaemia (p698). *Tests:* Bone marrow biopsy is diagnostic. *Treatment:* Mainly supportive in asymptomatic patients. Transfuse blood products as required and initiate neutropenic regimen if count $<0.5 \times 10^9$/L (p352). The treatment of choice in young patients with severe disease is allogeneic marrow transplantation from an HLA-matched sibling, which can be curative. Otherwise, immunosuppression with ciclosporin and antithymocyte globulin may be effective, although it is not curative in most. There is no clear role for G-CSF.

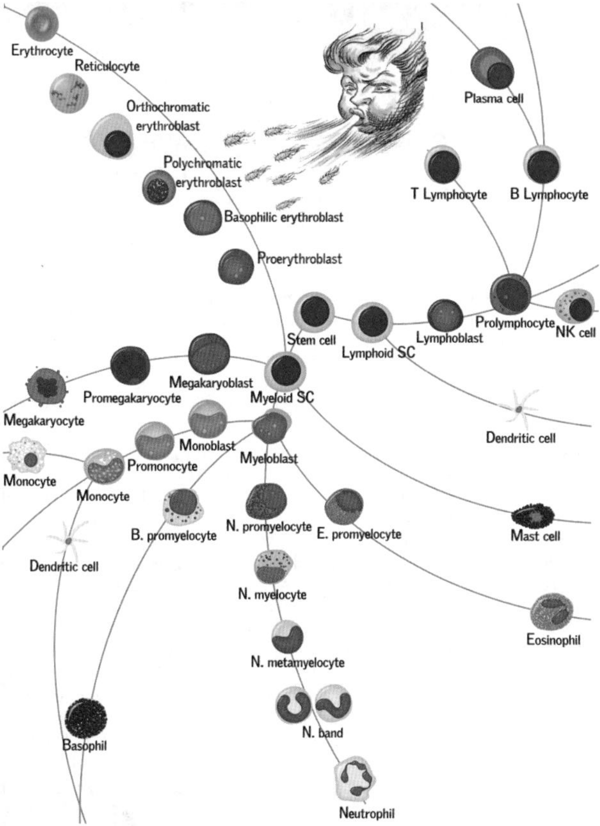

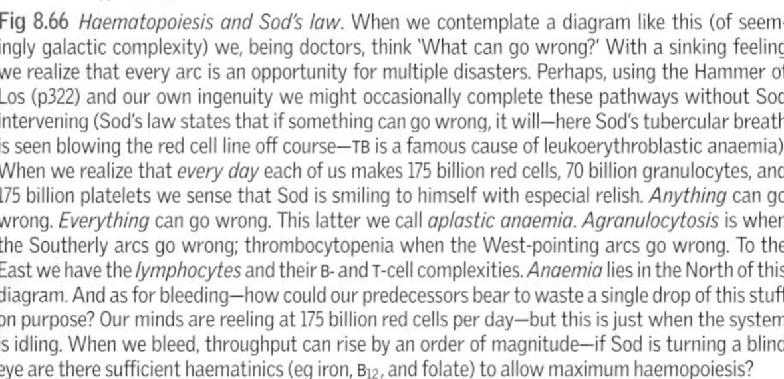

Fig 8.66 *Haematopoiesis and Sod's law.* When we contemplate a diagram like this (of seemingly galactic complexity) we, being doctors, think 'What can go wrong?' With a sinking feeling we realize that every arc is an opportunity for multiple disasters. Perhaps, using the Hammer of Los (p322) and our own ingenuity we might occasionally complete these pathways without Sod intervening (Sod's law states that if something can go wrong, it will—here Sod's tubercular breath is seen blowing the red cell line off course—TB is a famous cause of leukoerythroblastic anaemia). When we realize that *every day* each of us makes 175 billion red cells, 70 billion granulocytes, and 175 billion platelets we sense that Sod is smiling to himself with especial relish. *Anything* can go wrong. *Everything* can go wrong. This latter we call *aplastic anaemia*. *Agranulocytosis* is when the Southerly arcs go wrong; thrombocytopenia when the West-pointing arcs go wrong. To the East we have the *lymphocytes* and their B- and T-cell complexities. *Anaemia* lies in the North of this diagram. And as for bleeding—how could our predecessors bear to waste a single drop of this stuff on purpose? Our minds are reeling at 175 billion red cells per day—but this is just when the system is idling. When we bleed, throughput can rise by an order of magnitude—if Sod is turning a blind eye are there sufficient haematinics (eg iron, B_{12}, and folate) to allow maximum haemopoiesis?

Figure ©Aria Rad.

The myeloproliferative disorders

Caused by clonal proliferation of haematopoietic myeloid stem cells in the bone marrow. These cells retain the ability to differentiate into RBCs, WBCs, or platelets, causing an excess of one or more of these cell types (table 8.10).

Table 8.10 Classification of myeloproliferative disorders

By proliferating cell type		
RBC	→	Polycythaemia vera (PRV)
WBC	→	Chronic myeloid leukaemia (CML, p358)
Platelets	→	Essential thrombocythaemia
Fibroblasts	→	Myelofibrosis

Polycythaemia *Relative polycythaemia* (↓plasma volume, normal RBC mass) may be acute (due to dehydration) or chronic (associated with obesity, HTN, and a high alcohol and tobacco intake). *Absolute polycythaemia* (↑RBC mass) is classically measured by dilution of infused autologous radioactive chromium (^{51}Cr) labelled RBCs. Causes are primary (*polycythaemia vera*) or secondary due to hypoxia (eg high altitudes, chronic lung disease, cyanotic congenital heart disease, heavy smoking) or inappropriately ↑erythropoietin secretion (eg in renal carcinoma, hepatocellular carcinoma).

Polycythaemia vera The malignant proliferation of a clone derived from one pluripotent stem cell. A mutation in JAK2 (JAK2 V617F) is present in >95%. The erythroid progenitor offspring are unusual in not needing erythropoietin to avoid apoptosis. There is excess proliferation of RBCs, WBCs, and platelets, leading to hyperviscosity and thrombosis. Commoner if >60yrs old.

Presentation: May be asymptomatic and detected on FBC, or present with vague symptoms due to hyperviscosity (p372): headaches, dizziness, tinnitus, visual disturbance. Itching after a hot bath, and erythromelalgia, a burning sensation in fingers and toes, are characteristic. Signs: facial plethora and splenomegaly (in 60%). Gout may occur due to ↑urate from RBC turnover. Features of arterial (cardiac, cerebral, peripheral) or venous (DVT, cerebral, hepatic) thrombosis may be present.

Investigations: • FBC: ↑RCC, ↑Hb, ↑HCT, ↑PCV, often also ↑WBC and ↑platelets. • ↑B_{12}. • Marrow shows hypercellularity with erythroid hyperplasia. • Cytogenetics as required to differentiate from CML. • ↓Serum erythropoietin. • Raised red cell mass on ^{51}Cr studies and splenomegaly, in the setting of a normal P_aO_2, is diagnostic.

Treatment: Aim to keep HCT <0.45 to ↓risk of thrombosis. In younger patients at low risk, this is done by venesection. If higher risk (age >60yrs, previous thrombosis), hydroxycarbamide (=hydroxyurea) is used. α-interferon is preferred in women of childbearing age. Aspirin 75mg daily is also given.

Prognosis: Variable, many remain well for years. Thrombosis and haemorrhage (due to defective platelets) are the main complications. Transition to myelofibrosis occurs in ~30% or acute leukaemia in ~5%. Monitor FBC every 3 months.

Essential thrombocythaemia (fig 8.67) A clonal proliferation of megakaryocytes leads to persistently ↑platelets, often >1000 × 10^9/L, with abnormal function, causing bleeding or arterial and venous thrombosis, and microvascular occlusion—headache, atypical chest pain, light-headedness, erythromelalgia. Exclude other causes of thrombocytosis (see BOX). *Treatment:* aspirin 75mg OD. Hydroxycarbamide in high-risk patients.

Myelofibrosis There is hyperplasia of megakaryocytes which produce platelet-derived growth factor, leading to intense marrow fibrosis and haematopoiesis in the spleen and liver→massive hepatosplenomegaly. *Presentation:* Hypermetabolic symptoms: night sweats, fever, weight loss; abdominal discomfort due to splenomegaly; bone marrow failure (↓Hb, infections, bleeding). *Film:* Leukoerythroblastic cells (nucleated red cells, p328); characteristic teardrop RBCs (see fig 8.68). ↓Hb. Bone marrow trephine for diagnosis (fig 8.69). *Treatment:* Marrow support (see p364). Allogeneic stem cell transplant may be curative in young people but carries a high risk of mortality. *Prognosis:* Median survival 4-5 years.

Causes of thrombocytosis

↑Platelets >450 × 10^9/L may be a reactive phenomenon, seen with many conditions including:

- Bleeding
- Malignancy
- Post-surgery
- Infection
- Trauma
- Iron deficiency
- Chronic inflammation, eg collagen disorders.

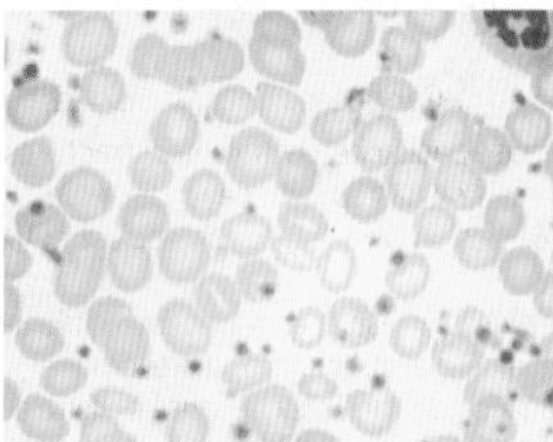

Fig 8.67 Essential thrombocythaemia: many platelets seen.

© Prof. Christine Lawrence.

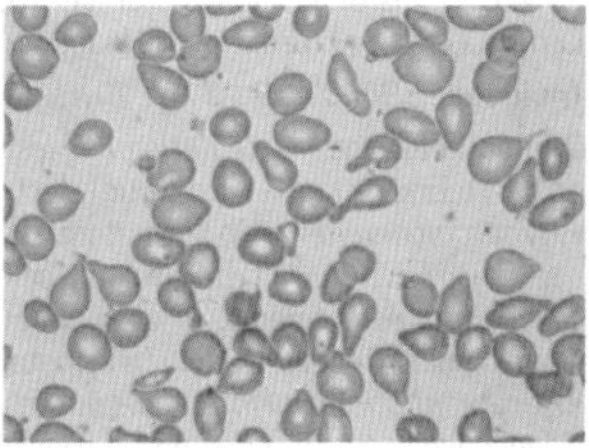

Fig 8.68 Teardrop cells, in myelofibrosis.

© Dr Nivaldo Medeiros.

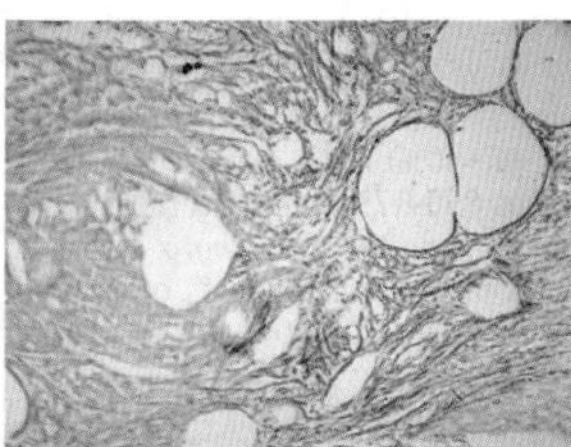

Fig 8.69 Marrow trephine in myelofibrosis: the streaming effect is caused by intense fibrosis. Other causes of marrow fibrosis: any myeloproliferative disorder, lymphoma, secondary carcinoma, TB, leukaemia, and irradiation.

© Prof. Christine Lawrence.

Myeloma: the chief plasma cell dyscrasia (PCD)

PCDs are due to an abnormal proliferation of a single clone of plasma or lymphoplasmacytic cells leading to secretion of immunoglobulin (Ig) or an Ig fragment, causing the dysfunction of many organs (esp kidney).The Ig is seen as a monoclonal band, or paraprotein, on serum or urine electrophoresis (see later in topic).

Classification Based on Ig product—IgG in ~⅔; IgA in ~⅓; a very few are IgM or IgD. Other Ig levels are low ('immunoparesis', causing ↑susceptibility to infection). In ~⅔, urine contains Bence Jones proteins, which are free Ig light chains of kappa (κ) or lambda (λ) type, filtered by the kidney.

Incidence 5/100 000. Peak age: 70yrs. ♂:♀≈1:1. Afro-Caribbeans:Caucasians≈2:1.

Clinical features • *Osteolytic bone lesions* cause backache, pathological fractures and vertebral collapse. ►Do serum electrophoresis on all >50 with new back pain.

- *Hypercalcaemia* may be symptomatic (p676). Lesions are due to ↑osteoclast activation, from signalling by myeloma cells.
- *Anaemia, neutropenia, or thrombocytopenia* may result from marrow infiltration by plasma cells, leading to symptoms of anaemia, infection, and bleeding.
- *Recurrent bacterial infections* due to immunoparesis, and also because of neutropenia due to the disease and from chemotherapy.
- *Renal impairment* due to light chain deposition (p314 & p370) is seen in up to 20% at diagnosis. The light chains have a toxic and inflammatory effect on the proximal tubule cells, but the damage is mainly caused by precipitation of light chains in the distal loop of Henle. Deposits may rarely be AL-amyloid (causing nephrotic syndrome, see p370). Monoclonal immunoglobulins also disrupt glomeruli.

Tests *Bloods:* FBC: normocytic normochromic anaemia. Film: rouleaux (p328). Persistently ↑ESR (p372). ↑Urea and creatinine, ↑Ca^{2+} (in ~40%). Alk phos usually ↔ unless healing fracture. *Bone marrow biopsy:* See figs 8.70–8.73. *Screening test:* Serum and/or urine electrophoresis. β_2-microglobulin (prognostic). *Imaging:* X-rays: lytic 'punched-out' lesions, eg pepper-pot skull, vertebral collapse, fractures, or osteoporosis. CT or MRI may be useful to detect lesions not seen on XR. *Diagnostic criteria:* See BOX 'Myeloma diagnosis'.

Treatment *Supportive:* • Analgesia for bone pain (avoid NSAIDs due to risk of renal impairment). Give all patients a bisphosphonate (clodronate, zolendronate, or pamidronate), as they reduce fracture rates and bone pain. Local radiotherapy can help rapidly in focal disease. Orthopaedic procedures (vertebroplasty or kyphoplasty) may be helpful in vertebral collapse. • Anaemia should be corrected with *transfusion*, and erythropoietin may be used. • Renal failure: rehydrate, and ensure adequate fluid intake of 3L/day to prevent further light chain-induced renal impairment. Dialysis may be needed in acute kidney injury. • Infections: Treat rapidly with broad-spectrum antibiotics until culture results are known. Regular IV *immunoglobulin infusions* may be needed if recurrent.

Chemotherapy: Induction therapy with, eg lenalidomide, bortezomib, and dexamethasone. In suitably fit patients this may be followed by autologous stem-cell transplantation. In those unsuitable for transplantation, induction therapy is typically continued for 12–18 months, or until serum paraprotein levels have plateaued. Treatment is then typically held until (inevitably) paraprotein levels start to rise again, at which point further chemotherapy or stem cell transplantation may be considered. NB: lenalidomide is a teratogenic immunomodulator which has multiple SE, notably neutropenia and thromboembolism: monitor for sepsis and consider aspirin or anticoagulation if risk ↑, eg hyperviscosity or other comorbidities.

Prognosis Worse if: >2 osteolytic lesions, β_2-microglobulin >5.5mg/L, Hb <11g/L; albumin <30g/L. Risk stratification increasingly based upon detection of specific cytogenetic abnormalities associated with high risk of progression. Causes of death infection, renal failure.

Myeloma diagnosis

Have a high index of suspicion, ►eg in bone pain or back pain which is not improving. Check blood film and electrophoresis. Diagnostic criteria:

1 Monoclonal protein band in serum or urine electrophoresis.
2 ↑Plasma cells on marrow biopsy.
3 Evidence of end-organ damage from myeloma:
   - Hypercalcaemia.
   - Renal insufficiency.
   - Anaemia.
4 Bone lesions: a skeletal survey after diagnosis detects bone disease: x-rays of chest; all of spine; skull; pelvis ± Tc-99m MIBI and PET (p739).

Causes of bone pain/tenderness

- Trauma/fracture (steroids ↑risk)
- Myeloma and other primary malignancy, eg plasmacytoma or sarcoma
- Secondaries (eg from breast, lung etc)
- Osteonecrosis, eg from microemboli
- Osteomyelitis/periostitis (eg syphilis)
- Hydatid cyst (bone is a rare site)
- Osteosclerosis, eg from hepatitis C
- Paget's disease of bone
- Sickle cell anaemia
- Renal osteodystrophy
- CREST syndrome/Sjögren's syndrome
- Hyperparathyroidism.

Tests: PSA, ESR, Ca^{2+}, LFT, electrophoresis.
Treatment: Treat the cause; bisphosphonates & NSAIDs may control symptoms.

Complications of myeloma

- *Hypercalcaemia* (p676). This occurs with active disease, eg at presentation or relapse. Rehydrate vigorously with IV saline 0.9% 4–6L/d (careful fluid balance). IV bisphosphonates, eg zolendronate or pamidronate, are useful for treating hypercalcaemia acutely.
- *Spinal cord compression* (p466). Occurs in 5% of those with myeloma. Urgent MRI if suspected. Treatment is with dexamethasone 8–16mg/24h PO and local radiotherapy.
- *Hyperviscosity* (p372) causes reduced cognition, disturbed vision, and bleeding. It is treated with plasmapheresis to remove light chains.
- *Acute renal injury* is treated with rehydration. Urgent dialysis may be needed.

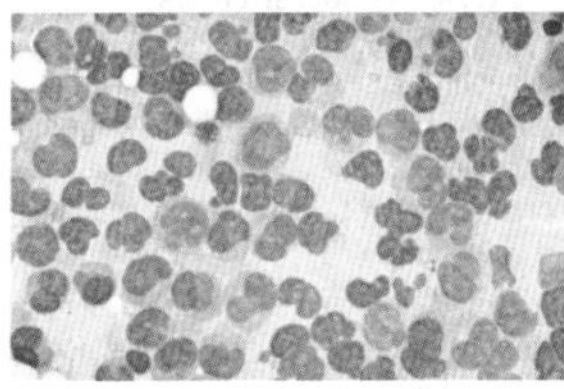

Fig 8.70 Myeloma bone marrow: many plasma cells with abnormal forms.

Courtesy of Prof. Christine Lawrence.

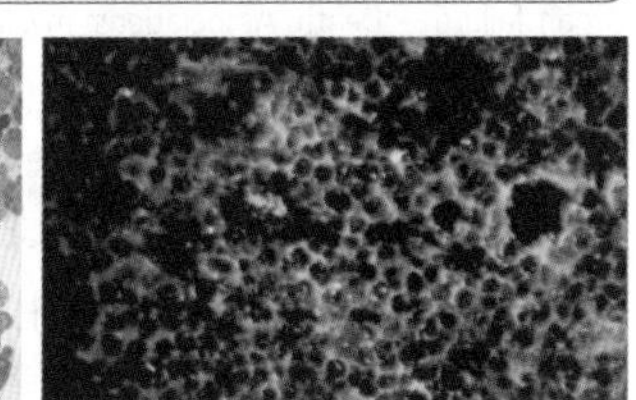

Fig 8.71 Marrow section in myeloma, stained with IGG kappa monoclonal antibody.

Courtesy of Prof. Christine Lawrence.

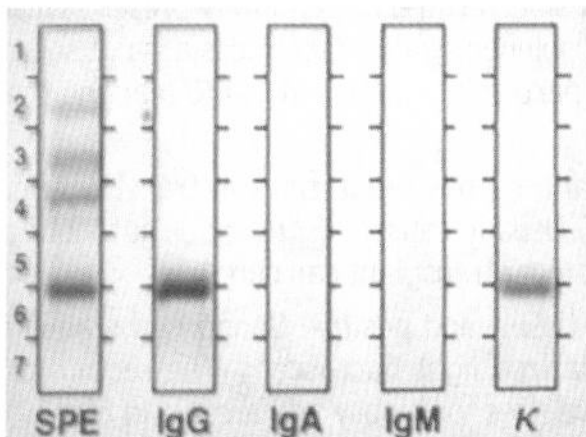

Fig 8.72 An IGG kappa paraprotein monoclonal band (immunofixation electrophoresis; a control sample has run on the left).

Courtesy of Prof. Christine Lawrence.

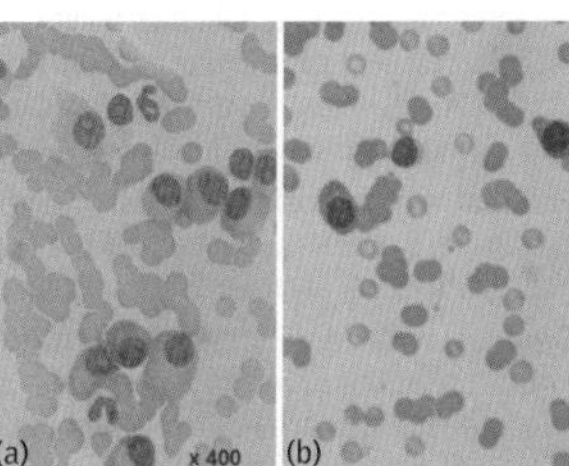

Fig 8.73 Plasma cells in myeloma. (a) marrow smear, (b) peripheral smear. Note rouleaux formation of red cells (p328 & p368).

Courtesy of Prof. Tangün & Dr Köroğlu.

Paraproteinaemia

Paraproteinaemia denotes the presence in the circulation of immunoglobulins produced by a single clone of plasma cells. The paraprotein is recognized as a monoclonal band (M band) on serum electrophoresis.[9] There are six major categories:

1 **Multiple myeloma** See p368.

2 **Waldenström's macroglobulinaemia** This is a lymphoplasmacytoid lymphoma producing a monoclonal IgM paraprotein. Hyperviscosity is common (p372), with CNS and ocular symptoms. Lymphadenopathy and splenomegaly are also seen. ↑ESR, with IgM paraprotein on serum electrophoresis. ℞: None if asymptomatic. Chlorambucil, fludarabine, or combination chemotherapy may be used. Plasmapheresis[9] for hyperviscosity (p372).

3 **Primary amyloidosis** See following topic.

4 **Monoclonal gammopathy of uncertain significance** (MGUS) is common (3% >70yrs). There is a paraprotein in the serum but no myeloma, 1° amyloid, macroglobulinaemia, or lymphoma, with no bone lesions, no Bence Jones protein, and a low concentration of paraprotein, with <10% plasma cells in the marrow. Some develop myeloma or lymphoma. Refer to a haematologist (?for marrow biopsy).

5 **Paraproteinaemia in lymphoma or leukaemia** Eg seen in 5% of CLL.

6 **Heavy chain disease** Neoplastic cells produce free Ig heavy chains. α chain disease is most important, causing malabsorption from infiltration of bowel wall (immunoproliferative small intestine disease—IPSID). It may progress to lymphoma.

Amyloidosis

This is a group of disorders characterized by extracellular deposits of a protein in abnormal fibrillar form, resistant to degradation. The following are the systemic forms of amyloidosis. Amyloid deposition is also a feature of Alzheimer's disease, type 2 diabetes mellitus, and haemodialysis-related amyloidosis.

AL amyloid (primary amyloidosis) Proliferation of plasma cell clone → Amyloidogenic monoclonal immunoglobulins → Fibrillar light chain protein deposition → Organ failure → Death. Associations: myeloma (15%); Waldenström's, lymphoma. Organs involved:

- Kidneys: glomerular lesions—proteinuria and nephrotic syndrome.
- Heart: restrictive cardiomyopathy (looks 'sparkling' on echo), arrhythmias, angina.
- Nerves: peripheral and autonomic neuropathy; carpal tunnel syndrome.
- Gut: macroglossia (big tongue), ↓malabsorption/weight, perforation, haemorrhage, obstruction, and hepatomegaly.
- Vascular: purpura, especially periorbital—a characteristic feature (fig 8.74).

℞: optimize nutrition; PO melphalan + prednisolone extends survival. High-dose IV melphalan with autologous stem cell transplantation may be better.

AA amyloid (secondary amyloidosis) Here amyloid is derived from serum amyloid A, an acute phase protein, reflecting chronic inflammation in rheumatoid arthritis, UC/Crohn's, familial Mediterranean fever, and chronic infections—TB, bronchiectasis, osteomyelitis. It affects kidneys, liver, and spleen (fig 8.75), and may present with proteinuria, nephrotic syndrome, or hepatosplenomegaly. Macroglossia is not seen; cardiac involvement is rare (ventricular hypertrophy and murmurs). ℞: manage the underlying condition optimally.

Familial amyloidosis (Autosomal dominant, eg from mutations in transthyretin, a transport protein produced by the liver.) Usually causes a sensory or autonomic neuropathy ± renal or cardiac involvement. Liver transplant can cure.

Diagnosis: Made with biopsy of affected tissue, and positive Congo Red staining with apple-green birefringence under polarized light microscopy. The rectum or subcutaneous fat are relatively non-invasive sites for biopsy and are +ve in 80%.

Prognosis: Median survival is 1-2 years. Patients with myeloma and amyloidosis have a shorter survival than those with myeloma alone.

9 Electro*phoresis* and plasma*pheresis* look as though they should share endings, but they do not: Greek *phoros* = *bearing* (*esis* = *process*), but *aphairesis* is Greek for *removal*.

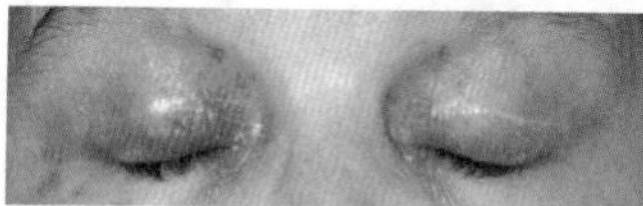

Fig 8.74 Periorbital purpura in amyloidosis.

©Prof. Christine Lawrence.

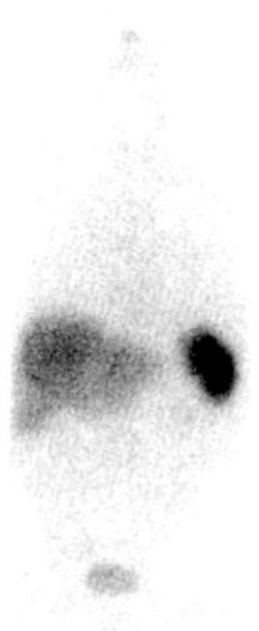

Fig 8.75 Areas of amyloid deposition in liver and spleen in amyloidosis (isotope scan).

Reproduced from Warrell *et al.*, *Oxford Textbook of Medicine*, 2010, with permission from Oxford University Press.

Erythrocyte sedimentation rate (ESR)

The ESR is a sensitive but non-specific indicator of the presence of disease. It measures how far RBCs fall through a column of anticoagulated blood in 1h. If certain proteins cover red cells, these cause RBCs to stick to each other in columns (the same phenomenon as rouleaux, p328) so they fall faster.

Causes of a raised ESR Any inflammation (eg infection, rheumatoid arthritis, malignancy, myocardial infarction), anaemia, and macrocytosis.

Caveats •ESR ↑ with age. The Westergren method is a rough guide to calculate the upper limit of normal in older patients: ♂: ESR=age ÷ 2; ♀: ESR=(age+10) ÷ 2.
•Some conditions *lower* the ESR, eg polycythaemia (due to ↑red cell concentration), microcytosis, and sickle-cell anaemia. Even a slightly raised ESR in these patients should prompt one to ask: '*What else is the matter?*'

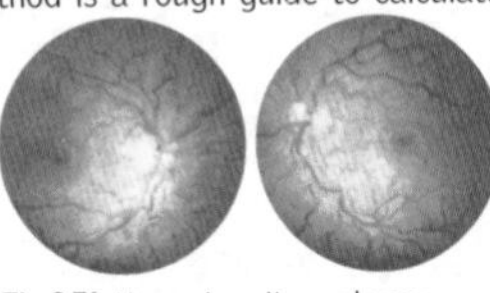

Fig 8.76 Hyperviscosity syndrome.

Management •In those with a slightly raised ESR, the best plan is probably to wait a month and repeat the test. •If the ESR is markedly raised (>100mm/h), this can have a 90% predictive value for disease, so such patients should be thoroughly investigated, even in the presence of non-specific symptoms. Take a full history, examine carefully and consider these tests: FBC, plasma electrophoresis, U&E, PSA, chest and abdominal imaging, ± biopsy of bone marrow or temporal artery.

Plasma viscosity (PV)

Normal range: 1.50-1.72mPa/s. In many labs, this has replaced the ESR, as it is less affected by anaemia and simpler to automate. PV is affected by the concentration of large plasma proteins and ↑ in the same conditions as the ESR—both PV and ESR ↑ in chronic inflammation and are less affected by acute changes (unlike CRP, p686).

Hyperviscosity syndrome

Symptoms Lethargy; confusion; ↓cognition; CNS disturbance; chest pain; abdominal pain (and sometimes spontaneous GI or GU bleeding); faints; visual disturbance (eg ↓vision, amaurosis fugax, retinopathy—eg engorged retinal veins, haemorrhages, exudates; and a blurred disc as seen in fig 8.76). The visual symptoms are like 'looking through a watery car windscreen'.

Causes of high blood viscosity Very high red cell count (haematocrit >50, eg polycythaemia vera), white cell count (>100×10^9/L, eg leukaemia), or plasma components—usually immunoglobulins, in myeloma or Waldenström's macroglobulinaemia (p370, as IgM is larger and so ↑ viscosity more than the same amount of IgG). Drugs: oral contraceptives, diuretics, IV IG, erythropoietin, chemotherapy, radio-contrast media.

Treatment Urgent treatment is needed which depends on the cause. Venesection is done in polycythaemia. Leukapheresis in leukaemias to remove white cells. Plasmapheresis in myeloma and Waldenström's: blood is withdrawn via a plasma exchange machine, the supernatant plasma from this is discarded, and the RBCs returned to the patient after being resuspended in a suitable medium.

The spleen and splenectomy

The spleen plays a vital immunological role by acting as a reservoir for lymphocytes, and in dealing with bacteraemias.

Causes of splenomegaly: (See also p604.) *Massive* (enlarged to the RIF): CML, myelofibrosis, malaria (hyperreactive malarial splenomegaly), visceral leishmaniasis, 'tropical splenomegaly' (idiopathic—Africa, south-east Asia), and Gaucher's syndrome. *Moderate:* • Infection (eg EBV, endocarditis, TB, malaria, leishmaniasis, schistosomiasis). • Portal hypertension (liver cirrhosis). • Haematological (haemolytic anaemia, leukaemia especially CML, lymphoma). • Connective tissue disease (RA, SLE). • Others: sarcoidosis, primary antibody deficiency (*OHCS* p198), idiopathic.

When is a mass in the left upper quadrant a spleen: (Main differential: enlarged left kidney.) The spleen: • Is dull to percussion. • Enlarges towards the RIF. • Moves down on inspiration. • You may feel a medial notch. • 'You can't get above it' (ie the top margin disappears under the ribs).

Tests: Image the spleen with abdominal USS or CT. Hunt for the cause of enlargement: look for lymphadenopathy and liver disease, eg: FBC, ESR, LFT ± liver, marrow, or lymph node biopsy.

Complications: Symptoms of anaemia, infection, or bleeding can occur as a result of hypersplenism: cells become trapped in the spleen's reticuloendothelial system causing pancytopenia. Splenectomy may be required if severe.

Splenectomy: Main indications: splenic trauma, hypersplenism, autoimmune haemolysis: in ITP (p345), warm autoimmune haemolytic anaemia (p338), or congenital haemolytic anaemias. Mobilize early post-splenectomy as transient ↑platelets predisposes to thrombi. A characteristic blood film is seen following splenectomy, with Howell-Jolly bodies, Pappenheimer bodies, and target cells (see p328).

►*The main problem post-splenectomy is lifelong increased risk from infection.* The spleen contains macrophages which filter and phagocytose bacteria. Post-splenectomy infection is caused most commonly by encapsulated organisms: *Streptococcus pneumoniae*, *Haemophilus influenzae*, and *Neisseria meningitidis*. Reduce this risk by giving:

1 Immunizations:
- Pneumococcal vaccine (p167), at least 2 weeks pre-op to ensure good response, or as soon as possible after emergency splenectomy, eg after trauma. Re-immunize every 5–10yrs. Avoid in pregnancy.
- *Haemophilus influenzae* type b vaccine (Hib, see p391).
- Meningococcal vaccination course, including Men B, Men C, and Men ACWY.
- Annual influenza vaccine (p396).

2 Life-long prophylactic oral antibiotics: phenoxymethylpenicillin (penicillin V) or erythromycin if penicillin allergic.

3 Pendants, bracelets, or patient-held cards to alert medical staff.

4 Advice to seek urgent medical attention if any signs of infection: will require admission for broad-spectrum antibiotics if infection develops.

5 If travelling abroad, warn of risk of severe malaria and advise meticulous prophylaxis, with nets, repellent, and medication.

The advice given here also applies to hyposplenic patients, eg in sickle-cell anaemia or coeliac disease.

Thrombophilia

Thrombophilia is an inherited or acquired coagulopathy that predisposes to thrombosis, usually venous: DVT or PE (venous thromboembolism: VTE). Special precautions are needed when there is an additional risk factor for thrombosis, eg *surgery, pregnancy*, or *enforced rest* (see BOX for other risk factors). Only ~50% of patients with thrombosis and a +ve family history have an identifiable thrombophilia on routine tests: others may have abnormalities that are as yet unidentified.

Inherited • *Activated protein C (APC) resistance/factor V Leiden:* Chief cause of inherited thrombophilia. Present in ~5% of the population, although most will not develop thrombosis. Usually associated with a single point mutation in factor V (factor V Leiden), so that this clotting factor is not broken down by APC. Risk of DVT or PE is raised 5-fold if heterozygous for the mutation (50-fold if homozygous). Thrombotic risk is increased in pregnancy and those on oestrogens (*OHCS* p33, p257 & p303).

• *Prothrombin gene mutation:* Causes high prothrombin levels and ↑thrombosis due to down-regulation of fibrinolysis, by thrombin-activated fibrinolysis inhibitor.

• *Protein C & S deficiency:* These vitamin K-dependent factors act together to cleave and so neutralize factors V & VIII. Heterozygotes deficient for either protein risk thrombosis. Skin necrosis also occurs (esp. if on warfarin). Homozygous deficiency for either protein causes neonatal purpura fulminans—fatal, if untreated.

• *Antithrombin deficiency:* Antithrombin is a co-factor of heparin, and inhibits thrombin. Less common, affects 1:500. Heterozygotes' thrombotic risk is greater than protein C or S deficiency by ~4-fold. Homozygosity is incompatible with life.

Acquired *Causes:* • Antiphospholipid syndrome (APL: p554)—serum antiphospholipid antibodies (lupus anticoagulant ± anticardiolipin antibody) predispose to venous *and* arterial thrombosis, thrombocytopenia, and recurrent fetal loss. In most it is a primary disease, but it is also seen in SLE. • Oral contraceptive pills/HRT (relative risk 2-4; related to both oestrogen and progesterone content/type). • Any cause of thrombocytosis or polycythaemia may also cause thrombosis (p366).

Which tests? Ask the lab. Do FBC, film, clotting (PT, thrombin time, APTT, fibrinogen) ± APC resistance test, lupus anticoagulant and anticardiolipin antibodies, and assays for antithrombin and proteins C & S deficiency (± DNA analysis by PCR for the factor V Leiden mutation if APC resistance test is +ve, and for prothrombin gene mutation). ►These tests should ideally be done when the patient is well, not pregnant, and off anticoagulation for 1 month.

Who? Test those with: • arterial thrombosis or MI at <50yrs old (eg for APL) • unprovoked VTE (ie at <40yrs with no risk factors) • VTE with oral contraceptives/pregnancy • unexplained recurrent VTE • unusual site, eg mesenteric or portal vein thrombosis • recurrent fetal loss (≥3) • neonatal thrombosis.

Who not? Those already on lifelong anticoagulation, 1st-degree relatives of people with a history of DVT/PE or thrombophilia except in special circumstances. ►There is often no benefit to testing (ie no change to management), it is expensive and may cause significant worry to patients: be sparing in requesting these tests.

Treatment Anticoagulate acute thrombosis (p350). If recurrence occurs with no other risk factors, consider lifelong anticoagulation. Recurrence whilst on treatment should be treated by increasing treatment intensity (eg ↑target INR to 3-4). In antithrombin deficiency, high doses of heparin may be needed; liaise with a haematologist. In protein C or S deficiency, monitor treatment closely as skin necrosis may occur with warfarin.

Prevention Lifelong anticoagulation is not needed in absence of VTE, but advise of ↑risk with the oral contraceptive pill or HRT, and counsel as regards to the best form of contraception. Warn about other risk factors for VTE. Prophylaxis may be needed in pregnancy, eg in antiphospholipid syndrome (get expert help: aspirin and, sometimes, prophylactic heparin are used as warfarin is teratogenic, see *OHCS* p33). Prophylactic SC heparin may also be indicated in high-risk situations, eg pre-surgery.

Other risk factors for thrombosis

Arterial:
- Smoking
- Hypertension
- Hyperlipidaemia
- Diabetes mellitus.

Venous:
- Surgery
- Trauma
- Immobility
- Pregnancy, oral contraceptive pill, HRT
- Age
- Obesity
- Varicose veins
- Other conditions: heart failure, malignancy, inflammatory bowel disease, nephrotic syndrome, paroxysmal nocturnal haemoglobinuria (p338).

For thrombophilia in pregnancy, see *OHCS* p32; for anticoagulant use in pregnancy and thromboprophylaxis, see *OHCS* p33.

As well as being used in leukaemias and cancers, immunosuppression is required in organ and marrow transplants, and plays a role in the treatment of many diseases: rheumatoid arthritis, psoriasis, autoimmune hepatitis, asthma, SLE, vasculitis, and IBD, to name a few.

Prednisolone Steroids can be life-saving, but bear in mind:

- Long-term steroids (>3 weeks, or repeated courses) *must not* be stopped suddently. ►►Risk of Addisonian crisis due to adrenal insufficiency, see p836. Plan a gradual taper over weeks (with the advice of an endocrinologist if needed).
- Certain conditions may be made worse by steroids, eg TB, hypertension, chickenpox, osteoporosis, diabetes: here careful monitoring is needed.
- Growth retardation may occur in young patients, and the elderly frequently get more SE from treatment.
- Interactions: efficacy is reduced by anti-epileptics (see later in topic) and rifampicin.
- Caution in pregnancy (may cause fetal growth retardation). See *BNF* for use in breastfeeding.

Side effects: Multiple and serious (see table 8.11): minimize these by using the lowest dose possible for the shortest period of time. Prescribe calcium and vitamin D supplements to reduce risk of osteoporosis (p682) or consider bisphosphonates. Before starting long-term treatment, explain *clearly* the potential SE to patients and ensure they are aware of the following:

- *Do not* stop steroids suddenly (p836).
- Consult a doctor if unwell; ↑steroid dose (eg if requiring antibiotics or surgery).
- Carry a steroid card stating dose taken, and the indication.
- Avoid over-the-counter drugs, eg NSAIDs: aspirin and ibuprofen (↑risk of DU).
- Exercise and smoking cessation help to prevent osteoporosis.

Azathioprine *SE:* Diarrhoea, abdominal pain, marrow suppression (anaemia, lymphopenia), nephritis, pancreatitis, transaminitis. *Interactions:* Mercaptopurine and azathioprine (which is metabolized to mercaptopurine) are metabolized by xanthine oxidase (XO). So toxicity results if full dose azathioprine co-administered with XO inhibitors (eg allopurinol). *Monitoring:* Local guidelines should be in place to guide; typically weekly FBC, U&E, creatine, LFT during initation then 1-3-monthly once stable.

Ciclosporin, tacrolimus Calcineurin inhibitors with important roles in reducing rejection in organ and marrow transplant. The main SE is dose-related nephrotoxicity: check blood levels.

- Other SE: gum hyperplasia (ciclosporin), tremor, ↑BP (stop if ↑↑), oedema, paraesthesiae, confusion, seizures, hepatotoxicity, lymphoma, skin cancer—avoid sunbathing.
- Monitor U&E and creatinine every 2 weeks for the first 3 months, then monthly if dose >2.5mg/kg/d (every 2 months if less than this). ►Reduce the dose if creatinine rises by >30% on two measurements *even if the creatinine is still in normal range*. Stop if the abnormality persists. Also monitor LFT.
- Interactions are legion: potentiated by: ketoconazole, diltiazem, verapamil, the Pill, erythromycin, grapefruit juice. Efficacy is reduced by: barbiturates, carbamazepine, phenytoin, rifampicin. Avoid concurrent nephrotoxics: eg gentamicin. Concurrent NSAIDs augment hepatotoxicity—monitor LFT.

Methotrexate An antimetabolite. Inhibits dihydrofolate reductase, which is involved in the synthesis of purines and pyrimidines. See p547.

Cyclophosphamide An alkylating agent. SE: marrow suppression (monitor FBC) nausea, infertility, teratogenic, haemorrhagic cystitis due to an irritative urinary metabolite. There is a slight ↑risk of later developing bladder cancer or leukaemia.

Table 8.11 Side-effects of steroid use

System	Adverse reactions
Gastrointestinal	Pancreatitis
	Candidiasis
	Oesophageal ulceration
	Peptic ulceration
Musculoskeletal	Myopathy
	Osteoporosis
	Fractures
	Growth suppression
Endocrine	Adrenal suppression
	Cushing's syndrome
CNS	Aggravated epilepsy
	Depression; psychosis
Eye	Cataracts; glaucoma
	Papilloedema
Immune	Increased susceptibility to and severity of infections, eg chickenpox
Steroids can also cause fever and ↑WCC; steroids only rarely cause leucopenia.	

9 Infectious diseases

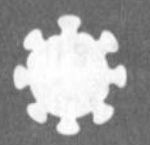

Contents

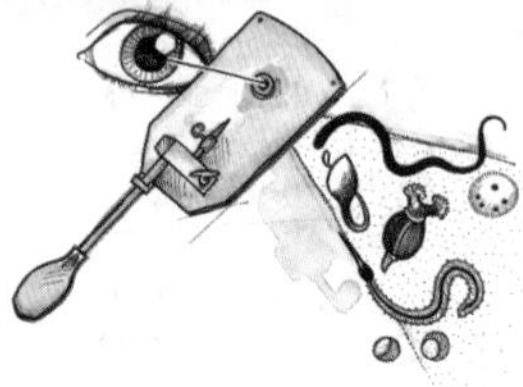

Fig 9.1 Leeuwenhoek's microscope. Antoni van Leeuwenhoek (1632-1723) was an unlikely scholar: a draper with no academic education. He mixed uncomfortably in a scientific world made up of those better educated, wealthier, and with more refined manners. He felt unworthy of publication but submitted hundreds of letters to the Royal Society, always asking his readers to account for his humble origins. Despite his self-deprecation, his microscopy was sophisticated. His surviving lens magnified ×266 and resolved down to 1.35μm, comparable to that of a modern compound microscope. With it he gained one of the first insights into the 'invisible' living creatures of the microscopic world. His microscopes were cheap and easy to produce—he made 500 for his personal use. He plated them in gold and silver to add a prestige that the scientific world felt they lacked. But that world failed to see beyond the end of its turned up nose. Bloodletting, purging, and emetics would continue to fail patients for a further 150 years.

We thank Dr Chris Conlon, our Specialist Reader for this chapter.

What is life?

By convention, life is anything which is organic and converts nutrients into progeny. Failure to meet this definition means non-living, dead, dying, or perhaps male. Life is a thing of dynamism, fragility, beauty, danger, and evanescence; gushing forth from a single source. But here the certainties end: what does it really take to be alive? Are viruses and prions living? How many branches are there on our tree? The harder we look, the more complexities we find. The Hillis plot is a circular phylogenetic tree, and a representation of humanity's place in nature. We are duly humbled by this challenge to our imagined self-importance, reminding us that we do not in reality occupy a privileged position in the hierarchy of the living, just a unique subunit RNA sequence (fig 9.2).

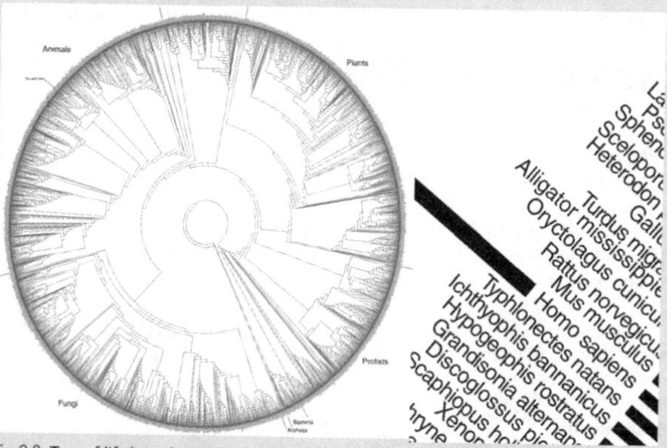

Fig 9.2 Tree of life based on subunit RNA sequences sampled from ~3000 species out of the 1.7 million species that are formally named. The image on the right is a close up of the 'animal' segment of the diagram (upper left quadrant) showing 'You are here'.

Copyright David M. Hillis, Derrick Zwickl and Robin Gutell, University of Texas.
http://www.zo.utexas.edu/faculty/antisense/downloadfilesToL.html

Because micro-organisms kill our friends we think of them as bad:

> *'I have no philosophy, nor piety, no art of reflection, no theory of compensation to meet things so hideous, so cruel, and so mad, they are just unspeakably horrible and irremediable to me and I stare at them with angry and almost blighted eyes.'*
>
> Henry James, 1915, describing the death of Rupert Brooke from septicaemia.

But this is a mistake. Kill off micro-organisms and the whole show fizzles out. Micro-organisms gave us the DNA and organelles needed for reading and digesting this page. Even killing a single pathogen might be a mistake: Sod's Law will probably ensure that something worse will come to inhabit the vacated ecospace. Prod one part of the system and events ripple out in an unending stream of unintended consequences, played out under the stars, which themselves are evolving, and which donate and receive our primordial elements.

Can we win against infectious diseases? No. But winning or losing is the wrong image: infectious diseases have made us who we are. All we can do is live with them. To help us do this in ways that are not too destructive we need robust public health surveillance, sound vector-control policies, political will, quarantine laws, openness, and cooperation. Most importantly, do not underestimate the importance of maintaining our infectious cohabitants in their apparent subordinate position. The speed and capacity for learning by ribonucleic malware and single-celled organisms is amazing. So do not inadvertently teach them. Preserve your precious warfare tactics. Expose them to antibiotic therapies only in a stand-off situation from which they cannot return to fight again.

Infectious disease: an overview

It is not possible for any ID chapter to be constructed so that it has the right balance throughout the world. Many of our readers come from communities where malaria is the primary differential, and AIDS-related deaths are common. In contrast, it is chest, GU, and ENT infections which predominate in the UK; and AIDS is considered only where there is failure of either the diagnosis or treatment of HIV, which are universally available and free at the point of care. Many of the diseases in this chapter cause multisystem pathology. For these infections, it may be helpful to classify by pathogen (table 9.1). However, infectious agents do not walk in the door and introduce themselves. Detective work may be necessary based on geography; or exposure: to vectors, animals, and contaminated water/food. And so other pages in this chapter have that as their (helpful) premise. When infection is organ specific, you may need to look elsewhere (table 9.2).

Table 9.1 Infectious disease by pathogen (illustrative, not exhaustive)

Bacteria	Viruses
Gram positive	**RNA viruses**
Staphylococci:	Picornavirus ('tiny RNA'):
• *Staph. aureus* (coagulase +ve)	• Rhinovirus
• *Staph. epidermidis* (coagulase −ve)	• Poliovirus
Streptococci:	Calicivirus ('cup'), eg norwalk
• α-haemolytic, eg *Strep. pneumoniae*	Flavivirus ('yellow'):
• β-haemolytic, eg *Strep. pyogenes*	• Dengue • Zika
Enterococci	• Yellow fever
Clostridium species:	Coronavirus ('crown'): URTI
• *C. botulinum* (botulism)	Rhabdovirus ('rod'), eg rabies
• *C. perfringens*(gas gangrene)	Filovirus ('thread'), eg Ebola/Marburg
• *C. tetani* (tetanus)	Paramyxovirus ('near mucus'), eg mumps
• *C. difficile* (diarrhoea)	
Gram negative	**DNA viruses**
Neisseria:	Hepadnavirus ('liver DNA'): hepatitis
• *N. meningitidis* (meningitis)	Parvovirus ('small'): gastroenteritis
• *N. gonorrheae* (gonorrhea)	Herpesvirus ('creeping'):
Helicobacter pylori	• HSV
Escherichia coli	• VZV
Shigella species	• CMV
Salmonella species	• EBV
Campylobacter jejuni	**Fungi**
Klebsiella pneumoniae	*Candida*
Pseudomonas aeruginosa	*Pneumocystis jirovecii*
Haemophilus influenzae	*Cryptococcus*
Bordetella pertussis (whooping cough)	**Parasites**
Vibrio cholerae (cholera)	**Protozoa**
Yersinia pestis (plague)	*Entamoeba histolytica*
Mycobacteria	*Giardia lamblia*
M. tuberculosis	*Cryptosporidium* species
M. leprae	*Toxoplasma gondii*
Intracellular bacteria	*Plasmodium* species (malaria)
Chlamydia	*Leishmania* species (leishmaniasis)
Rickettsia (rickettsial disease)	*Trypanosoma* species (trypanosomiasis)
Coxiella burnetii	**Nematodes**
Spirochaetes	Soil-transmitted helminths
Borrelia burgdorferi (Lyme disease)	Filarial disease
Treponema (syphilis, yaws)	**Trematodes**
Leptospira (Weil's disease)	*Schistosoma* (schistosomiasis), flukes
	Cestodes
	Hydatid disease, tapeworm

Table 9.2 Infectious disease by organ system

System	Infection	Page
Respiratory	Pneumonia	pp166-70
	Empyema—infected pleural effusion	p170
	Fungal infections of the lung	p177
GI	Peptic ulcer disease	p252
	Gastroenteritis	pp428-33
	Colitis, proctitis, diverticulitis, appendicitis	
	Viral hepatitis	p278
	Tropical liver disease	pp434-5
	Cholecystitis, cholangitis, gallbladder empyema	p634
	Peritonitis	p606
GU and gynaecology	Lower urinary tract infection, cystitis, pyelonephritis	pp296-7
	Cervicitis, vulvovaginitis	pp412-3
	Genital ulceration	pp412-3
	Genital warts	p406
	Pelvic inflammatory disease, endometritis	*OHCS* p286
Cardiovascular	Infective endocarditis	pp150-1
	Myocarditis	pp152-4
	Pericarditis	p154
Nervous system	Meningitis, encephalitis, subdural empyema	pp822-4
	Infective neuropathy	pp504-5
Skin and soft tissue	Skin ulcers, gangrene	pp660-1
	Tropical skin disease	pp422-3
	Surgical wound infection	p571, p576
Bone and joint	Osteomyelitis	*OHCS* p696
	Septic arthritis	p544
ENT	Pharyngitis, laryngitis, otitis media	*OHCS* p564
Eye	Tropical eye disease	pp438-9

The management of infectious disease includes prevention whenever possible. Tracing the source of disease and contacts are essential in the management of outbreaks. Notification to your local health protection team (see https://www.gov.uk/guidance/notifiable-diseases-and-causative-organisms-how-to-report) is a statutory duty for the following conditions (only clinical suspicion is required, accuracy of diagnosis is secondary):

- Acute encephalitis
- Acute infectious hepatitis
- Acute meningitis
- Acute poliomyelitis
- Anthrax
- Botulism
- Brucellosis
- Cholera
- Diphtheria
- Enteric fever
- Food poisoning
- HUS
- Infectious dysentery
- Invasive group A strep
- Legionnaire's disease
- Leprosy
- Malaria
- Measles
- Meningococcal sepsis
- Mumps
- Plague
- Rabies
- Rubella
- SARS
- Scarlet fever
- Small pox
- Tetanus
- Tuberculosis
- Typhus
- Viral haemorrhagic fever
- Whooping cough
- Yellow fever.

Infectious disease resources

The Hillis plot (fig 9.2, p379) tells us that ID chapters will always fail to be exhaustive. We therefore direct you to the following excellent resources:

- *Public Health England,* https://www.gov.uk/topic/health-protection/infectious-diseases
- *World Health Organization (WHO),* http://www.who.int/topics/en/
- *Centers for Disease Control and Prevention,* http://www.cdc.gov

Bacterial infection: an overview

Humans and bacteria are symbiotes, with each of us host to ten times as many bacterial cells as our own human cells. Our gut, skin, and mucosal linings are covered with bacteria. We rely on this for nutrition, functioning vitamin K, anti-inflammatory effects, and immune system regulation.

Bacterial disease results from a breach of the measures that limit bacteria to their 'normal' roles: skin commensals moved into the bloodstream by a cannula, antibiotics altering the commensal microflora, immune system evasion or dysfunction allowing organisms to stray beyond their usual boundaries, toxin production. When treating infections we should therefore remember to look beyond the offending organism and consider what factors may have aided pathogenesis: malnutrition, 'barrier' breach by cancer/plastic, immunosuppression.

►See 'Sepsis', p792.

Bacterial glossary

Bacteria: Prokaryotic micro-organism without a membrane-bound nucleus.

Classification of bacteria: By microscopy and culture of infected samples. Informs antibiotic choice. Includes:

- *Gram stain:* a staining technique. Bacteria with thick, exposed peptidoglycan layers will stain 'Gram positive' (purple/blue). Bacteria with a protected peptidoglycan layer will counterstain pink/red and are 'Gram negative' (fig 9.3).
- *Shape:* cocci = round; bacilli = rod-shaped; spirochaete = spiral.
- *Aerobes/anaerobes:* some bacteria cannot survive without oxygen (obligate aerobes), whilst others cannot grow in its presence (obligate anaerobes). Many more can survive in either environment (facultative anaerobes). Some types of infection are more likely to involve aerobic or anaerobic bacteria, eg GI infections are typically anaerobic.

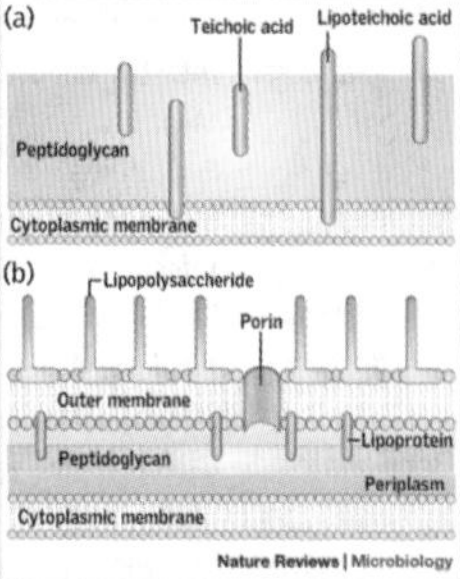

Fig 9.3 (a) Gram-positive versus (b) Gram-negative cell membranes.

Reprinted by permission from Macmillan Publishers Ltd: *Nature Reviews Microbiology*, Cabeen *et al*., 3(8), 601–610, copyright 2005.

Bacteraemia: Bacteria circulating in the bloodstream.

Bacteriocidal: Kills bacteria both in and out of the replication cycle.

Bacteriostatic: Stops replication without killing existing bacteria.

Capsulate bacteria: Bacteria with a thick outer capsule, eg *Haemophilus influenzae, Neisseria meningitidis*, and *Streptococcus pneumoniae*. These are destroyed in the spleen. Following splenectomy (or splenic infarction, eg sickle cell anaemia) there is an increased risk of infection by capsulate bacteria and prophylactic vaccination should be offered (p407).

Commensal: An organism that lives in/on a host without causing harm.

Endotoxin: A lipopolysaccharide complex found on the outer membrane of Gram-negative bacteria. Can elicit an inflammatory response. Activates complement via the alternative pathway.

Enterotoxin: Exotoxin that targets the gut, eg *Clostridium difficile* toxin (p411).

Exotoxin: Toxins secreted by bacteria acting at a site distant from bacterial growth. Production of an exotoxin can determine virulence, eg botulinum, tetanus, diphtheria, shiga toxins.

Flagella: A tail-like appendage that moves to propel the bacterium, eg *Helicobacter pylori*.

Nosocomial: Acquired in a hospital/healthcare setting (pp410–1).

Obligate intracellular: Bacteria that can only survive in host cells ∴ induce a cell-mediated immune response and will not grow on standard culture media.

Ziehl-Neelsen stain: Mycolic acid in the cell wall of mycobacteria resists Gram staining but will appear red with acid-fast techniques (= acid-fast stain).

Antibiotics: action and resistance

The antibiotic revolution began in 1928 when a extraordinary series of fortuitous events (including a cancelled holiday and an unpredictable British summer) led to Alexander Fleming's observation that a contaminating *Penicillium* colony caused lysis of staphylococci. Mass production and the 'golden age' of antibiotics followed, with the introduction of a variety of drugs selectively toxic to bacterial, but not mammalian cells. This is achieved by:

- utilizing a target unique to bacteria, eg cell wall
- selectively targeting bacterial-specific components, eg enzymes, ribosomes
- preventing transport of the drug into human cells, eg metronidazole can only be transported into anaerobic bacteria.

The mechanism of action of different classes of antibiotic is shown in fig 9.4.

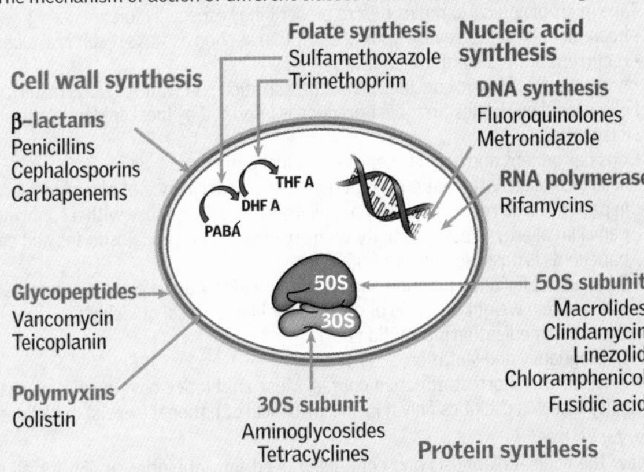

Fig 9.4 Classes of antibiotics and their bacterial cell targets.

This spectrum of available antibiotics revolutionized clinical practice and led to the declaration: *'It is time to close the book on infectious diseases, and declare the war against pestilence won'* (attributed in urban legend to Dr. William H Stewart, US Surgeon General, 1965–1969). Such confidence failed to consider that the capacity for a prokaryotic micro-organism to develop resistance far outstrips the human capacity to develop new antibiotic drugs.

Antibiotic resistance can be:

- Intrinsic: due to inherent structural or functional characteristics, eg vancomycin cannot cross the outer membrane of Gram-negative organisms.
- Acquired: bacteria have been evolving to resist antibacterial agents for billions of years through mutation and/or the transfer of resistance properties. This evolutionary phenomenon is accelerated by selection pressure from antibiotic use (including agriculture, aquaculture, and horticulture) which provides a competitive advantage for mutated, resistant strains.

Resistance has emerged for all known antibiotics causing morbidity, mortality, and a huge cost burden worldwide.[1] Misadventure is evident. Quinolones are synthetic, resistance cannot be acquired in nature, and yet it is epidemic.

Which brings us back to Alexander Fleming who, within 2 years of the mass-production of his 'miracle-mould', gave this sage warning in his Nobel lecture of 1945: *'Mr X has a sore throat. He buys some penicillin and gives himself, not enough to kill the streptococci, but enough to educate them to resist penicillin. He then infects his wife. Mrs X gets pneumonia and is treated with penicillin. As the streptococci are now resistant to penicillin the treatment fails. Mrs X dies. Who is primarily responsible for Mrs X's death? Why Mr X, whose negligent use of penicillin changed the nature of the microbe.'*

A guide to antibiotic prescribing

▸▸ Give antibiotics immediately in patients with a systemic inflammatory response to infection. See 'Sepsis', p792.

Start smart:

1 Do not prescribe[2] antibiotics in the absence of clinical evidence of bacterial infection, or for a self-limiting condition. Take time to discuss:
  - why an antibiotic is not the best option
  - alternative options, eg symptomatic treatment, delayed prescribing
  - the views and expectations of the patient
  - safety-netting advice: what the patient should do if their condition deteriorates.

2 Take microbiological samples *before* prescribing,[1] especially for:
  - hospital in-patients: review your prescription as soon as MC&S result is available
  - recurrent or persistent infection
  - non-severe infection: consider if your prescription can wait for MC&S results.

3 Follow local guidelines first: best practice is informed by local epidemiology and sensitivities.

4 Consider benefit and harm for each individual patient:
  - *Allergies:* clarify the patient's reaction—the true incidence of penicillin allergy in patients who report that they are allergic is <10%. In those with a confirmed penicillin allergy, cross-reactivity with 3rd-generation cephalosporins and carbapenems is possible but rare (<1%).
  - Dose adjust for renal function and weight: use ideal body weight in extremes of BMI (or ideal weight plus a % of excess weight—see local guidelines).
  - Check for medication interactions.
  - In pregnancy and lactation, see p17.

5 Prescribe the shortest effective course. Most antibiotics have good oral availability. Use IV antibiotics only if in line with local or national (sepsis) guidelines.

Then focus:

Review the clinical diagnosis and continuing need for antibiotics at 48h for all in-patients and all patients prescribed IV antibiotics:
- *Stop* antibiotics if there is no evidence of infection.
- Switch from IV to *oral* whenever possible.
- Change to a *narrower spectrum* antibiotic whenever possible.
- Continue regular clinical *review* whilst antibiotics are prescribed.

Antimicrobial stewardship

In England between 2010 and 2014, antibiotic prescribing rose by 4% in general practice, 12% in hospitals, and 32% in other healthcare settings; *E. coli* resistance to ciprofloxacin increased by 18%, to cephalosporins by 28%, and to gentamicin by 27%. 25 000 people in Europe die every year from antibiotic-resistant bacteria. Each year ~500 000 develop drug-resistant TB. Cost is the only barrier to buying carbapenems over-the-counter in Egypt, India, and Pakistan.

'This will be a post-antibiotic era. In terms of new replacement antibiotics, the pipeline is virtually dry, especially for Gram negative bacteria. The cupboard is nearly bare. Prospects for turning this situation around look dim.'

Dr M Chan, Director-General of WHO, March 2012.

Antimicrobial stewardship[2] is necessary in all healthcare settings:
- monitoring, evaluation, and feedback on antimicrobial prescribing, benchmarked against up-to-date local and national guidelines
- evaluation of high/low levels of prescribing and prescribing outside of guidelines
- review of patient safety events: avoidable infection, drug reactions, complications of antibiotic therapy, eg MRSA (p388), *C. difficile* (p259, p411)
- education and decision support systems for all antibiotic prescribers
- antibiotic pack sizes that correspond to appropriate course lengths
- regular review of all antimicrobial policy, treatment, and prophylaxis guidelines.

1 Clinical diagnosis of low-severity community-acquired pneumonia is an exception, see also UTI p296.

Inhibitors of cell wall synthesis

See fig 9.4. The bacterial cell wall is unique in nature and therefore acts as a selective target for antibiotics. Antibiotics which act on the cell wall include:

- β-lactam antibiotics
- others: glycopeptides, polymyxins.

β-lactams: penicillins, cephalosporins, carbapenems, monobactam

Contain a β-lactam ring which inhibits the formation of peptidoglycan cross-links in the bacterial cell wall. Resistance occurs when the bacteria (eg staphylococci) produce a β-lactamase enzyme.

Penicillins:

See table 9.3. Include natural penicillins (penicillin G and V) and synthetic penicillins which are chemically modified to extend their spectrum of activity, eg amoxicillin, piperacillin.

In an attempt to overcome β-lactamase resistance, penicillins have been combined with β-lactamase inhibitors to create β-lactam-β-lactamase inhibitor combinations eg co-amoxiclav (amoxicillin+clavulanic acid), Tazocin® (piperacillin+tazobactam).

Staphylococcal resistance is conventionally defined by stability to meticillin, an acid-labile and IV-only equivalent of flucloxacillin (see MRSA p388).

Cephalosporins:

See table 9.4. Contain a β-lactam ring attached to a six-membered nuclear structure (five in penicillin), which allows synthetic modification at two sites (one in penicillin). This means that cephalosporins are the largest groups of available antibiotics. Classification into 'generations' is not standardized: as a rough rule, the higher the generation, the wider the spectrum.

Carbapenems:

See table 9.5. Broadest spectrum of all β-lactam antibiotics. Seek expert microbiology advice before use.

Monobactam:

Aztreonam is only active against Gram-negative species including *Neisseria meningitidis, Haemophilus influenzae, Pseudomonas*. Given IV/IM. Inhaled preparation for chronic pulmonary *Pseudomonas* (cystic fibrosis). Dose adjust for renal function. SEs: N&V, GI bleed, rash, ↑LFTs, ↓plts, paraesthesia, seizures, bronchospasm.

Non-β-lactam cell wall inhibitors

See fig 9.4 and table 9.6. Includes glycopeptides, eg vancomycin, teicoplanin, and polymyxins, eg colistin.

Inhibitors of protein synthesis

See fig 9.4 and table 9.7. Includes:

- aminoglycosides
- macrolides
- tetracyclines and derivatives of tetracycline
- others: clindamycin, linezolid, chloramphenicol, fusidic acid.

Inhibitors of nucleic acid synthesis

See fig 9.4 and table 9.8. Includes:

- folate synthesis inhibitors: trimethoprim, co-trimoxazole
- fluoroquinolones
- others: metronidazole, rifampicin.

►Nitrofurantoin is unique. Metabolites interfere with cell growth via ribosomes, DNA, RNA, and cell wall. Multiple sites of attack means ↓resistance. Concentrates in the urine (but not if ↓GFR), used in uncomplicated UTI. SEs: haemolysis, pulmonary fibrosis, hepatotoxicity.

►Antibiotics for TB, see pp394–5.

Antibiotics: summary tables

Table 9.3 Penicillins

Antibiotic	Indications	Considerations
Penicillin G (benzylpenicillin, 'penicillin')	Gram +ve: streptococci (chest, throat, endocarditis, cellulitis), meningococcus, diphtheria, anthrax, leptospirosis, Lyme disease.	Give IV, poor oral absorption. Dose adjust for GFR. SE: allergy, rash, N&V, *C. difficile*, cholestasis.
Penicillin V (phenoxymethylpenicillin)	Prophylaxis: splenectomy/hyposplenism, rheumatic heart disease.	Oral bioavailability may vary.
Ampicillin/amoxicillin	Amino acid side chain extends penicillin spectrum to include enterobacteria (but ↓ activity against Gram +ve): URTI, sinusitis, chest, otitis media, UTI, *H. pylori*.	Ampicillin IV, amoxicillin PO. Dose adjust for GFR. SE: as per penicillin G, rash with EBV.
Amoxicillin+clavulanic acid (co-amoxiclav)	Used if resistance to narrower-spectrum antibiotics: chest, pyelonephritis, cellulitis, bone.	Dose adjust for GFR. SE: as per amoxicillin.
Piperacillin+tazobactam	Broad spectrum including Gram +ve, Gram −ve, *Pseudomonas:* neutropenic sepsis, hospital-acquired/complicated infection.	Tazobactam has ↓penetration of blood-brain barrier. Dose adjust for GFR. SE: as per penicillin G. Myelosuppression with prolonged use (rare).
Flucloxacillin	β-lactamase resistant, *Staphylococcus*: skin, bone, post-viral pneumonia.	Dose adjust for GFR. SE: allergy, rash, N&V, cholestasis.

Table 9.4 Cephalosporins

Antibiotic	Indications	Considerations
Cefalexin (1st generation)	Gram +ve infection: UTI, pneumonia.	↓First-line use in UK due to risk of *C. difficile*. Caution: false +ve urinary glucose and Coomb's test. SE: allergy, rash, N&V, cholestasis. Ceftriaxone can precipitate in urinary tract and biliary tree = pseudolithiasis.
Cefuroxime (2nd generation)	Gram +ve and Gram −ve (Enterobacteriaceae, *H. influenzae*): UTI, sinusitis, skin, wound.	
Cefotaxime (3rd generation)	Broad spectrum (not *Pseudomonas*, *Enterococcus* spp, *Bacteroides*).	
Ceftriaxone (3rd generation)	Meningococcus. Broad spectrum (not *Pseudomonas*, *Enterococcus* spp, *Bacteroides*).	
Ceftazidime (3rd generation)	Broad spectrum including *Pseudomonas* but ↓activity against Gram +ve: empirical treatment of neutropenic sepsis.	

Table 9.5 Carbapenems

Antibiotic	Indications	Considerations
Imipenem Meropenem Ertapenem	Broad spectrum (Gram +ve, Gram −ve, aerobes, anaerobes): hospital-acquired/ventilator-associated/complicated infection, neutropenic sepsis.	Dose adjust for GFR. Imipenem given with cilastatin to ↓renal metabolism. SE: N&V, *C. difficile*, rash, eosinophilia, ↓plts, ↑LFTs, seizures.

Table 9.6 Lipopeptides and polymyxins

Antibiotic	Indication	Considerations
Lipopeptides		
Vancomycin Teicoplanin	Complicated Gram +ve including MRSA. Oral for *C. difficile* (not absorbed).	Dose IV to trough serum concentration. SEs: nephrotoxic (monitor creatinine, care with other nephrotoxics) ototoxic, ↓plts.
Polymyxins		
Colistin, polymyxin B	Multi-resistant Gram −ve.	Nephrotoxicity in ~50%. Inhaled colistin for ventilator-associated pneumonia.

Table 9.7 Inhibitors of protein synthesis

Antibiotic	Indications	Considerations
Aminoglycosides		
Gentamicin Tobramycin Amikacin	Gram −ve infection (↓activity against most Gram +ve and anaerobes). Tobramycin has ↑activity against *Pseudomonas*. Amikacin has least resistance.	SEs: nephrotoxic (monitor drug levels and serum creatinine), vestibular toxicity, ototoxicity.
Macrolides		
Azithromycin Clarithromycin Erythromycin	Gram +ve cocci (not enterococci and staphylococci), syphilis, chlamydia.	SEs (↑ with erythromycin): GI, cholestasis, ↑QT. Cytochrome P450 inhibition (↓ with azithromycin): ↑warfarin, rhabdomyolysis with statins, ↑calcineurin inhibitor levels.
Tetracyclines and derivatives		
Tetracycline Doxycycline	Exacerbation COPD, chlamydia, Lyme disease, mycoplasma, rickettsiae, brucella, anthrax, syphilis, MRSA, malaria prophylaxis.	CI: pregnancy, <8y (teeth/bones). SEs: N&V, *C. difficile*, fatty liver, idiopathic intracranial hypertension.
Tigecycline	Gram +ve and Gram −ve including β-lactam-resistant strains.	Dose adjust in liver dysfunction. SEs: N&V, photosensitivity, ↑LFTs.
Other		
Clindamycin	Gram +ve cocci (not enterococci), MRSA, anaerobes.	↑ risk *C. difficile*.
Linezolid	Gram +ve cocci, MRSA, VRE, anaerobes, mycobacteria.	MAOI: check interactions, myelosuppression, optic neuropathy.
Chloramphenicol	Gram +ve, Gram −ve, anaerobes, mycoplasma, chlamydia, conjunctivitis (topical).	Systemic use limited by myelosuppression.
Fusidic acid	Staphylococci.	SEs: GI, ↑LFTs.

Table 9.8 Inhibitors of nucleic acid synthesis

Antibiotic	Indications	Considerations
Folate synthesis inhibitors		
Trimethoprim	Gram −ve: UTI, prostatitis.	Inhibits creatinine secretion: ↑serum creatinine without ↓GFR.
Co-trimoxazole (sulfamethoxazole+trimethoprim)	*Pneumocystis jirovecii*, GI infection (eg *Shigella, E. coli)*, protozoans (eg *Cyclospora*), listeria, nocardia, MRSA.	Synergistic combination. Good oral absorption and tissue/CSF penetration. SEs: folate deficiency, ↑K^+, rash, myelosuppression, haemolysis with G6PD deficiency.
Fluoroquinolones		
Ciprofloxacin Levofloxacin Moxifloxacin	Broad including *Pseudomonas*: UTI, prostatitis, atypical and hospital-acquired chest infection, infectious diarrhoea.	SEs: GI irritation, CNS effects (↓ seizure threshold, headache, drowsiness, mood change), peripheral neuropathy, tendinopathy (Achilles), ↑QT, *C. difficile*.
Others		
Metronidazole	Anaerobic infection: intra-abdominal, pelvic, oral, soft-tissue. Bacterial vaginosis. *C. difficile*.	Good oral absorption. Dose adjust for liver function. SEs: Disulfiram reaction with alcohol, inhibits warfarin metabolism.
Rifamycins: rifampicin, rifabutin, rifapentine	Mycobacteria (TB, atypical mycobacteria, leprosy), some staphylococci, *Legionella*, meningococcal prophylaxis.	SEs: hepatitis (monitor LFTs), GI, CNS effects, myelosuppression, red secretions (urine, saliva, sweat, sputum, tears).

Gram-positive bacteria

Gram-positive cocci

Staphylococci:

Staphylococci are skin/nasal commensals in ~80% of adults. They can also cause infectious disease. This produces a diagnostic challenge: are the detected organisms causing infection or a contaminating commensal? The answer may lie in the presence or absence of coagulase, an enzyme which coagulates plasma.

Coagulase-negative staphylococci: eg *Staphylococcus epidermidis* are less virulent. Pathogenicity is likely only if there is underlying immune system dysfunction or foreign material (prosthetic valve/joint, IV line, PD catheter, pacemaker).

Staphylococcus aureus is coagulase positive. *Presentation:*

1 Toxin release causes disease distant from infection. Includes:
- scalded skin syndrome—bullae and desquamation due to epidermolytic toxins (no mucosal disease, ↓skin loss compared to toxic epidermal necrolysis)
- preformed toxin in food—sudden D&V (p428)
- toxic shock—fever, confusion, rash, diarrhoea, ↓BP, AKI, multiorgan dysfunction. Tampon associated or occurs with (minor) local infection.

2 Local tissue destruction: impetigo, cellulitis, mastitis, septic arthritis, osteomyelitis, abscess, pneumonia, UTI.

3 Haematogenous spread: bacteraemia, endocarditis, 'metastatic' seeding.

Diagnosis: positive culture from relevant site of infection. *Treatment:* ►►Sepsis, see p792. Drain infected foci, antibiotic (topical/oral/IV) based on illness severity and risk factors. Consider local epidemiology of resistance. If systemic treatment indicated, use β-lactam whenever possible (may need to cover resistant strains until sensitivity available). Preformed toxin in food: supportive, antibiotics not usually indicated.

Resistant *Staphylococcus aureus:* MRSA, VISA, VRSA

Staph. aureus which produces β-lactamase, or an altered enzyme responsible for cell wall formation, will be resistant to β-lactam antibiotics (penicillins, cephalosporins, carbapenems, see p385). Resistance is usually defined by stability to meticillin, ie meticillin-resistant *Staph. aureus* (MRSA). Vancomycin resistance also exists and is classified according to the amount of vancomycin needed to inhibit bacterial growth: vancomycin-intermediate *Staph. aureus* (VISA) and vancomycin-resistant *Staph. aureus* (VRSA). Resistant staphylococci cause ↑ morbidity and mortality compared to sensitive strains. Risk factors for colonization include: antibiotic exposure, hospital stay, surgery, nursing home residence. Treatment of infection (not colonization): vancomycin (for MRSA), teicoplanin. Oral agents with activity against MRSA include clindamycin, co-trimoxazole, doxycycline, linezolid. *Prevention:* surveillance, barrier precautions, hand-hygiene, decolonization (mupirocin 2%, chlorhexidine, tea tree oil), antimicrobial stewardship. See p384, pp410–11.

Streptococci:

Classification based on Lancefield group persists in terminology (fig 9.5). Includes:
- *Streptococcus pyogenes* (β-haemolytic group A): colonizes throat, skin, anogenital tract. Range of infection: tonsillitis, pharyngitis, scarlet fever, impetigo, erysipelas, cellulitis, pneumonia, peripartum sepsis, necrotizing fasciitis. All can→streptococcal toxic shock = sudden-onset ↓BP, multiorgan failure. Post-infectious complications rare: rheumatic fever (p142), glomerulonephritis (p310). *Treatment:* penicillin.
- *Streptococcus agalactiae* (β-haemolytic group B): neonatal and peurperal infection, skin, soft tissue. Invasive disease (bacteraemia, endocarditis, osteomyelitis, septic arthritis, meningitis) usually has risk factors: DM, malignancy, chronic disease. *Treatment:* penicillin, macrolide, cephalosporin, chloramphenicol.
- *Streptococcus milleri:* if found in blood culture look for an abscess—mouth, liver lung, brain. *Treatment:* penicillin.
- *Streptococcus pneumoniae:* pneumonia (pp166–8), otitis media, meningitis, septicaemia. *Treatment:* penicillin. Vaccination: childhood, hyposplenism, >65y (p407).
- Viridans streptococci: commonest cause of oral/dental origin endocarditis (p150).
- *Streptococcus bovis:* bacteraemia→endocarditis. Look for colon/liver disease.

Enterococci:

Gut commensal. Resistance to cephalosporins and quinolones leads to nosocomial colonization and infection. Most common is *Enterococcus faecalis:* if found in blood culture, assume endocarditis until proven otherwise. Treatment: intrinsic and acquired resistance including vancomycin-resistant enterococci (VRE). Seek expert help.

Gram-positive bacilli

Listeria:

Caused by *Listeria monocytogenes* which lives in soil. Able to multiply at low temperatures. Found in pâté, raw vegetables/salad, unpasteurized milk/cheese. *Presentation:* most asymptomatic, or mild flu-like illness. In immunosuppressed (including elderly): gastroenteritis, local infection (abscess, osteomyelitis, septic arthritis, endocarditis, pneumonia), meningoencephalitis, life-threatening septicaemia. Listeria in pregnancy may cause mild disease in mother but transplacental infection→placentitis, amnionitis, preterm delivery, neonatal sepsis, intrauterine death. *Diagnosis:* culture: blood, placenta, amniotic fluid, CSF. PCR. Serology is non-specific. *Treatment:* ampicillin plus gentamicin (synergistic action) for systemic disease. Also co-trimoxazole (CNS disease), macrolides, tetracycline, rifampicin, vancomycin, carbopenem. ►Resistant to cephalosporins which are often 1st-line empirical treatment for meningitis so remember additional antimicrobial cover if listeria is a possibility.

Clostridia:

- *Clostridium difficile,* see p259, p411.
- *Clostridium perfringens:*
  - Gastroenteritis, see p430.
  - Gas gangrene due to exotoxin production (alpha toxin most common). Previously *Clostridium welchii. Presentation:* sudden, severe pain due to myonecrosis, tissue crepitus, systemic shock. Most post surgery (GI, biliary), or following soft-tissue trauma/open fracture. If spontaneous, look for malignancy. *Treatment:* early recognition, surgical debridement, protein synthesis inhibitors, eg clindamycin inhibit toxins >penicillins. Hyperbaric O_2 unproven in trials (fig 9.4, table 9.7).
- *Clostridium botulinum*, see p436.
- *Clostridium tetani*, see p436.

Diphtheria:

Caused by *Corynebacterium diphtheriae* toxin. Preventable with vaccine. *Presentation:* tonsillar pseudomembrane with fever, painful dysphagia, cervical lymphadenopathy (see *OHCS* p158). *Diagnosis:* culture, toxin detection, PCR. *Treatment:* antitoxin within 48h. Benzylpenicillin/erythromycin. Airway support.

Actinomycosis:

Due to *Actinomyces israelii,* a mucous membrane commensal. *Presentation:* subacute granulomatous/suppurative infection adjacent to mucous membrane. *Diagnosis:* culture. 'Sulphur' granules in pus/tissue are pathognomonic. *Treatment:* antibiotics covering actinomycetes and concomitant microbes.

Nocardia:

Rare cause of disease. *Presentation:* tropical skin abscess, lung/brain abscess, disseminated infection if immunosuppressed. *Treatment:* usually co-trimoxazole.

Anthrax: See p424.

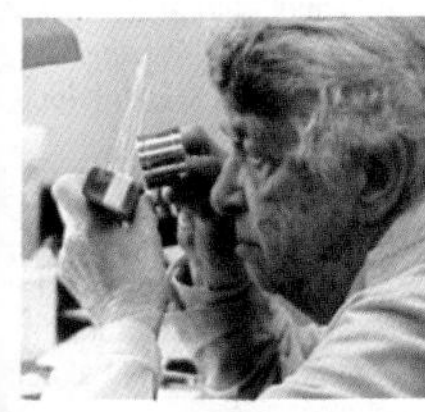

Fig 9.5 Streptococci are grouped by haemolytic pattern (α, β, or non-haemolytic), by Lancefield antigen (A–G), or by species. Rebecca Lancefield (1895–1981) is shown with her hand lens, typing streptococci with a variety of M protein-specific antibodies. Her lab became known as the 'Scotland Yard of Streptococcal Mysteries' after she found that the most grievous crimes of streptococci almost always involve M as a secret accomplice. Although she arrested M on many occasions, M outlived her, and still stalks our wards and clinics.

Gram-negative cocci

Neisseria:

Neisseria meningitidis (meningococcus) is an upper respiratory tract commensal in ~10% (~25% adolescents) adhering to non-ciliated epithelial cells in nasopharynx and tonsils. Person-to-person transmission via droplets or upper respiratory tract secretions. Most strains are harmless but induce immunity. Pathogenic, virulent strains are mostly encapsulated and have the potential to cause septicaemia and meningitis. Serogroups A, B, C, W and Y account for nearly all invasive forms. ↓Group C following introduction of vaccination in UK. ↑ in serotype W in UK since 2009. Incubation 2–7d. Peak ages: <2yr, ~18yr. Risk factors: complement system defects, hyposplenism, HIV.

Presentation:

1. Meningitis (~50% cases). Main proliferation of bacteria is in CSF. Insidious onset with malaise, nausea, headache, vomiting. May be misdiagnosed as gastroenteritis, URTI, or childhood viral illness. Later meningism: headache, vomiting, nuchal/back rigidity, photophobia, altered consciousness. Complications in up to 20%: sensorineural hearing loss, impaired vestibular function, epilepsy, diffuse brain injury.
2. Meningococcaemia. Symptoms/signs depends on amount of circulating bacteria. Mild disease presents with fever, macular rash (fig 9.6) but no signs of shock. High-grade meningococcaemia (~30% cases) causes pyrexia and septic shock within 6–12h due to rapidly escalating endotoxin levels: circulatory failure, coagulopathy with skin haemorrhage (fig 9.7), thrombosis of extremities/adrenals, AKI, ARDS. Meningism may be absent. Complications: amputation, skin necrosis, pericarditis, arthritis, ocular infection, pneumonia (especially serotypes Y and W), permanent adrenal insufficiency.

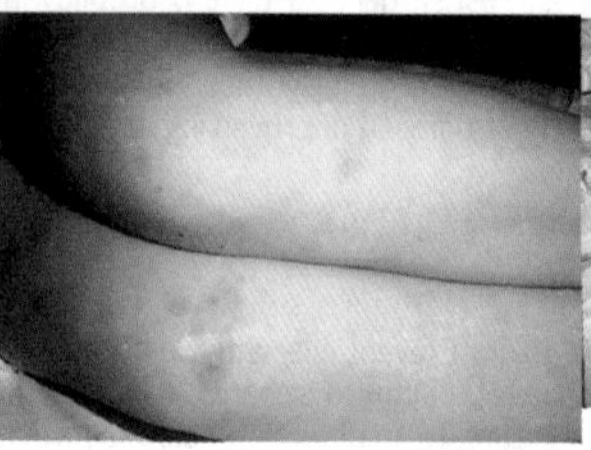

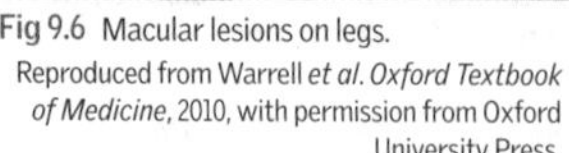

Fig 9.6 Macular lesions on legs.

Reproduced from Warrell *et al. Oxford Textbook of Medicine*, 2010, with permission from Oxford University Press.

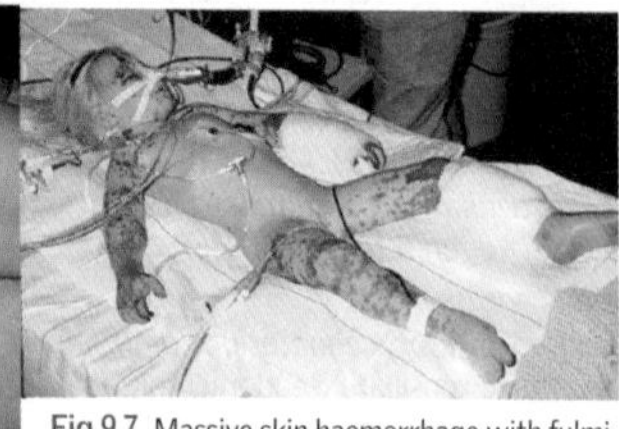

Fig 9.7 Massive skin haemorrhage with fulminant meningococcal septicaemia.

Reproduced from Warrell *et al. Oxford Textbook of Medicine*, 2010, with permission from Oxford University Press.

Diagnosis: ►►*Start treatment immediately if meningitis/meningococcal sepsis is a possible diagnosis*. Do not wait for confirmation: delay can be deadly. Intra- and extracellular diplococci on microscopy of CSF/blood/skin lesion. PCR of CSF/blood/skin lesion. *Treatment:* urgent antibiotic treatment: benzylpenicillin, ceftriaxone (see pp822–3). Cefotaxime, chloramphenicol, meropenem also bactericidal. *Prevention:* routine infant vaccination against capsular group C in UK. Capsular group B vaccine in UK infants since 2015: induces bacteriocidal antibodies, no population data, duration of protection unknown. Quadrivalent ACWY vaccine at age 14 and if high-risk travel. Additional B, C, ACWY doses if hyposplenism and complement deficiency. *Prophylaxis of contacts:* ciprofloxacin/ceftriaxone (single dose), or rifampicin 600mg BD for 48h.

Neisseria gonorrhoea: see pp412–3.

Moraxella catarrhalis:

Colonizes upper respiratory tract in children (↓ in adults). Resembles *Neisseria* commensal so may be overlooked. *Presentation*: pneumonia, exacerbation of COPD, up to 20% of acute otitis media, sinusitis. Bacteraemia is rare. *Diagnosis:* culture of sputum, ear effusion, sinus aspirate, blood. 'Hockey puck sign': colonies can be pushed along agar surface without disruption. *Treatment:* macrolide, cephalosporin.

Gram-negative bacilli

Enterobacteriaceae:

Enterobacteriaceae family is large: >50 genera, >170 named species. In the clinical setting, 3 species make up 80–95% of isolates:

1. *Escherichia coli:* part of normal colonic flora. Pathogenic forms can cause:
   Intestinal disease:
   Enterotoxigenic: a major cause of traveller's diarrhoea (pp428–9).
   Enterohaemorrhagic: diarrhoea, haemorrhagic colitis eg O157:H7 (p431).
   Enteropathogenic: infants in areas of poor sanitation.
   Enteroinvasive: dysentery-like syndrome.
   Enteroadherent: traveller's diarrhoea, chronic diarrhoea in children/HIV.
   Extra-intestinal disease: usually patient's own flora that is not pathogenic in the intestine but causes disease elsewhere: UTI (pp296–7); neonatal meningitis; nosocomial infection: pneumonia, meningitis, sepsis. Treat according to sensitivity: trimethoprim, ampicillin, cephalosporin, ciprofloxacin, aminoglycoside.
2. *Klebsiella pneumoniae:* colonizes skin, nasopharynx, GI tract, hospitalized patients. Associated with antibiotic exposure, in-dwelling catheters, immunosuppression. Causes pneumonia (necrotizing disease and sepsis if immunosuppressed). Also UTI, nasopharyngeal inflammation. Treat according to sensitivity: aminoglycoside, cephalosporin, carbapenem, quinolone.
3. *Proteus mirabilis:* gut commensal. Causes UTI (pp296–7). Stone formation due to urease production: breaks down urea to produce ammonia, struvite stones ('infection stones') then form in the presence of magnesium, calcium, and phosphate (pp638–9).

Other Enterobacteriaceae include *Salmonella, Shigella, Yersinia*: see enteric fever (p415), gastroenteritis (pp428–31), plague (p425).

Resistance: widespread antibiotic use has led to the development of highly virulent, multiple resistant *E. coli* and *Klebsiella* species including:

- extended-spectrum β-lactamase (ESBL) producing Enterobacteriaceae. Resistant to penicillins, cephalosporins, fluoroquinolones, trimethoprim, tetracycline, with possible extension to other antibiotic groups
- carbapenem-resistant Enterobacteriaceae (CRE).

Resistance requires antimicrobial stewardship (p384), surveillance, robust infection control, research into resistance risk and transmission (p383).

Pseudomonas aeruginosa:

Found in environment. Spread by contact/ingestion. *Presentation:* important cause of nosocomial infection. Infection if compromised tissue, eg wound, pneumonia with lung disease or ventilation, UTI with catheterization. Septicaemia if immunosuppressed. *Treatment:* options include ceftazidime/carbapenem, aminoglycoside, colistin. Combination may be needed. Impermeability of membrane and biofilm colonization lead to ↑antibiotic resistance. ↑Multidrug-resistance. ►Seek expert help.

Haemophilus influenzae:

Divided into encapsulated, typeable forms (a-f); and unencapsulated, non-typeable forms. Upper respiratory tract carriage, transmitted by droplets. *H. influenzae b* (Hib) causes meningitis, epiglottitis, otitis media, pneumonia, cellulitis, septic arthritis, and bacteraemia. Fatal in ~5%. Routine immunization in childhood and splenectomy/hyposplenism (p407). Non-typeable forms cause pneumonia and sinusitis. *Treatment:* amoxicillin, macrolide, cephalosporin, chloramphenicol, rifampicin.

Whooping cough:

Bordetella pertussis. Presentation: catarrhal phase 1–2wk, then paroxysmal coughing. 'Whoop' is a breath through partially closed vocal cords, seen mainly in children. Cough is prolonged ('100 day cough'). Infants have ↑complications/mortality. *Diagnosis:* PCR nasal/throat swab. Culture sensitivity 10–60%. *Treatment:* macrolides ↓infectivity, but may not alter disease course. Routine childhood vaccination. Vaccination in pregnancy ↑placental antibody transfer to protect neonate (p407).

Other:

Brucellosis (p424), cholera (p430), melioidosis (p414).

Tuberculosis (TB): presentation

Epidemiology

- 9.6 million new cases/yr of which 37% are unreported/undiagnosed (fig 9.8).
- 3.3% of new cases, and 20% of previously treated cases are drug resistant (p395).
- Co-infection with HIV in 12% of new cases.
- Leading cause of death worldwide, 1.5 million deaths/yr.
- Effective diagnosis and treatment saved 43 million lives between 2000 and 2014.
- *UK:* ~8000/yr, ~12 per 100 000. 73% born outside UK, 70% in deprived areas, 30% with pulmonary disease wait >4 months from symptoms to treatment.

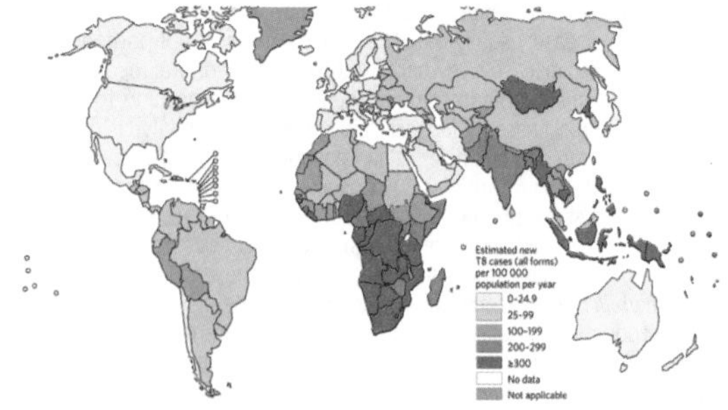

Fig 9.8 Estimated TB incidence rate worldwide.

Reproduced with permission from World Health Organization, *Global tuberculosis report 2016*. © World Health Organization 2016. http://www.who.int/tb/publications/global_report/en/

Pathophysiology

Caused by infection with *Mycobacterium tuberculosis.*

Active infection occurs when containment by the immune system (T-cells/macrophages) is inadequate. It can arise from primary infection, or re-activation of previously latent disease. Transmission of TB is via inhalation of aerosol droplets containing bacterium. This means only pulmonary disease is communicable.

Latent TB is infection without disease due to persistent immune system containment (ie granuloma formation prevents bacteria growth and spread). Positive skin/blood testing (p394) shows evidence of infection but the patient is asymptomatic and non-infectious (normal sputum/CXR). ~2 billion persons worldwide (~⅓ of world's population) are estimated to have latent TB. Lifetime risk of reactivation is 5-10%. Risk factors for reactivation: new infection (<2y), HIV, organ transplantation, immunosuppression (including corticosteroids), silicosis, illicit drug use, malnutrition, high-risk settings (homeless shelter, prison), low socio-economic status, haemodialysis.

Presentation

►TB, or not TB—that is the question. Maintain a high index of suspicion. TB can affect any organ in the body (table 9.9).

Table 9.9 UK TB case reports by site of disease

Site of disease	Number of cases in UK (%)
Pulmonary	4096 (52)
Extra-thoracic lymph nodes	1874 (24)
Intra-thoracic lymph nodes	916 (12)
Pleural	673 (9)
Gastrointestinal	432 (6)
Spine	353 (5)
Other bone	220 (3)
Miliary	211 (3)
Meningitis	172 (3)
Genitourinary	145 (2)

From: *Tuberculosis in the UK 2014 Report*, Public Health England. www.gov.uk/phe

Clinical features of TB

- *Systemic features:* Low-grade fever, anorexia, weight loss, malaise, night sweats, clubbing (bronchiectasis), erythema nodosum (p562).
- *Pulmonary TB:* Cough (in ~50%, >2-3 weeks, dry then productive), pleurisy, haemoptysis (uncommon, seen with bronchiectasis ∴ not always active disease), pleural effusion. An aspergilloma/mycetoma (p177) may form in the cavities. Presentation varies and may be silent or atypical, especially with immunosuppression, eg HIV, post-transplantation.
- *Tuberculous lymphadenitis:* (Usually) painless enlargement of cervical or supraclavicular lymph nodes. Axillary and inguinal node involvement less common. Coexisting systemic symptoms in 40–50%. Node is typically firm to touch and not acutely inflamed ('cold abscess'). Skin can adhere to the underlying mass with risk of rupture and sinus formation. Can occur with or without pulmonary disease. Investigate with fine-needle aspiration, AFB staining, and culture (p394).
- *Gastrointestinal TB:* Most disease is ileocaecal. Causes colicky abdominal pain and vomiting. Bowel obstruction can occur due to bowel wall thickening, stricture formation, or inflammatory adhesions. Biopsy is required for diagnosis. Caseation necrosis and an absence of transmural cracks/fissures distinguish from Crohn's disease.
- *Spinal TB:* Local pain and bony tenderness for weeks–months. Slow, insidious progression. May not present until deformity or neurological symptoms. Look for bony destruction, vertebral collapse, and soft tissue abscess (see Pott's vertebra p708).
- *Miliary TB:* Haematogenous dissemination leads to the formation of discrete foci (~2mm) of granulomatous tissue throughout the lung ('millet' seed appearance). CXR: fig 9.9. Dissemination is throughout the body with meningeal involvement in ~25%. Sputum may be negative for AFB as spread is haematogenous. Have a low threshold for LP. Untreated mortality is assumed to be close to 100%. Do not delay treatment while test results are pending.

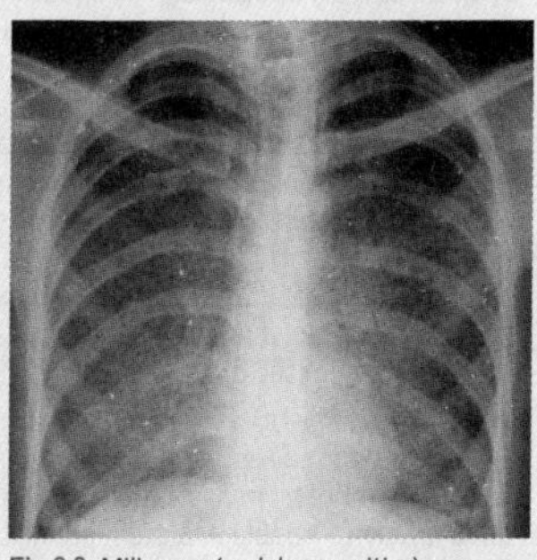

Fig 9.9 Miliary TB (nodular opacities).

- *CNS TB:* Haematogenous spread leading to foci of infection in brain and spinal cord. Foci can enlarge to form tuberculomas. Foci rupture leads to meningitis. ↑Risk with immune suppression, HIV, aged <3y. Headache, meningism, confusion, seizures, focal neurological deficit, and systemic symptoms. Needs LP and examination of CSF (leucocytosis, raised protein, CSF: plasma glucose <50%, AFB stain, PCR and culture). Look for TB elsewhere (CXR, etc), test for HIV. CT/MRI may show hydrocephalus, basal exudates. Tuberculomas are ring-enhancing. ►►All rapid diagnostic tests (p394) have ↓sensitivity, so treat on suspicion.
- *Genitourinary TB:* Symptoms may be chronic, intermittent, or silent. Include dysuria, frequency, loin pain, haematuria, sterile pyuria (see p296). Granuloma may cause fibrosis, strictures, infertility, and genital ulceration.
- *Cardiac TB:* Usually involves the pericardium: pericarditis, pericardial effusion, and/or constrictive pericarditis (p154). Check chest imaging for other TB pathology, eg pulmonary disease, mediastinal lymph nodes. Pericardiectomy may be indicated for persistent constriction despite anti-tuberculous treatment. Myocardial involvement (arrhythmias, heart failure, ventricular aneurysm, or outflow obstruction) is rare.
- *Skin:* Lupus vulgaris = persistent, progressive, cutaneous TB: red-brown, 'apple-jelly' nodules. Scrofuloderma: skin lesion extended from underlying infection eg lymph node, bone; causes ulceration and scarring.

Tuberculosis (TB): diagnosis and treatment

Diagnostic tests for TB

Latent TB:

Offer testing[3] to close contacts of those with pulmonary or laryngeal TB, those with immune dysfunction, healthcare workers, and high-risk populations, eg prison, homeless, vulnerable migrants.

- *Tuberculin skin testing (TST)* = Mantoux test. Intradermal injection of purified protein derivative (PPD) tuberculin. Size of skin induration is used to determine positivity depending on vaccination history and immune status (>5mm if risk factors, >15mm if no risk factors).
- *Interferon-gamma release assays (IGRAS)* diagnose exposure to TB by measuring the release of interferon-gamma from T-cells reacting to TB antigen. ↑Specificity compared to TST if history of BCG vaccination.

►Neither test can diagnose or exclude active disease (falsely negative in 20–25% of active disease): clinical evaluation is required.

►Immune-suppressed states reduce the sensitivity of both tests.

Active pulmonary TB:

- *CXR*. Fibronodular/linear opacities in upper lobe (typical), middle or lower lobes (atypical), cavitation, calcification, miliary disease (see fig 9.9), effusion, lymphadenopathy.
- *Sputum smear*. Sputum can be spontaneously produced or induced (with nebulized saline and precautions to prevent transmission). Three specimens are needed including an early-morning sample. It is stained for the presence of acid-fast bacilli (AFB). All mycobacteria are 'acid-fast' including *M. tuberculosis*. If AFB are seen, treatment should be commenced and the patient isolated (in hospital only if clinical indication, or public health reason for admission; or at home).
- *Sputum culture*. More sensitive than smear testing. Culture takes 1–3 weeks (liquid media) or 4–8 weeks (solid media). Can assess drug sensitivity.
- *Nucleic acid amplification test (NAAT)*. Direct detection of *M. tuberculosis* in sputum by DNA or RNA amplification. Rapid diagnosis (<8hrs). Can also detect drug resistance (see p395).

Extra-pulmonary TB:

- Investigate for coexisting pulmonary disease.
- Obtain material from aspiration or biopsy (lymph node, pleura, bone, synovium, GI/GU tract) to enable AFB staining, histological examination (caseating granuloma) and/or culture.
- NAAT can be carried out on any sterile body fluid, eg CSF, pericardial fluid.

►►Offer HIV test for all.

Treatment

Antibiotics used in the treatment[3] of TB are detailed in table 9.10.

Table 9.10 Antibiotics used in the treatment of TB

Antibiotic	Standard course for active disease	Notes
Rifampicin	2 months intensive 4 months continuation	Enzyme inducer: care with warfarin, calcineurin inhibitors, oestrogens, phenytoin; body secretions coloured orange-red (includes contact lens staining); altered liver function.
Isoniazid	2 months intensive 4 months continuation	Inhibits formation of active pyridoxine (Vit B_6) which causes a peripheral neuropathy (↑risk with DM, CKD, HIV, malnutrition) ∴ give with prophylactic pyridoxine; hepatitis.
Pyrazinamide	2 months intensive	Idiosyncratic hepatotoxicity, ↓dose if eGFR<30.
Ethambutol	2 months intensive	Colour blindness, ↓visual acuity, optic neuritis. Check visual acuity at start of treatment, monitor for symptoms. Monthly visual check if treatment > 2 months. Monitor levels if eGFR<30.

Latent TB

Balance the risk of development of active disease with the possible side-effects of treatment. Consider treatment in all at ↑risk of active disease: HIV, transplantation, chemotherapy, biological agents eg anti-TNFα (see p265), diabetes, CKD including dialysis, silicosis, bariatric surgery, and recent close contact with pulmonary/laryngeal TB. Offer HIV, hepatitis B and C testing prior to treatment.

Treat with 3 months of isoniazid (with pyridoxine) and rifampicin *OR* 6 months of isoniazid (with pyridoxine).

If concerns about hepatotoxicity then 3 months of isoniazid and rifampicin may be preferred. In severe liver disease, seek specialist advice. If interactions with rifamycins are a concern (eg HIV, transplant) then 6 months of isoniazid may be preferred.

Active TB

All forms of active TB are statutorily notifiable in UK. This includes both clinical and culture diagnoses. Notification is via your local public health protection team (www.gov.uk/health-protection-team).Treatment is given under the care of a specialist TB clinician/service according to table 9.10. Exceptions include:

- active CNS disease (including spinal cord involvement): continuation phase of treatment is extended from 4 to 10 months
- CNS and pericardial disease: use adjunctive high-dose steroids (with weaning and withdrawal during the intensive treatment period)
- drug-resistant TB.

Adherence is important for treatment to be effective and to prevent drug resistance. Directly observed therapy (DOT) should be considered if: previous treatment for TB, homelessness, drug/alcohol misuse, prison, psychiatric or cognitive disorder, multidrug resistant disease, patient request.

Universal access to diagnosis and treatment of TB is part of social justice. WHO has developed an 'End TB' strategy aiming to reduce TB deaths by 90% by 2030, and TB incidence by 90% by 2035 (www.who.int/tb/strategy/en).

Drug-resistant TB

NAAT (p394) for drug resistance should be requested for all patients with risk factors for drug-resistance: previous TB treatment, contact with drug-resistant disease, birth or residence in a country where ≥5% new cases are drug resistant (fig 9.10). Drug resistance may be:

- to any single agent in table 9.10.
- multidrug-resistant TB (MDR-TB): resistant to rifampicin and isoniazid.
- extensively drug-resistant TB (XDR-TB): resistant to rifampicin, isoniazid, one injectable agent (capreomycin, kanamycin or amikacin) and one fluoroquinolone.

If rifampicin resistance is detected, treat with at least six agents to which the mycobacterium is likely to be sensitive. Test for resistance to 2nd-line drugs. Remember infection control measures. Seek expert advice for all drug-resistant cases.

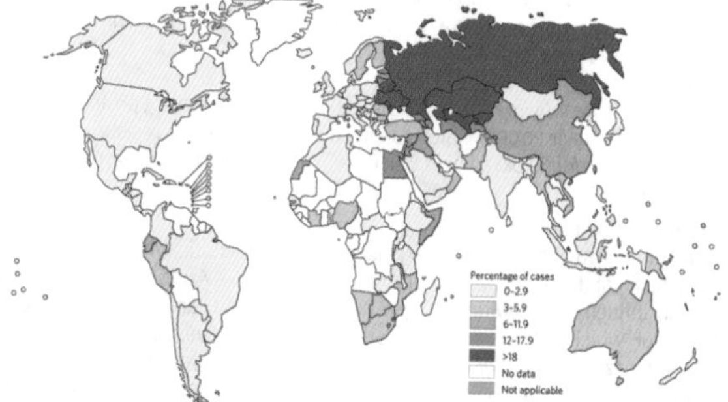

Fig 9.10 Percentage of new TB cases with multi-drug resistant TB.

Reproduced with permission from World Health Organization, *Global tuberculosis report 2016*. http://www.who.int/tb/publications/global_report/en/

Influenza

Influenza is common throughout the world, affecting ~5–10% of adults, and 20–30% of children each year. In most, it is a self-limiting illness. Complications can be life-threatening in the elderly, pregnant women, and those with chronic disease. There are ~4 million cases of severe influenza and ~500 000 deaths worldwide/yr.

Seasonal influenza

Acute viral infection of lungs and airways. Rapid person-to-person spread by aerosolized droplets and contact. Infectivity from 1d prior, to ~7d after symptoms. Includes three subtypes of virus: A, B, and C. Type A influenza is subdivided according to combinations of virus surface proteins eg A(H1N1), A(H3N2). Seasonal epidemics peak during the winter in temperate countries. Acquired immunity is specific to the virus subtype.

Presentation: Incubation: 1–4d. Fever, dry cough, sore throat, coryzal symptoms, headache, malaise, myalgia, conjunctivitis, eye pain ± photophobia. Complications include pneumonia, exacerbation of chronic lung disease, croup, otitis media, D&V, myositis, encephalitis, Reye syndrome (encephalopathy + fatty degenerative liver failure).

Diagnosis: Clinical: acute onset+cough+fever has positive predictive value >79%. Testing limited to outbreaks, and public health surveillance. Includes: viral PCR, rapid antigen testing, viral culture of clinical samples (throat swab, nasal swab, nasopharyngeal washings, sputum).

Treatment:

- *Uncomplicated influenza* symptomatic treatment eg paracetamol. Antivirals only if high risk:
  - Chronic disease: lung, heart, kidney, liver, CNS, DM
  - Immunosuppression: immunodeficiency, current or planned or within 6 months of immunosuppressive therapy, ↓CD4 (<200 in adults, <500 if child <5yr)
  - Pregnancy
  - >65yr
  - BMI>40
  - <6 months old.
- *Complicated influenza* includes lower respiratory tract infection, exacerbation of any underlying medical condition, all needing hospital admission. Give antiviral[4] inhibitors of influenza neuraminidase:
  1. Oseltamivir: PO or NG. Adult dose: 75mg BD. 5d course. 1st line in UK.
  2. Zanamivir: inhaled (10mg BD, 5d course, confirm technique), nebulized, or IV (respiratory disease affecting nebulizer delivery, ITU). Used if: oseltamivir resistance (eg A(H1N1)), poor clinical response to oseltamivir, concerns re GI absorption of oseltamivir.

Retrospective observational data, and animal studies of oseltamivir and zanamivir show no evidence of harm in pregnancy. Supportive treatment for all. Extracorporeal membrane oxygenation (ECMO) has been used to support gas exchange in severe acute lung injury due to influenza.

Prevention:

- *Post-exposure prophylaxis:* if high risk (see 'Treatment') *AND* not protected by vaccination: oseltamivir PO OD (inhaled zanamivir OD if oseltamivir resistance) for 10d.
- *Annual vaccination* in UK: all high risk (see 'Treatment'), children>2yrs, healthcare workers. See p407.

Pandemic influenza

Seasonal influenza is subject to antigenic drift: small genetic changes during replication which can be accounted for in the annual vaccine. Antigenic shift is a major change in influenza A resulting in new haemgglutinin (H) and neuraminidase proteins (N) for which there is no pre-existing immunity in the population. Any non-human influenza viruses which transfer to humans are novel. If they also have, or develop, capacity for rapid human-to-human transmission a pandemic results. Based on previous pandemics, up to 50% of the UK population may become infected leading to 20 000–750 000 excess deaths.

Sailing the choppy waters of pandemic influenza

Pandemic influenza is the stormy sea of clinical medicine. Like sailors, we know there are deadly challenges to come, but we cannot predict their exact timing or nature. To prepare a boat for the tempestuous waters ahead, the mast is key; without it the sails are unsupported and progress will flounder. The mast of pandemic influenza is a tall, vertical **spar** which produces maximum drive through the swell, and allows sailors to climb up high to see what the horizon has in store. When preparing for pandemic influenza, we must make for ourselves a **spar** of principles and plans fit for the storm ahead:

- **S**urveillance, planning, and communication: worldwide influenza virological surveillance has been conducted through the WHO for >50yr. It offers a global alert mechanism for viruses with pandemic potential and defines methodologies for assessing antiviral susceptibility. Cooperation between international and national public health bodies is required for an understanding of clinical characteristics and disease spread. Communication to the individual (public and social media) is needed with advice about self-isolation, when and how to seek medical help, personal hygiene.
- **P**rotect: vaccine development and production capacity (stockpiling), adequate personal protective equipment (apron, gloves, well-fitting mask), antiviral administration according to robust evidence and sensitivity.
- **A**nimals: limiting/eliminating the animal reservoir of virus by culling, restricting animal movement, vaccination of livestock.
- **R**esearch: virus characteristics, disease severity predictors, epidemiological risk factors, antiviral development, targeting of treatment and vaccination, increased-spectrum vaccines with longer-lasting immunity, effective healthcare worker protection, evidence-based social distancing measures.

Hide and seek

In 2009, there was justifiable global concern about a 'swine flu' pandemic. Based on a Cochrane review in 2008, which showed reduced complications with oseltamivir, billions were spent stockpiling the drug worldwide.

In fact, the positive conclusion was driven mainly by data from an industry-funded summary of 10 trials, of which only two had been published.[5] Cochrane needed access to these missing data. The ensuing fight for information was to take 5 years. The offer of a secret contract, with secret terms, and secrecy about methods, was declined. These are not acceptable methods for meta-analysis. Inconsistencies began to arise in conclusions about effectiveness. Were people seeing different data, or was this simply a close call with two sides separated by a very small fence? Either way, being able to see *all* the data started to become increasingly important. But even the largest phase three trial of the drug had never been published. And was self-reported pneumonia a useful outcome measure? In December 2009, Cochrane could only declare that paucity of data undermined previous findings.

This battle for data became part of 'Alltrials': a campaign for transparency in clinical trials. ~50% of all clinical trials remain unpublished. The hunt goes on to find them. You can run your own drug trial, choose what to publish, and watch how the data become skewed at: www.alltrials.net/news/the-economist-publication-bias.

After half a decade, under ceaseless demand, and with the withholding of data become increasingly indefensible, the clinical study reports were released. These are normally used to provide authorities with a detailed trial report. They are not easy fodder for meta-analysis. Assessing 160 000 pages was uncharted territory for Cochrane. And the conclusion: oseltamivir shortens symptoms by <1d and hospitalization is not reduced. Other complications were unreliably reported.

The WHO includes oseltamivir on its *WHO Model List of Essential Medicines* (19th edition, 2015) which means it is considered efficacious, safe, cost-effective, and a minimum requirement for basic healthcare. Does this stand up to independent scrutiny? The evidence base is certainly tarnished. But a pandemic is not a RCT. And the threshold of evidence to reverse policy decisions may be different from the threshold needed to introduce them. If a new pandemic looms, millions more will be thrown in, for now.

Human immunodeficiency virus (HIV): diagnosis

HIV is a retrovirus which infects and replicates in human lymphocytes (CD4 + T-cells) and macrophages. This leads to progressive immune system dysfunction, opportunistic infection, and malignancy = Acquired Immunodeficiency Syndrome (AIDS). The virus is transmitted via blood, sexual fluids, and breast milk. Virus subtypes include HIV1 (global epidemic) and HIV2 (↓ pathogenic, predominantly West Africa).

Epidemiology

~37 million adults and children are estimated to be living with HIV worldwide (fig 9.11), with 1.2 million deaths/yr. Africa has most of the disease (~26 million), most of the mortality (790 000/yr), and ~1% of the world's wealth.

UK: estimated ~100 000 living with HIV (=1.9/1000) including 5% of men who have sex with men (MSM). ~17% of those with HIV in UK are unaware of their infection.

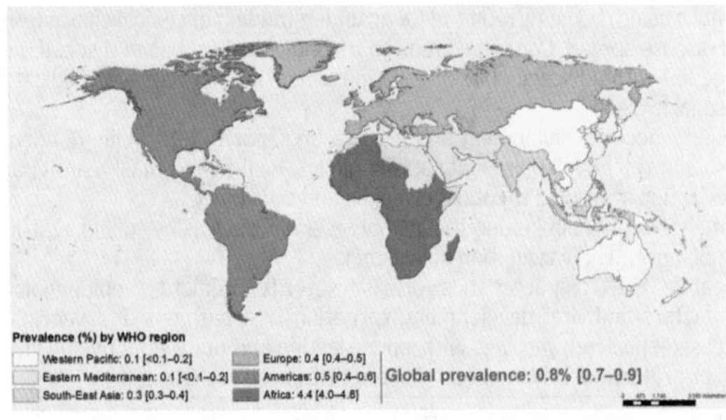

Fig 9.11 Adult HIV prevalence (15–49 years).

Pathophysiology

HIV binds, via its GP120 envelope glycoprotein, to CD4 receptors on helper T cells, monocytes, and macrophages. These 'CD4 cells' migrate to lymphoid tissue where the virus replicates, producing billions of new virions. These are released, and in turn infect new CD4 cells. As infection progresses, depletion or impaired function of CD4 cells leads to ↓immune function. HIV is a retrovirus: it encodes reverse transcriptase, allowing DNA copies to be produced from viral RNA. This is error prone, meaning a significant mutation rate, which contributes to treatment resistance.

Prevention

Sexual transmission: Consistent and correct use of (male and female) condoms ↓transmission by ~90%. Serosorting is the restriction of (unprotected) sex depending on HIV status. It is unsafe due to inaccuracies in HIV status (which is only as reliable as a person's last test) and failure to disclose. It does not consider transfer of treatment resistance, other STIs, or hepatitis.

Post-exposure prophylaxis (PEP): The short-term use of antiretroviral therapy (ART) after potential HIV exposure (sexual or occupational) should be considered an emergency method of HIV prevention. Can be given up to 72h (ideally <24h) after exposure. Not recommended if exposure is to a person on ART with a confirmed and sustained (>6 months) undetectable (<200 copies/mL) viral load. 1st-line PEP[6] in UK is Truvada® (tenofovir/emtricitabine) and raltegravir for 28 days (2015) (refer to local guidelines). Test for HIV 8-12 weeks after exposure.

Pre-exposure prophylaxis (PrEP): The use of ART in those at high risk of acquiring HIV including serodifferent relationships without suppression of viral load, condomless anal sex in MSM. Trials (PROUD, IPERGAY) show an 86% reduction in HIV incidence. A large scale trial of PrEP provision (2017–2020) will inform future NHS funding decisions.

Vertical transmission: All pregnant women with HIV should have commenced ART by 24 weeks' gestation. Caesarean delivery indicated if viral load >50 copies/mL. Neonatal PEP is given from birth to 4wks old with formula-feeding.

Presentation

With symptoms of early HIV infection:

- *Primary HIV infection* is symptomatic in ~80%, typically 2-4 weeks after infection (= seroconversion illness, acute retroviral syndrome). Maintain a high index of suspicion. Offer HIV testing to anyone (regardless of risk) presenting with flu-like symptoms and an eythematous/maculopapular rash. Consider primary HIV as a differential in any combination of fever, rash, myalgia, pharyngitis, mucosal ulceration, lymphadenopathy, and headache/aseptic meningitis. Diagnosis of primary HIV is a unique opportunity to prevent transmission (↑viral load and genital shedding). HIV antibody testing may be negative but HIV RNA levels are high—seek expert help regarding viral load testing (see HIV testing later in topic).
- *Persistant generalized lymphadenopathy* = swollen/enlarged lymph nodes >1cm in two or more non-contiguous sites (not inguinal) persisting for >3 months. Due to follicular hyperplasia caused by HIV infection. Exclude TB, infection, and malignancy.

In the asymptomatic, latent phase of chronic HIV infection:
In the UK there is universal testing in sexual health clinics, antenatal services, drug dependency programmes, and in patients with TB/hepatitis B/hepatitis C/lymphoma. Where HIV prevalence is >2/1000 universal testing by GPs and medical admissions units should be considered. Any request for a HIV test should be met.

With complications of immune system dysfunction: See pp400–1.

HIV testing

The prognosis for patients with HIV in the UK is much better than for many other serious illness for which doctors routinely test. HIV testing[6] should not be viewed differently. Any doctor can consent for a HIV test: explain the benefits of testing and detail how results will be given. Written consent is unnecessary. Arrange follow-up with a local HIV/GUM service within 2 weeks (preferably <48h) for patients testing positive for the first time.

- *ELISA for HIV antibody and antigen (p24):* 4th-generation assays test for HIV antibody and p24 antigen. This reduces the 'window period' (time of false-negative testing between infection and the production of measurable antigen/antibody) to average ~10 days. Diagnosis in UK is confirmed by a confirmatory assay.
- *Rapid point-of-care testing:* Immunoassay kit which gives a rapid result from a finger-prick or mouth swab. Only CE-marked kits should be used. Needs serological confirmation.
- *Viral load:* Quantification of HIV RNA. Used to monitor response to ART. Not diagnostic due to possibility of a false-positive result ∴ care if used to test for symptomatic primary HIV in the 'window period'—confirmation of seroconversion is still required.
- *Nucleic acid testing/viral PCR:* Qualitative test for the presence of viral RNA. Used to test for vertical transmission in neonates as placental transfer of maternal antibodies can affect ELISA antibody testing up to 18 months of age.
- *CD4 count:* Cannot diagnose HIV. Used to monitor immune system function and disease progression in patients with HIV. <200 cells/microlitre is one of the defining criteria for AIDS.

►See www.aidsmap.com for available HIV testing and country-specific resources.

Needle-stick injury

Risk of HIV transmission from a single needle-stick exposure from a person with HIV not on ART is ~1 in 300 (lower than risks of hepatitis B and C transmission).

Prevent:
- Use 'safer sharps' (incorporates a mechanism to minimize accidental injury).
- Do not recap unprotected medical sharps.
- When using sharps, ensure there is a disposal container nearby.

Manage:
- Encourage the wound to bleed, ideally under running water (do not suck).
- Wash with soap and running water, do not scrub.
- Seek advice from occupational health/infection control (or A&E outside of working hours) regarding source testing and post-exposure prophylaxis (p398).

Complications of HIV infection

Complications of HIV can be divided into:

- complications of immune dysfunction (opportunistic infection/malignancy)
- complicating comorbidity
- complications of treatment, ie adverse drug effects (see pp402-3).

The differential diagnosis for symptoms presenting in a person with HIV is given in table 9.11. This is not exhaustive. ►Do not forget your usual differentials, the presentation may not relate to the patient's HIV status.

Opportunistic disease

►ART is part of the treatment regimen of all opportunistic infections (see pp402-3).

- *Pneumocystis jirovecii:* ('yee-row-vet-zee') *Presentation:* progressive SOB on exertion, malaise, dry cough. Haemoptysis and pleuritic pain rare. *Examination:* ↑respiratory rate, often normal breath sounds. *Investigation:* SpO_2 (compare rest and exertion). CXR: classically perihilar infiltrates (fig 9.12), but may be normal. Induced sputum or BAL with staining or nucleic acid amplification. *Treatment:* IV co-trimoxazole (convert to oral if favourable response). 21-day course. Steroids in moderate-severe disease (P_aO_2 <9.3KPa/SpO_2 <92%). 2nd-line: clindamycin, pentamidine, atovaquone. *Prophylaxis:* co-trimoxazole if CD4 <200 cells/microlitre.
- *Candidiasis:* Oral or oesophageal. Pain in the tongue, dysphagia, odynophagia. Diagnosed clinically or endoscopically. Treated with systemic '-azole', eg fluconazole.
- *Cryptococcus neoformans:* Commonest systemic fungal infection in HIV (5–10% pre-ART). *Presentation:* meningitis: headache, fever, meningism variable. May be associated skin (molluscum-like papules) and lung disease. *Investigation:* LP with manometry. CSF stain (India ink), CSF/blood cryptococcal antigen. *Treatment:* induction with liposomal amphotericin B (SE: renal tubular damage and AKI). Addition of flucytosine has shown benefit in patients not on ART (SE: haematological toxicity). Maintenance treatment with fluconazole. Normalize ICP with repeat LPs/shunt.
- *Toxoplasma gondii:* Toxoplasma abscesses are commonest cause of intracranial mass lesions when CD4 <200 cells/microlitre. *Presentation:* focal neurological signs ± seizures. Headache and vomiting if raised ICP. *Investigation:* ring-enhancing lesions on MRI (ΔΔ lymphoma) with associated oedema. CSF PCR for *T. gondii* is specific but only moderately sensitive. Blood serology is not diagnostic as most cases are a reactivation of previous infection. *Treatment:* consider in any brain mass lesion with CD4 <200 cell/microlitre. Pyrimethamine, sulfadiazine, folinic acid.
- *Cytomegalovirus (CMV):* Severe primary or reactivated disease (see p405). *Presentation:* retinitis (blurred then loss of vision), encephalitis, GI disease (oesophagitis, colitis), hepatitis, bone marrow suppression, pneumonia. *Diagnosis:* serial CMV viral load, retinal lesions (p438), GI ulceration, 'owl's eye' inclusions on biopsy. *Treatment:* ganciclovir/valganciclovir. Side-effects: rash, diarrhoea, bone myelosuppression.
- *Cryptosporidium:* Common cause of chronic diarrhoea in HIV pre-ART. *Presentation:* acute or sub-acute non-bloody, watery diarrhoea. Also cholangitis, pancreatitis. *Investigation:* stool microscopy (multiple samples as oocyst excretion intermittent), PCR, enzyme immunoassay, direct fluorescent antibody. *Treatment:* supportive, ART.
- *Kaposi's sarcoma:* Most common tumour in HIV and AIDS defining. Caused by Kaposi sarcoma herpes virus (human herpesvirus 8, p405). *Presentation:* cutaneous or mucosal lesions: patch, plaque, or nodular. Visceral disease less common. *Investigation:* histological confirmation. *Treatment:* ART. Intralesional retinoids or vinblastine. Radiotherapy for cosmesis/pain. Chemotherapy (+ART) in advanced disease.
- *Lymphoma:* Increased risk of non-Hodgkin's lymphoma in HIV. Includes: diffuse large B-cell lymphoma, Burkitt's lymphoma, primary CNS lymphoma. *Presentation:* dependent upon area of involvement. Includes lymphadenopathy, cytopenia, CNS symptoms. *Treatment:* combined ART and chemotherapy. Rituximab for non-CNS disease. Whole-brain radiotherapy for CNS disease if excess toxicity with chemotherapy.

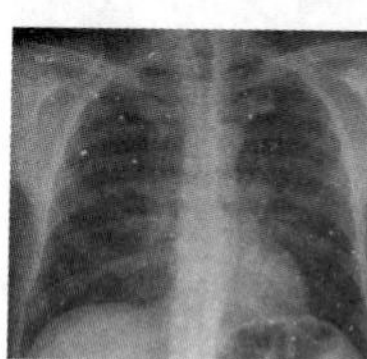

Fig 9.12 Bilateral interstitial infiltrates in *P. jirovecii*.
Reproduced from Lim, *Acute Respiratory Infections*, 2012, with permission from Oxford University Press.

Complicating comorbidity

- *Cardiovascular disease:* Increased risk of CVD in HIV. Includes individuals where risk traditionally lower: younger age, normotensive, no DM, non-obese. Contributing factors: dyslipidaemia caused by ART, acceleration of pro-atherosclerotic inflammatory processes by HIV. Management of CV risk factors although no outcome data to guide specific lipid and BP targets in HIV.
- *Bone disease:* Increased risk of low bone-mineral density and fragility fractures in HIV. Contributing factors: side effect of ART, increased prevalence of risk factors, eg poor nutrition, smoking, alcohol, low vitamin D levels. Risk assess and consider bisphosphonate.
- *TB:* All patients with TB and HIV need ART (as soon as TB treatment tolerated and within 2 weeks if CD4 <100 cells/microlitre). Seek expert advice and refer to local guidelines. Consider Truvada® plus efavirenz as 1st line in UK (serum levels of integrase inhibitors are decreased by rifampicin). See ART, pp402–3, TB, pp394–5.
- *Hepatitis B (HBV):* Co-infection requires an ART regimen including antivirals with anti-HBV activity, eg tenofovir plus emtricitabine (not lamivudine or emtricitabine as a single agent due to potential for emergence of HBV resistance).
- *Hepatitis C (HCV):* Assess all with HIV for HCV treatment. Pegylated interferon efficacy is less with lower CD4 count. Aim for CD4 >500 cells/microlitre with ART first.

Table 9.11 Differential diagnoses in HIV

Presentation	Differential diagnosis
Fever	Intraoral abscess, sinusitis, pneumonia, TB, endocarditis, meningitis, encephalitis, pyomyositis, lymphoma, immune-reconstitution after commencement of ART, any non-HIV cause.
Lymphadenopathy	Persistent generalized lymphadenopathy (p399), TB, syphilis, histoplasmosis, cryptococcus, lymphoma, Kaposi's sarcoma, local infection.
Rash	Drug reaction, herpes zoster, scabies, cutaneous cryptococcus or histoplasmosis, Kaposi's sarcoma, seborrhoeic dermatitis.
Cough/SOB	Community-acquired pneumonia, *Pneumocystis jirovecii,* TB, bronchial compression (TB, lymphoma, Kaposi's sarcoma), pulmonary Kaposi's sarcoma (uncommon), cardiac failure (HIV cardiomyopathy, infective pericardial effusion, HIV vasculopathy).
Diarrhoea	*Salmonella, Shigella, Clostridium difficile*, amoebiasis, *Giardia, Cryptosporidia,* CMV, HIV enteropathy is a diagnosis of exclusion.
Abdominal pain	TB, CMV colitis, pancreatitis (CMV, TB or secondary to ART). ►Do not forget a pregnancy test.
Dysphagia	Candidiasis, HSV.
↑Liver enzymes	Viral hepatitis (A, B, C, CMV, HSV, EBV), drug-induced liver injury (anti-TB or ART), HIV cholangiopathy, lymphoma, congestion due to cardiac disease (pericardial effusion?).
AKI	Pre-renal due to sepsis/dehydration, interstitial nephritis secondary to medication, HIV-associated nephropathy (proteinuria, CKD).
Headache/ seizures/focal neurology	Meningitis (bacterial, TB, cryptococcal, syphilis), empyema, space-occupying lesion (toxoplasmosis, lymphoma, tuberculoma), adverse drug reaction, HIV encephalopathy, progressive multifocal leukoencephalopathy (PML), stroke (HIV vasculopathy). See p517.
Eye disease	Herpes zoster, CMV retinitis. See pp438–9.
Peripheral neuropathy	ART, CMV, HIV neuropathy, nutritional deficiency.

HIV: antiretroviral therapy (ART)

▶▶ Antiretroviral therapy (ART)[7] is recommended for everyone with HIV, regardless of CD4 count.

Strategic Timing of AntiRetroviral Treatment (START) study, 2015

4685 participants (215 sites, 35 countries) with HIV, CD4 >500 cells/microlitre, no previous ART. Randomized to:
- immediate ART
- deferred ART until CD4 <350 cells/microlitre or AIDS-defining illness.

Study was terminated early when an independent interim analysis revealed benefit to immediate initiation of ART, and recommended that patients on the deferred group start ART. ▶Immediate initiation of ART reduced the risk of AIDS, serious non-AIDS events, or death by 57% (CI 38–70%) at 3 years.

Aims of ART To reduce the HIV viral load to a level undetectable by standard laboratory techniques leading to immunological recovery, reduced clinical progression, and reduced mortality. These aims should be met with the least possible side-effects.

Mechanism of action (See fig 9.13.)
- *CCR5 antagonists* inhibit the entry of the virus into the cell by blocking the CCR5 co-receptor.
- *Nucleos(t)ide and non-nucleoside reverse transcriptase inhibitors (NRTIs, NNRTIs)* inhibit reverse transcriptase and the conversion of viral RNA into DNA.
- *Integrase strand transfer inhibitors (INSTIs)* inhibit integrase and prevent HIV DNA integrating into the nucleus.
- *Protease inhibitors (PIs)* inhibit protease, an enzyme involved in the maturation of virus particles.
- *Pharmacokinetic enhancers/boosters* increase the effectiveness of antiretroviral drugs allowing lower doses eg cobicistat, ritonavir.

Starting treatment ▶Seek expert help.

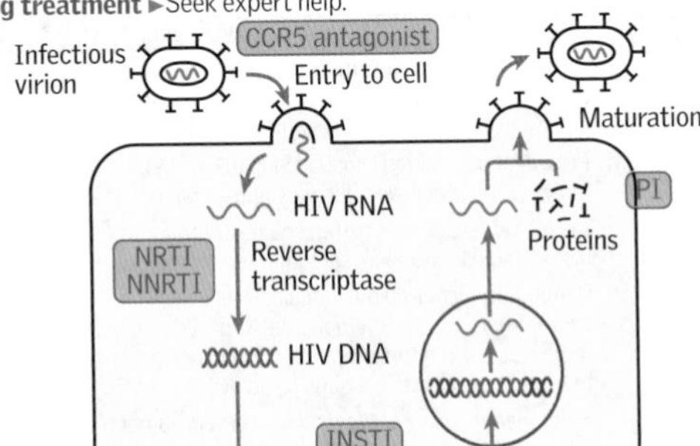

Fig 9.13 Mechanism of action of ART.

1. Counselling: HIV transmission and sexual health, benefits of therapy (not cure), adherence (life long), resistance, side-effects of treatment, necessary monitoring, disclosure to partner/family/friends, partner testing.
2. Screen for infections and malignancy (pp400–1). Includes TB, hepatitis B&C. Treat or offer prophylaxis with co-trimoxazole if CD4 <200 cells/microlitre. For latent TB see p395. Aim to start ART within 2 weeks of initiation of antimicrobial treatment for opportunistic or serious infection (seek expert advice if drug interactions or intracerebral disease).
3. Baseline tests: CD4, viral load, FBC, LFT, electrolytes, creatinine, pregnancy test, viral genotype for drug resistance.
4. Review usual medications for possible drug interactions. Advise the patient to check for drug interactions with any new medication.

   ▶See www.hiv-druginteractions.org

What to start

►Use local guidelines. ►Get expert help.

For a treatment-naive patient consider two nucleoside reverse transcriptase inhibitors (='NRTI backbone') plus one of:

- ritonavir-boosted protease inhibitor
- non-nucleoside reverse transcriptase inhibitor
- integrase inhibitor.

1st line drugs commonly used in the UK include:

- *NRTI backbone:* Tenofovir and emtricitabine (combination tablet=Truvada®), abacavir and lamivudine (combination tablet=Kivexa®). Side-effects: GI disturbance, anorexia, pancreatitis, hepatic dysfunction (severe lactic acidosis with hepatomegaly and hepatic steatosis reported, caution with hepatitis B/C), ↓bone-mineral density. Avoid abacavir if high risk of CVD. Avoid tenofovir if eGFR <30.
- *Protease inhibitors:* Atazanavir, darunavir. Side-effects: hyperglycaemia, insulin resistance (mainly 1st-generation drugs), dyslipidaemia, jaundice, and hepatitis.
- *NNTRI:* Rilpivirine (give with food, interaction with proton pump inhibitors), efavirenz (CNS toxicity, association with suicidality ∴ care in depression/anxiety, adverse lipid profile). Other side-effects: rash, GI disturbance.
- *Integrase inhibitor:* Dolutegravir, elvitegravir, raltegravir. Side-effects: rash, GI disturbance, insomnia.

Monitor: adherence (see BOX 'Adherence'), adverse effects (LFTs, glucose), virological response (viral load). CD4 counts guide prophylaxis of opportunistic infection (values may not correlate with virological response, use viral load preferentially).

Adherence

↓Adherence to ART is associated with drug resistance, disease progression, and death. Adherence support should be integral to ART provision.

Assess: Ask about adherence in a non-judgemental way. Do not blame. Explain the reasoning behind your questions. Is non-adherence due to practical problems or healthcare beliefs? Be ready to address both. What help would your patient like?

Intervene: Normalize the situation—doubts and concerns about ART are common. Find time for discussion/information. Address concerns. Simplify the dosage regimen, offer a multicompartment medication system. Link the taking of medication to a regular daily activity. Discuss side-effects: what are the risks/benefits to changing dose or ART regimen?

Resource-limited settings

In many resource-limited settings, universal access to ART remains an objective yet to be achieved. ~50% of those in need of treatment for HIV do not receive it. Interim prioritization of those with symptomatic HIV or CD4 count <350 cells/microlitre may be appropriate as these patients are at high risk of mortality and have most short-term benefit from ART.

Equality in the treatment of HIV requires:

- Effective, acceptable, and reliable methods to reduce HIV transmission, including treatment as prevention.
- Rapid, accurate, and low-cost diagnosis and monitoring.
- Standardization and simplification of ART regimens.
- Evidence-based ART to prevent the use of sub-standard protocols which compromise treatment and lead to the emergence of drug-resistant strains.
- Reduced ART costs and/or effective allocation of resources.

An HIV vaccine?

Vaccines are the most effective way to prevent infectious disease. They can also be therapeutic, clearing a virus after infection. HIV vaccines to date have failed to induce an immune response sufficient to confer protection. Research is ongoing into neutralizing HIV antibodies, peptides, genes, viral vectors, physiological 'boosters', and mechanisms to counter the mutational evolution of HIV. See www.hvtn.org

Herpes simplex virus (HSV) (human herpesvirus 1 and 2)

Includes HSV1 and HSV2. HSV1 infection in ⅔ of world's population (~3.7 billion <50yrs), and HSV2 in ~11% (~400 million). Viruses multiply in epithelial cells of mucosal surface producing vesicles or ulcers. Lifelong latent infection when virus enters sensory neurons at infection site. Can then reactivate, replicate, and infect surrounding tissue. Disseminated infection if impaired T-cell immunity: pneumonitis, hepatitis, colitis.

Presentation: Primary infection: subclinical or sensory nerve (tingling) prodrome, then vesicles, shallow ulcers. Systemic symptoms possible: fever, malaise, lymphadenopathy. Heals 8-12d. Reactivation: usually ↓severe unless immunosuppressed. Anatomy of infection:

- Herpes labialis: cold sore lesion at lip border, predominantly HSV1.
- Genital herpes: predominantly HSV2 (see p412).
- Gingivostomatitis: fever, sore throat followed by tender oropharyngeal vesicles.
- Keratoconjunctivitis: corneal dendritic ulcers. ►Avoid steroids. See *OHCS* p416.
- Herpetic whitlow: painful vesicles on distal phalanx due to inoculation through a break in the skin.
- Herpes encephalitis: most common treatable viral encephalitis. Transfer of virus from peripheral site to brain via neuronal transmission. Prodrome: fever, malaise, headache, nausea. Then encephalopathy: general/focal signs of cerebral dysfunction including psychiatric symptoms, seizure, focal neurology (temporal involvement in ~60%), memory loss. Predominantly HSV1 in immunocompetent patients.
- Secondary infection: eg HSV infection of eczematous skin—eczema herpeticum.

Diagnosis: Clinical diagnosis. Confirmation required in encephalitis, keratoconjunctivits, or immunosuppression: viral PCR of CSF, swab, or vesicle scraping. Also culture, immunofluorescence, serology.

Treatment: Aciclovir: ↓symptoms and viral shedding, will not prevent latent infection. ►Give empirical IV aciclovir as soon as HSV encephalitis is suspected, mortality ~70% in untreated disease (see p824).

Varicella zoster virus (VZV) (human herpesvirus 3)

Primary infection transmitted by respiratory droplets. Incubation 14–21d. Invades respiratory mucosa, replicates in lymph nodes. Disseminates via mononuclear cells to infect skin epithelial cells. Leads to virus containing vesicles = chicken pox. Virus then remains dormant in sensory nerve roots. Reactivation is dermatomal = shingles.

Presentation:

- *Chicken pox:* prodrome 1-2d: fever, malaise, headache, abdominal pain. Then rash (fig 9.14): pruritic, erythematous macules→vesicles, crust in ~48h. Infectious 1-2d pre-, to 5d post-rash development (lesions scabbed). Complications ↑ in immunosuppression: encephalitis (cerebellar ataxia), VZV pneumonia, transverse myelitis, pericarditis, purpura fulminans/DIC.

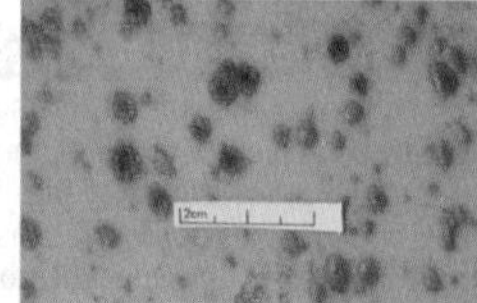

Fig 9.14 Chicken pox (VZV).

- *Shingles:* painful, hyperaesthetic area, then macular→vesicular rash in dermatomal distribution. Disseminated infection if immunosuppressed. Infectious until scabs appear. Chicken pox risk in non-immune contacts. Complications: post-herpetic neuralgia, Ramsay Hunt syndrome (p501).

Diagnosis: Clinical diagnosis unless immunosuppressed: viral PCR, culture, immunofluorescence.

Treatment: Oral aciclovir/valaciclovir for uncomplicated chicken pox/shingles in adults, aim to give within 48h of rash. IV aciclovir if pregnant, immunosuppressed, severe/disseminated disease (including ocular).

Prevention: Vaccination: not routine in children in UK, given at aged 70 to prevent shingles reactivation. VZV immunoglobulin if non-immune exposure in immunosuppression, pregnancy, neonates.

Epstein-Barr virus (EBV) (human herpesvirus 4)

Virus targets circulating B lymphocytes (lifelong latent infection) and squamous epithelial cells of oropharynx.

Presentation: Usually asymptomatic infection in childhood. Infectious mononucleosis in ~50% of primary infection in adults: sore throat, fever, anorexia, lymphadenopathy (esp. posterior triangle of neck), palatal petechiae, splenomegaly, hepatomegaly, jaundice. Malaise is prominent. Resolution of symptoms usually within 2 weeks. Chronic active infection and recurrence are rare. Oncogenicity: see BOX 'Oncogenic viruses'.

Diagnosis:

- Blood film: lymphocytosis. Atypical lymphocytes (large, irregular nuclei) also occur in other viral infection (CMV, HIV, parvovirus, dengue), toxoplasmosis, typhus, leukaemia, lymphoma, drug reactions, lead poisoning.
- Heterophile antibody tests (eg Monospot®, Paul-Bunnell) detect non-EBV heterophile antibodies which are present in ~85% of infectious mononucleosis sera. False positive: pregnancy, autoimmune disease, lymphoma/leukaemia.
- Serology: IgM to EBV viral capsid antigen in acute infection. IgG if past infection.
- Reverse transcriptase viral PCR.

Treatment: Supportive. ►Seek expert help if severe disease/immunosuppression: observational data on the use of antivirals and steroids.

Cytomegalovirus (CMV) (human herpesvirus 5)

50–100% of adults are seropositive depending on socioeconomic and sexual risk. Latent infection: periodic, asymptomatic (but infectious) viral shedding in bodily fluids including blood transfusion, transplantation (CMV+ve donor to CMV−ve recipient).

Presentation: Asymptomatic in most. Symptoms mimic infectious mononucleosis (see earlier in topic) or hepatitis. Severe disease in immunosuppressed (post-transplantation, HIV): oesophagitis, gastritis, colitis, retinitis (p438), pneumonitis, hepatitis. Infection in pregnancy is associated with congenital abnormality.

Diagnosis: Primary infection in immunocompetent: IgM. Immunosuppressed: quantitative nucleic acid amplification testing (QNAT) in blood greater than a defined threshold, or rising titre. Invasive disease: tissue QNAT, histopathology.

Treatment: Given in severe infection/immunosuppression. Ganciclovir, valganciclovir (↑oral bioavailability). Foscarnet and cidofovir: nephrotoxicity limit use. Pre-emptive treatment in transplant patients based on QNAT results. Risk/benefit for antivirals/immunoglobulin in pregnancy remains unclear. Use CMV−ve, irradiated blood for transfusion if immunosuppressed and at risk: transplant, HIV, leukaemia.

Other herpes viruses

Human herpesvirus 6 (HHV6): Roseola infantum, febrile illness without rash.

Human herpesvirus 8 (HHV8): Oncogenic (see BOX 'Oncogenic viruses'), Castleman's disease.

Oncogenic viruses

~12% of human cancers are caused by viruses, >80% of these occur in low- and middle-income countries (table 9.12).

Common traits of oncoviruses:

- Virus is necessary but not sufficient to cause cancer.
- Cancers appear in context of chronic infection, taking years-decades to appear.
- Immune system has variable role: cancers are associated with both immunosuppression and chronic inflammation.

Table 9.12 Oncogenic viruses

Virus	Cancers
EBV (HHV4)	Burkitt's lymphoma, Hodgkin's lymphoma, B-cell lymphoma in immunosuppression, gastric cancer, nasopharyngeal cancer, post-transplantation lymphoproliferative disease (PTLD)
HHV8	Kaposi's sarcoma (p400) and primary effusion lymphoma
HPV	Cancers of: cervix, anus, vulva, penis, head, neck, oropharynx (p406)
Hepatitis B and C	Hepatocellular carcinoma (p278)
HTLV-1	Human T-lymphotropic virus→adult T-cell leukaemia
MCV	Merkel cell polyomavirus→Merkel cell carcinoma

Other viruses

Respiratory tract viruses

Include rhinovirus, coronovirus, adenovirus, respiratory syncytial virus (RSV). Transmission by direct contact, infected fomites, airborne droplets. *Presentation:* Coryza, pharyngitis, croup, bronchiolitis, pneumonia. *Diagnosis:* Clinical. Viral culture, antigen detection, PCR. *Treatment:* None in uncomplicated disease/immunocompetent. Limited evidence for specific treatments in high-risk complicated disease, immunosuppression: cidofovir for adenovirus; aerosolized ribavarin, immunoglobulin, monoclonal antibody in RSV. For influenza see pp396-7.

Human papilloma virus (HPV)

>120 HPVs. Pathology:

- Skin warts, verrucas (HPV 1, 2). Treatment: none, topical salicylic acid, freezing.
- Anogenital warts (HPV 6, 11). Treatment: topical podophyllin, imiquimod; ablation.
- Cervical cancer (HPV 16, 18), other cancers (see p405).

Vaccination in UK: ♀ only, age 12–13, HPV 6, 11, 16, and 18 since 2012.

Polyomavirus

~100% exposure. Disease only with immunosuppression: BK virus causes renal transplant nephropathy; JC virus causes progressive multifocal leucoencephalopathy.

Measles

Transmitted by respiratory droplets. Incubation 10–18d. Highly contagious: >95% population coverage needed for 'herd' immunity. *Presentation:* Prodrome (2–4d): fever, conjunctivitis, coryza, diarrhoea, Koplik spots (white spots on red buccal mucosa, fig 9.15). Then generalized, maculopapular rash, classically face/neck→trunk→limbs (fig 9.16). Complications:

- Secondary infection: bacterial pneumonia, otitis media, ocular herpes simplex, oral/GI candidiasis.
- Acute demyelinating encephalitis: 1 in 1000, usually within 2wk of rash. Seizures, fever, irritability, headache, ↓conscious level.
- Subacute sclerosing panencephalitis: 5–10yr after infection, disturbances in intellect, personality, seizures, motor dysfunction, decerebration. No treatment available.

Diagnosis: Clinical. IgM. Antigen in saliva/urine. *Treatment:* Prevent with vaccination. Human immunoglobulin within 3d of exposure in non-immune. Supportive. No benefit shown for dexamethasone in encephalitis.

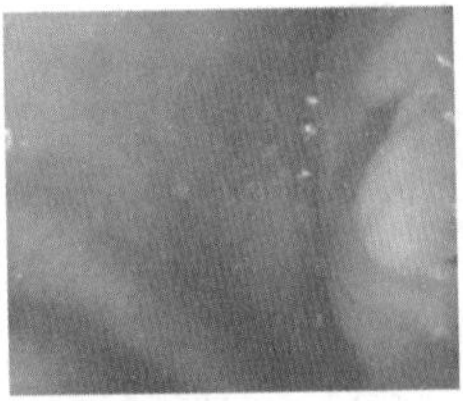

Fig 9.15 Koplik spots.
Courtesy of CDC.

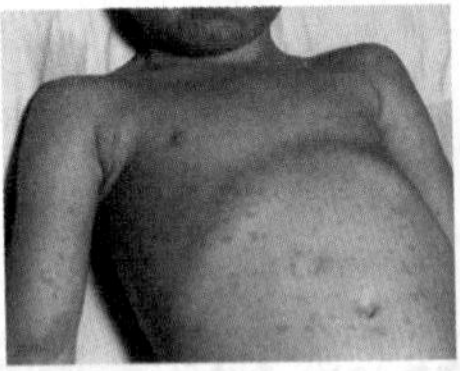

Fig 9.16 Measles rash.
Reproduced from Gardiner *et al.*, *Training in Paediatrics*, 2008, with permission from Oxford University Press.

Mumps

Respiratory droplet spread. Incubation 14–21d. Common cause of encephalitis pre-vaccination. *Presentation:* Can be subclinical. Prodrome: fever, myalgia, headache. Infection and tender swelling of salivary glands: parotid > submandibular. Complications: meningoencephalitis, epididymo-orchitis if pubertal/post-pubertal infection (warm, swollen, tender testes 4d–6wk after parotitis→subfertility in ~10%, infertility rare), oophoritis, pancreatitis, deafness. *Diagnosis:* Clinical. If confirmation needed eg meningitis/encephalitis: mumps specific IgM/IgA, PCR. *Treatment:* Supportive.

Rubella (German measles)

Respiratory droplet spread. *Presentation:* Usually mild/subclinical. Prodrome: fever, conjunctivitis, rhinorrhoea. Rash: generalized, pink, maculopapular. Lymphadenopathy: occipital, cervical, post-auricular. *Congenital infection:* Up to 90% risk of fetal malformation in 1st trimester, sensorineural hearing loss/retinopathy in 2nd trimester. Offer IgM/IgG testing. Immunoglobulin may ↓viraemia but will not prevent infection. ►Vaccinate *PRE*-pregnancy, live vaccines are contraindicated in pregnancy.

Immunization

Passive immunity uses pre-formed antibody to protect against infection. It offers immediate but short-lived protection. Natural passive immunity occurs in the placental transfer of maternal antibodies to the fetus; acquired passive immunity includes treatment with immunoglobulin eg hepatitis B, rabies, tetanus, varicella-zoster.

Active immunity follows exposure to an antigen, which generates an adaptive immune response. Natural active immunity occurs following infection. Acquired active immunity is provided by vaccination. Routine vaccinations in the UK are shown in table 9.13. Additional vaccines are offered to specific vulnerable groups (table 9.14).

Immunosuppression is a contraindication to live vaccines due to the risk of disseminated disease. Includes immunodeficiency, immunosuppressive treatment, HIV. Inactivated vaccines can be given but the antibody response may be less: aim to give >2wks prior to immunosuppressive therapy when possible (or vaccinate whilst on treatment and considered repeat re-immunization when/if treatment complete).

Table 9.13 UK vaccination summary (*=live vaccine)

Vaccination	Age (m=months, y=years)									
	2m	3m	4m	12m	>2y	3-5y	12y ♀	14y	>65y	70y
Diphtheria	+	+	+			+		+		
Tetanus	+	+	+			+		+		
Pertussis	+	+	+			+				
Poliomyelitis	+	+	+			+		+		
Haemophilus influenzae B (Hib)	+	+	+	+						
Pneumococcal	+		+	+						
Rotavirus*	+	+								
Meningitis B	+		+	+						
Meningitis C				+						
Measles, mumps, rubella*				+		+				
Influenza					+				+	
HPV 6, 11, 16, 18							+			
Meningitis ACWY								+		
Varicella zoster*										+

Table 9.14 Additional vaccination of specific groups in UK (*=live vaccine)

Vaccination	Offered to
BCG*	Infants/children where TB incidence >40/100 000 or parent/grandparent born in country where incidence >40/100 000, TB contacts.
Hib	Hyposplenism, complement disorders.
Meningitis B, ACWY	Hyposplenism, complement disorders.
Influenza	Hyposplenism, DM, chronic heart disease, chronic respiratory disease, CKD, chronic liver disease, chronic neurological disease, immunosuppression, pregnancy.
Pneumococcal	Hyposplenism, cochlear implants, complement disorders, DM, chronic heart disease, chronic respiratory disease, CKD, chronic liver disease, chronic neurological disease, immunosuppression.
Hepatitis A, B	Chronic liver disease, haemophilia, CKD (hepatitis B only).
Pertussis	Pregnancy 16–32 weeks (neonatal protection).

Travel

Travel advice (food/drink, insect repellent, malaria prophylaxis, condoms) is more important than vaccination. Check routine vaccinations are up to date. Vaccination depends upon area of travel and planned activities: BCG (live), rabies, yellow fever (live), hepatitis A/B, cholera, Japanese encephalitis, tick-borne encephalitis, typhoid. For up-to-date recommendations see http://www.fitfortravel.nhs.uk/destinations.

Fungi

Worldwide ↑ in fungal infection with new pathogenicity, ↑virulence, and new infective mechanisms. Incidence data limited by failures in recognition and diagnosis. Divided into superficial/cutaneous and systemic/invasive.

Superficial/cutaneous mycoses

- *Dermatophytosis:* Dermatophyte fungi digest keratin. Cause infection of skin and keratinized structures, eg hair, nails. *Presentation:* Scale and pruritus. Skin lesion may be annular with central healing, eg *ring worm, tinea corporis. Tinea pedis* affects up to 15% of healthy population: skin erosions and blisters in toe web spaces, dry scale on soles. *Fungal nail disease* = onychomycosis/tinea unguium: discolouration, nail thickening. *Tinea capitis:* scalp scaling, alopecia.
- *Superficial candidiasis:* Usually *Candida albicans* (fig 9.17), a commensal in mouth, vagina, and GI tract. Risk factors: immunosuppression, antibiotic treatment. *Presentation: Oropharyngeal:* white patches on erythematous background (plaque type); sore, inflamed areas (erythematous type). *GU:* soreness, white patches/discharge (fig 9.18). *Skin:* usually in folds/interdigital (fig 9.19).

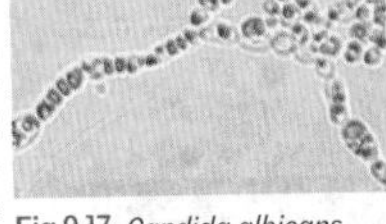

Fig 9.17 *Candida albicans.*
Courtesy of P-Y Guillaume.

- *Malassezia:* Commensals of greasy skin. *Presentation: Pityriasis versicolor:* scaly hypo/hyperpigmented rash with scaling (fig 9.20). *Seborrhoeic dermatitis:* scaling of face, scalp (dandruff), anterior chest. *Malassezia folliculitis:* itchy, follicular rash on back and shoulders (ΔΔ acne).

Diagnosis: Clinical, microscopy of skin scrapings. *Treatment:* All superficial mycoses: topical '-azole' antifungal or terbinafine 1–4wk. Also topical nystatin and amphotericin in superficial candidiasis. Tinea capitis: griseofulvin, terbinafine, itraconazole. Nail infection requires systemic treatment (terbinafine, itraconazole)∴ confirm diagnosis, and caution re side-effects including hepatotoxicity.

Systemic/invasive mycoses

- *Invasive candidiasis:* Typically occurs in immunocompromised, comorbidity, or ITU settings. Genetic susceptibility likely contributes. Estimated 250 000/yr with 50 000 deaths. Candidaemia in ~7/1000 ICU patients. *Presentation:* Risk factors for invasive fungal disease (see p409), febrile with no microbiological evidence of infection, new murmur, muscle tenderness, skin nodules. *Diagnosis:* (Repeated) blood/tissue culture. PCR. Candida in respiratory secretions alone is insufficient. *Treatment:* Remove all possible catheters. Echinocandins (caspofungin, anidulafungin, micafungin), fluconazole, amphotericin (liposomal for ↓renal toxicity). Consider fluconazole prophylaxis if risk factors for invasive disease (p403). Consider empirical treatment if persistent fever, unresponsive to other therapy (discuss with microbiologist, choice depends on local epidemiology, comorbidity).
- *Cryptococcus:* See HIV p400. Causes meningitis, pneumonia. *Presentation:* Usually immunosuppression, eg HIV, sarcoid, Hodgkin's, haematological malignancy, post-transplant. History may be long, non-specific. Headache, confusion, ataxia, focal neurological signs, fever, cough, pleuritic pain, SOB. *Diagnosis:* Indian ink CSF stain, culture blood/CSF/BAL, antigen testing in blood/CSF. *Treatment:* Amphotericin + flucytosine, fluconazole.
- *Histoplasmosis:* Worldwide distribution of *Histoplasma,* ↑ in soil contaminated with bird/bat faeces. Illness depends on host immunity, estimated ~1%. *Presentation:* Flu-like symptoms, fever, malaise, cough, headache, myalgia, pneumonia, lung nodules/cavitation, pericarditis, mediastinal fibrosis/granuloma (ΔΔ sarcoid, TB). *Diagnosis:* Serology, antigen testing. *Treatment:* Moderate-severe lung disease or any CNS involvement: amphotericin, itraconazole.
- *Blastomycosis: Blastomyces* in decomposing matter, mainly USA/Canada. *Presentation:* Fever, cough, night sweats, ARDS. ↑risk of extra-pulmonary disease with immunosuppression: skin, bone, GU, CNS. *Diagnosis:* Culture, antigen detection (cross-reacts with histoplasmosis). *Treatment:* Amphotericin, itraconazole.

►See also: Fungi and the lung p177, *Pneumocystis jirovecii* p400.

Invasive fungal infection

Invasion: fungus in normally sterile tissues.
Dissemination: infection of remote organs via haematogenous spread.
►Suspect an invasive fungal infection in:

1 Any patient with risk factors (see table 9.15).
2 Any systemically unwell patient who fails to respond to antibiotic therapy.
3 Any persistently febrile patient with no microbiological evidence of infection.

Table 9.15 Risk factors associated with invasive fungal infection.

Risk factor	Includes
Infection	HIV, CMV, TB, colonization/inadequate treatment of superficial fungal disease, broad-spectrum antibiotics, prior fungal infection.
Malignancy	Neutropenia, mucositis, haematological malignancy.
Critical illness	↑Mortality prediction score (eg APACHE), prolonged ITU admission, prolonged ventilation, severe trauma/pancreatitis.
Catheter	Central venous catheter, urinary catheter, dialysis access, TPN.
Transplantation	Immunosuppressant medication, recent rejection, graft-versus-host disease.
Genetic	Hereditary chronic granulomatous disease, abnormalities in tumour necrosis factor/interleukins/cytokines.
Surgical	Major surgery, GI perforation, anastomotic leak, length of transplant operation, delayed closure.
Other comorbidity	Any disease managed with immunosuppressive therapy, burns.

Data source: Ramana KV *et al.* Invasive fungal infections. *Am J Infectious Diseases and Microbiology* 2013, 1(4);64–69.

Investigations:

- Blood culture: three samples, different sites, same sitting, aim total 40–60mL blood.
- Microscopy+immunohistochemistry/fluorescence depending on site/risk.
- Other: antigen/antibody testing for general (eg mannan, galactomannan) and specific (eg cryptococcal) fungi; fungal metabolites; PCR: for typing/confirmation.

►Seek expert advice on empirical treatment, agent depends on local epidemiology.

Facts of life for 'budding' mycologists

To the uninitiated, fungi are like bacteria, but their chitin cell walls and their knack of mitosis puts them in their own kingdom. They are larger than bacteria (eg 8μm across), and mostly reproduce by budding of germ tubes (fig 9.21), not by fission. Yeasts occur as single cells or as clusters. Hyphae often occur in a mass of cells (called moulds). A hyphal cell with cross-walls is called a mycelium. Some yeasts are dimorphic: single cells at 37°C but forming structures called mycelia, containing fruiting bodies (hyphae), at room temperature.

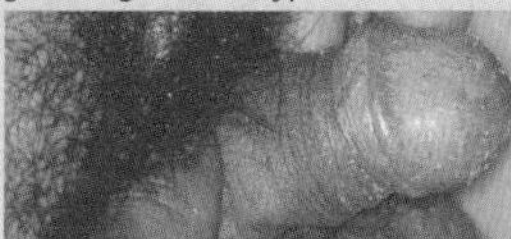

Fig 9.18 Candida of the glans.
Courtesy of P-Y Guillaume.

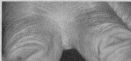

Fig 9.19 Web-space candida.
Courtesy of A Huntley.

Fig 9.20 Pityriasis versicolor.
Reproduced from Lewis-Jones (ed), *Paediatric Dermatology* 2010, with permission from Oxford University Press.

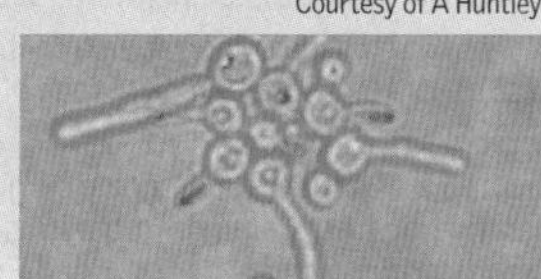

Fig 9.21 Germ tubes emerging from dimorphic *Candida albicans* blastospores.
Courtesy of P-Y Guillaume.

Healthcare-associated (nosocomial) infection

Healthcare-associated, or nosocomial, infections include diseases which occur:

- As a direct result of treatment or contact in a hospital or healthcare setting.
- As a result of healthcare delivered in the community.
- Outside a healthcare setting but are brought in by patients, staff, or visitors and transmitted to others.

7-25% of hospital admissions are complicated by a nosocomial infection resulting in morbidity, mortality, and cost. The causal microbe may be benign in normal circumstances, but is able to cause disease when the patient:

1 has been given broad-spectrum antibiotics (eg antibiotic-resistant organisms, *Clostridium difficile* colitis)
2 is unwell/immunosuppressed (opportunistic infection)
3 has compromised barriers (indwelling catheter/line, ventilation, surgery).

Healthcare-associated infection

Catheter-associated UTI:
A catheter is inserted in ~20% of hospitalized patients. UTI is the most common infection acquired as a result of healthcare, accounting for 19% of all healthcare-associated infection. ~50% of UTIs are associated with a urethral catheter. Risk of infection is related to method of catheter insertion, duration of catheter, quality of catheter care, and patient susceptibility.

To reduce risk, only catheterize if necessary: Is there obstruction? Do you need precise urine output monitoring? Remove as soon as possible. See UTI pp296–7.

Infections associated with the use of intravascular access devices:
Includes peripheral, central venous, and arterial catheters: tunnelled and non-tunnelled. >60% of bloodstream infections are associated with intravascular devices. Risk is higher with central catheters. Infection can result from introduction of microbes during insertion, access (eg when giving IV antibiotics), or from microbes elsewhere in the body seeding to the foreign material. Organisms include *Staphylococcus epidermidis* (p388), *Staphylococcus aureus* (including meticillin-resistant forms ►MRSA see p388), *Candida* species (p408), and enterococci (p389).

Ensure that vascular access devices are used only when clinically indicated. Switch to oral treatment (fluid, medication, nutrition) as soon as clinically appropriate. Treatment includes removal/exchange of the device whenever possible.

Ventilator-associated pneumonia (VAP):
VAP affects up to 20% of patients admitted to intensive care units. Occurs as the endotracheal tube interferes with protective upper airway reflexes and facilitates microaspiration. Risks ↓ with non-invasive ventilation. In critical illness, the oropharynx becomes contaminated with Gram−ve bacteria due to antibiotic exposure, altered host defences, and changes in mucosal adherence. Access to the airway occurs via folds in the endotracheal cuff and the bacterial biofilm is then propelled to the distal airways. Organisms include *Pseudomonas aeruginosa* (p391), Enterobacteriaceae (p391), and *Staphylococcus aureus* (p388).

Clinical diagnosis has ↓sensitivity and ↓specificity. Suspect if new/persistent infiltrates on CXR plus two or more of: purulent sputum, leucocytosis (>12×10^9/L), leucopenia (<4×10^9/L), temperature >38.3°C.

Prevent by reducing colonization (mouthwash, silver-coated endotracheal tubes), nurse at 45° to ↓ aspiration risk, wean off ventilator as soon as possible.

Surgical site infection:
Affects 5% of patients undergoing surgical procedures, contributes to >⅓ of post-operative deaths. Common organisms include *Staphylococcus aureus* (p388), *Streptococcus pyogenes* (p388), and Enterobacteriaceae when surgery involves entry to hollow viscera (p391). Prevention methods include hand hygiene, strict asepsis, MRSA screening and decolonization, hair removal, peri-operative normothermia, minimally disturbed low adherence/transparent dressings.

Clostridium difficile

Gram-positive anaerobic bacillus and most common healthcare-associated pathogen. Part of colonic flora in 2-5% of healthy adults, and 20-40% of hospitalized adults. Disease occurs when it converts to a vegetative (growth) state with production of enterotoxins A and B, causing colitis. Typically happens when inhibition by competing colonic flora is lost due to antibiotic exposure.

Presentation: Watery diarrhoea, mild→fulminant colitis (pseudomembranes on endoscopy='pseudomembranous colitis'), ileus, toxic megacolon. Consider in all diarrhoea associated with antibiotic use, especially if marked neutrophilia.

Diagnosis: Immunoassay for glutamate dehydrogenase (common antigen) detects all strains of *C. difficile*. Detection of toxin (toxin immunoassay, toxin gene nucleic acid amplification) distinguishes infection from carriage.

Management: SIGHT: Suspect, Isolate within 2h, Gloves and aprons, Hand wash with soap, Test immediately.

- Mild/moderate: metronidazole PO.
- Severe (WCC $>15\times10^9$/L or AKI or colitis or temperature >38.5°C): vancomycin PO (injection preparation can be given orally and is cheaper than capsules) or fidaxomicin (↑cost).
- Non-responders: high-dose vancomycin+IV metronidazole, fidaxomicin, IV immunoglubulin (no RCT data).
- Recurrence: (weaning) vancomycin, fidaxomicin, faecal transplantation.

Management of healthcare-associated infection

Identify: Screening (eg hospital admissions for MRSA) allows isolation and decolonization before harm. Be alert to new infections.

Protect: Isolate multi-antibiotic-resistant microbes (eg MRSA), highly transmissible infections (eg norovirus), and high-risk groups including reverse barrier nursing (avoids transmission to, rather than from, patients, eg neutropenia). Patients with high-risk infections may need negative-pressure rooms (to prevent potentially infected air leaving the room), or in severe immunosuppression, positive-pressure rooms (to prevent potentially infected air entering the room). When many patients have the same nosocomial infection (eg norovirus) they may be barrier nursed together in dedicated bays.

Treat: Refer to local guidelines, seek expert help. Initial antibiotic choice may differ for healthcare-associated infection.

Prevent: Modify risk factors, eg nutrition, post-operative incentive spirometry to reduce pneumonia risk. Use/convert to narrow-spectrum antibiotics whenever possible. Remove catheters, intravascular access devices, and wean off ventilators as soon as clinically appropriate. Take measures to ↓ person-to-person transmission:

1 *Hand hygiene.* Wash hands before and after each patient contact (fig 9.22). Alcohol-based gels are helpful but soap is needed to kill *C. difficile* spores.

2 *Personal attire.* In the UK there is a bare-below-the-elbows policy. Long hair should be tied back. In areas where infection risk is particularly high (theatre, ICU), staff change into scrubs on arrival.

3 *Personal protective equipment (PPE).* Used for isolated patients and during procedures. Includes gloves, aprons, caps, respiratory protection/mask according to risk, eg FFP3 respirators in aerosolized infection.

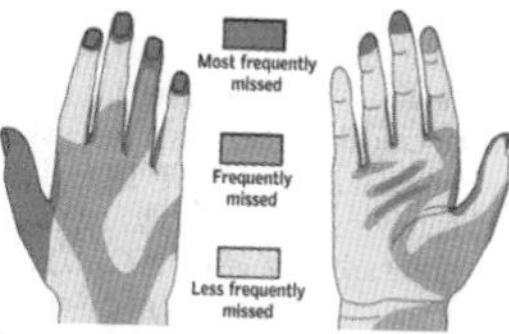

Fig 9.22 Areas commonly missed when washing hands.

Contains public sector information licensed under Open Government Licence v3.0, www.whatdotheyknow.com/request/21861/response/56086/attach/3/04072 Hand Hygiene 5 1.1.pdf

4 *Procedures.* Strict aseptic techniques for any procedure which breaches the body's defences including insertion/maintenance of invasive devices, IV infusions, wound care.

5 *Environment.* Should be clean and safe, with effective decontamination.

System interventions: Up-to-date infection guidelines, audit, education, training.[8]

Sexually transmitted infection (STI)

STIs[6] are common with increasing rates of diagnosis: ~×2 for *Chlamydia trachomatis, N. gonorrhoeae*, genital herpes, and syphilis since 2006. Prevalence highest in young adults (<25yr) and MSM. For HIV see pp398–403. For hepatitis B and C see p278.

Taking a sexual history
- *Symptoms:* ♂: urethral discharge, dysuria, genital skin problems, testicular pain/swelling, peri-anal or anal symptoms in MSM. ♀: unusual vaginal discharge, vulval skin problems, abdominal pain, dyspareunia, unusual vaginal bleeding (post-coital, intermenstrual, consider referral for urgent colposcopy).
- *Exposure:* Sexual contacts within last 3 months including sex of partner(s), type of contact (oral, vaginal, anal), contraceptive method (properly used?), type and duration of relationship, symptoms in partner(s), risk factors for HIV/hepatitis in partner(s), whether partner(s) can be contacted. STI history in all. Ask men whether they have ever had sex with another man.
- *Other:* Last menstrual period, menstrual pattern, date of last cervical cytology (smear). Current contraceptive, difficulties with use/supply. Current/recent antimicrobial therapy. HPV vaccine history. There may be disclosure of non-consensual sex, or intimate partner violence. Do not be afraid to ask for help: '*Everything you tell me today is confidential unless you tell me something that worries me about your safety, at which point I may need to discuss this with another professional in order to keep you safe.*'

Examination
♂: retract foreskin, inspect urethral meatus for discharge, scrotal contents/tenderness/swelling (stand patient up). ♀: vulval examination (lithotomy), speculum of vagina/cervix, bimanual examination for adnexal tenderness, abdomen/pelvis for masses. In all: genitoanal area, protoscopy if anal symptoms, inguinal lymph nodes, oral mucosa if orogenital sex. Use a chaperone and document their name.

Urethritis/vaginal discharge See table 9.16.

Genital warts Caused by human papilloma virus (HPV). See p406.

Genital ulcer(s)
- *Genital herpes:* HSV. *Presentation:* flu-like prodrome, then vesicles/papules around genitals, anus, throat. These burst, forming painful shallow ulcers. Also urethral discharge, dysuria, urinary retention, proctitis. *Diagnosis:* PCR. *Treatment:* analgesia, topical lidocaine. Antivirals within 5d: aciclovir, valaciclovir, famciclovir.
- *Syphilis: Treponema pallidum. Presentation:*
  1 Primary: <90d after innoculation (median 3wk). Macule→papule→typically painless ulcer (chancre). Central slough, defined rolled edge. Highly infectious.
  2 Secondary: dissemination ~4–10wks after chancre. Rash (maculopapular in 50–75%, on palms/soles in 11–70%), mucous patches, condyloma lata (raised, pale plaques, often flexural), fever, headache, myalgia, lymphadenopathy, hepatitis.
  3 Tertiary: 20–40yr after infection. *Neurosyphilis:* aseptic meningitis, focal neurological deficits, seizures, psychiatric symptoms, Argyll Robertson pupil (p72), tabes dorsalis (areflexia, extensor plantar reflex, dorsal column deficits, Charcot joints). *Gummatous syphilis:* destructive granulomata in skin, mucus membranes, bones, viscera. *Cardiovascular:* aortitis, aortic regurgitation/aneurysm.

  Diagnosis: PCR. Serology: non-specific (RPR, VDRL) sensitive in early infection then decline; specific (*T. pallidum* as antigen, eg TPHA, TPPA) reacts in early infection and persists. *Treatment:* parenteral benzylpenicillin (eg benzathine penicillin IM), duration depends on stage. Procaine benzylpenicillin boosted with probenicid in CSF disease
- *Lymphogranuloma venerum: Chlamydia trachomatis. Presentation:* mostly MSM in UK. Painless papule/ulcer→lymphadenopathy, fever, arthritis, pneumonitis. Direct transmission to rectal mucosa causes haemorrhagic proctitis: pain, rectal bleeding/discharge, tenesmus. *Diagnosis:* PCR. *Treatment:* doxycycline.
- *Tropical infections:* Chancroid (*Haemophilus ducreyi*), Donovanosis (*Klebsiella granulomatis*). *Presentation:* both cause genital ulceration, and lymphadenitis with spread of infection into overlying tissue (pseudobubo). *Diagnosis: H. ducreyi* PCR, Donovan bodies in tissue. *Treatment:* azithromycin, ceftriaxone.

Table 9.16 Overview of urethritis and vaginal discharge

STI	Presentation	Diagnosis	Treatment	Other
Chlamydia trachomatis	Often asymptomatic: detected on screening. ♀: dyspareunia, dysuria, post-coital/inter-menstrual bleeding, ↑vaginal discharge. ♂: dysuria, urethral discharge.	Nucleic acid amplification test (NAAT) on: ♀: vulvovaginal swab—can be done by patient. Endocervical swabs and urine samples less sensitive. ♂: first-pass urine. Oral/anal swabs if oral/anal sex.	Azithromycin 1g PO (single dose) or 100mg doxycycline BD for 7d. Partner tracing, screening, treatment. Avoid sexual intercourse until treatment complete.	Pharyngeal and rectal infection may be asymptomatic. Complications: ♀: pelvic inflammatory disease, salpingitis, infertility, ectopic pregnancy, reactive arthritis, perihepatitis (Fitz-Hugh-Curtis syndrome). ♂: epididymo-orchitis, reactive arthritis. Eye disease see p438.
Neisseria gonorrhoeae	Urethral/vaginal discharge, dysuria. Asymptomatic: 50% ♀, 10% ♂, most pharyngeal/rectal infection.	Nucleic acid amplification test (NAAT) on: ♀: vaginal swab or endocervical swab. Urine samples less sensitive. ♂: first-pass urine. Culture (endocervical/urethral swab prior to antibiotics) for sensitivity.	Ceftriaxone 500mg IM + azithromycin 1g PO. Complicated disease: add doxycycline ± metronidazole. Partner tracing, screening, treatment. Avoid sexual intercourse until treatment complete.	↑Antibiotic resistance. Complications: ♀: pelvic inflammatory disease: salpingitis, infertility, ectopic pregnancy. ♂: epididymitis, prostatitis, increased HIV transmission, reactive arthritis; infective endocarditis, disseminated gonococcal infection.
Non-gonococcal urethritis (NGU)	Urethral discharge, dysuria, urethral discomfort. Only assess symptomatic patients/visible discharge for urethritis.	↑Polymorphonuclear leucocytes on microscopy of urethral swab. Needs testing for chlamydia and gonorrhoea. Exclude UTI.	As for *Chlamydia trachomatis*. 5d course of azithromycin if patient/partner known to be positive for *Mycoplasma genitalium*.	NGU refers to a pattern of infection rather than a cause. The main causes are *Chlamydia trachomatis* (11–50%) and *Mycoplasma genitalium* (6–50%).
Trichomonas vaginalis	♀: vaginal discharge (~70%), itch. ♂: asymptomatic (~70%), discharge.	NAAT, culture, microscopy (mobile trichomonads).	Metronidazole (2g single dose or 5–7d course). Partner tracing, screening, treatment. Avoid sexual intercourse until treatment complete.	Pregnancy: ↑risk of preterm delivery, low birth weight. May enhance HIV transmission.
Bacterial vaginosis	Thin, white, fishy-smelling vaginal discharge. No itch or soreness. Asymptomatic in ~50%.	Gram stain to examine vaginal flora (predominance/absence of lactobacilli), clue cells, vaginal pH >4.5.	Oral or PV metronidazole or PV clindamycin.	Elevated vaginal pH alters vaginal flora: ↑anaerobic bacteria. Not sexually transmitted but associated with STI.
Genital candidiasis	Genital itch, burning, cottage cheese-like discharge, dyspareunia.	Microscopy and culture for *Candida* (see p408).	-azoles: pessary, eg clotrimazole, cream if vulval symptoms, oral fluconazole if severe.	Very common. No evidence for treatment of sexual partners. ↑Risk: pregnant, antibiotic therapy, DM, immunosuppressed.

Fever in the returning traveller

► Exclude malaria in all travellers from the tropics (p416–9).
► Exclude HIV in all (p398).
► Most travellers have self-limiting illnesses that could have been acquired in UK. Look for tropical infection[9] but don't forget your usual differentials.

History Detailed geography of travel (table 9.17)[9] including setting (rural/urban), time of onset of symptoms, duration of symptoms (table 9.18).[9] Ask about activities and events: bites, diet, fresh-water exposure (schistosomiasis, leptospirosis), dust exposure, sexual activity, game parks (tick typhus, anthrax, trypanosomiasis), farms, caves (histoplasmosis, rabies, Ebola), unwell contacts.

Associated symptoms:

- Respiratory: *S. pneumoniae, H. influenzae,* legionella, influenza, viral respiratory disease (SARS, MERS), TB, HIV-associated disease, melioidosis.[2]
- Neurological: malaria, meningococcal meningitis, HIV, syphilis, Lyme disease, leptospirosis, brucellosis, tick-borne encephalitis, relapsing fever, trypanosomiasis.

Table 9.17 Differential diagnosis by geography

Area of travel	Common	Occasional	Rare but do not miss
Sub-Saharan Africa	Malaria (pp416–9) HIV (pp398–403) Rickettsiae (p422)	Schistosomiasis (p434) Amoebiasis (p432) Brucellosis (p424) Dengue (p420) Enteric fever (p415) Meningococcus (p390)	Other arbovirus (p420) Trypanosomiasis (p423) VHF (pp426–7) Visceral leishmaniasis (p423)
South-East Asia	Malaria (pp416–9) Chikungunya (p420) Dengue (p420) Enteric fever (p415)	Leptospirosis (p425) Melioidosis[2]	Hanta virus (p426) Japanese encephalitis (p436) Rickettsiae (p422) Scrub typhus (p422)
South and Central Asia	Malaria (pp416–9) Dengue (p420) Enteric fever (p415)	Chikungunya (p420) Visceral leishmaniasis (p423)	VHF (CCHF) (pp426–7) Rickettsiae (p422) Japanese encephalitis (p436)
Middle East Mediterranean North Africa		Brucellosis (p424) Q-fever (p424) Zika (p421)	Visceral leishmaniasis (p423)
South America Caribbean	Malaria (pp416–9) Dengue (p420) Enteric fever (p415)	Brucellosis (p424) Leptospirosis (p425) Zika (p421)	Trypansomiasis (p423) Hanta virus (p426) Yellow fever (p420)
Eastern Europe Scandinavia		Lyme disease (p422)	Hanta virus (p426) Tick-borne encephalitis
Australia		Dengue (p420) Q fever (p424) Rickettsiae (p422)	Melioidosis[2]
North America		Lyme disease (p422) Rickettsiae (p422)	Melioidosis[2]

Table 9.18 Differential diagnosis according to incubation time

Incubation period	Infections
Short <10d	Dengue, chikungunya, gastroenteritis, relapsing fever, rickettsiae
Medium 10–21d	Malaria, HIV, brucellosis, enteric fever, leptospirosis, melioidosis, Q-fever, coccidioidomycosis, VHF, Chagas' disease, trypanosomiasis
Long >21d	Malaria, HIV, TB, viral hepatitis, brucellosis, schistosomiasis, amoebic liver abscess, trypanosomiasis, visceral leishmaniasis
Chronic fever <14d	TB, HIV plus opportunistic infection, pyogenic deep seated abscess, infective endocarditis, brucellosis, enteric fever, fungal infection, schistosomiasis, visceral leishmaniasis, PE

2 *Burkholderia pseudomallei* in tropical water/soil. Causes pneumonia, pleural effusions, pulmonary abscess. Systemic abscess if haematogenous spread: liver, spleen, skin, muscle. Treat with co-amoxiclav, doxycycline, co-trimoxazole. In severe disease: ceftazidime, meropenem.

Examination

Rash:

- *Maculopapular:* dengue, chikungunya, EBV, HIV seroconversion, VHF.
- *Purpuric:* dengue, meningococcal infection, plague, DIC, VHF.
- *Ulcer:* trypanosomiasis, *Yesinia pestis,* tick typhus, anthrax, tropical ulcer.

Jaundice: Viral hepatitis, severe falciparum malaria, enteric fever, leptospirosis, relapsing fever, typhus, VHF, bartonellosis

Hepatosplenomegaly: Viral hepatitis, HIV, enteric fever, brucellosis, leptospirosis, rickettsial infection, relapsing fever, schistosomiasis, amoebic liver abscess, trypanosomiasis, visceral leishmaniasis.

Investigation

Directed by travel history and examination. In undifferentiated fever:

- Malaria film/rapid diagnostic testing (p417).
- HIV test (p399).
- FBC: lymphopenia in viral infection including HIV; eosinophilia in parasitic/fungal eg soil-transmitted helminths, filiariasis, schistosomiasis, hydatid disease; ↓platelets in malaria, dengue, HIV, typhoid, severe sepsis.
- Blood culture ×2: prior to antibiotics.
- LFT.
- Consider: save serum, specific serology, or EDTA sample for PCR.

Support

- Local infectious diseases team (including on-call).
- Disease notification: www.gov.uk/health-protection-team.
- Public Health England imported fever service 0844 778 8990.
- National Travel Health Network and Centre (NaTHNaC)/TravelHealthPro www.travelhealthpro.org.uk (0845 602 6712).
- Hospital for Tropical Diseases 0203 456 7890.
- Travel fever diagnostic website: www.fevertravel.ch

Enteric fever: typhoid and paratyphoid

~20 million cases and 200 000 deaths per year worldwide, ~500/yr in UK mostly imported from India, Pakistan, and Bangladesh. Caused by related, Gram-negative strains of 'typhoidal' *Salmonella* spp:

- Typhoid (~75–90%): *Salmonella typhi.*
- Paratyphoid (~10–25%, less severe): *Salmonella paratyphi* serotype A>B>C.

The bacteria invade the intestinal mucosa. Dissemination occurs without a primary diarrhoeal response. This distinguishes 'typhoidal' from 'non-typhoidal' serovars of *Salmonella* which cause D&V (p428). Transmission is faecal-oral from contaminated water/food. Incubation 6–30d (most 10–20d). ~10 000 organisms are required to cause illness. Can be asymptomatic (but shed organism).

Symptoms: Fatigue, headache, anorexia. Marked fever, 'stepwise' (rising through each day with progressive peaks) in <20%. Abdominal pain, relative bradycardia (Faget's sign), cough, constipation. Rose spots in ~25% (salmon-coloured, 1–4cm, blanching, due to bacterial emboli to dermis). Diarrhoea ('pea-soup') and hepatosplenomegaly in 2nd week. Progressive toxicity and complicated disease in up to 10%: intestinal haemorrhage/perforation, myocarditis, hepatitis, pneumonia, DIC, CNS involvement (delirium, meningism, encephalitis, cerebellar signs, fits, coma), eye complications (corneal ulcer, uveitis, neuritis, thrombosis).

Diagnosis: Isolation of *S. typhi* from: blood (take multiple cultures of 10–15mL in first 10d to ↑ sensitivity), bone marrow, intestinal secretions, or stool (↑sensitivity after 1st week). Serology has ↓ sensitivity and specificity, not sufficient as sole diagnostic tool (Widal test is −ve in ~30% of culture-proven cases). ↑LFT. PCR (not routine).

Treatment: Azithromycin ± IV ceftriaxone. >70% imported from Asia are resistant to fluoroquinolones. Fever takes median 5–7d to respond due to intracellular niche of organism. Antipyretics, fluid management, nutrition. CNS disease: dexamethasone 3mg/kg IV then 1mg/kg/6h for 8 doses (limited data).

Vaccine: Ty21a (oral, live, CI: immunosuppression, pregnancy) or Vi (IM, capsular vaccine). ~50–80% effective for ~3yr. Limited/no protection against paratyphoid.

Epidemiology

- 3.2 billion people at risk in 95 countries = half the world's population (fig 9.23).
- 214 million/cases per year with 438 000 deaths.
- Sub-Saharan Africa: 88% of malaria cases, 90% of deaths (most age <5yr).
- Most common tropical disease imported into UK, ~2000 cases/yr.
- ~20% fever in travellers from Africa presenting to UK hospitals is due to malaria.
- *Plasmodium falciparum* is the most prevalent parasite in Africa and responsible for most malaria deaths worldwide (=~75% of malaria presenting in UK).
- *Plasmodium vivax* is the dominant parasite outside of sub-Saharan Africa.
- Preventable and treatable: incidence ↓ by 37% and deaths ↓ by 60% since 2000.

Malaria parasites

Malaria parasites belong to the genus *Plasmodium*. >100 species exist of which 5 cause human disease (see table 9.19). Transmission occurs through the bite of an infected *Anopheles* mosquito. Only female mosquitoes transmit *Plasmodium* as only females require a blood meal for egg development. Transmission in the absence of a mosquito is rare: vertical (congenital transfer from mother to child), transfusion, organ transplantation, needle-sharing.

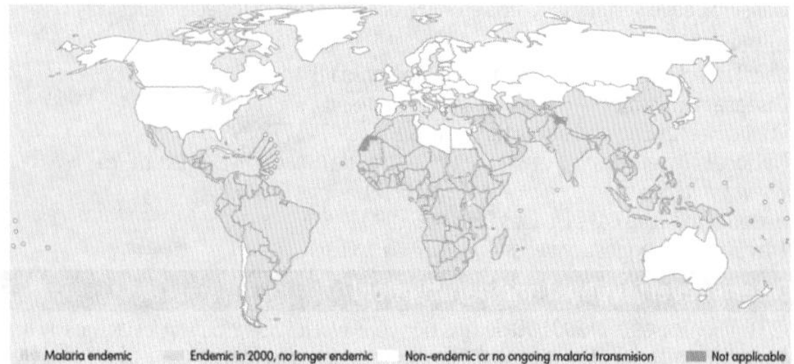

Fig 9.23 Countries with malaria transmission.

Reproduced with permission from World Health Organization, *World malaria report 2015*. © World Health Organization 2015. http://www.who.int/malaria/publications/world-malaria-report-2015/report/en/

Table 9.19 Malaria species in humans

Species	Average incubation (range)	Persistent liver stage	Distribution
P. falciparum (fig 9.24)	12 days (6 days–6 months)	No	Africa, India, South East Asia, Indonesia, Oceania, Central America, Middle East
P. vivax (fig 9.25)	14 days (days–years)	Yes	South Asia, South and Central America, Africa, Middle East
P. malariae (fig 9.26)	30 days (28 days–years)	No	Africa, South and Central America, South East Asia
P. ovale	11–16 days (years)	Yes	Africa
P. knowlesi	9–12 days	No	South East Asia

Reproduced from Detels *et al.*, *Oxford Textbook of Global Public Health*, 2015, with permission from Oxforc University Press

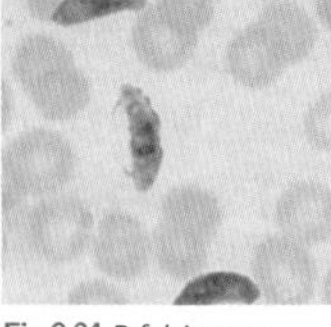

Fig 9.24 *P. falciparum* sausage-like gametocytes in RBC. ©S Upton, Kansas Univ.

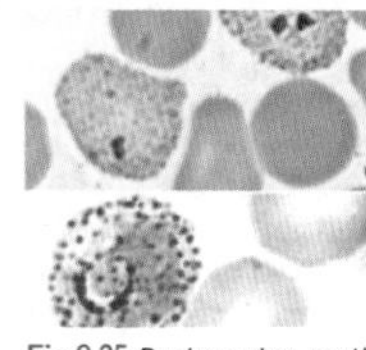

Fig 9.25 *P. vivax* ring partly hidden by Schuffner's dots. Stained and examined in the field by JML.

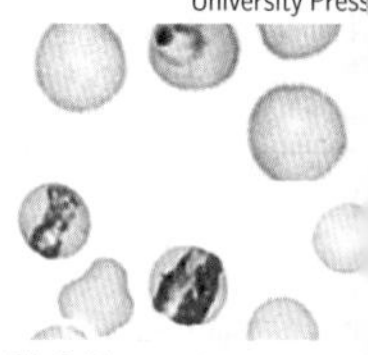

Fig 9.26 *P. malariae* ring ar band forms from 2 specimens ©S Upton, Kansas Uni

The life cycle of malaria is dependent on both humans and mosquitoes (fig 9.27). Sporozoites are transferred to a human host when an infected mosquito bites. These travel via the bloodstream to the liver where maturation occurs to form schizonts containing ~30 000 merozoite offspring. If a dormant stage exists (*vivax, ovale,* see table 9.19), and is inadequately treated, merozoites can be released from the liver weeks, months, or years later causing recurrent disease. The rupture of schizonts releases merozoites which enter RBCs (*'what a fantastic niche!'*). In the RBC, merozoites form larger trophozoites and erthrocytic schizonts (poor prognostic indicator if seen on blood film). The rupture of erthrocytic schizonts produces the clinical manifestations of malaria.

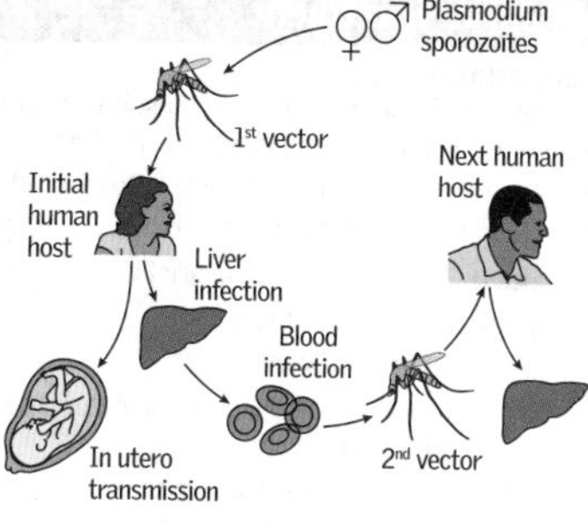

Fig 9.27 Malaria lifecycle.

Clinical features

►Consider in anyone with a fever who has previously visited a malarial area (fig 9.23), regardless of prophylaxis.

Presentation: P. falciparum has a minimum incubation of 6 days and most commonly occurs within 3 months of return from an endemic area. Take a careful travel history: country, area of travel, date of return. Do not forget to ask about stopovers. Symptoms are non-specific: fever, headache, malaise, myalgia, diarrhoea, cough. Fever patterns are described but only occur if rupture of infected RBCs is synchronized: alternate day for *P. falciparum, P. vivax, P. ovale ('tertian')*; every 3rd day for *P. malariae ('quartan')*. ►Most patients have no specific fever pattern.

Examination: Fever, otherwise unremarkable. If diagnosis is delayed or severe disease then may present with jaundice, confusion, seizures.

Diagnosis

Immediate blood testing is mandatory in UK:
- Microscopy of thick and thin blood smear. Sensitive and specific in experienced hands.
- Rapid diagnostic test (RDT) detection of parasite antigen. Used for initial screen if expert microscopy is unavailable, eg out-of-hours. Used in addition to (not instead of) blood film.

Results should be available within 4h. ►If malaria is suspected but blood film is negative: repeat at 12–24h and after further 24h. Malaria is unlikely if three expert serial blood films are negative. ΔΔ dengue, typhoid, hepatitis, meningitis/encephalitis, HIV, viral haemorrhagic fever. Care in pregnancy: thick films can be negative despite parasites in the placenta. Seek expert help.

If *P. falciparum* (or *P. knowlesi*) estimated % parasitized red cells should be given:
- >2% = ↑ chance of severe disease (indication for parenteral treatment see pp418–9).
- >10% = severe disease.

Other: FBC (anaemia, thrombocytopenia), creatinine and urine output (AKI), clotting (DIC), glucose (hypoglycaemia), ABG/lactate (acidosis), urinalysis (haemoglobinuria). Malaria is notifiable to public health: www.gov.uk/health-protection-team

Errors to avoid

- Failure to consider diagnosis
- Inadequate travel history
- Belief prophylaxis prevents all malaria
- Belief presents with a fever pattern
- Non-specific symptoms not recognized
- Delay in blood film/RDT
- No serial blood film if first test negative
- Inadequate treatment (pp418–9)
- Inappropriate treatment (pp418–9)
- Failure to anticipate/treat complications.

Reproduced from Beeching *et al.*, Returned travellers. In: *Principles and Practice of Travel Medicine*, 2013, John Wiley and Sons.

Malaria: treatment

Falciparum malaria

Risk of deterioration ∴ admit to hospital. Treatment[10] depends upon whether the disease is *uncomplicated*, or *severe*. Features of severe disease are:

- Impaired consciousness/seizures (consider LP)
- AKI (oliguria <0.4mL/kg/h, creatinine>265μmol/L)
- Shock (BP <90/60) = 'Algid malaria'
- Hypoglycaemia (<2.2mmol/L)
- Pulmonary oedema/ARDS
- Hb <80g/L
- Spontaneous bleeding/DIC
- Acidosis (pH <7.3)
- Haemoglobinuria
- Parasitaemia >10%.

Remember other poor prognostic indicators: peripheral blood schizonts (see p417), elevated serum lactate, ↑age.

Uncomplicated falciparum malaria:

Artemisinin combination therapies (ACT) achieve rapid clearance of parasites by combined action at different stages of the parasite cycle (p417):

1. Artemether-lumefantrine: 4 tablets at 0, 4, 8, 24, 36, 48, and 60h. 1st line in UK (including pregnant >13wks), take with high-fat food to ↑ absorption.
2. Dihydroartemisinin (DHA)-piperaquine: 4 tablets OD for 3d (if weight >60kg). Take >3h before and after food to prevent excessive peak levels. Possible ↑QT_c ∴ avoid in arrhythmia.

Options if ACT not available:

- Atovaquone-proguanil: 4 tablets OD for 3 days. Parasite clearance ~66% after 3d, GI side-effects in ~25%.
- Oral quinine sulphate 600mg TDS for 5-7d *plus* doxycycline 200mg OD (or clindamycin 450mg TDS if pregnant) for 7d. Parasite monitoring required. Can cause 'cinchonism': nausea, deafness, ringing in ears.

►Resistance to ACT is emerging in Asia.
►↑Failure rates with antifolate drugs mean Fansidar® is no longer used.
►Chloroquine is not used in the *treatment* of falciparum malaria.

Severe *P. falciparum* malaria

►►Give urgent parenteral treatment. *Artesunate is treatment of choice.* Meta-analysis shows reduction in mortality of 39% (CI: 25-50%) compared to quinine, preventing 94 deaths for every 1000 adults treated.[11] IV artesunate is stocked by many infectious disease units in the UK. It can be obtained from tropical disease centres in London (020 3456 7890) and Liverpool (0151 706 2000).

Artesunate regimen (adult): 2.4mg/kg IV at 0h, 12h, 24h and then daily for up to 5d. Converted to a full course of ACT (see uncomplicated falciparum earlier in topic) when able to tolerate oral medication. Side-effects: delayed haemolysis 7-21d post-treatment (usually self-limiting)—check Hb 14d post treatment.

If artesunate is not available immediately, treatment should be started with quinine. It is safe to overlap/combine with artensuate when it is available.

Quinine regimen (adult): Loading dose 20mg/kg over 4h. Then 10mg/kg every 8h for next 48h or until patient can swallow (dose every 12h if patient has renal failure or hepatic dysfunction or if IV needed >48h). Convert to 600mg PO TDS to total quinine course 5-7d. Give with 7d oral doxycycline (clarithromycin in children/pregnant). Side-effects: cinchonism (see earlier in topic), hyperinsulinaemia.

►Manage in a high dependency setting. ↑Capillary permeability so vulnerable to pulmonary oedema if over-filled. Lactate levels may reflect intravascular obstruction rather than circulating hypovolaemia. Monitor: blood glucose every 4h (2h if quinine infusion), Hb, clotting, electrolytes, creatinine. Daily parasite counts are sufficient NB: will fluctuate with the life cycle of the parasite (see p417) and an increase in first 36h of treatment may not indicate treatment failure. Given the rapid action of artesunate, exchange transfusion is no longer considered to offer any additional benefit.

Pregnancy: Little evidence on use/safety of artesunate. On balance of risk (pregnancy loss, pulmonary oedema, maternal mortality), artesunate should be given.

Non-falciparum malaria

P. vivax, P. ovale, P. malariae, P. knowlesi:

- If mixed infection with falciparum, treat as falciparum.
- If severe/complicated non-falciparum disease, treat as severe falciparum.
- If uncomplicated disease, treat with ACT as uncomplicated falciparum.

Chloroquine can be used for non-falciparum disease. Dosing in adult: 620mg base at 0h, 310mg base at 6–8h, 310mg base on day 2 and 3. *But:*

- do not use if *P. falciparum* cannot be excluded
- be aware that ACT may work more quickly on both fever and parasite count
- chloroquine resistance exists in *P. vivax* (Papua New Guinea, Indonesia).

►In addition to other treatment, *P. vivax* and *P. ovale* require eradication of liver hypnozoites with primaquine:

- *P. vivax:* adult 30mg (0.5mg/kg) daily for 14d.
- *P. ovale:* adult 15mg (0.25mg/kg) daily for 14d.

►Risk of haemolysis with primaquine in G6PD deficiency so screen prior to use. Seek expert advice for dosing/monitoring patients with G6PD deficiency, and in pregnancy.

Malaria prevention

Vector control for all people at risk of malaria. Includes:

- Source reduction by destruction of mosquito breeding sites (ie standing water).
- Long-lasting insecticidal nets. These should be provided free of charge and with equity of access. Nets last for ~3y, a lifespan of 5y could save ~$3.8bn. Insecticidal resistance is an increasing concern, should dual agents be used?
- Indoor residual spraying, effective for 3–6 months when >80% of houses included.
- Sterile male mosquito release. Estimated to initially require 20 males/human to be protected ∴ ~64 billion sterile mosquitoes worldwide.
- Genetic modification to develop mosquitoes that are not susceptible to malaria (and other) parasites. Requires modification that does not ↓ fertility or will not disperse in vector population. Requires acceptability, infrastructure, and money.

Chemoprophylaxis is the use of antimalarial drugs to prevent clinical disease. In high-transmission areas it is recommended for pregnant women (given at antenatal visits) and infants (given with routine vaccination).

Travellers from the UK to malaria areas should be given:

1. Bite prevention advice: insect repellents with 20–50% DEET (for all >2 months old including pregnant and breast-feeding). Apply after sunscreen with SPF >30 as DEET may ↓ sunscreen efficacy.
2. Chemoprophylaxis (table 9.20) according to area of travel. See www.fitfortravel.nhs.uk/destinations.aspx

Table 9.20 Prophylactic regimen against malaria in adults (refer to *BNF*)

Area	Regimen	Notes
No drug resistance	Chloroquine 310mg base/week *OR* proguanil 200mg OD	1wk before and 4wks after travel. Chloroquine: GI disturbance, headache. CI epilepsy. Proguanil: diarrhoea, antifolate (care if possibility of pregnancy).
Little chloroquine resistance	Chloroquine 310mg base/week *PLUS* proguanil 200mg OD	
Chloroquine-resistant *P. falciparum*	Mefloquine 250mg/week *OR*	2–3wks prior and 4wks after. Neuropsychiatric SE, dizziness.
	Doxyxcycline 100mg OD *OR*	1–2d prior, 4wks after, SE: hepatic impairment, teratogenic.
	Atovaquone-proguanil combination	1–2d prior, 1wk after, expert advice with HIV ART.

Malaria eradication is the permanent reduction of the incidence of malaria meaning that intervention is no longer required. It is dependent upon the social, demographic, and economic status of a country, the available healthcare system, and investment. It requires diagnosis and treatment to achieve parasitologic (as opposed to clinical) cure in order to eliminate asymptomatic transmission.

Mosquito-borne disease

Mosquito-borne diseases[12] are transmitted by the bite of a mosquito infected with a virus, bacteria, or parasite. The mosquito acts as the disease vector. Mosquitoes are arthropods (see table 9.21). Mosquito-borne diseases can therefore also be described as vector-borne or arthropod-borne disease. When a virus is transmitted by an arthropod it is termed an arbovirus (ARthropod-BOrne VIRUS).

►**Malaria** See pp416–9.

Dengue

Most important arbovirus in humans. Dengue viruses (*Flaviviruses* DENV1–4) are transmitted by day-biting *Aedes* mosquito. 120 countries (fig 9.28). Symptoms in 100 million/yr. UK: ~500 imported cases/yr.

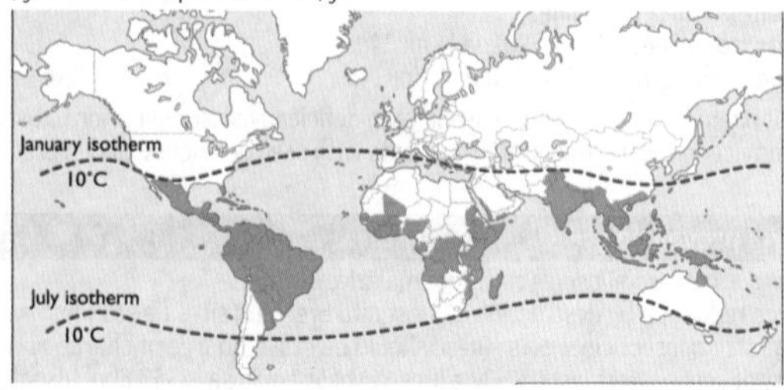

Fig 9.28 Countries at risk of dengue (dotted line = 10°C isotherm).

Reproduced from Johnson *et al.*, *Oxford Handbook of Expedition and Wilderness Medicine*, 2016, with permission from Oxford University Press.

Presentation: Incubation 3-14d. Fever (up to 40°C), N&V, headache, retro-orbital pain, myalgia, arthralgia, +ve tourniquet test (inflate BP cuff to midway between systolic and diastolic for 5 min→≥10 petechiae/inch^2). ►*Warning signs/critical phase* may occur 3-7d into illness and needs hospital admission: abdominal pain, persistent vomiting, fluid accumulation, mucosal bleeding, hepatomegaly, ↑haematocrit + ↓plt. ►*Severe disease:* shock (includes postural BP drop >20mmHg), respiratory distress, severe bleeding, organ involvement (transaminases >1000, ↓GCS, other organ failure). *Diagnosis:* PCR for virus/ELISA antigen[3] during viraemia (~1st 5d of fever). Serology (IgM, IgG) after 5d. Also ↓plt, ↓WCC, transaminitis. (ΔΔ: Chikungunya, Zika.) *Treatment:* Supportive: prompt but careful fluid balance due to potential for plasma leak. IV crystalloid, to maintain effective circulation, only in severe disease. 20mL/kg over 15-30min if hypotensive shock. Monitor clinically and via haematocrit. Reduce IV fluid as soon as stable. Beware: plasma leak maintains haemocrit unless bleeding Consider transfusion if ↓haematocrit without clinical improvement. Avoid NSAIDS.

Chikungunya

Arbovirus (*Alphavirus*) transmitted by *Aedes* mosquito. Widespread: Asia, Africa Europe, and Americas. Name derives from Kimakonde language meaning 'to become contorted' due to arthralgia. Blood-borne and vertical transmission possible, but rare. *Presentation:* Incubation 1-12d. Fever. Polyarthralgia: bilateral, symmetrical can be severe, persistent. Headache, myalgia, N&V, maculopapular rash. *Diagnosis.* Viral culture/PCR (~1st 8d), serology. *Treatment:* Supportive. Analgesia.

Yellow fever

Arbovirus (*Flavivirus*) spread by *Aedes* mosquitoes in Africa, South America. *Presentation:* Incubation ~3-6d. Viraemia ~3d with fever, headache, myalgia, anorexia N&V, relative bradycardia (ΔΔ: enteric fever p415). ~15% have remission followed by severe symptoms ~48h later: epigastric pain, jaundice, AKI, cardiac instability bleeding. Mortality 5%-30%. *Diagnosis:* Clinical and travel history. Virus/PCR in 1st 3d.[3] Serology: cross reacts with other flaviviruses, IgM can persist after vaccination *Treatment:* Supportive. Live vaccine, effective for life (certificate for 10yr).

West Nile and **Japanese encephalitis**, see Neurological disease pp436-7.

3 In UK testing done via Rare and Imported Pathogens Laboratory (RIPL): www.gov.uk/government/collections/rare-and-imported-pathogens-laboratory-ripl

Zika virus

Arbovirius (*Flavivirus*) transmitted by *Aedes* mosquito. First identified in Zika forest, Uganda, 1947. Human cases rare until outbreak in Pacific Islands (2007–2013), and Brazil (2015). Estimated 1.5 million cases in Brazil by 2016. Zika detected in sperm and blood products so transmission not limited to vector. Up-to-date geographic and clinical data available at: www.ecdc.europa.eu *Presentation:* Subclinical in ~80%. Mild illness in ~20%: fever, conjunctivitis, myalgia, rash. Severe acute illness and Guillian-Barré are rare. *Zika and birth defects:* Geographical and temporal relationship between infection and microcephaly. Zika detected in amniotic fluid is evidence of placental transfer. Specific fetal syndrome: microcephaly, intracranial calcification, eye pathology, redundant scalp skin. Small, uncontrolled studies show fetal abnormalities in up to 30% of pregnant women infected with Zika.[13] Absolute and relative risks unknown (2016). *Diagnosis*: PCR of viral DNA in blood/body fluid. *Treatment:* Vector control, avoid non-essential travel in pregnancy, condoms to prevent sexual transmission. Vaccine trials ongoing (2016).

Lymphatic filariasis (elephantiasis)

>40 million affected and disfigured. >1 billion at risk (80% in sub-Saharan Africa). Filarial parasites (nematodes) transmitted via mosquitoes which bite infected hosts and ingest microfilaria. These mature in the mosquito with infective larvae transferring to new hosts during feeding. Adult worms form nests in lymphatic vessels causing damage and lymphoedema. Transmission prevented by an annual dose of two drugs—5.63 billion treatments delivered by WHO since 2000.[12] Types of filarial worm:

- *Wuchereria bancrofti* (fig 9.29) ~90% of disease.
- *Brugia malaya* ~10%.
- *Brugia timori* possible cause of disease.

Presentation: Asymptomatic infection ± subclinical lymphatic damage. Acute episodes of local inflammation: pain, fever. Chronic damage: lymphoedema (fig 9.30), hydrocele, chylocele, scrotal/penile swelling. CKD: proteinuria, haematuria. Immune hyperreactivity →tropical pulmonary eosinophilia (cough, wheeze, fibrosis, ↑eosinophil counts, ↑IgE). *Diagnosis:* Microfilariae in blood smear (fig 9.29), antifilarial IgG, visualization of worms on USS/tissue sample. *Treatment:* Lymphoedema care. Prevention in high-risk populations: albendazole plus either diethylcarbamazine (DEC) or ivermectin. DEC is contraindicated in onchocerciasis (p439), care with ↑circulating Loa Loa (p439) due to risk of encephalopathy and renal failure. Household salt can be fortified with DEC.

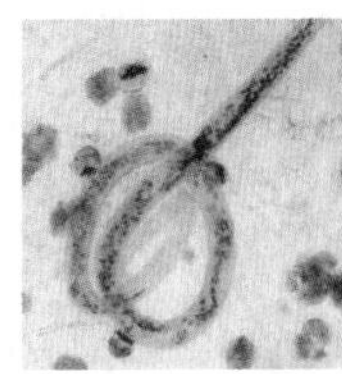

Fig 9.29 Blood smear of *W. bancrofti* (290×8.5μm). Courtesy of Prof. S. Upton, Kansas University.

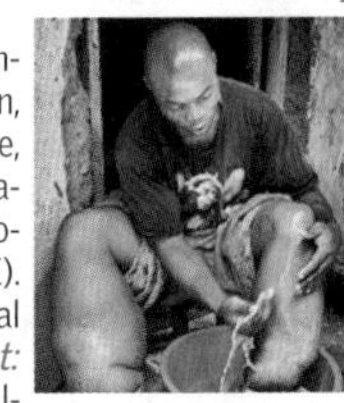

Fig 9.30 Lymphoedema. Reproduced with permission from World Health Organization. © World Health Organization. http://www.who.int/lymphatic_filariasis/disease/en/

The global advance of vector-borne disease?

Since 1990, five species of *Aedes* mosquito have become established in Europe. The adaptation of mosquitoes to a temperate environment, combined with future climate forecasts has led to models[14] that predict the UK will be suitable for:

- *Plasmodium falciparum* transmission by 2030–2080
- *Plasmodium vivax* transmission by 2030
- Chikungunya transmission in London by 2041
- Dengue transmission after 2100.

Of course, modelling is not simple. Socioeconomic development, urbanization, land-use change, migration, and globalization all come into play. Surveillance of mosquitoes at sea-ports, airports, and used-tyre companies remains uninteresting to date. But consider a time when a visit to South-East England offers an opportunity to explore the historical gems of our wonderful capital, and simultaneously becomes a pertinent question in your diagnostic sieve....

Vector-borne disease

Vector borne diseases are infections transmitted by the bite of infected arthropod species including mosquitoes, ticks, flies, and bugs (table 9.21).

Table 9.21 Vector-borne disease

Vector/arthropod		Disease	Page
Mosquito	*Anopheles*	Malaria	416-9
	Aedes	Dengue, Chikungunya, yellow fever, Zika	420-1
	Culex	Lymphatic filariasis, Japanese encephalitis, West Nile	421,436-7
Ticks		Lyme disease, rickettsial disease, relapsing fever, tick-borne encephalitis, Crimean-Congo haemorrhagic fever	422-3, 426-7
Bugs/Flies		Leishmaniasis, trypanosomiasis, onchocerciasis, loiasis	423, 439
Snails		Schistosomiasis	434

Lyme disease (Lyme borreliosis)

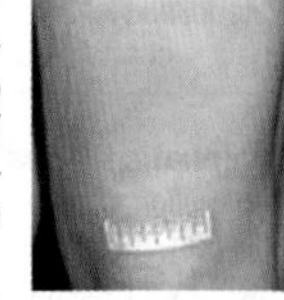

Fig 9.31 Erythema migrans: distinct advancing edge.

Reproduced from Lewis-Jones, *Paediatric Dermatology* 2010, with permission from Oxford University Press.

Tick-borne multisystem disease caused by the spirochaete *Borrelia burgdorferi* (or related *Borrelia* spp). ~All cases limited to northern hemisphere (mainly Europe and US). ~2000-3000 cases/yr in UK. Risk of infection from tick bite is 3-12% in Europe. *Presentation:* ►≤75% remember the tick bite. Peak infection with 48-72h of attachment. Disease stages:

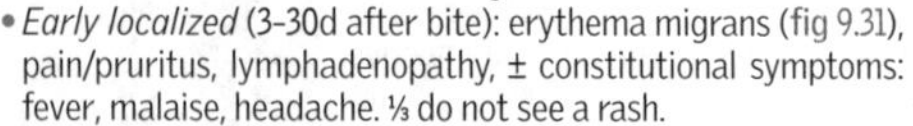

- *Early localized* (3-30d after bite): erythema migrans (fig 9.31), pain/pruritus, lymphadenopathy, ± constitutional symptoms: fever, malaise, headache. ⅓ do not see a rash.
- *Early disseminated* (wks-months): borrelial lymphocytoma = bluish-red plaque/nodule: check earlobes, nipples, genitals. Neuroborreliosis: lymphocytic meningitis, ataxia, amnesia, facial/cranial nerve palsies, neuropathy (severe pain, worse at night), encephalomyelitis. Carditis: acute onset 2nd/3rd-degree heart-block, myocarditis.
- *Late disseminated* (months-yr): acrodermatitis chronic atrophicans = focal inflammation then atrophic skin; Lyme arthritis.

Diagnosis: Clinical: erythema migrans with known exposure or evidence of infection. Borrelia culture (↓sensitivity: 40-70% for erythema migrans, <20% for CSF), PCR.[4] Two-tier serology due to false-positive reaction with other spirochaete infection: enzyme immunoassay/immunofluorescence + immunoblot. Sensitivity ↓ due to slow seroconversion: IgM 1-2wks (and may persist), IgG 4-6wks and background positivity 3-15%. *Treatment:* Erythema migrans: doxycycline 100mg BD PO for 10-21d (CI <8y, pregnant). Alternatives: amoxicillin, phenoxymethylpenicillin, azithromycin. Neuroborreliosis: ceftriaxone or IV benzylpenicillin or doxycycline for 10-30d. Arthritis/carditis: doxycyline or amoxicillin or ceftriaxone for 14-30d.[15] *Prevention:* Keep limbs covered; use insect repellent (DEET); inspect skin and remove ticks (use tweezers, hold close to head/mouth).

Rickettsial disease

Rickettsiae are obligate, intracellular coccobacillary forms lying between bacteria and viruses. Mammals and arthropods are natural hosts. ↑Risk with rural activities eg camping, hiking, hunting. Divided into:

- *Spotted fevers:* eg Rocky Mountain spotted fever (Americas); rickettsialpox (ΔΔ chicken-pox).
- *Typhus:* scrub typhus in Asia-Pacific regions; endemic (flea-borne) typhus in tropical areas; epidemic (louse-borne) typhus in homeless populations, eg refugees.
- *Other emerging illnesses:* eg *ehrlichia, anaplasma*.

Presentation: Incubation ~1-2wks. Fever, headache, malaise, rash (maculopapular, vesicular or petechial), N&V, myalgia. Check for local lymphadenopathy and an eschar at the site of the bite (scrub typhus). Wide variation in severity depending on aetiology. Fulminant, life-threatening infection possible with Rocky Mountain spotted fever, louse-borne typhus, scrub typhus. *Diagnosis:* Clinical: fever + rash + travel to an endemic area. Serology, culture/PCR of blood/skin biopsy. *Treatment:* Antibiotics in severe cases: doxycycline, azithromycin, chloramphenicol.

4 Specialist diagnostic service and advice in UK via Rare and Imported Pathogens Laboratory (RIPL): www.gov.uk/government/collections/rare-and-imported-pathogens-laboratory-ripl

Leishmaniasis

Caused by protozoan parasites of *Leishmania*[12] species, transmitted by infected female *phlebotomine* sandflies. 556 million at risk. Risk factors: poverty, malnutrition, displacement, deforestation, dam building/irrigation. *Presentation:*

- *Cutaneous,* most common form, ulceration (fig 9.56, p440).
- *Mucocutaneous* (fig 9.32): leads to tissue destruction of nose, mouth, throat. 90% occurs in Bolivia, Brazil, Peru.
- *Visceral leishmaniasis* (VL, kala-azar, 'black sickness') (fig 9.33): fever, weight loss, hepatosplenomegaly, anaemia. >95% mortality without treatment. Endemic in Indian subcontinent, East Africa. 90% of new cases occur in Bangladesh, Brazil, Ethiopia, India, South Sudan, Sudan. 300 000 cases/yr, 20 000 deaths/yr. Post kala-azar is a complication of *Leishmania donovani* = a hypopigmented macular/nodular rash (ΔΔ leprosy), 6 months–1yr after apparent cure, can heal but is a reservoir for parasites and maintains transmission.

Diagnosis: Clinical. Microscopy of tissue samples (skin, bone marrow) for parasite. Antibody detection in VL (indirect fluorescence, ELISA, western blot, direct agglutination test, or immunochromatographic test) is limited due to: **1** Ab levels detectable for years after cure, cannot distinguish VL relapse/active infection. **2** Tests are +ve in many with no history of VL. **3** Serology may be −ve if HIV+ve. *Treatment:* Liposomal amphoterin (single dose), oral miltefosine, pentavalent antimonials (resistance in India). The WHO Kala-azar Elimination Programme (including donated liposomal amphotericin) has achieved a 75% reduction in new cases of VL.

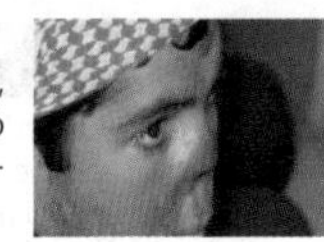

Fig 9.32 Mucocutaneous leishmaniasis.

Reproduced with permission from World Health Organization. © World Health Organization. http://www.who.int/leishmaniasis/mucocutaneous_leishmaniasis/en/

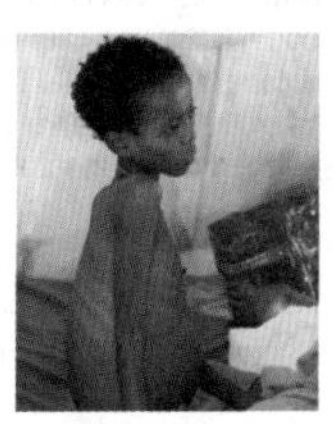

Fig 9.33 Visceral leishmaniasis.

Reproduced with permission from World Health Organization. © World Health Organization. http://www.who.int/leishmaniasis/visceral_leishmaniasis/en/

Human African trypanosomiasis (HAT, sleeping sickness)

Infection with *Trypanosoma* protozoan parasites[16], transmitted by the tsetse fly in sub-Saharan Africa. Divided into:

- *Rhodesiense HAT,* incubation <21d, high fever, GI disturbance, lymphadenopathy, headache. Chancre at bite site in ~84%, maculopapular rash. Progresses to myopericarditis, arrhythmias, and neurological symptoms.
- *Gambiense HAT,* chronic disease in African population, presents years after infection (can present with acute febrile illness in travellers). Low-grade fever. Sleep disorder: reversal of sleep-wake cycle, uncontrollable sleep episodes. Weakness, abnormal gait, psychiatric symptoms.

Diagnosis: ↓Hb, ↓plt, AKI, ↑LFTs, polyclonal ↑IgM. Microscopy of parasite (blood, lymph node, chancre, CSF). Serology and PCR if available. *Treatment:* According to disease type and stage. Available from WHO. Includes suramin, melarsoprol, pentamidine, nifurtimox-eflornithine. Seek specialist advice—side-effects from all.

Chagas' disease (American trypanosomiasis)

Life-threatening illness due to protozoan *Trypanosoma cruzi* transmitted by triatomine bugs. Endemic in Latin America: ~6–7 million infected. *Presentation: Acute phase* (~2 months): skin lesion (chagoma), fever, headache, myalgia, lymphadenopathy, unilateral conjunctivitis, periorbital oedema (Romaña's sign), myocarditis, meningoencephalitis. *Chronic phase* (yrs): cardiac: dilated cardiomyopathy; GI: mega-oesophagus (dysphagia, aspiration), mega-colon (abdominal distension, constipation); CNS symptoms. *Diagnosis: Acute:* trypomastigotes in blood, CSF, node aspirate. *Chronic:* serology (Chagas' IgG ELISA). *Treatment:* Benznidazole, nifurtimox. ↓effective in chronic disease.

Relapsing fever

Caused by spirochaete *Borrelia recurrentis* (louse-borne, sub-Saharan Africa, refugee camps) or other *Borrelia* (tick-borne, world-wide). *Presentation:* Intermittent fever 'crisis' due to antigenic variation (~3d fever, then afebrile ~7d), headache, myalgia, ↓BP. *Diagnosis:* Spirochaetes on blood smear, false +ve serology for Lyme disease. *Treatment:* Doxycyline/macrolides (single dose if louse-borne). Neuroborreliosis treatment if CNS disease (p422). Jarisch–Herxheimer reaction due to endotoxins (?TNFα) can mimic fever 'crisis': observe 1st ~4h treatment, use cooling/antipyretics.

Anthrax (*Bacillus anthracis*)

Gram-positive, aerobic bacillus found in soil worldwide. Humans exposed via infected livestock or animal products, eg hide, wool, tusks. Infection via inhalation, ingestion, contamination of broken skin (includes IV drug use). Bacteria secrete exotoxins: oedema toxin and lethal toxin. *Presentation:*

- *Cutaneous (~95%):* itchy papule→vesicle→necrotic eschar. Oedema may be striking. Regional lymphadenopathy, malaise.
- *Inhalation:* fever, cough, myalgia, SOB, pleural effusion (haemorrhagic mediastinitis), stridor, death.
- *GI (rare):* fever, abdominal pain, ascites, mucosal ulcers, GI perforation.

Diagnosis: Vesicular fluid culture (care, do not disseminate), blood culture, antibody ELISA, PCR. (NB: not pneumonic so sputum cultures are −ve). *Treatment:* Quinolone/doxycycline. Two agents if systemic disease, eg ciprofloxacin+clindamycin or linezolid (then narrow according to sensitivity). Consider anti-anthrax monoclonal antibody/immunoglobulin as adjunct in inhalational disease.

Bartonella

- *B. henselae (*cat-scratch disease): from infected cat fleas. Low-grade fever, regional lymphadenopathy. Encephalitis rare. Skin lesions mimic Kaposi's sarcoma.
- *B. quintana* (trench fever): from human body louse. Fever, headache, bone pain.
- *B. bacilliformis* (bartonellosis): from infected sandflies in Andes mountains. Oroya fever = fever, headache, myalgia, haemolysis. Later nodular→vascular skin lesions.

Diagnosis: Clinical, blood culture (fastiduous ∴ needs prolonged culture), serology. *Treatment:* Cat-scratch disease often self-limiting. Azithromycin, aminoglycoside.

Brucellosis

Most common zoonosis worldwide: 500 000 cases/yr. Gram −ve infection of cattle, swine, goats, sheep, dogs. Human infection via ingestion of infected meat/unpasteurized milk/cheese; or through inhalational/mucosal contact with animal body fluids (eg farmers, slaughterhouse workers, meat packers, hunters). ↑Risk in countries without animal health programmes. *Presentation:* Acute (<1 month), sub-acute (1-6 months), or chronic (>6 months). Non-specific: fever, anorexia, sweats, weight loss, malaise (ΔΔ TB). Localized infection: septic arthritis, spondylitis, meningitis, endocarditis, orchitis, abscess. *Diagnosis:* Culture with prolonged incubation due to slow doubling time.[17] Serology (four assays performed by Public Health England Brucella Reference Unit 0151 529 4900). *Treatment:* Doxycycline, rifampicin, aminoglycoside, ceftriaxone, co-trimoxazole. Needs prolonged course as intracellular with slow doubling time. Relapse usually due to inadequate dose/duration/adherence.

***Coxiella burnetii* (Q fever)**

Q fever is derived from the label 'query' fever attributed to an unexplained disease in Australian abattoir workers. *C. burnetii* is now recognized as the pathogenic agent. Sheep, goats, cattle are main sources of infection (also cats, dogs, rabbits, ducks, ticks). Occurs worldwide. Spores can survive in soil, animal products, and water for months-yr. Transmitted by contact, inhalation of dust, or consumption of raw milk products. *Presentation:* Incubation 3-30d. ~50% asymptomatic. Non-specific symptoms: fever (1-3wks), nausea, fatigue, headache. Pneumonia in 1-2%: typical or atypical, may have rapid progression. Also splenomegaly, granulomatous hepatitis, aseptic meningitis, encephalitis, osteomyelitis. Endocarditis is the most common form of chronic disease. *Diagnosis: Coxiella* cannot be cultured using routine lab methods.[17] PCR is rapid. Serology can take 2-6wks to become positive and detects variation in lipopolysaccharide (LPS) coat. Phase II LPS appears before phase I LPS ∴ acute infection = IgM/IgG to phase II LPS, chronic infection = IgG to phase I LPS. Serology on paired sera 2-4wks apart provides best diagnostic evidence. *Treatment:* Doxycycline. Also rifampicin, chloramphenicol, fluoroquinolone, macrolide. Hydroxychloroquine alkalinizes the phagosomes in which the bacteria resides and may ↑ bactericidal effect.

Leptospirosis (Weil's disease)

Pathogenic leptospire spirochaetes belonging to the subgroup *Leptospira interrogans*. >250 pathogenic serovars. Chronic renal infection of carrier animals: rodent, cattle, pigs. Spread by water/soil/food contaminated by infected animal urine. *Presentation:* Incubation ~7d (2–30d). 1st (acute/septicaemic) phase: fever, non-specific flu-like symptoms. Mild/subclinical in ~90%. Followed by recovery or 2nd (immune/leptospiruric) phase: conjunctival suffusion, myalgia (↑CK), jaundice, meningitis, uveitis, AKI, pulmonary haemorrhage, ARDS, myo/pericarditis. (Weil's disease described in 1886: fever, jaundice splenomegaly, renal failure, CNS symptoms. Term now applied to all severe disease.) *Diagnosis:* In UK[18] via National Leptospirosis Service (https://www.gov.uk/guidance/leptospira-reference-unit-services). Culture (blood/CSF) +ve during 1st phase. Serology. PCR. *Treatment:* Doxycycline, penicillin. Conflicting evidence of benefit for steroids in severe disease.

Yersinia pestis **(plague)**

Gram −ve, obligate intracellular pathogen transmitted by small animals and their fleas by bite, direct contact, inhalation or ingestion (rare). ~300 cases/yr worldwide. *Presentation:* Incubation: 3–7d. Flu-like symptoms, then one of three disease forms:

1 *Bubonic:* most common form. *Yersinia pestis* enters at bite and travels via lymphatics. Inflamed, painful lymph node is termed 'bubo' and can suppurate.
2 *Septicaemic:* direct spread without 'bubo', or advanced stage after 'bubo'.
3 *Pneumonic:* lung disease. Most virulent, least common. Usually from advanced bubonic form but can then transmit via droplets to other humans without fleas/animals.

Diagnosis: Culture bubo fluid, blood, sputum. Rapid antigen testing available. *Treatment:* Reduces mortality from 60% to <15%: streptomycin, tetracycline.[12]

Toxoplasmosis

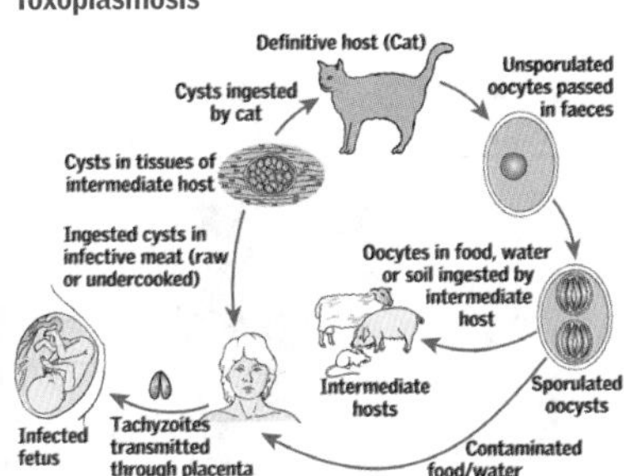

Fig 9.34 Oocysts in cat faeces can stay in the soil for months, where rats eat them. The rats get infected, and, under the direction of *Toxoplasma* in the amygdala, the rats lose their fear of cats, and so get eaten in turn. So the parasite ensure success by facilitating a jump from intermediate to definitive host. How does the parasite overwhelm the innate fear of cats? By causing a sexual attraction to normally aversive cat odour through limbic activity.

From Fernando Monroy: www2.nau.edu/~fpm/research/res.html

Caused by protozoan *Toxoplasma gondii.* Found worldwide. Life cycle (fig 9.34). Infection is lifelong (~⅓ of population). HIV may cause reactivation (p400). *Presentation:* Asymptomatic in ~90%. Self-limiting cervical lymphadenopathy, low-grade fever if normal immune system. Disseminated disease if immunosuppressed: cerebral abscess, encephalitis, choroidoretinitis, myocarditis, myositis, pneumonitis, hepatitis. Congenital infection: pregnancy loss, neurocognitive deficit, retinal damage. *Diagnosis:* In UK via Toxoplasma Reference Laboratory (0179 228 5058). Serology: IgG=previous exposure (high avidity IgG suggests infection >3–5 months ago, used in pregnancy); IgM=acute infection, false +ve or chronic infection with persistent IgM; IgA in cord serum=congenital infection. PCR: blood/CSF/urine/amniotic fluid/aqueous/vitreous humour. *Treatment:* If eye disease, immunosuppressed or neonate: pyrimethamine + sulfadiazine + folinic acid. Corticosteroids for eye inflammation. Spiramycin reduces vertical transmission. Prophylaxis: co-trimoxazole (see HIV, p400).

Echinococcosis (hydatid disease) p435. *Rabies* p437. *Hanta virus* p426.

Viral haemorrhagic fever (VHF)

Viral haemorrhagic fever (VHF) is a term used for severe, multi-organ disease in which the endothelium is damaged, and homeostasis is impaired. Haemorrhage complicates the disease course and can be life-threatening. VHF classification by viral subtype is shown in table 9.22.

Table 9.22 VHF classification (HF=haemorrhagic fever)

Virus family	Disease (virus subtype)	Details
Filovirus	Ebola	See Ebola, this page
	Marburg	See Marburg, p427
Arenavirus	Lassa fever (Lassa)	See Lassa, p427
	Argentinian HF (Junin) Bolivian HF (Chapare, Machupo) Brazilian HF (Sabia) Venezualan HF (Guanarito)	South American VHF are rare causes of infection in travellers. Incubation 2-16d. Resemble Lassa fever. Severe disease with bleeding in ~⅓. Supportive treatment. Live vaccine available for Junin virus.
Bunyavirus	Crimean-Congo HF	See CCHF, p427
	Hanta	Rodent host. Incubation 2d-8wk. Causes: 1 HF with renal syndrome: fever, headache, GI symptoms, and AKI. 2 Hanta virus pulmonary syndrome: bilateral interstitial pulmonary infiltrates, mortality 30-40%. Supportive treatment.
	Rift valley fever	Endemic in Africa. 80% asymptomatic or self-limiting febrile illness. <2% CNS involvement/haemorrhagic.
Flavivirus	Dengue	see p420
	Yellow fever	see p420

The Advisory Committee on Dangerous Pathogens (ACDP) classifies a pathogen as Group 4 (highest) when it causes severe human disease, with high risk of spread, and no effective prophylaxis or treatment. Ebola,[19] Marburg, Lassa, and Crimean-Congo haemorrhagic fever (CCHF) are all Hazard Group 4 haemorrhagic fever viruses. They are largely confined to Africa (fig 9.35), with the exception of CCHF which occurs in Africa, the Middle East, Eastern Europe, and Asia.

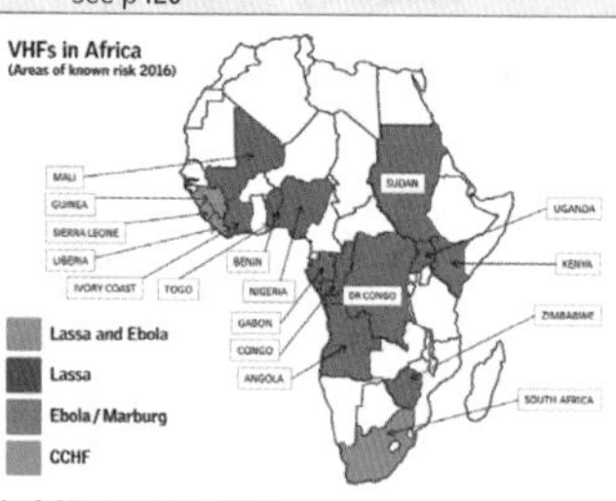

Fig 9.35 VHF risk in Africa.

Ebola

Incubation 2-21d (usually 3-12d). Evidence for fruit bats as reservoir. Outbreaks with ↑mortality. Largest epidemic (2014-16) due to Ebola virus (EBOV, formally Zaire ebolavirus): 28 646 cases and 11 323 deaths in Guinea, Liberia, and Sierra Leone. Cytokine activation→endothelial damage, oedema, coagulopathy, tissue necrosis, multi-organ failure. Transmission from index case via mucous membranes, or contact with body fluids (including burial contact), viral shedding in semen. *Presentation:*

- *Undifferentiated* (0-3d). Fever (>38°C axillary), myalgia, weakness, anorexia, headache, sore throat. May not look unwell.
- *GI* (4-10d). Epigastric/abdominal pain, liver tenderness, N&V, hiccups, diarrhoea, hypovolaemia.
- *Late organ stage* (>10d). Haemorrhagic: petechiae, ecchymoses, mucosal haemorrhage, GI bleeding, haemoptysis. Neurological: extreme weakness, confusion, agitation, bradypsychia, coma. Other: hypoglycaemia, electrolyte abnormalities, secondary infection, shock, DIC, multi-organ failure, death.

- *Post-infection:* arthralgia, hepatitis, orchitis, transverse myelitis, meningitis, uveitis, vision/hearing impairment, social isolation, psychological effects.

Diagnosis: ►PPE (see BOX 'Equipment') if high possibility (see 'Risk assessment'). ↓WCC, ↓plt, ↑AST>ALT. IgM (~day 3), IgG (~day 7), reverse transcriptase PCR on blood/urine/saliva/throat swab. ►Exclude malaria. *Treatment:* Supportive: fluid resuscitation, correct electrolytes/coagulation/glucose, treat secondary infection, nutrition. Ribavirin not effective. Trace contacts, support family. Experimental: anti-RNA agents, immunotherapy with blood/plasma from survivors, monoclonal antibodies (ZMapp™), Ebola vaccine (rVSV-ZEBOV, Ebola ça suffit! trial). *Ethics:* Randomization versus compassionate use: is it ethical to withhold even potentially beneficial therapy to a control group with a life-threatening condition? Is observational data gained through the compassionate use of experimental therapy sufficient to guide clinical decisions? Where should resources be directed to improve outcome: drug development or basic healthcare provision, eg would the capacity to check K^+ improve mortality?

Equipment

- Double gloves
- Fluid-repellent gown
- Full-length plastic apron
- Head cover (surgical cap)
- Fluid-repellent footwear
- Full face shield
- Full-repellent respirator
- Meticulous removal.

Marburg, Lassa, and CCHF

Differentiating features are given in table 9.23.

Table 9.23 Differentiation between VHF

VHF	Clinical features
Marburg	Incubation typically 5-9d. Clinically identical disease course to Ebola. Ebola/Marburg suggested by liver tenderness.
Lassa	~80% mild/asymptomatic. Haemorrhage in ~20%. Variable mortality in different epidemics 25–80%. Exudative pharyngitis. Convalescent hearing loss. Observational data shows response to ribavarin if given in first 6d.
CCHF	Tick-borne. Sudden onset prodrome. Haemorrhagic stage common, develops rapidly, but usually short-lived 2-3d. Ribavarin used in treatment (↓evidence).

Risk assessment for VHF in UK

Assess for possible transmission *and* fever.

- Transmission: **1** Travel to endemic area (rural for Lassa fever; caves/primates/antelopes/bats for Ebola/Marburg; tick/animal slaughter for CCHF). **2** Travel to known outbreak (http://www.promedmail.org). **3** Contact with infected specimen.
- Fever: >37.5°C in the past 24h.

If possible transmission *and* fever consider 'high possibility' (≠high probability), isolate, PPE (see BOX 'Equipment'). Inform local infectious disease team and contact the Imported Fever Service (0844 778 8990) for VHF investigation. ►Bruising, bleeding, and uncontrolled D&V also warrant isolation and discussion if relevant contact history.

Ebola and sacrifice

This page is dedicated to Dr Sam Brisbane, director of the emergency department in Monrovia, Liberia. Caring, light-hearted, intense, profane. In 2013, he expressed his greatest worry: an epidemic of VHF. A well-founded fear which would ultimately prove prophetic, in a hospital with a shortage of personnel, rationing of gloves, and limited soap. Universal precautions? Unaffordable, and not even close. He was also a coffee farmer. But not for him a deserved retirement to his plantation, surrounded by photographs of 8 children, 6 adopted children, and grandchildren to match. Unprotected, despite a lucky fedora and a gallows sense of humour, he contracted Ebola in 2014 at the age of 74 whilst manning the front line of the world's deadliest VHF epidemic to date. During his illness he told his doctors, '*When we find ourselves in the middle of the sea and there are rough waves, we should not give up. We should fight on to the end*'. A truly sagacious man whose life and doctoring transcends Western perspectives. We can never replicate your courage, because we will never know your fear. It is fittingly, the stuff of legend.

Gastroenteritis = diarrhoea (± vomiting) due to enteric infection with viruses, bacteria, or parasites.

Diarrhoea can be defined as:

- acute diarrhoea: ≥3 episodes partially formed or watery stool/day for <14d
- dysentery: infectious gastroenteritis with bloody diarrhoea
- persistent diarrhoea: acutely starting diarrhoea lasting >14d
- traveller's diarrhoea: starting during, or shortly after, foreign travel
- food poisoning: disease (infection or toxin) caused by consumption of food/water.
  ► Food poisoning is notifiable in the UK (www.gov.uk/health-protection-team).

Gastroenteritis can be classified according to infectious aetiology (table 9.24) or predominant clinical presentation (table 9.25, also see p259).

Table 9.24 Gastroenteritis by infectious aetiology

Infection	Organism	Incubation	Notes	Page
Virus ~50–60%	Norovirus	1d	Important cause of epidemic gastroenteritis. 600 000–1million cases/yr in UK.	430
	Rotavirus	1–3d	Affects nearly all children by age 5y. Routine, childhood (live) vaccine in UK.	430
	Astrovirus	4–5d	Often less severe than norovirus.	
	Adenovirus	3–10d	Enteric adenovirus. Mainly children.	
	Sapovirus	1–3d	Children. Not common in food-borne disease.	
	CMV	~3–12wks	Usually asymptomatic. If immunosuppression: colitis, hepatitis, retinitis, pneumonia.	400, 405
Bacteria ~30–40%	*Salmonella* (non-typhoidal)	12–72h	Under-cooked eggs, poultry, meat.	431
	Campylobacter	2–5d	Under-cooked meat, cross-contamination, unpasteurized milk, water.	431
	E. coli	1–10d (usually 3–4d)	Bloody diarrhoea if Shiga-toxin producing *E. coli* (STEC) eg 0157. Can cause HUS. Under-cooked beef, unpasteurized milk most common.	391, 429, 431
	Shigella	1–2d	*S. sonnei* most common. Deadly epidemics with *S. dysenteriae* in low-income countries.	431
	Staphylococcus aureus	30min–6h	Unpasteurized milk/cheese, uncooked food. Multiplication leads to toxin production.	388
	Clostridium perfringens	6–24h	Raw meat. Inadequately reheated food.	430
	Clostridium difficile		Antibiotic-associated diarrhoea. Spore-forming therefore persists: wash your hands.	411
	Listeria	3–70d	Cold meat, soft cheese, refrigerated pâté. Diarrhoea, fever, myalgia. ↑Severity in immunosuppression and pregnancy (bacteraemia, fetal loss).	389
	Vibrio cholerae	2h–5d	Human and aquatic reservoirs. Epidemics due to inadequate environmental management.	430
	Yersinia enterocolitica	4–7d	Main source is undercooked pork. Most infection in young children.	431
	Bacillus cereus	30min–15h	Leftover food, rice. Emetic or diarrhoeal toxins.	
Parasites <2%	*Giardia*	1–3wks	Intestinal parasite. Cyst transfer via infected faeces, eg contaminated water. Malabsorption.	432
	Cryptosporidium	1–12d	Transfer via infected faeces. Symptoms and ↑severity with immunosuppression, eg HIV.	400, 432
	Entamoeba histolytica	2–4wks (can be years)	Asymptomatic carrier, intestinal disease and/or extra-intestinal disease (liver, skin, lung, brain).	432
	Cyclospora cayetanensis	~1wk	Transfer via infected faeces. May have relapsing course.	433
	Trichinella	1–2d	Enteral at 1–2d. Parenteral at 2–8wks: larval migration, facial swelling, myocarditis, encephalitis.	433
	Trichuriasis	~3months	Whipworm. Dysentery with heavy infection.	433
	Intestinal flukes	4d–months	Eg *Fasciolopsis buski*.	

Table 9.25 Gastroenteritis by clinical presentation

Diarrhoea without blood (enteritis)	Diarrhoea with blood (dysentery)
Norovirus	Shigellosis (bacillary dysentery)*
Rotavirus	Enterohaemorrhagic *E. coli*
Astrovirus	*Campylobacter* enterocolitis*
Enteric adenovirus	*Salmonella* enterocolitis*
Enterotoxigenic *E. coli*	*Clostridium difficile*
Enteropathogenic *E. coli*	*Yersinia* enterocolitis
Toxin-producing *Staph. aureus*	*Entamoebic histolytica* (amoebic dysentery)
Cholera	Trichuriasis (whipworm)
Clostridium perfringens	CMV
Giardia	
Cryptosporidium	
Cyclospora cayetanensis	

*Milder disease may present as diarrhoea without blood.

Traveller's diarrhoea

Diarrhoea affects 20–60% of travellers.[20,21] High-risk areas: South Asia, Central and South America, Africa. Major cause = enterotoxigenic *E. coli*.

Prevention: Boil water, cook thoroughly, peel fruit and vegetables. Avoid ice, salads, shellfish. Drink with a straw. Hand washing with soap may ↓ risk.

Presentation: Most diarrhoea is during first week of travel. Symptoms are often unreliable indicators of aetiology but the following may be indicative:
- Enterotoxigenic *E. coli*: watery diarrhoea preceded by cramps and nausea.
- *Giardia lamblia*: upper GI symptoms, eg bloating, belching.
- *Campylobacter jejuni* and *Shigella*: colitic symptoms, urgency, cramps.

Duration of diarrhoea: most <1wk, 10%>1wk, 5% >2wks, 1%>30d.

Treatment:
- Oral rehydration. Clear fluid or oral rehydration salts. ►Home-made oral rehydration recipe: 6 level teaspoons of sugar + half level teaspoon salt in 1L clean, drinking water.
- Antimotility agents, eg loperamide, bismuth subsalicylates. Avoid if severe pain or bloody diarrhoea as may indicate invasive colitis.
- Antibiotics: usually not indicated. Considered if rapid cessation of diarrhoea needed and/or limited access to sanitation/healthcare. Reduce diarrhoea from ~3 to ~1.5 days. Choice depends on allergy, comorbidity, concomitant medication, and destination of travel: ciprofloxacin 500mg BD for 3d (care ↑quinolone resistance, eg SE Asia), rifaximin 200mg TDS for 3d, azithromycin 1g single dose or 500mg OD for 3d.

Prophylaxis: Not recommended as severe disease and long-term sequelae rare, risk of *C. difficile*. Consider in immunosuppressed (transplant, HIV, chemotherapy), GI pathology (IBD, ileostomy, short-bowel), ↑risk with dehydration (sickle cell, CKD). Care with interactions with usual medications.
- Ciprofloxacin 500mg OD (80–100% protection).
- Norfloxacin 400mg OD (75–95% protection).
- Rifaximin 200mg every 12–24h (72–77% protection).
- Bismuth subsalicylate 2 tablets QDS (62–65% protection, 1st line in US).

Persistent diarrhoea: Investigate if >14d or dysentery: FBC, U&E, LFT, inflammatory markers, stool microscopy for ova/cysts/parasites (historically 3 samples but may not actually improve diagnostic yield, time intensive), molecular testing for (pre-defined) microbes. ΔΔ of persistent diarrhoea = *Giardia* (most common diagnosis, send PCR), *Entamoeba histolytica, Shigella*. Post-infectious irritable bowel syndrome is a diagnosis of exclusion (in up to 30%).

►Do not forget: malaria, HIV.

Diarrhoea without blood

Norovirus: Single-stranded RNA virus. Highly infectious. Transmission by contact with infected people, environment, food (~10%). Most common cause of infectious GI disease, ~600 000 cases in England/yr. *Presentation:* 12–48h after exposure, lasting 24–72h: acute-onset vomiting, watery diarrhoea, cramps, nausea. Virus shed in stool even if asymptomatic. Numerous genotypes and unknown longevity of immunity ∴ repeat infection occurs. *Diagnosis:* clinical, stool sample reverse transcriptase PCR. *Treatment:* supportive, anti-motility agents, usually self-limiting.

Rotavirus: Double-stranded RNA virus. Wheel-like appearance on EM ∴ 'rota'. Commonest cause of gastroenteritis in children (~50%). Most infected by 5y. *Presentation:* incubation ~2d. Watery diarrhoea and vomiting for 3–8d, fever, abdominal pain. *Diagnosis:* clinical, antigen in stool. *Treatment:* supportive. Routine vaccination in UK (p407). Virus shed in stool post vaccine ∴ careful hygiene if immunosuppressed and changing nappies. Live vaccine ∴ delay vaccination if *in utero* biological agents with active transfer across placenta (eg infliximab, adalimumab).

Enterotoxigenic E. coli: Gram −ve anaerobe. Disease due to heat-stable or heat-labile toxin which stimulates Na^+, Cl^- and water efflux into gut lumen. ~20% of all infective diarrhoea, ~80% of traveller's diarrhoea. *Presentation:* incubation 1–3d. Watery diarrhoea, cramps. Lasts ~3–4d. *Diagnosis:* clinical, identification of toxin from stool culture. *Treatment:* supportive. See Traveller's diarrhoea p429.

Clostridium perfringens (type A): Gram +ve, anaerobe. Produces enterotoxin. Spores survive cooking and germinate during unrefrigerated storage. 2–30 outbreaks/yr in UK. *Presentation:* sudden-onset diarrhoea, cramps, usually lasts <24h. *Diagnosis:* stool toxin, quantification of faecal bacteria. *Treatment:* supportive. β-toxin of *C. perfringens* type C can cause a necrotizing enteritis with fulminant disease, pain, bloody diarrhoea, septic shock. β-toxin is sensitive to trypsin proteolysis so ↑ risk with trypsin inhibition by sweet potatoes, ascaris infection ∴ occurs in New Guinea ('pigbel'), central/south America, south-east Asia, China.

Cholera: Vibrio cholerae is a Gram −ve, aerobic, 'comma-shaped' flagellated motile vibrating/swarming rod. Found in faecally contaminated water. Serovars O1 and O139 cause disease. ~190 000 cases in 2014 (fig 9.36). Last indigenous case in UK in 1893. *Presentation:* incubation 2h–5d. ~75% asymptomatic but shed bacteria. Profuse (1L/h) diarrhoea ('rice-water' stool), vomiting, dehydration, metabolic acidosis, circulatory collapse, death. *Diagnosis:* Clinical: death due to dehydration from watery diarrhoea age >5y, or any watery diarrhoea age >5y during known epidemic. Identification of serovars O1 or O139 in stool. Rapid dipstick testing available but culture confirmation recommended. *Treatment:* ►►oral rehydration salts (WHO/UNICEF ORS sachet) will treat[12] up to 80%. Needs safe water. Adults may need 1L/hr initially: offer 100mL/5 min. NG if vomiting. IV fluids if severely dehydrated: Ringer's lactate or 0.9% saline *plus* ORS (beware ↓K^+) up to 200mL/kg in first 24h. Antibiotics in severe dehydration to ↓ diarrhoea: doxycycline (single dose 300mg) or tetracycline (3d course) guided by local susceptibility (azithromycin in children/pregnancy). Zinc shortens illness in children (10–20mg/24h). *Prevention:* cholera loves filth: clean water (and clean politics) abolishes it. Oral cholera vaccines (56–94% efficacy in adults) dependent on logistics, cost, production capacity. Antibiotic prophylaxis breeds resistance.

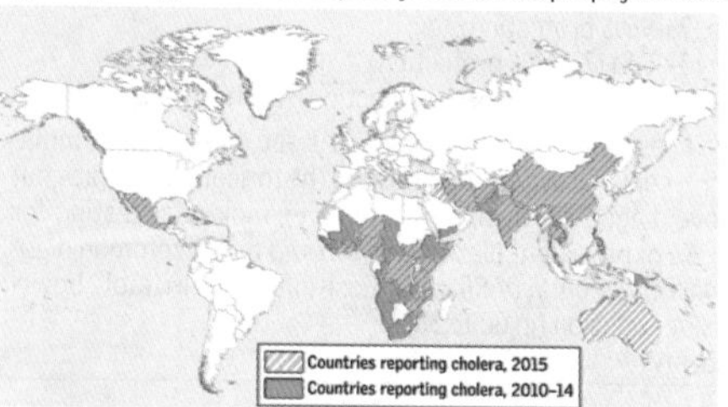

Fig 9.36 Cholera: areas reporting outbreaks 2010–2014.
Reproduced with permission from World Health Organization, *Countries reporting cholera, 2010–2015*. ©World Health Organization 2016. http://www.who.int/gho/epidemic_diseases/cholera/epidemics/en/

On the mode of communication of cholera

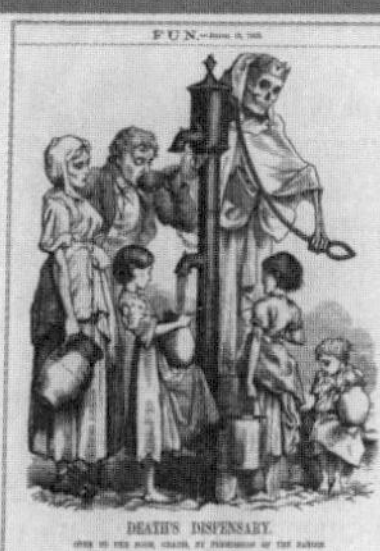

Fig 9.37 *Death's Dispensary,* George Pinwell, 1866.

In 1854, at 40 Broad St, London, a child became ill with diarrhoea, dying on 2 September. Her mother rinsed her soiled nappies into the house drains where faulty brickwork allowed mixing with the water supply of the Broad St pump (fig 9.37). From this confluence sprung the discipline of Public Health. The ensuing deaths from cholera clustered around the Broad St pump, as detailed by the local doctor, Dr John Snow. He used his now famous Voronoi diagram showing the deaths within a 'line of nearest pump' to motivate the parish vestry: 'In consequence of what I said, the handle of the pump was removed the following day', so inaugurating the control of cholera. These events illustrate a number of truths:

1 Knowledge of the microscopic cause of disease is not required for public health measures to succeed (*Vibrio cholerae* was identified by Robert Kock in 1883).
2 Even the most parochial are capable of life-saving action when assisted by a doctor in command of the facts.
3 Influential friends help. Snow remained largely unknown until the 1930s when *On the Mode of Communication of Cholera* was republished by Wade Hampton Frost, first professor of epidemiology at John Hopkins School.
4 Randomization (Broad St pump versus an alternative water supply) is king.

Diarrhoea with blood (dysentery)

Shigella (sonnei, flexneri, dysenteriae, boydii): Gram −ve anaerobe. *Presentation:* watery or bloody diarrhoea, pain, tenesmus, fever 1-2d after exposure. Lasts ~5-7d. ↑ in MSM. Complications: bacteraemia, reactive arthritis (~2% of *flexneri*), HUS (Shiga-toxin-producing *dysenteriae,* p315). *Diagnosis:* stool culture. PCR/enzyme immunoassay. *Treatment:* supportive. Nutrition: green bananas (↑short-chain fatty acids in colon), zinc if age <6y, vitamin A. Antibiotics if systemically unwell, immunosuppressed. Guided by local sensitivities (ciprofloxacin, azithromycin). Avoid antidiarrhoeal agents: risk of toxic dilatation.

Enterohaemorrhagic/Shiga-toxin producing E. coli (STEC), eg O157:H7: Gram −ve anaerobe. Produces veratoxins which are 'Shiga-like' due to similarity with *Shigella dysenteriae*. *Presentation:* incubation 3-8d. Diarrhoea, haemorrhagic colitis. HUS in up to 10% (p315). *Diagnosis:* stool culture. PCR/enzyme immunoassay for Shiga-toxin. *Treatment:* Supportive. Do not give antibiotics: ↑ risk of HUS.

Campylobacter: Gram −ve, spiral-shaped rod. *Presentation:* incubation 1-10d (usually 2-5d). Bloody diarrhoea, pain, fever, headache. Complications: bacteraemia, hepatitis, pancreatitis, miscarriage, reactive arthritis, Guillain-Barré. *Diagnosis:* stool culture. PCR/enzyme immunoassay. *Treatment:* supportive. Antibiotics only in invasive cases, refer to local sensitivities (macrolide, doxycycline, quinolone).

Salmonella enterocolitis (non-typhoidal): Gram −ve, anaerobic, motile bacilli. *Presentation:* diarrhoea, cramps, fever, usually within 12-36h of exposure. Invasive infection (<10%) can cause bacteraemia/sepsis, meningitis, osteomyelitis, septic arthritis. *Diagnosis:* stool culture. PCR. *Treatment:* supportive. Meta-analysis shows no evidence of benefit for antibiotics in healthy people. Consider in severe/extra-intestinal disease according to local sensitivities (quinolone, macrolide).

Yersinia enterocolitica: Gram −ve rod. *Presentation:* incubation 4-7d. Diarrhoea, fever, pain (may mimic appendicitis), vomiting. May last 1-3wk. Also erythema nodosum, reactive arthritis (~1 month after diarrhoea). *Diagnosis:* stool culture, agglutination titres. *Treatment:* antibiotics in severe disease depending on local sensitivities (aminoglycosides, co-trimoxazole, quinolone).

► See also: *Staph. aureus* pre-formed toxin (p388), *GI parasites* (pp432-3), *Clostridium difficile* (p411).

Giardiasis

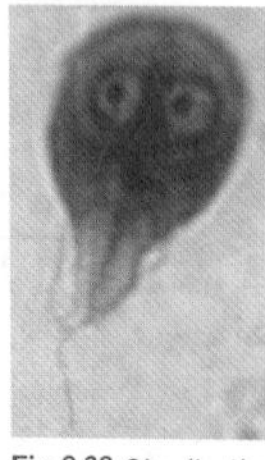

Fig 9.38 *Giardia:* the only diplomonadid to trouble us.

Giardia lamblia (fig 9.38) is a flagellate protozoan. Faecal-oral spread from infected drinking water/food/fomites. *Presentation:* Asymptomatic in the majority. Incubation 1-3wks. Diarrhoea, flatulence, bloating, pain, malabsorption. Duration of symptoms typically ~2-6wks. Most common diagnosis if persistent traveller's diarrhoea (p429). *Diagnosis:* Stool microscopy for cysts and trophozoites. Intermittent shedding so multiple samples (≳3) *may* ↑ sensitivity. Faecal immunoassay. PCR for diagnosis/subtype. Duodenal fluid aspirate analysis. *Treatment:* Hygiene to prevent transmission. Metronidazole (treatment failure in up to 20%), tinidazole (single dose), albendazole (↓ side-effects, simultaneous treatment of other parasites). Lactose-intolerance develops in 20–40%. No treatment for asymptomatic disease in endemic areas due to likelihood of re-infection.

Cryptosporidium

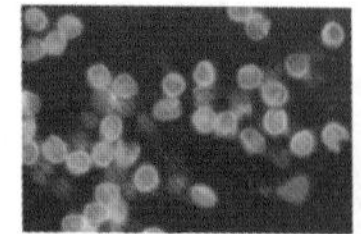

Fig 9.39 *Cryptosporidium* immunofluorescence.
© Prof. S Upton; Kansas Univ.

Apicomplexan protozoan (fig 9.39). Ingestion of oocytes in infected water. Asymptomatic or self-limiting diarrhoea in immunocompetent hosts. Chronic/severe diarrhoea with immunosuppression: HIV (p400), transplantation, hypogammaglobulinaemia, immunosuppressive therapy.

Amoebiasis

Protozoan *Entamoeba histolytica* (fig 9.40) ~10% world's population, mortality ~100 000/yr. Faecal-oral spread. Boil water to destroy cysts. *Presentation:*

- Asymptomatic passage of cysts in ~90% ('luminal amoebiasis').
- Intestinal amoebiasis: dysentery (often insidious onset/relapsing), pain, colitis, appendicitis, toxic megacolon. Amoeboma = inflammatory abdominal mass, usually caecal/RIF ± obstruction.
- Extra-intestinal (invasive) disease. Amoebic liver abscess in ~1%. Single mass containing 'anchovy-sauce' pus. High swinging fever, RUQ pain/tenderness. LFT normal or ↑ (cholestatic). 50% have no history of amoebic dysentery. Also peritonitis (rupture of colonic abscess), pleuropulmonary abscess, cutaneous/genital lesions.

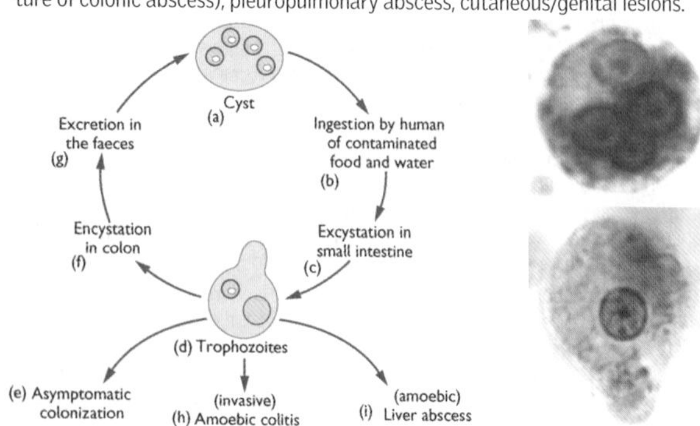

Fig 9.40 The lifecycle of *Entamoeba histolytica* is in two stages: cysts and trophozoites. Cysts (10–15μm across) typically contain four nuclei (upper right image). During excystation in the gut lumen, nuclear division is followed by cytoplasmic division, giving rise to eight trophozoites. Trophozoites (10–50μm across) contain one nucleus with a central karyosome (lower right image). Trophozoites inhabit the caecum and colon. Re-encystation of the trophozoites occurs in the colon, and excretion of cysts in faeces perpetuates the lifecycle.

Left hand image from Hutson C *et al.*, 'Molecular-based diagnosis of Entamoeba histolytica infection', *Expert Reviews in Molecular Medicine*, 1(9): 1–11, 1999, reproduced with permission from Cambridge University Press. Upper and lower right images courtesy of Prof. S Upton, Kansas University.

Diagnosis: Microscopy of stool (cysts and trophozoites, fig 9.40), aspirate or biopsy sample. Enzyme immunoassay: antigen detection as adjunct to microscopy, antibody detection in extra-intestinal disease. PCR can distinguish *E. histolytica* from morphologically identical but non-invasive *E. dispar*. *Treatment:* Metronidazole/tinidazole for amoebic dysentery and invasive disease. Diloxanide furoate: luminal agent, 10d course to destroy gut cysts, given in asymptomatic gut carriers and symptomatic disease, in addition to other treatment. Abscess may require (image-guided) drainage.

Cyclospora

Coccidean protozoan *Cyclospora cayetanensis*. ~50 imported cases/yr in UK. *Presentation:* Flu-like prodrome, watery diarrhoea, weight loss, marked fatigue, low-grade fever in ~25%. Self-limiting after 7–9wks in immunocompetent. *Diagnosis:* Autofluorescent oocytes in stool (appear blue-green under UV fluorescence fig 9.41), PCR. *Treatment:* Co-trimoxazole.

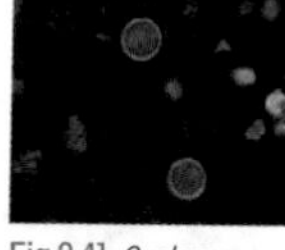

Fig 9.41 *Cyclospora* oocysts fluorescence.
Credit: CDC DPDx.

Nematodes (soil-transmitted helminths and *Trichinella*)

- Roundworm: *Ascaris lumbricoides* ~1 billion affected, *Trichinella spiralis* (contaminated meat source).
- Whipworm: *Trichuris trichiura*, 600–800 million affected.
- Hookworm: *Necator americanus*, *Ancylostoma duodenale* ~700 million affected.
- Threadworm: eg *Strongyloides stercoralis*, 30–100 million affected.

One of most common infections worldwide, affects poor and deprived (fig 9.42). Parasites live in intestines, producing 1000s egg/day in faeces. Humans infected by eggs (ascariasis, trichinosis) or larvae (*Ancylostoma*) in contaminated food; or via direct penetration of the skin (hookworm, *Strongyloides*). *Presentation:* Diarrhoea, abdominal pain, blood/protein loss, impaired growth/cognitive development. Pruritus/urticaria if migration involves skin (*Strongyloides* fig 9.42). Lung invasion (ascariasis, hookworm, *Strongyloides*) can lead to a Loeffler-like syndrome: cough, SOB, wheeze, haemoptysis, consolidation, eosinophilia. Other tissue invasion (trichinosis): myalgia, conjunctivitis, photophobia, meningitis, encephalitis, neuropathy. *Diagnosis:* Clinical, eggs in stool sample (fig 9.43). Eosinophilia. *Strongyloides* serology/PCR. *Treatment:* table 9.26.

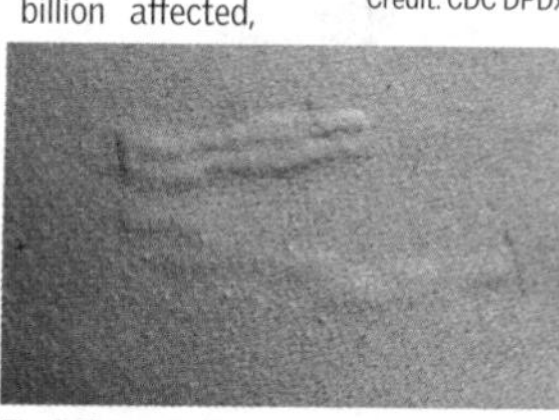

Fig 9.42 Larva currens: a serpinginous maculopapular rash pathognomonic of chronic strongyloidiasis. Oedema, an urticarial appearance, and speed of migration (>5cm/hr) distinguish this from cutaneous larva migrans which is caused by animal (dog/cat) hookworm.

Reproduced from Johnson *et al.*, *Oxford Handbook of Expedition and Wilderness Medicine*, 2016, with permission from Oxford University Press.

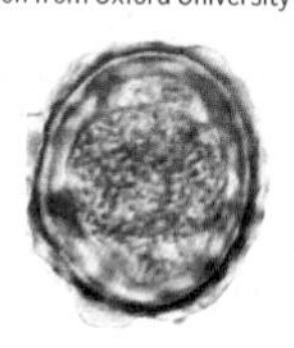

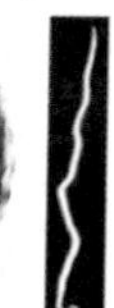

Fig 9.43 *Ascaris* eggs (45× 40μm) & ♂ worm (20cm).
Courtesy of Prof. S Upton; Kansas University.

Table 9.26 Anthelmintic drugs

Drug	Mechanism	Indication
Mebendazole	Irreversible block of glucose/nutrient uptake	Roundworm, whipworm, hookworm
Albendazole	↓ATP, immobilization and death of worm	Ascariasis, hookworm, (strongyloides)
Ivermectin	↑Cl^- permeability, hyperpolarization, paralysis	Strongyloides, ascariasis
Pyrantel pamoate	Depolarizing neuromuscular blockade causing spastic paralysis of worm	Single dose in threadworm, roundworm, hookworm
Piperazine	Flaccid paralysis of worm, expel live worm	(Ascariasis), pregnancy

Taeniasis (tapeworm)

Includes *Taenia solium* (pork, 2–8m, 50 000 eggs/worm), *Taenia saginata* (beef, 4–12m, 100 000 eggs/worm), *Taenia asiatica* (Asian, 4–8m, millions of eggs). *Presentation:* No or mild GI symptoms, tapeworm segments (proglottids) through anus/in faeces. *Diagnosis:* Eggs/proglottids in faeces. *Treatment:* Praziquantel, niclosamide.

►See also *toxoplasmosis* (p425), *schistosomiasis* (p434), *cysticercosis* (p437).

Schistosomiasis and liver disease

Schistosomiasis (bilharzia)

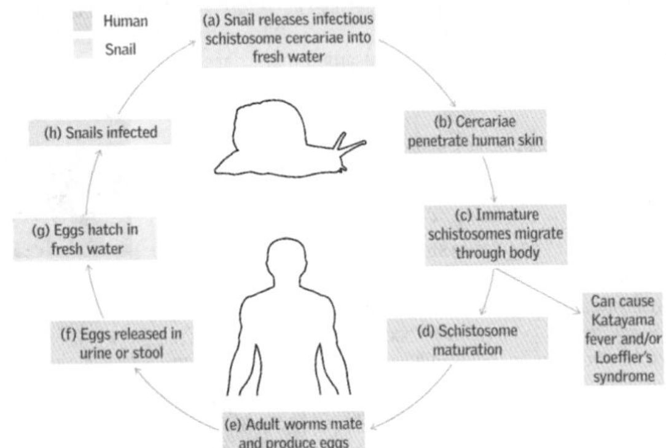

Fig 9.44 Schistosomiasis life cycle.

Caused by blood-flukes (trematode worms) of the genus *Schistosoma* (table 9.27). 258 million people in 78 countries required treatment in 2014. The life cycle is shown in fig 9.44. Disease develops after contact with contaminated freshwater (swimming, washing). Symptoms are due to an immune complex response to the migrating parasite (Katayama syndrome), or deposition of parasite eggs in body tissues.

Presentation: ~50% asymptomatic or non-specific symptoms. Clinical syndromes:

- Larval penetration: pruritic papular rash ('swimmer's itch').
- Migration of schistosomules: Katayama syndrome 2-8wks after exposure: fever, urticaria, diarrhoea, cough, wheeze, hepatosplenomegaly, eosinophilia.
- Host response to egg deposition:
  - Intestinal disease: pain, diarrhoea, blood in stool, (granulomatous) hepatomegaly, splenomegaly. Heavy chronic infection can cause bowel perforation, hyperplasia, polyposis, liver fibrosis, portal hypertension→varices.
  - Urogenital disease: haematuria, dysuria, ureteric fibrosis→hydronephrosis, CKD, bladder fibrosis/cancer, genital lesions, vaginal bleeding, dyspareunia, vulval nodules, haemospermia, prostatitis.
  - Lung disease: pulmonary hypertension and cor pulmonale.
  - CNS disease: rare, acute lower limb paraplegia, transverse ('traveller's') myelitis.

Diagnosis: Ova in urine (*S. haematobium*) or faeces (all other species) is specific, but sensitivity <50% if light infection. Serology for egg antigen becomes +ve once mature flukes lay eggs ∴ will be −ve in Katayama fever. Bowel/bladder histology. Chronic *S. haematobium*: bladder calcification on AXR, renal obstruction, hydronephrosis ± thick bladder wall on USS. *Treatment:* two doses of praziquantel 20mg/kg PO separated by 4h. Steroids for Katayama fever. If ↑eosinophils >3months after treatment look for other helminths (+ve serology can persist for years).

Table 9.27 Parasite species and geographical distribution

Disease form	Species	Geography
Intestinal	*S. mansoni*	Africa, Middle East, Caribbean, Brazil, Venezuela, Suriname
	S. japonica	China, Indonesia, Philippines
	Other	*S. mekongi*: Cambodia, Laos; *S. guineensis/ intercalatum*: rainforests of central Africa
Urogenital	*S. haematobium*	Africa, Middle East, France

Echinococcosis (hydatid disease)
Zoonotic disease caused by tapeworms of the genus *Echinococcus*. Clinically important disease forms in humans are:

- Cystic echinococcosis (hydatid disease, hydatosis): *E. granulosus*. Found worldwide. Usual host is dog. Also goats, swine, horses, cattle, camels, yaks.
- Alveolar echinococcosis: *E. multilocularis*. Found in northern hemisphere. Usual hosts are foxes and rodents.

Human ingest parasite eggs via food/water contaminated by animal faeces, or by handing animals which are infected with the tapeworm. Disease is due to the development of cyst-like larvae in viscera, usually liver/lungs. *Presentation:* Slow growing cysts may be asymptomatic for many years. Symptoms and signs depends on location:

- *Liver:* abdominal pain, nausea, hepatomegaly, obstructive jaundice, cholangitis, PUO.
- *Lung:* dyspnoea, chest pain, cough, haemoptysis.
- *CNS:* space-occupying signs.
- *Bone:* an interesting osteolytic cause of knee pain, cord compression.
- Silent disease in breast, kidney, adrenals, bladder, heart, psoas.

Diagnosis: USS/CT/MRI: avascular fluid-filled cysts ± calcification (ΔΔ benign cyst, TB, mycoses, abscess, neoplasm). Serology. Positive echinococcal antigen. *Treatment:* Get help (including surgical). Depends on cyst type, location, size, and complications. Prolonged treatment (months/years) with albendazole. **PAIR**: **P**uncture, **A**spirate, **I**nject (hypertonic saline/chemicals), **R**easpirate. Beware spillage of cyst contents: praziquantel can be given peri-operatively.

***Fasciola hepatica* (common liver fluke)**
Parasitic infection. ~2 million infected worldwide. Highest rates of infection in Bolivia and Peru. Infective larvae develop in aquatic snail hosts. Humans infected via contaminated water, waterplants eg watercress, or by eating the undercooked liver of another host animal eg sheep, goat. Disease caused by migration of parasite to bile ducts. *Presentation: Acute phase* with migration from intestine through liver (2–4 months): abdominal pain, nausea, fever, urticarial rash, eosinophilia. *Chronic phase* with egg production in the bile ducts: cholecystitis, cholangitis, pancreatitis, cirrhosis. *Diagnosis:* Serology in acute and chronic phase. Ova in stool/bile aspirate only in chronic phase. *Treatment:* Triclabendazole as a single dose. Treat all suspected cases in endemic areas.

Other liver flukes: opisthorchiasis and clonorchiasis
Opisthorchis and *clonorchis* are liver flukes acquired by eating contaminated fish, mainly in south-east Asia. Adult worms lodge in the small bile ducts and gallbladder. *Presentation:* Abdominal pain, GI disturbance, cholecystitis, cholangitis, cholangiocarcinoma. *Diagnosis:* Ova in stool. *Treatment:* Praziquantel.

Tropical liver disease

An overview of the differential diagnosis of tropical/imported liver disease is shown in table 9.28.

Table 9.28 Tropical liver disease by presentation[22]

Presentation	Differential diagnosis
Jaundice/hepatitis	Viral hepatitis, brucellosis, dengue, enteric fever, HIV, leptospirosis, malaria, rickettsial infection, sepsis, TB, viral haemorrhagic fever, yellow fever
Hepatomegaly	Amoebic/pyogenic liver abscess, echinococcosis, liver fluke, carcinoma
Massive hepatomegaly	Visceral leishmaniasis, tropical lymphoma, late-stage schistosomiasis
Fibrosis/cirrhosis	Chronic hepatitis, schistosomiasis, alcohol, non-alcoholic fatty liver disease

Consider liver toxicity: ackee fruit (Jamaica), aflatoxins (peanuts, corn, tropical countries without monitoring/regulation), death cap mushroom, iron, bush tea, methanol, copper, paraquat, pyrrolizidine alkaloids (herbal remedies).

Botulism

Neuroparalytic infection caused by neurotoxin from anaerobic, spore-forming *Clostridium botulinum* (rarely *C. butyricum, C. barattii*). Food-borne due to toxin production in food (*botulus* is Latin for sausage), or wound botulism due to spore germination in wound (includes IV drug use). Toxin blocks release of acetylcholine at neuromuscular junction causing flaccid paralysis. *Presentation:* Incubation up to 8d (usually 12-36h). Afebrile, descending, flaccid paralysis: diplopia, ptosis, dysarthria, dysphagia, progressive paralysis of limbs, respiratory failure. Autonomic signs: dry mouth, fixed/dilated pupils, urinary/cardiac/GI dysfunction. ►*No sensory signs. Diagnosis:* Clinical: do not delay treatment. Take samples (serum, faeces, wound swab) for later confirmation by culture/PCR. In UK contact GI Bacteria Reference Unit (020 8327 7887). *Treatment:* Get help. Admit to ITU. Botulinum antitoxin (from Public Health England, Colindale 020 8200 4400), benzylpenicillin, metronidazole.

Tetanus

Caused by anaerobic *Clostridium tetani* spores universally present in soil. Enters body via a breach in skin. Produces a neurotoxin (tetanospasmin) which disseminates via blood/ lymphatics and interferes with neurotransmitter release causing unopposed muscle contraction and spasm (tetanus = 'to stretch'). ~6 cases/yr in England and Wales (2015). Maternal and neonatal tetanus important cause of preventable mortality in low-middle income countries. *Presentation:* Site of entry may be trivial/unnoticed. Incubation ~3-21d. Prodrome: fever, malaise, headache. Trismus (lockjaw, Greek 'trismos' = grinding). Risus sardonicus = a grin-like posture of hypertonic facial muscles. Opisthotonus (fig 9.45). Muscular spasms induced by movement, injections, noise, then spontaneous. Dysphagia. Autonomic dysfunction: arrhythmias ± fluctuating BP. Respiratory arrest. *Diagnosis:* Clinical. Detection of tetanus toxin/isolation of *C. tetani*. *Treatment:* ►►Get help on ITU: level of supportive care predicts outcome. Tetanus immunoglobulin (TIG) IM (or equine antitetanus serum if not available). Take blood for detection of tetanus-toxin and anti-tetanus antibodies first. Wound debridement, metronidazole. Management of spasm: diazepam/lorazepam/midazolam (may need high doses IV), IV magnesium sulphate, baclofen (intra-thecal administration needed for penetration of blood-brain barrier ∴ only with ICU ventilatory support), dantrolene, botulinum toxin-A.[23] *Vaccination:* Routine in UK (p407). Prophylaxis following injury: TIG if heavy contamination. If vaccination history unknown/incomplete: TIG plus dose of vaccine in a different site. Precautionary travel booster if >10y since last dose.

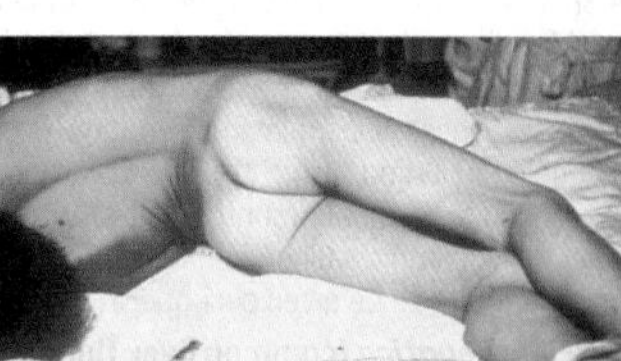

Fig 9.45 Spasm causing opisthotonus (arching of body with neck hyperextension). ΔΔ tetanus, rabies, cerebral malaria, neurosyphilis, acute cerebral injury, catatonia.

Poliomyelitis

A highly infectious picornavirus, transmitted via faeco-oral route or contaminated food/water. Replicates in intestine. Invades nervous system with destruction of anterior horn cells/brain stem→irreversible paralysis. Incidence ↓by 99% since formation of Global Polio Eradication Initiative in 1988. 74 cases in 2015. Remains endemic in Afghanistan and Pakistan (2016).[12] *Presentation:* Incubation 7-10d. Flu-like prodrome in ~25%. Pre-paralytic stage: fever, ↑HR, headache, vomiting, neck stiffness tremor, limb pain. ~1 in 200 progress to paralytic stage: LMN/bulbar signs ± respiratory failure. ►*No sensory signs*. Post-polio syndrome in ~40% of survivors (up to 40y later): new progressive muscle weakness, myalgia, fatigue.

Diagnosis: Viral culture of stool (most sensitive, 2 samples >24h apart), pharyngeal swabs, blood, CSF. PCR can differentiate wild-type from vaccine. Paired serology. *Treatment:* None. *Vaccination:* Salk (inactivated, IM) or Sabin (live, oral). In previously endemic areas 200 million volunteers have vaccinated 3 billion children preventing 1.5 million deaths in the last 20y.

Rabies

Rhabdovirus transmitted through saliva or CNS tissue, usually from the bite of an infected mammal, eg bat (in UK), dog (95% of transmissions to humans), cat, fox. Disease is fatal once symptoms appear. Worldwide distribution. ~50 000 deaths/yr, most in Africa/Asia. *Presentation:* Incubation ~9-90d. Prodrome: headache, malaise, odd behaviour, agitation, fever, paraesthesia at bite/wound site. Progresses to one of two disease forms:

- *'Furious rabies':* hyperactivity and terror (hydrophobia, aerophobia)
- *'Paralytic rabies':* flaccid paralysis in the bitten limb→coma→death.

Diagnosis: Clinical: potential exposure + signs of myelitis/encephalitis (non-progressive disease and disease >3wk are negative indicators). Viral PCR (saliva, brain, nerve tissue) or CSF antibodies may offer later (post-mortem) confirmation. *Treatment:* If bitten, or lick to broken skin, wash (>15min) with soap and seek urgent help. Post-exposure prophylaxis: vaccination ± rabies immunoglobulin. Experimental treatments: ribavirin, interferon alfa, ketamine. Preventable and elimination feasible with pre-exposure vaccination of all at risk. Vaccination of dogs can ↓ human cases.

Japanese encephalitis virus

Flavivirus spread by mosquitoes. Endemic transmission (~3 billion at risk) and common cause of viral encephalitis in Asia and west Pacific. Severe disease is rare (1 in 250) but leads to neurological or psychiatric sequelae in up to 50%, mortality up to 30%. *Presentation:* Incubation 5-15d. Most asymptomatic, or mild fever and headache only. Severe disease: high fever, headache, meningism, altered mental status, coma, seizures, spastic paralysis, death. *Diagnosis:* Clinical in endemic area. Serum/CSF serology, PCR.[7] *Treatment:* Supportive. Vaccination.

West Nile virus

Mosquito-borne flavivirus with transmission in Europe, Middle East, Africa, Asia, Australia, and Americas. *Presentation:* Incubation 2-14d. Asymptomatic in ~80%. West Nile fever in ~20%: fever, headache, N&V, lymphadenopathy. Neuroinvasive in ~1%: encephalitis, meningitis, flaccid paralysis, mortality ~10%. *Diagnosis:* Serum/CSF IgM, viral PCR. *Treatment:* Supportive. Vaccine awaited (2016).

Neurocysticercosis

Most common helminthic disease of the CNS and most frequent cause of preventable epilepsy (~50% of epilepsy in endemic areas, fig 9.46). Caused by pork tapeworm *Taenia solium*. Consumption of infected pork leads to intestinal infection (taeniasis) and the shedding of *T. solium* eggs in stool. Invasive disease occurs when the shed eggs are ingested via faeco-oral transmission. Neurocysticercosis is due to larval cysts infecting the CNS. *Presentation:* Determined by site and number of lesions (cysticerci) within the brain/spinal cord. Epilepsy in 70%. Focal neurology in ~20%: motor/sensory loss, language disturbance, involuntary movements. Also headache, visual loss, meningitis, hydrocephalus, cognitive impairment. *Diagnosis:* CT/MRI imaging plus serology. *Treatment:* Seizure control (↓evidence on drug choice, length of treatment or prophylaxis). Neurosurgical advice if hydrocephalus/↑ICP. Albendazole for non-calcified lesions (better penetration of CNS than praziquantel). Beware inflammatory response provoked by treatment—consider dexamethasone.

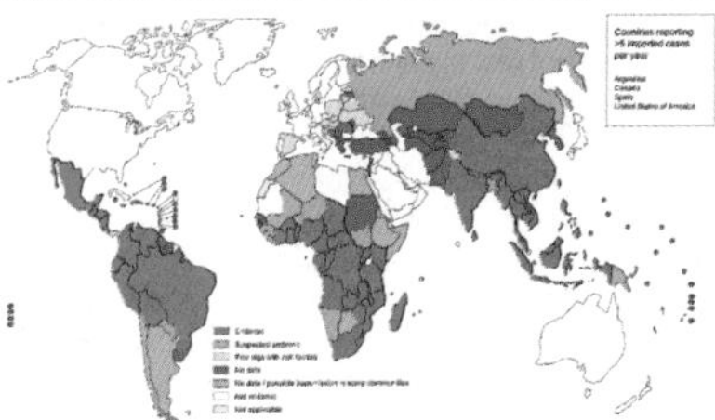

Fig 9.46 Endemicity (red) and suspected endemicity (orange) of *Taenia solium* 2015.

Reproduced with permission from WHO, *Endemicity of Taenia solium, 2015.* ©World Health Organization 2016. http://www.who.int/mediacentre/factsheets/Endemicity_Taenia_Solium_2015-1000x706.jpg?ua=1

Specialist diagnostic service and advice in UK via Rare and Imported Pathogens Laboratory (RIPL): www.gov.uk/government/collections/rare-and-imported-pathogens-laboratory-ripl

Conjunctivitis

Common in tropical areas. Vision is normal. Differentiation between common infectious causes is outlined in table 9.29.

Table 9.29 Common causes of conjunctivitis

Cause	Secretions	Features	Treatment
Bacterial	Purulent	Red and swollen	Topical antibiotics for 5d
Viral	Watery	± Corneal lesion	Symptomatic
Trachoma (chlamydial)	Mucopurulent	Follicles and papillae on lid	Azithromycin PO or topical tetracycline

Reproduced from Brent *et al.*, *Oxford Handbook of Tropical Medicine*, 2014, with permission from Oxford University Press.

Trachoma

Leading infectious cause of blindness worldwide: visual impairment/blindness in 1.9 million, 200 million at risk. Prevalence in endemic areas 60- 90% (Africa, Central and South America, Asia, Middle East). Caused by *Chlamydia trachomatis*. Human-to-human transmission with contact, or via flies which land on noses/eyes. *Presentation:* Active infection causes purulent discharge and follicular inflammation of the eyelid (fig 9.47a)→scarring (fig 9.47b)→eyelids turn inwards (entropion) and irritate the cornea (trichiasis) (fig 9.47c) leading to visual loss.

Treatment: WHO public health strategy **SAFE:** surgery to treat blinding disease (trichiasis), antibiotics (azithromycin) to clear infection (mass administration in endemic areas through International Trachoma Initiative), facial cleanliness, environmental improvement with access to water and sanitation.[12]

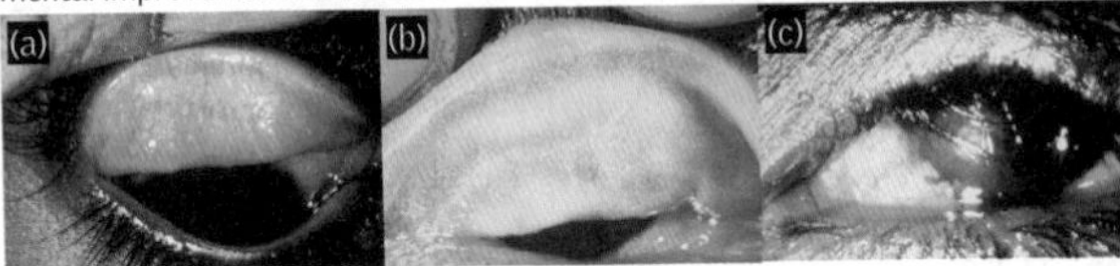

Fig 9.47 (a) Follicular trachoma. (b) Scarring. (c) Trichiasis.

Reproduced from Warrell *et al.*, *Oxford Textbook of Medicine*, 2010, with permission from Oxford University Press.

Immunosuppression and the eye

• *Herpes zoster ophthalmicus:*

Due to reactivation of latent varicella zoster virus (p404) in the ophthalmic branch of the trigeminal nerve. ↑ Risk of reactivation and ocular complications in immunosuppression: HIV, post-transplantation. *Presentation:* vesiculomacular skin rash and dysaesthesia in ophthalmic division of the trigeminal nerve (fig 9.48). Hutchinson's sign = lesion at tip/side of nose indicates involvement of nasociliary branch of V1 and ↑chance of eye involvement. Complications: corneal opacification, uveitis, ocular nerve palsy, eyelid deformity, optic neuritis, post-herpetic neuralgia. Can be sight-threatening ∴ recognition and urgent treatment are required. *Diagnosis:* clinical. Antibody staining/PCR of skin scrapings. *Treatment:* oral famciclovir/valacyclovir or systemic aciclovir reduce complications if given within 72h of symptoms. Analgesia. If retinitis IV cidofovir ± intravitreal ganciclovir or foscarnet.

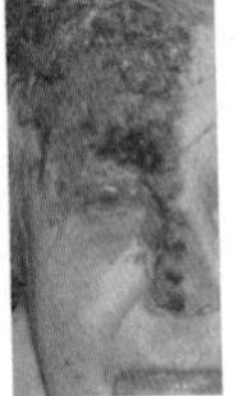

Fig 9.48 Herpes zoster ophthalmicus

©MN Oxman , University of California

• *CMV retinitis:*

Reactivation of CMV infection (p405). *Presentation:* floaters due to inflammatory cells in vitreous, flashing lights, scotomata, eye pain, visual loss. Peripheral lesions

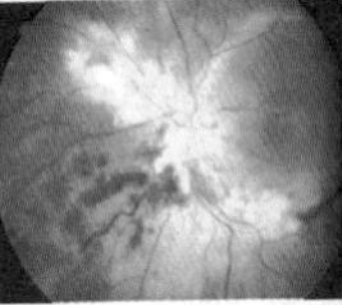

Fig 9.49 CMV retinitis (mozzarella pizza fundus).

©Prof Trob

may be asymptomatic. Routine examination for those at risk (CD4<100 cells/microlitre). *Diagnosis:* clinical. Fundoscopy: granular white dots, haemorrhage (fig 9.49). Can progress to an arcuate/triangular zone of infection, or can be linear following vessels/nerve fibres. *Treatment:* systemic valganciclovir (oral, IV). Also ganciclovir, foscarnet, cidofovir. ART if underlying HIV (see p402).

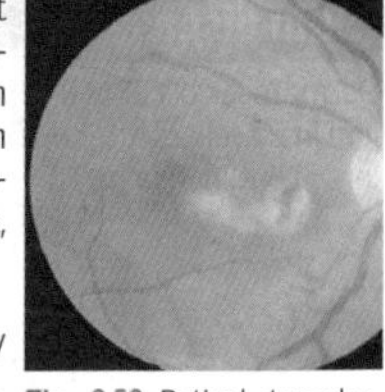

Fig 9.50 Retinal toxoplasmosis. ©Prof Trobe.

- *Ocular toxoplasmosis:*

Causes posterior uveitis. *Presentation:* blurred vision/floaters. *Diagnosis:* clinical. Fundoscopy (fig 9.50): focus of choroiditis, chorioretinal scar from previous infection, overlying vitreal haze due to inflammatory response. Multiple/bilateral/extensive lesions if ↑ immunosuppression. Serology. Ocular fluid PCR. *Treatment:* atovaquone (↓toxicity), sulfadiazine, and pyrimethamine.

Filarial infection

Onchocerciasis ('river blindness')

Caused by filarial worm, *Onchocerca volvulus*. Transmitted by the bite of infected black flies which breed in fast-flowing rivers and streams. Second most common infectious cause of blindness worldwide: predominantly sub-Saharan Africa, Brazil, Venezuela, Yemen. *Presentation:* A nodule forms at the site of the bite where larvae mature to adult worms. The female adult can release up to 1000 microfilariae/day causing:

- skin disease: altered pigmentation, lichenification, loss of elasticity, poor healing
- eye disease: keratitis, uveitis, cataract, fixed pupil, fundal degeneration, optic neuritis/atrophy, visual impairment/loss (fig 9.51)
- impaired lymphatic function: lymphadenopathy, elephantiasis.

Diagnosis: Visualization of microfilaria in eye or on skin snip biopsy: a fine shaving of clean skin is incubated in 0.9% saline to allow microfilariae to emerge for microscopic identification. Serology. *Treatment:* Ivermectin 150mcg/kg, one dose every 3-12 months (depending on likely re-exposure). CI if coexisting Loa-Loa due to risk of fatal encephalitic reaction. Or 6wk doxycycline. No vaccine available.

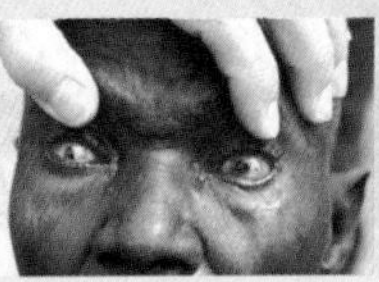

Fig 9.51 Bilateral sclerosing keratitis in onchocerciasis causing blindness.

Reproduced from Warrell *et al.* *Oxford Textbook of Medicine*, 2010, with permission from Oxford University Press.

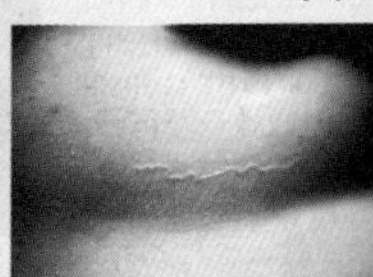

Fig 9.52 Migrating *Loa loa* in the skin.

Reproduced from Warrell *et al.* *Oxford Textbook of Medicine*, 2010, with permission from Oxford University Press.

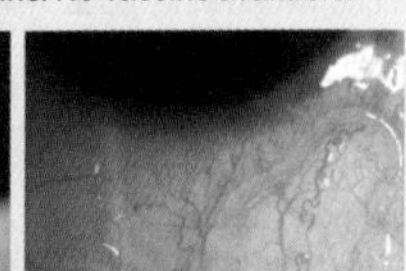

Fig 9.53 *Loa loa* crossing the conjunctiva.

Reproduced from Warrell *et al.* *Oxford Textbook of Medicine*, 2010, with permission from Oxford University Press.

Loiasis (African eye-worm)

Caused by parasitic worm *Loa loa*. Transmitted via bite of deerflies (=mangrove/mango flies) which breed in rainforests of west and central Africa. *Presentation:* Recurrent pruritic lesions due to angioedema ('Calabar swellings'), myalgia, arthralgia. The adult worm can migrate through subcutaneous (fig 9.52) and subconjunctival (fig 9.53) tissue: 'Something's wiggling in my eye, doctor'. This eerie eye trip causes intense conjunctivitis, which heals if left alone. (Don't treat until transmigration in the eye is over: on detecting your therapy the worm tends to panic.) Also causes glomerulonephritis, and encephalitis. *Diagnosis:* Microfilariae on blood smear, serology, PCR. Eosinophilia. *Treatment:* Diethylcarbamazine (DEC) kills both microfilariae and adult worms. Risk of encephalopathy is related to microfilarial load: albendazole can be used to ↓ microfilarial load prior to DEC (response may be slow).

►See also lymphatic filariasis p421.

Dermatoses occur in 8–23% of travellers and are the 3rd most common health problem in travellers after diarrhoea and fever. The differential of skin problems in travellers in outlined in fig 9.54.

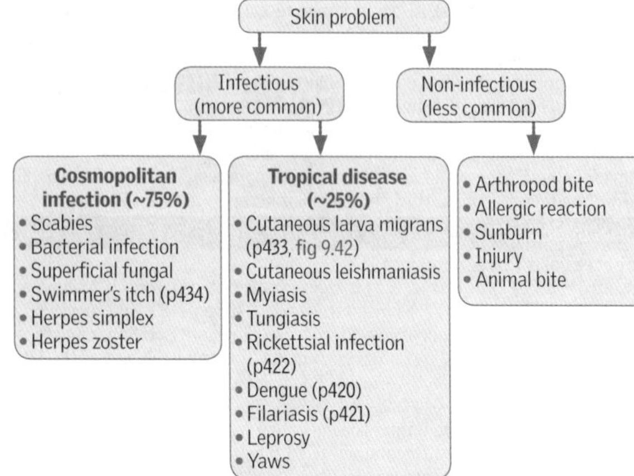

Fig 9.54 Skin problems in travellers.

Adapted from *Travel Medicine and Infectious Disease*, 7(3), O'Brien, BM, 'A practical approach to common skin problems in returning travellers', 125–46. Copyright 2009, with permission from Elsevier.

Scabies

Caused by microscopic mite *Sarcoptes scabiei*. Found worldwide, ~300 million cases/yr. Female mites burrow into the epidermis and deposit eggs. Symptoms due to an allergic reaction to the parasite. Transmission via direct and prolonged skin-to-skin contact. Epidemics linked to poverty, overcrowding, and poor water supply. *Presentation:* Severe (nocturnal) pruritus, papular/scaly rash, burrows may be visible (fig 9.55). Itch can lead to secondary bacterial infection. *Diagnosis:* Clinical. Skin scraping for mite/eggs/faeces. *Treatment:* Topical permethrin 5% or malathion 0.5%. Ivermectin given for filariasis (p421) may effectively treat concurrent scabies.

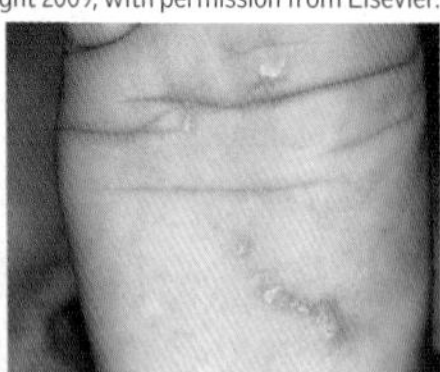

Fig 9.55 Scabies burrow.

Reproduced from Burge *et al.*, *Oxford Handbook of Medical Dermatology*, 2016, with permission from Oxford University Press.

Cutaneous leishmaniasis

Most common form of leishmaniasis. Estimated 0.7–1.3 million new cases/yr: Americas, Mediterranean basin, north Africa, Middle East, central Asia. *Presentation:* Lesions develop at the bite site, beginning as an itchy papule; crusts fall off to leave a painless ulcer with a well-defined, raised border and a crusted base = 'Chiclero's ulcer' (fig 9.56). *Diagnosis:* Skin biopsy + PCR. *Treatment:* Most heal in ~2–15 months with scarring (disfiguring if extensive). 'New World' disease (South America) needs treating due to risk of mucocutaneous disease: pentavalent antimony, eg meglumine antimoniate, sodium stibogluconate. (See p423.)

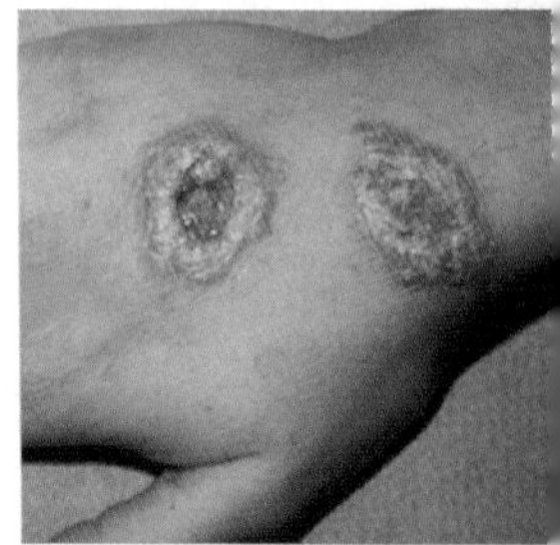

Fig 9.56 Cutaneous leishmaniasis with central crusting.

Reproduced from Lewis-Jones, *Paediatric Dermatology*, 2010, with permission from Oxford University Press.

Myiasis

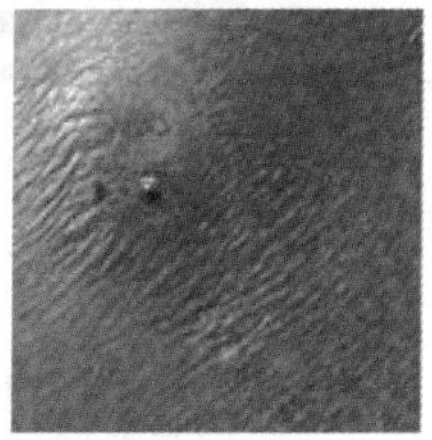

Fig 9.57 Myiasis.

Infection with fly larvae/maggot. Can affect living and necrotic tissue. In south and central America the human botfly lays its eggs on mosquitoes which deposit them when they bite. In sub-Sahran Africa the tumbu fly lays its eggs on clothing which then transfer to skin. *Presentation:* Painful swelling. May have sensation of movement within the lesion. May open to reveal larval breathing tubes (fig 9.57). *Diagnosis:* Clinical. Identification of larvae in lesion. *Treatment:* Petroleum or pork fat cause asphyxiation of the maggot causing it to protrude further out of the skin enabling removal with tweezers. Care: backward-facing spines in American disease may prevent complete removal unless done surgically. Ensure tetanus vaccination is up to date.

Tungiasis

Infection of the skin by the sand/jigger flea *Tunga penetrans*. Acquired (usually walking barefoot) in sandy soil, rainforests, and banana plantations in south and central America, sub-Saharan Africa, Asia, Caribbean. *Presentation:* Painful, itchy papule on the feet. May be visible extrusion of eggs. Black crusting when flea dies. *Diagnosis:* Clinical. *Treatment:* None, self-limiting.

Leprosy (Hansen's disease)

Caused by slow-growing, acid-fast *Mycobacterium leprae* which affects skin, nerves, and mucous membranes. Incubation 5-20y. Transmitted via droplets from nose/mouth during close and frequent contact. Classified as:

- Multibacillary ('lepromatous'): ↓immune response, ↑bacilli, +ve smear.
- Paucibacillary ('tuberculoid'): ↑immune response, granulomata with ↓bacilli, smears may be −ve.

Free treatment through WHO since 1995: prevalence ↓ by 99% to 176 000 in 2014 (5.2 million in 1985).[12] *Presentation:* Hypopigmented skin lesions (fig 9.58, less well demarcated than vitiligo), sensory loss, thickened nerves, nodules, plaques, nasal congestion, epistaxis, muscle weakness, paralysis, neuropathic ulcers. Eye involvement: chronic iritis, scleritis, episcleritis, ↓corneal sensation (V nerve palsy), ↓blinking and lagophthalmos (VII nerve palsy), trauma from eyelashes (trichiasis). *Diagnosis:* Clinical, +ve skin smear, skin biopsy. Serology unreliable. *Treatment:* WHO multidrug therapy:

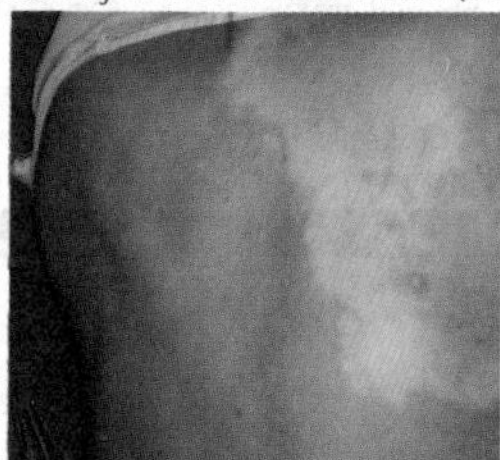

Fig 9.58 Leprosy: hypopigmented macules. Courtesy of Prof. Jayakar Thoma.

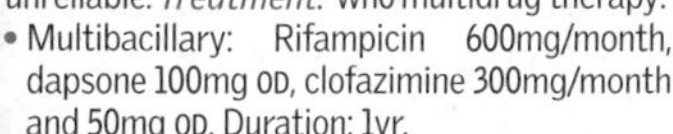

- Multibacillary: Rifampicin 600mg/month, dapsone 100mg OD, clofazimine 300mg/month and 50mg OD. Duration: 1yr.
- Paucibacillary: rifampicin 600mg/month, dapsone 100mg OD. Duration: 6 months. If single lesion: rifampicin 600mg+ofloxacin 400mg+minocycline 100mg (single dose).

Yaws

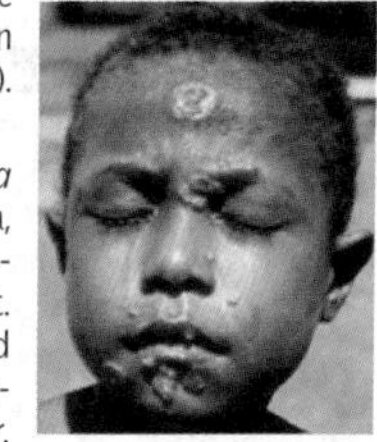

Fig 9.59 Ulceropapillomatous yaws.

Courtesy of Dr B Hudson, Sydney, Australia.

Chronic granulomatous disease caused by *Treponema pertenue*. Found in humid/rainforest areas in Africa, Asia, Latin American, Pacific. Associated with ↓socioeconomic conditions. Transmission via direct contact. *Presentation:* Primary disease = papilloma. If untreated will ulcerate (fig 9.59). Secondary disease: yellow skin lesions, dactylitis. CVS and CNS complications do not occur. *Diagnosis:* Serology is indistinguishable from syphilis (*Treponema pallidum*). Dual-path platform (DPP) assay can distinguish between current and past infection. PCR. *Treatment:* Single-dose azithromycin PO.

Pyrexia of unknown origin (PUO)

This chapter gives guidance on hundreds of pyrexia-causing infections; but what should you do if your patient has a fever that you cannot explain? Pyrexia of unknown origin (PUO)[24] has a differential of >200 diseases. 15-30% of these patients will eventually be given an infective diagnosis (depending on your corner of the globe). ~20% will remain undiagnosed, but in most of these the fever will resolve within 4wks.

Diagnostic criteria

Pyrexia >3wks with no identified cause after evaluation in hospital for 3d or ≥3 out-patient visits.

Fever may also be undiagnosed in specific subgroups despite appropriate evaluation for 3d, including negative cultures at ≥2 days:

- *Nosocomial PUO:* Patient hospitalized for >48h with no infection at admission.
- *Immunodeficient PUO:* Pyrexia in patient with <500 neutrophils/microlitre.
- *HIV PUO:* Pyrexia in HIV infection lasting 3d as an in-patient or >4wks as an outpatient.

History

Most PUO are due to common diseases with atypical presentation. Consider all details as potentially relevant. Include: travel (p414), diet, animal contact, changes in medication, recreational drug use, obstetric/sexual history, family history (table 9.30).

Examination

Confirm fever. Pattern of fever is rarely helpful (contrary to the textbooks, most malaria has no specific pattern). Do not forget: mouth, genitals, skin, thyroid, lymphatic system, eyes including retina, temporal arteries (table 9.30).

Investigation

►Extent of investigation depends on immune status and how well the patient is.

- *Blood tests:* FBC, U&E, LFT, CRP, ESR, electrophoresis, LDH, CK, ANA, ANCA, rheumatoid factor, HIV test, malaria smear, interferon-gamma release assay for TB (p394).
- *Microscopy and culture:* Blood ×3, urine, sputum (including AFB), stool, CSF.
- *Imaging:* CXR, abdominal/pelvic USS, venous Doppler. Consider: CT(PA), MRI, echo (TOE). Fluorodeoxyglucose-PET (FDG-PET) highlights areas of ↑glucose uptake including tumour and inflammation. It may aid/direct diagnosis in up to 50% of PUO.
- *Other:* Hepatitis serology, CMV, EBV, autoimmune screen, cryoglobulins, toxoplasmosis, brucellosis, *Coxiella*, lymph node biopsy, endoscopy, temporal artery biopsy.

Table 9.30 PUO differential according to history and examination findings

History	Differential
Animal contact	Brucellosis, toxoplasmosis, *Bartonella*, leptospirosis, Q fever, psittacosis
Cough	TB, PE, Q fever, enteric fever, sarcoidosis, legionnaire's disease
Nasal symptoms	Sinusitis, GPA, relapsing fever, psittacosis
Confusion	TB, *Cryptococcus*, sarcoid, carcinomatosis, brucellosis, enteric fever
Arthralgia	SLE, infective endocarditis, Lyme disease, brucellosis, TB, IBD
Weight loss	Malignancy, vasculitis, TB, HIV, IBD, thyrotoxicosis
Family history	Familial Mediterranean fever
Drug history	Drug-induced fever (~7-10d after new drug)
Examination	**Differential**
Conjunctivitis	Leptospirosis, relapsing fever, spotted fever, trichinosis
Uveitis	TB, sarcoid, adult Still's disease, SLE, Behçet's disease
Mouth	Dental abscess, Behçet's disease, CMV, IBD
Lymphadenopathy	Lymphoma, TB, EBV, CMV, HIV, toxoplasmosis, brucellosis, *Bartonella*
Rash	HIV, EBV, SLE, vasculitis, Still's disease, endocarditis
Hepatomegaly	TB, EBV, malignancy, malaria, enteric fever, granulomatous hepatitis, Q fever, visceral leishmaniasis
Splenomegaly	Leukaemia, lymphoma, TB, brucellosis, infective endocarditis, CMV, EBV, rheumatoid arthritis, sarcoid, enteric fever, relapsing fever
Renal	Chronic pyelonephritis, perinephric abscess, renal tumour
Epididymo-orchitis	TB, lymphoma, EBV, brucellosis, leptospirosis

Eliciting the weird and the wonderful

Listen to your patient You have two cultures to master: the host and the pathogen. Prolonged immersion in both may be needed.

Ask Do not expect to find apposite questions such as these in any other textbook:

1 *'Have you delivered any septic babies in the last year?'* Impress and cure your obstetrician friends who tell you that 'I'm so depressed about not being able to shake off this flu', and who have forgotten about transfer of brucellosis from baby to obstetrician.
2 *'Are your carp well at present?' Mycobacterium marinum* skin infection.
3 *'Could that be a Hyalomma tick bite from when you rode your ostrich in last week's race?'* Crimean-Congo haemorrhagic fever.
4 *'Who has been licking your face recently?' Pasteurella multocida.*
5 *'Has your dog been on holiday this year?'* Monkeypox from prairie dogs.
6 *'Has your pet hedgehog lost weight?' Salmonella.*
7 *'Did you develop your headache after you adopted your pet magpie?'* Zoonotic transmission of *Cryptococcus neoformans* causing meningitis.
8 *'Did you have a stray pig living under your house when the monsoon started?'* Pigs + standing water + mosquitoes = Japanese encephalitis.
9 *'Did you sample the local frog paella?'* Angiostrongyliasis causing eosinophilic meningitis.
10 *'Did your goat miscarry last year?' Coxiella burnetii.*
11 *'Did your depressed pig develop a purple snout?' Erysipelothrix rhusiopathiae* endocarditis via swine erysipelas.
12 *'Can I see your pet lobster: he may be the cause of your bad hand?'* Lobsterman's hand, an erysipeloid infection from *Erysipelothrix*. Pet lobsters have a grand pedigree. Gérard de Nerval used to take his pet lobster for walks, on a blue silk lead, beside the Seine (fig 9.60). A lobster, he said, is, 'serious-minded and quiet, doesn't scratch or bark like a dog, and knows all of the secrets of the deep'. His lobster's mission was to combat the Philistinism chaining us all to mediocrity.

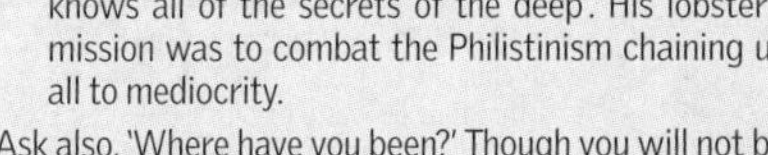

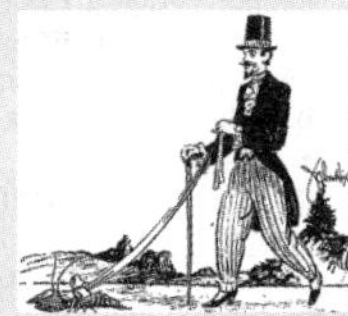

Fig 9.60 'Is your pet lobster well?' (Gérard de Nerval).

Ask also, 'Where have you been?' Though you will not be absolved of thought, even when the answer is, 'Southend'. It may be a question of amnesic stopovers. Or perhaps your patient is an airport baggage-handler, bitten by a hitch-hiking mosquito. And even when there has been no travel to the tropics, global warming is ensuring that the tropics are travelling to us. To the first writers of medical books, Paradise was just beyond the Far East, and the world was a disc surrounded by oceans of blue water. But the world moves on, tarnished, tawdry, and trashed; and Paradise appears to be evolving with ever more serpents in the garden, beguiling us with ambiguous answers to our great questions.

Don't give up If the culture is negative, tests may need repeating. Perhaps the organism is 'fastidious' in its nutritional requirement or requires a longer incubation? Even if culture is achieved, it may be that the organism grown is flora not pathogen. If culture fails, look for antibodies or antigen. PCR is increasingly used for identification, but it is far from infallible; beware of inhibitors, contamination, and a primer that is not as unique as your patient.

Remember Sherlock: *'My mind,' he said, 'rebels at stagnation. Give me problems, give me work, give me the most abstruse cryptogram or the most intricate analysis, and I am in my own proper atmosphere. I can dispense then with artificial stimulants. But I abhor the dull routine of existence. I crave for mental exaltation. That is why I have chosen my own particular profession, - or rather created it, for I am the only one in the world.'*

The Sign of the Four, Arthur Conan Doyle, 1890.

No, Sherlock, you are not; you have the infectious disease physicians for company.

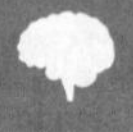

Contents

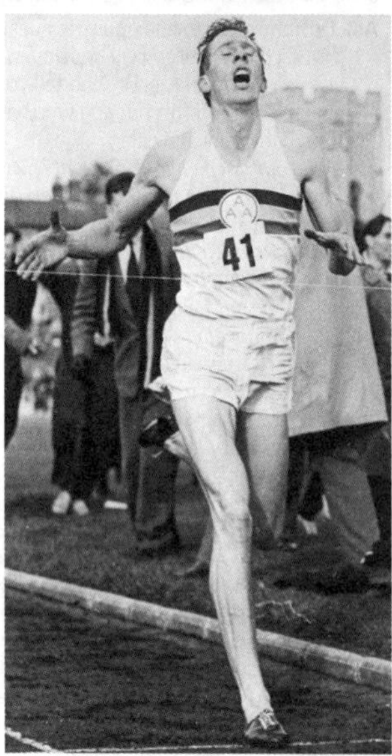

Fig 10.1 Sir Roger Bannister CBE ran the first ever sub-4 minute mile on 6 May 1954 at the age of 25. At that time he was a medical student at Oxford University, and graduated the following year. He went on to become a prominent academic neurologist, conducting research into the autonomic nervous system, which he regarded as his greatest achievement. Autonomic activity and running are, of course, intimately linked, as Bannister reflected in a more poetic manner than the usual 'fight or flight' cliché: 'As a child I ran barefoot along damp, fresh sand by the seashore. The air there had a special quality.... The sound of breakers shut out all others, and I was startled, almost frightened, by the tremendous excitement a few steps could create. It was an intense moment of discovery of a source of power and beauty that one previously hardly dreamt existed.' In 2014, Bannister spoke publicly of his sense of irony at being diagnosed with Parkinson's disease.

Bettmann / Bettmann collection / Getty Images.

We thank Dr Thomas Hughes, our Specialist Reader, for his contribution to this chapter.

I think, therefore I am

It is the brain, more than any other organ, that marks *Homo sapiens* apart from other animals. Our ability to be self-aware, to think, and to reason has formed the basis of scientific inquiry and philosophical speculation for millennia, as we attempt to rationalize and define this cognitive capability. What is the mind? Less tangible than other aspects of our being, throughout time humans have looked to explanations from philosophy, folklore, religion, and now science. The concept of the sense of self and being that defines us all—whether it be called the ego, nous, or the soul—remains intriguing yet elusive to explain. Aristotle held that the psyche (Greek: ψυχή=*soul*) was not separate to its housing body, as one could not exist without the other. This view was directly contradicted by the 17th-century French philosopher René Descartes. He proposed the theory of 'mind-body dualism' in which the mind, located in the pineal gland, is an entirely separate entity to the material being, and controls the avatar of the physical body like a puppeteer.

These conflicting viewpoints well illustrate the spectrum of neurological disease and its blurred boundaries with psychiatry and psychology. Jean Martin Charcot (1825-1893), often credited as the father of neurology, appeared to be more interested in this crossover than neuronal dysfunction: he spent two decades of his career studying hysteria in Paris, initially attributing symptoms of crying, fainting, and temporary blindness to an organic, inherited cause, before revising his view in later life to conclude that this was a psychological disease. His controversial work in this field inspired his student Sigmund Freud's psychoanalytical theories, and illustrated the very real power of the conscious, or sub-conscious, to produce physical symptoms, a phenomenon familiar to all physicians. Perhaps reflecting our frustration with this challenging area as much as his limited success, we remember Charcot for his more tangible outputs, for example, in giving the inaugural description of, among other things, multiple sclerosis, Parkinson's disease, amyotrophic lateral sclerosis (ALS), Charcot-Marie-Tooth disease, and of course his eponymous misshapen joint resulting from proprioceptive loss.

However, both Aristotle and Charcot would have surely agreed with Descartes' proposition of 'cogito ergo sum': I think, therefore I am. Whether mind and brain are dual or one, they are inextricably linked and the very nature of awareness proves its existence.

Where is the lesion?

This is an important first question to ask and depends on recognizing characteristic patterns of cognitive, cranial nerve, motor, and sensory deficits. Locating a focal lesion can be aided by features such as asymmetry (eg one pupil dilated, one upgoing plantar response) or a spinal level (effects may be symmetrical below the lesion). ►Note that sometimes there is no single lesion, rather, a *general insult* causing a falsely localizing sign, eg abducens nerve palsy in ↑ICP. Other generalized causes of specific local effects are: trauma, encephalitis, anoxia, poisoning, or post-ictal states.

Patterns of loss Are crucial in locating the lesion (see BOX 'From findings to neuroanatomy'):

Upper motor neuron (UMN): Patterns of weakness are caused by damage anywhere along the corticospinal (=pyramidal) tracts: pathways that carry motor information from the precentral gyrus of the frontal cortex up to the synapse with anterior horn cells in the spinal cord (via the internal capsule, brainstem, and cord).[1] •UMN weakness affects groups rather than individual muscles, typically in a '*pyramidal*' pattern: in the arm, extensors are predominantly affected; in the leg the opposite is true and the flexors are the weaker muscle group. •*Spasticity* develops in the stronger muscle groups (arm flexors and leg extensors). It manifests as ↑*tone* that is *velocity-dependent*, ie the faster you move the patient's muscle, the greater the resistance, until it finally gives way (like a 'clasp-knife').[2] •Muscle wasting is less prominent. • There is *hyperreflexia:* reflexes are brisk. • *Plantars are upgoing* (+ve Babinski sign) ± *clonus* (elicited by rapidly dorsiflexing the foot; ≤3 rhythmic, downward beats of the foot are normal). •*Loss of skilled fine finger movements* may be greater than expected from the overall grade of weakness (see BOX 'Muscle weakness grading'). ►UMN lesions can mimic LMN lesions in the first few hours before spasticity and hyperreflexia develop.

Lower motor neuron (LMN): Lesions are caused by damage anywhere from the anterior horn cells distally, including the nerve roots, plexuses, and peripheral nerves. The pattern of weakness corresponds to the muscles supplied by the involved neurons. •Affected muscles show *wasting ± fasciculation* (spontaneous involuntary twitching). •There is *hypotonia/flaccidity:* the limb feels soft and floppy, providing little resistance to passive stretch. •*Reflexes are reduced* or absent; the *plantars remain flexor*. ►The chief differential for LMN weakness is a primary muscle disease (p510)—but here there is symmetrical loss, reflexes are normal or lost late, and there is no sensory component.

Mixed LMN and UMN signs: Can occur, eg in MND, ↓B_{12}, taboparesis (see p466).

Sensory deficits: It is important to test individual modalities and remember the quirks of our normal wiring: correctly interpreted, the distribution of sensory loss and the modality involved (pain, T°, touch, vibration, joint-position sense) will help refine and increase your confidence in localizing the lesion (see BOX 'From findings to neuroanatomy'). Pain and T° sensations travel along small fibres in peripheral nerves and the *anterolateral (spinothalamic) tracts* in the cord and brainstem (p516), whereas joint-position and vibration sense travel in large fibres in peripheral nerves and the large *dorsal columns* of the cord.

Muscle weakness grading (MRC classification)

• Grade 0 No muscle contraction	• Grade 3 Active movement against gravity
• Grade 1 Flicker of contraction	• Grade 4 Active movement against resistance
• Grade 2 Some active movement	• Grade 5 Normal power (allowing for age)

Grade 4 covers a big range: 4−, 4, and 4+ denote movement against slight, moderate, and stronger resistance; avoid fudging descriptions—'strength 4/5 throughout' suggests a mild quadriparesis or myopathy. It is better to document 'poor effort' and the maximum grade for each muscle tested. ►Distribution of weakness tells us more than grade of weakness (grade does help document improvement).

1 Most of the fibres of the corticospinal (=pyramidal) tract decussate at the medullary pyramids, hence the name and the contralateral nature of symptoms. *Extrapyramidal* denotes damage to the basal ganglia and presents as parkinsonism (see p468, 494).

2 Whereas with *rigidity*, ↑ tone is not velocity-dependent but constant throughout passive movement.

From findings to neuroanatomy: localizing the lesions

Cortical lesions may cause a particularly localized problem with hand or foot movements, with normal or even ↓tone—but ↑reflexes more proximally in the arm or leg will point to this being an UMN rather than LMN lesion. Sensory loss may be confined to discriminative functions, eg stereognosis and two-point discrimination (p499). *Internal capsule* (p470) and *corticospinal tract* lesions cause contralateral hemiparesis (UMN signs). There is generalized contralateral sensory loss. A cranial nerve palsy (III–XII) contralateral to a hemiplegia implicates the *brainstem* on the side of the cranial nerve palsy. *Lateral brainstem* lesions show both dissociated and crossed sensory loss with pain and T° loss on the side of the face ipsilateral to the lesion, and contralateral arm and leg sensory loss. *Cord lesions* causing paraparesis (both legs) or quadriparesis/tetraplegia (all limbs) are suggested by finding a motor and reflex level (power is unaffected above the lesion, with LMN signs *at* the level of the lesion, and UMN signs *below* the lesion). A *sensory level* is the hallmark (albeit a rather unreliable one)—ie decreased sensation below the level of the lesion with normal sensation above. Hemi-cord lesions cause a Brown-Séquard picture (p696): dorsal column loss on the side of the lesion and contralateral spinothalamic loss. *Dissociated sensory loss* may occur, eg in *cervical cord lesions*—loss of fine touch and proprioception without loss of pain and temperature (or vice versa, eg syringomyelia, p516; or cord tumours). *Peripheral neuropathies:* (p502.) Most cause distal weakness, eg foot-drop; weak hand (note: although Guillain-Barré syndrome typically presents as distal weakness that ascends over time, some atypical forms of Guillain-Barré syndrome may present with proximal weakness due to nerve root involvement). Sensory loss is typically worse distally (may involve all sensory modalities or be selective, depending on nerve fibre size involved). Involvement of a single nerve (mononeuropathy) occurs with trauma or entrapment (carpal tunnel, p503); involvement of several nerves (mononeuritis multiplex) is seen, eg in DM or vasculitis. Sensory loss from individual nerve lesions will follow anatomical territories (dermatomes, p454), which are usually more sharply defined than those of root lesions.

Also ask

What is the lesion? Are the cells diseased, dysfunctional, disconnected (after a stroke), or under- or overexcited (migraine; epilepsy)? Is there loss of a specific type of nerve cell, as in MND or subacute combined degeneration of the cord (↓B_{12}, p334). Arteriopaths get strokes, tropical travellers get wormy lesions.

Why? Is there a systemic disease causing the neurology? Eg atrial fibrillation allowing an embolus to form, which then lodges in the patient's dominant hemisphere, causing an infarct that presents with dysphasia. Do a full systems examination and always beware the irregularly irregular pulse.

Drugs and the nervous system

The brain is a gland that secretes both thoughts and molecules: both products are modulated by neurotransmitter systems. Some target sites for drugs:

1 Precursor of the transmitter (eg levodopa).
2 Interference with the storage of transmitter in vesicles within the pre-synaptic neuron (eg tetrabenazine).
3 Binding to the post-synaptic receptor site (eg bromocriptine).
4 Binding to the receptor-modulating site (eg benzodiazepines).
5 Interference with the breakdown of neurotransmitter within the synaptic cleft (eg acetylcholinesterase inhibitors; monoamine oxidase inhibitors—MAOIs).
6 Reduce reuptake of transmitter from synaptic cleft into pre-synaptic cell (eg selective serotonin reuptake inhibitors—SSRIs, eg fluoxetine; or serotonin and noradrenaline reuptake inhibitors—SNRIs, eg mirtazapine).
7 Binding to pre-synaptic autoreceptors (eg pindolol, a β-blocker with partial 5HT autoreceptor antagonist effects, can be used to augment antidepressant therapy).

Important neurotransmitters (and some associated drugs) are listed in table 10.1.

Storms on the sea of neurotransmission

The complex and subtle mixture of chemicals that bathes our hundreds of trillions of synapses has been likened to a 'sea' of neurotransmitters. If so, it is surely a seascape of exquisite beauty, no matter how disturbed cognition may become by the storms that whip the waves on the surface. A well-chosen prescription may offer a lifeboat from such storms, but before prescribing any drug that modulates neurotransmission, consider that you are about to release a blunt and poorly understood force into a delicate environment. • The drug (or a metabolite) must be able to pass through the blood-brain barrier to have an effect. • The consequences of any sedative effects may be severe. • There will be short- and long-term SEs (eg tardive dyskinesia with neuroleptic drugs). • Most drugs affect many neurotransmitters, increasing therapeutic scope (and uncertainty) eg risperidone (blocks D_2, $5HT_2$, α_1 and α_2 receptors). • Metabolites of drugs may have equal or more important pharmacological effects resulting in clinically important interactions with drugs affecting eg hepatic metabolism. • One neurotransmitter may have many effects, eg dopaminergic neurons go awry in Parkinson's disease, schizophrenia, and addiction to drugs and gambling, by affecting motor control, motivation, effort, reward, analgesia, stress, learning, attention, and cognition.

Table 10.1 Major neurotransmitters and associated drugs

Drugs increasing activity (≈agonists)	Drugs decreasing activity (≈antagonists)
Dopamine Acts on receptors D_{1-5}; affects mood and reward-seeking behaviour.	
Pramipexole, ropinirole, levodopa, apomorphine (Parkinson's*) Cabergoline (hyperprolactinaemia; acromegaly).	Chlorpromazine (schizophrenia, *OHCS* p340) Metoclopramide (nausea) *Inhibition of dopamine signalling may lead to drug induced parkinsonism.*
Serotonin (5-hydroxytryptamine; 5HT) Many receptor types $5HT_{1-7}$; multiple effects.	
Lithium (mood stabilizer) Sumatriptan (migraine) Buspirone (partial agonist; anxiety) Fluoxetine, sertraline (reuptake inhibitors; depression).	Ondansetron (nausea) Mirtazapine (depression) Olanzapine, clozapine (schizophrenia)
Amino acids Glutamate and aspartate act as excitatory transmitters on NMDA and non-NMDA receptors—relevant in epilepsy and CNS ischaemia. γ-aminobutyric acid (GABA) is mostly inhibitory.	
Gabapentin, valproate (GABA agonists; epilepsy and neuropathic pain) Benzodiazepines (GABA agonists; sedation) Baclofen (GABA agonists; spasticity) Alcohol (GABA agonist)†	Memantine (glutamate antagonist; dementia)
Acetylcholine Multiple receptors classed into muscarinic and nicotinic types. Peripheral agonists used in glaucoma (pilocarpine); myasthenia (anticholinesterases). Peripheral antagonists used in asthma (ipratropium); incontinence; to dry secretions pre-op; to dilate pupils; to ↑ heart rate (atropine). Centrally acting drugs include:	
Donepezil, galantamine, rivastigmine (acetylcholinesterase inhibitors; dementia)	Procyclidine, trihexyphenidyl (drug-induced parkinsonism)
Histamine and purines (eg ATP)	
	Cyclizine (antihistamine; nausea) Purinergic receptor blockers (emerging role in chronic pain).
Neuropeptides Multiple and growing list; includes opioids and substance P	
Exogenous opioids (wide-ranging analgesic and mood-related effects).	Aprepitant (↓chemotherapy-related nausea by blocking substance P receptors).
Noradrenaline, adrenaline (=norepinephrine, epinephrine) 4 receptor types: α_{1-2}, β_{1-2}. Noradrenaline is more specific for α-receptors but both transmitters affect all receptors. In the periphery, α-receptors drive arteriolar vasoconstriction and pupillary dilation; β_1 stimulation leads to ↑ pulse and myocardial contractility; β_2 stimulation leads to bronchodilatation, uterine relaxation, and arteriolar vasodilation. Centrally acting drugs include:	
Clonidine (refractory hypertension) Tricyclic antidepressants and venlafaxine (5HT and noradrenaline reuptake inhibitors; depression) MAOIs	

*Agonism at D_3 receptor agonists may cause pathological behavioural patterns, eg hypersexuality, pathological gambling or hobbying, and disorders of impulse control in people having no history of these.
†In chronic alcohol use, GABA receptors are downregulated; acamprosate, used in alcoholism, may help to maintain GABA signalling after alcohol withdrawal.

Cerebral blood supply

Knowledge of the anatomy of the blood supply of the brain helps diagnosis and management of cerebrovascular disease (pp470–8). Always try to identify the area of brain that correlates with a patient's symptoms and identify the affected artery.

Internal carotid arteries Supply the majority of blood to the anterior two-thirds of the cerebral hemispheres and the basal ganglia (via the lenticulostriate arteries). At worst, internal carotid artery occlusion causes fatal total infarction of these areas. More often, the picture is like middle cerebral artery occlusion (see later in topic).

The circle of Willis (fig 10.2) An anastomotic ring at the base of the brain fed by the three arteries that supply the brain with blood: the internal carotids (anteriorly) and the basilar artery (posteriorly, formed by the joining of the vertebral arteries, which supply the brainstem). This arrangement may compensate for the effects of occlusion of a feeder vessel by allowing supply from unaffected vessels; however, the anatomy of the circle of Willis is variable and in many people it does not provide much protection.

Cerebral arteries Three pairs of arteries leave the circle of Willis to supply the cerebral hemispheres: the anterior, middle, and posterior cerebral arteries (figs 10.2, 10.3). The anterior and middle cerebrals are branches of the internal carotid arteries; in 80%, the basilar artery divides into the two posterior cerebral arteries. Ischaemia from occlusion of any one of them may be lessened by retrograde supply from leptomeningeal vessels.

Anterior cerebral artery: (fig 10.2) Supplies the frontal and medial part of the cerebrum. Occlusion may cause a weak, numb contralateral leg ± similar, if milder, arm symptoms. The face is spared. Bilateral infarction is a rare cause of paraplegia and an even rarer cause of akinetic mutism.

Middle cerebral artery: (fig 10.2) Supplies the lateral part of each hemisphere. Occlusion may cause contralateral hemiparesis, hemisensory loss (esp. face and arm), contralateral homonymous hemianopia due to involvement of the optic radiation, cognitive change including dysphasia with dominant hemisphere lesions, and visuospatial disturbance (eg cannot dress; gets lost) with non-dominant lesions.

Posterior cerebral artery: (figs 10.2, 10.4) Supplies the occipital lobe. Occlusion gives contralateral homonymous hemianopia (often with macula sparing).

Vertebrobasilar circulation Supplies the cerebellum, brainstem, occipital lobes; occlusion causes signs relating to any or all three: hemianopia; cortical blindness; diplopia; vertigo; nystagmus; ataxia; dysarthria; dysphasia; hemi- or quadriplegia; unilateral or bilateral sensory symptoms; hiccups; coma. Infarctions of the brainstem can produce various syndromes, eg *lateral medullary syndrome*, in which occlusion of one vertebral artery or the posterior inferior cerebellar artery causes infarction of the lateral medulla and the inferior cerebellar surface (→vertigo, vomiting, dysphagia, nystagmus, ipsilateral ataxia, soft palate paralysis, ipsilateral Horner's syndrome, and a crossed pattern sensory loss—analgesia to pin-prick on ipsilateral face and contralateral trunk and limbs). *Locked-in syndrome* is caused by damage to the ventral pons due to pontine artery occlusion. Patients are unable to move, but retain full cognition and awareness, communicating by blinking, electronic boards, or special computers. Right-to-die legislation may be invoked...as one sufferer blinked: 'My life is dull, miserable, demeaning, undignified, and intolerable.' Locked-in syndrome is different from other right-to-die conditions because patients need someone to do the act for them.

Subclavian steal syndrome: Subclavian artery stenosis proximal to the origin of the vertebral artery may cause blood to be *stolen* by retrograde flow down this vertebral artery down into the arm, causing brainstem ischaemia typically after use of the arm. Suspect if the BP in each arm differs by >20mmHg.

'Dizzy-plus' syndromes and arterial events

- SCA→dizzy
- AICA→dizzy and deaf
- PICA→dizzy and dysphagic and dysphonic.

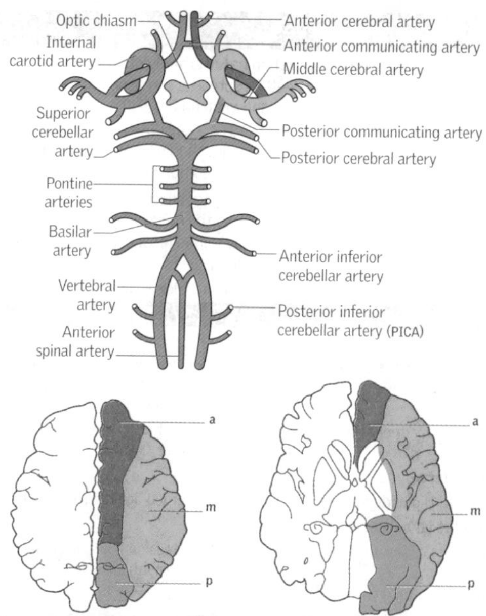

Fig 10.2 The circle of Willis at the base of the brain. See also **figs 10.17, 10.18.**

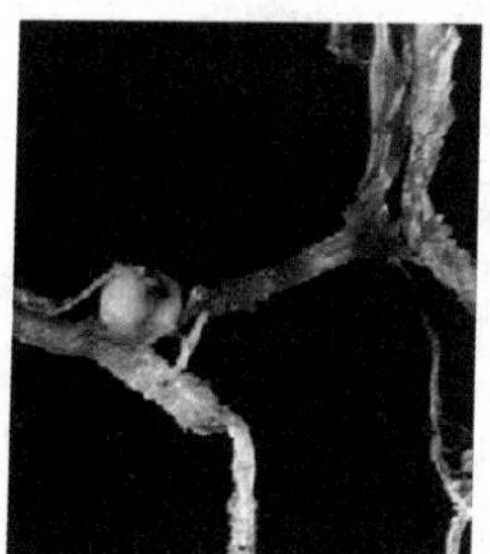

Fig 10.3 Berry aneurysm at junction of posterior communicating artery with internal carotid (p478). ©Dr D Hamoundi.

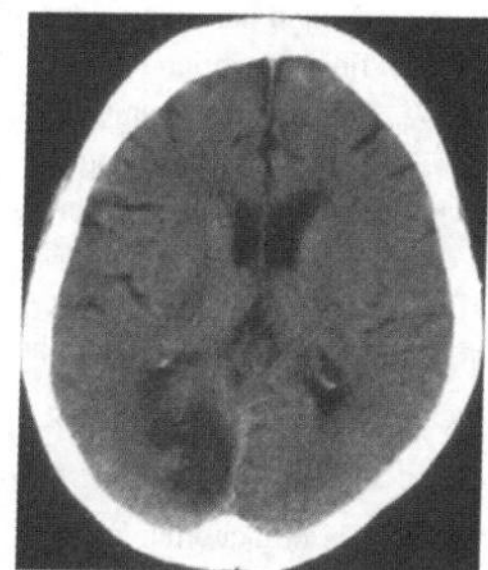

Fig 10.4 CT of stroke in posterior cerebral artery territory. ©J Trobe.

Thomas Willis

Thomas Willis (1621–1675) is one of those happy Oxford heroes who hold a bogus DM degree, awarded in 1646 for his Royalist sympathies while at Christ Church, the most loyally royal college in the University. He had a busy life inventing terms such as 'neurology' and 'reflex'. Not only has his name been given to his famous circle, but he was the first to describe myasthenia gravis, whooping cough, and the sweet taste of diabetic urine. He was the first person (few have followed him) to know the course of the spinal accessory nerve. He is unusual among Oxford neurologists in that he developed the practice of giving his lunch away to the poor. He also espoused iatrochemistry: a theory of medicine according to which all morbid conditions of the body can be explained by disturbances in the fermentations and effervescences of its humours.

Testing peripheral nerves

While there is some anatomical variation between individuals in ascribing particular nerve roots to muscles, tables 10.2–10.4 represent a reasonable compromise. Dermatomes and sensory nerve roots are shown in figs 10.5–10.9, pp454–5.

Remember to test proximal muscle power: ask the patient to sit from lying, to pull you towards him/herself, and to rise from squatting (if reasonably fit).

►Observe walking—easy to forget, even if the complaint is of difficulty walking!

►Don't be caught out by weakness secondary to musculoskeletal pathology—the traditional neurological examination relies on the musculoskeletal system being intact. Ruptured tendons and fractures may mimic focal neurological lesions (especially in patients who can't give a clear history).

Table 10.2 Assessment of peripheral nerve function in the lower limb

Nerve root	Muscle	Test by asking the patient to:
Femoral nerve		
L1, 2, 3	Iliopsoas (also supplied via L1, 2, & 3 spinal nerves)	Flex hip against resistance with knee flexed and lower leg supported: patient lies on back
L2, 3, 4	Quadriceps femoris	Extend at knee against resistance. Start with knee flexed
Obturator nerve		
L2, 3, 4	Hip adductors	Adduct leg against resistance
Inferior gluteal nerve		
L5, S1, S2	Gluteus maximus	Hip extension ('bury heel into the couch')—with knee in extension
Superior gluteal nerve		
L4, 5, S1	Gluteus medius and minimus	Abduction and internal hip rotation with leg flexed at hip and knee
Sciatic and common peroneal* nerves; sciatic and tibial nerves**		
*L4, 5	Tibialis anterior	Dorsiflex ankle
*L5, S1	Extensor digitorum longus	Dorsiflex toes against resistance
*L5, S1	Extensor hallucis longus	Dorsiflex hallux against resistance
*L5, S1	Peroneus longus and brevis	Evert foot against resistance
*L5, S1	Extensor digitorum brevis	Dorsiflex proximal phalanges of toes
(*)L5, S1, 2	Hamstrings (short head of biceps femoris is from the common peroneal nerve)	Flex knee against resistance
**L4, 5	Tibialis posterior	Invert plantarflexed foot
**S1, 2	Gastrocnemius	Plantarflex ankle or stand on tiptoe
**L5, S1, 2	Flexor digitorum longus	Flex terminal joints of toes
**S1, 2	Small muscles of foot	Make the sole of the foot into a cup

Table 10.3 Rapid screening tests for peripheral nerve roots

Shoulder	Abduction	C5	**Hip**	Flexion	L1–L2
	Adduction	C5–C7		Adduction	L2–3
Elbow	Flexion	C5–C6		Extension	L5–S1
	Extension	C7	**Knee**	Flexion	L5–S1
Wrist	Flexion	C7–8		Extension	L3–L4
	Extension	C7	**Ankle**	Dorsiflexion	L4
Fingers	Flexion	C8		Eversion	L5–S1
	Extension	C7		Plantarflexion	S1–S2
	Abduction	T1	**Toe**	Big toe extension	L5

Table 10.4 Assessment of peripheral nerve function in the upper limb

Nerve root	Muscle	Test by asking the patient to:
C3, 4	Trapezius	Shrug shoulder (via accessory nerve)
C5, 6, 7	Serratus anterior	Push arm forward against resistance; look for scapula winging (p511) if weak
C5, 6	Pectoralis major (P major) clavicular head	Adduct arm from above horizontal, and push it forward
C6, 7, 8	P major sternocostal head	Adduct arm below horizontal
C5, 6	Supraspinatus	Abduct arm the first 15°
C5, 6	Infraspinatus	Externally rotate semi-flexed arm, elbow at side
C6, 7, 8	Latissimus dorsi	Adduct arm from horizontal position
C5, 6	Biceps	Flex supinated forearm
C5, 6	Deltoid	Abduct arm between 15° and 90°
Radial nerve (p502)		
C6, 7, 8	Triceps	Extend elbow against resistance
C5, 6	Brachioradialis	Flex elbow with forearm half way between pronation and supination
C5, 6	Extensor carpi radialis longus	Extend wrist to radial side
C6, 7	Supinator	Arm by side, resist hand pronation
C7, 8	Extensor digitorum	Keep fingers extended at MCP joint
C7, 8	Extensor carpi ulnaris	Extend wrist to ulnar side
C7, 8	Abductor pollicis longus	Abduct thumb at 90° to palm
C7, 8	Extensor pollicis brevis	Extend thumb at MCP joint
C7, 8	Extensor pollicis longus	Resist thumb flexion at IP joint
Median nerve (p502)		
C6, 7	Pronator teres	Keep arm pronated against resistance
C6, 7	Flexor carpi radialis	Flex wrist towards radial side
C7, 8, T1	Flexor digitorum superficialis	Resist extension at PIP joint (with proximal phalanx fixed by the examiner)
C7, 8	Flexor digitorum profundus I & II	Resist extension at index DIP joint of index finger
C7, 8, T1	Flexor pollicis longus	Resist thumb extension at interphalangeal joint (fix proximal phalanx)
C8, T1	Abductor pollicis brevis	Abduct thumb (nail at 90° to palm)
C8, T1	Opponens pollicis	Thumb touches base of 5th fingertip (nail parallel to palm)
C8, T1	1st lumbrical/interosseus (median and ulnar nerves)	Extend PIP joint against resistance with MCP joint held hyperextended
Ulnar nerve (p502)		
C7, 8, T1	Flexor carpi ulnaris	Flex wrist to ulnar side; observe tendon
C7, C8	Flexor digitorum profundus III & IV	Resist extension of distal phalanx of 5th finger while you fix its middle phalanx
C8, T1	Dorsal interossei	Finger abduction: cannot cross the middle over the index finger (tests index finger adduction too)
C8, T1	Palmar interossei	Finger adduction: pull apart a sheet of paper held between middle and ring finger DIP joints of both hands; the paper moves on the weaker side*
C8, T1	Adductor pollicis	Adduct thumb (nail at 90° to palm)
C8, T1	Abductor digiti minimi	Abduct little finger
C8, T1	Flexor digiti minimi	Flex little finger at MCP joint

*Also, metacarpophalangeal joint flexion may be more on the affected side as flexor tendons are recruited—the basis of Froment's paper sign. Wartenberg's sign is persistent little finger abduction.

Dermatomes and peripheral nerves

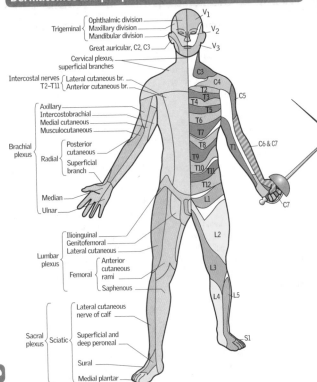

Trigeminal: Ophthalmic division; Maxillary division; Mandibular division
Great auricular, C2, C3
Cervical plexus, superficial branches
Intercostal nerves T2–T11: Lateral cutaneous br.; Anterior cutaneous br.
Brachial plexus: Axillary; Intercostobrachial; Medial cutaneous; Musculocutaneous; Radial (Posterior cutaneous; Superficial branch); Median; Ulnar
Lumbar plexus: Ilioinguinal; Genitofemoral; Lateral cutaneous; Femoral (Anterior cutaneous rami; Saphenous)
Sacral plexus: Sciatic (Lateral cutaneous nerve of calf; Superficial and deep peroneal; Sural; Medial plantar)

V1 V2 V3 C3 C4 C5 T2 T3 T4 T5 T6 T7 T8 T9 T10 T11 T12 T1 C6 & C7 C7 L1 L2 L3 L4 L5 S1

Fig 10.5 The white areas denote *terra incognita*: considerable inter-individual variation exists, and no single best option can be given.

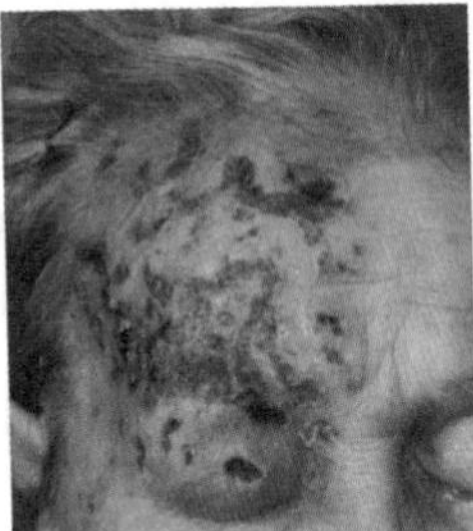

Fig 10.6 Pain in a dermatomal distribution suggests a problem with a cranial nerve or dorsal root ganglion (radiculopathy)—where the cell bodies of sensory fibres live. What is the dermatome? What is the lesion? See p404 for the answer.

Aim to keep a few key dermatomes up your sleeve (C5–T2)

C3–4	Clavicles
C6–7	Lateral arm/forearm
T1	Medial side of arm
C6	Thumb
C7	Middle finger
C8	Little finger
T4	Nipples
T10	Umbilicus
L1	Inguinal ligament
L2–3	Anterior and inner leg
L5	Medial side of big toe
L5, S1–2	Posterior and outer leg
S1	Lateral margin of foot and little toe
S2–4	Perineum

Rough approximations!

C2
C3
C4
C5
T2
T3
T4
T5
T6
T7
T8
T9
T10
T11
T12
L1
L2
L3
C7
T1
C6 & C7
C8
S3
S4
S5
S1
S2
L4

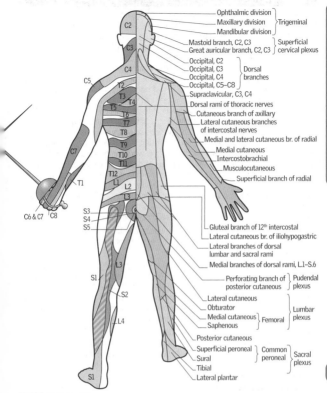

Ophthalmic division
Maxillary division
Mandibular division
Trigeminal
Mastoid branch, C2, C3
Great auricular branch, C2, C3
Superficial cervical plexus
Occipital, C2
Occipital, C3
Occipital, C4
Occipital, C5–C8
Dorsal branches
Supraclavicular, C3, C4
Dorsal rami of thoracic nerves
Cutaneous branch of axillary
Lateral cutaneous branches of intercostal nerves
Medial and lateral cutaneous br. of radial
Medial cutaneous
Intercostobrachial
Musculocutaneous
Superficial branch of radial
Gluteal branch of 12th intercostal
Lateral cutaneous br. of iliohypogastric
Lateral branches of dorsal lumbar and sacral rami
Medial branches of dorsal rami, L1–S.6
Perforating branch of posterior cutaneous
Pudendal plexus
Lateral cutaneous
Obturator
Medial cutaneous
Saphenous
Femoral
Lumbar plexus
Posterior cutaneous
Superficial peroneal
Sural
Common peroneal
Tibial
Lateral plantar
Sacral plexus

Fig 10.7 Posterior view.

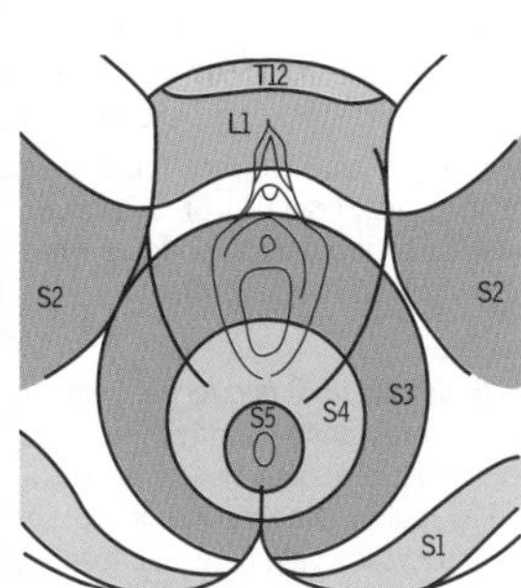

Fig 10.8 The anterior ⅓ of the scrotum is L1; the posterior ⅔ is S3. The penis is S2/3 (L1 at its root).

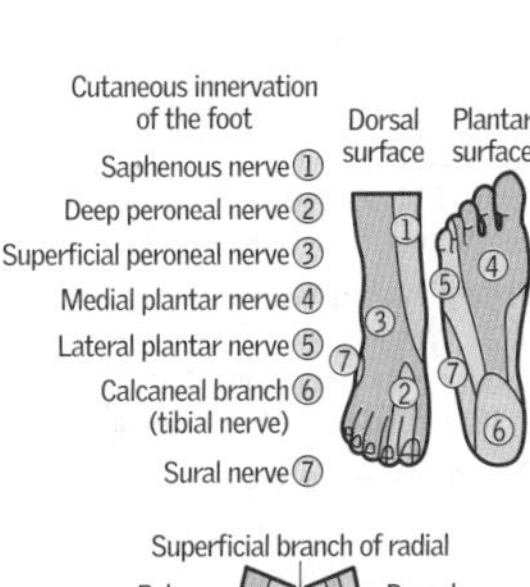

Fig 10.9 Feet and hands.

Headache

Every day, *thousands* of people visit the doctor complaining of headache. Tension headaches are the most common, but beware the disabling and treatable (migraine, cluster headache), and the sinister (space-occupying lesions, meningitis, subarachnoid haemorrhage). A good history is the key. Ask about:

Onset *Rapid onset* headaches are concerning; the key diagnosis to rule out here is •*subarachnoid haemorrhage* (SAH, p478), *sudden*-onset, 'worst ever' headache, often occipital, stiff neck, focal signs, ↓consciousness. Other differentials include: •*Meningitis* (p822): fever, photophobia, stiff neck, purpuric rash, coma. May be associated with neck stiffness (≈meningeal irritation). Do an LP, start antibiotics. •*Encephalitis* (p824): fever, odd behaviour, fits, or reduced consciousness. Do an urgent CT head and LP to look for signs of infection. •*Post-coital headache.*
Subacute/gradual onset headaches: •*Venous sinus thrombosis* (p480): subacute headache, papilloedema. •*Sinusitis:* dull, constant ache over frontal or maxillary sinuses, with tenderness ± postnasal drip. Pain is worse on bending over. Ethmoid or sphenoid sinus pain is felt deep in the midline at the root of the nose. Common with coryza (p406). The pain lasts ~1-2 wks. CT can confirm diagnosis but is rarely needed. •*Tropical illness:* eg malaria: travel history, flu-like illness (p416); typhus (p415). •*Intracranial hypotension:* CSF leakage, eg iatrogenic after LP or epidural anaesthesia. Suspect if headaches worse on standing; treat with epidural blood patch over leak, if conservative management with IV fluids and caffeine fails.

Character Tight band? Think *tension headache* (the usual cause of bilateral, non-pulsatile headache ± scalp muscle tenderness). Throbbing/pulsatile/lateralizing? Think *migraine* (p458).

Frequency Headaches that recur tend to be benign: • *Migraine:* p458. • *Cluster headache:* (see BOX 'Cluster headache') • *Trigeminal neuralgia:* (see BOX 'Trigeminal neuralgia') • *Recurrent (Mollaret's) meningitis:* suspect if fever/meningism with each headache. Send CSF for herpes simplex PCR (HSV2). Is there access to subarachnoid spaces via a skull fracture, or a recurring cause of aseptic meningitis (SLE, eg abducens nerve palsy, Behçet's, sarcoid)?

Duration Chronic, progressive headaches can indicate ↑ICP. Typically worse on waking, lying, bending forward, or coughing. Also: vomiting, papilloedema, seizures, false localizing signs, or odd behaviour. Do imaging to exclude a space-occupying lesion, and consider idiopathic intracranial hypertension. ►LP is contraindicated until after imaging.

Associated features *Eye pain ± reduced vision:* Think *acute glaucoma.* Typically elderly, long-sighted people. Constant pain develops rapidly around one eye, radiating to the forehead with markedly reduced vision, visual haloes, and a red, congested eye (p561). ►Seek expert help at once. If delay in treatment of >1h is likely, give eye drops (eg 0.5% timolol maleate ± 2% pilocarpine) and acetazolamide 500mg PO. *Jaw claudication tender with thickened, pulseless temporal arteries: Giant cell arteritis:* (p556) Subacute-onset headache with ESR >40mm/h. ►Exclude in all >50yrs old with a headache that has lasted a few weeks: prompt diagnosis and steroids avoid blindness.

Precipitating causes *Head trauma:* Commonly causes localized pain but can be more generalized. It lasts ~2wks; often resistant to analgesia. Do CT to exclude subdural or extradural haemorrhage if drowsiness ± lucid interval, or focal signs (p482). *Also ask about:* Analgesia, sex, food (eg chocolate, cheese, coffee).

Red flags See p780.

Drug history *Exclude medication overuse (analgesic rebound) headache:* Culprits are mixed analgesics (paracetamol+codeine/opiates), ergotamine, and triptans. This is a common reason for episodic headache becoming chronic daily headache. Analgesia must be withdrawn—aspirin or naproxen may mollify the rebound headache. A preventive may help once off other drugs (eg tricyclics, valproate, gabapentin; p504). Limit use of over-the-counter analgesia (no more than 6d per month).

Social history Ask about stress or recent life events; may not explain the pathology, but will help you appreciate the context in which symptoms are experienced.

Cluster headache

Cluster headache may be the most disabling of the primary headache disorders. The cause (unknown ♂:♀ ≥5:1; onset at any age; commoner in smokers).

Symptoms Rapid-onset of excruciating pain around one eye that may become watery and bloodshot with lid swelling, lacrimation, facial flushing, rhinorrhoea, miosis ± ptosis (20% of attacks). Pain is strictly unilateral and almost always affects the same side. It lasts 15-180min, occurs once or twice a day, and is often nocturnal. Clusters last 4-12wks and are followed by pain-free periods of months or even 1-2yrs before the next cluster. Sometimes it is chronic, not episodic.

Treatment *Acute attack:* 'Keep calm... carry oxygen': give 100% O_2 for ~15min via non-rebreathable mask (not if COPD); sumatriptan SC 6mg at onset (or zolmitriptan nasal spray 5mg).

Preventives *Avoid triggers:* Eg alcohol. *Medication:* Consider: corticosteroids (short term only; many SE); verapamil 360mg, lithium 900mg (monitor carefully).

Trigeminal neuralgia

Symptoms: Paroxysms of intense, stabbing pain, lasting seconds, in the trigeminal nerve distribution. It is unilateral, typically affecting mandibular or maxillary divisions. The face screws up with pain (*hence tic douloureux*). *Triggers:* Washing affected area, shaving, eating, talking, dental prostheses. *Typical patient:* ♂ >50yrs old; in Asians ♀:♂ ≈ 2:1. *Secondary causes:* Compression of the trigeminal root by anomalous or aneurysmal intracranial vessels or a tumour, chronic meningeal inflammation, MS, zoster, skull base malformation (eg Chiari). *MRI:* Is necessary to exclude secondary causes (~14% of cases). *℞:* Carbamazepine (start at 100mg/12h PO; max 400mg/6h; lamotrigine; phenytoin 200-400mg/24h PO; or gabapentin (p504). If drugs fail, surgery may be necessary. This may be directed at the peripheral nerve, the trigeminal ganglion, or the nerve root. *Microvascular decompression:* Anomalous vessels are separated from the trigeminal root. Stereotactic gamma knife surgery can work, but length of pain relief and the time to treatment response are limiting factors. *Facial pain ΔΔ:* p65.

Migraine

15% of us suffer from migraines, (♀:♂ ≈3:1); the economic costs extend to £billions/yr.

Symptoms *Classically:* •Visual or other aura (see below) lasting 15–30min followed within 1h by unilateral, throbbing headache. Or: •Isolated aura with no headache; •Episodic severe headaches without aura, often premenstrual, usually unilateral, with nausea, vomiting ± photophobia/phonophobia ('*common migraine*'). There may be allodynia—all stimuli produce pain: 'I can't brush my hair, wear earrings or glasses, or shave, it's so painful.' *Prodrome:* Precedes headache by hours/days: yawning, cravings, mood/sleep change. *Aura:* • *Visual:* chaotic distorting, 'melting' and jumbling of lines, dots, or zigzags, scotomata or hemianopia; • *Somatosensory:* paraesthesiae spreading from fingers to face; • *Motor:* dysarthria and ataxia (basilar migraine), ophthalmoplegia, or hemiparesis; • *Speech:* (8% of auras) dysphasia or paraphasia.

Partial triggers Seen in 50%: **CHOCOLATE** or: **c**hocolate, **h**angovers, **o**rgasms, **c**heese/caffeine, **o**ral contraceptives, **l**ie-ins, **a**lcohol, **t**ravel, or **e**xercise.

Associations Obesity, family history.

Diagnosis Clinical, based on the history. ***Diagnostic criteria if no aura:*** ≥5 headaches lasting 4–72h + nausea/vomiting (or photo/phonophobia) + any 2 of: • Unilateral • Pulsating • Impairs (or worsened by) routine activity.

Differentials Cluster or tension headache, cervical spondylosis, ↑BP, intracranial pathology, sinusitis/otitis media, dental caries. TIAs may mimic migraine aura.

Management ►Avoid identified triggers and ensure analgesic rebound headache is not complicating matters (p456). ***Prophylactic treatment:*** Can achieve ~50%↓ in attack frequency in most patients; consider after risks and benefits discussion. 1st line: Propranolol 40–120mg/12h or topiramate 25–50mg/12h (teratogenic, can interfere with Pill efficacy). Amitriptyline 10–75mg nocte can be used, though this is off-licence. ►Patients may be on previously-recommended prophylactic agents (eg valproate, pizotifen, pregabalin or ACE-i): if achieving good control then continue as required. 12-weekly botulinum toxin type A injections are a last resort in chronic migraine. ***Treatment during an attack:*** NICE recommends an oral triptan (or nasal in 12–17y) combined with either an NSAID or paracetamol.[1] Monotherapy with any of the above (or aspirin 900mg) can also be considered. Anti-emetics may help even in the abscence of nausea and vomiting. Triptans are CI if IHD, coronary spasm, uncontrolled ↑BP, recent lithium, SSRIs, or ergot use. Rare SE: arrhythmias or angina ± MI, even if no pre-existing risk. ***Non-pharmacological therapies:*** Warm or cold packs to the head, or rebreathing into paper bag (↑P_aCO_2) may help abort attacks. Butterbur extracts or riboflavin supplementation may have a role. NICE recommend 10 sessions of acupuncture over 5–8 weeks if both topiramate and propranolol are unsuitable or ineffective. Transcutaneous nerve stimulation may help.

Considerations in females Incidence of migraine (especially with aura) + ischaemic stroke is increased by use of a combined OCP. Use progesterone-only or non-hormonal contraception in migraine + aura, though a low dose combined OCP can be used in those *without* aura. Further ↑risk: • Smoking • Age >35yrs • BP↑ • Obesity (body mass index >30) • Diabetes mellitus • Hyperlipidaemia • Family history of arteriopathy <45yrs. ►Warn patients to stop OCP at once if they develop aura or worsening migraine; see *OHCS* p301. *Perimenstrual migraine:* If uncontrolled with standard treatment and the onset of headache is predictable then consider frovatriptan 2.5mg BD or zolmitriptan 2.5mg BD/TDS on the days migraine is expected. *Pregnancy:* Migraine often improves; if not, get help—worsening headaches in pregnancy are associated with a greater risk of pre-eclampsia and cardiovascular complications. Offer paracetamol 1st line. Triptans and NSAIDs can be used but discuss risks and benefits with patients first. Don't use aspirin if breastfeeding. Anti-emetic: cyclizine or promethazine. *Prophylaxis:* seek specialist advice.

What is going on in migraine?

Despite the high prevalence of migraines, the underlying pathophysiology is poorly understood. The previously favoured theory of dilatation of cerebral and meningeal arteries has been largely disproven, so what is the cause? • MRI during attacks shows episodic cerebral oedema, dilatation of intracerebral vessels, and ↓water diffusion not respecting vascular territories, so the primary event may be neurological. • PET suggests migraine is a subcortical disorder affecting the modulation of sensory processing • Magneto-encephalographic (MEG) studies have shown resting (interictal) hyperexcitability at least in the visual cortex, suggesting a failure of inhibitory circuits. • Hormones play a role: the incidence of migraine in both pre-pubertal and post-menopausal women is equal to men, yet increases to 3:1 during reproductive years, with 50% of females reporting synchrony of migraines with the menstrual cycle. • Elevated levels of 5-HT metabolites in the urine of patients during migraine attacks was first reported in 1972, and while its exact significance is controversial, the efficacy of triptans ($5HT_{1B/1D}$ agonists) support its role in migraine. • Triptans also inhibit release of substance P and pro-inflammatory neuropeptides, blocking transmission from the trigeminal nerve and implicating trigeminal nerve dysfunction.

The bigger picture

Vincent Van Gogh suffered from 'sick headaches', widely believed to have been migraines. Could his swirling, cascading starry night (fig 10.10) be a visual aura? ►Just as with the fragile mental health of Van Gogh, migraine often co-exists with other chronic conditions—and the combined negative impact on physical and mental health is immense. Don't treat each disease in isolation. Rather, attempt to restore a good relationship with the self—and the recovery of the purpose of life through dialogue. This is the hardest but the most rewarding task, and may save some ears.

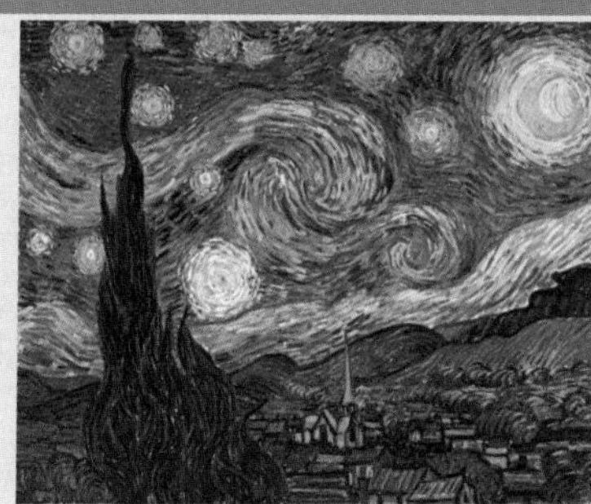

Fig 10.10 'The Starry Night' Vincent Van Gogh 1889
World History Archive/Ann Ronan Collection / Age Fotostock

Blackouts

Causes of collapse ± loss of consciousness (LOC) are many; take a careful history (BOX).

Vasovagal (neurocardiogenic) syncope Occurs due to reflex bradycardia ± peripheral vasodilation provoked by emotion, pain, or standing too long (it cannot occur when lying down). Onset is over seconds (*not* instantaneous), and is often preceded by pre-syncopal symptoms, eg nausea, pallor, sweating, and narrowing of visual fields. Brief clonic jerking of the limbs may occur due to cerebral hypoperfusion, but there is no tonic/clonic sequence. Urinary incontinence is uncommon, and there is no tongue-biting. Unconsciousness usually lasts for ~2min and recovery is rapid.

Situation syncope Symptoms as for vasovagal syncope but with a clear precipitant: *cough syncope* occurs after a paroxysm of coughing; *effort syncope* is brought on by exercise; there is usually a cardiac cause, eg aortic stenosis, HCM; *micturition syncope* happens during or after urination: mostly men, at night.

Carotid sinus syncope Hypersensitive baroreceptors cause excessive reflex bradycardia ± vasodilation on minimal stimulation (eg head-turning, shaving).

Epilepsy (p490) Features suggestive of this diagnosis include: attacks when asleep or lying down; aura; identifiable triggers (eg TV); altered breathing; cyanosis; typical tonic-clonic movements; incontinence of urine; tongue-biting; prolonged post-ictal drowsiness, confusion, amnesia, and transient focal paralysis (Todd's palsy).

Stokes-Adams attacks Transient arrhythmias (eg bradycardia due to complete heart block) cause ↓cardiac output and LOC. The patient falls to the ground (often with *no* warning except palpitations; injuries are common), and is pale, with a slow or absent pulse. Recovery is in seconds: the patient flushes, the pulse speeds up, and consciousness is regained. As with vasovagal syncope, anoxic clonic jerks may occur in prolonged LOC. Attacks may happen several times a day and in any posture.

Other causes *Hypoglycaemia:* (p214) Tremor, hunger, and perspiration herald light-headedness or LOC; rare in non-diabetics. *Orthostatic hypotension:* Unsteadiness or LOC on standing from lying in those with inadequate vasomotor reflexes: the elderly; autonomic neuropathy (p505); antihypertensive medication; overdiuresis; multisystem atrophy (MSA; p494). *Anxiety:* Hyperventilation, tremor, sweating, tachycardia, paraesthesiae, light-headedness, and no LOC suggest a panic attack. *Drop attacks:* Sudden fall to the ground *without* LOC. Mostly benign and due to leg weakness but may also be caused by hydrocephalus, cataplexy, or narcolepsy. *Factitious blackouts:* Pseudoseizures, Münchausen's (p706).

Examination Cardiovascular, neurological. Measure BP lying and standing.

Investigation All with recurrent syncope (or falls) need cardiac assessment—urgently if associated with palpitations, arrhythmias, 3rd-degree AV block, or prolonged QT interval (p711). ECG ± 24h ECG (arrhythmia, long QT, eg Romano-Ward, p96); U&E, FBC, Mg^{2+}, Ca^{2+}, glucose; tilt-table test;[3] EEG, sleep EEG; echocardiogram; CT/MRI brain; ABG if practical (↓P_aCO_2 in attacks suggests hyperventilation as the cause).

►While the cause is being elucidated, advise against driving (see p158).

3 Patient is subject to continuous ECG and BP monitoring while strapped to a table and moved rapidly from resting horizontal position to vertical. Induction of symptoms with inappropriate BP drop >30mmHg or bradycardia suggests neurally mediated syncope. Consider pacing.

Blackout history

It is vital to establish exactly what patients mean by 'blackout': loss of consciousness?—a fall to the ground without loss of consciousness?—vertigo or visual disturbance? Talk to the patient *and* witnesses and let them tell you as much as possible without prompting or leading. Ask:

- Does the patient lose awareness?
- Does the patient injure themselves?
- Does the patient move? Are they stiff or floppy? (A tonic phase preceding clonic jerking points towards epilepsy.)
- Is there incontinence? (More common in epilepsy, but can occur with syncope.)
- Does their complexion change? (Pale/cyanosis suggests epilepsy; very pale/white suggests syncope or arrhythmia.)
- Does the patient bite the side of their tongue? (Suggests epilepsy.)
- Are there associated symptoms eg palpitations, sweats, pallor, chest pain, dyspnoea (see fig 10.11)?
- How long does the attack last?

Before the attack:

- Is there any warning?—Eg typical epileptic aura or cardiac pre-syncope.
- In what circumstances do attacks occur? (If watching TV, consider epilepsy).
- Can the patient prevent attacks?

After the attack:

- How much does the patient remember about the attack?
- Is there muscle ache? (Suggests a tonic-clonic seizure.)
- Is the patient confused or sleepy? (Suggests epilepsy.)

Background to attacks:

- When did they start?
- Are they getting more frequent?
- Is anyone else in the family getting them? Sudden arrhythmic death may leave no evidence at postmortem, or there may be hereditary cardiomyopathy (refer those with a relative who has had a sudden unexplained death <40yrs old).

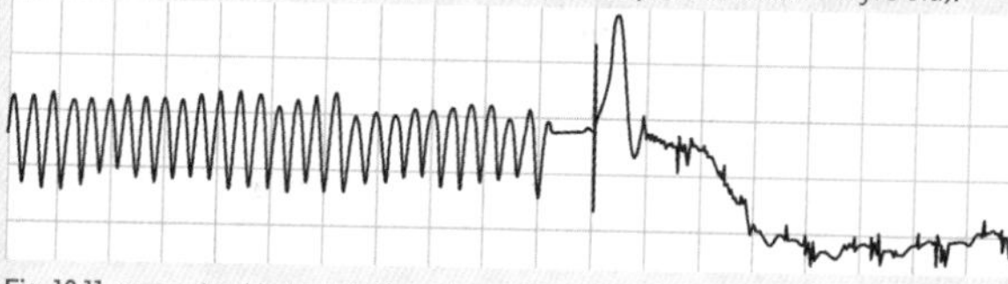

Fig 10.11 VT causing blackout in Brugada syndrome (p695). This patient had been treated with an implantable defibrillator (see p132).

Vertigo and dizziness

Is this vertigo? Complaints of 'dizzy spells' are very common and are used by patients to describe many different sensations. True vertigo is a *hallucination of movement*, often rotatory, of the patient or their surroundings. In practice, simple 'spinning' is rare—the floor may tilt, sink, or rise. The key to diagnosis is to find out exactly what the patient means by 'dizzy:' if this is not vertigo or if atypical symptoms are present consider other causes, eg if there is loss of awareness, think of epilepsy or syncope; if there is faintness, lightheadedness, or palpitations, think of anaemia, dysrhythmia, anxiety, or hypotension.

Associated symptoms: Difficulty walking or standing (may fall suddenly to the ground), relief on lying or sitting still (vertigo is almost always worsened by movement); nausea, vomiting, pallor, sweating. Associated hearing loss or tinnitus implies labyrinth or VIIIth nerve involvement.

Causes

Benign positional vertigo: Occurs on head movement due to disruption of debris in the semicircular canal of the ears (canalolithiasis). Fatiguable nystagmus on performing the Hallpike manoeuvre is diagnostic; Epley manoeuvres clear the debris (*OHCS* p555).

Acute labyrinthitis (vestibular neuronitis): Abrupt onset of severe vertigo, nausea, vomiting ± prostration. No deafness or tinnitus. Causes: virus; vascular lesion. Severe vertigo subsides in days, complete recovery takes 3-4wks. ℞: reassure. Sedate.

Ménière's disease: Increased pressure in the endolymphatic system of the inner ear causes recurrent attacks of vertigo lasting >20min, fluctuating (or permanent) sensorineural hearing loss, and tinnitus (with a sense of aural fullness ± falling to one side). ℞: bed rest and reassurance in acute attacks. An antihistamine (eg cinnarizine) is useful if prolonged, or buccal prochlorperazine if severe, for up to 7d.

Ototoxicity: Aminoglycosides, loop diuretics, or cisplatin can cause deafness±vertigo.

Acoustic neuroma: (figs 10.12, 10.13) Doubly misnamed: it is a Schwannoma (not neuroma) arising from the vestibular (not auditory) nerve. They account for 80% of cerebellopontine angle tumours and often present with unilateral hearing loss, with vertigo occurring later. Growth rate is slow (usually 1-2 mm/year) and can be predicted by serial MRIs. With progression, ipsilateral Vth, VIth, IXth, and Xth nerves may be affected (also ipsilateral cerebellar signs). Signs of ↑ICP occur late, indicating a large tumour. Commoner in ♀ and neurofibromatosis (esp. NF2, p514).

Traumatic damage: If trauma affects the petrous temporal bone or the cerebellopontine angle then the auditory nerve may be damaged, causing vertigo, deafness, and/or tinnitus.

Herpes zoster: Herpetic eruption of the external auditory meatus; facial palsy ± deafness, tinnitus, and vertigo (Ramsay Hunt syndrome, see p501).

Others: Vertiginous epilepsy; MS; stroke/TIA; migraine; motion sickness; alcohol intoxication.

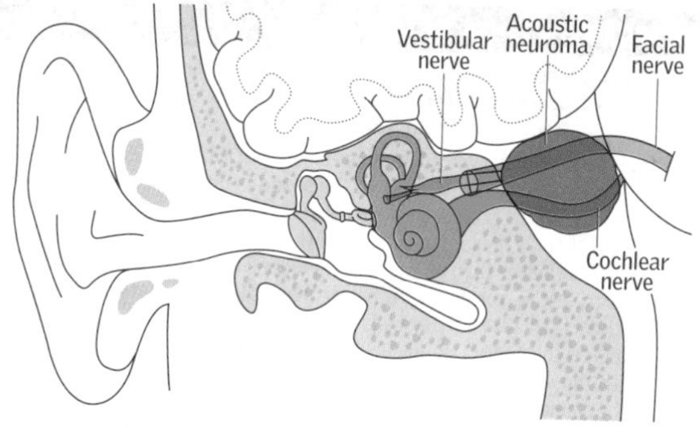

Fig 10.12 An acoustic neuroma (vestibular schwannoma) growing dangerously near the facial nerve.

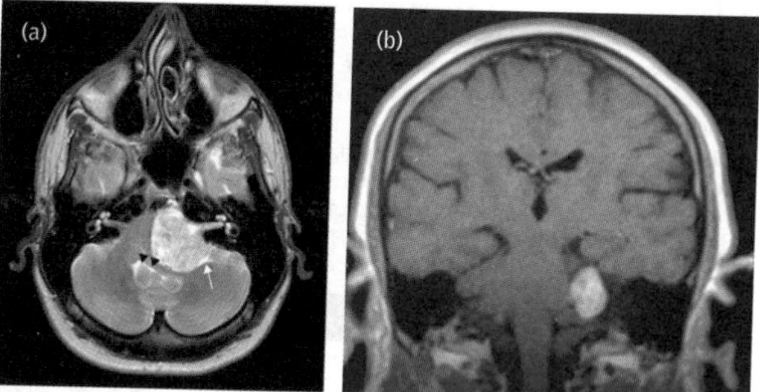

Fig 10.13 Large vestibular schwannoma: axial T2W (a) and contrast-enhanced coronal MRI (b).

Reproduced from Manji *et al.*, *Oxford Handbook of Neurology*, 2007, with permission from Oxford University Press.

Hearing loss

Whisper test A simple but effective crude assessment of hearing: whisper numbers in one ear while blocking the other. Ask your patient to repeat the number. Make sure that failure is not from misunderstanding.

Tuning fork tests *Rinne:* Hold a vibrating tuning fork (512Hz or 256Hz) on the mastoid to test bone conduction (BC). When the sound is no longer audible move it in front of the ear with the prongs perpendicular to the auditory canal to test air conduction (AC). If there is no conductive deficit (ie in normal hearing or sensorineural hearing loss), AC is better than BC and the patient will be able to hear the note again. This is a 'Rinne positive' result. If BC is better than AC (Rinne negative), this indicates conductive deafness >20dB. A false-negative may occur in severe sensorineural hearing loss (SNHL) as the contralateral cochlea picks up the sound by bone conduction. *Weber:* With the vibrating tuning fork on the vertex or forehead, ask the patient which ear the sound is louder in. Sound localizes to the affected ear with conductive loss (>10dB loss), to the contralateral ear in SNHL, and to the midline if both ears are normal (or if bilateral SNHL).

Conductive deafness *Causes:* Wax (remove, eg by syringing with warm water after softening with olive oil drops), otosclerosis, otitis media, or glue ear (*OHCS* p546).

Chronic sensorineural deafness Often due to accumulated environmental noise toxicity, presbyacusis, or inherited disorders. *Presbyacusis:* Loss of acuity for high-frequency sounds starts before 30yrs old. We do not usually notice it until hearing of speech is affected. Hearing is most affected in the presence of background noise. Hearing aids are the usual treatment.

Sudden sensorineural deafness ►Get an ENT opinion *today* (steroids may cure)! *Causes:* Noise exposure; gentamicin/other toxin; mumps; acoustic neuroma; MS; stroke; vasculitis; TB. *Tests:* ESR, FBC, LFT, pANCA, viral titres and TB (see BOX 'Diagnostic tests for TB', p394); evoked response audiometry; CXR; MRI; lymph node and nasopharyngeal biopsy for culture.

Tinnitus

This ringing or buzzing in the ears is common, and may cause depression or insomnia. ►Investigate unilateral tinnitus fully to exclude an acoustic neuroma (p462).

Causes Inner ear damage and hearing loss (leading to auditory cortex hyper-excitability), wax, excess noise, head injury, otitis media, post-stapedectomy, Ménière's, anaemia (if pulsatile then think of carotid artery stenosis or dissection, AV fistulae, and glomus jugulare tumours). *Drugs:* Aspirin (reversible), loop diuretics, aminoglycosides. *Mean age at onset:* 40–50yrs. ♂:♀≈1:1.

Management Exclude serious causes. ►Psychological support is very important: reassure that tinnitus does not mean madness or serious disease and that it often improves in time. *Cognitive therapy* helps, as do 'tinnitus coping training' and patient support groups. *Drugs* are disappointing: anticonvulsants (eg carbamazepine) are not of benefit; misoprostol appears to help (small-scale trials only); hypnotics at night may be of some benefit. Avoid tranquillizers, particularly if depressed (use tricyclic antidepressants here). If Ménière's disease is the cause, betahistine helps only a few. *Masking* may give relief: white noise (like an off-tuned radio) is given via a noise generator worn like a post-aural hearing aid. *Hearing aids* may help by amplifying desirable sounds. *Cochlear nerve section* is a drastic option that can relieve disabling tinnitus in 25% but at the expense of deafness.

Bittersweet symphony

German composer Ludwig van Beethoven (1770-1827) began to lose his hearing from his early 30s—first high-frequency sounds were lost, associated with debilitating tinnitus: 'My ears sing and buzz continually, day and night. I can truly say that I am living a wretched life...in my profession it is a frightful state.' However, despite becoming profoundly deaf by the age of 44, he continued to compose and perform throughout his auditory decline. As deafness crept into the ears of the French composer, Gabriel Fauré (1845-1924), he composed less, but only after losing his hearing did he manage to overcome his previous fear of writing a string quartert, telling his wife 'This is a genre which Beethoven in particular made famous, and causes all those who are not Beethoven to be terrified of it'. They are not the only masters of their field to overcome auditory impairment; so did cardiologist Helen Taussig (see p92).

Acute bilateral leg weakness

It is crucial to establish a diagnosis quickly to avoid permanent disability. Look for specific patterns (see later in topic) and ask these questions to help elicit the diagnosis:

1 *Where is the lesion?* • Are the legs flaccid or spastic? (ie LMN or UMN?) • Is there sensory loss? A sensory *level* usually means spinal cord disease. • Is there loss of bowel or bladder control? (Lesion more likely to be in the conus medullaris or cauda equina.)

2 *What is the lesion?* • Was onset sudden or rapidly progressive? ►This is an emergency; it suggests cord compression so get urgent help (see next paragraph). • Are there any signs of infection (eg tender spine, ↑T°, ↑WCC, ↑ESR, ↑CRP: extradural abscess)?

Cord compression (See also p528.) ***Symptoms:*** Bilateral leg weakness (arm weakness—often less severe—suggests a cervical cord lesion, see p508) a sensory level ± preceding back pain (see p542). Bladder (and anal) sphincter involvement is late and manifests as hesitancy, frequency, and, later, as painless retention. ***Signs:*** Look for a motor, reflex, and sensory level, with normal findings above the level of the lesion, LMN signs at the level (especially in cervical lesions), and UMN signs *below* the level (but remember tone and reflexes are usually reduced in *acute* cord compression; *OHCS* p756). ***Causes:*** Secondary malignancy (breast, lung, prostate, thyroid, kidney) in the spine is commonest. Rarer: infection (epidural abscess), cervical disc prolapse, haematoma (warfarin), intrinsic cord tumour, atlanto-axial subluxation, myeloma. ΔΔ: Transverse myelitis, MS, carcinomatous meningitis, cord vasculitis (PAN, syphilis), spinal artery thrombosis or aneurysm, trauma, Guillain–Barré syndrome (p702). ***Investigations:*** ►Do not delay imaging at any cost. Spinal x-rays are unreliable; MRI is the definitive modality. Biopsy or surgical exploration may be needed to identify the nature of any mass. Do a CXR (primary lung malignancy, lung secondaries, TB). Bloods: FBC, ESR, B_{12}, syphilis serology, U&E, LFT, PSA, serum electrophoresis. ***Treatment:*** Give urgent dexamethasone in malignancy (p528) while considering more specific therapy, eg radiotherapy or chemotherapy ± decompressive laminectomy; which is most appropriate depends on tumour type, quality of life, and likely prognosis. Epidural abscesses must be surgically decompressed and antibiotics given.

Cauda equina and conus medullaris lesions The big difference between these lesions and those high up in the cord is that leg weakness is flaccid and areflexic, not spastic and hyperreflexic. ***Causes:*** As above, plus congenital lumbar disc disease and lumbosacral nerve lesions. ***Signs:*** *Conus medullaris lesions* feature mixed UMN/LMN signs, leg weakness, early urinary retention and constipation, back pain, sacral sensory disturbance and erectile dysfunction. *Cauda equina lesions* feature back pain and radicular pain down the legs; asymmetrical, atrophic, areflexic paralysis of the legs; sensory loss in a root distribution; and ↓sphincter tone; do PR.

Other patterns of leg weakness

Unilateral foot drop: DM, common peroneal nerve palsy, stroke, prolapsed disc, MS.

Weak legs with no sensory loss: MND, polio, parasagittal meningioma (an exception to the rule that weak legs mean cord or distal lesion).

Chronic spastic paraparesis: MS, cord primary malignancy/metastasis, MND, syringomyelia, subacute combined degeneration of the cord (p334), hereditary spastic paraparesis, taboparesis (tertiary syphilis, see p412), histiocytosis X, parasites (eg schistosomiasis).

Chronic flaccid paraparesis: Peripheral neuropathy, myopathy.

Absent knee jerks and extensor plantars: (Ie combined LMN or UMN signs.) Combined cervical and lumbar disc disease, conus medullaris lesions, MND, myeloradiculitis, Friedreich's ataxia, subacute combined degeneration of the cord, taboparesis.[4]

4 Tertiary syphilis (p412): in tabes dorsalis the afferent pathways from muscle spindles are lost, with reduced tone and tendon reflexes (without weakness). Later, additional involvement of the pyramida tracts causes taboparesis—a spastic paraparesis with the peculiar combination of extensor plantars (from the taboparesis) and absent tendon reflexes (from the tabes dorsalis).

Gait disorders

Spastic: Stiff, circumduction of legs ± scuffing of the toe of the shoes: UMN lesions.
Extrapyramidal: Flexed posture, shuffling feet, slow to start, postural instability, eg Parkinson's disease.

Apraxic: Pathognomonic 'gluing-to-the-floor' on attempting walking or a wide-based unsteady gait with a tendency to fall, like a novice on an ice-rink. Seen in normal pressure hydrocephalus and multi-infarct states.

Ataxic: Wide-based; falls; cannot walk heel-to-toe. Caused by cerebellar lesions (eg MS, posterior fossa tumours, alcohol, phenytoin toxicity); proprioceptive sensory loss (eg sensory neuropathy, ↓B_{12}). Often worse in the dark or with eyes closed.
Myopathic: Waddling gait, cannot climb steps or stand from sitting due to hip girdle weakness.

Psychogenic: Suspect if there is a bizarre gait not conforming to any pattern of organic gait disturbance and without any signs when examined on the couch.
Tests Spinal X-rays; MRI; FBC; ESR; syphilis serology; serum B_{12}; U&E; LFT; PSA; serum electrophoresis; CXR; LP; EMG; muscle ± sural nerve biopsy.

Non-neurological considerations in paralysed patients

Avoid pressure sores by turning and review weight-bearing areas often. Use appropriate pressure-relieving mattresses/cushions. Prevent thrombosis in paralysed limbs by frequent passive movement, pressure stockings, and LMWH (p350). Bladder care is vital; catheterization is only one option (do not control incontinence by decreasing fluid intake). Bowel evacuation may be manual or aided by suppositories; increasing dietary fibre intake may help. Exercise of unaffected or partially paralysed limbs is important to avoid unnecessary loss of function.

Abnormal involuntary movements (dyskinesia)

These are characterized by impairment of the planning, control, or execution of movement. They can have multiple manifestations:

Tremor Note frequency, amplitude, and exacerbating factors (stress; fatigue).

- *Rest tremor:* Abolished on voluntary movement. *Cause:* parkinsonism (p494).
- *Intention tremor:* Irregular, large-amplitude, worse at the end of purposeful acts, eg finger-pointing or using a remote control. *Cause:* cerebellar damage (eg MS, stroke).
- *Postural tremor:* Absent at rest, present on maintained posture (arms outstretched) and may persist (but is not worse) on movement. *Causes:* benign essential tremor (autosomal dominant; improves with alcohol), thyrotoxicosis, anxiety, β-agonists.
- *Re-emergent tremor:* Postural tremor developing after a delay of ~10s. *Causes:* Parkinson's disease (don't mistake for essential tremor).

Chorea Non-rhythmic, jerky, purposeless movements flitting from one place to another—eg facial grimacing, raising the shoulders, flexing/extending the fingers. *Causes:* Huntington's disease, Sydenham's chorea (rare complication of group A streptococcal infection). Worsened by levodopa.

Hemiballismus Large-amplitude, flinging hemichorea (affects proximal muscles) contralateral to a vascular lesion of the subthalamic nucleus (often elderly diabetics). Recovers spontaneously over months.

Athetosis Slow, sinuous, confluent, purposeless movements (especially digits, hands, face, tongue), often difficult to distinguish from chorea. *Causes:* Commonest is cerebral palsy (*OHCS* p214). Most other 'athetoid' patterns may now be better classed as dystonias. *Pseudoathetosis:* Caused by severe proprioceptive loss.

Tics Brief, repeated, stereotyped movements which patients may suppress for a while. Tics are common in children (and usually resolve). In Tourette's syndrome (p700), motor and vocal tics occur. Consider psychological support, clonazepam or clonidine if tics are severe (haloperidol may help but risks tardive dyskinesia).

Myoclonus Sudden involuntary focal or general jerks arising from cord, brainstem, or cerebral cortex, seen in metabolic problems, neurodegenerative disease (eg lysosomal storage enzyme defects), CJD (p696), and myoclonic epilepsies (infantile spasms). *Benign essential myoclonus:* Childhood onset with frequent generalized myoclonus, without progression. Often autosomal dominant. It may respond to valproate, clonazepam, or piracetam. *Asterixis ('metabolic flap'):* Jerking (~1-2 jerks/sec) of outstretched hands, worse with wrists extended, from loss of extensor tone—ie incoordination between flexors and extensors (='negative myoclonus'). *Causes:* Liver or kidney failure, ↓Na^+, ↑CO_2, gabapentin, thalamic stroke (consider if unilateral).

Tardive syndromes Delayed onset yet potentially irreversible symptoms occuring after chronic exposure to dopamine antagonists (eg antipsychotics, antiemetics). *Classification:* •*Tardive dyskinesia:* orobuccolingual, truncal, or choreiform movements, eg vacuous chewing and grimacing movements. •*Tardive dystonia:* sustained, stereotyped muscle spasms of a twisting or turning character, eg retrocollis and back arching/opisthotonic posturing. •*Tardive akathisia:* sense of restlessness or unease ± repetitive, purposeless movements (stereotypies, eg pacing). •*Tardive myoclonus.* •*Tardive tourettism* (p700). •*Tardive tremor.* *Treating tardive dyskinesia:* Gradually withdraw neuroleptics and wait 3–6 months. Tetrabenazine may help. Quetiapine, olanzapine, and clozapine are examples of atypical antipsychotics that are less likely to cause tardive syndromes.

Dystonia

Dystonia describes prolonged muscle contractions causing abnormal posture or repetitive movements.

Idiopathic generalized dystonia: Childhood-onset dystonia often starting in one leg with ipsilateral progression over 5-10yrs. Autosomal dominant inheritance is common (DYT1 deletion). Exclude Wilson's disease and dopa-responsive dystonia (needs an L-dopa trial). Anticholinergics and muscle relaxants may help. Deep brain stimulation for refractory, disabling symptoms.

Focal dystonias: Confined to one part of the body, eg *spasmodic torticollis* (head pulled to one side), *blepharospasm* (involuntary contraction of orbicularis oculi, *OHCS* p417), *writer's cramp*. Focal dystonias in adults are typically idiopathic, and rarely generalize. They are worsened by stress. Patients may develop a *geste antagoniste* to try to resist the dystonic posturing (eg a touch of the finger to the jaw in spasmodic torticollis). Injection of botulinum toxin into the overactive muscles is usually effective.

Acute dystonia: (fig 10.14) May occur on starting many drugs, including neuroleptics and some anti-emetics (eg metoclopramide, cyclizine). There is torticollis (head pulled back), trismus (oromandibular spasm), and/or oculogyric crisis (eyes drawn up). You may mistake this for tetanus or meningitis, but such reactions rapidly disappear after a dose of an anticholinergic, see p843.

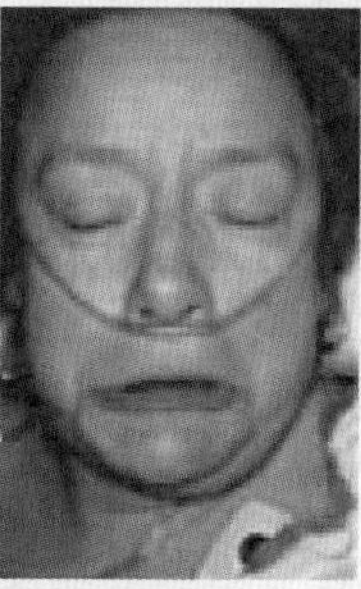
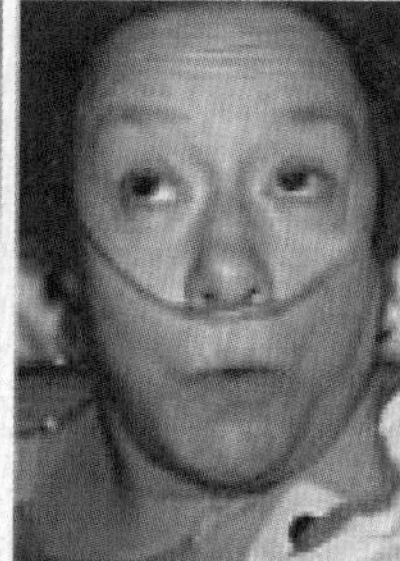
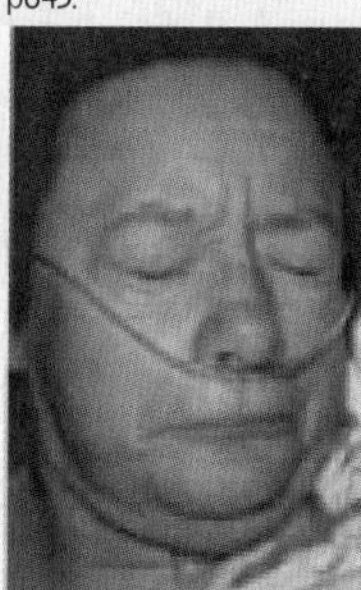

Fig 10.14 Oromandibular/oculogyric crisis in acute dystonia.

St Vitus's dance

Throughout the middle ages, Europe was plagued by epidemics of 'dancing mania', in which afflicted individuals were described to have danced wildly, displaying strange contortions and convulsions until they collapsed from exhaustion. If the afflicted touched a relic of St Vitus they were miraculously cured: observing this, Paracelsus, 16th-century Swiss-German physician and philosopher, described the phenomenon of *chorea Sancti Viti* ('St Vitus's dance'). There may have been an infectious component, although mass hysteria induced by religious cults that swept across medieval Europe seems a more likely cause. Chorea was subsequently used as a general term for large-amplitude involuntary movements before being further refined by physicians such as Sydenham (though he did not connect his eponymous chorea seen in rheumatic fever with an infectious trigger) and Charcot. Nowaways, a more frequent cause of involuntary movements with behavioural disturbance is NMDA-receptor antibody encephalitis, the impact of which was documented in Susannah Cahalan's excellent 2012 autobiography *Brain on Fire: My Month of Madness*.

Stroke: clinical features and acute management

Infarction or bleeding into the brain manifests with sudden-onset focal CNS signs. Someone in the UK has a stroke every 3.5 minutes; 1 in 4 of those will die within a year and half of survivors will have a permanent disability.

Causes • Small vessel occlusion/cerebral microangiopathy or thrombosis *in situ*. • Cardiac emboli (AF; endocarditis; MI—see BOX 'Cardiac causes of stroke', p473). • Atherothromboembolism (eg from carotids). • CNS bleeds (↑BP, trauma, aneurysm rupture, anticoagulation, thrombolysis). *Other causes:* ►Consider in younger patients: sudden BP drop by ≥40mmHg (most likely to affect the boundary zone between vascular beds), carotid artery dissection (spontaneous, or from neck trauma or fibromuscular dysplasia), vasculitis, subarachnoid haemorrhage (p478), venous sinus thrombosis (p480), antiphospholipid syndrome, thrombophilia (p374), Fabry disease (p698), CADASIL.[5]

Differentials Head injury, hypo/hyperglycaemia, subdural haemorrhage, intracranial tumours, hemiplegic migraine, post-ictal (Todd's palsy), CNS lymphoma, Wernicke's encephalopathy, hepatic encephalopathy, encephalitis, toxoplasmosis, cerebral abscesses, mycotic aneurysm, drug overdose (if comatose).

Modifiable risk factors ↑BP, smoking, DM, heart disease (valvular, ischaemic, AF), peripheral vascular disease, ↑PCV, carotid bruit, combined OCP, ↑lipids, ↑alcohol use, ↑clotting (eg ↑plasma fibrinogen, ↓antithrombin III, p374), ↑homocysteine, syphilis.

Signs Worst at onset. *Pointers to bleeding (unreliable!):* meningism, severe headache, coma. *Pointers to ischaemia:* carotid bruit, AF, past TIA, IHD. *Cerebral infarcts:* (50%.) Depending on site there may be contralateral sensory loss or hemiplegia—initially flaccid (floppy limb, falls like a dead weight when lifted), becoming spastic (UMN); dysphasia; homonymous hemianopia; visuo-spatial deficit. *Brainstem infarcts:* (25%.) Varied; include quadriplegia, disturbances of gaze and vision, locked-in syndrome (aware, but unable to respond). *Lacunar infarcts:* (25%). Basal ganglia, internal capsule, thalamus, and pons.) Five syndromes: ataxic hemiparesis, pure motor, pure sensory, sensorimotor, and dysarthria/clumsy hand. Cognition/consciousness are intact except in thalamic strokes.

Acute management ► *Protect the airway:* This avoids hypoxia/aspiration.

- *Maintain homeostasis:* Blood glucose: keep between 4-11 mmol/L. Blood pressure: only treat if there is a hypertensive emergency (eg encephalopathy or aortic dissection) or thrombolysis is considered (ideally aim for ≤185/110) as treating even very high BPs may impair cerebral perfusion.
- *Screen swallow:* 'Nil by mouth' until this is done (but keep hydrated).
- *CT/MRI within 1h:* Essential if: thrombolysis considered, high risk of haemorrhage (↓GCS, signs of ↑ICP, severe headache, meningism, progressive symptoms, bleeding tendency or anticoagulated), or unusual presentation (eg fluctuating consciousness, fever). Otherwise imaging less urgent (aim <24h). Diffusion-weighted MRI is most sensitive for an acute infarct, but CT helps rule out primary haemorrhage (fig 10.15).
- *Antiplatelet agents:* Once haemorrhagic stroke is excluded, give aspirin 300mg (continue for 2 weeks, then switch to long-term antithrombotic treatment, p472).
- *Thrombolysis:* Consider this as soon as haemorrhage has been excluded, provided the onset of symptoms was ≤4.5h ago.[2] The benefits of thrombolysis outweigh the risks within this window, though best results are within 90min. Alteplase is the agent of choice and must be given by trained staff, ideally within an expert acute stroke team. ► Always do CT 24h post-lysis to identify bleeds.[6] CI to thrombolysis • Major infarct or haemorrhage on CT. • Mild/non-disabling deficit. • Recent surgery, trauma, or artery or vein puncture at uncompressible site. • Previous CNS bleed. • AVM/aneurysm. • Severe liver disease, varices, or portal hypertension. • Seizures at presentation. • Blood glucose (<3 or >22). • Stroke or serious head injury in last 3 months. • GI or urinary tract haemorrhage in the last 21 days. • Known clotting disorder. • Anticoagulants or INR >1.7. • Platelets $<100 \times 10^9$/L. • History of intracranial neoplasm. • Rapidly improving symptoms. • BP >180/105.
- *Thrombectomy:* Intra-arterial mechanical thrombectomy provides additional benefit for those with large artery occlusion in the proximal anterior circulation.

► Admit to an acute stroke unit: multidisciplinary care improves outcomes (p474).

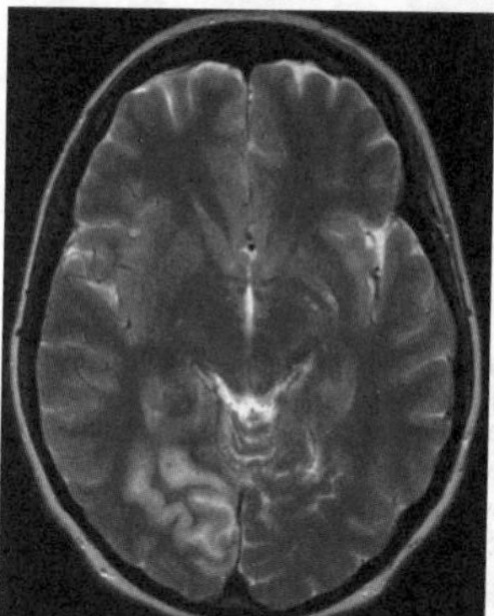

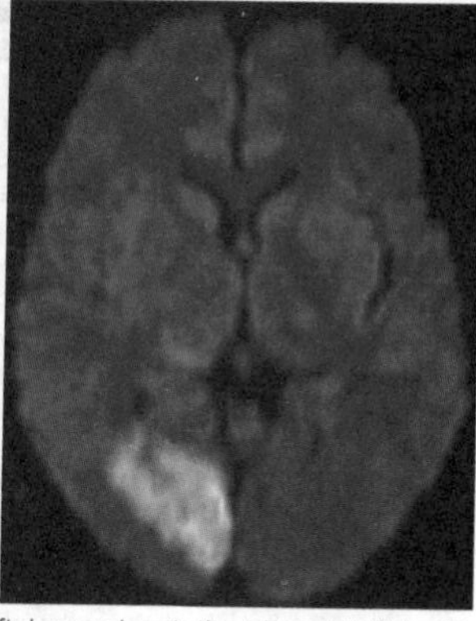

Fig 10.15 The T2-weighted (p746) image on the left shows oedema in the right occipital lobe. Differentials: infarct (right PCA), inflammation, or tumour. The diffusion-weighted image on the right shows limited diffusion in the region, indicating this is an infarct. ©Prof Peter Scally.

Act FAST

Several public health measures have aimed to increase awareness of stroke and the seriousness of the condition: the relabelling of stroke as a 'brain attack,' and via the graphic mass media FAST campaign = Facial asymmetry, Arm/leg weakness, Speech difficulty, Time to call 999. The publicity surrounding this acronym has increased recognition of the symptoms of stroke and emphasized the urgency of seeking medical help; following the introduction of the campaign in 2011 the NHS in England saw a 24% rise in stroke-related 999 calls.

5 Cerebral Autosomal Dominant Arteriopathy with Subcortical Infarcts & Leucoencephalopathy: the main genetic cause of stroke (there is also an autosomal recessive form).

6 If +ve, register at SITS, www.sitsinternational.org

Stroke: investigation and prevention

Primary prevention (Ie before any stroke.)
Control risk factors (p470): look for and treat hypertension, DM, ↑lipids (p690), cardiac disease (see BOX 'Cardiac causes of stroke') and help quit smoking (see p93). Exercise helps (↑HDL, ↑glucose tolerance). Use *lifelong anticoagulation* in AF (see BOX 'Cardiac causes of stroke') and prosthetic heart valves. • For prevention post-TIA see p476.

Secondary prevention (Ie preventing further strokes.)
Control risk factors (as *Primary prevention* mentioned above): there is a considerable advantage from lowering blood pressure and cholesterol (even if not particularly raised). *Antiplatelet agents after stroke:* (See BOX 'Antiplatelets'.) If no primary haemorrhage on CT, give 2 weeks of aspirin 300mg, then switch to long-term clopidogrel monotherapy. If this is CI or not tolerated then give low dose aspirin plus slow-release dipyridamole. *Anticoagulation after stroke from AF:* See BOX 'Cardiac causes of stroke'.

Tests (See p470 for imaging.) Investigate promptly to identify risk factors for further strokes, but consider whether results will affect management. Look for:

- *Hypertension.* Look for retinopathy (p560), nephropathy, or cardiomegaly on CXR.
- *Cardiac source of emboli.* (See BOX 'Cardiac causes of stroke'.) 24h ECG to look for AF (p130). CXR may show an enlarged left atrium. Echocardiogram may reveal mural thrombus due to AF or a hypokinetic segment of cardiac muscle post-MI. It may also show valvular lesions in infective endocarditis or rheumatic heart disease. Transoesophageal echo is more sensitive than transthoracic.
- *Carotid artery stenosis.* Do carotid Doppler US ± CT/MRI angiography. Benefits and risks of revascularization should be individualized by an expert but generally most with ≥70% stenosis and life expectancy ≥5yrs will benefit while some (especially ♂) will benefit with 50–69% stenosis[7] (see p476). Carotid endarterectomy is the procedure of choice; endovascular carotid artery angioplasty with stenting is an alternative for those unfit for surgery and achieves similar long-term outcomes but has higher peri-procedure stroke and mortality rates.
- *Hypoglycaemia, hyperglycaemia, dyslipidaemia,* and *hyperhomocysteinaemia.*
- *Vasculitis.* ↑ESR, ANCA (p556). VDRL to look for active, untreated syphilis (p412).
- *Prothrombotic states,* eg thrombophilia (p374), antiphospholipid syndrome (p554).
- *Hyperviscosity,* eg polycythaemia (p366), sickle-cell disease (p340).
- *Thrombocytopenia* and other bleeding disorders.
- *Genetic tests.* CADASIL (p470); Fabry disease (p698).

Prognosis *Overall mortality:* 60 000/yr; UK 20% at 1 month, then ≲10%/yr. *Full recovery:* ≤40%. Drowsiness≈poor prognosis. Avoid pressure ulcers (fig 10.16).

7 Interventions for 50–69% stenoses can be justifiable; individualize risk and check local guidelines. In particular, check which criteria used to estimate degree of stenosis since NASCET (North American Symptomatic Carotid Endarterectomy Trial) criteria tend to include some more severe lesions in 50–69% range as compared to the ECST (European Carotid Surgery Trialists' Collaborative Group) criteria.

Cardiac causes of stroke

Cardioembolic causes are the source of stroke in >30% of patients, and may be hinted at if there are bilateral infarcts on imaging.

Non-valvular atrial fibrillation: (p130) Associated with an overall risk of stroke of 4.5%/yr, and ischaemic strokes in AF carry a worse prognosis.

- *CHA_2DS_2VASc score* (p131) can be used to calculate risk of stroke in patients with AF. Offer anticoagulation in patients with a score of 2 or above. ►Take bleeding risk into account: calculate the risk of major bleeding using the HAS-BLED score. Caution and regular review of oral anticoagulants are required if the HAS-BLED score >3. ► Do not offer stroke prevention therapy in patients with AF if <65y and CHA_2DS_2VASc score is 0 for men or 1 for women.
- *Anticoagulation* (see p350) can be commenced 2wks after a stroke (or from 7–10d if clinically and radiologically small). Offer a direct oral anticoagulant (DOAC) or warfarin (p350), following a discussion of risks and benefits.

Other cardiac sources of emboli: • Cardioversion. • Prosthetic valves. • Acute myocardial infarct with large left ventricular wall motion abnormalities on echocardiography. • Patent foramen ovale/septal defects. • Cardiac surgery. • Infective endocarditis (gives rise to septic emboli; 20% of those with endocarditis present with CNS signs).

Antiplatelets: mechanism of action

Aspirin: Inhibits COX-1, suppressing prostaglandin and thromboxane synthesis.

Clopidogrel: A thienopyridine that inhibits platelet aggregation by modifying platelet ADP receptors, preventing further strokes and MIs.

Dipyridamole: ↑cAMP and ↓thromboxane A2.

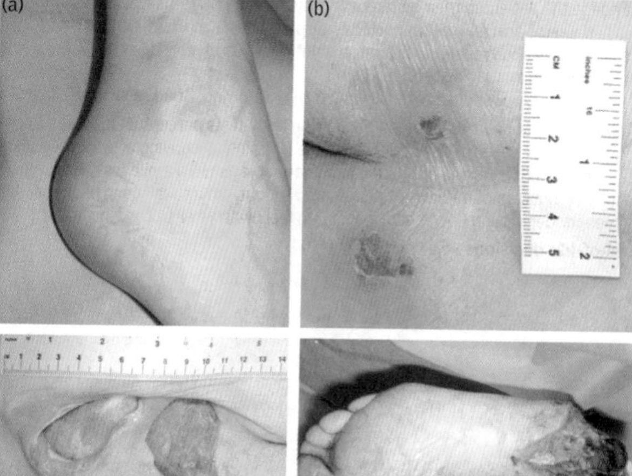

Fig 10.16 Categorization of pressure ulcers. (a) Stage 1: non-blanchable redness of intact skin, typically over a bony prominence. (b) Stage 2: partial thickness loss of dermis presenting as a shallow open ulcer with a red/pink wound bed, without slough. May also present as an intact or open/ruptured sero-sanguinous blister. (c) Stage 3: full thickness skin loss with visible subcutaneous fat. Bone, tendon, or muscle are not exposed. (d) Stage 4: full thickness tissue loss wth exposed bone, tendon, or muscle.

Re-enablement after stroke

Coordinated multidisciplinary care on a specialized stroke unit is essential, and leads to better patient outcomes. Rehabilitation must be started early post-stroke in order to maximize improvement and prevent complications related to immobility such as pressure sores, aspiration pneumonia, constipation, and contractures. Ongoing input after discharge consolidates inpatient gains and helps align the individual with their previous capability. It also helps with depression—both in the patient and their carer.
►Setting achievable goals and acknowledging the patient's own agenda is key.

Imperatives for re-enablement

- Watch the patient swallow a small volume of water; if signs of aspiration (a cough or voice change) make *nil by mouth* until formal assessment by a speech therapist. Use IV fluids, then semi-solids (eg jelly; avoid soups and crumbly food). Avoid early NG tube feeds; these may be needed to safeguard nutrition in those with swallowing problems that persist beyond the first 2-3d. If swallowing fails to recover, consider benefits of enteral feeding tube placement (p759). Speech therapists skilled in assessing swallowing difficulties are invaluable here.
- Avoid further injury: minimize falls risk and take care when lifting the patient not to damage their shoulders.
- Ensure good bladder and bowel care through frequent toileting. Avoid early catheterization which may prevent return to continence.
- Position to minimize spasticity (occurs in ~40%). Get prompt physiotherapy. Splints and botulinum toxin injections are helpful for focal spasticity.
- Monitor progress: eg measure time taken to sit up and transfer to chair.
- Monitor mood: in pseudo-emotionalism/emotional lability (sobbing unprovoked by sorrow, from failure of cortical inhibition of the limbic system), tricyclics or fluoxetine may help.
- Engage the patient in their own recovery by making physiotherapy fun. Swimming (a hemiplegic arm may be supported on a special float), music, and video games are all enjoyable and ↑ recovery through promoting cerebral reorganization. Constraint of the good arm may be helpful.

►Involve the carer/spouse with all aspects of care-giving. Good rehab saves lives.

Tests Asking to point to a named part of the body tests perceptual function. Copying matchstick patterns tests spatial ability. Dressing or copying a clock face tests for *apraxia* (p86). Picking out and naming easy objects from a pile tests for agnosia (acuity OK, but cannot mime use; guesses are way-out, semantically, and phonetically). Screen for depression (low mood; inability to feel pleasure or to concentrate).

End-of-life decisions ►See p13.

Neurology

Assessing dependence in daily life

Handicap entails inability to carry out social functions. 'A disadvantage for a given individual, resulting from an impairment or disability, that limits or prevents the fulfilment of a role.' Two people with the same *impairment* (eg paralysed arm) may have different *disabilities* (table 10.5, eg one may be able to dress but the other cannot). Disabilities are likely to determine quality of future life. Treatment is often best aimed at reducing disability, not curing disease. For example, Velcro® fasteners in place of buttons may enable a person to dress.

Table 10.5 Barthel's index of activities of daily living

Bowels	0	Incontinent (or needs to be given enemas)
	1	Occasional accidents (once a week)
	2	Continent
Bladder	0	Incontinent, or catheter inserted but unable to manage it
	1	Occasional accidents (up to once per 24h)
	2	Continent (for more than 7 days)
Grooming	0	Needs help with personal care: face, hair, teeth, shaving
	1	Independent (implements provided)
Toilet use	0	Dependent
	1	Needs some help but can do some things alone
	2	Independent (on and off, wiping, dressing)
Feeding	0	Unable
	1	Needs help in cutting, spreading butter, etc.
	2	Independent (food provided within reach)
Transfer	0	Unable to get from bed to commode: the vital transfer to prevent the need for 24-hour nursing care
	1	Major help needed (physical, 1–2 people), can sit
	2	Minor help needed (verbal or physical)
	3	Independent
Mobility	0	Immobile
	1	Wheelchair-independent, including corners, etc.
	2	Walks with help of one person (verbal or physical)
	3	Independent
Dressing	0	Dependent
	1	Needs help but can do about half unaided
	2	Independent (including buttons, zips, laces, etc.)
Stairs	0	Unable
	1	Needs help (verbal, physical, carrying aid)
	2	Independent up and down
Bath/shower	0	Dependent
	1	Independent (must get in and out unaided and wash self)

Mahoney FI, Barthel DW: Functional evaluation: the Barthel Index. *Maryland State Medical Journal*. 1965; 14:61–65.

Barthel's paradox

The more we contemplate Barthel's eulogy of independence, the more we see it as a mirage reflecting a greater truth about human affairs: ►there is no such thing as independence—only *interdependence*—and in fostering this interdependence lies our true vocation:

> *No man is an Island, intire of it selfe; every man is a peece of the Continent, a part of the maine; if a Clod bee washed away by the Sea, Europe is the lesse, as well as if a promontorie were, as well as if a Mannor of thy friends or of thine owne were. Any man's death diminishes me, because I am involved in mankinde; And therefore never send to know for whom the bell tolls: It tolls for thee.*

John Donne 1572–1631; *Meditation* XVII.

Transient ischaemic attack (TIA)

This is an ischaemic (usually embolic) neurological event with symptoms lasting <24h (often much shorter). ► Without intervention, more than 1 in 12 patients will go on to have a stroke within a week, so prompt management is imperative.

Signs Specific to the arterial territory involved (p450). *Amaurosis fugax* occurs when the retinal artery is occluded, causing unilateral progressive vision loss 'like a curtain descending'. *Global* events (eg syncope, dizziness) are *not* typical of TIAs. Attacks may be single or many; multiple highly stereotyped attacks ('crescendo' TIAS) suggest a critical intracranial stenosis (commonly the superior division of the MCA).

Causes (See p470.) • *Atherothromboembolism* from the carotid is the chief cause: listen for bruits (though not a sensitive test). • *Cardioembolism:* mural thrombus post-MI or in AF, valve disease, prosthetic valve (p473). • *Hyperviscosity:* eg polycythaemia, sickle-cell anaemia, myeloma. • *Vasculitis* is a rare, non-embolic cause of TIA symptoms (eg cranial arteritis, PAN, SLE, syphilis, etc.).

Differentials Hypoglycaemia, migraine aura (p458), focal epilepsy (symptoms spread over seconds and often include twitching and jerking), hyperventilation, retinal bleeds. *Rare mimics of TIA:* Malignant hypertension, MS (paroxysmal dysarthria), intracranial tumours, peripheral neuropathy, phaeochromocytoma, somatization.

Tests FBC, ESR, U&Es, glucose, lipids, CXR, ECG, carotid Doppler ± angiography, CT or diffusion-weighted MRI, echocardiogram.

Treatment

- *Control cardiovascular risk factors:* Optimize: BP (cautiously lower; aim for <140/85mmHg, p140); hyperlipidaemia (p690); DM (p206); help to stop smoking (p93).
- *Antiplatelet drugs:* As with stroke, give aspirin 300mg OD for 2wks, then switch to clopidogrel 75mg OD. If this is contraindicated or not tolerated, give aspirin 75mg OD combined with slow-release dipyridamole.
- *Anticoagulation indications:* Cardiac source of emboli (see p473).
- *Carotid endarterectomy:* Perform within 2wks of first presentation if 70-99% stenosis[8] and operative risk is acceptable (higher risk in: ♀, >75y, ↑systolic BP, contralateral artery occluded; ipsilateral carotid syphon/external carotid stenosed). Do not stop aspirin preoperatively. Surgery is preferred to endovascular carotid artery angioplasty with stenting in those fit enough to tolerate due to higher peri-procedure stroke and mortality rates with stenting.

Driving Prohibited for at least 1 month, see p158.

Prognosis Long-term risks of stroke or cardiovascular events following TIAs are dependent on underlying vascular risk factors: calculate using the ABCD^2 score (see BOX and table 10.6).

8 Interventions for 50-69% stenoses can be justifiable; individualize risk and check local guidelines. In particular, check which criteria used to estimate degree of stenosis since NASCET (North American Symptomatic Carotid Endarterectomy Trial) criteria tend to include some more severe lesions in 50-69% range as compared to the ECST (European Carotid Surgery Trialists' Collaborative Group) criteria.

When should TIA lead to emergency referral?

The ABCD² score is a helpful tool to stratify which patients are at higher risk of having a stroke following a suspected TIA (table 10.6).

Table 10.6 The ABCD² score

Age ≥60 yrs old	1 point
Blood pressure ≥140/90	1 point
Clinical features	
Unilateral weakness	2 points
Speech disturbance without weakness	1 point
Duration of symptoms	
Symptoms lasting ≥1h	2 points
Symptoms lasting 10–59min	1 point
Diabetes	1 point

A score of ≥4 indicates that the patient is at high risk of an early stroke, and must be assessed by a specialist within 24h. A score of ≥6 strongly predicts a stroke (8.1% within 2 days, 35.5% in the next week). Other factors that suggest increased risk are: • AF • >1 TIA in a week • TIA while anticoagulated. Crucially, risk is lowest if the patient is treated in a specialized stroke unit (p474).

ABCD² score reprinted from *The Lancet*, 366, Rothwell *et al.*, 'A simple score (ABCD) to identify individuals at high early risk of stroke after transient ischaemic attack', 29–36. 2003, with permission from Elsevier.

Subarachnoid haemorrhage (SAH)

Spontaneous bleeding into the subarachnoid space, often catastrophic (table 10.7).

Incidence 9/100 000/yr; typical age: 35–65.

Symptoms Sudden-onset excruciating headache, typically occipital—like a 'thunderclap'. Vomiting, collapse, seizures, and coma often follow. Coma/drowsiness may last for days. Some patients report a preceding, 'sentinel' headache, perhaps due to a small warning leak from the offending aneurysm (~6%).

Signs Neck stiffness; Kernig's sign (takes 6h to develop); retinal, subhyaloid and vitreous bleeds (=Terson's syndrome; ↑mortality × 5). Focal neurology at *presentation* may suggest site of aneurysm (eg pupil changes indicating a IIIrd nerve palsy with a posterior communicating artery aneurysm) or intracerebral haematoma. Later deficits suggest complications (see later in topic).

Causes • *Berry aneurysm rupture (80%).* Common sites: junctions of posterior communicating with the internal carotid (see fig 10.3, p451) or of the anterior communicating with the anterior cerebral artery, or bifurcation of the middle cerebral artery (fig 10.17). 15% are multiple. •*Arterio-venous malformations (15%).*• *Other causes;* encephalitis, vasculitis, tumour (invading blood vessels), idiopathic.

Risk factors Previous aneurysmal SAH (new aneurysms form, old ones get bigger), smoking, alcohol misuse, ↑BP, bleeding disorders, SBE (mycotic aneurysm), family history (3–5x ↑risk of SAH in close relatives). Polycystic kidneys, aortic coarctation, and Ehlers-Danlos syndrome (p149) are all associated with berry aneurysms.

Differentials Meningitis (p822), migraine (p458), intracerebral bleed, cortical vein thrombosis (p480), dissection of a carotid or vertebral artery, benign thunderclap headache (triggered by Valsalva manoeuvre, eg cough, coitus).

Tests • *Urgent CT:* Detects >95% of SAH within the 1st 24h (fig 10.18). • *Consider LP:* If CT −ve but the history is very suggestive of SAH (and no CI: p768). This needs to be done >12h after headache onset to allow breakdown of RBCs so that a positive sample is xanthrochromic (yellow, due to bilirubin: differentiaties between old blood from SAH vs a 'bloody tap').

Management ►Refer all proven SAH to neurosurgery immediately.

- *Re-examine CNS* often; chart BP, pupils, and GCS (p788). Repeat CT if deteriorating.
- *Maintain cerebral perfusion* by keeping well hydrated, but aim for SBP <160mmHg.
- *Nimodipine* (60mg/4h PO for 3wks, or 1mg/h IVI) is a Ca^{2+} antagonist that reduces vasospasm and consequent morbidity from cerebral ischaemia.
- *Surgery:* endovascular coiling vs surgical clipping (requiring craniotomy): the decision depends on the accessibility and size of the aneurysm, though coiling is preferred where possible (fewer complications, better outcomes). Do catheter or CT angiography to identify single *vs* multiple aneurysms *before* intervening. Newer techniques such as balloon remodelling and flow diversion can be helpful in anatomically challenging aneurysms.

Complications *Rebleeding* is the commonest cause of death, and occurs in 20%, often in the 1st few days. *Cerebral ischaemia* due to vasospasm may cause a permanent CNS deficit, and is the commonest cause of morbidity. If this happens, surgery is not helpful at the time but may be so later. *Hydrocephalus,* due to blockage of arachnoid granulations, requires a ventricular or lumbar drain. *Hyponatraemia* is common but should not be managed with fluid restriction. Seek expert help.

Table 10.7 Mortality in subarachnoid haemorrhage

Grade	Signs	Mortality: %
I	None	0
II	Neck stiffness and cranial nerve palsies	11
III	Drowsiness	37
IV	Drowsy with hemiplegia	71
V	Prolonged coma	100

Most mortality occurs in 1st month. 90% of survivors of the 1st month, survive >1 year.

Unruptured aneurysms: 'the time-bomb in my head'

Bear in mind the old adage: 'if it ain't broke, don't fix it'—usually, risks of *preventive* intervention outweigh any benefits, except perhaps in •young patients (more years at risk, and surgery is twice as hazardous if >45yrs old) who have •aneurysms >7mm in diameter, especially if located at the •junction of the internal carotid and the posterior communicating cerebral artery, or at the •rostral basilar artery bifurcation, and especially if there is •uncontrolled hypertension or a •past history of bleeds. Data from the 2003 International Study of Unruptured Intracranial Aneurysms (ISUIA) show that relative risk of rupture for an aneurysm 7-12mm across is 3.3 compared with aneurysms <7mm across; if the diameter is >12mm, the relative risk is 17.

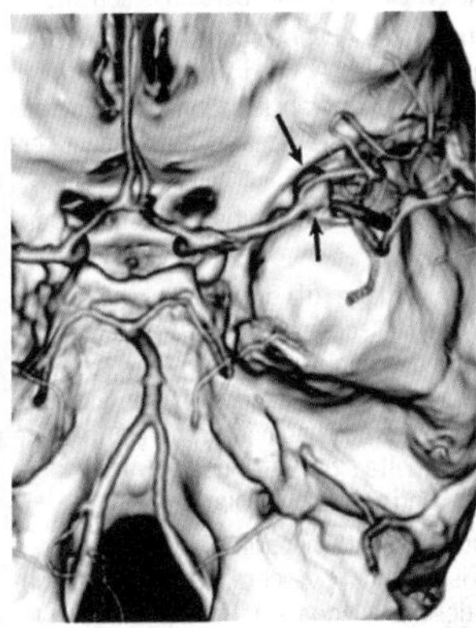

Fig 10.17 CT images can be manipulated to show only high-density structures such as bones and arteries containing contrast. Here is a middle cerebral artery aneurysm.

We thank Prof. Peter Scally for these CT images and the commentaries on them.

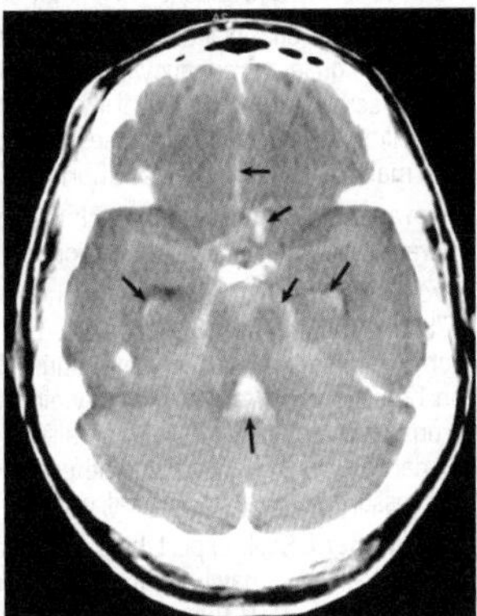

Fig 10.18 Blood from a ruptured aneurysm occupies the interhemispheric fissure (top arrow), a crescentic intracerebral area presumably near the aneurysm (2nd arrow), the basal cisterns, the lateral ventricles (temporal horns), and the 4th ventricle (bottom arrow).

We thank Prof. Peter Scally for these CT images and the commentaries on them.

Intracranial venous thrombosis (IVT)

Thrombosis of the cerebral sinuses or veins causes cerebral infarction, though much less commonly than arterial disease. Seizures are common and focal; they can complicate diagnosis and post-ictal drowsiness may impair GCS assessment. Although ~80% will make a good functional recovery, death is mainly due to transtentorial herniation from mass effect or oedema.[9]

Dural venous sinus thrombosis Most commonly sagittal sinus thrombosis (figs 10.19, 10.20; 47% of all IVT) or transverse sinus thrombosis (35%). Sagittal sinus thrombosis often coexists if other sinuses are thrombosed. Symptom onset is gradual (over days or weeks). Features are dependent on the sinus affected:

- *Sagittal sinus:* Headache, vomiting, seizures, ↓vision, papilloedema.
- *Transverse sinus:* Headache ± mastoid pain, focal CNS signs, seizures, papilloedema.
- *Sigmoid sinus:* Cerebellar signs, lower cranial nerve palsies.
- *Inferior petrosal sinus:* vth and vith cranial nerve palsies, with temporal and retro-orbital pain (Gradenigo's syndrome, suggesting otitis media is the cause).
- *Cavernous sinus:* Often due to spread from facial pustules or folliculitis, causing headache, chemosis, oedematous eyelids, proptosis, painful ophthalmoplegia, fever.

Cortical vein thrombosis (CVT) Usually occurs with a sinus thrombus as it extends into the cortical veins, causing infarction in a venous territory (fig 10.21). These infarcts give rise to stroke-like focal symptoms that develop over days. There are often seizures, and an associated headache which may come on suddenly (thunderclap headache).

Causes Numerous, including anything that promotes a hypercoagulable state (p374). *Common causes:* Pregnancy/puerperium, combined OCP, head injury, dehydration, blood dyscrasias, tumours (local invasion/pressure), extracranial malignancy (hypercoagulability), recent LP. *Other causes:* Infection (meningitis, abscesses, otitis media, cerebral malaria, TB), Drugs (eg antifibrinolytics, androgens), SLE, vasculitis, Crohn's or UC.

Differential diagnosis Subarachnoid haemorrhage, meningitis, encephalitis, intracranial abscess, arterial infarction.

Investigations Exclude subarachnoid haemorrhage (if thunderclap headache, p478) and meningitis (p822). *Bloods:* Thrombophilia screen. *Imaging:* CT/MRI venography may show the absence of a sinus (fig 10.19), though an absent transverse sinus can be a normal variant. MRI T2-weighted gradient echo sequences can visualize thrombus directly (fig 10.20), and also identify haemorrhagic infarction. CT may be normal early, but show a filling defect at ~1wk (delta sign). *LP* (if no CI): raised opening pressure. CSF may be normal, or show RBCs and xanthochromia.

Management Seek expert help. Anticoagulation with heparin or LMWH and then warfarin (INR 2–3) may benefit even if there is secondary cerebral haemorrhage (unless otherwise CI). If there is deterioration despite adequate anticoagulation, endovascular thrombolysis or mechanical thrombectomy may provide limited benefit (but not in those with large infarcts and impending herniation). ↑ICP requires prompt attention (p830); decompressive hemicraniectomy may prevent impending herniation.

9 Predictors of poor prognosis include: GCS score on admission <9, deep CVT location, CNS infection, malignancy, intracranial haemorrhage, mental status abnormality, age >37 years, and ♂.

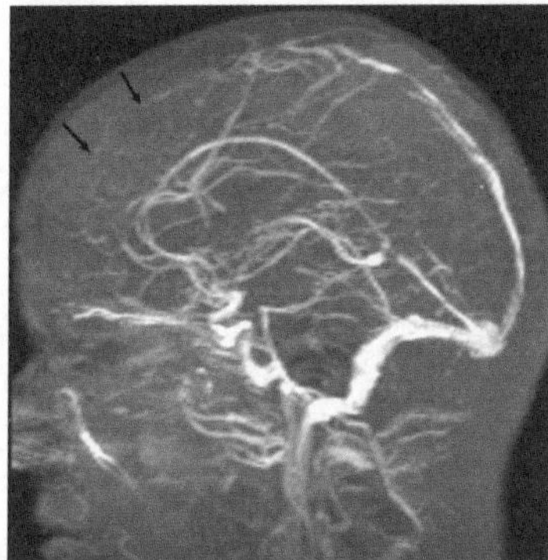

Fig 10.19 This magnetic resonance venogram (MRV) could look normal at first glance: the hardest thing to see in imaging is often that which is not there. Much of the superior sagittal sinus is not seen because it is filled with clot—a superior sagittal sinus thrombosis. The arrows point to where it should be seen. Posteriorly, the irregularity of the vessel indicates non-occlusive clot.

Image and commentary courtesy of Prof. P. Scally.

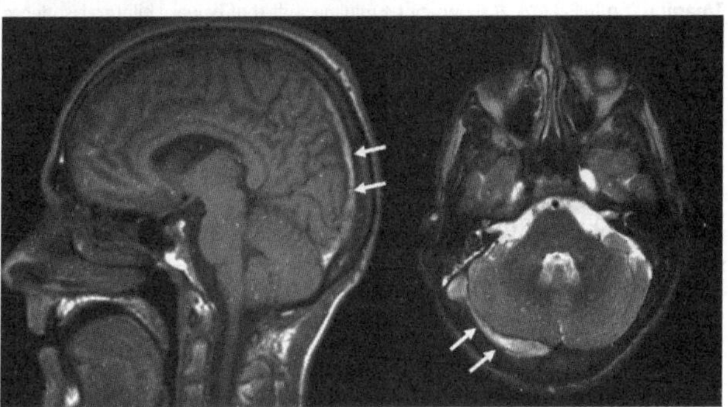

Fig 10.20 MRI showing thrombus (arrows) in the sagittal sinus (sagittal T1-weighted image, LEFT), and in the right transverse sinus (axial T2-weighted image, RIGHT). Often more than one sinus is involved.

Image courtesy of Dr David Werring.

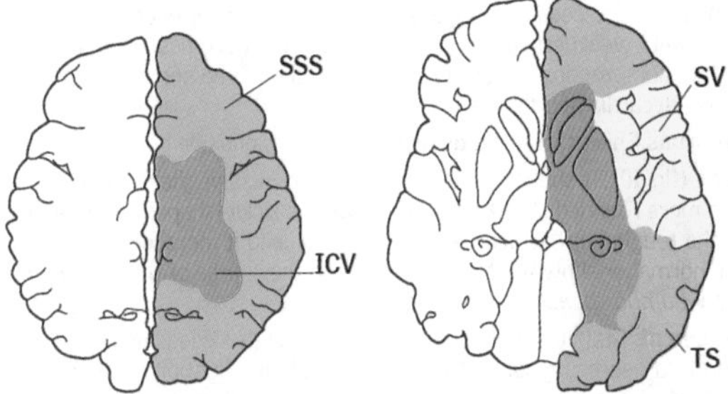

Fig 10.21 Venous territories (compare with arterial territories on p451). SSS—superior sagittal sinus; TS—transverse sinus; SV—Sylvian veins; ICV—internal cortical veins.

There is much greater variation in venous anatomy between individuals than there is in arterial anatomy, so this diagram is only a rough guide. The key point is to realize that infarction that crosses boundaries between arterial territories may be venous in origin.

Subdural haematoma

►Consider this very treatable condition in all whose conscious level fluctuates, and also in those having an 'evolving stroke', especially if on anticoagulants. Bleeding is from bridging veins between cortex and venous sinuses (vulnerable to deceleration injury), resulting in accumulating haematoma between dura and arachnoid. This gradually raises ICP, shifting midline structures away from the side of the clot and, if untreated, eventual tentorial herniation and coning. Most subdurals are from trauma but the trauma is *often forgotten as it was so minor or so long ago* (up to 9 months). It can also occur without trauma (eg ↓ICP; dural metastases). The elderly are most susceptible, as brain atrophy makes bridging veins vulnerable. *Other risk factors:* falls (epileptics, alcoholics); anticoagulation.

Symptoms Fluctuating level of consciousness (seen in 35%) ± insidious physical or intellectual slowing, sleepiness, headache, personality change, and unsteadiness.

Signs ↑ICP (p830), seizures. Localizing neurological symptoms (eg unequal pupils, hemiparesis) occur late, often >1 month after the injury.

Differentials Stroke, dementia, CNS masses (eg tumours, abscesses).

Imaging (fig 10.22) CT/MRI shows clot ± midline shift (but beware bilateral isodense clots). Look for crescent-shaped collection of blood over 1 hemisphere. The sickle-shape differentiates subdural blood from extradural haemorrhage.

Management Reverse clotting abnormalities urgently. Surgical management depends on the size of the clot, its chronicity, and the clinical picture: generally those >10mm or with midline shift >5mm need evacuating (via craniotomy or burr hole washout). Address the cause of the trauma (eg falls, abuse).

Extradural (epidural) haematoma

► Beware deteriorating consciousness after any head injury that initially produced no loss of consciousness or after initial drowsiness post injury seems to have resolved. This *lucid interval* pattern is typical of extradural bleeds.

Cause ►Suspect after any traumatic skull fracure. Often due to a fractured temporal or parietal bone causing laceration of the middle meningeal artery and vein, typically after trauma to a temple just lateral to the eye. Any tear in a dural venous sinus will also result in an extradural bleed. Blood accumulates between bone and dura.

Clinical features The lucid interval may last a few hours to a few days before a bleed declares itself by ↓GCS from rising ICP. Increasingly severe headache, vomiting, confusion, and seizures follow, ± hemiparesis with brisk reflexes and an upgoing plantar. If bleeding continues, the ipsilateral pupil dilates, coma deepens, bilateral limb weakness develops, and breathing becomes deep and irregular (brainstem compression). Death follows a period of coma and is due to respiratory arrest. Bradycardia and ↑BP are late signs.

Differentials Epilepsy, carotid dissection, carbon monoxide poisoning.

Tests CT (fig 10.23) shows a haematoma (often biconvex/lens-shaped; the blood forms a more rounded shape compared with the sickle-shaped subdural haematoma as the tough dural attachments to the skull keep it more localized). Skull X-ray may be normal or show fracture lines crossing the course of the middle meningeal vessels. ►*Lumbar puncture is contraindicated.*

Management Stabilize and transfer urgently (with skilled medical and nursing escorts) to a neurosurgical unit for clot evacuation ± ligation of the bleeding vessel. Care of the airway in an unconscious patient and measures to ↓ICP often require intubation and ventilation (+ mannitol IVI, p831).

Prognosis Excellent if diagnosis and operation early. Poor if coma, pupil abnormalities, or decerebrate rigidity are present pre-op.

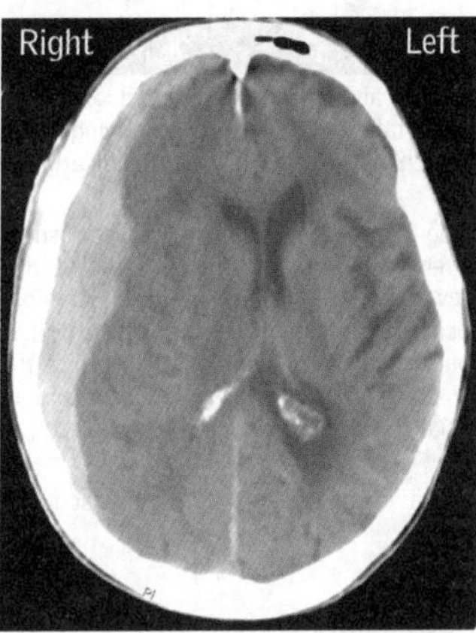

Fig 10.22 This image explains the cause as well as the pathology. On the patient's left, cerebral sulci are prominent and prior to this adverse event would have been even larger. The brain had shrunk within the skull as a result of atherosclerosis, and poor perfusion, leaving large subarachnoid spaces. A simple, quick rotation of the head is enough to tear a bridging vein, causing this *acute subdural haematoma*.

We thank Prof. Peter Scally for these CT images and commentary.

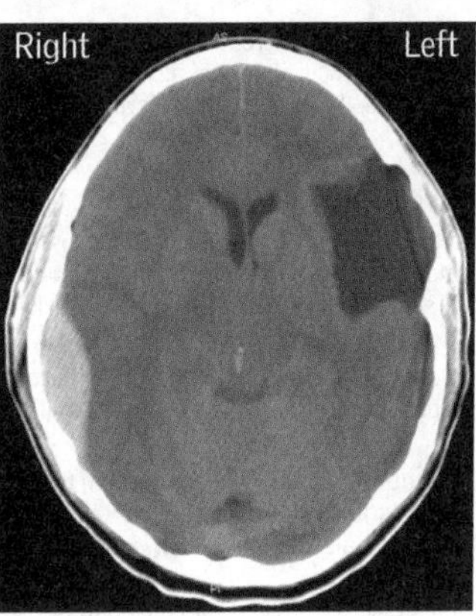

Fig 10.23 The blood (high attenuation, fusiform or biconvex collection) on the right side is limited anteriorly by the coronal suture and posteriorly by the lambdoid suture. This is therefore an *extradural haematoma*. The low-attenuation CSF density collection on the left is causing scalloping of the overlying bone. It is in the typical location of an arachnoid cyst; an incidental finding of a congenital abnormality.

We thank Prof. Peter Scally for these CT images and commentary.

Delirium (acute confusional state)

Delirium[10] affects up to 50% of inpatients >65y, and is associated with a longer admission, more complications, and higher mortality. ►Look for an underlying cause in *any* acute fluctuating, baffling behaviour change; it may be an early indication of treatable pathology (eg UTI).

Clinical features Globally impaired cognition, perception, and consciousness which develops over hours/days, characterized by a marked memory deficit, disordered or disorientated thinking, and reversal of the sleep-wake cycle. Some patients experience tactile or visual hallucinations. Delirium can be: •*hyperactive,* with restlessness, mood lability, agitation, or aggression •*hypoactive* in which the patient becomes slow and withdrawn or •*mixed.* ►Hypoactive and mixed delirium are much harder to recognize: it is crucial to compare current behaviour to the patient's baseline (see BOX).

Risk factors >65y, dementia/previous cognitive impairment, hip fracture, acute illness, psychological agitation (eg pain).

Causes

- Surgery/post-GA.
- Systemic infection: pneumonia, UTI, malaria, wounds, IV lines.
- Intracranial infection or head injury.
- Drugs/drug withdrawal: opiates, levodopa, sedatives, recreational.
- Alcohol withdrawal (2–5d post-admission; ↑LFTs, ↑MCV; history of alcohol abuse).
- Metabolic: uraemia, liver failure, Na^+ or ↑↓glucose, ↓Hb, malnutrition (beriberi, p268).
- Hypoxia: respiratory or cardiac failure.
- Vascular: stroke, myocardial infarction.
- Nutritional: thiamine, nicotinic acid, or B_{12} deficiency.

Differentials Dementia (see BOX), anxiety, epilepsy: ►non-convulsive status epilepticus is an underdiagnosed cause of impaired cognition and odd behaviour: consider an EEG. Primary mental illness (eg schizophrenia) can also mimic delirium, but this is rare on the wards (especially if no past history).

Tests Look for the cause (eg UTI, pneumonia, MI): do FBC, U&E, LFT, blood glucose, ABG, septic screen (urine dipstick, CXR, blood cultures); also consider ECG, malaria films, LP, EEG, CT.

Management As well as identifying and treating the underlying cause, aim to:[3]

- Reorientate the patient: explain where they are and who you are at each encounter. Hunt down hearing aids/glasses. Visible clocks/calendars may help.
- Encourage visits from friends and family.
- Monitor fluid balance and encourage oral intake . Be vigilant for constipation.
- Mobilize and encourage physical activity.
- Practise sleep hygeine: restrict daytime napping, minimize night-time disturbance.
- Avoid or remove catheters, IV cannulae, monitoring leads and other devices (they increase infection risk and may get pulled out).
- Watch out for infection and physical discomfort/distress.
- Review medication and discontinue any unnecessary agents. Only use sedation if the patient is a risk to their own/other patients' safety (never use physical restraints). Consider haloperidol 0.5–2mg, or chlorpromazine 50–100mg, PO if they will take it, IM if not (p15). Wait 20min to judge effect—further doses can be given if needed. NB: avoid chlorpromazine in the elderly and in alcohol withdrawal (p280); avoid antipsychotics in those with Parkinson's disease or Lewy body dementia.

►Be aware that delirium may persist beyond the duration of the original illness by several weeks in the elderly. Do not assume this must be dementia—provide support and reassess 1–2 months later.

10 Delirium, from the Latin *de* (from) and *lira* (ridge between furrows), meaning 'out of one's furrow'.

Delirium vs dementia

One is often mistaken for the other, yet perhaps the interconnectedness of these two conditions is greater than we realize: not only is dementia the leading risk factor for delirium, but delirium itself confers a greater risk of subsequently developing dementia.[4] It is likely that this is due to a number of factors: delirium is a marker of vulnerability of the brain, and may also emphasize previously unrecognized dementia symptoms. Furthermore, there may be direct causation through the noxious insults incurred during an episode of delirium, which can lead to permanent neuronal damage.

In distinguishing the two conditions (not always an easy task) the presence of inattention, distractibility, and disorganized thinking will all point you towards delirium. But the fundamental question is 'Has there been an *acute* change from the patient's cognitive baseline?' Family or carer collateral reports are invaluable, but may not always be available. Document cognition in all patients >65y admitted to hospital (eg AMTS, p64, many admission proformas allow for this). This will then allow you to compare their admission score with subsequent assessments and track any improvements, deteriorations, or fluctuations in cognition throughout the admission.

Dementia

A neurodegenerative syndrome with progressive decline in several cognitive domains. The initial presentation is usually of memory loss over months or years (►look for other causes if over days/weeks). Prevalence increases with age: 20% of people >80yrs are known to have dementia, yet probably only half of cases are diagnosed.

Diagnosis Is made by: *History* from the patient with a thorough collateral narrative—ask about the timeline of decline and the domains affected. Non-cognitive symptoms such as agitation, aggression, or apathy indicate late disease.[5] *Cognitive testing:* Use a validated dementia screen such as the AMTS (p64) or similar, plus short tests of executive function and language. Carry out a mental state examination to identify anxiety, depression, or hallucinations. *Examination* may identify a physical cause, risk factors (eg for vascular dementia), or parkinsonism. *Medication review* is important to exclude drug-induced cognitive impairment.

Investigations Look for reversible/organic causes: ↑TSH/↓B_{12}/↓folate (treat low-normals, p334), ↓thiamine (eg alcohol), ↓Ca^{2+}. Check MSU, FBC, ESR, U&E, LFT, and glucose. An MRI (preferred to CT) can identify other reversible pathologies (eg subdural haematoma, p482; normal-pressure hydrocephalus[11]), as well as underlying vascular damage or structural pathology. Functional imaging (FDG, PET, SPECT) may help delineate subtypes where diagnosis is not clear. Consider EEG in: suspected delirium, frontotemporal dementia, CJD, or a seizure disorder. If clinically indicated then check autoantibodies, syphilis, HIV, CJD, or other rare causes (see later in topic).

Subtypes • *Alzheimer's disease (AD):* See p488. • *Vascular dementia:* (~25%.) Cumulative effect of many small strokes: sudden onset and stepwise deterioration is characteristic (but often hard to recognize). Look for evidence of arteriopathy (↑BP, past strokes, focal CNS signs). ►Do not use acetylcholinesterase inhibitors or memantine in these patients. • *Lewy body dementia:* (15-25%.) Fluctuating cognitive impairment, detailed visual hallucinations, and later, parkinsonism (p494). Histology is characterized by Lewy bodies (eosinophilic intracytoplasmic inclusion bodies) in brainstem and neocortex. ►Avoid using antipsychotics in Lewy body dementia (↑↑risk of SE, see p489). • *Fronto-temporal dementia:* Frontal and temporal atrophy with loss of >70% of spindle neurons. Patients display executive impairment; behavioural/personality change; disinhibition; hyperorality, stereotyped behaviour, and emotional unconcern. Episodic memory and spatial orientation are preserved until later stages. *Pick's disease* refers to the few fronto-temporal dementia patients who have Pick inclusion bodies on histology (spherical clusters of tau-laden neurons).

Other causes Alcohol/drug abuse; repeated head trauma; pellagra (p268), Whipple's disease (p716); Huntington's (p702); CJD (p696); Parkinson's (p494); HIV; cryptococcosis (p408); familial autosomal dominant Alzheimer's; CADASIL (p470).

Management ►Refer suspected or diagnosed dementia to integrated memory services for further assessment and management. *Medication:* (p489). Avoid drugs that impair cognition (eg neuroleptics, sedatives, tricyclics). *Non-pharmacological interventions:* Non-cognitive symptoms (eg agitation) may respond to measures such as aromatherapy, multisensory stimulation, massage, music, and animal-assisted therapy.

Other considerations • *Depression:* Common. Try an SSRI (eg citalopram 10-20mg OD) or, if severe, mirtazapine (15-45mg at night if eGFR >40). Cognitive behavioural therapy can help with social withdrawal and catastrophic thinking. • *Capacity:* Can the patient make decisions regarding medical or financial affairs? Wherever possible, allow them to. Suggest making an advanced directive or appointing a Lasting Power of Attorney in the early stages of the disease.

11 Dilated ventricles *without* enlarged sulci. *Signs:* gait apraxia, incontinence, dementia; CSF shunts help.

Who will care for the carers?

Our ageing population and improvements in medicine mean that we not only have an increasing number of people with dementia in the UK, but that those people are living longer with the disease in more advanced stages. Their needs become more complex and they become increasingly dependent. Currently, informal (mostly family) carers of people with dementia save the UK £11 billion a year. Yet this is not an easy task: most dementia sufferers display behavioural or psychological symptoms, which can be particularly distressing for the carer. Carer stress is inevitable and causes ↑morbidity and mortality. Ameliorate this with:

- *A care coordinator* (via Social Services or the local Old Age Community Mental Healthcare Team); vital to coordinate the various teams and services available:
  - Laundry services for soiled linen
  - Car badge giving priority parking
  - Help from occupational therapist, district nurses, and community psychiatric nurses
  - Attendance allowance
  - Respite care in hospital
  - Council tax rebate (forms from local council office).
- *Day services* can be invaluable for stimulating patients and providing regular, much-needed breaks for carers.
- *Moral support* Support groups, telephone helplines, and charities can all ease the burden, eg UK Alzheimer's Disease Society.
- *Combatting challenging behaviour:* First rule out pain, infection, and depression. Then consider trazodone (50–300mg at night) or lorazepam (0.5–1mg/12–24h PO). Haloperidol (0.5–4mg) can be useful in the short term.

Alzheimer's disease (AD)

This leading cause of dementia is *the* big neuropsychiatric disorder of our times, dominating the care of the elderly and the lives of their families who give up work, friends, and ways of life to support relatives through the long final years as they exit into their '*worlds of preoccupied emptiness*'. Suspect AD in adults >40yrs with persistent,[12] progressive, and *global* cognitive impairment: visuo-spatial skill, memory, verbal abilities, and executive function (planning) are all affected, unlike other dementias which may affect certain domains but not others (identify which with neuropsychometric tests). There is also anosognosia—a lack of insight into the problems engendered by the disease, eg missed appointments, misunderstood conversations or plots of films, and mishandling of money. Later there may be irritability; mood disturbance (depression or euphoria); behavioural change (eg aggression, wandering, disinhibition); psychosis (hallucinations or delusions); agnosia (may not recognize self in the mirror). There is no standard natural history. Cognitive impairment is progressive, but non-cognitive symptoms may come and go over months. Eventually many patients become sedentary, taking little interest in anything.

Cause Environmental and genetic factors both play a role. Accumulation of β-amyloid peptide, a degradation product of amyloid precursor protein, results in progressive neuronal damage, neurofibrillary tangles, ↑numbers of amyloid plaques, and loss of the neurotransmitter acetylcholine (fig 10.24). Neuronal loss is selective—the hippocampus, amygdala, temporal neocortex, and subcortical nuclei are most vulnerable. Vascular effects are also important—95% of AD patients show evidence of vascular dementia.

Risk factors 1st-degree relative with AD; Down's syndrome (in which AD is inevitable, often <40yrs); homozygosity for apolipoprotein E (ApoE) E4 allele (see BOX 'Genetics and the future'); PICALM, CL1 & CLU variants; vascular risk factors (↑BP, diabetes, dyslipidaemia, ↑homocysteine, AF); ↓physical/cognitive activity; depression; loneliness (↑risk × 2; simply living alone is not a risk factor); smoking.

Management ►See p486 for a general approach to management in dementia. • Refer to a specialist memory service. • Acetylcholinesterase inhibitors (see BOX 'Pharmacological treatment'). • BP control (in heart failure there is a 2x ↑risk of AD; extra risk halves with BP control).

Prevention in the context of AD's time-course: Changes in CSF β-amyloid are seen ~25yrs before onset of unequivocal symptoms (USy) and its deposition is detected 15yrs before USy. CSF tau protein and brain atrophy are also detected 15yrs before USy. Cerebral hypometabolism and impaired episodic memory occur 10yrs before USy. Global cognitive impairment occurs 5yrs before USy. Prevention will probably be most effective before any of this starts—though there is currently insufficient evidence to recommend any specific interventions (BOX 'Genetics and the future'). Ultimately, there is no simple relationship between brain structure, neurofibrillary tangles, and function.

Prognosis Mean survival = 7yrs from USy.

12 'Enduring' doesn't mean unfluctuating: cognition comes and goes, allowing poetic insights, as in Iris Murdoch's poignant self-diagnosis: 'I am sailing into the dark'.

Pharmacological treatment of cognitive decline

There is overlap between Lewy body dementia, AD, and Parkinson's disease (PD), complicating treatment decisions: L-dopa (p495) can precipitate delusions, and antipsychotic drugs worsen PD. Rivastigmine may help all three.

Acetylcholinesterase (AChE) inhibitors: Donepezil, rivastigmine, and galantamine are all modestly effective in treating AD and are recommended by NICE.[6] There is also some evidence for their efficacy in the dementia of Parkinson's disease, and rivastigmine may improve behavioural symptoms in Lewy body dementia—▶though none should be used in mild disease and they should be discontinued if there is no worthwile effect on symptoms. Doses:

- Donepezil: initially 5mg PO, eg doubled after 1 month.
- Rivastigmine: 1.5mg/12h initially, ↑ to 3–6mg/12h. Patches are also available.
- Galantamine: initially 4mg/12h, ↑ to 8–12mg/12h PO.

►The cholinergic effects of acetylcholinesterase inhibitors may exacerbate peptic ulcer disease and heart block. Ask about symptoms and do an ECG first.

Antiglutamatergic treatment: Memantine (an NMDA antagonist, p449) is reasonably effective in late-stage AD, and is recommended in patients with severe disease or those with moderate disease in which AChE inhibitors are not tolerated/CI. *Dose:* 5mg/24h initially, ↑ by 5mg/d weekly to 10mg/12h. *SE:* hallucinations, confusion, hypertonia, hypersexuality.

Antipsychotics: Consider in severe, non-cognitive symptoms only (eg psychosis or extreme agitation). ►Possible increased risk of stroke/TIA so discuss risks and assess cerebrovascular risk factors. Avoid in mild-to-moderate: Lewy body dementia (risk of neuroleptic sensitivity reactions), AD, and vascular dementia.

Vitamin supplementation: Trials of dietary and vitamin supplements have been mixed and disappointing. Perhaps the best evidence exists for vitamin E (2000IU OD) which may confer a modest benefit in delaying functional progression in mild to moderate AD, but with no effect on cognitive performance.

Genetics and the future

Possession of the APOE4 allele on chromosome 19 is the leading genetic cause of AD; homozygosity increases risk of developing the disease 12x. Yet while identifying this risk could enable a person to make lifestyle changes, there is little else to be done but anticipate one's impending cognitive decline (just one of the dilemmas raised by genetic testing). While the proteins that make up the plaques and neurofibrillary tangles seen in AD were identified in the early 1980s, progress has since been slow. So much so that in 2013, world leaders pledged to have a drug that would halt dementia within the next 10 years. Now a second-generation tau aggregation inhibitor called LMTX just might do the job, having shown success in phase III clinical trials in patients with mild/moderate AD, with clinical improvement and a slowing of atrophy on MRI. Perhaps in the imminent future, identifying those at greater risk of developing AD through genetic testing will have a role.

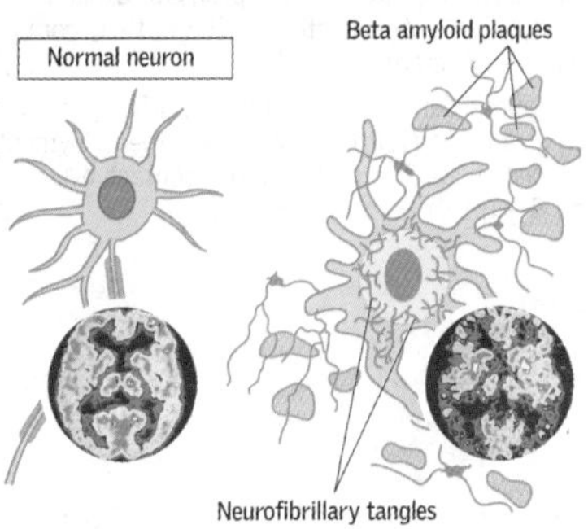

Fig 10.24 Normal neuron (left) and one exhibiting senile plaques and neurofibrillary tangles (right). The corresponding changes on functional neuroimaging are also shown.

Epilepsy: diagnosis

Epilepsy is a recurrent tendency to spontaneous, intermittent, abnormal electrical activity in part of the brain, manifesting as *seizures*. *Convulsions* are the motor signs of electrical discharges.

Elements of a seizure Some patients may experience a preceding *prodrome* lasting hours or days in which there may be a change in mood or behaviour. An *aura* implies a focal seizure, often, but not necessarily, from the temporal lobe. It may be a strange feeling in the gut, an experience such as *déjà vu* or strange smells or flashing lights. *Post-ictally* there may be headache, confusion, and myalgia; or temporary weakness after a focal seizure in the motor cortex (Todd's palsy, p712), or dysphasia following a focal seizure in the temporal lobe.

Causes ⅔ are idiopathic. *Structural:* Cortical scarring (eg head injury years before onset), developmental (eg dysembryoplastic neuroepithelial tumour or cortical dysgenesis), space-occupying lesion, stroke, hippocampal sclerosis (eg after a febrile convulsion), vascular malformations. *Others:* Tuberous sclerosis, sarcoidosis, SLE, PAN, antibodies to voltage-gated potassium channels.

Diagnosis Can be difficult due to the heterogenous nature of the disease (there are >40 different types of epilepsy). NICE estimate 5-30% of people with 'epilepsy' have been wrongly diagnosed. ► All patients with a seizure must be referred for specialist assessment and investigation in <2 wks.

Take a thorough history: Including a detailed description from a witness. Ask specifically about tongue-biting and a slow recovery. If this is a first seizure, enquire about past funny turns/odd behaviour. Déjà vu and odd episodic feelings of fear may well be relevant. Are there any triggers (eg alcohol, stress, flickering lights/TV)? Triggered attacks tend to recur.

Establish the type of seizure: See BOX 'Seizure classification'.[7] NB: if a seizure begins with focal features, it is a partial seizure, however rapidly it then generalizes. ►Don't forget non-epileptic attack disorder (='pseudo' seizures—psychogenic): this is not uncommon. (Suspect if seizures have a gradual onset, prolonged duration, and abrupt termination and are accompanied by closed eyes ± resistance to eye opening, rapid breathing, fluctuating motor activity, and episodes of motionless unresponsiveness. CNS exam, CT, MRI, and EEG are normal. It may coexist with true epilepsy.)

Rule out provoking causes: Most people would have a seizure given sufficient provocation (eg reflex anoxic seizures in faints) but would not be classed as epileptic: only 3-10% of provoked seizures recur; generally when the provocation is irreversible. *Causes:* trauma; stroke; haemorrhage; ↑ICP; alcohol or benzodiazepine withdrawal; metabolic disturbance (hypoxia, ↑↓Na^+, ↓Ca^{2+}, ↑↓glucose, uraemia, liver disease); infection (eg meningitis, encephalitis); ↑T°; drugs (tricyclics, cocaine). ►Unprovoked seizures have a recurrence rate of 30-50%.

Investigations Look for provoking causes. *Consider* an EEG: it cannot exclude epilepsy and can be falsely +ve, so don't do one if simple syncope is the likely diagnosis. Only do *emergency* EEGs if non-convulsive status is the problem. Other tests: MRI (structural lesions); drug levels (if on anti-epileptics: is the patient compliant?); drugs screen; LP (eg if infection suspected).

Counselling After any 'fit', advise about dangers, eg swimming, driving, heights until the diagnosis is known; then give *individualized* counselling on employment, sport, insurance, and conception (*OHCS* p28). The patient must contact DVLA and avoid driving until seizure-free for >1yr (p159).

Seizure classification

Focal seizures Originating within networks linked to one hemisphere and often seen with underlying structural disease. Various subclasses include:

- *Without impairment of consciousness:* (Previously described as 'simple'.) Awareness is unimpaired, with focal motor, sensory (olfactory, visual, etc.), autonomic, or psychic symptoms. No post-ictal symptoms.
- *With impairment of consciousness:* (Previously described as 'complex'.)Awareness is impaired—either at seizure onset or following a simple partial aura. Most commonly arise from the temporal lobe, in which post-ictal confusion is a feature.
- *Evolving to a bilateral, convulsive seizure:* (Previously described as 'secondary generalized'.) In ⅔ of patients with partial seizures, the electrical disturbance, which starts focally, spreads widely, causing a generalized seizure, which is typically convulsive.

Generalized seizures Originating at some point within, and rapidly engaging bilaterally distributed networks leading to simultaneous onset of widespread electrical discharge with no localizing features referable to a single hemisphere. Important subtypes include:

- *Absence seizures:* Brief (≤10s) pauses, eg suddenly stops talking in mid-sentence, then carries on where left off. Presents in childhood.
- *Tonic-clonic seizures:* Loss of consciousness. Limbs stiffen (tonic), then jerk (clonic). May have one without the other. Post-ictal confusion and drowsiness.
- *Myoclonic seizures:* Sudden jerk of a limb, face, or trunk. The patient may be thrown suddenly to the ground, or have a violently disobedient limb: one patient described it as '*my flying-saucer epilepsy*', as crockery which happened to be in the hand would take off.
- *Atonic (akinetic) seizures:* Sudden loss of muscle tone causing a fall, no LOC.
- *Infantile spasms:* (*OHCS* p206) Commonly associated with tuberous sclerosis.

NB: the classification of epileptic syndromes is separate to the classification of seizures, and is based on seizure type, age of onset, EEG findings, and other features such as family history.

Localizing features of focal seizures

Temporal lobe •Automatisms—complex motor phenomena with impaired awareness, varying from primitive oral (lip smacking, chewing, swallowing) or manual movements (fumbling, fiddling, grabbing) , to complex actions. •Dysphasia. •*Déjà vu* (when everything seems strangely familiar), or *jamais vu* (everything seems strangely unfamiliar). •Emotional disturbance, eg sudden terror, panic, anger, or elation, and derealization (out-of-body experiences).• Hallucinations of smell, taste, or sound. •Delusional behaviour. • Bizarre associations—eg 'Canned music at Tesco always makes me cry and then pass out'.

Frontal lobe •Motor features such as posturing or peddling movements of the legs. •Jacksonian march (a spreading focal motor seizure with retained awareness, often starting with the face or a thumb). •Motor arrest. •Subtle behavioural disturbances (often diagnosed as psychogenic). •Dysphasia or speech arrest. •Post-ictal Todd's palsy (p712).

Parietal lobe •Sensory disturbances—tingling, numbness, pain (rare). •Motor symptoms (due to spread to the pre-central gyrus).

Occipital lobe •Visual phenomena such as spots, lines, flashes.

Epilepsy: management

Living with epilepsy creates many problems: inability to drive and drug side-effects to name a few. Good management of the condition by an integrated specialized team is therefore of utmost importance.

Anti-epileptic drugs (AEDs) Should only be commenced by a *specialist*, after confirmed epilepsy diagnosis, ≥2 seizures (unless risk of recurrence is high, eg structural brain lesion, focal CNS deficit, or unequivocal epileptiform EEG), and following a detailed discussion of treatment options with the patient. AED choice depends on seizure type and epilepsy syndrome, comorbidities, lifestyle, and patient preference:

- *Focal (partial) seizures:* 1st line: carbamazepine or lamotrigine. 2nd line: levetiracetam, oxcarbazepine, or sodium valproate.[13]
- *Generalized tonic-clonic seizures:* 1st line: sodium valproate[13] or lamotrigine. 2nd line: carbamazepine, clobazam, levetiracetam, or topiramate.
- *Absence seizures:* 1st line: sodium valproate[13] or ethosuximide. 2nd line: lamotrigine.
- *Myoclonic seizures:* 1st line: sodium valproate.[13] 2nd line: levetiracetam, or topiramate (but ↑SE). Avoid carbamazepine and oxcarbazepine—may worsen seizures.
- *Tonic or atonic seizures:* Sodium valproate[13] or lamotrigine.

Treat with *one* drug and with *one* doctor in charge only. Slowly build up doses over 2-3 months (see BOX 'Anti-epileptic drugs (AEDs)') until seizures are controlled or maximum dosage is reached. If ineffective or not tolerated, switch to the next most appropriate drug. To switch drugs, introduce the new drug slowly, and only withdraw the 1st drug once established on the 2nd. Dual (adjunct) therapy is necessary in <10% of patients—consider if all appropriate drugs have been tried singly at the optimum dose.

Stopping AEDs: May be done *under specialist supervision* if the patient has been seizure-free for >2yrs and after assessing risks and benefits for the individual (eg the need to drive). The dose must be decreased slowly: over at least 2-3 months, or >6 months for benzodiazepines and barbiturates.

Other interventions *Psychological therapies:* Eg relaxation, CBT. May benefit some, but do not improve seizure frequency so only use as an adjunct to medication. *Surgical intervention:* Can be considered if a single epileptogenic focus can be identified (such as hippocampal sclerosis or a small low-grade tumour). Neurosurgical resection offers up to 70% chance of seizure resolution, but carries the risk of causing focal neurological deficits. Alternatives: vagal nerve stimulation, deep brain stimulation (DBS).

Sudden unexpected death in epilepsy (SUDEP) More common in uncontrolled epilepsy, and may be related to nocturnal seizure-associated apnoea or asystole. Those with epilepsy have 3x ↑mortality. >700 epilepsy-related deaths are recorded/yr in the UK; up to 17% are SUDEPs. The charity SUDEP Action may be of some help to families.

13 Sodium valproate is associated with significantly ↑risk of birth and developmental defects in children born to exposed mothers. Use in women of childbearing potential with caution and only after counselling.

Anti-epileptic drugs (AEDs): typical adult doses and side-effects

Carbamazepine: (As slow-release.) Initially 100mg/12h, increase by 200mg/d every 2wks up to max 1000mg/12h. *SE:* leucopenia, diplopia, blurred vision, impaired balance, drowsiness, mild generalized erythematous rash, SIADH (rare; see p673).

Lamotrigine: As monotherapy, initially 25mg/d, ↑ by 50mg/d every 2wks up to 100mg/12h (max 250mg/12h). ►Halve monotherapy dose if on valproate; double if on carbamazepine or phenytoin (max 350mg/12h). *SE:* maculopapular rash—occurs in 10% (but 1/1000 develop *Stevens-Johnson syndrome* or *toxic epidermal necrolysis*) typically in 1st 8wks, especially if on valproate; warn patients to see a doctor at once if rash or flu symptoms develop; Other SEs: diplopia, blurred vision, photosensitivity, tremor, agitation, vomiting, aplastic anaemia.

Levetiracetam: Initially 250mg/24h, increase by 250mg/12h every 2wks up to max 1.5g/12h (if eGFR >80). *SE:* psychiatric side-effects are common, eg depression, agitation. Other SEs: D&V, dyspepsia, drowsiness, diplopia, blood dyscrasias.

Sodium valproate: Initially 300mg/12h, increase by 100mg/12h every 3d up to max 30mg/kg (or 2.5g) daily. *SE:* teratogenic. Nausea is very common (take with food). Other SEs: liver failure (watch LFT especially during 1st 6 months), pancreatitis, hair loss (grows back curly), oedema, ataxia, tremor, thrombocytopenia, encephalopathy (hyperammonaemia).

Phenytoin: No longer 1st line due to toxicity (nystagmus, diplopia, tremor, dysarthria, ataxia) and *SE:* ↓intellect, depression, coarse facial features, acne, gum hypertrophy, polyneuropathy, blood dyscrasias. Blood levels required for dosage.

►Carbamazepine, phenytoin, and barbiturates are liver enzyme inducing.

Epilepsy and pregnancy

Epilepsy carries a 5% risk of fetal abnormalities, so good seizure control prior to conception and during pregnancy is vital. Yet some anti-epileptics are teratogenic: the patient must be given accurate information and counselling about contraception, conception, pregnancy, and breastfeeding in order to make informed decisions. In particular:

- Advise women of child-bearing age to take folic acid 5mg/d.
- Strictly avoid sodium valproate and polytherapy prior to conception and during pregnancy (lamotrigine is preferred but transition needs to be planned).
- Advise that most AEDs except carbamazepine and valproate are present in breast milk. Lamotrigine is not thought to be harmful to infants.
- Discuss contraceptive methods, bearing in mind that: enzyme-inducing AEDs make progesterone-only contraception unreliable, and oestrogen-containing contraceptives lower lamotrigine levels—an increased dose may be needed to achieve seizure control.

Parkinsonism

This is the extrapyramidal triad of:

1 *Tremor.* Worse at rest; often 'pill-rolling' of thumb over fingers (see p468).
2 *Hypertonia.* Rigidity + tremor gives 'cogwheel rigidity', felt by the examiner during rapid pronation/supination.
3 *Bradykinesia.* Slow to initiate movement; actions slow and decrease in amplitude with repetition, eg ↓blink rate, micrographia. Gait is festinant (shuffling, pitched forward, fig 10.25) with ↓arm-swing and freezing at obstacles or doors (due to poor *simultaneous* motor and cognitive function). Expressionless face.

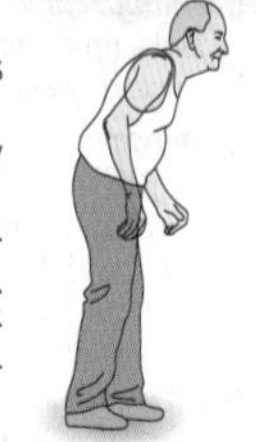

Fig 10.25 *'Marche à petit pas.'*

Causes

Parkinson's disease (PD): Loss of dopaminergic neurons in the substantia nigra, associated with Lewy bodies in the basal ganglia, brainstem, and cortex. Most cases are sporadic, though multiple genetic loci have been identified in familial cases. Mean age at onset is 60yrs. *Prevalence:* ↑ with age: 3.5% at 85–89yrs. *Clinical features:* The parkinsonian triad, plus non-motor symptoms such as: autonomic dysfunction (postural hypotension, constipation, urinary frequency/urgency, dribbling of saliva), sleep disturbance, and reduced sense of smell. Neuropsychiatric complications, such as depression, dementia, and psychosis, are common and debilitating. *Diagnosis:* Is clinical and based on the core features of bradykinesia with resting tremor and/or hypertonia; cerebellar disease and fronto-temporal dementia should be excluded; a clinical response to dopaminergic therapy is supportive. ►Signs are invariably worse on one side—if symmetrical look for other causes. If an alternative cause is suspected then consider MRI to rule out structural pathology. Functional neuroimaging (DaTscan™, PET) is playing an emerging role. *Treatment:* Focuses on symptom control and does not slow disease progression (see BOX). Non-pharmacological options include deep brain stimulation (DBS, may help those who are partly dopamine-responsive) and surgical ablation of overactive basal ganglia circuits (eg subthalamic nuclei).

Parkinson's plus syndromes *Progressive supranuclear palsy:* (PSP, Steele-Richardson-Olszewski syndrome.) Early postural instability, vertical gaze palsy ± falls; rigidity of trunk >limbs; symmetrical onset; speech and swallowing problems; little tremor. *Multiple system atrophy:* (MSA; Shy-Drager.) Early autonomic features, eg impotence/incontinence, postural ↓BP; cerebellar + pyramidal signs; rigidity > tremor. *Cortico-basal degeneration:* (CBD.) Akinetic rigidity involving one limb; cortical sensory loss (eg astereognosis); apraxia (even autonomous interfering activity by affected limb—the 'alien limb' phenomenon). *Lewy body dementia:* See p486.

Secondary causes *Vascular parkinsonism:* (2.5–5% of parkinsonism, also called 'lower limb' parkinsonism). Eg diabetic/hypertensive patient with postural instability and falls (rather than tremor, bradykinesia, and festination). *Other secondary causes:* Drugs (neuroleptics, metoclopramide, prochlorperazine), toxins (manganese), Wilson's disease (p285), trauma (*dementia pugilistica*), encephalitis, neurosyphilis.

Management Requires input of a a multidisciplinary team (GP, neurologist, nurse specialist, social worker, carers, physio- and occupational therapist) to boost quality of life. Assess disability and cognition objectively and regularly, and monitor mood—depression is common. Involve palliative care services early on. Postural exercises and weight lifting may help. ►Don't forget the carers (p487): offer respite care.

Pharmacological therapy in Parkinson's disease

A key decision is when to start supplementation of dopaminergic signalling with levodopa. Efficacy of this therapy reduces with time, requiring larger and more frequent dosing, with worsening SEs and response fluctuations (such as unpredictable freezing and pronounced end-of-dose reduced response: ~50% at 6yrs). Starting late may therefore be wise, eg when >70yrs or when PD seriously interferes with life: discuss pros and cons with the patient. ►Do not withdraw medication suddenly—risks acute akinesia and neuroleptic malignant syndrome. Be aware of situations where malabsorption could also have this effect (eg abdominal surgery, gastroenteritis).

Levodopa: Dopamine precursor, given combined with a dopa-decarboxylase inhibitor in co-beneldopa or co-careldopa. SEs: dyskinesia, painful dystonia. Non-motor SEs: psychosis; visual hallucinations, nausea and vomiting (give domperidone). Modified-release preparations should only be used in late disease.

Dopamine agonists (DAs): Ropinirole and pramipexole monotherapy can delay starting levodopa in early stages of PD, and allow lower doses of levodopa as PD progresses. Rotigotine transdermal patches are available as mono- or additive. SEs: drowsiness, nausea, hallucinations, compulsive behaviour (gambling, hypersexuality, p449). Ergot-derived DA-agonists (bromocriptine, pergolide, cabergoline) can cause fibrotic reactions, and are not favoured. Amantadine (weak DA) is used for drug-induced dyskinesias in late PD.

Apomorphine: Potent DA agonist used with continuous SC infusion to even out end-of-dose effects, or as a rescue-pen for sudden 'off' freezing. SE: injection-site ulcers.

Anticholinergics: (Eg benzhexol, orphenadrine.) Cause confusion in the elderly and have multiple SEs—limit to younger patients (but not 1st line).

MAO-B inhibitors: (Eg rasagiline, selegiline.) An alternative to dopamine agonists in early PD. SEs include postural hypotension and atrial fibrillation.

COMT inhibitors: (Eg entacapone, tolcapone.) May help motor complications in late disease. Lessen the 'off' time in those with end-of-dose wearing off. Tolcapone has better efficacy, but may cause severe hepatic complications and requires close monitoring of LFT.

Multiple sclerosis (MS)

Inflammatory plaques of demyelination in the CNS *disseminated in space and time*; ie occuring at multiple sites, with ≥30d in between attacks. Demyelination heals poorly, eventually causing axonal loss; >80% of patients develop progressive disability. The exact cause of the disease remains unknown; it is most likely a combination of genetic and environmental factors. There is >30% concordance in identical twins, and unusual geographical distribution, with increasing incidence with latitude in some parts of the world (NB: adult migrants take their risk with them; children acquire the risk of where they settle)—leading to hypotheses of the roles of vitamin D and infection. *Mean age of onset* is 30yrs. ♀:♂ ≥3:1.

Presentation Usually monosymptomatic: ~20% present with unilateral optic neuritis (pain on eye movement and ↓rapid central vision). Corticospinal tract and bladder involvement are also common, and symptoms may worsen with heat (eg hot bath or exercise). Other symptoms/signs see table 10.8.

Diagnosis This is clinical, made by a consultant neurologist using established criteria (eg McDonald, see table 10.9) and after alternative diagnoses have been excluded. ►Early diagnosis and treatment reduce relapse rates and disability so refer to neurology as soon as MS is suspected.

Tests Depending on presenting symptoms, some patients may need extra supporting information to make a diagnosis (as per the McDonald criteria). *MRI:* Sensitive but not specific for plaque detection. It may also exclude other causes, eg cord compression. *CSF:* Oligoclonal bands of IgG on electrophoresis that are not present in serum suggest CNS inflammation. Delayed visual, auditory, and somatosensory *evoked potentials*.

Progression Most patients follow a relapsing-remitting course, with initial recovery in between relapses. With time, remission becomes incomplete, so disability accumulates (secondary progression). 10% of patients display steadily progressive disability in the absence of relapses (primary progressive MS), while a minority of patients experience no progressive disablement at all. *Poor prognostic signs:* Older ♂; motor signs at onset; many early relapses; many MRI lesions; axonal loss. *Pregnancy:* Does not alter the rate of progression: relapses may reduce during pregnancy and increase 3-6 months afterwards, but return to their previous rate thereafter.

Management As with all neurological conditions, requires the coordinated care of a multidisciplinary team and full involvement of the patient in all decisions.[8]

Lifestyle advice: Regular exercise, stopping smoking and avoiding stress may help.

Disease-modifying drugs: Dimethyl fumarate is an option for mild/moderate relapsing-remitting MS. The monoclonal antibodies alemtuzumab (acts against T cells) and natalizumab (acts against VLA-4 receptors that allow immune cells to cross the blood-brain barrier) are also approved for relapsing-remitting disease. Interferon beta and glatiramer are not recommended by NICE on the balance of clinical and cost-effectiveness. Azathioprine is not recommended due to its SE profile.

Treating relapses: Methylprednisolone, eg 0.5-1g/24h IV/PO for 3-5d shortens acute relapses; use sparingly (≲twice/yr; steroid SE, p377). It doesn't alter overall prognosis.

Symptom control: Spasticity: offer baclofen or gabapentin. Tizanidine or dantrolene are 2nd line; if these fail consider benzodiazepines. *Tremor:* botulinum toxin type A injections improve arm tremor and functioning. *Urgency/frequency:* if post-micturition residual urine >100mL, teach intermittent self-catheterization; if <100mL, try tolterodine. *Fatigue:* amantadine, CBT, and exercise may help.

Table 10.8 Clinical features of MS

Sensory:	• Dysaesthesia • Pins and needles • ↓Vibration sense • Trigeminal neuralgia	*GI:* Swallowing disorders; constipation. *Eye:* Diplopia; hemianopia; optic neuritis; visual phenomena (eg on exercise); bilateral internuclear ophthalmoplegia (p73); pupil defects.
Motor:	• Spastic weakness • Myelitis	*Cerebellum:* Trunk and limb ataxia; intention tremor; scanning (ie monotonous) speech; falls.
Sexual/GU:	• Erectile dysfunction • Anorgasmia; urine retention; incontinence	*Cognitive/visuospatial decline:* ►A *big* cause of unemployment, accidents, amnesia, ↓mood, ↓executive functioning.
NB ↑T°, malaise, nausea, vomiting, positional vertigo, seizures, aphasia, meningism, bilateral optic neuritis, CSF leucocytosis and ↑CSF protein are rare in MS, and may suggest non-MS recurrent demyelinating disease, eg vasculitis or sarcoidosis.		

Diagnostic criteria for MS

Table 10.9 McDonald criteria for diagnosing MS (2010)

Clinical presentation	Additional evidence needed for diagnosis
≥2 attacks (relapses) with ≥2 objective clinical lesions	None
≥2 attacks with 1 objective clinical lesion	• MRI: spatially disseminated lesions, or • +ve CSF *and* ≥2 MRI lesions, or • 2nd attack at a new site
1 attack with ≥2 objective clinical lesions	Dissemination in time: • new lesion on repeat MRI after >3 months or • 2nd attack
1 attack with 1 objective clinical lesion (monosymptomatic presentation)	Dissemination in space: • MRI *or* +ve CSF if ≥2 MRI lesions consistent with MS • *and* dissemination in time (by MRI *or* a 2nd clinical attack)
Insidious neurological progression suggestive of primary progressive MS	+ve CSF *and* dissemination in space on MRI/VEP *or* continued progression for ≥1yr

►A careful history may reveal past episodes, eg brief unexplained visual loss, and detailed examination may show more than 1 lesion.
Attacks must last >1h, with >30d between attacks.

Six MS eponyms

Devic's syndrome: (=Neuromyelitis optica, NMO.) MS variant with transverse myelitis, (loss of motor, sensory, autonomic, reflex, and sphincter function below the level of a lesion), optic atrophy, and anti-aquaporin 4 antibodies (p698).
Lhermitte's sign: Neck flexion causes 'electric shocks' in trunk/limbs. (Also +ve in cervical spondylosis, cord tumours and ↓B_{12}.)
Uhthoff's phenomenon: Worsening of symptoms with heat, eg in bath.
Charles Bonnet syndrome: (Rare.) ↓Acuity/temporary blindness ± complex visual hallucinations of faces, as well as animals, plants, and trees.
Pulfrich effect: Unequal eye latencies, causing disorientation in traffic as straight trajectories seem curved and distances are misjudged on looking sideways.
Argyll Robertson pupil: See p72.

Space-occupying lesions (SOL)

Signs •↑*ICP:* (See p830.) Headache worse on waking, lying down, bending forward, or with coughing (p456); vomiting; papilloedema (only in 50% of tumours); ↓GCS.

- *Seizures:* Seen in ≤50%. Exclude SOL in all adult-onset seizures, especially if focal, or with a localizing aura or post-ictal weakness (Todd's palsy, p712).
- *Evolving focal neurology:* See BOX for localizing signs. ↑ICP causes *false localizing signs*: VIth nerve palsy is commonest (p70) due to its long intracranial course.
- *Subtle personality change:* Irritability, lack of application to tasks, lack of initiative, socially inappropriate behaviour.

Causes Tumour (primary or metastatic, later in topic), aneurysm, abscess (25% multiple); chronic subdural haematoma, granuloma (p197, eg tuberculoma), cyst (eg cysticercosis). *Tumours:* 30% are metastatic (eg breast, lung, melanoma). *Primaries:* astrocytoma, glioblastoma multiforme, oligodendroglioma, ependymoma. Also meningioma, primary CNS lymphoma (eg as non-infectious manifestation of HIV), and cerebellar haemangioblastoma.

Differentials Stroke, head injury, venous sinus thrombosis, vasculitis, MS, encephalitis, post-ictal, metabolic, or idiopathic intracranial hypertension.

Tests CT ± MRI (good for posterior fossa masses). Consider biopsy. Avoid LP before imaging (risks *coning*, ie cerebellar tonsils herniate through the foramen magnum).

Tumour management *Benign:* Remove if possible but some may be inaccessible. *Malignant:* Excision of gliomas is hard as resection margins are rarely clear, but surgery does give a tissue diagnosis, it debulks pre-radiotherapy, and makes a cavity for inserting carmustine wafers (delivers local chemotherapy). If a tumour is inaccessible but causing hydrocephalus, a ventriculo-peritoneal shunt can help. Chemo-radiotherapy is used post-op for gliomas or metastases, and as sole therapy if surgery is impossible. Oligodendroglioma with 1p/19q deletions is especially sensitive. In glioblastoma, temozolomide (alkylating agent) ↑survival. Seizure prophylaxis (eg phenytoin) is important, but often fails. Treat headache (eg codeine 60mg/4h PO). *Cerebral oedema:* Dexamethasone 4mg/8h PO; mannitol if ↑ICP acutely (p831). Plan meticulous palliative treatment (p534).

Prognosis Poor but improving (<50% survival at 5yrs) for CNS primaries; 40% 20yr survival for cerebellar haemangioblastoma; benign tumours are curable by excision.

Third-ventricle colloid cysts These congenital cysts declare themselves in adult life with amnesia, headache (often positional), obtundation (blunted consciousness), incontinence, dim vision, bilateral paraesthesiae, weak legs, and drop attacks. ℞: Excision or ventriculo-peritoneal shunting.

Idiopathic intracranial hypertension

Think of this in those presenting as if with a mass (headache, ↑ICP, and papilloedema)—*when none is found*. Most commonly seen in obese females in 3rd decade, who present with narrowed visual fields, blurred vision ± diplopia, VIth nerve palsy, and an enlarged blind spot, if papilloedema is present (it usually is). Consciousness and cognition are preserved.

Associations Endocrine abnormalities (Cushing's syndrome, hypoparathyroidism, ↑↓TSH), SLE, CKD, IDA, PRV, drugs (tetracycline, steroids, nitrofurantoin, and oral contraceptives).

Management Weight loss, acetazolamide or topiramate, loop diuretics, and prednisolone (start at ~40mg/24h PO; more SE than diuretics). Consider optic nerve sheath fenestration or lumbar-peritoneal shunt if drugs fail and visual loss worsens.

Prognosis Often self-limiting. Permanent significant visual loss in 10%.

Localizing features

Temporal lobe: •Dysphasia (p86). •Contralateral homonymous hemianopia (or upper quadrantanopia if only Meyer's loop affected). •Amnesia. •Many odd or seemingly inexplicable phenomena, p491.

Frontal lobe: •Hemiparesis. •Personality change (indecent, indolent, indiscreet, facetious, tendency to pun). •Release phenomena such as the grasp reflex (fingers drawn across palm are grasped), significant only if unilateral. •Broca's dysphasia (p86), or more subtle difficulty with initiating and planning speech with intact repetition and no anomia—but loss of coherence. •Unilateral anosmia (loss of smell). •Perseveration (unable to switch from one line of thinking to another). •Executive dysfunction (unable to plan tasks). •↓Verbal fluency.

Parietal lobe: •Hemisensory loss. •↓2-point discrimination. •Astereognosis (unable to recognize an object by touch alone). •Sensory inattention. •Dysphasia (p86). •Gerstmann's syndrome (p700).

Occipital lobe: •Contralateral visual field defects. •Palinopsia (persisting images once the stimulus has left the field of view). •Polyopia (seeing multiple images).

Cerebellum: Remember DANISH: **d**ysdiadochokinesis (impaired *rapidly alternating* movements, p67) and **d**ysmetria (past-pointing); **a**taxia (limb/truncal—but if truncal ataxia is worse on eye closure, blame the dorsal columns); **n**ystagmus; **i**ntention tremor; **s**lurred speech (dysarthria); **h**ypotonia.

Cerebellopontine angle: (Eg acoustic neuroma/vestibular Schwannoma; p462.) Ipsilateral deafness, nystagmus, ↓corneal reflex, facial weakness (rare), ipsilateral cerebellar signs (above), papilloedema, VIth nerve palsy (p70).

Midbrain: (Eg pineal tumours or midbrain infarction.) Failure of up or down gaze; light-near dissociated pupil responses (p72), nystagmus on convergent gaze.

Bell's palsy (idiopathic facial nerve palsy)

Affects 15–40/100 000/yr, ♂≈♀. Risk ↑ in pregnancy (×3) and in diabetes (×5).

Clinical features Abrupt onset (eg overnight or after a nap) with complete unilateral facial weakness at 24–72h; ipsilateral numbness or pain around the ear; ↓taste (ageusia); hypersensitivity to sounds (from stapedius palsy). On examination the patients will be unable to wrinkle their forehead, confirming LMN pathology (see p70), or whistle (tests buccinator). *Other symptoms of VIIth palsy (from any cause):* • Unilateral sagging of the mouth. • Drooling of saliva. • Food trapped between gum and cheek. • Speech difficulty. • Failure of eye closure may cause a watery or dry eye, ectropion (sagging and turning-out of the lower lid), injury from foreign bodies, or conjunctivitis.

Other causes of VIIth palsy Account for ~30% of facial palsies. Think of these if: rashes, bilateral symptoms, UMN signs, other cranial nerve involvement, or limb weakness. *Infective:* Ramsay Hunt syndrome (BOX), Lyme disease, meningitis, TB, viruses (HIV, polio). *Brainstem lesions:* Stroke, tumour, MS. *Cerebellopontine angle tumours:* Acoustic neuroma, meningioma. *Systemic disease:* DM, sarcoidosis, Guillain-Barré. *Local disease:* Orofacial granulomatosis, parotid tumours, otitis media or cholesteatoma, skull base trauma.

►Lyme disease, Guillain-Barré, sarcoid, and trauma often cause bilateral weakness.

Tests Rule out the other causes: *Blood:* ESR; glucose; ↑*Borrelia* antibodies in Lyme disease, ↑VZV antibodies in Ramsay Hunt syndrome (BOX). *CT/MRI:* Space-occupying lesions; stroke; MS; *CSF:* (Rarely done) for infections.

Prognosis *Incomplete paralysis* without axonal degeneration usually recovers completely within a few weeks. Of those with *complete paralysis* ~80% make a full spontaneous recovery, but ~15% have axonal degeneration (~50% in pregnancy) in which case recovery is delayed, starting after ~3 months, and may be complicated by aberrant reconnections: *synkinesis,* eg eye blinking causes synchronous upturning of the mouth; misconnection of parasympathetic fibres (red in fig 10.26) can produce *crocodile tears* (gusto-lacrimal reflex) when eating stimulates unilateral lacrimation, not salivation.

Management *Drugs:* If given within 72h of onset, prednisolone (eg 60mg/d PO for 5d, tailing by 10mg/d) speeds recovery, with 95% making a full recovery. Antivirals (eg aciclovir) don't help; although some cases are thought to be associated with HSV-1, no one has shown actively replicating virus. There are little data to guide treatment if presenting after 72h of onset, but corticosteroids are widely used (though SE, p377). No advice on the use of steroids is universally agreed in pregnancy. *Protect the eye:* • Dark glasses and artificial tears (eg hypromellose) if evidence of drying. • Encourage regular eyelid closure by pulling down the lid by hand. • Use tape to close the eyes at night. *Surgery:* Consider if eye closure remains a long-term problem (lagophthalmos) or ectropion is severe.

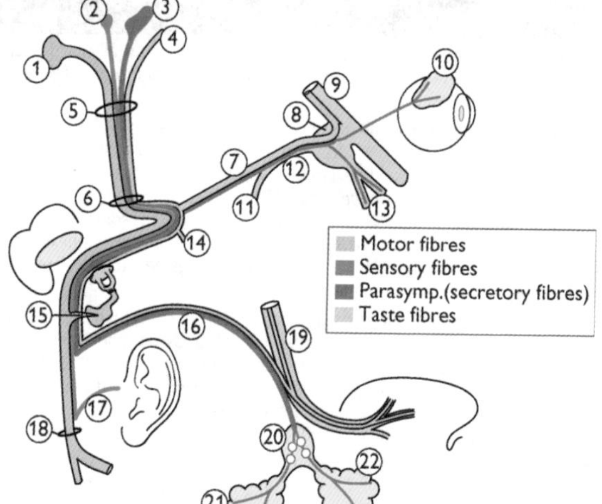

1 Facial nerve nucleus, deep in reticular formation of lower pons
2 Spinal nucleus of V
3 Superior salivary nuc.
4 Solitary tract
5 Porus acusticus internus
6 Meatal foramen
7 Large petrosal nerve
8 Sphenopalatine ganglion
9 Superior maxillary nerve
10 Lacrimal gland
11 Large deep petrosal nerve
12 Vidian nerve
13 Nose/palate gland nerves
14 Small petrosal nerve at geniculate ganglion
15 Stapedial nerve
16 Chorda tympani
17 Auricular branch
18 Stylomastoid foramen
19 Lingual nerve—and taste VII and general sensory from tongue (V^3)
20 Submandibular ganglion (and gland, **21**)
22 Sublingual gland

Fig 10.26 Facial nerve branches. The motor part moves the muscles of the face, scalp, and ears—also buccinator (puffs out the cheeks), platysma, stapedius, and the posterior belly of the digastric. It also contains the sympathetic motor fibres (vasodilator) of the submaxillary and sublingual glands (via the chorda tympani nerve). The sensory part contains the fibres of taste for the anterior ⅔ of the tongue and a few somatic sensory fibres from the middle ear region.

Ramsay Hunt syndrome

Latent varicella zoster virus reactivating in the geniculate ganglion of the VIIth cranial nerve. *Symptoms:* Painful vesicular rash on the auditory canal ± on drum, pinna, tongue palate, or iris (→hyphaema, ie blood under the cornea) with ipsilateral facial palsy, loss of taste, vertigo, tinnitus, deafness, dry mouth and eyes. The rash may be subtle or even absent (*'herpes sine herpete'*=herpes without herpes). *Incidence:* ~5/100 000 (higher if >60yrs). *Diagnosis:* Clinical, as antiviral treatment is thought to be most effective within the 1st 72h, while the virus is replicating. ℞: Antivirals (eg *aciclovir* 800mg PO 5× daily for 7d) + *prednisolone*, as for Bell's palsy. *Prognosis:* If treated within 72h, ~75% recover well; if not, ~⅓ make a good recovery, ⅓ a reasonable recovery, and ⅓ a poor recovery.

Mononeuropathies

Lesions of individual peripheral or cranial nerves. Causes are usually local, such as trauma,or entrapment (eg tumour), except for carpal tunnel syndrome (see BOX 'Carpal tunnel syndrome').

Median nerve C6-T1 The median nerve is the nerve of precision grip—muscles involved are easier to remember if you use your '**LOAF**' (two **l**umbricals, **o**pponens pollicis, **a**bductor pollicis brevis, and **f**lexor pollicis brevis). The clinical features depend on the location of the lesion: *At the wrist:* (Eg see BOX 'Carpal tunnel syndrome'.) Weakness of abductor pollicis brevis and sensory loss over the radial 3½ fingers and palm. *Anterior interosseous nerve lesions:* (Eg trauma.) Weakness of flexion of the distal phalanx of the thumb and index finger. *Proximal lesions:* (Eg compression at the elbow.) May show combined defects.

Ulnar nerve C7-T1 Vulnerable to elbow trauma. *Signs:* Weakness/wasting of medial (ulnar side) wrist flexors, interossei (cannot cross the fingers in the good luck sign), and medial two lumbricals (claw hand, more marked in wrist lesions with digitorum profundus intact); hypothenar eminence wasting, weak 5th digit abduction, and 4th and 5th DIP joint flexion; sensory loss over medial 1½ fingers and ulnar side of the hand. *Treatment:* see BOX 'Managing ulnar mononeuropathies from entrapments'.

Radial nerve C5-T1 This nerve opens the fist. It may be damaged by compression against the humerus. *Signs:* Test for wrist and finger drop with elbow flexed and arm pronated; sensory loss is variable—the dorsal aspect of the root of the thumb (the anatomical snuff box) is most reliably affected. Muscles involved: ('**BEAST**') **b**rachioradialis; **e**xtensors; **a**bductor pollicis longus; **s**upinator; **t**riceps.

Brachial plexus Pain/paraesthesiae and weakness in the affected arm in a variable distribution. *Causes:* Trauma, radiotherapy (eg for breast carcinoma), prolonged wearing of a heavy rucksack, cervical rib, thoracic outlet compression (also affects vasculature), or neuralgic amyotrophy (Parsonage-Turner syndrome: unilateral sudden, severe pain, followed over hours by profound weakness, resolving completely over days. May rarely involve the phrenic or lower cranial nerves.)

Phrenic nerve C3-5 C3, 4, 5 keeps the diaphragm alive: lesions cause orthopnoea with a raised hemidiaphragm on CXR. *Causes:* Lung cancer, TB, paraneoplastic syndromes, myeloma, thymoma, cervical spondylosis/trauma, thoracic surgery, infections (HZV, HIV, Lyme disease), muscular dystrophy.

Lateral cutaneous nerve of the thigh L2-L3 *Meralgia paraesthetica* is anterolateral burning thigh pain from entrapment under the inguinal ligament.

Sciatic nerve L4-S3 Damaged by pelvic tumours or fractures to pelvis or femur. Lesions affect the hamstrings and all muscles below the knee (foot drop), with loss of sensation below the knee laterally.

Common peroneal nerve L4-S1 Originates from sciatic nerve just above knee. Often damaged as it winds round the fibular head (trauma, sitting cross-legged). *Signs:* Foot drop, weak ankle dorsiflexion/eversion, sensory loss over dorsal foot.

Tibial nerve L4-S3 Originates from sciatic nerve just above knee. Lesions lead to an inability to stand on tiptoe (plantarflexion), invert the foot, or flex the toes, with sensory loss over the sole.

Mononeuritis multiplex Describes the involvement of two or more peripheral nerves. Causes tend to be systemic: DM, connective tissue disorders (rheumatoid, SLE), vasculitis (granulomatosis with polyangiitis formerly Wegener's granulomatosis, PAN), and more rarely sarcoidosis, amyloid, leprosy. Electromyography (EMG) helps define the anatomic site of lesions.

Carpal tunnel syndrome: the commonest mononeuropathy

The median nerve and nine tendons compete for space within the wrist. Compression is common, especially in women who have narrower wrists but similar-sized tendons to men.

Clinical features: Aching pain in the hand and arm (especially at night), and paraesthesiae in thumb, index, and middle fingers: relieved by dangling the hand over the edge of the bed and shaking it (remember 'wake and shake'). There may be sensory loss and weakness of abductor pollicis brevis ± wasting of the thenar eminence. Light touch, 2-point discrimination, and sweating may be impaired.

Causes: Anything causing swelling or compression of the tunnel: myxoedema; prolonged flexion (eg in a Colles' splint); acromegaly; myeloma; local tumours (lipomas, ganglia); rheumatoid arthritis; amyloidosis; pregnancy; sarcoidosis.

Tests: Neurophysiology helps by confirming the lesion's site and severity (and likelihood of improvement after surgery). Maximal wrist flexion for 1 min (*Phalen's test*) may elicit symptoms, and tapping over the nerve at the wrist can induce tingling (*Tinel's test*) but both are rather non-specific.

Treatment: Splinting, local steroid injection ± decompression surgery.

NB: There is also *tarsal* tunnel syndrome: unilateral burning sole pain following tibial nerve compression.

Managing ulnar mononeuropathies from entrapments

The ulnar nerve asks for trouble in at least five places at the elbow, starting proximally at the arcade of Struthers (a musculofascial band ~8cm proximal to the medial epicondyle), and ending distally where it exits the flexor carpi ulnaris muscle in the forearm. Most often, compression occurs at the *epicondylar groove* or at the point where the nerve passes between the two heads of flexor carpi ulnaris (true *cubital tunnel syndrome*). Trauma can easily damage the nerve against its bony confines (the medial condyle of the humerus—the 'funny bone'). Normally, stretch and compression forces on the ulnar nerve at the elbow are moderated by its ability to glide in its groove. When normal excursion is restricted, irritation ensues. This may cause a vicious cycle of perineural scarring, consequent loss of excursion, and progressive symptoms—without antecedent trauma. Compressive ulnar neuropathies at the wrist (*Guyon's canal*—between the pisiform and hamate bones) are less common, but they can also result in disability.

Treatment centres on rest and avoiding pressure on the nerve, but if symptoms continue, night-time soft elbow splinting (to prevent flexion >60°) is warranted. A splint for the hand may help prevent permanent clawing of the fingers. For chronic neuropathy associated with weakness, or if splinting fails, a variety of *surgical procedures* have been tried. For moderately severe neuropathies, decompressions *in situ* may help, but often fail. Medial *epicondylectomies* are effective in ≤50% (but many will recur). Subcutaneous *nerve re-routing* (transposition) may be tried.

Polyneuropathies

Motor and/or sensory disorder of multiple peripheral or cranial nerves: usually symmetrical, widespread, and often worse distally ('glove and stocking' distribution). They can be classified by: chronicity, function (*sensory, motor, autonomic, mixed*), or pathology (*demyelination, axonal degeneration*, or *both*). For example, Guillain-Barré syndrome (p702) is an acute, predominantly motor, demyelinating neuropathy, whereas chronic alcohol abuse leads to a chronic, initially sensory then mixed, axonal neuropathy.

Diagnosis The history is vital: be clear about the time course, the precise nature of the symptoms, and any preceding or associated events (eg D&V before Guillain-Barré syndrome; ↓weight in cancer; arthralgia from a connective tissue disease). Ask about travel, alcohol and drug use, sexual infections, and family history. If there is palpable nerve thickening think of leprosy or Charcot-Marie-Tooth. Examine other systems for clues to the cause, eg alcoholic liver disease.

Tests FBC, ESR, glucose, U&E, LFT, TSH, B_{12}, electrophoresis, ANA, ANCA, CXR, urinalysis, consider LP ± specific genetic tests for inherited neuropathies, lead level, antiganglioside antibodies. Nerve conduction studies distinguish demyelinating from axonal causes.

Sensory neuropathy: (Eg DM, CKD, leprosy.) Numbness; pins and needles, paraesthesiae; affects 'glove and stocking' distribution. Difficulty handling small objects such as buttons. Signs of trauma (eg finger burns) or joint deformation may indicate sensory loss. Diabetic and alcoholic neuropathies are typically painful.

Motor neuropathy: (Eg Guillain-Barré syndrome, lead poisoning, Charcot-Marie-Tooth syndrome.) Often progressive (may be rapid); weak or clumsy hands; difficulty in walking (falls, stumbling); difficulty in breathing (↓vital capacity). Signs: LMN lesion: wasting and weakness most marked in the distal muscles of hands and feet (foot or wrist drop). Reflexes are reduced or absent.

Cranial nerves: Swallowing/speaking difficulty; diplopia.

Autonomic system: See BOX.

Management *Treat the cause* (table 10.10). Involve physio and OT. Foot care and *shoe choice* are important in sensory neuropathies to minimize trauma. Splinting joints helps prevent contractures in prolonged paralysis. In Guillain-Barré and chronic inflammatory demyelinating polyradiculoneuropathy (CIDP: autoimmune demyelination of peripheral nerves), IV immunoglobulin helps. For vasculitic causes, steroids/immunosuppressants may help. Treat neuropathic pain with amitriptyline, duloxetine, gabapentin or pregabalin.

Table 10.10 Causes of polyneuropathy

Metabolic	Vasculitides	Malignancy	Inflammatory
Diabetes mellitus Renal failure Hypothyroidism Hypoglycaemia Mitochondrial disorders	Polyarteritis nodosa Rheumatoid arthritis GPA	Paraneoplastic syndromes Polycythaemia rubra vera	Guillain-Barré syndrome Sarcoidosis; CIDP*
Infections	**Nutritional**	**Inherited syndromes**	**Drugs**
Leprosy HIV Syphilis Lyme disease	↓Vit B_1 ↓Vit B_{12}/folate ↑Vit B_6 ↓Vit E	Charcot-Marie-Tooth Refsum's syndrome Porphyria Leucodystrophy	Vincristine Cisplatin Isoniazid Nitrofurantoin Phenytoin Metronidazole
Others			
Paraproteinaemias, amyloidosis, lead, arsenic			

*Chronic inflammatory demyelinating polyradiculoneuropathy (CIDP): autoimmune demyelination of peripheral nerves (distal onset of weakness/sensory loss in limbs + nerve enlargement + ↑CSF protein).

Autonomic neuropathy

Sympathetic and parasympathetic neuropathies may be isolated or part of a generalized sensorimotor peripheral neuropathy.

Causes DM, amyloidosis, Guillain-Barré and Sjögren's syndromes, HIV, leprosy, SLE, toxic, genetic (eg porphyria), or paraneoplastic, eg paraneoplastic encephalomyeloneuropathies and Lambert-Eaton myasthenic syndrome (LEMS, p512).

Signs *Sympathetic:* Postural hypotension, ↓sweating, ejaculatory failure, Horner's syndrome (p702). *Parasympathetic:* Constipation, nocturnal diarrhoea, urine retention, erectile dysfunction, Holmes-Adie pupil (p72).

Autonomic function tests

- *BP: Postural drop* of ≥20/10mmHg is abnormal.
- *ECG:* A variation of <10bpm with respiration is abnormal (check R-R interval).
- *Cystometry:* Bladder pressure studies.
- *Pupils:* Instil 0.1% adrenaline (dilates if post-ganglionic sympathetic denervation, not if normal); 2.5% cocaine (dilates if normal; not if sympathetic denervation); 2.5% methacholine (constricts if parasympathetic lesion)—rarely used.
- *Paraneoplastic antibodies:* Anti-HU, anti-YO, anti-RI, anti-amphiphysin, anti-CV2, anti-MA2. *Other Ab:* Antiganglionic acetylcholine receptor antibody presence shows that the cause may be autoimmune autonomic ganglionopathy.

Primary autonomic failure Occurs alone (autoimmune autonomic ganglionopathy), as part of multisystem atrophy (MSA, p494), or with Parkinson's disease, typically in a middle-aged/elderly man. Onset: insidious; symptoms as listed previously.

Motor neuron disease (MND)

MND is a cluster of neurodegenerative diseases affecting 6/100 000 (♂:♀≈3:2), characterized by selective loss of neurons in motor cortex, cranial nerve nuclei, and anterior horn cells. Upper and lower motor neurons can be affected but there is *no* sensory loss or sphincter disturbance, thus distinguishing MND from MS and polyneuropathies. MND never affects eye movements, distinguishing it from myasthenia (p512). There are four clinical patterns:

1 *ALS/amyotrophic lateral sclerosis.* (Archetypal MND; up to 80%.) Loss of motor neurons in motor cortex *and* the anterior horn of the cord, so combined UMN + LMN signs (p446). Worse prognosis if: bulbar onset, ↑age; ↓FVC.

2 *Progressive bulbar palsy.* (10–20%.) Only affects cranial nerves IX–XII. See BOX 'Bulbar and corticobulbar ('pseudobulbar') palsy'.

3 *Progressive muscular atrophy.* (<10%.) Anterior horn cell lesion, so LMN signs only. Affects distal muscle groups before proximal. Better prognosis than ALS.

4 *Primary lateral sclerosis.* (Rare.) Loss of Betz cells in motor cortex: mainly UMN signs, marked spastic leg weakness and pseudobulbar palsy. No cognitive decline.

Presentation Think of MND in those >40yrs (median UK age at onset is 60) with stumbling spastic gait, foot-drop ± proximal myopathy, weak grip (door-handles don't turn) and shoulder abduction (hair-washing is hard), or aspiration pneumonia. Look for UMN signs: spasticity, brisk reflexes, ↑plantars; and LMN signs: wasting, fasciculation of tongue, abdomen, back, thigh. Is speech or swallowing affected (bulbar signs)? Fasciculation is not enough to diagnose an LMN lesion: look for weakness too. Frontotemporal dementia occurs in ~25% (see BOX 'Dignity and Dignitas').

Diagnostic criteria (See BOX 'Revised El Escorial diagnostic criteria for ALS'). There is no diagnostic test. Brain/cord MRI helps exclude structural causes, LP helps exclude inflammatory ones, and neurophysiology can detect subclinical denervation and help exclude mimicking motor neuropathies.[14]

Prognosis Poor, <3yrs post onset in half of patients.

Management Adopt a multidisciplinary approach: neurologist, palliative nurse, hospice, physio, OT, speech therapist, dietician, social services—all orchestrated by the GP. Riluzole, an inhibitor of glutamate release and NMDA receptor antagonist, is the only medication shown to improve survival. Mulitple other drugs that have shown promise in animal models have failed to prove benefit in clinical trials, including neurotrophic factors, anti-apoptotic agents, antioxidants, and immunomodulatory drugs. For supportive/symptomatic treatment: *Excess saliva:* Advise on positioning, oral care, and suctioning. Try an antimuscarinic (eg propantheline) or glycopyrronium bromide (can be given SC). Botulinum toxin A may help. *Dysphagia:* Blend food. Gastrostomy is an option—discuss early on. *Spasticity:* Exercise, orthotics. See MS for drugs (p496). *Communication difficulty:* Provide 'augmentative and alternative' communication equipment. *End-of-life care:* ►Involve palliative care team from diagnosis (p532). Consider opioids to relieve breathlessness and discuss non-invasive ventilation (see BOX 'Dignity and Dignitas').

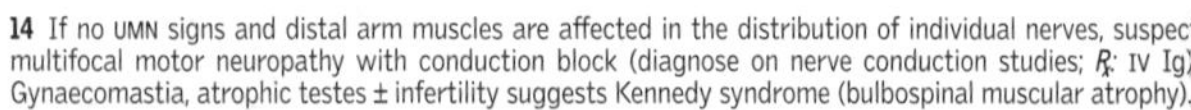
14 If no UMN signs and distal arm muscles are affected in the distribution of individual nerves, suspect multifocal motor neuropathy with conduction block (diagnose on nerve conduction studies; ℞: IV Ig). Gynaecomastia, atrophic testes ± infertility suggests Kennedy syndrome (bulbospinal muscular atrophy).

Bulbar and corticobulbar ('pseudobulbar') palsy

Bulbar palsy denotes diseases of the nuclei of cranial nerves IX–XII in the medulla. *Signs:* An *LMN lesion* of the tongue and muscles of talking and swallowing: flaccid, fasciculating tongue (like a sack of worms); jaw jerk is normal or absent, speech is quiet, hoarse, or nasal. *Causes:* MND, Guillain-Barré, polio, myasthenia gravis, syringobulbia (p516), brainstem tumours, central pontine myelinolysis (p672).

Corticobulbar palsy *UMN lesion* of muscles of swallowing and talking due to bilateral lesions above the mid-pons, eg corticobulbar tracts (MS, MND, stroke, central pontine myelinolysis). It is commoner than bulbar palsy. *Signs:* Slow tongue movements, with slow deliberate speech; ↑jaw jerk; ↑pharyngeal and palatal reflexes; pseudobulbar affect (PBA)—weeping unprovoked by sorrow or mood-incongruent giggling (emotional incontinence *without* mood change is also seen in MS, Wilson's, and Parkinson's disease, dementia, nitrous oxide use, and head injury). In some countries, dextromethorphan + quinidine is licensed for PBA.

Revised El Escorial diagnostic criteria for ALS

Definite Lower + upper motor neuron signs in 3 regions.
Probable Lower + upper motor neuron signs in 2 regions.
Probable with lab support Lower + upper motor neuron signs in 1 region, or upper motor neuron signs in ≥1 region + EMG shows acute denervation in ≥2 limbs.
Possible Lower + upper motor neuron signs in 1 region.
Suspected Upper or lower motor neuron signs only—in 1 or more regions.

Dignity and Dignitas

ALS is closely linked with frontotemporal dementia (FTD, p486) by increasing clinical, genetic, and molecular evidence (nucleotide repeat expansions in gene C9orf72 have been described in familial and sporadic ALS and in FTD). However, patients with MND often have no cognitive impairment in the early stages of the disease, and witness their inorexable physical decline with terrified awareness. For this reason it is imperative to plan for the future early: discuss their wishes for end-of-life care and in the eventuality of respiratory decline before it is too late for wishes to be communicated. These discussions are crucial but not binding: the patient can change their mind at any point, and also refuse any life-prolonging treatment, knowing the consequence is death. However, in most countries, including the UK, we cannot traverse that line that lies between management of a supported death following withdrawal of life-prolonging (or death-prolonging) interventions, and acting with the intention of causing death. Court battles ensue, with requests for assisted suicide that may frustrate and challenge ethicists, physicians, politicians, and the judiciary, but above all, patients and their families. Faced with such conflicting passions, perhaps our role is to be clear that we stand beside our patients, come what may.

Cervical spondylosis

Degeneration of the cervical spine with age is inevitable, and has a wide clinical spectrum, ranging from asymptomatic to progressive spastic quadriparesis and sensory loss due to compression of the cord (myelopathy).

Pathogenesis Degeneration of the annulus fibrosus (the tough coating of the intervertebral discs), combined with osteophyte formation on the adjacent vertebra leads to narrowing of the spinal canal and intervertebral foramina (figs 10.27, 10.28). As the neck flexes and extends, the cord is dragged over these protruding bony spurs anteriorly and indented by a thickened ligamentum flavum posteriorly.

Presenting complaint Neck stiffness (but common in anyone >50yrs old), crepitus on moving neck, stabbing or dull arm pain (brachialgia), forearm/wrist pain.

Signs Limited, painful neck movement ± crepitus (examine gently). Neck flexion may produce tingling down the spine (Lhermitte's sign, p497). NB: this does not distinguish between cord or roots (or both) involvement.
Root compression (radiculopathy): Pain/'electrical' sensations in arms or fingers at the level of the compression (table 10.11), with numbness, dull reflexes, LMN weakness, and eventual wasting of muscles innervated by the affected root. NB: UMN signs below level of the affected root suggests cord compression.
►*Features of cord compression:* Progressive symptoms (eg ↑weak, clumsy hands; gait disturbance); UMN leg signs (spastic weakness, ↑plantars); LMN arm signs (wasting, hyporeflexia); incontinence, hesitancy, and urgency are late features.
Which nerve root is affected? See table 10.11.

ΔΔ MS; nerve root neurofibroma; subacute combined degeneration of the cord (↓B_{12}); compression by bone or cord tumours.

Management ►Urgent MRI and specialist referral guided by red flag symptoms (see p542). Bear in mind that although these are stressed in virtually every set of guidelines, no two lists are alike and review of evidence suggests that the accuracy of these features is low. ►Don't make referral decisions based upon the presence or absence of a single feature, but use these to inform your judgement. Otherwise: give analgesia (as per WHO ladder) and encourage gentle activity. Cervical collars may give respite during brief periods of increased pain, but restrict mobility, so may prolong symptoms: avoid where possible. If no improvement in 4–6 weeks then MRI and consider neurosurgical referral for: interlaminar cervical epidural injections, transforaminal injections or surgical decompression (via *anterior approach*, eg discectomy or *posterior approach*, eg laminectomy—fig 10.29, or laminoplasty—fig 10.30). There is no consensus or high-quality evidence to guide selection of approach or of patients, though interventions may be best reserved for those with progressive deterioration, myelopathy causing disabling neurologic deficits, or those at risk for deterioration (eg severe spinal cord compression on MRI).

Table 10.11 Clinical patterns of nerve root impingement

Typical motor and sensory deficits from individual root involvement (C5-8)		
Nerve root	**Motor and sensory deficit**	**Pain pattern**
C5 (C4/C5 disc)	Weak deltoid & supraspinatus; ↓supinator jerks; numb elbow.	Pain in neck/shoulder that radiates down front of arm to elbow.
C6 (C5/C6 disc)	Weak biceps & brachioradialis; ↓biceps jerks; numb thumb & index finger.	Pain in shoulder radiating down arm below elbow.*
C7 (C6/C7 disc)	Weak triceps & finger extension; ↓triceps jerks; numb middle finger.	Pain in upper arm and dorsal fore-arm.
C8 (C7/T1 disc)	Weak finger flexors & small muscles of the hand; numb 5th & ring finger.	Pain in upper arm and medial fore-arm.
►*Worrying symptoms:* Night pain, ↓weight, fever.		

*Passive head turning may exacerbate C6 radicular pain but not carpal tunnel syndrome (Spurling's manoeuvre).

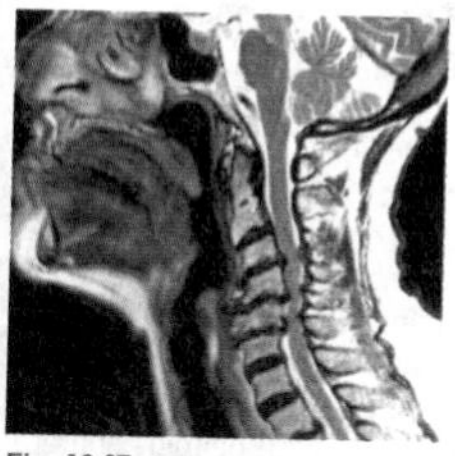

Fig 10.27 A T2-weighted MRI (∴ CSF looks bright). The cord is compressed between osteophytes anteriorly and the ligamentum flavum posteriorly.

©Prof P Scally.

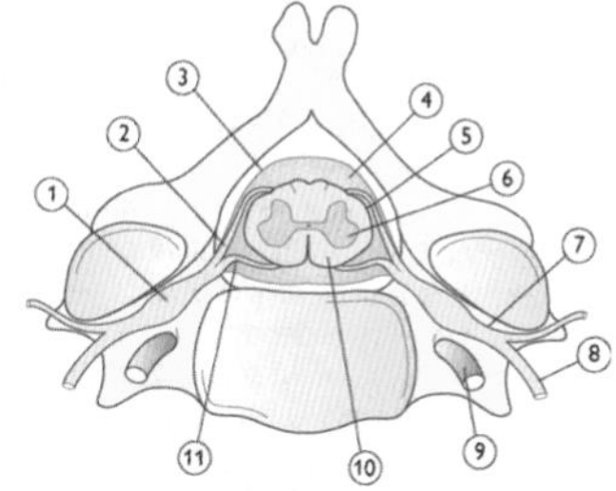

Fig 10.28 Cervical vertebra. **1** Dorsal root ganglion; **2** Dorsal root; **3** Dura mater; **4** Subarachnoid space; **5** Pia mater; **6** Grey matter; **7** Spinal nerve; **8** Ventral ramus; **9** Vertebral artery in the transverse foramen; **10** White matter; **11** Ventral spinal nerve.

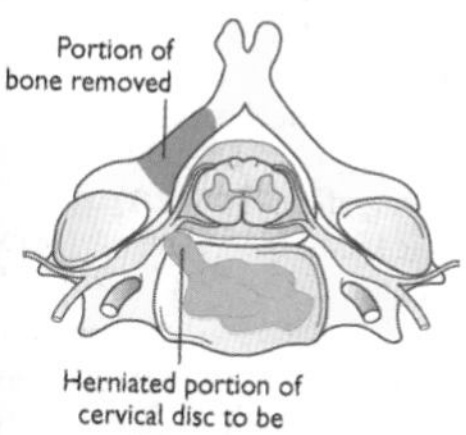

Fig 10.29 Laminectomy.

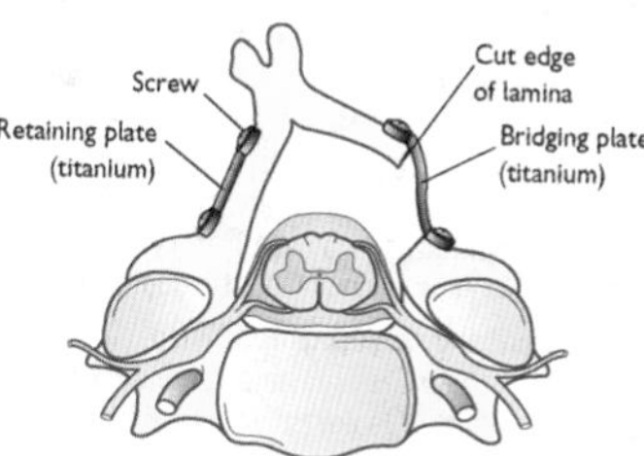

Fig 10.30 Laminoplasty (screws and plates).

Myopathy

Primary disorder of muscle with gradual-onset symmetrical weakness; it may be confused clinically with neuropathy. *In favour of myopathy:* •Gradual onset of symmetric *proximal* weakness—difficulty combing hair and climbing stairs (NB: weakness is also *distal* in myotonic dystrophy). •Specific muscle groups affected (ie *selective* weakness on first presentation). •Preserved tendon reflexes. •No paraesthesiae or bladder problems. •No fasciculation (suggests anterior horn cell or root disease).

Rapid onset suggests a toxic, drug, or metabolic myopathy (or a neuropathy). *Excess fatigability* (↑weakness with exercise) suggests myasthenia (p512). Spontaneous *pain* at rest and local tenderness occurs in inflammatory myopathies. Pain on exercise suggests ischaemia or metabolic myopathy (eg McArdle's disease). *Oddly firm* muscles (due to infiltrations with fat or connective tissue) suggest pseudohypertrophic muscular dystrophies (eg Duchenne's).

Tests ESR, CK, AST, and LDH may be raised. Do EMG and tests relevant to systemic causes (eg TSH, p216). Muscle biopsy and genetic testing may help reach a diagnosis.

Muscular dystrophies A group of genetic diseases (see table 10.12) with progressive degeneration and weakness of specific muscle groups. The primary abnormality may be in the muscle membrane. There may be unusually firm muscles due to infiltration by fat or connective tissue, and marked variation in size of individual muscle fibres on histology. • *Duchenne's muscular dystrophy:* The commonest (3/1000 male live births). Presents at ~4yrs old with clumsy walking, then difficulty in standing, and respiratory failure. Pseudohypertrophy is seen, especially in the calves. Serum creatine kinase ↑ >40-fold. There is no specific treatment. Some survive beyond 20yrs. Home ventilation improves prognosis. Genetic counselling is vital. • *Becker's muscular dystrophy:* (~0.3/1000 ♂ births.) Presents similarly to Duchenne's but with milder symptoms, at a later age, and with a better prognosis. • *Facioscapulohumeral muscular dystrophy:* (FSHD, Landouzy-Dejerine.) Almost as common as Duchenne's. Onset is ~12-14yrs old, with inability to puff out the cheeks and difficulty raising the arms above the head. *Signs:* weakness of face ('ironed out' expression), shoulders, and upper arms (often asymmetric with deltoids spared), foot-drop, scapular winging (fig 10.31), scoliosis, anterior axillary folds, and horizontal clavicles. ≤20% need a wheelchair by 40yrs.

Myotonic disorders Cause tonic muscle spasm (myotonia), and demonstrate long chains of central nuclei within muscle fibres on histology. The commonest is *myotonic dystrophy* which is, in fact, clinically and genetically heterogeneous, with two major forms (DM1 and DM2—see table 10.12), both showing abnormal trinucleotide repeat expansions in regulatory (non-coding) genetic regions. DM1 is the commoner, more severe, and typically presents between 20–40 yrs old with *distal* weakness (hand/foot drop), weak sternomastoids, and myotonia. Facial weakness and muscle wasting give a long, haggard appearance. *Also:* cataracts, male frontal baldness, diabetes, testis/ovary atrophy, cardiomyopathy, and ↓cognition. Most DM1 patients die in late middle age of respiratory or cardiac complications. Mexiletine may help with disabling myotonia. Genetic counselling is important.

Inflammatory myopathies There may be spontaneous muscle pain at rest and local tenderness on palpation. *Inclusion body myositis* is the chief example if aged >50yrs. Weakness starts with quadriceps, finger flexors, or pharyngeal muscles. Ventral extremity muscle groups are more affected than dorsal or girdle groups. Response to therapy is poor and patients typically progress over a decade to require assistance with activites of daily living. Histology shows ringed vacuoles + intranuclear inclusions. *Polymyositis* and *dermatomyositis*, see p552.

Metabolic myopathies Eg *McArdle's disease* (glycogen storage disorder). Presents with muscle pain and weakness after exercise.

Acquired myopathies of late onset Often part of systemic disease—eg hyperthyroidism, malignancy, Cushing's, hypo- and hypercalcaemia.

Drug causes Alcohol; statins; steroids; chloroquine; zidovudine; vincristine; cocaine

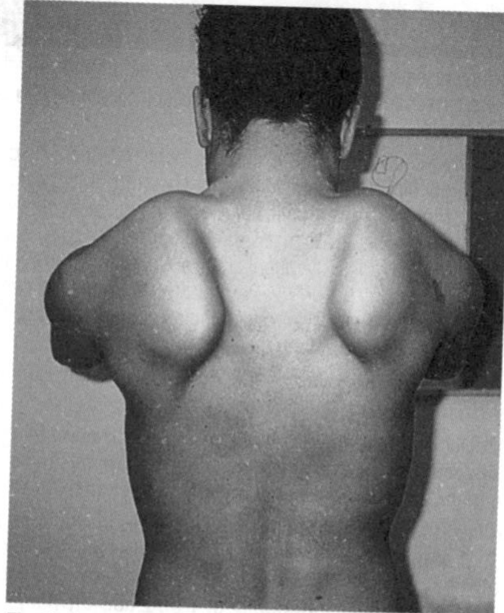

Fig 10.31 Winging of both scapulae in facioscapulohumeral muscular dystrophy, due to weakness of thoracoscapular muscles.

Table 10.12 Genetics of some commoner congenital myopathies

Condition	Inheritance	Chr	Gene	Pathogenesis
Duchenne's muscular dystrophy	X-linked recessive	X	Dystrophin (stabilizes muscle fibres)	Partial deletions or duplications in dystrophin render *non*-functional
Becker's muscular dystrophy	X-linked recessive	X	Dystrophin	Partial deletions or duplications in dystrophin render *hypo*-functional
FSHD type 1	Autosomal dominant	4	DUX4 (transcriptional activator)	Partial deletion of D4Z4 repeating unit releases normal repression of DUX4 expression
FSHD type 2	Autosomal dominant	4	DUX4 (transcriptional activator)	Hypomethylation of D4Z4 releases normal repression of DUX4 expression
DM type 1	Autosomal dominant	19	DMPK (serine-threonine kinase)	Expansion of short repetitive sequences of nucleotides; in both forms this expanded sequence is transcribed into RNA which then misfolds and sequesters other RNA binding proteins
DM type 2	Autosomal dominant	3	ZNF9 (transcriptional regulator)	

Myasthenia gravis (MG)

MG is an autoimmune disease mediated by antibodies to nicotinic acetylcholine receptors (AChR) on the post-synaptic side of the neuromuscular junction (fig 10.32). Both B and T cells are implicated.

Presentation Slowly increasing or relapsing muscular fatigue. Muscle groups affected, in order: extraocular; bulbar (swallowing, chewing); face; neck; limb girdle; trunk. *Signs:* Ptosis, diplopia, myasthenic snarl on smiling, 'peek sign' of orbicularis fatigability (eyelids begin to separate after manual opposition to sustained closure). On counting to 50, the voice fades (dysphonia is a rare presentation). Tendon reflexes are normal. *Symptoms exacerbated by:* Pregnancy, ↓K^+, infection, over-treatment, change of climate, emotion, exercise, gentamicin, opiates, tetracycline, quinine, β-blockers.

Differentials Polymyositis/other myopathies (p510); SLE; Takayasu's arteritis (fatigability of the extremities); botulism (see BOX).

Associations Include autoimmune disease (especially rheumatoid arthritis and SLE). If <50yrs, it is commoner in ♀ and associated with thymic hyperplasia; >50, it is commoner in men, and associated with thymic atrophy or thymic tumour.

Tests •*Antibodies:* ↑Anti-AChR antibodies in 90% (70% in MG variant confined to ocular muscles). If anti-AChR −ve look for MuSK antibodies (muscle-specific tyrosine kinase; especially in ♀). •*EMG:* Decremental muscle response to repetitive nerve stimulation ± ↑single-fibre jitter. •*Imaging:* CT to exclude thymoma (68% 5yr survival). •*Other:* Ptosis improves by >2mm after ice application to the eyelid for >2min—a neat, non-invasive test (but not diagnostic). The Tensilon® (edrophonium) test may not give clear answers and has dangers, so is rarely used.

Treatment •*Symptom control:* Anticholinesterase, eg pyridostigmine (60–120mg PO up to 6×daily; max 1.2g/d). Cholinergic SE: ↑salivation, lacrimation, sweats, vomiting, miosis. Other SE: diarrhoea, colic (controllable with propantheline 15mg/8h). • *Immunosuppression:* Treat relapses with prednisolone—start at 5mg on alternate days, ↑ by 5mg/wk up to 1mg/kg on each treatment day. ↓Dose on remission (may take months). Give osteoporosis prophylaxis. SE: weakness (hence low starting dose). Azathioprine, ciclosporin, and mycophenolate mofetil may also be used. • *Thymectomy:* Has beneficial effects, even in patients without a thymoma: consider especially in younger patients with onset <5yrs previously and poor response to medical therapy. A recent randomized controlled trial shows improved symptom scores sustained over 3yrs, with reduced need for immunosuppression. Surgery also prevents local invasion if thymoma is present.

Myasthenic crisis Life-threatening weakness of respiratory muscles during a relapse. ►Can be difficult to differentiate from cholinergic crisis (ie overtreatment—but this is rare, and usually only occurs in doses of pyridostigmine >960mg/d). Monitor forced vital capacity. *Ventilatory support* may be needed. Treat with plasmapheresis (removes AChR antibodies from the circulation) or IVIg and identify and treat the trigger for the relapse (eg infection, medications).

Lambert-Eaton myasthenic syndrome (LEMS)

LEMS can be paraneoplastic (50% are associated with malignancies, in particular small-cell lung cancer) or autoimmune. Unlike MG, antibodies are to voltage-gated Ca^{2+} channels on *pre*-synaptic membrane (see fig 10.33; anti-P/Q type VGCC antibodies are +ve in 85–95%).

Clinical features •Gait difficulty before eye signs. •Autonomic involvement (dry mouth, constipation, impotence). •Hyporeflexia and weakness, which improve after exercise. •Diplopia and respiratory muscle involvement are rare. •EMG shows similar changes to MG except amplitude increases greatly post-exercise.

Treatment Pyridostigmine, 3,4-diaminopyridine or IVIg (get specialist help). ►Do regular CXR/high-resolution CT as symptoms may precede the cancer by >4yrs.

How synapses work—the neuromuscular junction

1 Before transmission can occur, neurotransmitter must be packed into synaptic vesicles. At the neuromuscular junction (NMJ) this is acetylcholine (ACh). Each vesicle contains ~8000 ACh molecules.

2 When an action potential arrives at the pre-synaptic terminal, depolarization opens voltage-gated Ca^{2+} channels (VGCCs). In *Lambert-Eaton* syndrome, anti-P/Q type VGCC antibodies disrupt this stage of synaptic transmission.[15]

3 Influx of Ca^{2+} through the VGCCs triggers fusion of synaptic vesicles with the pre-synaptic membrane (a process that *botulinum toxin* interferes with), and neurotransmitter is released from the vesicles into the synaptic cleft.

4 Transmitter molecules cross the synaptic cleft by diffusion and bind to receptors on the post-synaptic membrane, causing depolarization of the post-synaptic membrane (the end-plate potential). This change in the post-synaptic membrane triggers muscle contraction at the NMJ, or onward transmission of the action potential in neurons. In *myasthenia gravis*, antibodies block the post-synaptic ACh receptors, preventing the end-plate potential from becoming large enough to trigger muscle contraction—and muscle weakness ensues.

5 Transmitter action is terminated by enzyme-induced degradation of transmitter (eg acetylcholinesterase), uptake into the pre-synaptic terminal or glial cells, or by diffusion away from synapse. Anticholinesterase treatments for myasthenia gravis, such as *pyridostigmine*, reduce the rate of degradation of ACh, increasing the chance that it will trigger an end-plate potential.

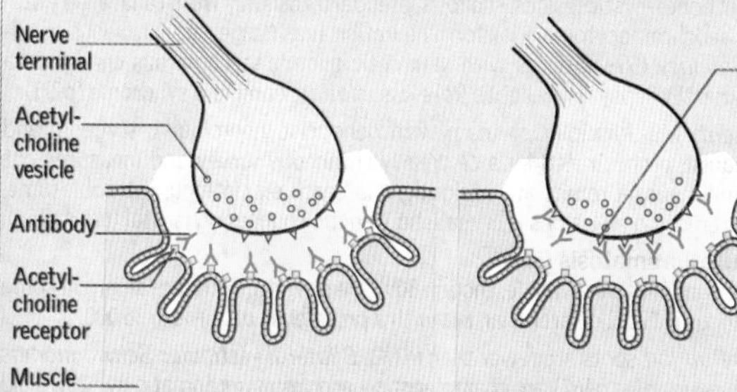

Fig 10.32 Myasthenia gravis features *post-synaptic* AChR antibodies. Tendon reflexes are normal because the synapses do not have time to become fatigued with such a brief muscle contraction. Ocular palsies are common (it's not exactly clear why).

Fig 10.33 Lambert-Eaton syndrome features pre-synaptic Ca^{2+}-channel antibodies. Depressed tendon reflexes are common, because less transmitter is released, but reflexes may ↑ after maximum voluntary contraction due to a build of transmitter in the synaptic cleft (post-tetanic potentiation).

Disruption of pre-synaptic transmission affects release of ACh in autonomic nervous system as well as neuromuscular junction, explaining the prominence of dysautonomia in LEMS unlike in MG.

Neurofibromatosis

Type 1 neurofibromatosis (NF1, von Recklinghausen's disease)
Autosomal dominant inheritance (gene locus 17q11.2). Expression of NF1 is variable, even within a family. *Prevalence:* 1 in 2500, ♀:♂≈1:1; no racial predilection.

Signs: Café-au-lait spots: flat, coffee-coloured patches of skin seen in 1st year of life (clearest in UV light), increasing in size and number with age. Adults have ≥6, >15mm across. They do *not* predispose to skin cancer. *Freckling:* typically in skin-folds (axillae, groin, neck base, and submammary area), and usually present by age 10. *Dermal neurofibromas:* small, violaceous nodules, gelatinous in texture, which appear at puberty, and may become papillomatous. They are not painful but may itch. Numbers increase with age. *Nodular neurofibromas* arise from nerve trunks. Firm and clearly demarcated, they can give rise to paraesthesiae if pressed. *Lisch nodules* (fig 10.34) are tiny harmless regular brown/translucent mounds (hamartomas) on the iris (use a slit lamp) ≤2mm in diameter. They develop by 6yrs old in 90%. Also short stature and macrocephaly.

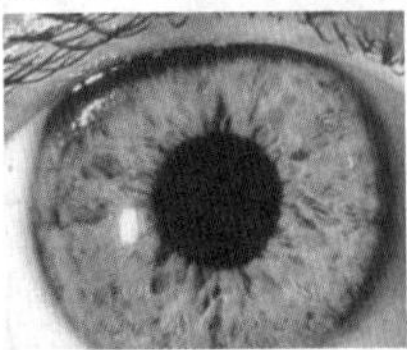

Fig 10.34 Multiple brown Lisch nodules on the iris. ©Jon Miles.

Complications: Occur in 30%. Mild learning disability is common. *Local effects of neurofibromas:* nerve root compression (weakness, pain, paraesthesiae); GI—bleeds, obstruction; bone—cystic lesions, scoliosis, pseudarthrosis. ↑BP from renal artery stenosis or phaeochromocytoma. Plexiform neurofibromas (large, subcutaneous swellings). *Malignancy* (5% patients with NF1): optic glioma, sarcomatous change in a neurofibroma. ↑Epilepsy risk (slight). *Rare association:* carcinoid syndrome (p271).

Management: Multidisciplinary team with geneticist, neurologist, surgeon, and physiotherapist, orchestrated by a GP. Yearly cutaneous survey and measurement of BP. Dermal neurofibromas are unsightly, and catch on clothing; if troublesome, excise, but removing all lesions is unrealistic. Genetic counselling is vital (*OHCS* p154).

Type 2 neurofibromatosis (NF2)
Autosomal dominant inheritance, though 50% are *de novo*, with mosaicism in some (NF2 gene locus is 22q11). Rarer than NF1 with a prevalence of only 1 in 35 000.

Signs: Café-au-lait spots are fewer than in NF1. *Bilateral vestibular Schwannomas* (= acoustic neuromas; p462) are characteristic, becoming symptomatic by ~20yrs old when sensorineural hearing loss is the 1st sign. There may be tinnitus and vertigo. The rate of tumour growth is unpredictable and variable. The tumours are benign but cause problems by pressing on local structures and by ↑ICP. They may be absent in mosaic NF2. *Juvenile posterior subcapsular lenticular opacity* (a form of cataract) occurs before other manifestations and can be useful in screening those at risk

Complications: Tender Schwannomas of cranial and peripheral nerves, and spina nerve roots. Meningiomas (45% in NF2, often multiple). Glial tumours are less commor Consider NF2 in any young person presenting with one of these tumours in isolation

Management: Hearing tests yearly from puberty in affected families, with MRI brai if abnormality is detected. A normal MRI in the late teens is helpful in assessing ris to any offspring. A clear scan at 30yrs (unless a family history of late onset) indicates that the gene has not been inherited. Treatment of vestibular Schwannomas neurosurgical and complicated by hearing loss/deterioration and facial palsy. Mea survival from diagnosis is ~15yrs.

Schwannomatosis Multiple tender cutaneous Schwannomas without the bila eral vestibular Schwannomas that are characteristic of NF2. Indistinguishable fro mosaic NF2, where vestibular Schwannomas are also absent, except by genet analysis of tumour biopsies. There is typically a large tumour load, assessable on by whole-body MRI. Mutations in the tumour suppressor genes SMARCB1 and LZT and spontaneous NF2 mutations have all been described. Life expectancy is norma

Diagnostic criteria for neurofibromatosis

NF1 (von Recklinghausen's disease):
Diagnosis is made if 2 of the following are found:

1 ≥6 *café-au-lait* macules >5mm (pre-pubertal) or >15mm (post-pubertal)
2 ≥2 neurofibromas of any type or 1 plexiform
3 Freckling in the axillary or inguinal regions
4 Optic glioma
5 ≥2 Lisch nodules
6 Distinctive osseous lesion typical of NF1, eg sphenoid dysplasia
7 First-degree relative with NF1 according to the above-listed criteria.

Differential: McCune-Albright syndrome (*OHCS* p650), multiple lentigines, urticaria pigmentosa.

NF2:
Diagnosis is made if either of the following are found:

1 Bilateral vestibular Schwannomas seen on MRI or CT
2 First-degree relative with NF2, and either:
a) Unilateral vestibular Schwannoma; or
b) One of the following:
- Neurofibroma
- Meningioma
- Glioma
- Schwannoma
- Juvenile cataract (NF2 type).

Differential: NF1, Schwannomatosis.

Causes of café-au-lait spots: Normal (eg up to 5); NF1 (↑melanocyte density vs 'normal' *café-au-lait* spots); NF2; rare syndromes: Gaucher's; McCune-Albright; Russell-Silver; tuberous sclerosis; Wiskott-Aldrich.

Syringomyelia

A syrinx is a tubular cavity in or close to the central canal of the cervical cord. *Mean age of onset:* 30yrs. *Incidence:* 8/100 000/yr. Symptoms may be static for years, but then worsen fast—eg on coughing or sneezing, as ↑pressure causes extension, eg into the brainstem (syringobulbia, see later in topic).

Causes *Typically,* blocked CSF circulation (without 4th ventricular communication), with ↓flow from basal posterior fossa to caudal space, eg Arnold-Chiari malformation (cerebellum herniates through foramen magnum); basal arachnoiditis (after infection, irradiation, subarachnoid haemorrhage); basilar invagination (in which the top of the odontoid process of C2 migrates upwards, causing foramen magnum stenosis ± medulla oblongata compression); masses (cysts, rheumatoid pannus, encephalocoele, tumours). *Less commonly,* a syrinx may develop after myelitis, cord trauma, or rupture of an AV malformation, or within spinal tumours (ependymoma or haemangioblastoma) due to fluid secreted from neoplastic cells or haemorrhage.

Signs *Dissociated sensory loss* (absent pain and T° sensation, with preserved light touch, vibration, and joint-position sense) due to pressure from the syrinx on the decussating anterolateral pathway (fig 10.35) in a root distribution reflecting the location of the syrinx (eg for typical cervical syrinx then sensory loss is over trunk and arms); *wasting/weakness* of hands ± *claw-hand* (then arms→shoulders→respiratory muscles). Anterior horn cells are also vulnerable. *Other signs:* Horner's syndrome (can be bilateral and therefore more difficult to spot); UMN leg signs; body asymmetry, limb hemihypertrophy, or unilateral odo- or chiromegaly (enlarged hand or foot), perhaps from release of trophic factors via anterior horn cells; Charcot's joints in the shoulder/wrist due to lost joint proprioception (see fig 5.11, p213).

Syringobulbia (Brainstem involvement.) Nystagmus, tongue atrophy, dysphagia, pharyngeal/palatal weakness, Vth nerve sensory loss.

MRI imaging How big is the syrinx? Any base-of-brain (Chiari) malformation?

Surgery Don't wait for gross deterioration to occur. Decompression at the foramen magnum may be tried in Chiari malformations to promote free flow of CSF, and so prevent syrinx dilatation. Surgery may reduce pain and progression.

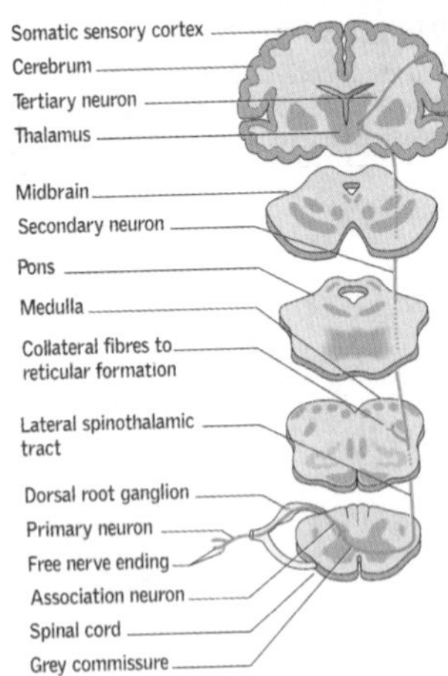

Fig 10.35 The anterolateral system.

HIV and AIDS (p398.) Can have multiple neurological manifestations: these conditions are part of the differential diagnosis of meningitis, intracranial mass lesions, dementia, encephalomyelitis, cord problems, and peripheral neuropathies.

Acute infection: May be associated with transient aseptic meningoencephalitis (typically self-limiting), myelopathy, and neuropathy.

Opportunistic infections: Arise during low CD4 counts, which allow unusual or atypical organisms to infect the nervous system: • *Toxoplasma gondii* (p400) is the main CNS pathogen in AIDS, causing cerebral abscesses which present with focal signs, eg seizures, hemiparesis. CT/MRI shows ring-shaped contrast-enhancing lesions. Treat with pyrimethamine (+folinic acid) + sulfadiazine or clindamycin for 6 months. Continue secondary prophylaxis until CD4 count >200. Pneumocystis prophylaxis also protects against toxoplasmosis. • *Cryptococcus neoformans* (fig 10.36) causes a chronic meningitis with fever and headache (neck stiffness may be absent). Cognition alters slowly, seizures and coma may follow. Treat with amphotericin followed by fluconazole. • *Cytomegalovirus (CMV)* can cause encephalopathy. • *Progressive multifocal leukoencephalopathy (PML)* is caused by the JC virus. There is progressive white matter inflammation. Mortality even with antiretroviral therapy is around 50% at 1yr. • Syphilis and TB may also cause meningitis.

Tumours: Affecting the CNS include primary cerebral lymphoma (associated with EBV) and B-cell lymphoma. CSF JC virus PCR is useful in distinguishing PML from lymphoma.

Neuropathies: Common in HIV, and may be a result of the disease itself or antiretroviral therapy. Up to 30% of patients have a peripheral neuropathy, which is painful and predominantly sensory. Other clinical pictures include polyradiculopathy, mononeuritis multiplex, and proximal myopathy.

Chronic HIV-associated neurocognitive disorder (HAND): While antiretroviral therapy (ART) has decreased the incidence of CNS complications in HIV/AIDS, people are living longer with the disease, and chronic complications such as HIV-associated dementia are increasing. This occurs in 7–15%, late in the disease, and usually when the CD4 count is <200. Progressive behavioural changes are seen along with subcortical features: memory loss, poor attention, and bradykinesia. Various encephalopathies may also contribute to this, eg PML.

Human T-cell lymphotrophic virus (HTLV-1) Is another retrovirus with neurological manifestations, though much more rarely than HIV (~0.5%). It causes: *Tropical spastic paraplegia,* a slowly progressing myelopathy, typically affecting the thoracic area. There may be paraesthesiae, sensory loss, and disorders of micturition. *Demyelinating polyneuropathy* and *ataxia* may also occur.

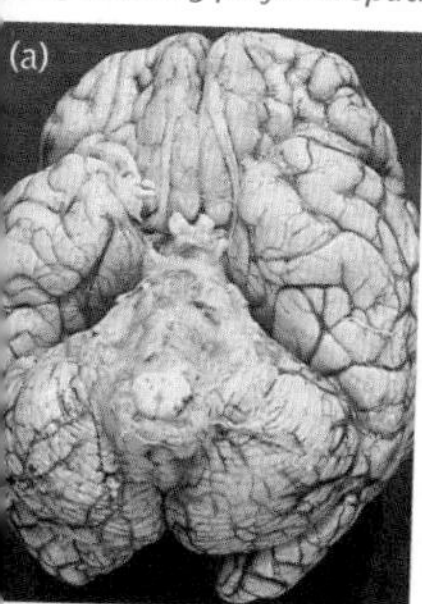

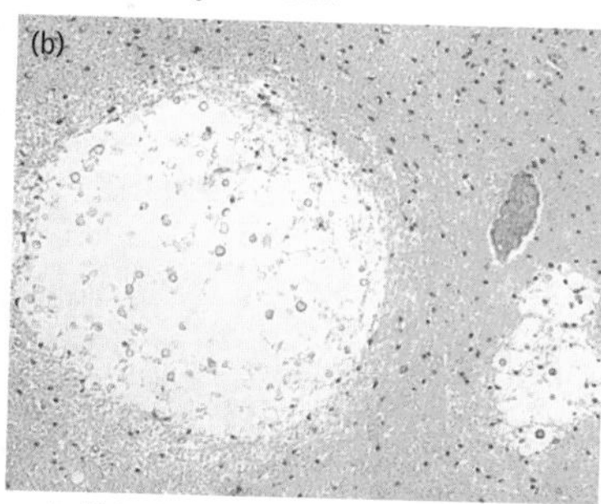

Fig 10.36 Cryptococcosis: (a) Chronic meningitis involving the basal leptomeningitis with multiple small intraparenchymal cysts seen in the cerebral cortex. (b) Under the microscope we see these cysts as dilatation of the perivascular space to form cavities filled with colonies of cryptococci, which appear as round basophilic structures.

Reproduced from Gray *et al.*, *Escourelle and Poirier's Manual of Basic Neuropathology*, 2013, by permission of Oxford University Press, USA.

11 Oncology and palliative care

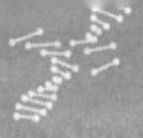

Contents

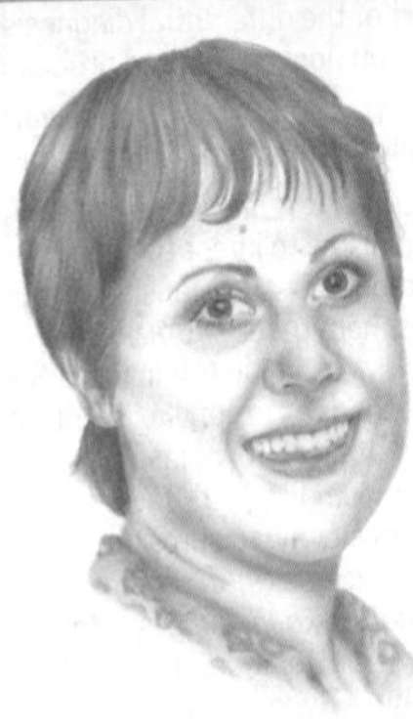

Fig 11.1 How not to break bad news. The third day of admission brings me some examples of doctor's communication skills being the worst I could possibly imagine under the most painful of circumstances...I'm laid in a hospital bed sobbing and scared, about at the most vulnerable a patient could be...a young gynaecology SHO I have never met enters my room...I can tell he has pulled the short straw... He nervously sits down next to me and out of the blue, after a cursory introduction tells me, 'Your MRI shows evidence of spread'. I am quite astounded at the lack of quality communication given the circumstances.

The Other Side, by Kate Granger MBE, FRCP, 1981–2016.

Kate Granger, a medical registrar then consultant geriatrician, was diagnosed with a desmoplastic small round cell tumour at the age of 29. This is a cancer that medical science has no answer to. But Kate had her own answer. She turned her terminal diagnosis on its head and began a dialogue on death and dying, offering her experience as an inspirational lesson in compassion and care. Before you are a patient, before you have cancer, but most importantly, before you are a doctor, you are simply a human being. And if your humanity is lost or forgotten then you cannot care, even if medical science is able to provide an answer. hellomynameis.org.uk #hellomynameis

Image and text reproduced courtesy of the family of Dr Kate Granger, MBE.

We thank Professor Max Watson and Dr Antonia Field-Smith, our Specialist Readers, for their contribution to this chapter.

Looking after people with cancer

Cancer will affect 50% of people born after 1960 and >25% of all deaths in the UK are from cancer.[1] While many may not appreciate the poor prognosis attached to diagnoses such as liver failure or heart failure, 'cancer' has a widespread association with suffering and death. Yet 'cancer' is not a homogenous disease but a group of conditions with prognoses ranging from very good (98% 10yr survival for testicular cancer) to extremely poor (21% 1yr survival for pancreatic cancer).[1]

Communication[2] is the first step on a cancer pathway and underpins whatever that diagnosis may subsequently entail for the individual. A range of overwhelming feelings can surface upon receiving a cancer diagnosis: shock, numbness, denial, panic, anger, resignation ('I knew all along...'). Preconceptions, possibly derived vicariously from friends and family, may be deeply embedded leading to despair or inappropriate optimism. Without an understanding of your patient's starting point, you may fail to be effective in your guidance and support.

Tips for the discussion of a cancer diagnosis

1. Set the environment up carefully. Choose a quiet place where you will not be disturbed. Make sure family or friends are present according to your patient's wishes. Anticipate likely questions and be sure of your facts.
2. Find out what the patient already knows and believes (often a great deal). 'What are you worried about today?'
3. Give some warning: 'There is some bad news for us to address'.
4. Ascertain how much the person wants to know. 'Are you someone who likes to know all the details about your condition?' Although information is a priority for the majority of cancer patients, this may change with the individual, and the course of the disease. 'Monitors' will seek information, 'blunters' will distract themselves.
5. Share information about diagnosis and treatments. Specifically list supporting people (oncology multidisciplinary team) and institutions (hospices). Break information down into manageable chunks and check understanding for each.
6. Invite questions patients may feel they cannot ask. 'Is there anything else you want me to explain?' Do not hesitate to go over the same ground repeatedly. Allow denial, don't force the pace, give time. Listen to any concerns raised, encourage the airing of feelings. Empathize.
7. Address prognosis. Be honest. Doctors are often too optimistic. Encourage an appropriate level of hope (see BOX 'Spiritual pain', p535), refer to an expert.
8. Make a plan. The desire to be involved in decisions about treatment is variable: your patient's locus of control can be internal (desire control of their own destiny) or external (passive acceptance). Decision-making can be immediate, deferred, panicked, or rationally deliberated. Time may be required to facilitate any style of decision-making: your plan may be simply to come back and talk again.
9. Summarize, and offer availability. Record details of your conversation including the language used.
10. Follow through. ►Leave your patient with the knowledge that you are with them, and that your unwritten contract will not be broken.

No rules guarantee success. Use whatever your patient gives you—closely observe both verbal and non-verbal cues. Getting to know your patient, seeking out the right expert for each stage of treatment, and making an agreed management plan, are all required.

For any situation which involves the communication of bad news, consider **SPIKES**:[3]

- **S**etting up the interview.
- Assess the patient's **P**erception of the situation.
- Obtain an **I**nvitation (asking the patient's permission to explain).
- Give **K**nowledge and information to the patient.
- Address the **E**motional response with **E**mpathy.
- **S**trategy and **S**ummary: aim for consensus with patient and family.

How cancers develop

Human life requires cells which are capable of dividing millions of times. These cells need to be able to adapt and change so that different tissues and organs can be formed. They need to command their own blood supply. Without extensive mechanisms to control cell growth and prevent the replication of abnormal cells, these requirements for life become the basis for the development of a cancer. Failure of control mechanisms causes cancer.

Cancer is a genetic disease. Genetic changes occur in pathways associated with cell growth, cell differentiation, and cell death. Mutations can be inherited or acquired. Acquired or somatic errors occur due to age, exposure to carcinogens, and in unchecked rapid cell turnover. Mutations result in:

- 'gain of function' *oncogenes* that have pathological activity in the absence of a relevant signal. For example, ras is a protein involved in signal transduction. It is mutated in ~30% of human cancers. Oncogenes behave in a dominant manner: mutation to one allele results in unchecked activation.
- 'loss of function' *tumour suppressor genes* no longer act as inhibitors of pro-malignant processes. In most cases, mutations to both alleles must occur for a cancer phenotype. This can occur either as two separate somatic events, or in the case of predisposition genes, the first 'hit' is inherited and the second occurs somatically. Tumours therefore occur earlier and more frequently in familial cancers. p53 is a tumour suppressor gene mutated in ~50% of human cancers.

Most cancers arise from multiple mutations. This is perhaps best represented in the stepwise accumulation of mutations in colorectal cancer (fig 11.2). An understanding of the molecular biology of cancer facilitates drug development (fig 11.3).

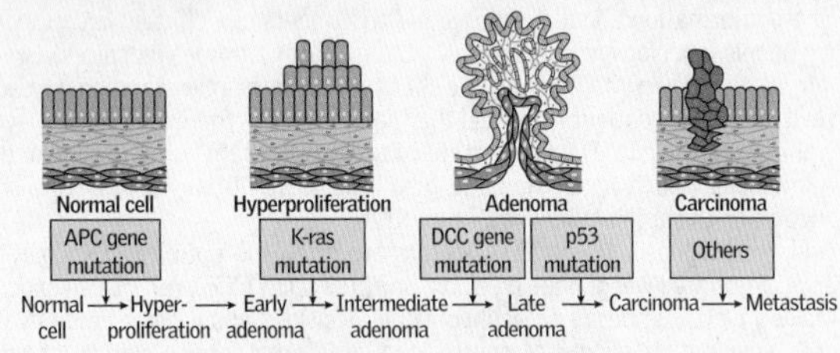

Fig 11.2 Cellular mutations and contributing genes in the development of colorectal cancer.

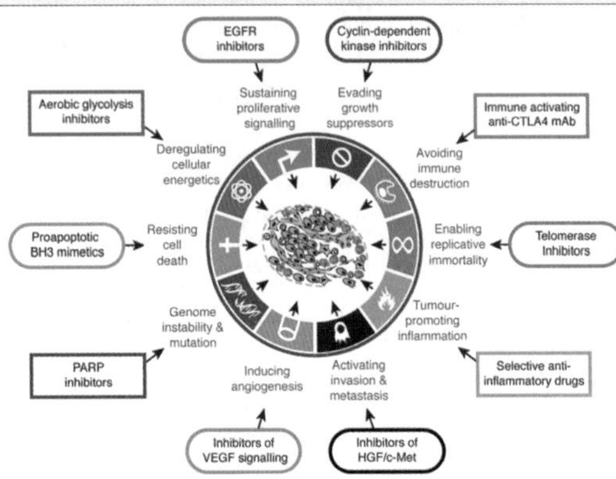

Fig 11.3 Therapeutic targeting in cancer.

Hereditary cancer syndromes

A hereditary cancer[4] is suggested by:

- unusual early age or presentation (eg male breast cancer)
- multiple primary cancers or bilateral/multifocal cancers
- clustering of cancers in relatives
- cancers in multiple generations
- rare tumours (eg retinoblastoma) or histology (medullary thyroid cancer, p223)
- ethnicity (eg Ashkenazi heritage and breast cancer).

Genetic testing is appropriate if the sensitivity and specificity of the test are good enough, and if the result of the test will impact diagnosis and management (see p27).

Breast/ovarian cancer

~5-10% of breast cancers are due to mutations in BRCA1 (17q) or BRCA2 (13q).[4,5] Both genes function as tumour suppressors although they are dominant: a cancer phenotype can be seen when one copy of the gene is normal. A BRCA1 mutation confers a 55-65% lifetime risk of breast cancer and a 39% risk of ovarian cancer. For BRCA2, the risk of breast cancer is 45% (6% in affected males), and 11% for ovarian cancer. Mutations are also linked to prostate, peritoneal, and pancreatic cancers. TP53 mutations (somatic >inherited) also confer a risk of breast cancer. Refer if:

- 1st-degree relative with: breast cancer <40yrs, male breast cancer, bilateral breast cancer <50yrs
- 1st- and 2nd-degree relative with breast cancer or ovarian cancer
- three 1st- or 2nd-degree relatives with breast cancer
- risk assessment calculation of >3% risk in 10yrs or lifetime risk ≥17%
- other: Ashkenazi ancestry, sarcoma <45yrs, multiple cancers at a young age.

Genetic counselling and testing for BRCA1, BRCA2, and TP53 mutations is offered if calculated risk of mutation is >10%. If known BRCA1/2 mutation, offer women annual MRI 30–49yrs and annual mammograpy 50–69yrs (MRI 20–69yrs if TP53 mutation). Prophylactic tamoxifen or raloxifene may be appropriate depending on tolerance and VTE/endometrial cancer risk. Surgical management (mastectomy/oophorectomy) should only be via a specialist MDT.

Colorectal cancer

~25% have a family history. ~5% have identified mutations. Refer to specialist genetic service if: two 1st-degree relatives with colorectal cancer at average age <60yrs, or if criteria for an autosomal dominant colorectal cancer syndrome is met:

- *Lynch syndrome (hereditary non-polyposis colorectal cancer (HNPCC)):* 1-3% of colorectal cancer. Autosomal dominant due to mutations in mismatch repair genes. Lifetime risk of colorectal cancer up to ~80%. Increased risk of other 'Lynch cancers': endometrium, ovary, urinary tract, stomach, small bowel, hepatobiliary tract. Suspect if ≥3 affected relatives (one 1st-degree), from two successive generations, of whom one was affected <50yrs old. Colonoscopic surveillance (at least biennial) from 25–75yrs.
- *Familial adenomatous polyposis:* Due to mutations in the APC tumour suppressor gene (5q) (fig 11.2). <1% of colorectal cancer. Causes multiple colorectal adenomas (>100 in classical disease) which undergo malignant transformation. Gene penetrance approaches 100% by 50yrs. Surveillance sigmoidoscopy from 12yrs, with prophylactic surgery usually <25yrs guided by polyp number, size, and dysplasia.
- *Peutz-Jeghers syndrome:* 1 in 25000-280000. Hamartomatous polpys. 10-20% risk of colorectal cancer, ~50-60% risk of GI cancer, ~60% risk of breast cancer. Due to germline mutations in STK11, a tumour suppressor gene (19p14). Surveillance in all (see p708).

Prostate cancer

5-10% (~50% disease <55yrs) estimated to be due to inherited factors. Genes include BRCA1, BRCA2, mismatch repair, and HOXB13 which interacts with androgen receptor. Age and race contribute. See p530 for screening.

Other familial cancer syndromes Von Hippel-Lindau (p320, p712), Carney complex (p223), MEN (p223), neurofibromatosis (p514).

Cancer diagnosis

A variety of clinical signs and symptoms should alert you to the possible presence of malignancy. The following list is based on clinical features with a 3% positive predictive value for cancer.[6] It is by no means exhaustive and does not negate the value of clinical judgement. Urgent = within 2 weeks.

Lung
- Admit if: symptomatic superior vena caval obstruction (p528), stridor.
- Urgent referral if: >40yrs with unexplained haemoptysis, CXR suggestive of cancer.
- Urgent CXR if >40yrs and:
  - persistent/recurrent chest infection
  - finger clubbing
  - supraclavicular/cervical lymphadenopathy
  - thrombocytosis
  - two of: cough, fatigue, SOB, chest pain, weight loss, ↓appetite, smoker, asbestos.

Upper GI
- Urgent endoscopy if: dysphagia, or >55yrs with weight loss and upper abdominal pain/reflux/dyspepsia.
- Urgent referral if: >40yrs plus jaundice, or upper abdominal mass.
- Urgent CT of the pancreas if >60yrs plus weight loss plus any of: diarrhoea, back pain, abdominal pain, nausea, constipation, new-onset diabetes.
- Non-urgent endoscopy if:
  - >55yrs and one of: treatment-resistant dyspepsia, upper abdominal pain plus low Hb, ↑plts, or N&V plus upper GI symptoms/weight loss
  - haematemesis.

Lower GI
PR examination and FBC in all.
- Urgent referral if: positive faecal occult blood, >40yrs with abdominal pain plus weight loss, >50yrs with unexplained rectal bleeding, >60yrs with iron-deficient anaemia or change in bowel habit.
- Consider urgent referral if: rectal/abdominal mass, anal ulceration, <50yrs with rectal bleeding plus lower GI symptoms or weight loss or iron-deficiency anaemia.
- Faecal occult blood testing if: >50yrs plus abdominal pain or weight loss, <60yrs with change in bowel habit or iron-deficiency anaemia, >60yrs and anaemia.

Gynaecological
- Urgent referral if: ascites, pelvic mass (fibroid excluded), >55yrs with post-menopausal bleeding.

Breast
- Urgent referral if: >30yrs with unexplained breast lump, >50yrs with symptoms or change to one nipple.
- Consider urgent referral if: skin changes, >30yrs with axillary lump.

Urology
- Urgent referral if:
  - irregular prostate on PR, abnormal age-specific PSA (see p530)
  - >40yrs with unexplained visible haematuria, >60yrs with unexplained non-visible haematuria plus dysuria or ↑WCC
  - non-painful enlargement or change in shape/texture of testicle.

Central nervous system
- Urgent MRI in progressive, sub-acute loss of central neurological function.

►Unexplained weight loss, ↓appetite, and DVT can be non-specific signs of cancer. Assess for any additional risk factors, symptoms, signs, and refer accordingly.

See also *haematology* (p352); *thyroid* (p600); *skin* (p596).

Cancer and the multidisciplinary team

The care of all patients diagnosed with cancer is formally reviewed by a multidisciplinary team (MDT). The aim of the MDT is to coordinate high-quality diagnosis, treatment, and care. The MDT should make a recommendation on the best initial treatment for cancer. Note: an MDT can only 'recommend'; the decision must be made in consultation with the patient. The MDT is made up of healthcare professionals with expertise in treating and supporting patients with cancer. Members should include, but are not limited to:

- lead clinician and lead nurse specialist
- radiologists (see BOX 'Interventional oncology', p527)
- histopathologists
- expert surgeons, eg upper GI, colorectal, breast, plastics
- oncologists (medical and clinical)
- palliative care physicians
- nominated member to support ongoing clinical trials
- patient representative
- administrative support.

Cancer staging

Staging systems are used to describe the extent of a cancer. This is vital to determine the most appropriate treatment, to assess prognosis, and to identify relevant clinical trials. A cancer is always referred to by the stage given at diagnosis. The TNM system is most widely used and is based on the extent of tumour (T), spread to lymph nodes (N), and the presence of metastases (M) (table 11.1).

Table 11.1 TNM cancer staging

Tx	Primary tumour cannot be measured	**Nx**	Nodes cannot be assessed
T0	Primary tumour cannot be found	**N0**	No node involvement
T_{is}	Carcinoma *in situ* (abnormal cells present)	**N1–3**	Number/location of node metastases
T1–4	Size and/or extent of primary tumour (1=small tumour /minimal invasion; 4=large tumour/extensive invasion)	**M0**	No distant spread
		M1	Distant metastases

Other prefixes may also be used: c refers to clinical stage; p is the stage after pathological examination; y refers to stage after neoadjuvant therapy; r is used if a tumour is re-staged after a disease-free interval; a indicates stage at autopsy.

The TNM staging may be converted to an overall, less detailed classification of cancer stage: 0–IV. Stage 0 refers to carcinoma *in situ;* Stages I–III describe the size of cancer and/or nearby spread; Stage IV indicates metastatic disease.

Some cancers may have alternative staging systems such as Duke's classification for colorectal cancer (p616). See also lung cancer (p176); breast cancer (p602); oesophageal cancer (p618); bladder cancer (p647).

Cancer imaging

Imaging is essential in oncology for diagnosis, prognosis, and to inform and guide treatment. As well as plain radiographs, ultrasound scans, CT, and MRI; there is a wealth of more specialist imaging including:

PET-CT: PET uses a non-specific radioactive tracer (FDG) which highlights areas of increased metabolism, cell proliferation, or hypoxia. It therefore accumulates in cancer cells >non-cancer cells. PET-CT is a powerful combination of anatomical (CT) and functional (PET) information allowing diagnosis, increased accuracy of staging, and assessment of treatment response.

Monoclonal antibodies: Radio-labelled tumour antibodies specific to the tumour under investigation, eg prostate specific membrane antigen, somatostatin (neuroendocrine tumours), oestrogen receptor (breast). They can offer better specificity than standard PET images. (For monoclonal antibodies in treatment see p524.)

Bone scintigraphy (bone scan): Detects abnormal metabolic activity in bones including bone metastases.

Cancer treatment: medicine and surgery

Chemotherapy

Chemotherapy[7] is the use of any chemical substance to treat disease. In modern-day use, the term refers primarily to the use of cytotoxic drugs in the treatment of cancer. The aim is to deliver enough cytotoxic drug to a cancer-cell target which is expressed differently compared to normal tissue. Cytotoxic drugs are given at intervals (cycles of treatment) to allow recovery of normal tissue. Chemotherapy is the only systemic treatment for cancer (surgery and radiotherapy are local treatments). This is important as most cancers are considered to be systemic either due to metastases, or the potential to metastasize in the future. ►*Chemotherapy should be prescribed and given only under expert guidance by people trained in its use.* Includes:

- *Single-agent:* Rarely curative as genetically resistant cells are selected out.
- *Combination chemotherapy:* A combination of drugs with different mechanisms of action and different side-effect profiles reduces the likelihood of resistance and toxicity. The drugs used should have:
  - cytotoxic activity for that tumour, preferentially able to induce remission
  - different mechanisms of action, ideally additive or synergistic effects
  - non-overlapping toxicity to maximize benefit of full therapeutic doses
  - different mechanisms of resistance.
- *Adjuvant:* After other initial treatment to reduce the risk of relapse, eg following surgical removal of, eg breast, bowel cancer.
- *Neoadjuvant:* Used to shrink tumours prior to surgical or radiological treatment. May allow later treatment to be more conservative.
- *Palliative:* No curative aim, offers symptom relief, may prolong survival.

Classes of cytotoxic drugs

- *Alkylating agents:* Anti-proliferative drugs that bind via alkyl groups to DNA leading to apoptotic cell death, eg cyclophosphamide, chlorambucil, busulfan.
- *Angiogenesis inhibitors:* Eg bevacizumab, aflibercept, sunitinib.
- *Antimetabolites:* Interfere with cell metabolism including DNA and protein synthesis, eg methotrexate, 5-fluorouracil.
- *Antioestrogens:* Aromatoase inhibitors (eg letrozole, anastrozole), oestrogen receptor antagonists (eg tamoxifen, raloxifene) used in breast cancer treatment.
- *Antitumour antibiotics:* Interrupt DNA function, eg dactinomycin, doxorubicin, mitomycin, bleomycin.
- *Monoclonal antibodies:* Antibodies to a specific tumour antigen can slow tumour growth by enhancing host immunity, or be conjugated with chemotherapy/radioactive isotopes to allow targeted treatment. Expect more of these in future.
- *Topoisomerase inhibitors:* Interrupt regulation of DNA winding, eg etoposide.
- *Vinca alkaloids and taxanes:* 'Spindle poisons' which target mechanisms of cell division, eg vincristine, vinblastine, docetaxel.

Side-effects

Due to cytotoxic effects on non-cancer cells. Greatest effect seen on dividing cells, ie gut, hair, bone marrow, gametes (see BOX 'Fertility and cancer', p525).

- *Vomiting:* Prophylaxis given with most cytotoxic regimens (see p251).
- *Alopecia:* May profoundly impact quality of life. Consider 'cold-cap', wig services.
- *Neutropenia:* Most commonly seen 7-14d after chemotherapy. ►►Neutropenic sepsis is life-threatening and needs urgent assessment and empirical treatment (p352).

Extravasation of chemotherapy

Extravasation[8] = inadvertent infiltration of a drug into subcutaneous/subdermal tissue. *Presentation:* Tingling, burning, pain, redness, swelling, no 'flashback'/resistance from cannula. *Management:* Stop and disconnect infusion. Aspirate any residual drug before cannula removed. Follow local policies (ask for the 'extravasation kit'). Follow any drug-specific recommendations. For DNA-binding drugs (anthracyclines, alkylating agents, antitumour antibiotics), use a dry cold compress to vasoconstrict and ↓ drug spread. For non-DNA-binding drugs (vinca alkaloids, taxanes, platin salts), use a dry warm compress to vasodilate and ↑ drug distribution.

Surgery

- *Prevention:* Risk-reducing surgery, eg thyroidectomy in MEN (p223), colectomy in FAP (p521).
- *Screening:* Endoscopy, colposcopy.
- *Diagnosis and staging:* Fine needle aspiration, core needle biopsy, vacuum-assisted biopsy, excisional/incisional biopsy, sentinel lymph node biopsy, endoscopy, diagnostic/staging laparoscopy, laparascopic ultrasound.
- *Treatment:* Resection of solid tumour (may be combined with chemo/radiotherapy).
- *Reconstruction:* Eg following treatment for breast, head and neck cancers.
- *Palliation:* Bypass, stoma, stenting, pathological fractures.

Clinical trials

- *Advantages:* Possibility of more effective treatment than currently available, close monitoring with direct access to a research team, reassurance from increased number of clinical encounters, gain from altruism.
- *Disadvantages:* Possibility of receiving therapy that is no better or worse than standard therapy, unknown toxicity from new agents, time-consuming, anxiety from increased number of clinical encounters.

You may look after patients who are participating in clinical trials. For many of these, you will not be familiar with the trial therapy or even know which therapy the patient is receiving: a new therapy, an old therapy, or placebo. ►Contact the research team to discuss any clinical concerns or change in treatment. Contact details should be recorded in the patient's notes. Look in the notes for, or ask the patient if they have a copy of the 'Participant Information Sheet' which is mandatory for all UK research studies.

Information on relevant trials for your patient is available:

- Cancer Research UK (www.cancerresearchuk.org/about-cancer/find-a-clinical-trial).
- UK Clinical Trials Gateway (www.ukctg.nihr.ac.uk).

Fertility and cancer

Chemotherapy and radiotherapy may:

- damage spermatogonia causing impaired spermatogenesis or male sterility
- hasten oocyte depletion leading to premature ovarian failure.

If cancer treatment carries a risk of infertility, fertility preservation techniques[9] should be discussed prior to treatment being given.

- *Men:* Semen cryopreservation should be offered before treatment due to the risk of genetic damage in sperm after initiation of chemotherapy. Intracytoplasmic sperm injection means that even a small amount of banked sperm can be used successfully in the future.
- *Women:* Cryopreservation of:
  1. Embryos
  2. Oocytes: if ethical objections to embryo preservation or no partner
  3. Ovarian tissue: no ovarian stimulation required, experimental technique.

Ovarian transposition (oophoropexy) may be possible prior to pelvic radiotherapy but protection is not guaranteed due to radiation scatter.

Beau's lines

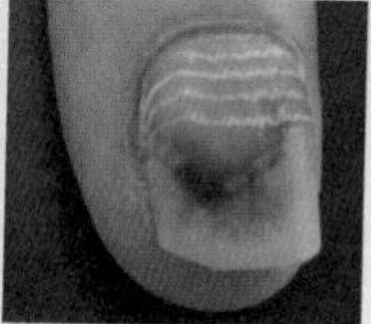

Fig 11.4 Beau's lines.

Beau's lines (fig 11.4) are horizontal depressions in the nail plate that run parallel to the moon-shaped portion of the nail bed. They result from a sudden interruption of nail keratin synthesis and may be due to local infection/trauma, systemic illness, or from medication (p76). Each line in this photo coincided with a round of chemotherapy for breast cancer.

Cancer treatment: radiotherapy

Radiotherapy[10] is used in >50% of all cancer and forms part of treatment in 40% of those considered cured. It uses ionizing radiation to cause damage to DNA. This prevents cell division and leads to cell death. The aim of radiotherapy treatment is to inactivate cancer cells without causing a severe reaction in normal tissue.

Radical treatment Given with curative intent. Total dose ranges from 40-70 gray (Gy) in up to 40 fractions. Some regimens involve several smaller fractions a day with a gap of 6-8h. Combined chemoradiation is used in some sites, eg anus and oesophagus, to increase response rate.

Palliative radiotherapy Aims to relieve symptoms, may not impact on survival. Doses are smaller and given in fewer fractions to offer short-term tumour control with minimal side-effects. Palliation is used for brain metastases, spinal cord compression, visceral compression, and bleeding, eg haemoptysis, haematuria. Bone pain from metastases can be reduced or eliminated in 60% of cases.

Early reactions

Occur ~2 weeks into treatment, peak ~2-4 weeks after treatment.

- *Tiredness:* ~80%. Improves ~4 weeks after treatment completed but chronic in ~30%. Advise patients to stay as active as possible.
- *Skin reactions:* Include erythema, dry desquamation, moist desquamation, and ulceration. Aqueous cream can be used on unbroken areas.
- *Mucositis:* All patients receiving head and neck treatment should have a dental check-up before therapy. Avoid smoking. Antiseptic mouthwashes may help. Aspirin gargle and other soluble analgesics can be tried. Treat oral thrush with fluconazole 50mg/24h PO, nystatin may exacerbate nausea.
- *Nausea and vomiting:* Occur when stomach, liver, or brain treated. Try metoclopramide 10mg/8h PO (dopamine antagonist), domperidone 10mg/8h PO (blocks the central chemoreceptor trigger zone), or ondansetron 4-8mg/8h PO/IV (serotonin $5HT_3$ antagonist) (see p251).
- *Diarrhoea:* Usually after abdominal or pelvic treatments. Maintain good hydration. Avoid high-fibre agents. Try loperamide 2mg PO after loose stools (max 16mg/24h).
- *Dysphagia:* Following thoracic treatments. Speech and language input, nutrition.
- *Cystitis:* After pelvic treatments. Drink plenty of fluid.

Late reactions

Months-years after treatment.

- CNS/PNS: *Somnolence:* 4-6wks after brain radiotherapy. Consider ↑steroid dose. *Spinal cord myelopathy:* progressive weakness. MRI to exclude cord compression. *Brachial plexopathy:* numb, weak, or painful arm after axillary radiotherapy.
- *Lung: Pneumonitis* can occur 6-12wks after thoracic treatment causing dry cough ± dyspnoea. Bronchodilators and tapered steroids may help.
- *GI: Xerostomia* = reduced saliva. Dental care and nutrition important. Treat with water, saliva substitutes, salivary stimulants. *Benign strictures* of oesophagus or bowel. Treat with dilatation. Seek a specialist surgical opinion regarding *fistulae*. *Radiation proctitis* may be a problem after prostate irradiation.
- *GU: Urinary frequency:* small fibrosed bladder after pelvic treatment. *Vaginal stenosis, dyspareunia, erectile dysfunction* can occur after pelvic radiotherapy. *↓fertility:* due to pelvic radiotherapy (see p525).
- *Endocrine: Panhypopituitarism* following radical treatment involving pituitary fossa. Check hormone profile in children: growth hormone replacement may be required. *Hypothyroidism* in ~50% after neck treatment: check TFTs annually.
- *Secondary cancers:* Risk (2-4 per 10000 person-years) is usually insignificant compared to recurrence/death from primary lesion. More important for younger patients after curative treatment. Women <35yrs receiving radiotherapy for Hodgkin's lymphoma should be offered breast screening from 8yrs after treatment.

►↑ Cancer survival means ↑ numbers living with poor health or disability after treatment (~625000 in UK). Remember the emotional and physical impact of cancer extends beyond the prescribed course of radiotherapy/chemotherapy.

Methods of delivering radiotherapy

Conventional external beam radiotherapy (EBRT): Is the most common form of treatment. Delivers beams of ionizing radiation to the patient from an external linear accelerator.

Stereotactic radiotherapy is a highly accurate form of EBRT used to target small lesions with great precision—most frequently in treating intracranial tumours. It is often referred to by the manufacturer's name, eg *Gamma Knife®*, *Truebeam®*.

Brachytherapy involves a radiation source being placed within or close to a tumour, allowing a high local radiation dose. Implants may be placed within a cavity (eg uterus, post-surgical space) or within tissue (eg prostate, breast).

Radioisotope therapy uses tumour-seeking radionuclides to target specific tissues. For example, ^{131}I (radioiodine) to ablate remaining thyroid tissue after thyroidectomy for thyroid cancer.

Interventional oncology

Interventional oncology (IO) refers to interventional radiology procedures used in the treatment or palliation of patients with cancer. IO can be divided into disease-modifying and symptomatic procedures.

Disease-modifying IO:
Intended to modify cancer progression and/or to improve prognosis. Includes:
- Image-guided ablation, eg radiofrequency ablation, cryoablation, irreversible electroporation.
- Embolization, eg transarterial embolization, chemoembolization, selective internal radiation therapy.
- Image-guided brachytherapy.
- Isolated perfusion chemotherapy: uses occlusion techniques to protect normal tissue from high doses of chemotherapy.

Symptomatic IO:
Provides relief from cancer-related symptoms, but does not modify the underlying disease process. The techniques (table 11.2) can offer significantly improved quality of life, reduce admissions, and increase time spent outside of hospital.

Table 11.2 Interventional techniques available for cancer symptom control

Clinical problem	Interventional treatment option
Ascites	Temporary/permanent image-guided ascitic drain
Pleural effusion	Temporary/permanent image-guided pleural drain
Superior vena cava obstruction (p528)	Superior vena cava stenting
Oesophageal obstruction	Oesophageal stenting
Large bowel obstruction	Colonic stenting
Tumour-related haemorrhage	Transarterial embolization
Jaundice	Biliary drainage and stenting
Renal tract obstruction	Nephrostomy, ureteric stenting
Bone metastases	Image-guided ablation

►Talk to your interventional radiologist.

Oncology emergencies

Emergencies[11,12] in oncology include:

Neutropenic sepsis

Temperature >38°C and neutrophil count <0.5×10^9/L. Suspect in all patients who are unwell and within 6wks of receiving chemotherapy. Localizing signs may be absent. Examine indwelling catheter sites. ►►Immediate treatment saves lives. Use local guidelines or treat empirically with piperacillin/tazobactam (see p352).

Spinal cord compression

3-5% of cancer patients have spinal metastases. ~15% of those with advanced cancers develop metastatic spinal cord compression. Most commonly associated with lung, prostate, breast, myeloma, melanoma. ►►Urgent treatment is required to preserve neurological function and relieve pain.

Causes: Collapse or compression of a vertebral body due to metastases (common), direct extension of a tumour into vertebral column (rare).

Signs and symptoms: Back pain in ~95%. Ask about nocturnal pain and pain with straining. Worry if there is cervical/thoracic pain. Also limb weakness, difficulty walking, sensory loss, bowel/bladder dysfunction. Maintain a high index of suspicion.

Management: Admit for bed rest and arrange urgent (within 24h) MRI of the whole spine. Give dexamethasone 16mg/24h PO with prophylatic gastroprotection, eg PPI, and blood glucose monitoring. If reduced mobility consider thromboprophylaxis (compression stockings, LMWH). Refer urgently to clinical oncology/cancer MDT. Radiotherapy is the commonest treatment and should be given within 24 hours of MRI diagnosis. Decompressive surgery ± radiotherapy may be appropriate depending on prognosis. Patients with loss of motor function after >48h are unlikely to recover function. (See also p466.)

Superior vena cava (SVC) syndrome

Reduced venous return from head, neck, and upper limbs. Due to extrinsic compression (most common), or venous thrombosis (consider if current or past central venous access). ►►SVC syndrome with airway compromise requires urgent treatment.

Causes: >90% of SVC syndrome results from malignancy. Most common cancers: lung (~75%), lymphoma, metastatic (eg breast), thymoma, germ cell.

Signs and symptoms: Diagnosis is made clinically. SOB, orthopnoea, stridor, plethora/cyanosis, oedema of face and arm, cough, headache, engorged neck veins (non-pulsatile ↑JVP), engorged chest wall veins. *Pemberton's test:*[1] elevation of the arms to the side of the head causes facial plethora/cyanosis.

Management: Prop up. Assess for hypoxia (pulse oximetry, blood gas) and give oxygen if needed. Dexamethasone 16mg/24h. CT is used to define the anatomy of the obstruction. Balloon venoplasty and SVC stenting provide the most rapid relief of symptoms (see BOX 'Interventional oncology', p527). Treat with radiotherapy or chemotherapy depending on the sensitivity of the underlying cancer.

Malignancy-associated hypercalcaemia

Most common metabolic abnormality in cancer patients: ~10-20% of patients with cancer, ~40% of myeloma. It is a poor prognostic sign: 75% mortality within 3 months. Calcium is highly protein-bound and needs correcting to the serum albumin concentration. PTH levels should be suppressed (see pp676-7).

Causes: PTH-related protein produced by the tumour (see p529), local osteolysis, eg myeloma, tumour production of calcitriol.

Signs and symptoms: Weight loss, anorexia, nausea, polydipsia, polyuria, constipation, abdominal pain, dehydration, weakness, confusion, seizure, coma.

Management: Aggressive rehydration. Bisphosphonates (if eGFR ≥30), eg zoledronic acid IV, usually normalize calcium within 3 days and can be given as a repeated infusion. Calcitonin produces a more rapid (2h) but short-term effect and tolerance can develop. Long-term treatment is by control of the underlying malignancy.

1 Pemberton described this 'useful' sign of venous obstruction due to a goitre in 1946.

Brain metastases

Affect up to ~40% of patients with cancer. Most commonly: lung, breast, colorectal, melanoma. Poor prognosis: median survival 1–2 months; better prognosis with single lesion, breast cancer (see also p830).

Signs and symptoms: Headache (~50%, often worse in the morning, when coughing or bending), focal neurological signs (~30%), ataxia (~21%), fits (~18%), nausea, vomiting, papilloedema.

Management: Urgent CT/MRI depending on underlying diagnosis, disease stage, and performance status. Dexamethasone 16mg/24h to reduce cerebral oedema. Stereotactic radiotherapy (see p527). Discuss with neurosurgery, especially if large lesion or associated hydrocephalus.

Tumour lysis syndrome

Chemotherapy for rapidly proliferating tumours (leukaemia, lymphoma, myeloma) leads to cell death and ↑urate, ↑K^+, ↑phosphate, ↓calcium. Risk of arrhythmia and renal failure (see p314).

Management: Prevent with hydration and uricolytics, eg rasburicase, allopurinol.

Paraneoplastic syndromes

Paraneoplastic syndromes[13] (table 11.3) consist of symptoms attributable to a malignancy mediated by hormones, cytokines, or the cross-reaction of tumour antibodies. They do not correlate with stage/prognosis and may pre-date other cancer symptoms.

Table 11.3 Examples of paraneoplastic syndromes

Paraneoplastic syndrome	Comment	Malignancies	See
Hypercalcaemia	Parathyroid hormone-related protein secreted by tumour	Lung, oesophagus, skin, cervix, breast, kidney	p528
SIADH	Excessive antidiuretic hormone (ADH) secretion causing ↓Na^+	Lung, pancreas, lymphomas, prostate	p673
Cushing's syndrome	Tumour secretes ACTH or CRF, causing adrenal to produce high levels of corticosteroid	Lung, pancreas, thymus, carcinoid	p224
Neuropathy	Antibody-mediated neuronal degeneration: peripheral, autonomic, cerebellar	Lung, breast, myeloma, Hodgkin's, GI	p504
Lambert-Eaton myasthenic syndrome	Antibody to voltage-gated ion channel on pre-synaptic membrane causes weakness (proximal leg most common)	Mostly lung. Also GI, breast, thymus	p512
Dermatomyositis & polymyositis	Inflammation of the muscles +/- heliotrope rash	Lung, breast, ovary, GI	p552
Acanthosis nigricans	Velvety, hyperpigmented skin (usually flexural)	GI	p562
Pemphigus	Blisters to skin/mucous membranes	Lymphoma, thymus, Kaposi's sarcoma	
Hypertrophic osteoarthropathy	Periosteal bone formation, arthritis, and finger clubbing	Lung	

Trousseau's sign

Trousseau (fig 11.5) was probably the first to discover a paraneoplastic syndrome. He noticed that many patients with migratory thrombophlebitis ('Trousseau's sign') developed gastric cancer. Unfortunately, he developed migratory thrombophlebitis himself and correctly predicted his own death from GI malignancy.

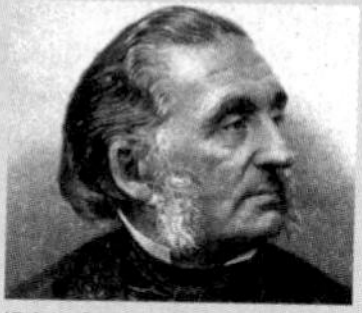

Fig 11.5 Armand Trousseau 1801–1867.
Wellcome Library, London. Armand Trousseau. Lithograph by JBA Lafosse, 1866, after P Petit.

Tumour markers

Tumour markers[14] are specific molecules (usually glycoproteins) that may be found in higher concentrations in the serum, tissue, or urine in patients with certain cancers.

Tumour markers in diagnosis

► *Tumour markers are insufficiently sensitive or specific to be diagnostic in isolation.*

- Many tumour markers are ↑ in several cancers and benign conditions (table 11.4).
- Measuring ≥1 tumour marker is unlikely to aid diagnosis unless suspecting a germ cell tumour.
- Do not make opportunistic requests for panels of tumour markers in patients with non-specific symptoms: they are not helpful and lead to potentially unnecessary investigation. This includes testing PSA in women and CA 125 in men.
- In carefully selected patients, in whom cancer is suspected, highly raised levels of a tumour marker may be helpful:
  - α-fetoprotein (αFP) and human chorionic gonadotrophin (hCG) in testicular/germ cell tumours.
  - CA 125 in combination with USS and menopausal status.
  - αFPin those at high risk of hepatocellular carcinoma.
  - PSA >100ng/mL usually indicates metastatic prostate cancer.

Tumour markers in monitoring

The main value of tumour markers is in monitoring patients known to have cancer. This includes the course of the disease, the effectiveness of treatment, and the detection of cancer recurrence. The following markers may be useful:

- αFP and hCG in testicular/germ cell tumours.
- CEA in colorectal cancer.
- CA 125 in ovarian cancer.
- A cautious interpretation of PSA within the limits of its specificity and sensitivity.

Screening for cancer

The UK has several well-established cancer screening programmes. Women are invited for mammography every 3yrs (50–70yrs) and offered cervical smear tests every 3–5yrs (25–64yrs). Men and women aged 60–74yrs are offered faecal occult blood testing every 2yrs.

Screening tests aim to pick out those who need further investigation to rule out or diagnose a cancer, in the hope that earlier diagnosis and treatment result in better outcomes. All screening tests come with risk: anxiety, harm/discomfort from the test, cost, false positives resulting in further invasive tests, false negatives conferring inappropriate reassurance when symptoms arise. When considering screening an asymptomatic population the potential risks and benefits need to be weighed carefully and the Wilson criteria (see p23) should be satisfied.

Should PSA be used to screen for prostate cancer?

Most men with prostate cancer will have a high prostate-specific antigen (PSA). The higher the PSA, the more likely cancer is. However, PSA is non-specific and also raised in benign prostatic disease, BMI <25, recent ejaculation, recent rectal examination, prostatitis, and UTI. 76% of patients with a raised PSA do not have cancer. Following screening tests (see PROMIS study, 2017, for use of multi-parametric MRI), prostate biopsy is required for diagnosis. This has an inherent risk of complications including bleeding, infection, and urinary retention. ~1% will require hospital admission.

The risks of PSA testing and subsequent biopsy need to be counterbalanced by benefits from screening.[15] ~1 in 800 men avoid death from prostate cancer as a result of PSA screening. But screening picks up many cancers that will never become fatal. This 'overdiagnosis' is thought to occur in ~40% of positive screens with significant risks from treatment including urinary incontinence, erectile dysfunction, and IHD. This balance of risk versus benefit means that population screening for prostate cancer using PSA is not recommended. Despite this, any patient >50yrs (or >45yrs if high risk) can request PSA testing in primary care. ► Interpret any PSA result in conjunction with digital rectal examination and other risk factors.

Summary of tumour markers

Tumour marker	Relevant cancer	Use	Other associated cancers	Associated benign conditions
Alpha-fetoprotein (αFP)	Germ cell/testicular Hepatocellular	Diagnosis, monitoring treatment, detecting recurrence	Colorectal; gastric; hepatobiliary; lung	Cirrhosis; pregnancy; neural tube defects
Calcitonin	Medullary thyroid	Diagnosis, monitoring treatment, detecting recurrence	None known	C-cell hyperplasia
Cancer antigen (CA)125	Ovarian	Monitoring ovarian cancer. Prognosis after chemotherapy	Breast; cervical; endometrial; hepatocellular; lung; non-Hodgkin's lymphoma; pancreatic; medullary thyroid carcinoma; peritoneal; uterine	Liver disease; cystic fibrosis; pancreatitis; urinary retention; diabetes; heart failure; pregnancy; SLE; sarcoid; RA; diverticulitis; IBS; endometriosis; fibroids
CA19–9	Pancreatic	Monitoring pancreatic cancer	Colorectal; gastric; hepatocellular; oesophageal; ovarian	Acute cholangitis; cholestasis; pancreatitis; diabetes; IBS; jaundice
CA15–3	Breast	Monitoring breast cancer	Hepatocellular; pancreatic	Cirrhosis; benign breast disease; in normal health
Carcinoembryonic antigen (CEA)	Colorectal	Monitoring adenocarcinomas	Breast; gastric; lung; mesothelioma; oesophageal; pancreatic	Smoking; chronic liver disease; chronic kidney disease; diverticulitis; jaundice
Human chorionic gonadotrophin (hCG)	Germ cell/testicular, gestational trophoblastic	Diagnosis, prognosis, monitoring of germ cell tumours	Lung	Pregnancy
Paraproteins	Myeloma	Diagnosis, monitoring treatment, detecting recurrence	None known	None known
Thyroglobulin	Thyroid (follicular/papillary)	Monitoring treatment, detecting recurrence	None known	None known

Source data from 'Serum tumour markers: how to order and interpret them', Sturgeon C M, Lai L C, Duffy M J, 2012, BMJ Publishing Ltd.

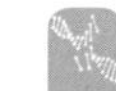

Palliative care: principles and pain

You matter because you are you and you matter to the last moment of your life. We will do all we can to help you, not only to die peacefully, but to live until you die.

Dame Cicely Saunders (1918–2005), founder of the modern hospice.

Palliative care is the active, holistic care of patients with advanced progressive illness. It combines management of pain and other symptoms, with the provision of psychological, social, and spiritual support.

►*Palliative care is not just for the end of life and it is not just for patients with cancer.*

Palliative care should run in parallel with other medical treatments. Good symptom control is important in any disease for improving quality of life and may even prolong survival.[16] Take time to find out exactly what is troubling your patient using a problem-based approach. Consider:
- physical
- psychological
- spiritual
- social.

Remember, each person comes with a set of emotions, preconceptions, and a family already attached. ►Most hospitals now have a dedicated palliative care team for help and advice (including out of hours). Use their expertise.

Assessment of pain

Pain is one of the most feared sequelae of a terminal diagnosis and yet it is not inevitable. However, pain is a complex phenomenon. While the aim of management is for the patient to be pain free, this may not be achievable in all cases so do not promise this.

Do not assume a cause: detailed history and examination are needed to understand aetiology, which will guide subsequent treatment, eg pain from nerve infiltration or local pressure may respond better to agents other than opioids. History and examination are essential for all patients, including those at the end of life. Evaluate severity, nature, functional deficit, and psychological state as all of these contribute to the symptom burden.

Management of pain

Aim to modify the underlying pathology where possible, eg radiotherapy, chemotherapy, surgery. Use analgesia to relieve background pain and provide additional PRN doses for 'breakthrough' pain. Effective analgesia is possible in the majority of patients by combining five principles:

1 *By the mouth*—give orally whenever possible.
2 *By the clock*—give at fixed intervals to offer continuous relief.
3 *By the ladder*—following the WHO stepwise approach (see fig 13.5, p575).
4 *For the individual*—there are no standard doses for opioids, needs vary.
5 *Attention to detail*—communicate, set times carefully, warn of side-effects.

The WHO analgesic ladder

Increase and decrease the analgesia required according to the 'steps' on the ladder[17] (fig 13.5, p575):

1 Non-opioid, eg paracetamol.
2 Opioid for mild to moderate pain, eg codeine.
3 Opioid for moderate to severe pain, eg morphine, diamorphine, oxycodone.

- Persisting/increasing pain and side-effects inform the decision to step up and step down. Take one step at a time to achieve pain relief without toxicity (except in new, severe pain when step 2 may be omitted).
- Paracetamol (PO/PR/IV) at step 1 may have an opiate-sparing effect, and should be continued at steps 2 and 3. Stop step 2 opioids if moving to step 3.
- Use laxatives and anti-emetics with strong opioids.
- Adjuvants which can be added at all steps include: NSAIDs, amitriptyline, pregabalin, corticosteroids, nerve block, transcutaneous electrical nerve stimulation (TENS), radiotherapy.

Opioids

The amount of opioid required to relieve pain varies and should be titrated on an individual basis. Oral morphine is 1st-line. If the oral route is unavailable, use morphine or diamorphine SC (see table 11.5, and tables 11.6, 11.7, p536). *Explanation and regular review are important.* Prescribe anti-emetics and laxatives for all patients.

Start low, go slow: For an opioid-naïve patient with moderate to severe pain, consider oral morphine 5mg every 4 hours plus 5mg PRN (maximum hourly). Consider a lower starting dose if elderly, ↓BMI, or renal impairment. If pain is not controlled, ↑ dose by 30–50% every 24h.

Convert to modified release: When pain is controlled, calculate the total daily dose *including PRN* and divide into two 12h doses of a modified-release preparation (eg MST Continus® 12h). Transdermal preparations are available: seek expert help for dose, check adhesion, and rotate site.

Use a PRN dose for breakthrough pain: 1/10th–1/6th of the total daily dose as an immediate-release preparation, eg Oramorph® or Sevredol®.

Side-effects: Drowsiness, nausea/vomiting (usually ↓ after 5 days), constipation, dry mouth. If difficulty tolerating morphine, or pain plus toxicity, consider an opioid switch (eg oxycodone) and ↓ dose by 25–30%.

Toxicity: Sedation, respiratory depression, visual hallucinations, myoclonic jerks, delirium. Be alert: recognizing toxicity early usually means naloxone is avoided. Monitor pulse oximetry, give oxygen if required. Consider ΔΔ: intracranial bleed, renal failure. ↓Opioids and sedating drugs. Consider hydration. Seek expert help if remains opioid-toxic or in pain. ►Naloxone is only indicated for life-threatening respiratory depression (see p842). In patients on regular opiates it can precipitate a pain crisis and potentially fatal acute withdrawal.[18]

Renal failure: Patients with renal impairment (eGFR <30) are at risk of toxicity due to accumulation of renally excreted opioids and metabolites. Monitor closely. Fentanyl, alfentanil, and buprenorphine have predominantly hepatic metabolism —seek expert advice.

Concerns: Patients may shrink from using opioids. Misconceptions are common: they are addictive, for the dying, if they use morphine now it will not work when they really need it. Respiratory depression is very rare when opioids are correctly titrated but opioids often get blamed when a patient deteriorates. *Reassure patients that opioids are effective and safe when used appropriately.*

Morphine-resistant pain: Seek expert help. Consider methadone, ketamine, and adjuvants such as NSAIDs, steroids, muscle relaxants, anxiolytics, nerve blocks. If neuropathic pain is suspected, try amitriptyline, pregabalin, or topical lidocaine. Consider the effect of psychological and spiritual well-being on pain (see p535).

Rapid analgesia: Most PRN medication takes time to have an effect. If this is a problem, seek expert help regarding rapid-release preparations (eg sublingual, intranasal, or buccal fentanyl). Try to pre-empt times of high pain (eg dressing changes) and give analgesia in advance.

Table 11.5 Opioid dose equivalents: conversions are not exact, potency can vary. If in doubt, use a dose below your estimate. Practice is variable: always defer to local guidelines first.

	Relative potency	4h dose (mg)	24h dose (mg)
Morphine PO	1	5	30
Morphine SC	2	2.5	15
Diamorphine SC	3	1.5–2	10
Oxycodone PO	2	2.5	15
Oxycodone SC	4	1.25	7.5
Alfentanil SC	30	Too short-acting	1
Codeine PO	0.1	60 (6h dose)	240
Tramadol PO	0.1	100 (6h dose)	400
Fentanyl patch	25mcg/h approximates to 60mg/24h oral morphine		

Non-pain symptoms[19] include:

Nausea and vomiting

Causes: Chemotherapy, constipation, hypercalcaemia, oral candidiasis, GI obstruction, drugs, severe pain, infection, renal failure.

Management: Treat reversible causes, eg laxatives for constipation, analgesia for pain, hypercalcaemia (see p528), fluconazole for oral candidiasis. Anti-emetic choice should be based on the likely mechanism of nausea. Consider the site of anti-emetic action, especially when using a combination of drugs. Oral absorption may be poor so consider alternative routes (SC/IV/PR). Options include the following:

- Cyclizine 50mg/8h: antihistamine, anticholinergic, central action so good for intracranial disorders.
- Metoclopramide 10–20mg/8h: blocks central chemoreceptor trigger zone, peripheral prokinetic effects so good in gastroparesis, monitor for extra-pyramidal side-effects.
- Domperidone 10–20mg/8h PO: peripheral antidopaminergic so no dystonic effects.
- Haloperidol 1.5mg PO initially 1–2 times daily: dopamine antagonist, effective in drug- or metabolically induced nausea, use lower doses IV/SC as twice as potent.
- Ondansetron 4–8mg/8h: serotonin antagonist, good for chemo/radiotherapy-related nausea, may cause constipation.
- Levomepromazine 6.25mg, initially 1–2 times daily: broad spectrum, but can sedate, may be very effective if fear/anxiety are contributing to symptoms.

Antisecretory drugs, such as hyoscine butylbromide or octreotide may be required for patients with vomiting and bowel obstruction: seek expert advice.

Constipation

Causes: Very common side-effect of opioids. Better to prevent than treat so prescribe laxatives for all patients starting opioids. Also hypercalcaemia (see p528), dehydration, drugs, or intra-abdominal disease.

Treatment: Treat reversible causes. Good fluid intake. Ensure privacy and access to toilet. Medication options include the following:

- Stimulant (eg senna 2–4 tablets or bisacodyl 5–10mg) at night ± a softener (eg sodium docusate 100mg BD).
- Osmotic laxative (eg macrogol).
- Rectal treatments: bisacodyl/glycerol suppositories, phosphate enema.

Breathlessness

Causes: Look for reversible causes including infection, effusion, anaemia, arrhythmia, thromboembolism. If stridor or signs of superior vena cava syndrome, treat urgently (see p528).

Treatment: Treat reversible causes as appropriate. Consider thoracocentesis ± pleurodesis for a pleural effusion. Recurrent pleural effusions may warrant a radiologically placed permanent drain (see p527). If the patient remains distressed, consider a trial of low-dose opioids. These reduce respiratory drive and the sensation of breathlessness. If opioid-naive, start with 2.5mg of an immediate-release morphine every 4h. If already taking an opioid, use the appropriate breakthrough dose (see p533). Benzodiazepines may help if associated anxiety, eg lorazepam 500mcg SL every 4–6h.

Oral problems

Causes: Poor oral hygiene, radiation, drugs (anticholinergics, chemotherapy, diuretics), infection (candidiasis, herpes simplex).

Treatment: Oral candidiasis: topical miconazole, oral fluconazole 50mg OD but check for interactions (eg warfarin). Nystatin is often ineffective and may exacerbate nausea. Herpes simplex: oral gan/aciclovir. Good mouth care maintains comfort and the ability to communicate. Maintain fluid intake with frequent, small drinks. Simple measures are often ↑ effective: sugar-free chewing gum, normal saline mouthwashes, soft toothbrush. Products containing alcohol may sting. Salivary stimulants (rather than substitutes) can be helpful for dry mouth, eg pilocarpine eye drops 4%, 3 drops in the floor of mouth QDS. Severe mucositis may need admission and systemic opioids.

Insomnia

Causes: Terminally ill patients may experience physical and emotional exhaustion. Often multifactorial. Poor sleep can increase symptom burden.
Treatment: Simple steps may make a big difference: appropriate room temperature, darkness, and quiet during the night (request a side room for in-patients). Give prescribed glucocorticoids in the morning. Avoid waking patients for late medications and routine observations. Discuss and address psychosocial issues. In some cases zopiclone or benzodiazepines may be used to help patients rest and re-establish normal sleep-wake cycles (may exacerbate delirium).

Pruritus

Causes: Systemic disease (renal failure, hepatitis, polycythaemia), cancer-related (cholestasis, lymphoma, leukaemia, hepatoma, myeloma, paraneoplastic), primary-skin disease, drug reaction (opioids, SSRI, chemotherapy).
Treatment: Underlying causes where possible: cholestasis (biliary stenting, colestyramine, sertraline, rifampicin), opioid-induced (antihistamine, opioid switch), paraneoplastic (paroxetine). Topical emollients regularly and as a soap substitute. Avoid topical antihistamines due to risk of contact dermatitis.

Venepuncture

Repeated venepuncture with the risk of painful extravasation and phlebitis may be avoided by use of a central catheter (eg Hickman® tunnelled line or PICC). Problems: infection, blockage (flush with 0.9% saline or dilute heparin every week), axillary thrombosis, and line slippage.

Agitation See 'Care in the last days of life', p536.

Respiratory tract secretions See 'Care in the last days of life', p536.

Spiritual pain

'The spiritual aspects of an illness concerns the human experiences of sickness (or 'dis-ease') and the search for meaning within it.'

Peter W Speck

Spirituality is a means of experiencing life. It relates to the way in which people understand and live their lives. It is comprised of elements including meaning, purpose, and something greater than 'self'. It is distinct from faith, which is a religious experience, that may or may not be part of spirituality. Spiritual pain[20,21] or suffering is common when people are facing death. It can include feelings of hopelessness, guilt, isolation, meaninglessness, and confusion. Consider:

- the past: painful memories, guilt
- the present: isolation, anger
- the future: fear, hopelessness.

Reminiscence helps address the past, provides context, and offers recognition of the patient as an individual. Anger should be acknowledged. Fear of the imagined future may not change, but is potentially reduced through discussion. The nature of hope may need to be modified. If hope for a cure is inappropriate, it should not be the main or only hope. Realistic hopes include discharge from hospital, seeing family members happy, being remembered. Making a will, handing over responsibilities, and dealing with unfinished business facilitate control and may allow a sense of completion.

►Remember the whole person: history, coping mechanisms, state of well-being. Elements such as these will alter how disease affects the patient and how the patient responds to disease.

►Companionship is essential in spiritual support. At times a doctor needs to modify their role to simply accompany the dying patient. This is manageable within established professional boundaries and therapeutic. If you cannot do this, find someone who can: palliative care teams, Macmillan nurses, and chaplains (a listening ear for patients of all faiths and none) are all valuable resources.

►Spiritual pain is exacerbated by physical symptoms. These must be addressed if spiritual support is to be effective.

Palliative care: care in the last days of life

Once it is recognized that a patient is entering the final days of their illness (see 'Diagnosing dying', p12), the focus of care should be the relief of distressing symptoms.[22]

►An individualized care plan should be made and discussed with your patient, their family, and relevant medical staff.

Continue to treat reversible problems as appropriate (eg urinary retention). Stop observations and blood tests (unless you are going to act on them). Rationalize medications but keep any that provide ongoing symptom benefit.

Prescribe as required subcutaneous end of life drugs. Prescribe PRN SC medications before they are needed, in anticipation of symptoms (see table 11.6).

Start a syringe driver when symptom control drugs are needed regularly (see table 11.7). Practice is variable, some drugs may be used outside of licensed indications. Always defer to local guidelines first. If pain relief is insufficient, review regular dose and recalculate the PRN requirement (1/10th–1/6th of 24h dose).

Anticipatory end of life medication

Table 11.6 Typical anticipatory medications.

Indication	Drug	Subcutaneous dose
Pain	Morphine	2.5mg SC or 5mg PO (maximum every 1h) If established on opioids use 1/10th–1/6th of daily dose (see p533 and table 11.5)
Agitation + N&V	Haloperidol	2.5mg SC (maximum every 1h)
Agitation + anxiety	Midazolam	2.5mg SC (maximum every 1h)
N&V	Levomepromazine	6.25mg SC TDS
Troublesome respiratory secretions	Glycopyrronium	200mcg SC every 4–8h

Syringe drivers

Syringe drivers (table 11.7) allow a continuous SC infusion of drugs, avoiding repeated cannulation and injection when the oral route is no longer feasible. Some medications should not be put in the same syringe—check interactions. Take into account regular doses when calculating requirements. If in doubt, seek expert help. Do not forget anticipatory prescribing in addition (table 11.6).

Table 11.7 Symptom control medication by SC infusion. Practice is variable, defer to local guidelines first.

Indication	Drug	Subcutaneous dose
Pain	Morphine	If opioid naïve: 10–15mg/24h If on opioids calculate daily opioid dose (consider reducing by 25–30%) then convert (table 11.5) to SC morphine over 24h
Anxiety, agitation, delirium	Midazolam	5–20mg/24h
	Levomepromazine	25–75mg/24h
	Haloperidol	2–10mg/24h
N&V	Cyclizine	150mg/24h
	Haloperidol	1–3mg/24h
	Levomepromazine	6.25–12.5mg/24h (sedation at higher doses)
Respiratory secretions	Hyoscine butylbromide	60–120mg/24h. Also used for bowel colic
	Glycopyrronium	600–1200mcg/24h
Seizures	Seizure prophylaxis: midazolam 20–30mg/24h (may sedate). Dexamethasone, midazolam and levetiracetam can be given by SC infusion.	

Manage agitation. Look for reversible causes (pain, dehydration, urinary retention). Use an antipsychotic agent (eg haloperidol) to manage agitated delirium (see tables 11.6, 11.7). Try a benzodiazepine such as midazolam if there is a large element of anxiety. *Opioids should not be used to sedate a dying patient.* Seek early advice from palliative care if agitation is escalating or a significant problem.

Manage excessive secretions. Noise is generated by turbulent air flow and pooling of saliva in the hypopharynx. This may be more distressing for relatives and staff than the patient. There is little evidence that pharmacological agents are beneficial, though they are commonly used. Repositioning and intermittent suctioning may help. If you think the patient is distressed, consider a trial of an antisecretory drug (glycopyrronium or hyoscine butylbromide: see tables 11.6, 11.7).

Hydration. Many patients approaching the end of life are unable to eat/drink or have a very poor appetite for food/fluid. Helping to take sips and good mouth care may suffice. Fluid via non-oral routes (NG, SC, IV) is given for symptomatic benefit; the effect on survival is unknown. Any potential benefit must be weighed against the risk of symptomatic fluid overload. Discuss this with patients and families, explaining the pros and cons of hydration and the uncertainty of the effect of hydration on survival:[23] relatives may assume the patient is dying faster because of dehydration or that they will be suffering with thirst. Make decisions about giving fluids on a case-by-case basis. Review a patient's hydration status at least daily.

Plan for death. Ensure that a 'Do not attempt resuscitation' or 'Allow natural death', order has been made. Discuss this with the patient (where appropriate), their family, and/or others of importance to them. Document everything clearly. Do they want to die at home? This can usually be arranged at very short notice with help from district nursing teams and community palliative care. Discuss transfer to a hospice or nursing home if appropriate.

Respond to changes in the clinical situation. Patients who are thought to be at the end of their life occasionally improve. Be alert to signs of improvement, and be prepared to switch back to active treatment when appropriate.

Communicate.[23] *The importance of clear and regular written and verbal communication with dying patients and their families cannot be overemphasized.* Find out what is important to your patient. How much information do they know and want to know about their situation and prognosis? Be sensitive to social, religious, and cultural issues.

On wanting to die

Physician-assisted suicide is the provision of drugs by a doctor for self-administration by a person to terminate their own life. This is distinct from euthanasia where a doctor administers the lethal drug. There have been repeated attempts to introduce physician-assisted dying (physician-assisted suicide only of the terminally ill) into UK law, but all have been rejected by Parliament.

Consider autonomy. Should competent patients have the right to determine their death, especially if their situation is unbearable, without prospect of improvement? It is a powerful argument. But bearable is subjective and prognosis is an inexact science. And beneficence is divided: is it merciful, or is it abandonment, to end suffering through death? And what of consent? Consent is key. Yet consent is complex. Could a legal process help? Not without a unique understanding of each patient and the means by which they experience life. A combination of law and medicine may offer false comfort without full accountability by either. Protection for the vulnerable is a valid concern for doctors and society.

Requests to hasten death are complex and include personal, psychological, spiritual, social, cultural, and demographic factors. ~10% of terminally ill patients will consider euthanasia or physician-assisted suicide. These wishes may or may not be fixed, with ~50% of patients changing their mind within 6 months. Discuss this. Ask your patient how they feel today and what they are afraid of feeling tomorrow. Listen. Answer questions. Offer palliative care. Palliative care is never futile. A wish to die is associated with a need for information, reassurance, and competence in symptom control. Provide these, or find someone who can.

12 Rheumatology

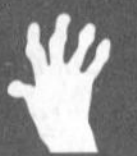

Contents

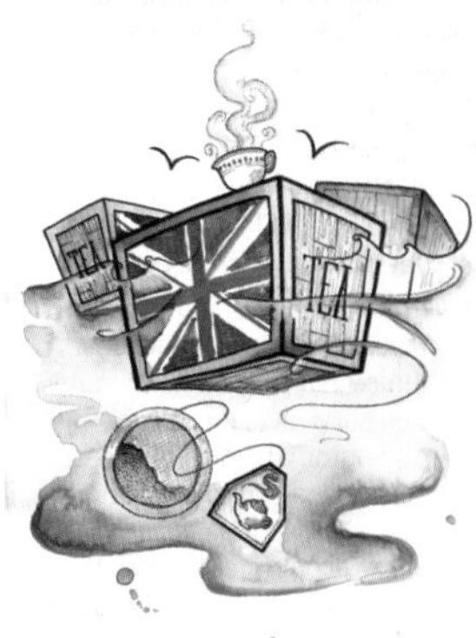

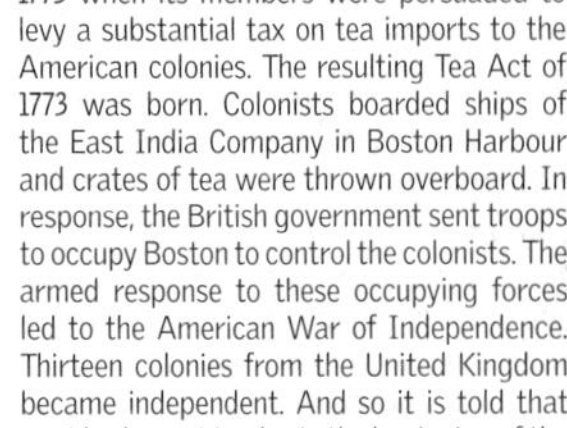

Fig 12.1 When William Pitt the Elder, British statesman, was struck by yet another attack of gout he was absent from Parliament in 1773 when its members were persuaded to levy a substantial tax on tea imports to the American colonies. The resulting Tea Act of 1773 was born. Colonists boarded ships of the East India Company in Boston Harbour and crates of tea were thrown overboard. In response, the British government sent troops to occupy Boston to control the colonists. The armed response to these occupying forces led to the American War of Independence. Thirteen colonies from the United Kingdom became independent. And so it is told that gout had a part to play in the beginning of the American Revolution!

A rapidly advancing speciality

Rheumatology originates from the Greek word 'rheuma' meaning that which 'flows as a river or stream'. The British Society of Rheumatology defines rheumatology as a 'multidisciplinary branch of medicine that deals with the investigation, diagnosis and management of patients with arthritis and other musculoskeletal conditions...incorporating over 200 disorders affecting joints, bones, muscles and soft tissues, including inflammatory arthritis and other systemic autoimmune disorders, vasculitis, soft tissue conditions, spinal pain and metabolic bone disease'. Rheumatological diseases affect over 10 million UK adults and 12 000 children. Recent advances owe largely to new discoveries about the immunology of these disorders and the discovery of biologic DMARDs.

We thank Professor Kevin Davies, our Specialist Reader, for his contribution to this chapter. We also thank Dr Susie Higgins for her contribution to this chapter.

The rheumatological history

In the assessment of an arthritic presentation, pay particular attention to the distribution of joint involvement (including spine) and the presence of symmetry. Also look for disruption of joint anatomy, limitation of movement (by pain or contracture), joint effusions and peri-articular involvement (see p540 for a fuller assessment). Ask about, and examine for, *extra-articular features:* skin and nail (see p76) involvement (include scalp, hairline, umbilicus, genitalia, and natal cleft—psoriasis can easily be missed); eye signs (see p560); lungs (eg fibrosis) (see p198); kidneys (see p314); heart; GI (eg mouth ulcers, diarrhoea); GU (eg urethritis, genital ulcers); and CNS.

Three screening questions for musculoskeletal disease

1 Are you free of any pain or stiffness in your joints, muscles, or back?
2 Can you dress yourself without too much difficulty?
3 Can you manage walking up and down stairs?

If *yes* to all three, serious inflammatory muscle/joint disease is unlikely.

Presenting symptoms:
- Pattern of involved joints.
- Symmetry (or not).
- Morning stiffness >30min (eg RA).
- Pain, swelling, loss of function, erythema, warmth.

Extra-articular features:
- Rashes, photosensitivity (eg SLE).
- Raynaud's (SLE; systemic sclerosis; polymyositis and dermatomyositis).
- Dry eyes or mouth (Sjögren's).
- Red eyes, iritis (eg AS).
- Diarrhoea/urethritis (reactive arthritis).
- Nodules or nodes (eg RA; TB; gout).
- Mouth/genital ulcers (eg Behçet's, SLE).
- Weight loss (eg malignancy, any systemic inflammatory disease).

Related diseases:
- Crohn's/UC (in ankylosing spondylitis), preceding infections, psoriasis.

Current and past drugs:
- NSAIDs, DMARDs (p547).
- Biological agents (eg TNFα inhibitors).

Family history:
- Arthritis, psoriasis, autoimmune disease.

Social history:
- Age.
- Occupation.
- Sexual history.
- Ethnicity (eg SLE is commoner in African-Caribbeans and Asians).
- Ability to function (eg dressing, grooming, writing, walking).
- Domestic situation, social support, home adaptations.
- Smoking (may worsen RA).
- IBD.

Arthritides

The pattern of joint involvement can provide clues to the underlying cause (table 12.1).

Table 12.1 Patterns of presentation of arthritis

Monoarthritis	Oligoarthritis (≤5 joints)	Polyarthritis (>5 joints involved)	
Septic arthritis	Crystal arthritis	**Symmetrical**	**Asymmetrical**
Crystal arthritis (gout, CPPD)	Psoriatic arthritis	Rheumatoid arthritis	Reactive arthritis
Osteoarthritis	Reactive arthritis, eg *Yersinia, Salmonella, Campylobacter*	Osteoarthritis	Psoriatic arthritis
Trauma (haemarthrosis)	Ankylosing spondylitis	Viruses (eg hepatitis A, B, & C; mumps)	
	Osteoarthritis	Systemic conditions* (can be either)	

*Connective tissue disease (eg SLE and relapsing polychondritis), sarcoidosis, malignancy (eg leukaemia), endocarditis, haemochromatosis, sickle-cell anaemia, familial Mediterranean fever, Behçet's.

▸▸Exclude septic arthritis in any acutely inflamed joint, as it can destroy a joint in under 24h (p544). Inflammation may be less overt if immunocompromised (eg from the many immunosuppressive drugs used in rheumatological conditions) or if there is underlying joint disease. Joint aspiration (p541) is the key investigation, and if you are unable to do it, find someone who can.

Assessing the locomotor system

This aims to screen for rheumatological conditions primarily affecting mobility (as a consequence of underlying joint disease). It is based on the GALS locomotor screen (Gait, Arms, Legs, Spine).[1]

Essence 'Look, feel, and move' (active and passive). If a *joint looks normal* to you, *feels normal* to the patient, and has *full range of movement*, it usually is normal. Make sure the patient is comfortable, and obtain their consent before examination. The GALS screening examination should be done in light underwear.

Spine: Observe from behind: is muscle bulk normal (buttocks, shoulders)? Is the spine straight? Are paraspinal muscles symmetrical? Any swellings/deformities? *Observe from the side:* is cervical and lumbar lordosis normal? Any kyphosis? '*Touch your toes, please*': is lumbar spine flexion normal, eg Schober's test?[1] *Observe from in front: 'Tilt your head'* (without moving the shoulders)—tests lateral neck flexion. Palpate for typical fibromyalgia tender points (see p558).

Arms: 'Try putting your hands behind your head'—tests functional shoulder movement. *'Arms out straight'*—tests elbow extension and forearm supination/pronation. Examine the hands: any deformity (fig 12.2), wasting, or swellings? *Squeeze across 2nd-5th metacarpophalangeal joints.* Pain may denote joint or tendon synovitis. *'Put your index finger on your thumb'*—tests pincer grip. Assess dexterity, eg fastening a button or picking up a coin.

Legs: Observe legs: normal quadriceps bulk? Any swelling or deformity? *With patient lying supine:* any leg length discrepancy? *Internally/externally rotate each hip in flexion. Passively flex knee and hip to the full extent.* Is movement limited? Any crepitus? *Find any knee effusion* using the patella tap test. If there is fluid, consider aspirating and testing for crystals or infection. *With patient standing: observe feet:* any deformity? Are arches high or flat? Any callosities? These may indicate an abnormal gait of some chronicity. *Squeeze across metatarsophalangeal joints:* see as for arms. Also: although not in the GALS system, *palpate the heel and Achilles tendon* to identify plantar fasciitis and Achilles tendonitis often associated with seronegative rheumatological conditions. *Examine the patient's shoes* for signs of uneven wear.

Gait: Observe walking: is the gait smooth? Good arm swing? Stride length OK? Normal heel strike and toe off? Can they turn quickly?

Range of joint movement Is noted in degrees, with anatomical position being the neutral position—eg elbow flexion 0°-150° normally, but with fixed flexion and limited movement, range may be reduced to 30°-90°. A valgus deformity deviates laterally (away from the mid-line, fig 12.3); a varus deformity points towards the mid-line.

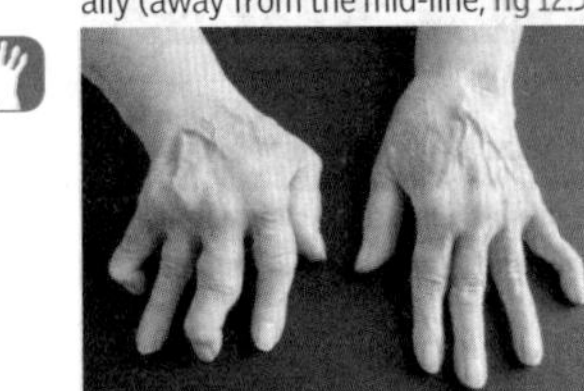

Fig 12.2 Swan-neck deformity.

Reproduced from Watts *et al.*, *Oxford Textbook of Rheumatology*, 2013, with permission from Oxford University Press.

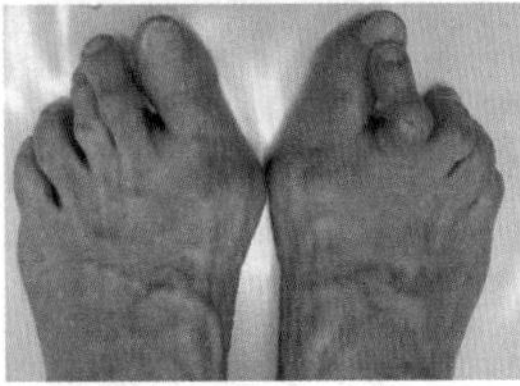

Fig 12.3 Bilateral hallux valgus.

Reproduced from *British Medical Journal*, 'Hallux valgus', R Choa, R Sharp, K R Mahtani, 2010, with permission from BMJ Publishing Group Ltd.

1 Schober's test: make a mark on the lumbar spine at the level of the posterior iliac spine. Measure out a line from 5cm below to 10cm above the mark. Ask to bend forward as far as they can. If the line does not lengthen by at least 5cm in flexion, there is reduced lumbar flexion, eg in ankylosing spondylitis.

Some important rheumatological investigations

Joint aspiration: The most important investigation in any monoarthritic presentation (table 12.2, see also *OHCS* p706). Send synovial fluid for urgent white cell count, Gram stain, polarized light microscopy (for crystals, p548), and culture. The risk of inducing septic arthritis, using sterile precautions, is <1:10 000.[2] Look for blood,[3] pus, and crystals (gout or CPPD crystal arthropathy; p548). ►Do not attempt joint aspiration through inflamed and potentially infected skin (eg through a psoriatic plaque or overlying cellulitis).

Table 12.2 Synovial fluid in health and disease

	Appearance	Viscosity	WBC/mm³	Neutrophils
Normal	Clear, colourless	↔	≲200	None
Osteoarthritis	Clear, straw	↑	≲1000	≲50%
Haemorrhagic*	Bloody, xanthochromic	Varies	≲10 000	≲50%
Acutely inflamed				
• *RA*	Turbid, yellow	↓	1000–50 000	Varies
• *Crystal*	Turbid, yellow	↓	5000–50 000	~80%
Septic	Turbid, yellow	↓	10 000–100 000	>90%

*Eg trauma, tumour, or haemophilia.

Blood tests: FBC, ESR, urate, U&E, CRP. Blood culture for septic arthritis. Consider rheumatoid factor, anti-CCP, ANA, other autoantibodies (p553), and HLA B27 (p551)—as guided by presentation. Consider causes of reactive arthritis (p551), eg viral serology, urine chlamydia PCR, hepatitis and HIV serology if risk factors are present.

Radiology: Look for erosions, calcification, widening or loss of joint space, changes in underlying bone of affected joints (eg periarticular osteopenia, sclerotic areas, osteophytes). Characteristic X-ray features for various arthritides are shown in figs 12.4–12.6. Irregularity of the sacroiliac joints is seen in spondyloarthritis. Ultrasound and MRI are more sensitive in identifying effusions, synovitis, enthesitis and infection than plain radiographs—discuss further investigations with a radiologist. Do a CXR for RA, vasculitis, TB, and sarcoid.

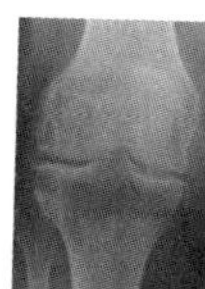

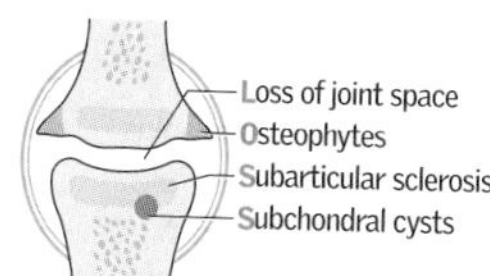

Fig 12.4 X-ray features of osteoarthritis.
Courtesy of Dr DC Howlett.

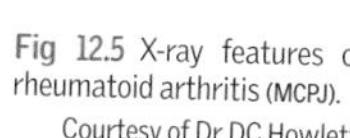

Fig 12.5 X-ray features of rheumatoid arthritis (MCPJ).
Courtesy of Dr DC Howlett.

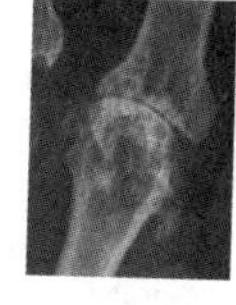

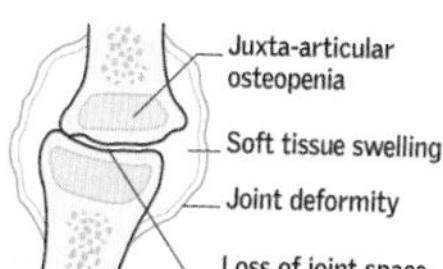

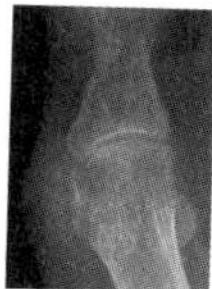

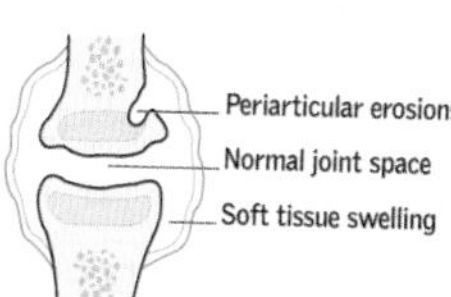

Fig 12.6 X-ray features of gout (1st MTPJ).
Courtesy of Dr DC Howlett.

Back pain

Back pain is very common, and often self-limiting, but *be alert to sinister causes*, ie malignancy, infection, or inflammatory causes.

Red flags for sinister causes of back pain	
►Aged <20yrs or >55yrs old	►Thoracic back pain
►Acute onset in elderly people	►Morning stiffness
►Constant or progressive pain	►Bilateral or alternating leg pain
►Nocturnal pain	►Neurological disturbance (incl. sciatica)
►Worse pain on being supine	►Sphincter disturbance
►Fever, night sweats, weight loss	►Current or recent infection
►History of malignancy	►Immunosuppression, eg steroids/HIV
►Abdominal mass	►Leg claudication or exercise-related leg weakness/numbness (spinal stenosis).

Examination

1. With the patient standing, gauge the extent and smoothness of lumbar forward/lateral flexion and extension (see p540).
2. *Test for sacroiliitis:* palpate posteriorly down the length of the spine, including over spinous processes, paraspinal muscles, and the sacroiliac joints; examining for tenderness.
3. Neurological deficits (see BOX): test lower limb sensation, power, and deep tendon and plantar reflexes. Digital rectal examination for perianal tone and sensation.
4. Examine for nerve root pain (table 12.3): this is distributed in relevant dermatomes, and is worsened by coughing or bending forward. *Straight leg test* (L4, L5, S1): positive if raising the leg with the knee extended causes pain below the knee, which increases on foot dorsiflexion (Lasègue's sign). It suggests irritation to the sciatic nerve. The main cause is lumbar disc prolapse. Also *femoral stretch test* (L2–L4): pain in front of thigh on lifting the hip into extension with the patient lying face downwards and the knee flexed.
5. Signs of generalized disease—eg malignancy. Examine other systems (eg abdomen) as pain may be referred.

Causes Age determines the most likely causes:

15–30yrs: Prolapsed disc, trauma, fractures, ankylosing spondylitis (AS; p550), spondylolisthesis (a forward shift of one vertebra over another, which is congenital or due to trauma), pregnancy.

30–50yrs: Degenerative spinal disease, prolapsed disc, malignancy (primary or secondary from lung, breast, prostate, thyroid, or kidney ca).

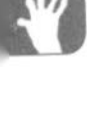

>50yrs: Degenerative, osteoporotic vertebral collapse, Paget's (see p685), malignancy, myeloma (see p368), spinal stenosis.

Rarer: Cauda equina tumours, psoas abscess, spinal infection (eg discitis, usually staphylococcal but also *Proteus*, *E. coli*, *S. typhi*, and TB—there are often no systemic signs).

Investigations Arrange relevant tests if you suspect a specific cause, or if red flag symptoms: FBC, ESR, and CRP (myeloma, infection, tumour), U&E, ALP (Paget's), serum/urine electrophoresis (myeloma), PSA. *X-rays*—imaging may not always be necessary but can exclude bony abnormalities and fractures. Correlation between radiographic abnormalities and clinical features can be poor. *MRI* is the image of choice and can detect disc prolapse, cord compression (fig 12.7), cancer, infection, or inflammation (eg sacroiliitis).

Management ►►Urgent neurosurgical referral if any neurological deficit (see BOX). Keep the diagnosis under review. For non-specific back pain, focus on *education* and *self-management*. Advise patients to continue normal activites and be active. Regular paracetamol ± NSAIDs ± codeine. Consider low-dose amitriptyline/duloxetine if these fail (not SSRIs for pain). Offer *physiotherapy*, *acupuncture*, or an *exercise programme* if not improving.[4] Address *psychosocial issues*, which may predispose to developing chronic pain and disability (see p559). Referral to pain clinic or surgical options for patients with intractable symptoms.

Neurosurgical emergencies

►*Acute cauda equina compression* Alternating or bilateral root pain in legs, saddle anaesthesia (perianal), loss of anal tone on PR, bladder ± bowel incontinence.
►*Acute cord compression* Bilateral pain, LMN signs (p446) at level of compression, UMN and sensory loss below, sphincter disturbance.
Immediate urgent treatment prevents irreversible loss, eg laminectomy for disc protrusions, radiotherapy for tumours, decompression for abscesses.
Causes (same for both): bony metastasis (look for missing pedicle on x-ray), large disc protrusion, myeloma, cord or paraspinal tumour, TB (p392), abscess.

Table 12.3 Nerve root lesions

Nerve root	Pain	Weakness	Reflex affected
L2	Across upper thigh	Hip flexion and adduction	Nil
L3	Across lower thigh	Hip adduction, knee extension	Knee jerk
L4	Across knee to medial malleolus	Knee extension, foot inversion and dorsiflexion	Knee jerk
L5	Lateral shin to dorsum of foot and great toe	Hip extension and abduction Knee flexion Foot and great toe dorsiflexion	Great toe jerk
S1	Posterior calf to lateral foot and little toe	Knee flexion Foot and toe plantar flexion Foot eversion	Ankle jerk

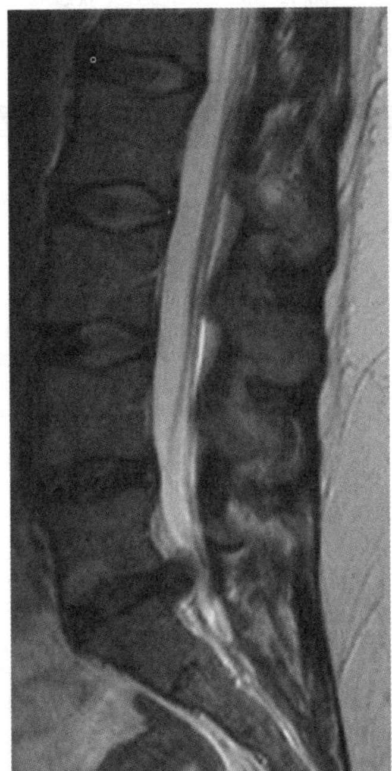

Fig 12.7 Sagittal T2-weighted MRI of the lumbar spine showing a herniated L5-S1 disc.

Courtesy of Norwich Radiology Department.

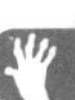

Osteoarthritis (OA)

Osteoarthritis is the most common joint condition worldwide, with a clinically significant impact on >10% of persons aged >60 years.[5] It is usually primary (generalized), but may be secondary to joint disease or other conditions (eg haemochromatosis, obesity, occupational).

Signs and symptoms *Localized disease* (often knee or hip): Pain and crepitus on movement, with background ache at rest. Worse with prolonged activity. Joints may 'gel' (brief stiffness after rest, usually 10-15 minutes or so). Joints may feel unstable, with a perceived lack of power due to pain. *Generalized disease:* 'Nodal OA' (typically DIP, PIP, CMC joints, and knees in post-menopausal females). There may be joint tenderness, derangement and bony swelling (Heberden's at DIP and Bouchard's at PIP), reduced range of movement and mild synovitis. Assess effect of symptoms on occupation, family duties, hobbies, and lifestyle expectations.

Tests Plain radiographs show: Loss of joint space, Osteophytes, Subarticular sclerosis and Subchondral cysts (fig 12.4 p541). CRP may be slightly elevated.[6]

Management *Core treatments:* Exercise to improve local muscle strength and general aerobic fitness (irrespective of age, severity, or comorbidity). Weight loss if overweight.[7] *Analgesia:* Regular paracetamol ± topical NSAIDs. If ineffective use codeine or short-term oral NSAID (+PPI)—see BOX. Topical capsaicin (derived from chillies) may help. Intra-articular steroid injections temporarily relieve pain in severe symptoms. Intra-articular hyaluronic acid injections (viscosupplementation) are not NICE approved[8] Glucosamine and chondroitin products are not recommended, although patients may try them if they wish (can be bought over the counter). *Non-pharmacological:* Use a multidisciplinary approach, including physiotherapists and occupational therapists. Try heat or cold packs at the site of pain, walking aids, stretching/manipulation or TENS. *Surgery:* Joint replacement (hips, or knees) is the best way to deal with severe OA that has a substantial impact on quality of life.

Septic arthritis

►►Consider septic arthritis in any acutely inflamed joint, as it can destroy a joint in under 24h and has a mortaility rate up to 11%. Inflammation may be less overt if immunocompromised (eg from medication) or if there is underlying joint disease. The knee is affected in >50% cases.

Risk factors Pre-existing joint disease (especially rheumatoid arthritis); diabetes mellitus, immunosuppression, chronic renal failure, recent joint surgery, prosthetic joints (where infection is particularly difficult to treat), IV drug abuse, age >80yrs.[9]

Investigations Urgent joint aspiration for synovial fluid microscopy and culture is the key investigation (p541), as plain radiographs and CRP may be normal. The main differential diagnoses are the crystal arthropathies (p548). Blood cultures are essential (prior to antibiotics).

Ask yourself 'How did the organism get there?' Is there immunosuppression, or another focus of infection, eg from indwelling IV lines, infected skin, or pneumonia (present in up to 50% of those with pneumococcal arthritis)?[10]

►►**Treatment** If in doubt start empirical IV antibiotics (after aspiration) until sensitivities are known. Common causative organisms are *Staph. aureus*, streptococci, *Neisseria gonococcus*, and Gram −ve bacilli. Follow local guidelines for antibiotic choice and contact microbiology for advice for all complex cases/immunosuppressed patients (eg HIV). Consider flucloxacillin 2g QDS IV (clindamycin if penicillin allergic); Vancomycin IV plus 2nd- or 3rd-generation cephalosporin, eg cefuroxime if MRSA risk; 2nd- or 3rd-generation cephalosporin if Gram −ve organisms suspected.[11] For suspected gonococcus or meningococcus, consider ceftriaxone. Antibiotics are required for a prolonged period, conventionally ~2 weeks IV, then if patient improving 2-4 weeks PO.[12] Consider orthopaedic review for arthrocentesis, washout, and debridement; ►►always urgently refer patients with prosthetic joint involvement.

Prescribing NSAIDs: benefit vs risk profiling

Around 60% of patients will respond to any NSAID, but there is considerable variation in response and tolerance—if one isn't effective, try another. Mainly act as analgesics rather than modifying the disease process *per se*.

►►NSAIDs caused ~2000 UK deaths in 2011.[13] Individualized risk: benefit analysis for each patient (including indication, dose, proposed duration of use, and comorbidity) is crucial and needs careful and experienced thought. Follow local recommendations and national guidelines where available.

NSAID side effects: ►The main serious side effects are GI bleeding (and ulcers and perforation), cardiovascular events (MI and stroke), and renal injury. The risks are dose related, starting with the first dose, so always aim to use the lowest possible dose for the shortest period of time. Risks increase considerably with age, polypharmacy, history of peptic ulcers, and renal impairment.

GI side effects: NICE recommends co-prescription of PPI for any patient aged >45 years, and those with other risk factors for GI bleeding. Drug interactions can increase bleeding risks—avoid concomitant prescribing of anticoagulants, antiplatelet agents, SSRI, spironolactone, steroids, and bisphosphonates. Coxibs are slightly lower risk than non-selective NSAIDS.

Cardiovascular side effects: NSAIDs—all are associated with a small increased risk of MI and stroke (independent of cardiovascular risk factor or duration of use).[14] Risks are higher in those with concomitant IHD risk factors, eg diabetes and hypertension. Coxibs and diclofenac are higher risk, and are contraindicated if prior history of MI, PVD, stroke, or heart failure. Naproxen has the lowest cardiovascular risk. Low-dose celecoxib may be considered for patients on low-dose aspirin (if NSAID is required) as it does not interact with it.[15]

Renal risks: Higher for patients already on diuretics, ACE, or ARB. Risks are also increased in the elderly, those with hypertension and T2DM. Overall, naproxen (<1000mg/day) or ibuprofen (<1200mg/day) plus PPI may be the safest options.

Alternatives to NSAIDs: Paracetamol, topical NSAIDs, opioids. Strengthening exercises may be more beneficial than mild oral analgesics.

Counselling patients: Make sure patients understand about the drugs they are taking: *bleeding is more common in those who know less about their drugs.*[16]

- Only to take NSAIDs when they need them.
- Stop NSAIDs and seek urgent medical review if they develop abdominal pain or any symptoms of GI bleeding (eg report black stools ± faints immediately).
- Do not mix prescription NSAIDs with over-the-counter formulations: mixing NSAIDs can increase risks 20-fold.
- Smoking and alcohol increase risk profile of NSAIDs.

Rheumatoid arthritis (RA)

RA is a chronic systemic inflammatory disease, characterized by a symmetrical, deforming, peripheral polyarthritis. It increases the risk of cardiovascular disease by 2-3 fold. **Epidemiology** Prevalence is ~1% (↑ in smokers). ♀:♂ >2:1. Peak onset: 5th-6th decade. HLA DR4/DR1 linked (associated with ↑severity).

Presentation *Typically:* Symmetrical swollen, painful, and stiff small joints of hands and feet, worse in the morning. This can fluctuate and larger joints may become involved. *Less common presentations:* •Sudden onset, widespread arthritis. •Recurring mono/polyarthritis of various joints (*palindromic RA*).[2] •Persistent monoarthritis (knee, shoulder, or hip). •Systemic illness with extra-articular symptoms, eg fatigue, fever, weight loss, pericarditis, and pleurisy, but initially few joint problems (commoner in ♂). •Polymyalgic onset—vague limb girdle aches. •Recurrent soft tissue problems (eg frozen shoulder, carpal tunnel syndrome, de Quervain's tenosynovitis).

Signs *Early:* (Inflammation, no joint damage.) Swollen MCP, PIP, wrist, or MTP joints (often symmetrical). Look for tenosynovitis or bursitis. *Later:* (Joint damage, deformity.) Ulnar deviation and subluxation of the wrist and fingers. Boutonnière and swan-neck deformities of fingers (fig 12.2 on p540) or Z-deformity of thumbs occur. Hand extensor tendons may rupture. Foot changes are similar. Larger joints can be involved. Atlanto-axial joint subluxation may threaten the spinal cord (rare).

Extra-articular manifestations Affect ~40% of RA patients. *Nodules:* Elbows, lungs, cardiac, CNS, lymphadenopathy, vasculitis. *Lungs:* Pleural disease, interstitial fibrosis, bronchiolitis obliterans, organizing pneumonia. *Cardiac:* IHD, pericarditis, pericardial effusion; carpal tunnel syndrome; peripheral neuropathy; splenomegaly (seen in 5%; only 1% have Felty's syndrome: RA + splenomegaly + neutropenia, see p698). *Eye:* Episcleritis, scleritis, scleromalacia, keratoconjunctivitis sicca (p560); osteoporosis; amyloidosis is rare (p370).[17,18]

Investigations Rheumatoid factor (RhF) is positive in ~70% (p553). High titres associated with severe disease, erosions, and extra-articular disease. Anticyclic citrullinated peptide antibodies (anti-CCP) are highly specific (~98%) for RA with a reasonable sensitivity (70-80%); they may also predict disease progression.[19] Anaemia of chronic disease, ↑platelets, ↑ESR, ↑CRP. *X-rays* show soft tissue swelling, juxta-articular osteopenia and ↓joint space. Later there may be bony erosions, subluxation, or complete carpal destruction (see fig 12.5 on p541). Ultrasound and MRI can identify synovitis more accurately, and have greater sensitivity in detecting bone erosions than conventional X-rays.[20]

Diagnostic criteria See table 12.4.

Management ►Refer early to a rheumatologist (before irreversible destruction).
- Disease activity is measured using the DAS28.[3] Treatment should be escalated until satisfactory control is achieved: 'treat to target'.
- Early use of DMARDs and biological agents improves long-term outcomes (see BOX 'Influencing biological events in RA').
- Steroids rapidly reduce symptoms and inflammation. Avoid starting unless appropriately experienced. Useful for acute exacerbations, eg IM depot *methylprednisolone* 80-120mg. Intra-articular steroids have a rapid but short-term effect (*OHCS* pp706-9). Oral steroids (eg *prednisolone* 7.5mg/d) may control difficult symptoms, but side effects preclude routine long-term use.
- NSAIDs (see p545) are good for symptom relief, but have no effect on disease progression. Paracetamol and weak opiates are rarely effective.
- Offer specialist physio- and occupational therapy, eg for aids and splints.
- Surgery may relieve pain, improve function, and prevent deformity.
- There is ↑risk of cardiovascular and cerebrovascular disease, as atherosclerosis is accelerated in RA.[21] Manage risk factors (p93). Smoking also ↑ symptoms of RA.

2 In rheumatological palindromes, arthritis lasting hours or days runs to and fro, visiting and revisiting three or more sites, typically knees, wrists, and MCP joints. It may presage RA, SLE, Whipple's, or Behçet's disease. Remissions are (initially) complete, leaving no radiological mark.
3 28-joint Disease Activity Score—assesses tenderness and swelling at 28 joints (MCPs, PIPs, wrists, elbows, shoulders, knees), ESR/CRP, and patient's self-reported symptom severity.

Table 12.4 Criteria for diagnosing RA[22]

	When to suspect RA? Those with ≥1 swollen joint and a suggestive clinical history, which is not better explained by another disease. Scores ≥6 are diagnostic.		
A	*Joint involvement* (swelling or tenderness ± imaging evidence)		
	1 large joint =0	2–10 large joints =1	1–3 small* joints† =2
	4–10 small* joints† =3	>10 joints (at least 1 small joint) =5	
B	*Serology* (at least 1 test result needed)		
	Negative RF *and* negative anti-CCP =0	Low +ve RF *or* low +ve anti-CCP =2	
	High +ve RF *or* high +ve anti-CCP =3		
C	*Acute phase reactants* (at least 1 test result needed)		
	Normal CRP and normal ESR =0	Abnormal CRP or abnormal ESR =1	
D	*Duration of symptoms:* <6 weeks =0 ≥6 weeks =1		

*= MCPJ, PIPJ, 2nd–5th MTPJ, wrists, and thumb IPJ; †= with or without involvement of large joints.

Quality of life

Depression, disability, and pain are important quality of life predictors. Be mindful of the impact of disease on relationships, work, and hobbies and acknowledge and explore this with your patients. Patients may wish to investigate complementary therapies and may find benefit from support groups .

Influencing biological events in RA

The chief biological event is inflammation. Over-produced cytokines and cellular processes erode cartilage and bone, and produce the systemic effects seen in RA.
Disease-modifying antirheumatic drugs (DMARDs) are 1st line and should ideally be started within 3 months of persistent symptoms. They can take 6–12 weeks for symptomatic benefit. Best results are often achieved with a combination of methotrexate, sulfasalazine, and hydroxychloroquine.[23] Leflunomide is another option. ►*Immunosuppression* is a potentially fatal SE of treatment (especially in combination with methotrexate) which can result in pancytopenia, ↑susceptibility to infection (including atypical organisms), and neutropenic sepsis (p352). Regular FBC, LFT monitoring.[24]
Other SE •Methotrexate—pneumonitis (pre treatment CXR), oral ulcers, hepatotoxicity, teratogenic. •Sulfasalazine—rash, ↓sperm count, oral ulcers, GI upset. •Leflunomide—teratogenicity (♂ and ♀), oral ulcers, ↑BP, hepatotoxicity. •Hydroxychloroquine—can cause retinopathy; pre treatment and annual eye screen required.
Biological agents and NICE guidance Initiated by specialists, for patients with active disease despite adequate trial of at least 2 DMARDs. Pre treatment screening for TB, hepatitis B/C, HIV essential.
1 *TNFα inhibitors:* Eg infliximab (p265), etanercept, adalimumab, are approved by NICE as 1st-line agents. Where methotrexate is contraindicated, can be used as monotherapy. Clinical response can be striking, with improved function and health outcomes, although response may be inadequate/unsustained.[25]
2 *B-cell depletion:* Eg rituximab, used in combination with methotrexate and approved by NICE for severe active RA where DMARDs and a TNFα blocker have failed.[26]
3 *IL-1 and IL-6 inhibition:* Eg tocilizumab (IL-6 receptor blocker), approved by NICE in combination with methotrexate where TNFα blocker has failed (or is contraindicated).[27] Monitor for hypercholesterolaemia.
4 *Inhibition of T-cell co-stimulation:* Eg abatacept—licensed for active RA where patients have not responded to DMARDs or TNFα blocker.[28]

Side effects of biological agents Serious infection, reactivation of TB (∴ screen and consider prophylaxis) and hepatitis B; worsening heart failure; hypersensitivity; injection-site reactions and blood disorders. ANA and reversible SLE-type illness may evolve. Data suggests there is no increased risk of solid organ tumours but skin cancers may be more common.[29] TNF inhibitors do not appear to be associated with a further increase in the already elevated lymphoma occurrence in RA.[30]

Crystal arthropathies: gout

Gout[31] typically presents with an acute monoarthropathy with severe joint inflammation (fig 12.8). >50% occur at the metatarsophalangeal joint of the big toe (fig 12.12) (podagra). Other common joints are the ankle, foot, small joints of the hand, wrist, elbow, or knee. It can be polyarticular. It is caused by deposition of monosodium urate crystals in and near joints. Attacks may be precipitated by trauma, surgery, starvation, infection, or diuretics. It is associated with raised plasma urate. In the long term, urate deposits (= tophi, eg in pinna, tendons, joints; see fig 12.9) and renal disease (stones, interstitial nephritis) may occur. *Prevalence:* ~1%. ♂:♀ ≈ 4:1.

Differential diagnoses Exclude septic arthritis in any acute monoarthropathy (p544). Then consider reactive arthritis, haemarthrosis, CPPD (see following topic) and palindromic RA (p546).

Risk factors *Reduced urate excretion:* Elderly, men, post-menopausal females, impaired renal function, hypertension, metabolic syndrome, diuretics, antihypertensives, aspirin. *Excess urate production:* Dietary (alcohol, sweeteners, red meat, seafood), genetic disorders, myelo- and lymphoproliferative disorders, psoriasis, tumour-lysis syndrome, drugs (eg alcohol, warfarin, cytotoxics). *Associations:* Cardiovascular disease, hypertension, diabetes mellitus, and chronic renal failure (see p680).[31] Gout is an independent risk factor for mortality from cardiovascular and renal disease. Screen for and treat CKD, hypertension, dyslipidaemia, diabetes.

Investigations Polarized light microscopy of synovial fluid shows *negatively birefringent* urate crystals (fig 12.10). Serum urate (SUA) is usually raised but may be normal.[32] Radiographs show only soft-tissue swelling in the early stages. Later, well-defined 'punched out' erosions are seen in juxta-articular bone (see fig 12.6 on p541). There is no sclerotic reaction, and joint spaces are preserved until late.

Treatment of acute gout High-dose NSAID (see BOX, p545) or if CI use colchicine (500mcg BD) which is effective but slower to work (*BNF* states max 6mg per course although rheumatologists will often use more).[33] NB: in renal impairment, NSAIDs and colchicine are problematic. Steroids (oral, IM, or intra-articular) may also be used.[34] Rest and elevate joint. Ice packs and 'bed cages' can be effective.

Prevention Lose weight, avoid prolonged fasts, alcohol excess, purine-rich meats, and low-dose aspirin. *Prophylaxis:* Start if >1 attack in 12 months, tophi, or renal stones. The aim is to ↓ attacks and prevent damage caused by crystal deposition. Use *allopurinol* and titrate from 100mg/24h, increasing every 4 weeks until plasma urate <0.3mmol/L (max 300mg/8h). SE: rash, fever, ↓WCC. Allopurinol may trigger an attack so wait 3 weeks after an acute episode, and cover with regular NSAID (for up to 6 weeks) or colchicine (0.5mg/12h PO for up to 6 months). Avoid stopping allopurinol in acute attacks once established. *Febuxostat* (80mg/24h) is an alternative if allopurinol is CI or not tolerated. It ↓ uric acid by inhibiting xanthine oxidase (SE: ↑LFTs) and is more effective at reducing serum urate than allopurinol (number of acute attacks the same).[35] Uricosuric drugs ↑ urate excretion.

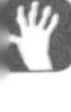

Calcium pyrophosphate deposition (CPPD)

- **Acute CPPD crystal arthritis** Acute monoarthropathy usually of larger joints in elderly. Usually spontaneous but can be provoked by illness, surgery, or trauma.
- **Chronic CPPD** Inflammatory RA-like (symmetrical) polyarthritis and synovitis.
- **Osteoarthritis** with CPPD chronic polyarticular osteoarthritis with superimposed acute CPP attacks.

Risk factors Old age, hyperparathyroidism (see p222), haemochromatosis (see p288), hypophosphataemia (see p679). **Tests** Polarized light microscopy of synovial fluid shows weakly positively birefringent crystals (fig 12.11). It is associated with soft tissue calcium deposition on x-ray. **Management** Acute attacks: cool packs, rest, aspiration, and intra-articular steroids. NSAIDs (+PPI) ± colchicine 0.5–1.0mg/24h (used with caution) may prevent acute attacks. Methotrexate and hydroxychloroquine may be considered for chronic CPP inflammatory arthritis.[36]

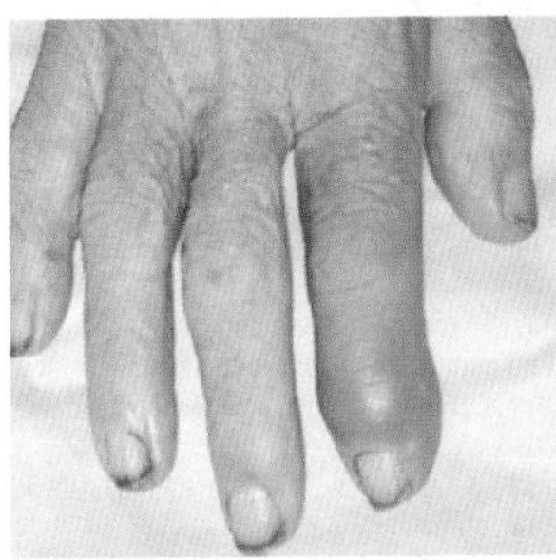

Fig 12.8 Acute monoarthritis in gout.

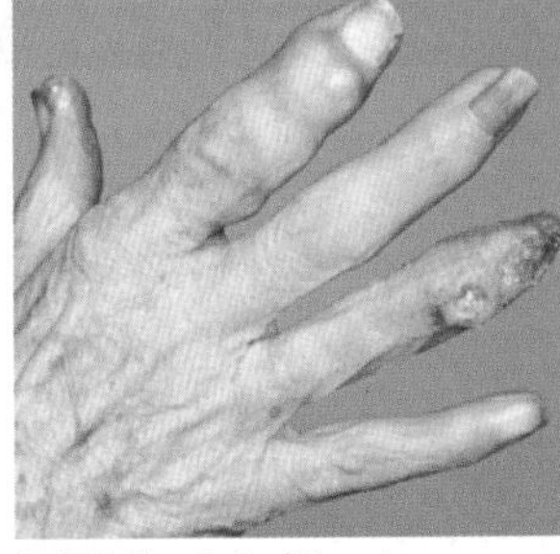

Fig 12.9 Ulcerated tophi in gout.

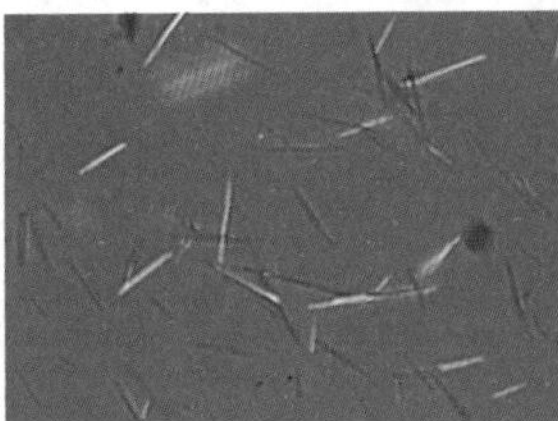

Fig 12.10 **N**eedle-shaped monosodium urate crystals found in gout, displaying **N**egative birefringence under polarized light.

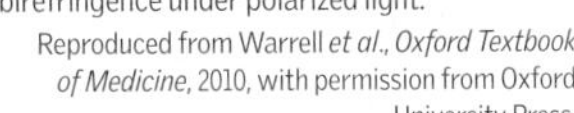

Reproduced from Warrell *et al*., *Oxford Textbook of Medicine*, 2010, with permission from Oxford University Press.

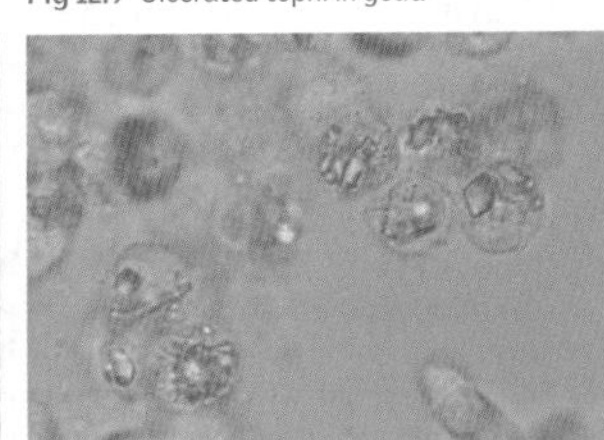

Fig 12.11 Rhomboid-shaped calcium pyrophosphate dihydrate crystals in **P**seudogout, showing **P**ositive birefringence in polarized light.

Image courtesy of Prof. Eliseo Pascual, Sección de Reumatología, Hospital General Universitario de Alicante.

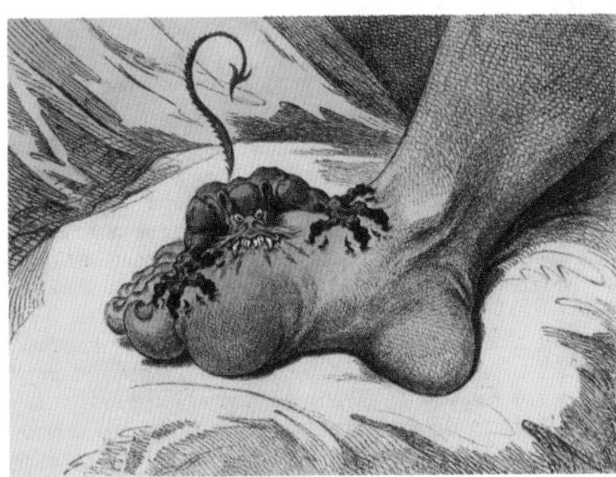

Fig 12.12 Don't underestimate the severity of pain caused by gout—as illustrated by satirical artist and gout sufferer James Gillray (1756–1815).

© Lordprice collection / Alamy Stock Photo.

Spondyloarthritides

The spondyloarthropathies (SpA) are a group of related chronic inflammatory conditions. They tend to, although not always, affect the axial skeleton with shared clinical features:

1. Seronegativity (= rheumatoid factor −ve).
2. HLA B27 association—see BOX.
3. 'Axial arthritis': pathology in spine (spondylo-) and sacroiliac joints.
4. Asymmetrical large-joint oligoarthritis (ie <5 joints) or monoarthritis.
5. Enthesitis: inflammation of the site of insertion of tendon or ligament into bone, eg plantar fasciitis, Achilles tendonitis, costochondritis.
6. Dactylitis: inflammation of an entire digit ('sausage digit'), due to soft tissue oedema, and tenosynovial and joint inflammation.
7. Extra-articular manifestations: eg iritis (anterior uveitis), psoriaform rashes (psoriatic arthritis), oral ulcers, aortic valve incompetence, inflammatory bowel disease.

NB: Behçet's syndrome (p694) can also present with uveitis, skin lesions, and arthritis and is not always associated with gross oral or genital ulcerations.

1. **Ankylosing spondylitis (AS)** A chronic inflammatory disease of the spine and sacroiliac joints, of unknown aetiology (likely strong genetic/environmental interplay). *Prevalence:* 0.25–1%. *Men present earlier:* ♂:♀ ~6:1 at 16yrs old, and ~2:1 at 30yrs old. ~90% are HLA B27 +ve (see BOX). *Symptoms and signs:* The typical patient is a man <30yrs old with gradual onset of low back pain, worse during the night with spinal morning stiffness relieved by exercise. Pain radiates from sacroiliac joints to hips/buttocks, and usually improves towards the end of the day. There is progressive loss of spinal movement (all directions)—hence ↓thoracic expansion. See pp540–2 for tests of spine flexion and sacroiliitis. The disease course is variable; a few progress to kyphosis, neck hyperextension (question-mark posture; fig 12.13), and spino-cranial ankylosis. Other features include *enthesitis* (see BOX), especially Achilles tendonitis, plantar fasciitis, at the tibial and ischial tuberosities, and at the iliac crests. Anterior mechanical chest pain due to costochondritis and fatigue may feature. *Acute iritis* occurs in ~⅓ of patients and may lead to blindness if untreated (but may also have occurred many years before, so enquire directly). AS is also associated with osteoporosis (up to 60%), aortic valve incompetence (<3%), and pulmonary apical fibrosis. *Tests:* Diagnosis is clinical, supported by imaging.[4] MRI allows detection of active inflammation (bone marrow oedema) as well as destructive changes such as erosions, sclerosis, and ankylosis. X-rays can show SI joint space narrowing or widening, sclerosis, erosions, and ankylosis/fusion. Vertebral syndesmophytes are characteristic (often T11–L1 initially): bony proliferations due to enthesitis between ligaments and vertebrae. These fuse with the vertebral body above, causing ankylosis. In later stages, calcification of ligaments with ankylosis lead to a 'bamboo spine' appearance. *Also:* FBC (normocytic anaemia), ↑ESR, ↑CRP, HLA B27 +ve (+ve in 90–95% of cases but only 5% of patients HLA B27 +ve have AS). *Management: Exercise*, not rest, for backache, including intense exercise regimens to maintain posture and mobility—ideally with a specialist physiotherapist. NSAIDs usually relieve symptoms within 48h, and may slow radiographic progression.[37] *TNFα BLOCKERS* (eg etanercept, adalimumab) are indicated in severe active AS.[38] Local steroid injections provide temporary relief. Surgery includes hip replacement to improve pain and mobility if the hips are involved, and rarely spinal osteotomy. There is ↑risk of osteoporotic spinal fractures (consider bisphosphonates). *Prognosis:* There is not always a clear relationship between the activity of arthritis and severity of underlying inflammation (as for all the spondyloarthritides). Prognosis is worse if ESR >30; onset <16yrs; early hip involvement or poor response to NSAIDs.[39]
2. **Enteric arthropathy** *Associations:* Inflammatory bowel disease, GI bypass, coeliac and Whipple's disease (p716). Arthropathy often improves with the treatment of bowel symptoms (beware NSAIDs). Use DMARDs for resistant cases.

4 Sacroiliitis on imaging plus ≥1 SpA feature or HLA B27 positive plus ≥2 SpA features.

3 **Psoriatic arthritis** (*OHCS* p594.) Occurs in 10–40% with psoriasis and can present before skin changes. Patterns are: •symmetrical polyarthritis (like RA) •DIP joints •asymmetrical oligoarthritis •spinal (similar to AS) •psoriatic arthritis mutilans (rare, ~3%, severe deformity). *Radiology:* Erosive changes, with 'pencil-in-cup' deformity in severe cases. Associated with nail changes in 80%, synovitis (dactylitis), acneiform rashes and palmo-plantar pustulosis. *Management:* NSAIDs, sulfasalazine, methotrexate. Anti-TNF agents are also effective.

4 **Reactive arthritis** A condition in which arthritis and other clinical manifestations occur as an autoimmune response to infection elsewhere in the body—typically GI or GU, although the preceding infection may have resolved or be asymptomatic by the time the arthritis presents. *Other clinical features:* Iritis, keratoderma blenorrhagica (brown, raised plaques on soles and palms), circinate balanitis (painless penile ulceration secondary to *Chlamydia*), mouth ulcers, and enthesitis. Patients may present with a triad of urethritis, arthritis, and conjunctivitis (Reiter's syndrome). *Tests:* ↑ESR & ↑CRP. Culture stool if diarrhoea. Infectious serology. Sexual health review. X-ray may show enthesitis with periosteal reaction. *Management:* There is no specific cure. Splint affected joints acutely; treat with NSAIDs or local steroid injections. Consider sulfasalazine or methotrexate if symptoms >6 months. Treating the original infection may make little difference to the arthritis.

HLA-B27 disease associations

The HLA system plays a key role in immunity and self-recognition. More than one hundred HLA B27 disease associations have been made[40], yet the actual role of HLA B27 in triggering an inflammatory response is not fully understood. ~5% of the UK population are HLA B27 positive—most do not have any disease. The chance of an HLA B27 positive person developing spondyloarthritis or eye disease is 1 in 4. Common associations include:

Ankylosing spondylitis: 85-95% of all those with AS are HLA B27 positive.
Acute anterior uveitis: 50-60% are HLA B27 positive.
Reactive arthritis: 60-85% are HLA B27 positive.
Enteric arthropathy: 50-60% are HLA B27 positive.
Psoriatic arthritis: 60-70% are HLA B27 positive.

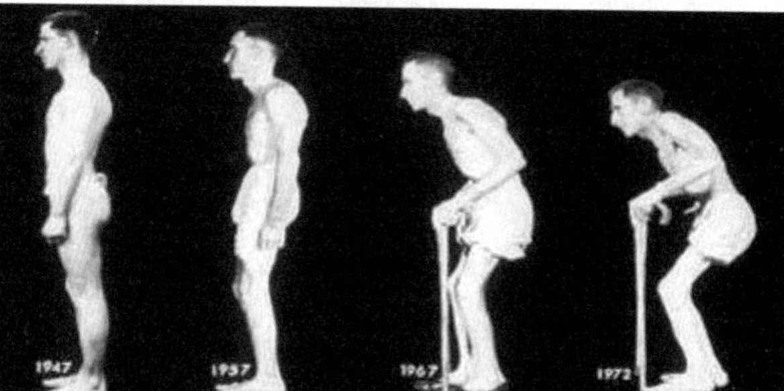

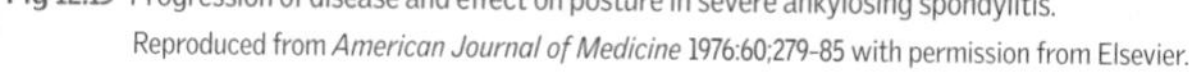

Fig 12.13 Progression of disease and effect on posture in severe ankylosing spondylitis.

Reproduced from *American Journal of Medicine* 1976:60;279–85 with permission from Elsevier.

Autoimmune connective tissue diseases

Included under this heading are SLE (p554), systemic sclerosis, Sjögren's syndrome (p710), idiopathic inflammatory myopathies (myositis—see following topic), mixed connective tissue disease, relapsing polychondritis, and undifferentiated connective tissue disease and overlap syndromes. They overlap with each other, affect many organ systems, and often require immunosuppressive therapies (p376). Consider as a differential in unwell patients with multi-organ involvement, especially if no infection.

Systemic sclerosis Features scleroderma (skin fibrosis), internal organ fibrosis, and microvascular abnormalities. Severe cases have a 40–50% mortality at 5 years. 90% are ANA positive and 30–40% have anticentromere antibodies (see BOX). Skin disease is limited or diffuse. *Limited* involves the face, hands, and feet (formally CREST syndrome). It is associated with anticentromere antibodies in 70–80%. Pulmonary hypertension is often present subclinically, and can become rapidly life-threatening, so should be looked for (℞: sildenafil, bosentan). *Diffuse* can involve the whole body. Antitopoisomerase-1 (SCL-70) antibodies in 40% and anti-RNA polymerase in 20%. Prognosis is often poor. Control BP meticulously. Perform annual echocardiogram and spirometry. Both limited and diffuse have the potential for organ fibrosis: lung, cardiac, GI, and renal (p314) but this occurs later in limited sub-set.

Management: Currently no cure. Immunosuppressive regimens, including IV cyclophosphamide, are used for organ involvement or progressive skin disease. Trials of antifibrotic tyrosine kinase inhibitors are ongoing.[41] Monitor BP and renal function. Regular ACE-i or A2RBs ↓ risk of renal crisis (p314). *Raynaud's phenomenon:* (see p708).

Mixed connective tissue disease Combines features of systemic sclerosis, SLE, and polymyositis and the presence of high titres of anti-U1-RNP antibodies.

Relapsing polychondritis Rare condition with recurrent episodes of cartilage inflammation and destruction. Affects pinna (floppy ears), nasal septum, larynx (stridor), tracheobronchial tree (infections), and joints. *Associations:* Aortic valve disease, polyarthritis, and vasculitis. 30% have underlying rheumatic or autoimmune disease. Diagnosis is clinical. ℞: Steroids, DMARDs or CPAP/tracheostomy for airway involvement.

Polymyositis and dermatomyositis

Rare conditions characterized by insidious onset of progressive symmetrical proximal muscle weakness and autoimmune-mediated *striated* muscle inflammation (myositis), associated with myalgia ± arthralgia. Muscle weakness may also cause dysphagia, dysphonia (ie poor phonation, *not* dysphasia), or respiratory weakness. The myositis (esp. in dermatomyositis) may be a paraneoplastic phenomenon, commonly from lung, pancreatic, ovarian, or bowel malignancy. Screen for cancers.

Dermatomyositis Myositis plus skin signs: •Macular rash (*shawl sign* is +ve if over back and shoulders). •Lilac-purple (*heliotrope*) rash on eyelids often with oedema (fig 12.26, p563). •Nailfold erythema (*dilated capillary loops*). •*Gottron's papules:* roughened red papules over the knuckles, also seen on elbows and knees (pathognomonic if ↑CK + muscle weakness). Malignancy in 30% cases.

Extra-muscular signs In both conditions include fever, arthralgia, Raynaud's, interstitial lung fibrosis and myocardial involvement (myocarditis, arrhythmias).

Tests Muscle enzymes (ALT, AST, LDH, CK, & aldolase) ↑ in plasma; EMG shows characteristic fibrillation potentials; muscle biopsy confirms diagnosis (and excludes mimicking conditions). MRI shows muscle oedema in acute myositis. *Autoantibody associations:* (see BOX) anti-Mi2, anti-Jo1—associated with acute onset and interstitial lung fibrosis that should be treated aggressively.

Differential diagnoses Carcinomatous myopathy, inclusion-body myositis, muscular dystrophy, PMR, endocrine/metabolic myopathy (eg steroids), rhabdomyolysis, infection (eg HIV), drugs (penicillamine, colchicine, statins, or chloroquine).

Management Start prednisolone. Immunosuppressives (p376) and cytotoxics are used early in resistant cases. Hydroxychloroquine/topical tacrolimus for skin disease.

Plasma autoantibodies (Abs): disease associations

►Always interpret in the context of clinical findings: Different antibodies have different disease asssociations.

Rheumatological: Rheumatoid factor (RhF) positive in:

Sjögren's syndrome	≤100%	Mixed connective tissue disease	50%
Felty's syndrome	≤100%	SLE	≤40%
RA	70%	Systemic sclerosis	30%
Infection (SBE/IE; hepatitis)	≤50%	Normal	2-10%

Anticyclic citrullinated peptide Ab (anti-CCP):[5] rheumatoid arthritis (~96% specificity)

Antinuclear antibody (ANA) positive by immunofluorescence in:

SLE	>95%	Systemic sclerosis	96%
Autoimmune hepatitis	75%	RA	30%
Sjögren's syndrome	68%	Normal	0-2%

ANA titres are expressed according to dilutions at which antibodies can be detected, ie 1:160 means antibodies can still be detected after the serum has been diluted 160 times. Titres of 1:40 or 1:80 may not be significant. The pattern of staining may indicate the disease (although these are not specific):

• *Homogeneous*	SLE	• *Nucleolar*	Systemic sclerosis
• *Speckled*	Mixed CT disease	• *Centromere*	Limited systemic sclerosis

Anti-double-stranded DNA (dsDNA): SLE (60% sensitivity, but highly specific).
Antihistone Ab: drug-induced SLE (~100%).
Antiphospholipid Ab (eg anti-cardiolipin Ab): antiphospholipid syndrome, SLE.
Anticentromere Ab: limited systemic sclerosis.
Anti-extractable nuclear antigen (ENA) antibodies (usually with +ve ANA):

• Anti-Ro (SSA)	SLE, Sjögren's syndrome, systemic sclerosis. Associated with congenital heart block.
• Anti-La (SSB)	Sjögren's syndrome, SLE (15%).
• Anti-Sm	SLE (20–30%).
• Anti-RNP	SLE, mixed connective tissue disease.
• Anti Jo-1; Anti-Mi-2	Polymyositis, dermatomyositis.
• Anti-Scl70	Diffuse systemic sclerosis.

Gastrointestinal: (For liver autoantibodies, see p284.)
Antimitochondrial Ab (AMA): primary biliary cholangitis (>95%), autoimmune hepatitis (30%), idiopathic cirrhosis (25–30%).
Anti-smooth muscle Ab (SMA): autoimmune hepatitis (70%), primary biliary cholangitis (50%), idiopathic cirrhosis (25–30%).
Gastric parietal cell Ab: pernicious anaemia (>90%), atrophic gastritis (40%), 'normal' (10%).
Intrinsic factor Ab: pernicious anaemia (50%).
α-gliadin Ab, antitissue transglutaminase, anti-endomysial Ab: coeliac disease.

Endocrine: Thyroid peroxidase Ab: Hashimoto's thyroiditis (~87%), Graves' (>50%). *Islet cell Ab (ICA), glutamic acid decarboxylase (GAD) Ab:* type 1 diabetes mellitus (75%).
Renal: Glomerular basement membrane Ab (anti-GBM): Goodpasture's disease (100%).
Antineutrophil cytoplasmic Ab (ANCA):

- *Cytoplasmic (cANCA)*, specific for *serine proteinase-3 (PR3 +ve).* Granulomatosis with polyangiitis (Wegener's) (90%); also microscopic polyangiitis (30%), polyarteritis nodosa (11%).
- *Perinuclear (pANCA)*, specific for *myeloperoxidase (MPO +ve).* Microscopic polyangiitis (45%), Churg-Strauss, pulmonary-renal vasculitides (Goodpasture's).

Unlike immune-complex vasculitis, in ANCA-associated vasculitis no complement consumption or immune complex deposition occurs (ie pauci-immune vasculitis).[42]
ANCA may also be +ve in UC/Crohn's, sclerosing cholangitis, autoimmune hepatitis, Felty's, RA, SLE, or drugs (eg antithyroid, allopurinol, ciprofloxacin).
Neurological: Acetylcholine receptor Ab: myasthenia gravis (90%)(see p512).
Anti-voltage-gated K^+-channel Ab: limbic encephalitis.
Anti-voltage-gated Ca^{2+}-channel Ab: Lambert-Eaton syndrome (see p512).
Anti-aquaporin 4: neuromyelitis optica (Devic's disease, p698).

5 Most centres now use anti-CCP antibodies for the initial workup of suspected RA.

Systemic lupus erythematosus (SLE)

SLE is a multisystemic autoimmune disease. Autoantibodies are made against a variety of autoantigens (eg ANA) which form immune complexes. Inadequate clearance of immune complexes results in a host of immune responses which cause tissue inflammation and damage. Environmental triggers play a part (eg EBV p405).[43]

Prevalence ~0.2%. ♀:♂≈9:1, typically women of child-bearing age. Commoner in African-Caribbeans, Asians, and if HLA B8, DR2, or DR3 +ve. ~10% of patients have a 1st- or 2nd-degree relative with SLE.

Clinical features See BOX. Remitting and relapsing illness of variable presentation and course. Features often non-specific (malaise, fatigue, myalgia, and fever) or organ-specific and caused by active inflammation or damage. Other features include lymphadenopathy, weight loss, alopecia, nail-fold infarcts, non-infective endocarditis (Libman-Sacks syndrome), Raynaud's (30%; see p708), stroke, and retinal exudates.

Immunology >95% are ANA +ve. A high anti-double-stranded DNA (dsDNA) antibody titre is highly specific, but only +ve in ~60% of cases. ENA (p553) may be +ve in 20–30% (anti-Ro, anti-La, anti-Sm, anti-RNP); 40% are RhF +ve; antiphospholipid antibodies (anticardiolipin or lupus anticoagulant) may also be +ve. SLE may be associated with other autoimmune conditions: Sjögren's (15–20%), autoimmune thyroid disease (5–10%).

Diagnosis See BOX. **Monitoring activity** *Three best tests:* **1** Anti-dsDNA antibody titres. **2** Complement: ↓C3, ↓C4 (denotes consumption of complement, hence ↓C3 and ↓C4, and ↑C3d and ↑C4d, their degradation products). **3** ESR. *Also:* BP, urine for casts or protein (lupus nephritis, below), FBC, U&E, LFTs, CRP (usually normal) ►*think of SLE whenever someone has a multisystem disorder and ↑ESR but CRP normal.* If ↑CRP, think instead of infection, serositis, or arthritis. Skin or renal biopsies may be diagnostic.

Drug-induced lupus Causes (>80 drugs) include isoniazid, hydralazine (if >50mg/24h in slow acetylators), procainamide, quinidine, chlorpromazine, minocycline, phenytoin, anti-TNF agents. It is associated with antihistone antibodies in >95% of cases. Skin and lung signs prevail (renal and CNS are rarely affected). The disease remits if the drug is stopped. Sulfonamides or the oral contraceptive pill may worsen idiopathic SLE.

Management Refer: complex cases should involve specialist SLE/nephritis clinics.

- *General measures:* High-factor sunblock. Hydroxychloroquine, unless contraindicated, reduces disease activity and improves survival. Screen for co-morbidities and medication toxicity. For skin flares, first trial topical steroids.
- *Maintenance:* NSAIDs (unless renal disease) and hydroxychloroquine for joint and skin symptoms. Azathioprine, methotrexate, and mycophenolate as steroid-sparing agents. Belimumab (monoclonal antibody) used as an add-on therapy for autoantibody positive disease where disease activity is high.[44] (See BOX.)

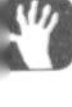

- *Mild flares:* (No serious organ damage.) Hydroxychloroquine or low-dose steroids.
- *Moderate flares:* (Organ involvement.) May require DMARDs or mycophenolate.

►►*Severe flares: If life- or organ-threatening,* eg haemolytic anaemia, nephritis, severe pericarditis or CNS disease; urgent high-dose steroids, mycophenolate, rituximab, cyclophosphamide. MDT working vital for neuropsychiatric lupus (psychometric testing, lumbar puncture may be indicated).

Lupus nephritis: (p314.) May require more intensive immunosuppression with steroids and cyclophosphamide or mycophenolate. BP control vital (e.g. ACE-i). Renal replacement therapy (p306) may be needed if disease progresses; nephritis recurs in ~50% post-transplant, but is a rare cause of graft failure.[45]

Prognosis: ~80% survival at 15 years.[43] There is an increased long-term risk of CVD and osteoporosis.

Antiphospholipid syndrome Can be associated with SLE (20–30%). Often occurs as a primary disease. Antiphospholipid antibodies (anticardiolipin & lupus anticoagulant, anti-β 2 glycoprotein 1) cause **CLOTS**: **C**oagulation defect (arterial/venous), **L**ivedo reticularis (p557), **O**bstetric (recurrent miscarriage), **T**hrombocytopenia. Thrombotic tendency affects cerebral, renal, and other vessels. *Dx:* Persistent antiphosphlolipid antibodies with clinical features. ℞: Anticoagulation; seek advice in pregnancy.[46]

Systemic Lupus International Collaborating Clinics Classification

A favourite differential diagnosis, SLE mimics other illnesses, with wide variation in symptoms that may come and go unpredictably. Diagnose SLE[47] in an appropriate clinical setting if ≥4 criteria (at least 1 clinical and 1 laboratory) *or* biopsy-proven lupus nephritis with positive ANA or anti-DNA.

Clinical criteria

1 *Acute cutaneous lupus:* Malar rash/butterfly. Fixed erythema, flat or raised, over the malar eminences, tending to spare the nasolabial folds (fig 12.14). Occurs in up to 50%. Bullous lupus, toxic epidermal necrolysis variant of SLE, maculopapular lupus rash, photosensitive lupus rash, or subacute cutaneous lupus (non-indurated psoriasiform and/or annular polycyclic lesions that resolve without scarring).
2 *Chronic cutaneous lupus:* Discoid rash, erythematous raised patches with adherent keratotic scales and follicular plugging ± atrophic scarring (fig 12.15). Think of it as a three-stage rash affecting ears, cheeks, scalp, forehead, and chest: erythema→pigmented hyperkeratotic oedematous papules→atrophic depressed lesions.
3 *Non scarring alopecia:* (In the absence of other causes.)
4 *Oral/nasal ulcers:* (In the absence of other causes.)
5 *Synovitis:* (Involving two or more joints *or* two or more tender joints with >30 minutes of morning stiffness.)
6 *Serositis:* a) Lung (pleurisy for >1 day, or pleural effusions, or pleural rub; b) pericardial pain for >1 day, or pericardial effusion, or pericardial rub, or pericarditis on ECG.
7 *Urinanalysis:* Presence of proteinuria (>0.5g/d) *or* red cell casts.
8 *Neurological features:* Seizures; psychosis; mononeuritis multiplex; myelitis; peripheral or cranial neuropathy; cerebritis/acute confusional state in absence of other causes.
9 *Haemolytic anaemia.*
10 *Leucopenia:* (WCC <4.) At least once, or lymphopenia (lymphocytes <1) at least once.
11 *Thrombocytopenia:* (Platelets <100.) At least once.

Laboratory criteria

1 +ve ANA (+ve in >95%).
2 Anti-dsDNA.
3 Anti-Smith antibodies present.
4 Antiphospholipid Abs present.
5 Low complement (C3, C4, or C50).
6 +ve Direct Coombs test.

Adapted from 'Derivation and validation of the Systemic Lupus International Collaborating Clinics classification criteria for systemic lupus erythematosus'. Petri M *et al., Arthritis and Rheumatism,* vol 64, issue 8 (2012) 2677–2686.

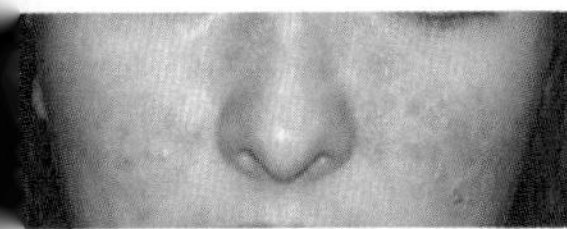

Fig 12.14 Malar rash, with sparing of the nasolabial folds.

Courtesy of David F. Fiorentino, MD, PhD; by kind permission of *Skin & Aging*.

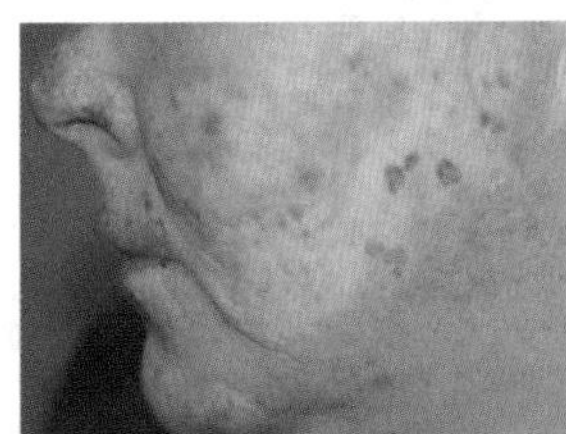

Fig 12.15 Discoid rash.

Courtesy of Amy McMichael, MD; by kind permission of *Skin & Aging*.

Vasculitis

The vasculitides are inflammatory disorders of blood vessels; commonly classified using the modified Chapel Hill criteria.[48] They can affect any organ, and presentation depends on the organs involved. It may be a primary condition or secondary to other diseases, eg SLE, RA, hepatitis B & C, HIV. Categorized by size of blood vessels affected.

- **Large** Giant cell arteritis, Takayasu's arteritis (see p712).
- **Medium** Polyarteritis nodosa, Kawasaki disease (*OHCS* p646).
- **Small** • ANCA-associated: microscopic polyangiitis; granulomatosis with polyangiitis (Wegener's granulomatosis); and eosinophilic granulomatosis with polyangiitis (Churg Strauss syndrome; 40–60% are ANCA positive). • Immune complex vasculitis: Goodpasture's disease; cryoglobulinaemic vasculitis; IgA vasculitis (Henoch-Schonlein purpura).
- **Variable vessel vasculitis** Behçet's (p694) and Cogan's syndrome.

Symptoms Different vasculitides preferentially affect different organs, causing different patterns of symptoms (see BOX 'Features of vasculitis'), Often only overwhelming fatigue with ↑ESR/CRP. ►►*Consider vasculitis in any unidentified multisystem disorder.* If presentation does not fit clinically or serologically into a specific category consider malignancy-associated vasculitis. A severe vasculitis flare is a medical emergency. If suspected, seek urgent help, as organ damage may occur rapidly (eg critical renal failure <24h). **Tests** ↑ESR/CRP. ANCA may be +ve. ↑Creatinine if renal failure. Urine: proteinuria, haematuria, casts on microscopy. Angiography ± biopsy may be diagnostic. **Management** Large-vessel: steroids in most cases, may add steroid-sparing agents later. Medium/small: immunosuppression (steroids, ± another agent, eg cyclophosphamide if severe, or methotrexate/azathioprine depending on features).

►►**Giant cell arteritis (GCA) = temporal arteritis** Common in the elderly—consider Takayasu's if under 55yrs (p712). Associated with PMR in 50%. *Symptoms:* Headache, temporal artery and scalp tenderness (eg when combing hair), tongue/jaw claudication, amaurosis fugax, or sudden unliateral blindness. Extracranial symptoms: malaise, dyspnoea, weight loss, morning stiffness, and unequal or weak pulses.[49] The risk is irreversible bilateral visual loss, which can occur suddenly if not treated—ask an ophthalmologist. *Tests:* ESR & CRP are ↑↑, ↑platelets, ↑ALP, ↓Hb. Temporal artery biopsy within 14 days of starting steroids, or FDG-PET. Skip lesions occur, so don't be put off by a negative biopsy (up to 10%). *Management:* Start prednisolone 60mg/d PO *immediately* or IV methylprednisolone if evolving visual loss or history of amaurosis fugax.[50] *Prognosis:* Typically a 2-year course, then complete remission. Reduce prednisolone once symptoms have resolved and ↓ESR; ↑dose if symptoms recur. Main cause of death and morbidity in GCA is long-term steroid treatment so balance risks! Give PPI, bisphosphonate, calcium with colecalciferol, and consider aspirin.[6; 51]

Polyarteritis nodosa (PAN) PAN is a necrotizing vasculitis that causes aneurysms and thrombosis in medium-sized arteries, leading to infarction in affected organs with severe systemic symptoms. ♂:♀≈2:1. It may be associated with hepatitis B, and is rare in the UK. *Symptoms:* See BOX. Systemic features, skin (rash, 'punched out' ulcers, nodules), renal (main cause of death, renal artery narrowing, glomerular ischaemia, insufficiency, HTN), cardiac, GI, GU, neuro involvement. Usually spares lungs. Coronary aneurysms occur in Kawasaki disease (*OHCS* p646). *Tests:* Often ↑WCC, mild eosinophilia (in 30%), anaemia, ↑ESR, ↑CRP, ANCA −ve. Renal or mesenteric angiography (see fig 12.16), or renal biopsy can be diagnostic. *Treatment:* Control BP and refer. Steroids for mild cases and steroid-sparing agents if more severe. Hepatitis B should be treated (p278) after initial treatment with steroids.[52]

Microscopic polyangiitis A necrotizing vasculitis affecting small- and medium-sized vessels. *Symptoms:* Rapidly progressive glomerulonephritis usually features; pulmonary haemorrhage occurs in up to 30%; other features are rare. *Tests:* pANCA (MPO) +ve (p553). *Treatment:* Steroids plus eg methotrexate. For maintenance: methotrexate, rituximab, or azathioprine.

Hypocomplementaemic urticarial vasculitis A lupus-like illness with urticaria and antibodies to complement (C1q).

6 Low-dose aspirin has been shown to decrease the rate of visual loss and cerebrovascular accidents in GCA but there are also conflicting reports regarding its efficacy at preventing ischaemic events in GCA.

Features of vasculitis

The presentation of vasculitis will depend on the organs affected:

Systemic: Fever, malaise, weight loss, arthralgia, myalgia.
Skin: Purpura, ulcers, livedo reticularis (fig 12.17), nailbed infarcts, digital gangrene.
Eyes: Episcleritis, scleritis, visual loss.
ENT: Epistaxis, nasal crusting, stridor, deafness.
Pulmonary: Haemoptysis and dyspnoea (due to pulmonary haemorrhage).
Cardiac: Angina or MI (due to coronary arteritis), heart failure, and pericarditis.
GI: Pain or perforation (infarcted viscus), malabsorption (chronic ischaemia).
Renal: Hypertension, haematuria, proteinuria, casts, and renal failure (renal cortical infarcts; glomerulonephritis in ANCA +ve vasculitis).
Neurological: Stroke, fits, chorea, psychosis, confusion, impaired cognition, altered mood. Arteritis of the vasa nervorum (arterial supply to peripheral nerves) may cause mononeuritis multiplex or a sensorimotor polyneuropathy.[53]
GU: Orchitis—testicular pain or tenderness.

Polymyalgia rheumatica (PMR)

PMR is not a true vasculitis and its pathogenesis is unknown. PMR and GCA share the same demographic characteristics and, although separate conditions, the two frequently occur together.

Features: Age >50yrs; subacute onset (<2 weeks) of bilateral aching, tenderness, and morning stiffness in shoulders, hips, and proximal limb muscles ± fatigue, fever, ↓weight, anorexia, and depression. There may be associated mild polyarthritis, tenosynovitis, and carpal tunnel syndrome (10%). Weakness is not a feature.

Investigations: ↑CRP, ESR typically >40 (but may be normal); AlkP is ↑ in 30%. Note creatinine kinase levels are normal (helping to distinguish from myositis/myopathies).

Differential diagnoses: Recent-onset RA, polymyositis, hypothyroidism, primary muscle disease, occult malignancy or infection, osteoarthritis (especially cervical spondylosis, shoulder OA), neck lesions, bilateral subacromial impingement (*OHCS* p666), spinal stenosis (*OHCS* p676).

Management: Prednisolone 15mg/d PO. Expect a dramatic response within 1 week and consider an alternative diagnosis if not. ↓ dose slowly, eg by 1mg/month (according to symptoms/ESR). Investigate apparent 'flares' during withdrawal—attributable to another condition? Most need steroids for ≥2yrs, so give bone protection. Addition of methotrexate may be considered, under specialist supervision, for patients at risk of relapse/prolonged therapy. NSAIDs are not effective. Inform patients to seek urgent review if symptoms of GCA develop.

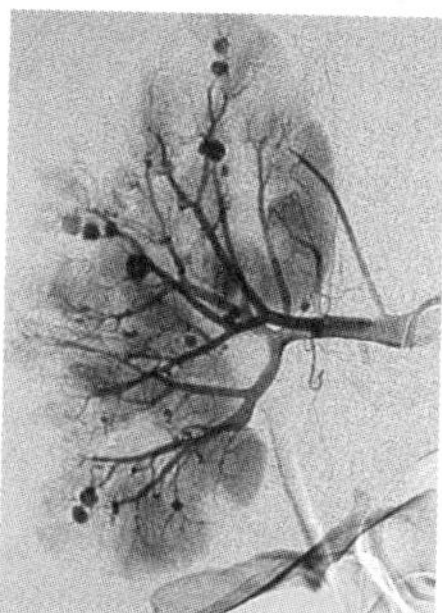

Fig 12.16 Renal angiogram showing multiple aneurysms in PAN.

Courtesy of Dr William Herring.

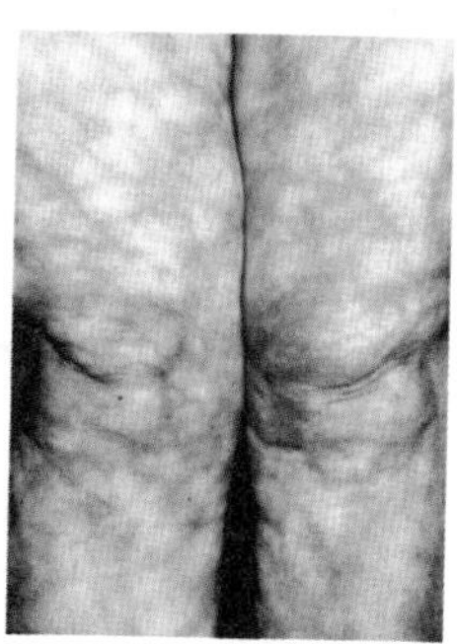

Fig 12.17 Livedo reticularis: pink-blue mottling caused by capillary dilatation and stasis in skin venules. Causes: physiological, cold, or vasculitis.

Fibromyalgia and chronic fatigue syndrome

Fibromyalgia and chronic fatigue syndrome are part of a diffuse group of overlapping syndromes, sharing similar demographic and clinical characteristics, in which chronic symptoms of fatigue and widespread pain feature prominently. Their existence as discrete entities is controversial, especially in the absence of clear pathology, and some find such dysfunctional diagnoses frustrating. However, a correct diagnosis enables the doctor to give appropriate counselling and advise appropriate therapies, and allows the patient to begin to accept and deal with their symptoms.

Fibromyalgia

Fibromyalgia comprises up to 10% of new referrals to the rheumatology clinic.[54]

Prevalence: 0.5–4%. ♀:♂≈6:1 but varies depending on which diagnostic criteria are used .

Risk factors: BOX 'Risk factors'. Female sex, middle age, low household income, divorced, low educational status.

Associations: Other somatic syndromes such as chronic fatigue syndrome, irritable bowel syndrome (p266), and chronic headaches syndromes (see *OHCS* p502). Also found in ~25% of patients with RA, AS, and SLE.

Features: Diagnosis depends on pain that is *chronic* (>3 months) and widespread (involves left and right sides, above and below the waist, and the axial skeleton). Profound fatigue is almost universal with complaint of unrefreshing sleep and significant fatigue and pain with small increases in physical exertion. *Additional features:* morning stiffness (~80–90%), paraesthesiae (without underlying cause), headaches (migraine and tension), poor concentration, low mood, and sleep disturbance (~70%). Widespread and severe tender points.

Investigations: All normal. Diagnosis is clinical. Over-investigation can consolidate illness behaviour; but exclude other causes of pain and/or fatigue (eg RA, PMR see p557, vasculitis see p556, hypothyroidism see p220, myeloma see p368).

Management: Multidisciplinary with optimal results coming from full engagement of the patient who should be encouraged to remain as active as they feel able, and ideally to continue to participate in the workforce. New symptoms should be fully reviewed to exclude an alternative diagnosis. Patients should be advised that there is no one specific treatment that is guaranteed to work, but any of the following may help: graded exercise programmes, including both aerobic and strength-based training. Pacing of activity is vital to avoid over-exertion and consequent pain and fatigue. Long-term *graded exercise programmes* improve functional capacity.[55,56] Relaxation, rehabilitation and physiotherapy may also help. *Cognitive-behavioural therapy* (CBT) aims to help patients develop coping strategies and set achievable goals.[57]

Pharmacotherapy: Low-dose amitriptyline (eg 10–20mg at night) has been shown to help relieve pain and improve sleep. Pregabalin (150–300mg/12h PO) can be used if amitriptyline is ineffective. Duloxetine or an SSRI can be used for fibromyalgia with comorbid anxiety and depression. Steroids or NSAIDs are not recommended because there is no inflammation (if it does respond, reconsider your diagnosis!).

Chronic fatigue syndrome (AKA myalgic encephalomyelitis)

Chronic fatigue syndrome[58] is defined as persistent disabling fatigue lasting >6 months, affecting mental and physical function, present >50% of the time, plus ≥4 of: myalgia (~80%), polyarthralgia, ↓memory, unrefreshing sleep, fatigue after exertion >24h, persistent sore throat, tender cervical/axillary lymph nodes. Management principles are similar to fibromyalgia and include graded exercise and CBT. No pharmacological agents have yet been proved effective for chronic fatigue syndrome (see also *OHCS* p502).

Risk factors: yellow flags

Psychosocial risk factors for developing persisting chronic pain and long-term disability have been termed 'yellow flags':[59]

- Belief that pain and activity are harmful.
- Sickness behaviours such as extended rest.
- Social withdrawal.
- Emotional problems such as low mood, anxiety, or stress.
- Problems or dissatisfaction at work.
- Problems with claims for compensation or time off work.
- Overprotective family or lack of support.
- Inappropriate expectations of treatment, eg low active participation in treatment.

An existential approach to difficult symptoms

The manner in which management is discussed is almost as important as the management itself, which should focus on education of the patient *and their family* and on developing coping strategies. Such a diagnosis may be a relief or a disappointment to the patient. *Explain* that fibromyalgia is a relapsing and remitting condition, with no easy cures, and that they will continue to have good and bad days. *Reassure* them that there is no serious underlying pathology, that their joints are not being damaged, and that no further tests are necessary, but be sympathetic to the fact that they may have been seeking a physical cause for their symptoms.

We all at some stage come across a patient with difficult symptoms and an exasperating lack of pathology to explain them. Investigations are all normal, and medications do not seem to work. It is tempting to dismiss such patients as malingerers, but often this conclusion comes from the clinician approaching the problem from the wrong angle. The patient has symptoms that are real and disabling to them, and that will not improve without help. Perhaps a more pragmatic approach is to take advice from the Danish philosopher Kierkegaard who wrote to a friend in 1835, '*What I really lack is to be clear in my mind what I am to do, not what I am to know ... The thing is to understand myself ... to find a truth which is true for me.*' Listen to the patient and accept their story. Then help them to focus on what they can *do* to improve their situation, and to move away from dwelling on finding a physical answer to their symptoms.

Pathogenesis of fibromyalgia

The current hypothesis is that fibromyalgia is caused by aberrant peripheral and central pain processing. Two key features of the condition are *allodynia* (pain in response to a non-painful stimulus) and *hyperaesthesia* (exaggerated perception of pain in response to a mildly painful stimulus), examined for by palpation of tender points. Research is beginning to suggest that certain antidepressants can relieve pain and other symptoms, and especially those that have both serotonergic and noradrenergic activity (tricyclics and venlafaxine). Those acting on serotonergic receptors only are less effective. There is also some evidence to support the use of alternative therapies such as acupuncture and spa therapies, which have been postulated to act through similar spinal pain-modulatory pathways.[60] Thus far, trials have involved relatively small numbers of patients or short time periods, and lack the power to draw strong conclusions. However, it is interesting to note that the CSF of patients with fibromyalgia appears to have increased levels of substance P, while levels of noradrenaline and serotonin metabolites are decreased. All three are neurotransmitters involved in descending pain-modulatory pathways in the spinal cord.[61,62] Evidence from PET imaging suggests that patients with fibromyalgia may have an abnormal central dopamine response to pain.[63] The critical question is: is this cause or effect?

Systemic conditions causing eye signs

The eye is host to many diseases: the more you look, the more you'll see, and the more you'll enjoy, not least because the eye is as beautiful as its signs are legion.

Behçet's (p694.) Systemic inflammatory disorder, HLA B27 association. Causes a uveitis amongst other systemic manifestations. Cause unknown.

Granulomatous disorders Syphilis, TB, sarcoidosis, leprosy, brucellosis, and toxoplasmosis may inflame either the front chamber (anterior uveitis/iritis) or back chamber (posterior uveitis/choroiditis). Refer to an ophthalmologist.

Systemic inflammatory diseases May manifest as *iritis* in ankylosing spondylitis and reactive arthritis; *uveitis* in Behçet's; *conjunctivitis* in reactive arthritis; *scleritis* or *episcleritis* in RA, vasculitis, and SLE. Scleritis in RA and granulomatosis with polyangiitis (Wegener's) may damage the eye. ►►Refer urgently if eye pain. GCA causes optic nerve ischaemia presenting as sudden blindness.

Keratoconjunctivitis sicca A reduction in tear formation, tested by the Schirmer filter paper test (<5mm in 5min). It causes a gritty feeling in the eyes, and a dry mouth (xerostomia from ↓saliva production). It is found on its own (Sjögren's syndrome), or with other diseases, eg SLE, RA, sarcoidosis. ℞: Artificial tears/saliva.

Hypertensive retinopathy ↑BP damages retinal vessels. Hardened arteries are shiny ('silver wiring'; fig 12.18) and 'nip' veins where they cross (AV nipping; fig 12.19). Narrowed arterioles may become blocked, causing localized retinal infarction, seen as cotton-wool spots. Leaks from these in severe hypertension manifest as hard exudates or macular oedema. Papilloedema (fig 12.20) or flame haemorrhages suggest accelerated hypertension (p138) requiring urgent treatment.

Vascular occlusion *Emboli* passing through the retinal vasculature may cause *retinal artery occlusion* (global or segmental retinal pallor) or *amaurosis fugax* (p476). Roth spots (small retinal infarcts occur in infective endocarditis. In dermatomyositis, there is orbital oedema with retinopathy showing cotton-wool spots (micro-infarcts). *Retinal vein occlusion* is caused by ↑BP, age, or hyperviscosity (p372). Suspect in any acute fall in acuity. If it is the central vein, the fundus is like a stormy sunset (those angry red clouds are haemorrhages). In branch vein occlusion, changes are confined to a wedge of retina. Get expert help.

Haematological disorders *Retinal haemorrhages* occur in leukaemia; comma-shaped *conjunctival haemorrhages* and retinal new vessel formation may occur in sickle-cell disease. *Optic atrophy* is seen in pernicious anaemia (and also MS).

Metabolic disease Diabetes mellitus: p210. Hyperthyroid exophthalmos: p219. Lens opacities are seen in hypoparathyroidism. Conjunctival and corneal calcification can occur in hypercalcaemia. In gout, conjunctival urate deposits may cause sore eyes.

Systemic infections Septicaemia may seed to the vitreous causing endophthalmitis. Syphilis can cause iritis (+ pigmented retinopathy if congenital). Systemic fungal infections may affect the eye, eg in the immunocompromised or in IV drug users, requiring intra-vitreal antibiotics. **AIDS and HIV** CMV retinitis (pizza-pie fundus—a mixture of cotton-wool spots, infiltrates, and haemorrhages, p438) may be asymptomatic but can cause sudden visual loss. If present, it implies AIDS (CD4 count <100 × 10^6/L; p398). Cotton-wool spots on their own indicate HIV retinopathy and may occur in early disease. Kaposi's sarcoma may affect the lids (non-tender purple nodule) or conjunctiva (red fleshy mass).

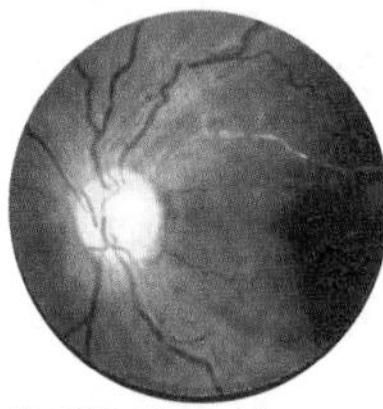

Fig 12.18 Silver wiring.
©Prof Jonathan Trobe.

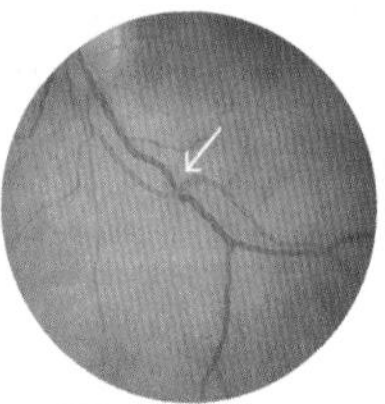

Fig 12.19 AV nipping.
©Prof Jonathan Trobe.

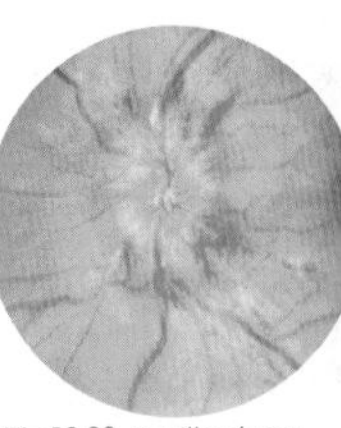

Fig 12.20 Papilloedema.
©Prof Jonathan Trobe.

Table 12.5 Differential diagnosis of a red eye

	Conjunctiva	Iris	Pupil	Cornea	Anterior chamber	Intraocular pressure	Treatment	Appearance
Acute glaucoma	Both ciliary and conjunctival vessels injected. Entire eye is red. See *OHCS* p430.	Injected	Dilated, fixed, oval	Steamy, hazy	Very shallow	Very high	Refer. IV acetazolamide + pilocarpine drops (miotic); peripheral iridotomy.	
Anterior uveitis (iritis)	Redness most marked around cornea, which doesn't blanch on pressure. Usually unilateral. *Causes:* AS, RA, Reiter's sarcoidosis, herpes simplex, herpes zoster, and Behçet's disease. NB: a similar scleral appearance but without papillary or anterior chamber involvement may be *scleritis* (eg RA, SLE, vasculitis).	Injected	Small, irregular due to adhesions between the anterior lens and the pupil margin	Normal	Turgid	Normal	Refer. Steroid eye drops (eg 0.5% prednisolone) + mydriatic (eg cyclopentolate 0.5%).	
Conjunctivitis	Often bilateral. Conjunctival vessels injected, greatest toward fornices, but blanching on pressure. Mobile over sclera. Purulent discharge.	Normal	Normal	Normal	Normal	Normal	Most do not require treatment. Consider chloramphenicol ointment or drops.	
Subconjunctival haemorrhage	Bright red sclera with white rim around limbus. *Causes:* ↑BP; leptospirosis; bleeding disorders; trauma; snake venom; haemorrhagic fevers.	Normal	Normal	Normal	Normal	Normal	Looks alarming but resolves spontaneously. Check BP if elderly; refer if traumatic; on warfarin?	

Images courtesy of Prof. Jonathan Trobe.

Skin manifestations of systemic diseases

Erythema nodosum (fig 12.21) Painful, blue-red, raised lesions on shins (± thighs/arms). *Causes:* sarcoidosis, drugs (sulfonamides, contraceptive pill, dapsone), streptococcal infection. *Less common:* IBD, BCG vaccination, leptospirosis, *Mycobacterium* (TB, leprosy), *Yersinia*, or various viruses and fungi. Cause unknown in 30–50%.

Erythema multiforme (See *OHCS* p588.) (fig 12.22) 'Target' lesions: symmetrical ± central blister, on palms/soles, limbs, and elsewhere. *Stevens-Johnson syndrome* (p710): a rare, severe variant with fever and mucosal involvement (mouth, genital, and eye ulcers), associated with a hypersensitivity reaction to drugs (NSAIDs, sulfonamides, anticonvulsants, allopurinol), or infections (herpes, *Mycoplasma*, orf). Also seen in collagen disorders. 50% of cases are idiopathic. Get expert help in severe disease.

Erythema migrans (fig 12.23) Presents as a small papule at the site of a tick bite which develops into a spreading large erythematous ring, with central fading. It lasts from 48h to 3 months and there may be multiple lesions in disseminated disease. *Cause:* the rash is pathognomonic of Lyme disease and occurs in ~80% of cases (p422).

Erythema marginatum Pink coalescent rings on trunk which come and go. It is seen in rheumatic fever (or rarely other causes, eg drugs). See fig 3.42, p143.

Pyoderma gangrenosum (fig 12.24) Recurring nodulo-pustular ulcers, ~10cm wide, with tender red/blue overhanging necrotic edge, purulent surface, and healing with cribriform scars on leg, abdomen, or face. *Associations:* IBD, autoimmune hepatitis, granulomatosis with polyangiitis (Wegener's), myeloma, neoplasia. ♀>♂. *Treatment:* get help. Oral steroids ± ciclosporin should be 1st-line therapy.[64]

Vitiligo (fig 12.25) *Vitellus* is Latin for *spotted calf:* typically white patches ± hyperpigmented borders. Sunlight makes them itch. *Associations:* autoimmune disorders; premature ovarian failure. Treat by camouflage cosmetics and sunscreens (± steroid creams ± dermabrasion). UK Vitiligo Society: 0800 018 2631.

Specific diseases and their skin manifestations

Crohn's Perianal/vulval/oral ulcers; erythema nodosum; pyoderma gangrenosum.

Dermatomyositis Gottron's papules (rough red papules on the knuckles/extensor surfaces); shawl sign; heliotrope rash on eyelids (fig 12.26). It may be associated with lung, bowel, ovarian, or pancreatic malignancy (p552).

Diabetes mellitus Ulcers, *necrobiosis lipoidica* (shiny yellowish area on shin ± telangiectasia; fig 12.27), *granuloma annulare* (*OHCS* p586), *acanthosis nigricans* (pigmented, rough thickening of axillary, neck, or groin skin with warty lesions; fig 12.28).

Coeliac disease *Dermatitis herpetiformis:* Itchy blisters, in groups on knees, elbows, and scalp. The itch (which can drive patients to suicide) responds to *dapsone* 25-200mg/24h PO within 48h—and this may be used as a diagnostic test. The maintenance dose may be as little as 50mg/wk. A gluten-free diet should be adhered to, but in 30% dapsone will need to be continued. SE (dose-related): haemolysis (CI: anaemia, G6PD-deficiency), hepatitis, agranulocytosis (monitor FBC and LFTs). There is an ↑ risk of small bowel lymphoma with coeliac disease *and* dermatitis herpetiformis—so surveillance is needed.

Hyperthyroidism *Pretibial myxoedema:* Red oedematous swellings above lateral malleoli, progressing to thickened oedema of legs and feet, *thyroid acropachy*—clubbing + subperiosteal new bone in phalanges. *Other endocrinopathies:* p203.

Liver disease Palmar erythema; spider naevi; gynaecomastia; decrease in pubic hair; jaundice; bruising; scratch marks.

Malabsorption Dry pigmented skin, easy bruising, hair loss, leuconychia.

Neoplasia *Acanthosis nigricans:* (See 'Diabetes mellitus' and fig 12.28.) Associated with gastric cancer. *Dermatomyositis:* see earlier in topic. *Thrombophlebitis migrans:* Successive crops of tender nodules affecting blood vessels throughout the body, associated with pancreatic cancer (especially body and tail). *Acquired ichthyosis:* Dry scaly skin associated with lymphoma. *Skin metastases:* Especially melanoma, and colonic, lung, breast, laryngeal/oral, or ovarian malignancy.

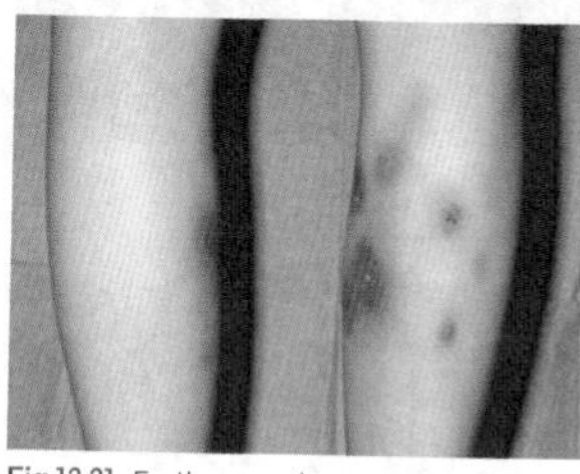
Fig 12.21 Erythema nodosum.

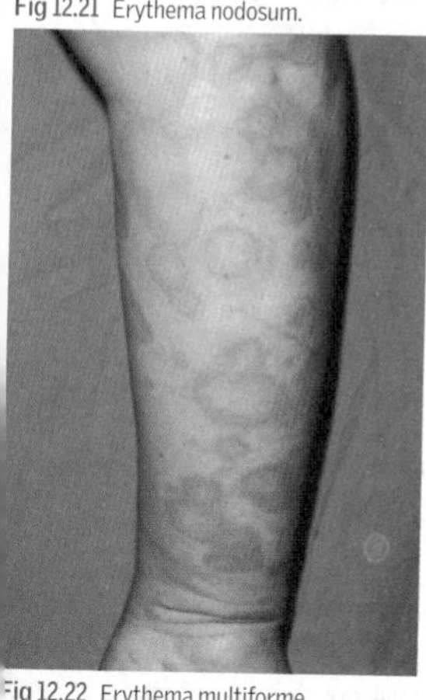
Fig 12.22 Erythema multiforme.

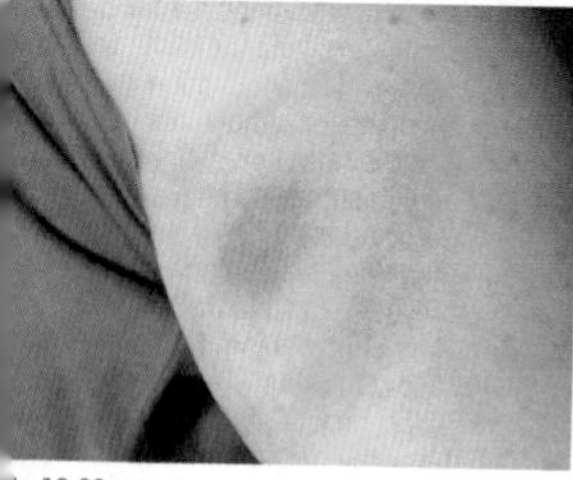
Fig 12.23 Erythema migrans.
Courtesy of CDC/James Gathany.

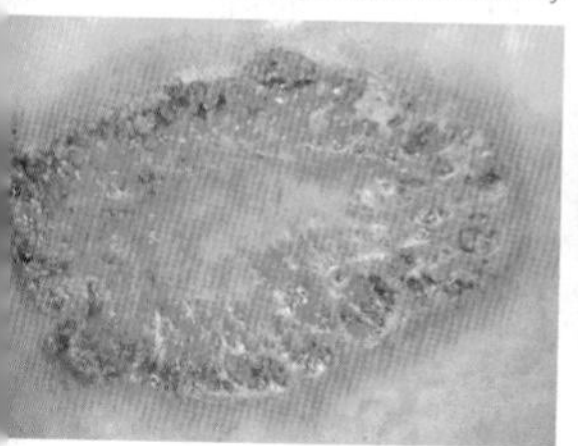
Fig 12.24 Pyoderma gangrenosum.
Reproduced from *BMJ*, 'Diagnosis and treatment of pyoderma gangrenosum', Brooklyn *et al.*, 333: 181-4, 2006; with permission from BMJ Publishing Group Ltd.

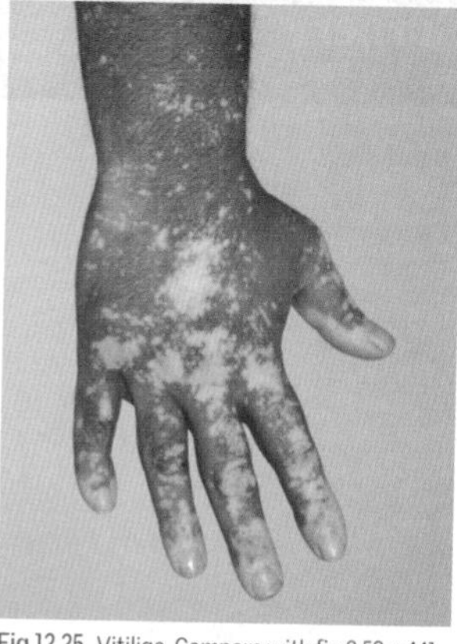
Fig 12.25 Vitiligo. Compare with fig 9.58, p441.

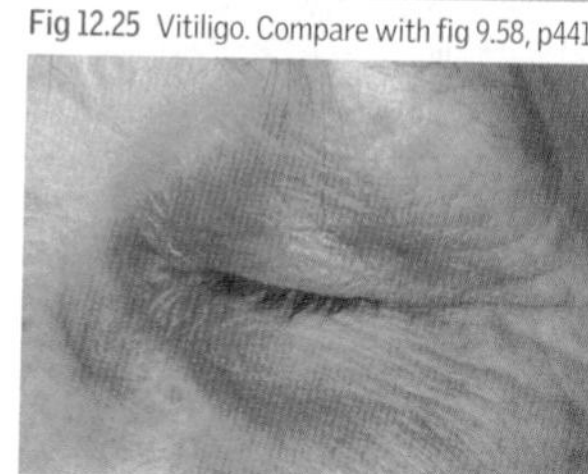
Fig 12.26 Heliotrope rash.
Courtesy of Nick Taylor, East Sussex Hospitals Trust.

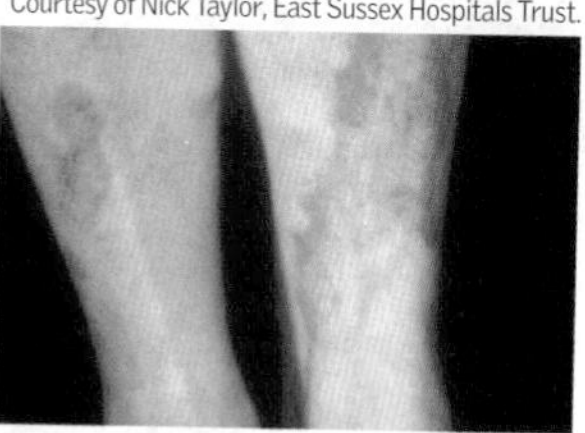
Fig 12.27 Necrobiosis lipoidica.
Reproduced from Warrell *et al.*, *Oxford Textbook of Medicine*, 2010, with permission from Oxford University Press.

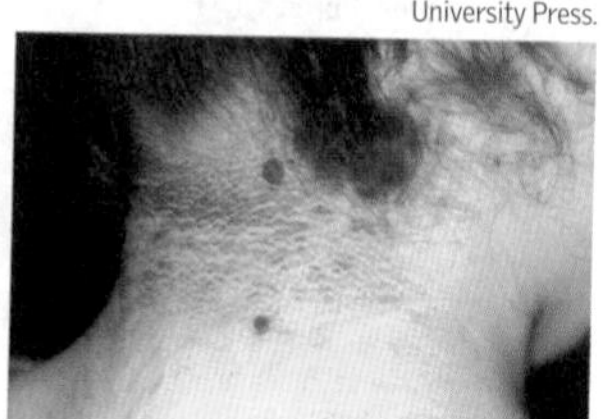
Fig 12.28 Acanthosis nigricans.
Reproduced from Lewis-Jones, *Paediatric Dermatology*, 2010, with permission from Oxford University Press.

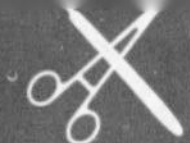

Contents

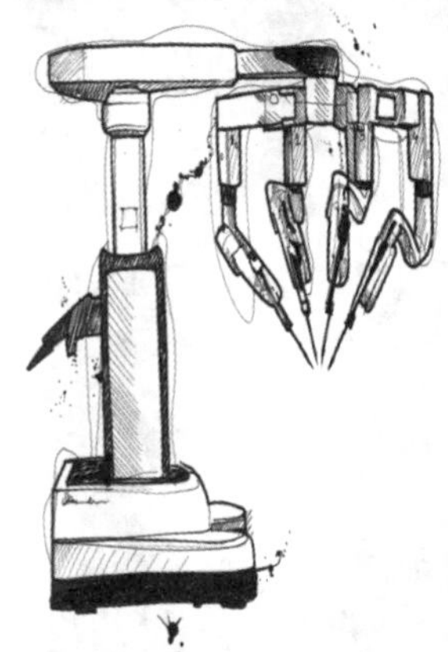

Fig 13.1 The Da Vinci robot, the first robotic surgery system to receive regulatory approval. With 4 arms, tiny, wristed tremor-free joints with multiple axes of rotation and high-resolution 3D imaging, the system offers the potential for significant advances in minimally invasive surgery, which are currently being realized across a range of fields. But where is the surgeon in this picture? At first glance, this technological *tour de force* may appear to supplant the skill of the human surgeon—yet the machine must still possess an operator who must train and achieve all of the skills necessary to perform this challenging surgery. The history of surgery is one of adaptation of surgical skill to new technologies, from anaesthesia and asepsis to organ transplantation and laparoscopy. How can training pathways adapt in turn to allow for acquisition of these new skills without unacceptable patient risk? And whatever the surgical approach, the old maxim remains the same: the art of surgery lies in selecting the right operation at the right time for the right patient.

We thank Mr Antonio Foliaki, our Specialist Reader for this chapter, and Mr William Breakey, for th contribution to this chapter.

The language of surgery

1 Right upper quadrant (RUQ) or hypochondrium.
2 Epigastrium.
3 Left upper quadrant (LUQ) or hypochondrium.
4 Right flank (merges posteriorly with right loin, p57).
5 Periumbilical or central area.
6 Left flank (merges posteriorly with left loin, p57).
7 Right iliac fossa (RIF).
8 Suprapubic area.
9 Left iliac fossa (LIF).

Fig 13.2 Abdominal areas.

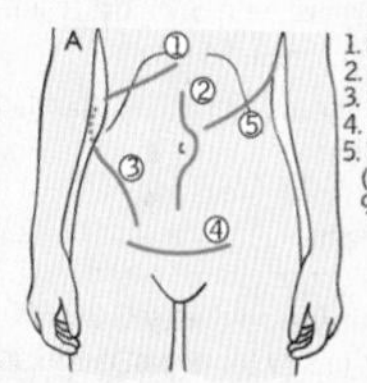

1. Kocher
2. Midline
3. Muscle splitting (ureter)
4. Pfannenstiel
5. Thoraco-abdominal (oesophagectomy 9th or 10th ICS)

Paramedian 1.
McBurney 2.
Lanz 3.
Muscle-cutting transverse 4.
Roof-Top 5.
McEvedy (femoral hernia) 6.
Inguinal hernia incision 7.

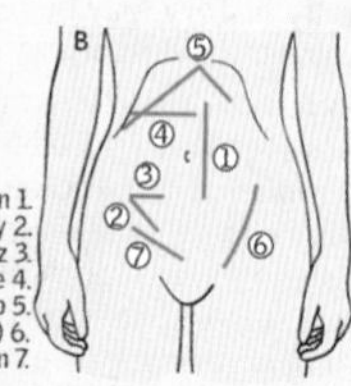

Fig 13.3 Incisions.

-ectomy Cutting something out.
-gram A radiological image.
-pexy Anchoring of a structure to keep it in position.
-plasty Surgical refashioning in order to regain function/cosmesis.
-scopy Procedure with instrumentation for looking into the body.
-stomy An artificial union between a conduit and the outside or another conduit.
-tomy Cutting something open to the outside world.
-tripsy Fragmentation of an object.

angio-	Tube or vessel	lith-	Stone
appendic-	Appendix	mast-	Breast
chole-	Relating to gall/bile	meso-	Mesentery
colp-	Vagina	nephr-	Kidney
cyst-	Bladder	orchid-	Testicle
-doch-	Ducts	oophor-	Ovary
enter-	Small bowel	phren-	Diaphragm
eschar-	Dead tissue, eg from burn	pyloro-	Pyloric sphincter
gastr-	Stomach	pyel-	Renal pelvis
hepat-	Liver	proct-	Anal canal
hyster-	Uterus	salping-	Fallopian tube
lapar-	Abdomen	splen-	Spleen

abscess A cavity containing pus. Remember: *if there is pus about, let it out.*
colic Intermittent pain from over-contraction/obstruction of a hollow viscus.
cyst Fluid-filled cavity lined by epi/endothelium.
fistula An abnormal connection between two epithelial surfaces. Fistulae often close spontaneously, but will not in the presence of malignant tissue, distal obstruction, foreign bodies, chronic inflammation, and the formation of a muco-cutaneous junction (eg stoma).
hernia The protrusion of a viscus/part of a viscus through a defect of the wall of its containing cavity into an abnormal position.
ileus Used in this book as a term for adynamic bowel.
sinus A blind-ending tract, typically lined by epithelial or granulation tissue, which opens to an epithelial surface.
stent An artificial tube placed in a biological tube to keep it open.
stoma (p582) An artificial union between conduits or a conduit and the outside.
ulcer (p660) Interruption in the continuity of an epi/endothelial surface.
volvulus (p611) Twisting of a structure around itself. Common GI sites include the sigmoid colon and caecum, and more rarely the stomach.

epi-	Upon	pan-	Whole	peri-	Around
end-	Inside	para-	Alongside	sub-	Beneath
mega-	Enlarged	per-	Going through	trans-	Across

Pre-operative care

Aims To provide diagnostic and prognostic information. Ensures the patient understands the nature, aims, and expected outcome of surgery. To allay anxiety and pain:

- Ensure that the right patient gets the right surgery. Have the symptoms and signs changed? If so, inform the surgeon.
- Assess/balance risks of anaesthesia, and maximize fitness. Comorbidities? Drugs? Smoker? Optimizing oxygenation *before* major surgery improves outcome.
- Obtain informed consent (p568).
- Check proposed anaesthesia/analgesia with anaesthetist.

Family history May be relevant, eg in malignant hyperpyrexia (p572); dystrophia myotonica (p510); porphyria; cholinesterase problems; sickle-cell disease.

Drugs Any drug/plaster/antiseptic allergies? ►Inform the anaesthetist about *all* drugs even if 'over-the-counter'. ►Steroids: see p590; diabetes: see p588.

- *Antibiotics:* Tetracycline and neomycin may ↑ neuromuscular blockade.
- *Anticoagulants:* ►*Tell the surgeon*. Avoid epidural, spinal, and regional blocks. *Aspirin* should probably be continued unless there is a major risk of bleeding. Discuss stopping *clopidogrel* therapy with the cardiologists/neurologists. See p590.
- *Anticonvulsants:* Give as usual pre-op. Post-op, give drugs IV (or by NGT) until able to take orally. Valproate: give usual dose IV. Phenytoin: give IV slowly (<50mg/min, on cardiac monitor). IM phenytoin absorption is unreliable.
- *β-blockers:* Continue up to and including the day of surgery as this precludes a labile cardiovascular response.
- *Contraceptive pill:* See *BNF*. Stop 4wks before major/leg surgery; ensure alternative contraception is used. Restart 2wks after surgery, provided patient is mobile.
- *Digoxin:* Continue up to and including morning of surgery. Check for toxicity (ECG; plasma level); do plasma K^+ and Ca^{2+} (suxamethonium can ↑K^+ and lead to ventricular arrhythmias in the fully digitalized).
- *Diuretics:* Beware hypokalaemia, dehydration. Do U&E (and bicarbonate).
- *Eye-drops:* β-blockers get systemically absorbed.
- *HRT:* As with contraceptive pill there may be an increased risk of DVT/PE.
- *Levodopa:* Possible arrhythmias when patient under GA.
- *Lithium:* Get expert help; may potentiate neuromuscular blockade and cause arrhythmias. See *OHCS* p349.
- *MAOIs:* Get expert help as interactions may cause hypotensive/hypertensive crises.
- *Thyroid medication:* see p600.
- *Tricyclics:* These enhance adrenaline (epinephrine) and arrhythmias.

Preparation ►Starve patient; NBM ≥2h pre-op for clear fluids and ≥6h for solids.[1]

- Is any bowel or skin preparation needed, or prophylactic antibiotics (p570)?
- Start DVT prophylaxis as indicated, eg graduated compression stockings (CI in peripheral arterial disease); LMWH (p350): eg moderate risk, 20mg ~2h pre-op then 20mg/24h; high risk (eg orthopaedic surgery), 40mg 12h pre-op then 40mg/24h or heparin 5000U SC 2h pre-op, then every 8–12h SC for 7d or until ambulant.
- Ensure necessary premedications (p572), regular medications, analgesia, antiemetics, antibiotics are all prescribed as appropriate. Confirm NBM.
- Book any pre-, intra-, or post-operative x-rays or frozen sections.
- Book post-operative physiotherapy.
- If needed, site IV cannula, catheterize (p762), and/or insert a Ryle's tube (p759).
- Meta-analyses have shown no benefit to patients from mechanical bowel cleansing before colonic surgery—this is no longer considered good practice. There is also no evidence for the use of enemas prior to rectal surgery.

Pre-operative history, examination, and tests

It is the anaesthetist's responsibility to assess suitability for anaesthesia. The ward doctor assists with a good history and examination, should anticipate necessary tests, and can also reassure and inform the patient. The surgical team should consent the patient.

►The World Health Organization 'Surgical Safety Checklist' should be completed for every patient undergoing a surgical procedure, ensuring pre-operative preparation, intra-operative monitoring, and post-operative review.

History Assess past history of: MI[1], diabetes, asthma, hypertension, rheumatic fever, epilepsy, jaundice. Existing illnesses, drugs, and allergies? Be alert to chronic lung disease, ↑BP, arrhythmias, and murmurs. Assess any specific risks, eg is the patient pregnant? Is the neck/jaw immobile and teeth stable (intubation risk)? Has there been previous anaesthesia? Were there any complications (eg nausea, DVT)?

Examination Assess cardiorespiratory system, exercise tolerance. Is the neck unstable (eg arthritis complicating intubation)? ►Is DVT/PE prophylaxis needed (p578)? ►For 'unilateral' surgery, mark the correct arm/leg/kidney (surgeon).

Tests Be guided by the history and examination and local/NICE protocols.

- *U&E, FBC, and finger-prick blood glucose in most patients.* If Hb <100g/L tell anaesthetist. Investigate/treat as appropriate. U&E are particularly important if the patient is starved, diabetic, on diuretics, a burns patient, has hepatic or renal disease, has an ileus, or is parenterally fed.
- *Crossmatch:* Blood type is identified and units are allocated to the patient. *Group and save (G&S):* Blood type is identified and held, pending crossmatch (if required). Contact your lab to discuss requirements—this decreases wastage and allows increased efficiency of blood stocks.
- *Specific blood tests:* LFT in jaundice, malignancy, or alcohol abuse. Amylase in acute abdominal pain. Blood glucose if diabetic (p588). Drug levels as appropriate (eg digoxin, lithium). Clotting studies in liver or renal disease, DIC (p352), massive blood loss, or if on valproate, warfarin, or heparin. HIV, HBsAg in high-risk patients, after counselling. Sickle test in those from Africa, West Indies, or Mediterranean—and if origins are in malarial areas (including most of India). Thyroid function tests in those with thyroid disease.
- *CXR* if known cardiorespiratory disease, pathology, or symptoms or >65yrs old. Remember to check the film prior to surgery.
- *ECG* if >55yrs old or poor exercise tolerance, or history of myocardial ischaemia, hypertension, rheumatic fever, or other heart disease.
- *Echocardiogram* may be performed if there is a suspicion of poor LV function.
- *Pulmonary function tests* in known pulmonary disease/obesity.
- *Lateral cervical spine X-ray* (flexion and extension views) if history of rheumatoid arthritis/ankylosing spondylitis/Down's syndrome, to warn of difficult intubations.
- *MRSA screen:* Screen and decolonize nasal carriers according to local policy (eg nasal mupirocin ointment). Colonization is *not* a contraindication to surgery. Place patients last on the list to minimize transmission to others and cover with appropriate antibiotic prophylaxis, eg vancomycin or teicoplanin. Consider and document major blood-borne virus risk (HIV/HBV/HCV) according to local policies.

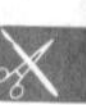

American Society of Anesthesiologists (ASA) classification

Class I	Normally healthy patient.
Class II	Mild systemic disease.
Class III	Severe systemic disease that limits activity but is not incapacitating.
Class IV	Incapacitating systemic disease which poses a constant threat to life.
Class V	Moribund: not expected to survive 24h even with operation.

You will see a space for an ASA number on most anaesthetic charts. It is a health index at the time of surgery. The suffix E is used in emergencies, eg ASA 2E.

[1] If within the last 6 months, the perioperative risk of re-infarction (up to 40%) makes most elective surgery too risky. ECHO, and stress testing (+ exercise ECG or MUGA scan, p741) should be done.

In which of the following situations would you seek 'informed written consent' from a patient? **1** Feeling for a pulse. **2** Taking blood. **3** Inserting a central line. **4** Removing a section of small bowel during a laparotomy for division of adhesions. **5** Orchidectomy after a failed operation for testicular torsion.

English law states that *any* intervention or treatment needs consent—ie all of the above—yet, for different reasons. In fact, *written* consent itself is not required by law, but it does constitute 'good medical practice' in the best interests of the patient and practitioner. Sometimes actions and words can imply valid consent, eg by simply entering into conversation or holding out an arm. If the consequences are not clear and the patient has *capacity* to give consent, you should seek informed written consent as a record of your conversation.

For consent to be valid

- It can be given any time before the intervention/treatment is initiated. Earlier is better as this will give the patient time to think about the risks, benefits, and alternatives—he or she may even bring forward questions on issues that you had not considered relevant. Think of consent as an ongoing process throughout the patient's time with you, not just the moment of signing the form.
- The proposed treatment or test must be clearly understood by the patient, taking into account the benefits, risks (including complication rates if known), additional procedures, alternative courses of action, and their consequences.
- It must be given *voluntarily*. This can be difficult to evaluate—eg when live organ donation is being considered—see BOX 'Special circumstances for consent' for other difficult situations.
- The doctor providing treatment or undertaking the test needs to ensure that the patient has given valid consent. The act of seeking consent is ultimately the responsibility of the doctor looking after the patient, though the task may be delegated to another health professional, as long as they are suitably trained and qualified.

Capacity relates to the ability to **1** understand, **2** retain, and **3** weigh up relevant information and **4** communicate the decision. Capacity is not a fixed state, but is specific to any given time and decision—a person may lack capacity to be involved in a particular complex decision but retain capacity to decide other aspects of their care, or recover capacity as they recover from acute illness. Therefore, do not label anyone as unable to make a decision unless you have taken all practicable steps to help them to do so without success—non-urgent decisions should always be deferred if there is a chance to recover capacity. When acting on behalf of a person who lacks capacity, do so in their best interests and involve family members or an appointed surrogate where clinical urgency allows.

When taking consent

- Does the patient currently have capacity for the decision in question?
- Are you the right person to be obtaining consent?[2]
- Use words the patient understands and avoid jargon and abbreviations.
- Ensure that they believe your facts and can retain 'pros' and 'cons' long enough to inform their decision. Fact sheets/diagrams for individual operations help.
- Make sure their choice is free from pressure from others, and explain that they can withdraw consent at any time after the form is signed. Some patients may view the consent form as a contract from which they cannot *renege*.
- If the patient is illiterate, a witnessed mark does endorse valid consent. Similarly, if the patient is willing but physically unable to sign the consent form, then a witnessed entry into the medical notes stating so is valid.
- Remember to discuss further procedures that may become necessary during the proposed treatment. This avoids waking up to a nasty surprise (eg a missing testicle as in scenario 5 earlier in this topic).

Special circumstances for consent

Consent is complex, but remember that it exists for the benefit of the patient *and* the doctor, giving you an opportunity to revisit expectations and involve the patient in their own care. There are some areas of treatment or investigation for which it may be advisable to seek specialist advice if it is not part of your regular practice[2]:

- Photography of a patient.
- Innovative or novel treatment.
- Living organ donation.
- Storage, use, or removal of human tissue (for any length of time).
- The storage, loss, or use of gametes.
- The use of patient records or tissue in research or teaching.
- In the presence of an advanced directive or living will, expressly refusing a particular treatment, investigation, or action.
- Consent if <16yrs (consent form 3 in NHS). In the UK, those >16yrs can give valid consent. Those <16yrs can give consent for a medical decision provided they understand what it involves—the concept of *Gillick* competence. It is still good practice to involve the parents in the decision, if the child is willing. If *<18yrs and refusing life-saving surgery*, talk to the parents and your senior; the law is unclear. You may need to contact the duty judge in the High Court.
- Consent in the incapacitated (NHS consent form 4). No one (parents, relatives, or even members of a healthcare team) is able to give consent on behalf of an adult in England, and the High Court may be required to give a ruling on the matters of lawfulness of a proposed procedure. Proceeding in a patient's best interest is decided by the clinician overseeing their care, with involvement of family members or a nominated advocate.

The right to refuse treatment

Theirs not to make reply,
Theirs not to reason why,
Theirs but to do and die. Alfred, Lord Tennyson from *The Charge of the Light Brigade*, 1854.

The rights of a patient are something of an antithesis to this military macabre of Tennyson, and it is our responsibility to respect the legal and ethical rights of those we treat. We do this not only for the sake of the individual, but also for the sake of an enduring trust between the patient and doctor, remembering that it is the patient's right to refuse treatment (if a fully competent adult) even when this may result in the death of the patient, or even the death of an unborn child, whatever the stage of pregnancy. The only exceptions apply to treatment of mental health disorders (see eg in England and Wales the Mental Health Act 2007).

If in any doubt, turn to: your senior/consultant; your employing organization; your legal defence organization; your national medical association; your local research ethics committee.

Prophylactic antibiotics in surgery

Prophylactic antibiotics are given to counter the risk of wound infection (see table 13.1), which occurs in ~20% of elective GI surgery (up to 60% in emergency surgery). Antibiotics are also given if infection elsewhere, although unlikely, would have severe consequences (eg when prostheses are involved). A single dose given before surgery has been shown to be just as good as more prolonged regimens in biliary and colorectal surgery. Additional doses may be given if high-risk/prolonged procedures, or if major blood loss. ►Wound infections are not necessarily trivial since sepsis may lead to haemorrhage, wound dehiscence, and initiate a fatal chain of events, so take measures to minimize the risk of wound infection:

- Time administration correctly (eg IV prophylaxis should be given 30min prior to surgery to maximize skin concentration; metronidazole PR is given 2h before).
- Use antibiotics which will kill anaerobes and coliforms.
- Consider use of peri-operative supplemental oxygen. This is a practical method of reducing the incidence of surgical wound infections.
- Practise strictly sterile surgical technique. (Ask for a hand with scrubbing up if you are not sure—theatre staff will be more than pleased to help!)

Antibiotic regimens ►Adhere to local guidelines. BNF examples include:

- *Appendicectomy; colorectal resections and open biliary surgery:* A single dose of IV piperacillin/tazobactam 4.5g/8h *or* gentamicin 1.5mg/kg + metronidazole 500mg *or* co-amoxiclav 1.2g alone.
- *Oesophageal or gastric surgery:* 1 dose of IV gentamicin *or* piperacillin/tazobactam *or* co-amoxiclav (doses as for appendicectomy).
- *Vascular surgery:* 1 dose of IV piperacillin/tazobactam *or* flucloxacillin 1-2g + gentamicin. Add metronidazole if risk of anaerobes (eg amputations, gangrene, or diabetes).
- *MRSA:* For high-risk patients add teicoplanin or vancomycin to the above-listed regimens.

Table 13.1 Classification of surgical procedures and wound infection risk

Category	Description	Infection risk
Clean	Incising uninfected skin without opening a viscus	<2%
Clean-contaminated	Intra-operative breach of a viscus (but not colon)	8-10%
Contaminated	Breach of a viscus + spillage or opening of colon	12-20%
Dirty	The site is already contaminated with pus or faeces, or from exogenous contagion, eg trauma	25%

Data from *MRCS Core Modules: Essential Revision Notes*, S. Andrews, Pastest

Sutures

Sutures are central to the art of surgery. No single suture fits the bill for every occasion, and so suture selection (including size) depends on the job in hand (see tables 13.2, 13.3). In their broadest sense they are absorbable or non-absorbable, synthetic or natural, and their structure may be divided into monofilament, twisted, or braided. Monofilament sutures are quite slippery but minimize infection and produce less reaction. Braided sutures have plaited strands and provide secure knots, but they may allow infection to occur in surrounding tissue between their strands. Twisted sutures have 2 twisted strands and similar qualities to braided sutures. Sizes are denoted according to a scale running down from #5 (heavy braided suture). Most common modern sutures are smaller than size #0, hence rising numbers with a -0 suffix correspond to progressively finer grades of suture up to 11-0 (fine ophthalmic monofilaments). 3-0 or 4-0 are the best sizes for skin closure. Timing of suture removal depends on site and the general health of the patient. Face and neck sutures may be removed after 5d (earlier in children), scalp and back of neck after 5d, abdominal incisions and proximal limbs (including clips) after ~10d, distal extremities after 14d. In patients with poor wound healing, eg steroids, malignancy, infection, cachexia (p35), the elderly, or smokers, sutures may need ~14d.

Some commonly encountered suture materials

Absorbable

Table 13.2 Absorbable suture materials

Name	Material	Construction	Use
Monocryl®	Poliglecaprone	Monofilament	Subcuticular skin closure
PDS®	Polydioxanone	Monofilament	Closing abdominal wall
Vicryl®	Polyglactin	Braided multifilament	Tying pedicles; bowel anastomosis; subcutaneous closure
Dexon®	Polyglycolic acid	Braided multifilament	Very similar to Vicryl®

Non-absorbable

Table 13.3 Non-absorbable suture materials

Name	Material	Construction	Use
Ethilon®	Polyamide	Monofilament	Closing skin wounds
Prolene®	Polypropylene	Monofilament	Arterial anastomosis
Mersilk®N	Silk	Braided multifilament	Securing drains
Metal	Eg steel	Clips or monofilament	Skin wound/sternotomy closure

N = natural; other natural materials (eg cotton and catgut) are rarely used these days.

Surgical drains in the post-operative period

The decision when to insert and remove drains may seem to be one of the great surgical enigmas—but there are basically three types to get a grip of:

1. To drain the area of surgery and are often put under suction or −ve pressure (Redivac® uses a 'high vacuum'). These are removed when they stop draining. They protect against collection, haematoma, and seroma formation (in breast surgery this can cause overlying skin necrosis).
2. To protect sites where leakage may occur in post-operative period, eg bowel anastomoses. These form a tract and are removed after about 1wk.
3. To collect red blood cells from the site of the operation, which can then be autotransfused within 6h, protecting from the hazards of allotransfusion—it is used commonly in orthopaedics. (eg Bellovac®).

'Shortening a drain' means withdrawing it (eg by 2cm/d) to allow the tract to seal, bit by bit. ►Check the surgeon's wishes before altering a drain. ►If a drain 'falls out' on the ward, avoid re-siting it because it is now covered in skin flora. Put a collecting bag over the wound and contact surgical registrar.

Anaesthesia

Before anaesthesia, explain to the patient what will happen and where they will wake up, otherwise the recovery room or ITU will be frightening. Explain that they may feel ill on waking. The premedication aims to allay anxiety and to make the anaesthesia itself easier to conduct (see BOX). Typical regimens might include:

- *Anxiolytics:* Benzodiazepines, eg lorazepam 2mg PO; temazepam 10–20mg PO. In children, use oral premeds as first choice, eg midazolam 0.5mg/kg (tastes bitter so often put in paracetamol suspension). Give oral premedication 2h before surgery (1h if IM route used).
- *Analgesics:* See p574. Pre-emptive analgesia is not often used and effects are hard to determine. The aim is to dampen pain signals before they arrive. In children or anxious adults, local anaesthetic cream may be used on a few sites before inserting an IVI (►the anaesthetist may prefer to site the cannula themselves!).
- *Anti-emetics:* Post-operative nausea and vomiting is experienced by ~25% of all patients. $5HT_3$ antagonists (eg ondansetron 4mg IV/IM) are the most effective agents; others, eg metoclopramide 10mg/8h IV/IM/PO, are also used—see p251.
- *Antacids:* Ranitidine 50mg IV or omeprazole 40mg PO/IV if aspiration risk.
- *Antisialogues:* Glycopyrronium (200–400mcg in adults, 4–8mcg/kg in children; given IV/IM 30–60min before induction) is sometimes used to decrease secretions that may cause respiratory obstruction in smaller airways.
- *Antibiotics:* See p570.

Side-effects of anaesthetic agents

- *Hyoscine, atropine:* Anticholinergic, ∴ tachycardia, urinary retention, glaucoma, sedation (especially in the elderly).
- *Opioids:* Respiratory depression, ↓cough reflex, nausea and vomiting, constipation.
- *Thiopental:* (Induction agent.) Laryngospasm.
- *Propofol:* (Induction agent.) Respiratory/cardiac depression, pain on injection.
- *Volatile agents, eg isoflurane:* Nausea and vomiting, cardiac depression, respiratory depression, vasodilation, hepatotoxicity (see *BNF*).

The complications of anaesthesia are due to loss of:

- *Pain sensation:* Urinary retention, pressure necrosis, local nerve injuries (eg radial nerve palsy from arm hanging over the table edge).
- *Consciousness:* Cannot communicate 'wrong leg/kidney'. NB: in some patients (eg 0.15%) *retained* consciousness is the problem. Awareness under GA sounds like a contradiction of terms, but remember that anaesthesia is a process rather than an event. Such awareness can lead to ill-defined, delayed neuroses and post-traumatic stress disorder (*OHCS* p353).
- *Muscle power:* Corneal abrasion (∴ tape the eyes closed), no respiration, no cough (leads to pneumonia and atelectasis—partial lung collapse causing shunting ± impaired gas exchange: it starts minutes after induction, and may be related to the use of 100% O_2, supine position, surgery, age, and to loss of power).

Local/regional anaesthesia If unfit/unwilling to undergo general anaesthesia, local nerve blocks (eg brachial plexus) or spinal blocks (contraindication: anticoagulation, local infection) using long-acting local anaesthetics such as bupivacaine may be indicated. See table 13.4 for doses and toxicity effects.

Drugs complicating anaesthesia ►Inform anaesthetist. See p566 for lists of specific drugs, and actions to take.

Malignant hyperpyrexia This is a rare complication, precipitated by any volatile agent, eg halothane, or suxamethonium. It exhibits autosomal dominant inheritance. There is a rapid rise in temperature (>1°C every 30min); masseter spasm may be an early sign. Complications include hypoxaemia, hypercarbia, hyperkalaemia, metabolic acidosis, and arrhythmias. ►Get expert help immediately. Prompt treatment with dantrolene[3] (skeletal muscle relaxant), active cooling and ITU care can reduce mortality significantly.

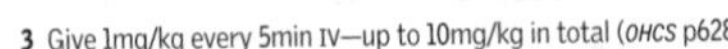

3 Give 1mg/kg every 5min IV—up to 10mg/kg in total (*OHCS* p628).

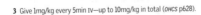

Principles and practical conduct of anaesthesia

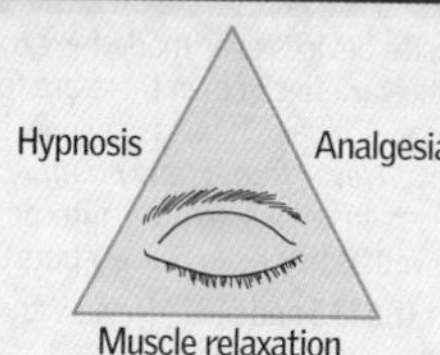

Fig 13.4 Principles of anaesthesia.

The conduct of anaesthesia (fig 13.4) typically involves:

- *Induction:* Either intravenous (eg propofol 1.5–2.5mg/kg IV at a rate of 20–40mg every 10s; thiopental is an alternative) or, if airway obstruction or difficult IV access, gaseous (eg sevoflurane or nitrous oxide, mixed in O_2).
- *Airway control:* Either using a facemask, an oropharyngeal (Guedel) airway or by intubation. The latter usually requires muscle relaxation with a depolarizing/non-depolarizing neuromuscular blocker (*OHCS* p622).
- *Maintenance of anaesthesia:* Either a volatile agent added to N_2O/O_2 mixture, or high-dose opiates with mechanical ventilation, or IV infusion anaesthesia (eg propofol 4–12mg/kg/h IVI).
- *Recovery:* Change inspired gases to 100% oxygen only, then discontinue any anaesthetic infusions and reverse muscle paralysis. Extubate once spontaneously breathing, place patient in recovery position, and give oxygen by facemask.
- For further details, see the *Anaesthesia* chapter in *OHCS* (p612).

⚠ Local anaesthetic toxicity and maximum doses

Anaesthetists are masters of the drug dose by weight! It is important to remember the maximum doses for local anaesthetics, not least because we use them so frequently, but because the effects of overdose can be lethal.

Handy to remember (though it can be worked out with a pen, paper, and SI units) is that a 1% concentration is equivalent to 10mg/mL. Local anaesthetics are also basic, and so do not work well in acidic environments, eg abscesses.

Table 13.4 Example of maximum doses for local anaesthetic

% concⁿ	Lidocaine concⁿ (mg/mL)	Approx. allowable volume (mL/kg)	Approx. allowable volume for 70kg adult (mL)
0.25%	2.5	1.12	≤80
0.5%	5	0.56	≤40
1%	10	0.28	≤20
2%	20	0.14	≤10

Local anaesthetic toxicity starts with peri-oral tingling and paraesthesiae, progressing to drowsiness, seizures, coma, and cardiorespiratory arrest. If suspected (the patient feels 'funny' and develops early signs) then stop administration immediately and commence ABC resuscitation as required. ►►Treatment is with lipid emulsion. Find out where this is stored in your hospital.

The control of pain

Humans are the most exquisite devices ever made for experiencing pain: the richer our inner lives, the greater the varieties of pain there are for us to feel, and the more resources we have for dealing with pain. If we can connect with patients' inner lives we may make a real difference. *Never forget how painful pain* is, nor how fear magnifies pain. Try not to let these sensations, so often interposed between your patient and recovery, be invisible to you as he or she bravely puts up with them.

Approach to management (fig 13.5 and p532.) Review and chart each pain carefully and individually.

- Identify and treat the underlying pathology wherever possible.
- Give *regular* doses rather than on an 'as-required' basis.
- Choose the best route: PO, PR, IM, epidural, SC, inhalation, or IV.
- Explanation and reassurance contribute greatly to analgesia.
- Allow the patient to be in charge. This promotes wellbeing, and does not lead to overuse. Patient-controlled continuous IV morphine delivery systems are useful.
- Liaise with the Acute Pain Service, if possible.

Non-narcotic (simple) analgesia Paracetamol 0.5–1.0g/4h PO (up to 4g daily; 15mg/kg/4h IV over 15min in children <50kg; up to 60mg/kg/d). Caution in liver impairment. NSAIDs, eg ibuprofen 400mg/8h PO (see *BNFc* for dosing in children) are good for musculoskeletal pain and renal or biliary colic. CI: peptic ulcer, clotting disorders, anticoagulants. Cautions: asthma, renal or hepatic impairment, heart failure, IHD, pregnancy, and the elderly. Aspirin is contraindicated in children due to the risk of Reye's syndrome (*OHCS* p652).

Opioid drugs for severe pain Morphine (eg 10–15mg/2–4h IV/IM) or diamorphine (5–10mg/2–4h PO, SC, or slow IV, but you may need much more) are best. NB: these are 'controlled' drugs. For palliative care, see p532. Alternative delivery routes include transdermal (once baseline requirements are established) or sublingual. *Side-effects of opioids:* These include nausea (so give with an anti-emetic, p251), respiratory depression, constipation, cough suppression, urinary retention, ↓BP, and sedation (do not use in hepatic failure or head injury). Dependency is rarely a problem. *Naloxone* (eg 100–200mcg IV, followed by 100mcg increments, eg every 2min until responsive) may be needed to reverse the effects of excess opioids (p842).

Epidural analgesia Opioids and anaesthetics are given into the epidural space by infusion or as boluses. Ask the advice of the Pain Service. SEs are thought to be less, as the drug is more localized: watch for respiratory depression and local anaesthetic-induced autonomic blockade (↓BP).

Adjuvant treatments Eg radiotherapy for bone cancer pain; anticonvulsants, antidepressants, gabapentin or steroids for neuropathic pain, antispasmodics, eg hyoscine butylbromide[4] (Buscopan® 10–20mg/8h PO/IM/IV) for intestinal or renal tract colic. If brief pain relief is needed (eg for changing dressings or exploring wounds), try inhaled nitrous oxide (with 50% O_2—as Entonox®) with an 'on-demand' valve. Transcutaneous electrical nerve stimulation (TENS), local heat, local or regional anaesthesia, and neurosurgical procedures (eg excision of neuroma) may be tried but can prove disappointing. Treat conditions that exacerbate pain (eg constipation, depression, anxiety).

4 Not to be confused with *hyoscine hydrobromide*; used for drying secretions and in motion sickness.

WHO's Pain relief ladder

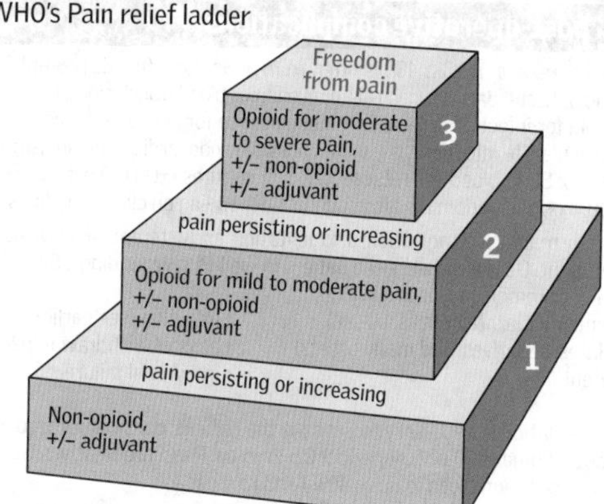

Fig 13.5 World Health Organization pain ladder.

General post-operative complications

Pyrexia Mild pyrexia in the 1st 48h is often from atelectasis (needs prompt physio, not antibiotics), tissue damage/necrosis, or even from blood transfusions, but still have a low threshold for infection screen. Consider evidence for peritonism, chest, urinary, wound, or cannula site infections, as well as possible endocarditis, meningism, or DVT (also causes ↑°T). Send blood for FBC, U&E, CRP, and cultures (±LFT). Dipstick the urine. Consider MSU, CXR, and abdominal ultrasound/CT depending on clinical findings.

Confusion may manifest as agitation, disorientation, and attempts to leave hospital, especially at night. Gently reassure the patient in well-lit surroundings. See p484 for a full work-up. Common causes are:

- hypoxia (pneumonia, atelectasis, LVF, PE)
- drugs (opiates, sedatives, and many others)
- urinary retention
- MI or stroke
- infection (see earlier)
- alcohol withdrawal (p280)
- liver/renal failure.

Occasionally, sedation is necessary to examine the patient; consider lorazepam 1mg PO/IM (antidote: flumazenil) or haloperidol 0.5–2mg IM. Reassure relatives that post-op confusion is common (seen in up to 40%) and reversible.

Dyspnoea or hypoxia Any previous lung disease? Sit patient up and give O_2, monitor peripheral O_2 sats by pulse oximetry (p162). Examine for evidence of: •pneumonia, pulmonary collapse, or aspiration •LVF (MI; fluid overload) •pulmonary embolism (p190) •pneumothorax (p190; due to CVP line, intercostal block, or mechanical ventilation). *Tests:* FBC; ABG; CXR; ECG. Manage according to findings.

↓BP If severe, tilt bed head-down and give O_2. Check pulse and BP yourself; compare it with pre-op values. Post-op ↓BP is often from hypovolaemia resulting from inadequate fluid input, so check fluid chart and replace losses. Monitor urine output (may need catheterization). A CVP line can help monitor fluid resuscitation (normal is 0–5cmH_2O relative to sternal angle). Hypovolaemia may also be caused by haemorrhage so review wounds, drains, and abdomen. If unstable, return to theatre for haemostasis. Beware cardiogenic and neurogenic causes and look for evidence of MI or PE. Consider sepsis and anaphylaxis. *Management:* p790.

↑BP may be from pain, urinary retention, idiopathic hypertension (eg missed medication), or inotropic drugs. Oral cardiac medications (including antihypertensives) should be continued throughout the perioperative period even if NBM. Treat the cause, consider increasing the regular medication, or if not absorbing orally try 50mg labetalol IV over 1min (see p140).

↓Urine output (oliguria) Aim for output of >30mL/h in adults (or >0.5mL/kg/h). *Anuria* may reflect a blocked or malsited catheter (see p763) rather than AKI. Flush or replace catheter. *Oliguria* is usually due to too little replacement of lost fluid. Treat by increasing fluid input. ►Acute kidney injury may follow shock, drugs, transfusion, pancreatitis, or trauma (see p300 for classification and management of AKI).

- Review fluid chart and examine for signs of volume depletion.
- Urinary retention is also common, so examine for a palpable bladder.
- Establish normovolaemia (a CVP line may help); you may need 1L/h IVI for 2–3h. A 'fluid challenge' of 250–500mL over 30min may also help.
- Catheterize bladder (for accurate monitoring)—see p762; check U&E.
- If intrinsic renal failure is suspected, stop nephrotoxic drugs (eg NSAIDs, ACE-i) and refer to a nephrologist early.

Nausea/vomiting Any mechanical obstruction, ileus, or emetic drugs (opiates, digoxin, anaesthetics)? Consider AXR, NGT, and an anti-emetic (►*not* metoclopramide because of its prokinetic property). See p251 for choice of anti-emetics.

↓Na^+ Pre-op level? Excess IV fluids may exacerbate the situation. Correct slowly (p672). SIADH (p673) can be precipitated by pain, nausea, opioids, and chest infection.

Post-operative bleeding

Primary haemorrhage: Continuous bleeding, starting during surgery. Replace blood loss. If severe, return to theatre for adequate haemostasis. Treat shock vigorously (p790–804).

Reactive haemorrhage: Haemostasis appears secure until BP rises and bleeding starts. Replace blood and re-explore wound.

Secondary haemorrhage (caused by infection) occurs 1–2wks post-op.

Talking about post-op complications...

When asked to give your thoughts on the complications of an operation—maybe with an examiner or a patient—a good starting point is to divide them up accordingly (and for each of the following stratify as immediate, early, and late):

- *From the anaesthetic:* (p572.) Eg respiratory depression from induction agents.
- *From surgery in general:* (p576.) Eg wound infection, haemorrhage, neurovascular damage, DVT/PE.
- *From the specific procedure:* Eg saphenous nerve damage in stripping of the long varicose vein.

Tailor the discussion towards the individual who, eg if an arteriopath, may have a significant risk of cardiac ischaemia during hypotensive episodes while under the anaesthetic. For some other post-op complications, see:
• Pain (p574) • DVT (p578) • Pulmonary embolus (p190; massive, p818) • Wound dehiscence (p580) • Complications in post-gastric surgery (p622) • Other complications of specific operations (p580).

Deep vein thrombosis (DVT)

DVTs occur in 25–50% of surgical patients, and many non-surgical patients. All hospital inpatients should be assessed for DVT/PE risk and offered prophylaxis if appropriate. 65% of below-knee DVTs are asymptomatic; these rarely embolize to the lung.

Risk factors ↑Age, pregnancy, synthetic oestrogen, trauma, surgery (especially pelvic/orthopaedic), past DVT, cancer, obesity, immobility, thrombophilia (p374).

Signs •Calf warmth/tenderness/swelling/erythema. •Mild fever. •Pitting oedema.

ΔΔ Cellulitis; ruptured Baker's cyst. Both may coexist with a DVT.

Tests ►Calculate Wells score (see table 13.5) before ordering *D-dimer.* D-dimer is sensitive but not specific for DVT (also ↑ in infection, pregnancy, malignancy, and post-op).

Wells score: *≤1 point = DVT unlikely:* Perform D-dimer. If negative, DVT excluded. If positive, proceed to USS (if USS negative, DVT excluded; if positive, treat as DVT).

≥2 points = DVT likely: Do D-dimer and USS. If both negative, DVT excluded. If USS positive, treat as DVT. If D-dimer positive and USS negative, repeat USS in 1 week.

Do *thrombophilia tests* (p374) *before* commencing anticoagulant therapy if there are no predisposing factors, in recurrent DVT, or if DVT in unusual site. Look for *underlying malignancy:* Urine dip; FBC, LFT, Ca^{2+}; CXR ± CT abdomen/pelvis (and mammography in ♀) if >40yrs.

Prevention •Stop the oral contraceptive pill 4wks pre-op. •Mobilize early. •LMWH eg enoxaparin 20mg/24h SC, ↑ to 40mg for high-risk patients (p375) (caution if eGFR less than 30mL/min/1.73m²). •Graduated compression stockings ('thromboembolic deterrent (TED) stockings'; CI: ischaemia) and intermittent pneumatic compression devices ↓ risk of DVT by ~70% in surgical patients.•Fondaparinux (a factor Xa inhibitor) ↓ risk of DVT over LMWH in eg major orthopaedic surgery without ↑ risk of bleeding.

Treatment LMWH (eg enoxaparin 1.5mg/kg/24h SC) or fondaparinux. LMWH is superior to unfractionated heparin (used in renal failure or if ↑risk of bleeding; dose guided by APTT, p350). Cancer patients should receive LMWH for 6 months (then review). In others, start warfarin simultaneously with LMWH (warfarin is prothrombotic for the first 48h). Stop heparin when INR is 2-3; treat for 3 months in most (longer in some cases—see p351). *Direct oral anticoagulants* (DOACs p190), eg dabigatan, apixaban, rivoraxaban, are newer alternatives licensed for the treatment of DVT with benefits relating to simpler dosing and monitoring and ↓ bleeding risk. *Inferior vena caval filters* may be used in active bleeding, or when anticoagulants fail, to minimize risk of PE. *Post-phlebitic change* (pain, swelling, and skin changes) can be seen in 10-30%—graduated compression stockings may help.

Pretest clinical probability scoring for DVT: the Wells score

In patients with symptoms in both legs, the more symptomatic leg is used.

Table 13.5 Wells score

Clinical features	Score
Active cancer (treatment within last 6 months or palliative)	1 point
Paralysis, paresis, or recent plaster immobilization of leg	1 point
Recently bedridden for >3d or majory surgery in last 12wks	1 point
Local tenderness along distribution of deep venous system	1 point
Entire leg swollen	1 point
Calf swelling >3cm compared with asymptomatic leg (measured 10cm below tibial tuberosity)	1 point
Pitting oedema (greater in the symptomatic leg)	1 point
Collateral superficial veins (non-varicose)	1 point
Previously documented DVT	1 point
Alternative diagnosis at least as likely as DVT	−2 points

Swollen legs

Bilateral oedema implies systemic disease with ↑venous pressure (eg right heart failure) or ↓intravascular oncotic pressure (any cause of ↓albumin, so test the urine for protein). It is *dependent* (distributed by gravity), which is why legs are affected early, but severe oedema extends above the legs. In the bed-bound, fluid moves to the new dependent area, causing a sacral pad. The exception is the local increase in venous pressure occurring in IVC obstruction: the swelling neither extends above the legs nor redistributes. *Causes:* •Right heart failure (p134). •↓Albumin (p686, eg renal or liver failure). •Venous insufficiency: acute, eg prolonged sitting, or chronic, with haemosiderin-pigmented, itchy, eczematous skin ± ulcers. •Vasodilators, eg *nifedipine, amlodipine*. •Pelvic mass (p57, p604). •Pregnancy—if ↑BP + proteinuria, diagnose pre-eclampsia (*OHCS* p48): find an obstetrician urgently. In all the above, both legs need not be affected to the same extent.

Unilateral oedema Pain ± redness implies DVT or inflammation, eg cellulitis or insect bites (any blisters?). Bone or muscle may be to blame, eg tumours; necrotizing fasciitis (p660); trauma (check for sensation, pulses, and severe pain esp. on passive movement: ►a *compartment syndrome* with ischaemic necrosis needs prompt fasciotomy). Impaired mobility suggests trauma, arthritis, or a Baker's cyst (p694). *Non-pitting oedema* is oedema you cannot indent: see p35.

Nine questions to ask

1 Is it *both* legs?	**2** Is she pregnant?	**3** Is she mobile?
4 Any trauma?	**5** Any pitting (p35)?	**6** Past diseases/on drugs?
7 Any pain?	**8** Any skin changes?	**9** Any oedema elsewhere?

Tests ►Look for proteinuria (+hypoalbuminaemia ≈nephrotic syndrome). CCF?

Treatment of leg oedema Treat the cause. Diuretics for all is not an answer. Elevating legs for dependent oedema (ankles higher than hips—do not just use footstools); raise the foot of the bed. Graduated support stockings may help (CI: ischaemia).

Travel and DVT

Long-distance travel appears to be a risk factor for the development of venous thromboembolism (VTE). Data suggests this is not confined to air travel, increases with the duration of travel, and results in clinical thrombosis more often in travellers with pre-existing risk factors. Dehydration, immobilization, decreased oxygen tension, and prolonged sitting have all been suggested as contributory factors. The risk of developing a DVT from a long-distance flight has been estimated at 1 in 10 000 to 1 in 40 000 for the general population.

- The incidence of DVT in *high-risk* groups has been shown to be 4–6% for flights >10h. Travellers with ≥1 risk factor should consider compression stockings. For high-risk individuals consider a single dose of prophylactic LMWH for flights >6h.
- There is ↑risk of PE associated with long-distance air travel.
- Compression stockings may ↓ risk of DVT.
- There is no evidence to support the use of prophylactic aspirin.
- Risk reduction measures: leg exercises, increased water intake, and refraining from alcohol or caffeine during the journey.

Specific post-operative complications

Laparotomy Wound may break down from a few days to a few weeks post-op (incidence ≈3.5%). Particular risk in the elderly, malnourished (eg cancer, IBD), if infection, uraemia, or haematoma is present, or in repeat laparotomies. Warning sign is a pink serous discharge. Always assume the defect involves the whole of the wound. Wound dehiscence may lead to a 'burst abdomen' with evisceration of bowel (mortality 15-30%). If you are on the ward when this happens, call your senior, put the viscera back into the abdomen, place a sterile dressing over the wound, and give IV antibiotics (eg piperacillin/tazobactam; see local guidelines). Allay anxiety, give parenteral pain control, set up an IVI, and return patient to theatre. *Incisional hernia* is a common late problem (20%), repairable by mesh insertion (if necessary).

Biliary surgery *Early:* Iatrogenic bile duct injury, cholangitis, bile leakage, bleeding into the biliary tree (haemobilia—may lead to melaena or haematemesis); pancreatitis. Retained stones may be removed by ERCP (p742); if this is not available a 'T-tube' left in the bile duct at the time of closure allows free drainage to the exterior; unrelieved distal obstruction of the bile duct may result in fistula formation and chronic leakage of bile. If jaundiced, maintain a good urine output, monitor coagulation, and consider antibiotics. *Late:* Bile duct stricture; post-cholecystectomy syndrome (symptoms arising from alterations in bile flow due to loss of the reservoir function of the gallbladder).

Thyroid surgery *Early:* Recurrent (± superior) laryngeal nerve palsy (→hoarseness) can occur permanently in 0.5% and transiently in 1.5%—warn the patient that *their voice will be different* for a few days post-op because of intubation and local oedema (NB: pre-operative fibreoptic laryngoscopy should be performed to exclude pre-existing vocal cord dysfunction); thyroid storm (symptoms of severe hyperthyroidism—see p834); tracheal obstruction due to haematoma in the wound: ►►relieve by immediate removal of stitches or clips using the cutter/remover that should remain at the beside; may require urgent surgery; hypoparathyroidism (p222); ►check plasma Ca^{2+} daily; transient drops in serum concentration are common, permanent in 2.5%. *Late:* Hypothyroidism; recurrent hyperthyroidism.

Mastectomy Arm lymphoedema in up to 20% of those undergoing axillary node sampling or dissection. The risk of lymphoedema increases with the level of axillary dissection: risk is lower with level 1 dissection (remains inferior to *pec. minor*) compared to level 3 dissection (goes superior to *pec. minor*, rarely done); skin necrosis.

Arterial surgery Bleeding; thrombosis; embolism; graft infection; MI; AV fistula formation. *Complications of aortic surgery:* Gut ischaemia; renal failure; respiratory distress; trauma to ureters or anterior spinal artery (leading to paraplegia); ischaemic events from distal emboli from dislodged thrombus; aorto-enteric fistula.

Colonic surgery *Early:* Sepsis; ileus; fistulae; anastomotic leak (11% for radical rectal surgery); haemorrhage; trauma to ureters or spleen. *Late:* Adhesional obstruction (BOX).

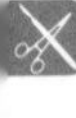

Small bowel surgery Short gut syndrome (best defined *functionally*, as malabsorption due to insufficient residual small bowel; adults with ≤150cm at risk). Diarrhoea and malabsorption (particularly of fats) lead to a number of metabolic abnormalities including deficiency in vitamins A, D, E, K, and B_{12}, hyperoxaluria (causing renal stones), and bile salt depletion (causing gallstones). The management of short bowel syndrome is complex, aiming to correct metabolic abnormalities, optimize residual bowel function, and support nutrition (using parenteral route if necessary).

Tracheostomy Mediastinitis; surgical emphysema. Later: stenosis.

Splenectomy (p373.) Acute gastric dilatation (a serious consequence of not using a NGT, or to check that the one in place is working); thrombocytosis; sepsis. ►Lifetime sepsis risk is partly preventable with pre-op vaccines—ie *Haemophilus* type B, meningococcal, and pneumococcal (p407 & p167) and prophylactic penicillin.

Genitourinary surgery Septicaemia (from instrumentation in the presence of infected urine)—consider a stat dose of gentamicin; urinoma—rupture of a ureter or renal pelvis leading to a mass of extravasated urine.

Gastrectomy See p622. **Prostatectomy** p642. **Haemorrhoidectomy** p632.

Adhesions—legacy of the laparotomy, bane of the surgeon

When re-operating on the abdomen, the struggle against adhesions tests the farthest and darkest boundaries of patience of the abdominal surgeon and the assistant. The skill and persistence required to gently and atraumatically tease apart these fibrous bands that restrict access and vision makes any progression, no matter how slight, cause for subdued celebration. Perseverance is the name of this game.

Surgical division of adhesions is known as *adhesiolysis*. Any surgical procedure that breaches the abdominal or pelvic cavities can predispose to the formation of adhesions, which are found in up to 90% of those with previous abdominal surgery; this is why we do not rush to operate on small bowel obstruction: the operation predisposes to yet more adhesions. Handling of the serosal surface of the bowel causes inflammation, which over weeks to years can lead to the formation of fibrous bands that tether the bowel to itself or adjacent structures—though adhesions can also form secondary to infection, radiation injury, and inflammatory processes such as Crohn's disease. Their main sequelae are intestinal obstruction (the cause in ~60% of cases—see p610) and chronic abdominal or pelvic pain. Studies have shown that adhesiolysis may help relieve chronic pain, though for a small proportion of patients the pain never improves or even worsens after directed intervention.

As far as prevention is concerned, the best approach is to avoid operating; laparoscopy compared with laparotomy reduces the rate of local adhesions. Insertion of synthetic films (eg hyaluronic acid/carboxymethyl membrane) to prevent adhesions to the anterior abdominal wall reduces incidence, extent, and severity of adhesions, but not incidence of obstruction or operative re-intervention.

Stoma care

A stoma (Greek=*mouth*) is an artificial union between a conduit and the outside world—eg a colostomy, in which faeces are made to pass through an opening in the abdominal wall when a loop of colon is brought out onto the skin. NB: a stoma can also be made between two internal conduits (eg a choledochojejunostomy).

Colostomies (Usually left illiac fossa and flush with the skin—fig 13.8.) May be temporary or permanent. Are they suitable for a laparoscopic operation?

- *Loop colostomy:* A loop of colon is exteriorized and partially divided, forming two stomas that are joined together (the proximal end passes stool, the distal end passes mucus, see fig 13.6). A rod under the loop prevents retraction and may be removed after 7d. A loop colostomy is often temporary and performed to protect a distal anastomosis, eg after anterior resection.
- *End colostomy:* The bowel is divided and the proximal end brought out as a stoma; the distal end may be: 1 *resected*, eg abdominoperineal (AP) resection (inspect the perineum for absent anus when examining a stoma) 2 *closed* and left in the abdomen (Hartmann's procedure) 3 *exteriorized*, forming a 'mucous fistula'.
- *Paul-Mikulicz colostomy:* A double-barrelled colostomy in which the colon is divided completely (eg to excise a section of bowel). Each end is exteriorized as two separate stomas.

Output: Colostomies ideally pass 1-2 formed motions/day into an adherent plastic pouch. Some may be managed with irrigation, thus avoiding a pouch.
Incidence: 21000 stomas/yr in UK (>50% are permanent). Most manage their stomas well. The cost for appliances is ~£1500/yr. If there is a skin reaction to the adhesive or pouch, a change of device may be all that is needed. Contact the stoma nurse.

Ileostomies (Usually right illiac fossa.) Protrude from the skin and emit frequent fluid motions which contain active enzymes (so the skin needs protecting—see fig 13.7). Loop ileostomies can be formed to defunction the colon as a temporary measure eg during control of difficult perianal Crohn's disease. End ileostomy follows total or subtotal colectomy, eg for UC; subsequent formation of *ileal pouch-anal anastomosis* (pouch of ileum is joined to the upper anal canal) can allow for stoma reversal.

Alternative (non-stoma forming) surgery *Low/ultralow anterior resection:* All or part of the rectum is excised and the proximal colon anastomosed to the top of the anal canal (the lower the level of anastomosis, the higher the risk of complication). *Transanal endoscopic microsurgery:* Allows excision of small tumours within the rectum with preservation of sphincter function.

Urostomies are fashioned after total cystectomy, bringing urine from the ureters to the abdominal wall via an *ileal conduit* that is usually incontinent. Formation of a catheterizable valvular mechanism may retain continence. Advances in urological surgery have seen an increase in continence-saving procedures such as orthotopic neobladder reconstruction, with good long-term continence rates.

When choosing a stoma site, avoid:

- Bony prominences (eg anterior superior iliac spine, costal margins).
- The umbilicus.
- Old wounds/scars—there may be adhesions beneath.
- Skin folds and creases.
- The waistline.
- The site should be assessed pre-operatively by the stoma nurse, with the patient both lying and standing.

Complications of stomas

►Liaise early with the stoma nurse, starting pre-operatively.

Early:
- Haemorrhage at stoma site.
- Stoma ischaemia—colour progresses from dusky grey to black.
- High output (can lead to ↓K^+)—consider loperamide ± codeine to thicken output.
- Obstruction secondary to adhesions (see p581).
- Stoma retraction.

Delayed:
- Obstruction (failure at operation to close lateral space around stoma).
- Dermatitis around stoma site (worse with ileostomy).
- Stoma prolapse.
- Stomal intussusception.
- Stenosis.
- Parastomal hernia (risk increases with time). NB: prophylactic mesh insertion at the time of stoma formation reduces this risk.
- Fistulae.
- Psychological problems.

Psychological aspects of stoma care

The physical and psychological aspects of stoma care must not be undervalued. Be alert to any vicious cycle in which a skin reaction leads to leakage and precipitates a fear of going out, or a fear of eating. This in turn may lead to poor nutrition and further skin reactions, resulting in further leakage and depression. These cycles can be circumvented by the *stoma nurse*, who is *the* expert in fitting secure, odourless devices and providing patients with a wealth of physical and psychological support, both pre and post operative (explaining what is going to happen, what the stoma will be like, and troubleshooting post-op problems). ►*Early referral prevents problems.* Without input from the stoma nurse, a patient may reject their colostomy, never attend to it, and develop deep-seated psychological and psychiatric problems.

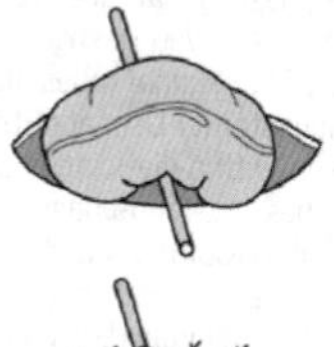

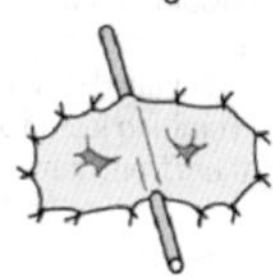

Fig 13.6 A loop colostomy with double-barrelled stoma and supporting ostomy rod.

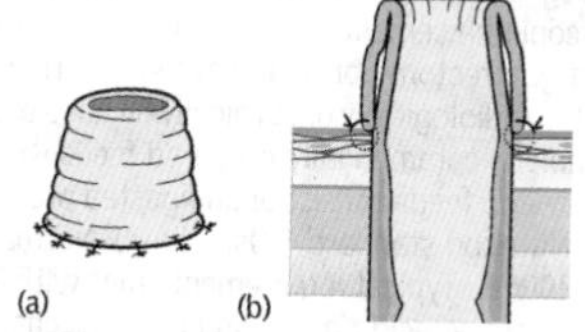

Fig 13.7 An ileostomy sits proud, has prominent mucosal folds, and is often right-sided.

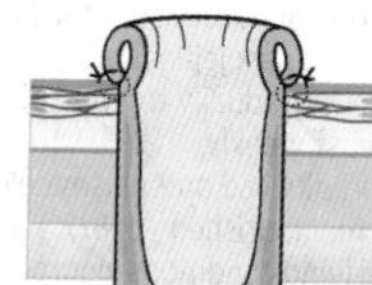

Fig 13.8 A colostomy sits flush with the skin and is typically sited in the left iliac fossa.

Nutritional support in hospital

►Over 25% of hospital inpatients may be malnourished. Hospitals can become so focused on curing disease that they ignore the foundations of good health—malnourished patients recover more slowly and experience more complications. See table 13.6.

Why are so many hospital patients malnourished?

1 Increased nutritional requirements (eg sepsis, burns, surgery).
2 Increased nutritional losses (eg malabsorption, output from stoma).
3 Decreased intake (eg dysphagia, nausea, sedation, coma).
4 Effect of treatment (eg nausea, diarrhoea).
5 Enforced starvation (eg prolonged periods nil by mouth).
6 Missing meals (eg due to investigations—minimize meal time disruption).
7 Difficulty with feeding (eg lost dentures; no one available to assist).
8 Unappetizing food.

Identifying at-risk patients Assess nutrition state (using eg Malnutrition Universal Screening Tool[3]) and weight on admission; reassess weekly thereafter. Involve dieticians early in those at risk.

- *History:* Recent ↓weight (>20%, accounting for fluid balance); recent reduced intake; diet change (eg recent change in consistency of food); nausea, vomiting, pain, diarrhoea which might have led to reduced intake.
- *Examination:* State of hydration (p666): dehydration can go hand-in-hand with malnutrition, and overhydration can mask malnutrition. Evidence of malnutrition: skin hanging off muscles (eg over biceps); no fat between fold of skin; hair rough and wiry; pressure sores; sores at corner of mouth. Calculate body mass index (p244); BMI <18.5kg/m^2 suggests malnourishment. Anthropomorphic indices, eg mid-arm circumference, skin fold measures, and grip strength are also used.
- *Investigations:* Generally unhelpful. Low albumin suggestive, but is affected by many things other than nutrition. ↑Albumin can be helpful in monitoring recovery.

Enteral nutrition (Ie nutrition given into gastrointestinal tract.) If at all possible, give nutrition by mouth. An all-fluid diet can meet requirements (but get advice from dietician). If danger of choking or aspiration (eg after stroke), consider semi-solid diet. Early post-op enteral nutrition has been shown to benefit patients (eg after GI surgery) and may reduce complications. *Tube feeding:* Liquid nutrition via a tube: Nasogastric typically placed without guidance (p759); nasojejunal tubes require endoscopic placement (used if gastric outlet obstruction, delayed gastric emptying, post-gastrectomy, or pancreatitis). Alternatively, gastric or jejunal tubes may be inserted radiologically or surgically (ie gastrostomy/jejunostomy). Use for nutritionally complete, commercially prepared feeds. ►Close liaison with a dietician is essential. *Polymeric* feeds consist of undigested proteins, starches, and long-chain fatty acids (eg Nutrison standard®, Osmolite®). Normally contain ~1kCal/mL and 4-6g protein per 100mL. Typical requirements met with 2L/24h. *Elemental* feeds consist of individual amino acids, oligo- and monosaccharides needing minimal digestion. Feed is typically initiated at a slow, continuous rate (nausea and vomiting less problematic) but patients may build up to shorter, bolus feeds, freeing them from pumps between.

Guidelines for success

- Use fine-bore (9Fr) nasogastric feeding tube when possible.
- Check position of nasogastric tube (pH testing) before starting feeding (p759); the positioning of a nasojejunal tube can be checked on abdominal X-ray.
- Build up feeds gradually to avoid diarrhoea and distension.
- Weigh at least weekly.
- Check blood glucose and plasma electrolytes (monitor for refeeding syndrome if previously malnourished—p587).
- Treat underlying conditions vigorously, eg sepsis may impede +ve nitrogen balance.

Nil by mouth (NBM) before theatre

If in doubt about what is acceptable oral intake prior to induction for general anaesthesia (eg for GI surgery), it is best to liaise with the anaesthetist concerned. However, guidelines have been published by many colleges and societies to outline what is safe in the perioperative period:

- For *adult elective surgery* in healthy patients without GI comorbidity:
  - Water or clear fluids (eg black tea/coffee) are allowed up to 2h beforehand.
  - All other intake up to 6h beforehand.
- In *emergency surgery*, ≥6h NBM prior to theatre is best—but poor scheduling of an emergency list is not an excuse for starving patients for days.

Table 13.6 Daily energy and nutritional requirements

Substance	Requirement (/kg/d)	Notes
Energy	20-40kCal	Normal adult requirements will be 2000-2500kCal/d; even catabolic patients rarely require >2500kCal/d.
	84-168kJ	Multiply kCal by a factor of 4.2.
Nitrogen	0.2-0.4g	6.25g of enteral protein gives 1g of nitrogen. Considering nitrogen balance is important because although catabolism is inevitable, replenishment is vital.
Protein	0.5g	Contains 5kCal/g.
Fat	3g	Contains 10kCal/g.
Carbohydrate	2g	Contains 4kCal/g.
Water	25-30mL	+500mL/d for each °C of pyrexia.
Na/K/Cl	1.0mmol each	Electrolytes need to be considered, even if not on IVI.

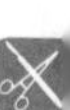

Parenteral (intravenous) nutrition

Do not undertake parenteral feeding lightly: it has risks. Specialist advice is vital. It should only be considered if the patient is likely to become malnourished without it—this normally means that the gastrointestinal tract is not functioning (eg bowel obstruction), and is unlikely to function for at least 7d. Parenteral feeding may supplement other forms of nutrition (eg in short bowel syndrome or active Crohn's disease, when nutrition cannot be sufficiently absorbed in the gut) or it can be used alone (total parenteral nutrition—TPN). ►Even if there is GI disease, studies show that enteral nutrition is safer, cheaper, and at least as efficacious as parenteral nutrition in the perioperative period.[5]

Administration Nutrition must be given via a dedicated central venous line (or peripherally inserted central catheter—PICC line) or via a dedicated lumen of a multi-lumen catheter (see figs 13.9 and 13.10).

Requirements There are many different regimens for parenteral feeding. Most provide 2000kCal and 10-14g nitrogen in 2-3L; this usually meets a patient's daily requirements (see table 13.6, p585). ~50% of calories are provided by fat and ~50% by carbohydrate. Regimens comprise vitamins, minerals, trace elements, and electrolytes; these will normally be included by the pharmacist.

Complications

- *Sepsis:* (eg *Staphylococcus epidermidis* and *Staphylococcus aureus; Candida; Pseudomonas;* infective endocarditis.) Look for spiking pyrexia and examine wound at tube insertion point. Stop PN, take line *and* peripheral cultures and give antibiotics via the line. If central venous line-related sepsis is suspected, the safest course of action is always to remove the line. Do not attempt to salvage a line when *Staph. aureus* or *Candida* infection has been identified.
- *Thrombosis:* Central vein thrombosis may occur, resulting in pulmonary embolus or superior vena caval obstruction (p528).
- *Metabolic imbalance:* Electrolyte abnormalities—see BOX 'Refeeding syndrome'; deranged plasma glucose; hyperlipidaemia; deficiency syndromes (table 6.9, p268); acid-base disturbance (eg hypercapnia from excessive CO_2 production).
- *Mechanical:* Pneumothorax; embolism of IV line tip.

Guidelines for success

►Liaise closely with line insertion team, nutrition team, and pharmacist.

- Meticulous sterility. Do not use central venous lines for uses other than nutrition. Remove the line if you suspect infection. Culture its tip.
- Review fluid balance at least twice daily, and requirements for energy and electrolytes daily.
- Check weight, fluid balance, and urine glucose daily during establishment of parenteral nutrition. Check plasma glucose, creatinine and electrolytes (including calcium and phosphate), and FBC daily until stable. Check LFT and lipid clearance three times a week until stable. Check zinc and magnesium weekly.
- Do not rush. Achieve the maintenance regimen in small steps.
- Treat underlying conditions vigorously—eg sepsis may impede +ve nitrogen balance.

5 Enteral feeding promotes integrity of the gut mucosal barrier, thus preventing bacterial and endotoxin translocation across the gut wall, which can lead to multiple organ dysfunction and perpetuation of a systemic inflammatory response—even when the gut is not the primary source of pathology.

Refeeding syndrome

►This is a life-threatening metabolic complication of refeeding via any route after a prolonged period of starvation. At-risk patients include those initiating artificial feeding (enteral or parenteral) after prolonged starvation, or with malignancy, anorexia nervosa, or alcoholism. As the body turns to fat and protein metabolism in the starved state, there is a drop in the level of circulating insulin (because of the paucity of dietary carbohydrates). The catabolic state also depletes intracellular stores of phosphate, although serum levels may remain normal (0.85–1.45mmol/L). When refeeding begins, the level of insulin rises in response to the carbohydrate load, and one of the consequences is to increase cellular uptake of phosphate.

A hypophosphataemic state (<0.50mmol/L) normally develops within 4d and is mostly responsible for the features of '*refeeding syndrome*', which include: rhabdomyolysis; red and white cell dysfunction; respiratory insufficiency; arrhythmias; cardiogenic shock; seizures; sudden death.

Prevention Give high-dose Pabrinex® during re-feeding window. Identify at-risk patients, assess and monitor closely during refeeding (glucose, lipids, sodium, potassium, phosphate, calcium, magnesium, and zinc). Close involvement of a nutritionist is required.

Treatment is of the complicating features and includes parenteral phosphate administration (eg 18mmol/d) in addition to oral supplementation.

The venous system at the thoracic outlet

When trying to judge the position of a central venous line tip on CXR (see fig 13.10) it helps to know the anatomical landmarks of the venous system (fig 13.9). The subclavian veins join the internal jugular veins behind the sternoclavicular joints to form the brachiocephalic veins. These come together behind the right 1st sternocostal joint to form the superior vena cava (SVC), which runs from this point to the right 3rd sternocostal joint. The right atrium starts here.

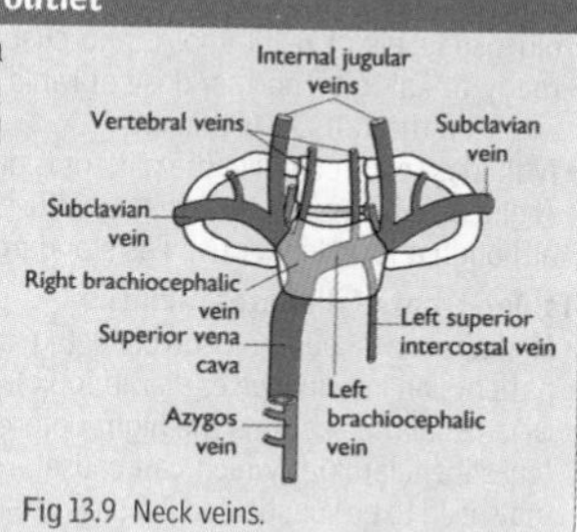

Fig 13.9 Neck veins.

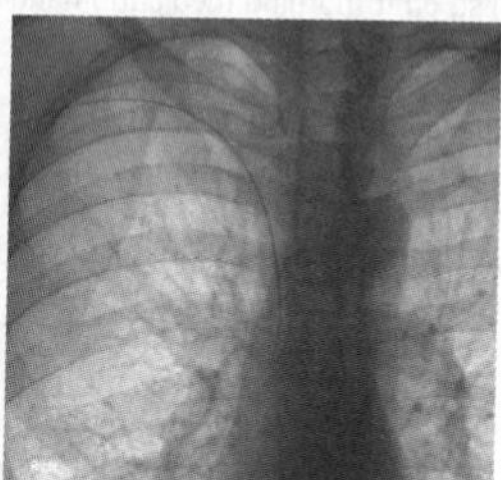

Fig 13.10 Right arm PICC (peripherally inserted central catheter) still with a wire in the lumen. This is a radiograph at the time of insertion to determine if placement is correct. The tip lies in the SVC—ie good positioning for TPN or long-term antibiotic therapy. The tip of a Hickman line, for cytotoxic administration, is better in the right atrium, to avoid possible irritation of the SVC and consequent thrombosis or stenosis. NB: this image was acquired in the angiography room, where radio-opaque material appears black (it is easier to see contrast media against a white background). A similar effect may be achieved by digitally inverting a standard X-ray.

Image courtesy of Prof. Peter Scally.

Diabetic patients undergoing surgery

Over 10% of surgical patients will have diabetes. This group face a greater risk of post-operative infection and cardiac complications. Tight glycaemic control is therefore essential and improves outcome. Aim to achieve an HbA1c of <69mmol/mol prior to elective surgery. Patients are often well informed about their diabetes—involve them fully in managing their diabetic care. Check your hospital's policy for managing diabetic patients who will be NBM before surgery. A general guide follows.

Insulin-treated diabetes mellitus

- Try to place the patient first on the list in order to minimize the fasting period.
- Give all usual insulin the night before surgery.
- Long-acting (basal) insulin is usually continued at normal times (eg glargine; detemir), even when patients are on a variable rate intravenous insulin infusion (VRIII)—previously known as a 'sliding scale' (see BOX).
- If on AM list, ensure no subcutaneous rapid-acting (bolus) or mixed insulin is given on the morning of surgery. If PM list, give the normal morning bolus insulin, or half the mixed insulin dose.
- If eating and drinking post-operatively, resume the usual insulin with evening meal. If AM list (or early PM) and eating a late lunch, give half the morning insulin dose with this meal. If not eating until evening, a VRIII may be needed if the capillary glucose readings are high.
- Omit all rapid-acting and mixed insulin while the patient is on a VRIII.
- It not eating or drinking post-op, start a VRIII 2 hrs prior to surgery. Aim for serum glucose levels of 6-10mmol/L and check finger-prick glucose every 2 hrs. When ready to eat, give normal dose of rapid acting or mixed insulin with the 1st meal and stop the VRIII 30–60min later.
- IV fluid is required while the patient is on a VRIII: see BOX.
- A glucose-potassium-insulin (GKI) infusion can be used as an alternative to a VRIII, although it is no longer used as standard in the UK.

Tablet-treated diabetes mellitus

- If diabetes is poorly controlled (eg fasting glucose >10mmol/L), treat as for patients on insulin (see earlier in topic).
- Give usual medications the night before surgery, except long-acting sulfonylureas (eg glibenclamide) which can cause prolonged hypoglycaemia when fasting and may need to be substituted 2–3 days pre-operatively. Discuss with the diabetes team.
- If eating and drinking post-operatively: on AM list, omit morning medication and take any missed drugs with lunch, after surgery. If PM list, take normal medications with breakfast, omit midday doses, and take any missed drugs with a late lunch. The dose of these may need reducing, depending on dietary intake.
- If not eating or drinking post-op, start a VRIII 2 hours prior to surgery. Once eating and drinking, oral hypoglycaemics can be restarted.
- Some patients may need a phase of subcutaneous insulin following major surgery—refer to the diabetes team if serum glucose levels are persistently raised.
- *Metformin and iodine IV contrast:* Metformin can be continued after IV contrast in patients with normal serum creatinine and/or eGFR >60mL/min. To minimize the risk of nephrotoxicity, if serum creatinine is raised or eGFR <60mL/min, stop metformin for 48h after contrast and check renal function has returned to baseline before restarting.

Diet-controlled diabetes There are usually no problems; patients should be treated as if not diabetic (and do not need to be first on the list). Check capillary blood glucose peri-operatively. Avoid 5% glucose IVI as this increases blood glucose levels.

Peri-operative morbidity and mortality Diabetes mellitus is classed as an intermediate risk factor for increased peri-operative cardiovascular risk by the American Heart Association, so screen for the presence of asymptomatic cardiac and renal disease (p567) and be aware of possible 'silent' myocardial ischaemia. Long-term post-op survival has been found to be poorer for patients with diabetes; however, peri-operative cardiovascular morbidity and mortality were only increased in the presence of congestive heart failure and haemodialysis—ie *not* diabetes alone.

How to write up a variable rate intravenous insulin infusion (VRIII)

Variable rate intravenous insulin infusion (VRIII) is more accurate a term than the previously used 'sliding scale'. Prescribe 50 units of short-acting insulin in 50mL of 0.9% saline to infuse at the rate shown in table 13.7 (according to blood glucose levels). NB: this is a guide only—infusions may vary between institutions and no one infusion rate is suitable for all patients.

Table 13.7 Guide to VRIII according to blood glucose levels

Capillary blood glucose (mmol/L)	IV soluble insulin (rate of infusion)
<4.0	0.5 units/h (0.0 if long-acting insulin continued)
4.1–7.0	1 unit/h
7.1–9.0	2 units/h
9.1–11.0	3 units/h
11.1–14.0	4 units/h
14.1–17.0	5 units/h
17.1–20	6 units/h
>20	6 units/h; request urgent diabetic review

Fluids should be prescribed to run with the VRIII (through the same cannula via a non-return valve). Ideally use 0.45% sodium chloride with 5% glucose *and* either 0.15% potassium chloride (KCl) (=20mmol/L) or 0.3% KCl (=40mmol/L). This provides a constant supply of substrate, but it is not widely available.

Alternatively, use 10% glucose + KCl. This has a lower risk of hypoglycaemia and hyponatraemia than 5% glucose. If capillary glucose >15mmol/L when starting the VRIII use 0.9% saline until <15mmol/L, then use 10% glucose.

Fluid should infuse at 83–125mL/h (ie 1L over 8–12 hours). Omit potassium if there is renal impairment or hyperkalaemia and slow the rate of infusion in heart failure.

Jaundiced patients undergoing surgery

Avoid operating in patients with obstructive jaundice—consider prior ERCP to relieve. There is ↑risk of bleeding, peri-operative infection, and renal failure.

Coagulopathy Vitamin K↓ in obstruction (requires bile in order to be absorbed. If no history of chronic liver disease, give parenteral vitamin K (consider even if clotting is normal). FFP may be required in liver disease or active bleeding.

Sepsis ↑Risk due to •↑bacterial translocation •bacterial colonization of biliary tree •↓neutrophil function. If cholangitis present, give antibiotics. Antibiotic prophylaxis for ERCP not recommended unless biliary decompression fails, or there is a history of biliary disorders; liver transplantation; presence of a pancreatic pseudocyst; or neutropenia, in which case give oral ciprofloxacin or IV gentamicin (check local policy).

Renal failure ↑Risk post-op due to ↑intestinal absorption of endotoxin (normally limited by the detergent effect of bile). This causes ↑renal vasoconstriction and acute tubular necrosis (see p298). The use of lactulose or bile salts pre-op may help. Ensure adequate IV fluids pre- and post-operatively to maintain good urine output. Monitor urine output every 2h. Consider central line, inotropes, and furosemide if output poor despite adequate hydration. Measure and correct U&E daily.

Surgery in those on anticoagulants

►Inform the surgeon and anaesthetist. Risks and benefits must be individualized.
Warfarin *Minor surgery* can be undertaken without stopping (if INR <3.5 it may be safe to proceed). In *major surgery*, stop for 3-5d pre-op. Vitamin K ± FFP or Beriplex® may be needed for emergency reversal of INR. One elective option is conversion to heparin (stop 6h prior to surgery, and monitor APTT perioperatively). When re-warfarinizing, give LMWH until INR is therapeutic, as warfarin is initially prothrombotic.
DOACs Decision to stop will be based upon the patient's risk of having a thromboembolic event and bleeding risk associated with the procedure.[4] Where procedure has *no clinically important bleeding risk* it can be performed just before the next DOAC dose/18-24h after last dose and dosing restarted 6h post-op. *Low bleeding risk procedure*, omit DOAC 24h pre-op. *High bleeding risk procedure*,omit DOAC 48h pre-op. ►If renal function impaired, may require longer periods of omission pre-op.
Antiplatelets Decision to stop is complex and best discussed with the treating team (eg cardiologist or neurologist). Premature discontinuation of clopidogrel in patients with drug-eluting stents can lead to stent thrombosis. The bleeding effects of aspirin are reversed 5d after stopping—check local policy to see if cessation required.

Surgery in those on steroids

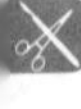

Patients on steroids may not be able to mount an appropriate adrenal response to meet the stress of surgery due to suppression of the hypothalamic-pituitary-adrenal (HPA) axis. Extra corticosteroid cover may be required, depending on the type of surgery. Consider cover for any patient taking >5mg/d of prednisolone (or equivalent) for more than 2 weeks or any patient who has had their long-term steroid reduced in the last 2-4 weeks. There is also potential for HPA suppression in patients taking long-term, high-dose inhaled or topical corticosteroids. A guide to supplementation follows. Patients should take their normal morning steroid dose.

- *Minor procedures under local anaesthetic:* No supplementation required.
- *Moderate procedures:* (Eg joint replacement.) Give 50mg hydrocortisone before induction and 25mg every 8h for 24h. Resume normal dose thereafter.
- *Major surgery:* Give 100mg hydrocortisone before induction and 50mg every 8h for 24h. After 24h, halve this dose each day until the level of maintenance.

Patients with primary adrenal insufficiency will need extra cover—discuss with an endocrinologist. The major risk with adrenal insufficiency is hypotension, so if this is encountered without an obvious cause, consider a stat dose of hydrocortisone. ►See p836 for treatment of Addisonian crisis and *BNF* section 6.3 for steroid dose equivalents.

This page intentionally blank

Minimally invasive and day case surgery

Laparoscopy was developed within gynaecology and is now in widespread use for diagnostic purposes and surgical procedures such as appendicectomy, fundoplication, splenectomy, adrenalectomy, hernia repair, colectomy, prostatectomy, and nephrectomy. Minimally invasive surgery is also used for thyroidectomy and parathyroidectomy.

As a rule of thumb, whatever can be done by laparotomy can also be done with the laparoscope. This does not mean that it *should* be done, but if the surgeon is adequately trained, and the patient feels better sooner, has less post-operative pain, can return to work earlier, and has fewer complications, then there are obvious advantages. Pre-procedure counselling should always discuss the complications of laparoscopic surgery (eg accidental damage to other intra-abdominal organs) as well as the risk of conversion to an open procedure.

Challenges of minimal access surgery The 2-dimensional visual representation and different surgical approach alters the normal appearance of familiar anatomy. Palpation is impossible and it may be harder to locate lesions prior to resection. As a result, pre-operative imaging may need to be more extensive. A new skill has to be learned and taught.

Day-case surgery Advances in surgical techniques as well as perioperative care mean better results for the patient (shorter waiting lists, fewer infections, fewer days off work, and ↑patient satisfaction). Many operations can now be performed as day cases. Theoretically any procedure is suitable, provided the time under general anaesthetic does not exceed ~1h. The use of regional anaesthesia helps to avoid the SE of nausea and disorientation that may accompany a general anaesthetic, thus facilitating discharge.

Bear in mind that the following groups of patients may not be suitable for day-case surgery: •Severe dementia. •Severe learning difficulties. •Living alone (and no helpers). •Children if supervision difficult—changes in expectation, delays, and pain relief can be problematic. •BMI >32 (p244). •ASA category ≥III (p567) thus potentially unstable comorbidities—discuss with the anaesthetist. •Infection at the site of the operation.

Exposing patients to our learning curves? The jury is still out...

All surgeons get better over time (for a while), as they perform new techniques with increasing ease and confidence. When Wertheim did his first hysterectomies, his first dozen patients died—but then one survived. He assumed it was a good operation, and pressed ahead. He was a brave man, and thousands of women owe their lives to him. But had he tried to do this today, he would have been stopped. The UK's General Medical Council (GMC) and other august bodies tell us that we must protect the public by reporting doctors whose patients have low survival rates. The reason for this is partly ethical, and partly to preserve self-regulation.

We have the toughest codes of practice and disciplinary procedures of any group of workers. It is assumed that doctors are loyal to each other out of self-interest, and that this loyalty is bad. This has never been tested formally, and is not evidence-based. We can imagine two clinical worlds: one of constant 'reportings' and recriminatory audits, and another of trust and team-work. Both are imperfect, but we should not assume that the first world would be better for our patients.

When patients are sick with fear, they do not, perhaps, want to know everything. We may tell to protect ourselves. We may *not* tell to protect ourselves. Perhaps what we should do is, in our hearts, appeal to those 12 dead women-of-Wertheim—a jury as infallible as sacrificial—and try to hear their reply. And to those who complain that in doing so we are playing God, it is possible to reply with some humility that, whatever it is, it does not seem like play.

'*It is amazing what little harm doctors do when one considers all the opportunities they have.*' M. Twain.

This page intentionally blank

Lumps

►Examine the regional lymph nodes as well as the lump. If the lump is a node, examine its area of drainage. Always examine the circulation and nerve supply distal to any lump.

History How long has it been there? Does it hurt? Any other symptoms, eg itch? Any other lumps? Is it getting bigger? Ever been abroad? Otherwise well?

Physical exam Remember the 6 **S**'s: **s**ite, **s**ize, **s**hape, **s**moothness (consistency), **s**urface (contour/edge/colour), and **s**urroundings. *Other questions:* Does it transilluminate (see next paragraph)? Is it fixed/tethered to skin or underlying structures (see BOX)? Is it fluctuant/compressible? Temperature? Tender? Pulsatile (US duplex may help)?

Transilluminable lumps After eliminating as much external light as possible, place a bright, thin 'pen' torch on the lump, from behind (or at least to the side), so the light is shining through the lump towards your eye. If the lump glows red it is said to transilluminate—a fluid-filled lump such as a hydrocele is a good example.

Lipomas These benign fatty lumps, occurring wherever fat can expand (ie *not* scalp or palms), have smooth, imprecise margins, a hint of fluctuance, and are not fixed to skin or deeper structures. Symptoms are only caused via pressure. Malignant change very rare (suspect if rapid growth/hardening/vascularization). Multiple scattered lipomas, which may be painful, occur in Dercum's disease, typically in postmenopausal women.

Sebaceous cysts Refer to either *epidermal* (fig 13.11) or *pilar cysts* (they are not of sebaceous origin and contain keratin, not sebum). They appear as firm, round, mobile subcutaneous nodules of varying size. Look for the characteristic central punctum. Infection is quite common, and foul pus exits through the punctum. They are common on the scalp, face, neck, and trunk. *Treatment:* Excision of cyst and contents.

Lymph nodes Causes of enlargement: *Infection:* Glandular fever; brucellosis; TB; HIV; toxoplasmosis; actinomycosis; syphilis. *Infiltration:* Malignancy (carcinoma, lymphoma); sarcoidosis.

Cutaneous abscesses Staphylococci are the most common organisms. Haemolytic streptococci only common in hand infections. *Proteus* is a common cause of non-staphylococcal axillary abscesses. Below the waist, faecal organisms are common (aerobes and anaerobes). *Treatment:* Incise and drain. *Boils (furuncles)* are abscesses involving a hair follicle and associated glands. A *carbuncle* is an area of subcutaneous necrosis which discharges itself on to the surface through multiple sinuses. Think of *hidradenitis suppurativa* if recurrent inguinal or axillary abscesses.

Rheumatoid nodules (fig 13.12) Collagenous granulomas which appear in established rheumatoid arthritis on the extensor aspects of joints—especially the elbows (fig 13.12).

Ganglia Degenerative cysts from an adjacent joint or synovial sheath commonly seen on the dorsum of the wrist or hand and dorsum of the foot. May transilluminate. 50% disappear spontaneously. Aspiration may be effective, especially when combined with instillation of steroid and hyaluronidase. For the rest, treatment of choice is excision rather than the traditional blow from your bible (the *Oxford Textbook of Surgery*)! See fig 13.13.

Fibromas These may occur anywhere in the body, but most commonly under the skin. These whitish, benign tumours contain collagen, fibroblasts, and fibrocytes.

Dermoid cysts Contain dermal structures and are found at the junction of embryonic cutaneous boundaries, eg in the midline or lateral to the eye. See fig 13.14.

Malignant tumours of connective tissue Fibrosarcomas, liposarcomas, leiomyosarcomas (smooth muscle), and rhabdomyosarcomas (striated muscle). These are staged using modified TNM system including tumour grade. Needle-core (Trucut®) biopsies of large tumours precede excision. Any lesion suspected of being a sarcoma should not be simply enucleated. ►Refer to a specialist.

Neurofibromas See p514.

Keloids Caused by irregular hypertrophy of vascularized collagen forming raised edges at sites of previous scars that extend outside the scar (fig 13.15). Common in dark skin. Treatment can be difficult. Intralesional steroid injections are a mainstay.

In or under the skin?

Intradermal	Subcutaneous
• Sebaceous cyst	• Lipoma
• Abscess	• Ganglion
• Dermoid cyst	• Neuroma
• Granuloma.	• Lymph node.

If a lump is intradermal, you cannot draw the skin over it, while if the lump is subcutaneous, you should be able to manipulate it independently from the skin.

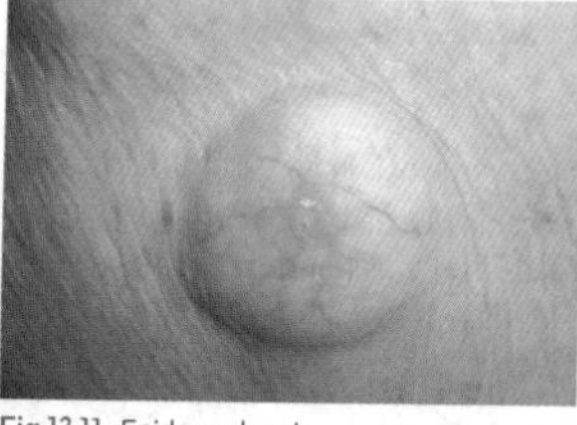

Fig 13.11 Epidermal cyst.

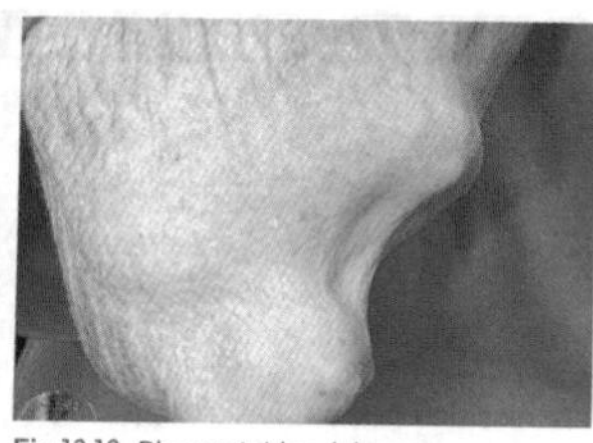

Fig 13.12 Rheumatoid nodule.

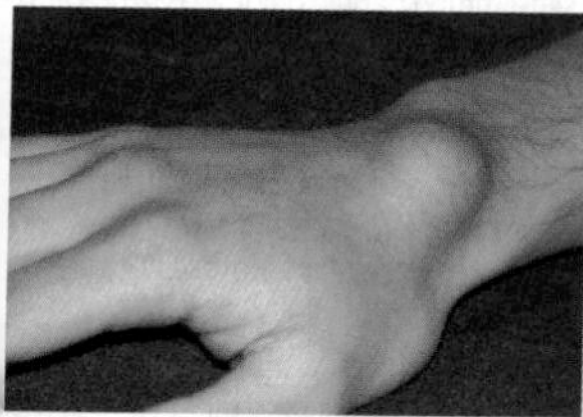

Fig 13.13 Ganglion.

Courtesy of John M Erikson, MD, Raleigh Hand Centre.

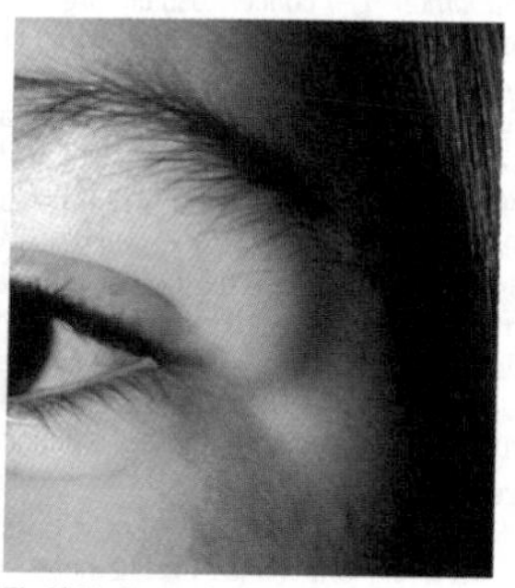

Fig 13.14 Dermoid cyst.

Reproduced from Lewis-Jones, *Paediatric Dermatology*, 2010, with permission from Oxford University Press.

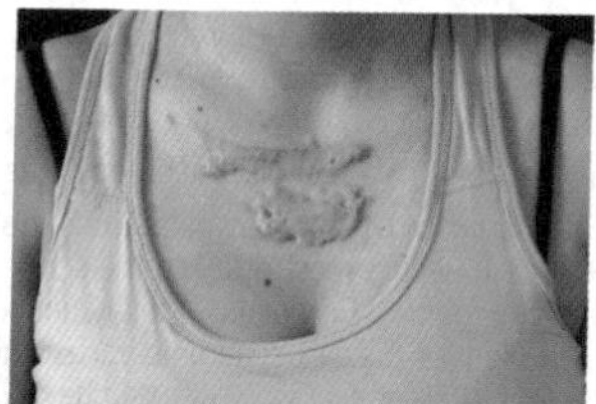

Fig 13.15 Keloid scar.

Courtesy of East Sussex Hospitals Trust.

Skin diagnoses not to be missed

Malignant tumours

1 *Malignant melanoma:* (See fig 13.16.) ♀:♂ ≈ 1.3:1. UK incidence: ≥10:100 000/yr (up ≥200% in last 20yrs). Commonly affects younger patients ∴ early diagnosis is vital. Short periods of intense UV exposure is a major cause, particularly in the early years. May occur in pre-existing moles. If smooth, well-demarcated, and regular, it is unlikely to be a melanoma but diagnosis can be tricky. Most melanomas have features described by Glasgow 7-point checklist (table 13.8) and ABCDE critera (BOX), but not all. ►If in doubt, refer.

Table 13.8 Glasgow 7-point checklist (refer if ≥3 points, or with 1 point if suspicious)

Major (2 pts each)	Minor (1 pt each)	
• Change in size	• Inflammation	• Crusting or bleeding
• Change in shape	• Sensory change	
• Change in colour	• Diameter >7mm (►unless growth is in the vertical plane)	

Superficial spreading melanomas (70%) grow slowly, metastasize later, and have better prognosis than *nodular melanomas* (10–15%) which invade deeply and metastasize early. Nodular lesions may be amelanotic in ~5%. *Others: acral melanomas* occur on palms, soles, and subungual areas; *lentigo maligna melanoma* evolves from pre-exisiting lentigo maligna. Breslow thickness (depth in mm), tumour stage, and presence of ulceration are important prognostic factors. *℞:* urgent excision can be curative. Chemotherapy gives a response in 10–30% with metastatic disease (*OHCS* p592). Ipilimumab, a human monoclonal antibody that blocks CTLA-4, an inhibitory T-cell receptor, has been shown to improve survival in patients with metastatic melanoma.[5,6]

2 *Squamous cell cancer:* Usually presents as an ulcerated lesion, with hard, raised edges, in sun-exposed sites. May begin in solar keratoses (see later in topic), or be found on the lips of smokers or in long-standing ulcers (=Marjolin's ulcer). Metastasis to lymph nodes is rare, local destruction may be extensive. *℞:* excision + radiotherapy to treat recurrence/affected nodes. See fig 13.17. NB: the condition may be confused with a keratoacanthoma—a fast-growing, benign, self-limiting papule plugged with keratin.

3 *Basal cell carcinoma:* (AKA *rodent ulcer*) *Nodular:* typically a pearly nodule with rolled telangiectatic edge, on the face or a sun-exposed site. May have a central ulcer. See fig 13.18. Metastases are very rare. It slowly causes local destruction if left untreated. *Superficial:* lesions appear as red scaly plaques with a raised smooth edge, often on the trunk or shoulders. *Cause:* (most frequently) UV exposure. *℞:* excision; cryotherapy; for superficial BCCs topical flurouracil or imiquimod (see as for 'Solar keratoses').

Pre-malignant tumours

1 *Solar (actinic) keratoses* appear on sun-exposed skin as crumbly, yellow-white crusts. Malignant change to squamous cell carcinoma may occur after several years. *Treatment:* cryotherapy; 5% fluorouracil cream or 5% imiquimod—work by causing: erythema → vesiculation → erosion → ulceration → necrosis → healing epithelialization, leaving healthy skin unharmed. Warn patients of expected inflammatory reaction. See *BNF* for dosing. Alternatively: diclofenac gel (3%, use thinly twice-daily for ≤90d).

2 *Bowen's disease:* Slow-growing red/brown scaly plaque, eg on lower legs. *Histology:* full-thickness dysplasia (carcinoma *in situ*). It infrequently progresses to squamous cell cancer. Penile Bowen's disease is called Queyrat's erythroplasia. *Treatment:* cryotherapy, topical fluorouracil (see as for 'Solar keratoses') or photodynamic therapy.

3 *See also* Kaposi's sarcoma (p702); Paget's disease of the breast (p708).

Others •*Secondary carcinoma:* Most common metastases to skin are from breast kidney, or lung. Usually a firm nodule, most often on the scalp. See also acanthosis nigricans (p562). •*Mycosis fungoides:* Cutaneous T-cell lymphoma usually confined to skin. Causes itchy, red plaques (Sézary syndrome-variant also associated with erythroderma). •*Leucoplakia:* This appears as white patches (which may fissure) on oral or genital mucosa (where it may itch). Frank carcinomatous change may occur. •*Leprosy:* Suspect in any anaesthetic hypopigmented lesion (p441). •*Syphilis:* Any genital ulcer is syphilis until proved otherwise. Secondary syphilis: papular rash—including, unusually, on the palms (p412).

ABCDE criteria for diagnosis of melanoma
Asymmetry
Border—irregular
Colour—non-uniform
Diameter >7mm
Elevation

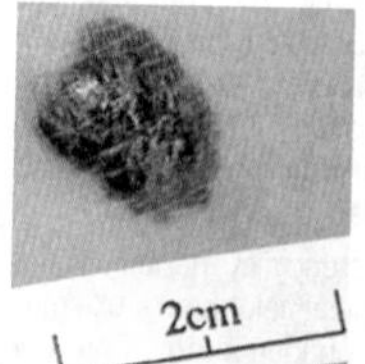

Fig 13.16 Melanoma.

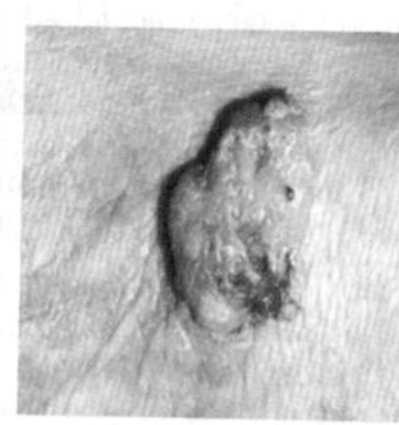

Fig 13.17 Squamous cell cancer.

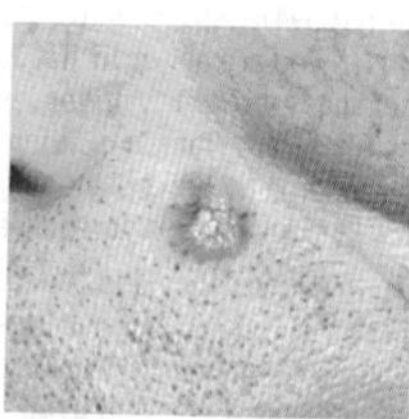

Fig 13.18 Basal cell carcinoma (BCC).

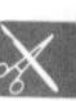

Lumps in the neck

►Don't biopsy lumps until tumours within the head and neck have been excluded by an ENT surgeon. Culture all biopsied lymph nodes for TB.

Diagnosis (See fig 13.19.) First, ask how long the lump has been present. If <3wks, self-limiting infection is the likely cause and extensive investigation is unwise. Next ask yourself where the lump is. Is it intradermal—eg sebaceous cyst with a central punctum (p594)? Is it a lipoma (p594)? If the lump is not intradermal, and is not of recent onset, you are about to start a diagnostic hunt over complicated terrain. 85% of neck swellings are *lymph nodes* (examine areas which they serve). Consider TB, viruses such as HIV or EBV (infectious mononucleosis), any chronic infection, or, if >20yrs, consider lymphoma (hepatosplenomegaly?) or metastases (eg from GI or bronchial or head and neck neoplasia), 8% are goitres (p600), and other diagnoses account for 7%.

Tests Do virology and TB tests (p394). US shows lump consistency: cystic, solid, complex, vascular. CT defines masses in relation to their anatomical neighbours. CXR may show malignancy or, in sarcoid, reveal bilateral hilar lymphadenopathy. Consider fine-needle aspiration (FNA).

Midline lumps •If patient is <20yrs old, likely diagnosis is *dermoid cyst* (p594). •If it moves *up* on tongue protrusion and is below the hyoid, likely to be a *thyroglossal cyst*, a fluid-filled sac resulting from incomplete closure of the thyroid's migration path. ℞: Surgery; they are the commonest congenital cervical cystic lump. •If >20yrs old, it is probably a *thyroid isthmus* mass. •If it is bony hard, the diagnosis may be a *chondroma* (benign cartilaginous tumour).

Submandibular triangle (Bordered by the mental process, mandible, and the line between the two angles of the mandible.) •If <20yrs, self-limiting lymphadenopathy is likely. If >20yrs, exclude *malignant lymphadenopathy* (eg firm and non-tender). ►Is TB likely? •If it is not a node, think of submandibular *salivary stone*, *sialadenitis*, or *tumour* (see BOX for *Salivary gland pathology*).

Anterior triangle (Between midline, anterior border of sternocleidomastoid, and the line between the two angles of the mandible.) •*Branchial cysts* emerge under the anterior border of sternocleidomastoid where the upper third meets the middle third (age <20yrs). Due to non-disappearance of the cervical sinus (where 2nd branchial arch grows down over 3rd and 4th). Lined by squamous epithelium, their fluid contains cholesterol crystals. Treat by excision. There may be communication with the pharynx in the form of a fistula. •If lump in the supero-posterior area of the anterior triangle, is it a *parotid tumour* (more likely if >40yrs)? •*Laryngoceles* are an uncommon cause of anterior triangle lumps. They are painless and may be made worse by blowing. These cysts are classified as external, internal, or mixed, and may be associated with laryngeal cancer. If pulsatile may be: •*Carotid artery aneurysm*, •*Tortuous carotid artery*, or •*Carotid body tumours* (chemodectoma). These are very rare, move from side to side but not up and down, and splay out the carotid bifurcation. They are usually firm and occasionally soft and pulsatile. They do not usually cause bruits. They may be bilateral, familial, and malignant (5%). Suspect in any mass just anterior to the upper third of sternomastoid. Diagnose by duplex USS (splaying at the carotid bifurcation) or digital computer angiography. ℞: Extirpation by vascular surgeon.

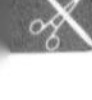

Posterior triangle (Behind sternocleidomastoid, in front of trapezius, above clavicle.) •*Cervical ribs* may intrude into this area. These are enlarged costal elements from C7 vertebra. The majority are asymptomatic but can cause Raynaud's syndrome by compressing subclavian artery and neurological symptoms (eg wasting of 1st dorsal interosseous) from pressure on lower trunk of the brachial plexus. •*Pharyngeal pouches* can protrude into the posterior triangle on swallowing (usually left-sided). •*Cystic hygromas* (usually infants) arise from jugular lymph sac. These macrocystic lymphatic malformations transilluminate brightly. Treat by surgery or hypertonic saline sclerosant injection. Recurrence can be troublesome. •*Pancoast's tumour* (see p708). •*Subclavian artery aneurysm* will be pulsatile.

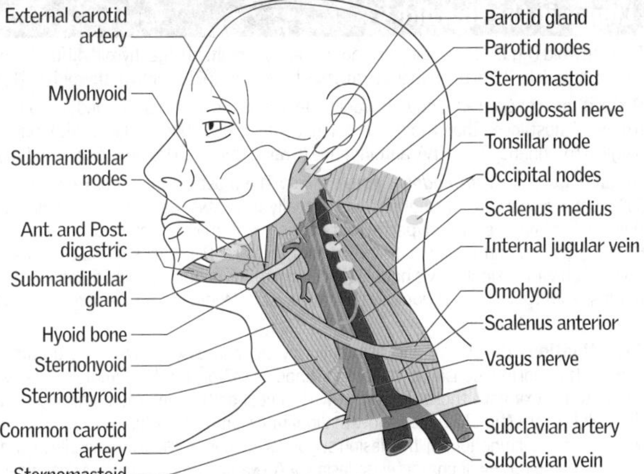

Fig 13.19 Important structures in the head and neck.

Salivary gland pathology

There are three pairs of major salivary glands: parotid, submandibular, and sublingual (there are many minor glands). *History:* Lumps; swelling related to food; pain. *Examination:* Note external swelling; look for secretions; bimanual palpation for stones. Examine VIIth nerve and regional lymph nodes. *Cytology:* Do FNA.

Acute swelling Think of mumps and HIV. *Recurrent unilateral pain and swelling* is likely to be from a stone. 80% are submandibular. The classical story is of pain and swelling on eating—with a red, tender, swollen, but uninfected gland. The stone may be seen on plain X-ray or by sialography (fig 13.20). Distal stones are removed via the mouth but deeper stones may require excision of the gland. *Chronic bilateral symptoms* may coexist with dry eyes and mouth and autoimmune disease, eg hypothyroidism, Mikulicz's or Sjögren's syndrome (p706 & p710)—also bulimia or alcohol excess. *Fixed swelling* may be from a tumour/ALL (fig 8.49, p355), sarcoid, amyloid, granulomatosis with polyangiitis , or be idiopathic.

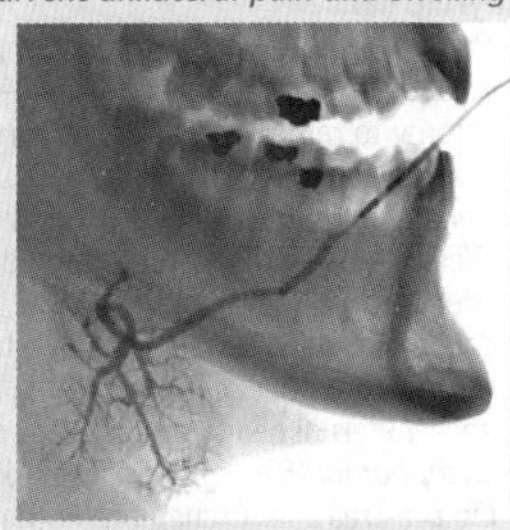

Fig 13.20 Normal sialogram of the submandibular gland. Wharton's (submandibular) duct opens into the mouth near the frenulum of the tongue.

Salivary gland tumours (table 13.9) '80% are in the parotid, 80% of these are pleomorphic adenomas, 80% of these are in the superficial lobe.' Deflection of the ear outwards is a classic sign. ►Remove any salivary gland swelling for assessment if present for >1 month. VIIth nerve palsy means malignancy.

Table 13.9 Types of salivary gland tumours

Benign or malignant	Malignant	Malignant
Cystadenolymphoma	Mucoepidermoid	Squamous or adeno ca
Pleomorphic adenoma	Acinic cell	Adenoid cystic ca

Pleomorphic adenomas often present in middle age and grow slowly. Remove by superficial parotidectomy. Adenolymphomas (Warthin's tumour): usually older men; soft; treat by enucleation. Carcinomas: rapid growth; hard fixed mass; pain; facial palsy. Treatment: surgery + radiotherapy.

Lumps in the thyroid

If the thyroid (fig 13.21) is enlarged (=goitre), ask yourself: **1** Is the thyroid diffusely enlarged or nodular? **2** Is the patient euthyroid, thyrotoxic (p218), or hypothyroid (p220)?

Diffuse goitre: *Causes:* Endemic (iodine deficiency); congenital; secondary to goitrogens (substances that ↓ iodine uptake); acute thyroiditis (de Quervain's); physiological (pregnancy/puberty); autoimmune (Graves' disease; Hashimoto's thyroiditis).

Nodular goitre: •*Multinodular goitre (MNG):* The most common goitre in the UK. 50% who present with a single nodule actually have MNG. Patients are usually euthyroid, but may become hyperthyroid ('toxic'). MNG may be retro- or substernal. Hypothyroidism and malignancy within MNG are rare. Plummer's disease is hyperthyroidism with a single toxic nodule (uncommon). •*Fibrotic goitre:* Eg Reidel's thyroiditis. •*Solitary thyroid nodule:* typically cyst, adenoma, discrete nodule in MNG or malignant (~10%).

Investigations Check TSH and USS (solid, cystic, complex or part of a group of lumps). If abnormal consider: •T_4, autoantibodies (p216, eg if Hashimoto's/Graves', suspected). •CXR with thoracic inlet view (tracheal goitres and metastases?). •Radionuclide scans (fig 13.22) may show malignant lesions as hypofunctioning or 'cold', whereas a hyperfunctioning 'hot' lesion suggests adenoma. •FNA (fine-needle aspiration) and cytology—will characterize lesion. ►A FNA finding of a follicular neoplasm can be challenging (15–30% malignant)—discuss with cytopathologist and perform molecular diagnostics where available; if any doubt, refer for surgery.

What should you do if high-resolution ultrasound shows impalpable nodules? Such thyroid nodules can usually be observed provided they are:

- <1cm across (which accounts for most; ultrasound can detect lumps <2mm; such 'incidentalomas' occur in 46% of routine autopsies) and are asymptomatic.
- There is no past history of thyroid cancer or neck irradiation.
- No family history of medullary cancer (if present, do USS-guided FNA).

Thyroid cancer

1 *Papillary:* (60%.) Often in younger patients. Spread: lymph nodes and lung (jugulodigastric node metastasis is the so-called lateral aberrant thyroid). ℞: total thyroidectomy to remove non-obvious tumour ± node excision ± radioiodine (^{131}I) to ablate residual cells. Give levothyroxine to suppress TSH. Prognosis: better if young and ♀.
2 *Follicular:* (≤25%.) Occurs in middle-age and spreads early via blood (bone, lungs). Well-differentiated. ℞: total thyroidectomy + T_4 suppression + radioiodine ablation.
3 *Medullary:* (5%.) Sporadic (80%) or part of MEN syndrome (p223). May produce calcitonin which can be used as a tumour marker. They do not concentrate iodine. ►Perform a phaeochromocytoma screen pre-op. ℞: thyroidectomy + node clearance. External beam radiotherapy may prevent regional recurrence.
4 *Lymphoma:* (5%.) ♀:♂≈3:1. May present with stridor or dysphagia. Do full staging pre-treatment (chemoradiotherapy). Assess histology for mucosa-associated lymphoid tissue (MALT) origin (associated with a good prognosis).
5 *Anaplastic:* Rare. ♀:♂≈3:1. Elderly, poor response to any treatment. In the absence of unresectable disease, excision + radiotherapy may be tried.

Thyroid surgery Plays a significant role in the management of thyroid disease. Operations include partial lobectomy or lobectomy (for isolated nodules); and thyroidectomy (for cancers, MNG, or Graves'). *Indications:* Pressure symptoms, relapse hyperthyroidism after >1 failed course of drug treatment, carcinoma, cosmetic reasons, symptomatic patients planning pregnancy. *Pre-operative management:* Render euthyroid pre-op with antithyroid drugs (eg carbimazole up to 20mg/12h PO or propylthiouracil 200mg/12h PO but stop 10d prior to surgery as these increase vascularity). Propranolol up to 80mg/8h PO can be used to control tachycardia or tremor associated with hyperthyroidism (continue for 5d post-op). Check vocal cords by indirect laryngoscopy pre- and post-op (risk of recurrent laryngeal nerve injury). Check serum Ca^{2+} (and PTH if abnormal). *Complications:* see p580.

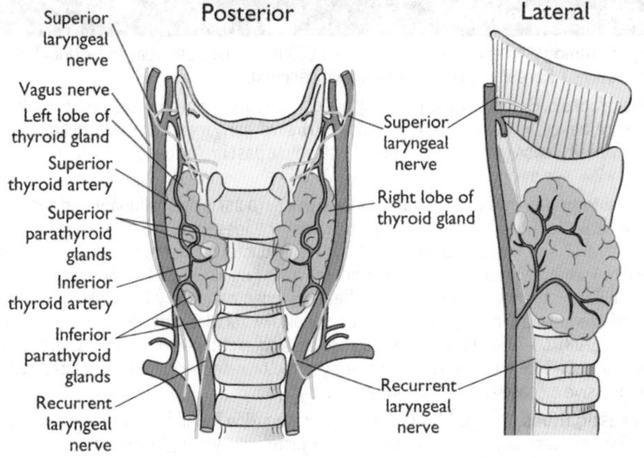

Fig 13.21 The anatomy of the region of the thyroid gland. The important structures that must be considered when operating on the thyroid gland include:
- Recurrent laryngeal nerve
- Superior laryngeal nerve
- Parathyroid glands
- Trachea
- Common carotid artery
- Internal jugular vein (not depicted—see fig 13.23).

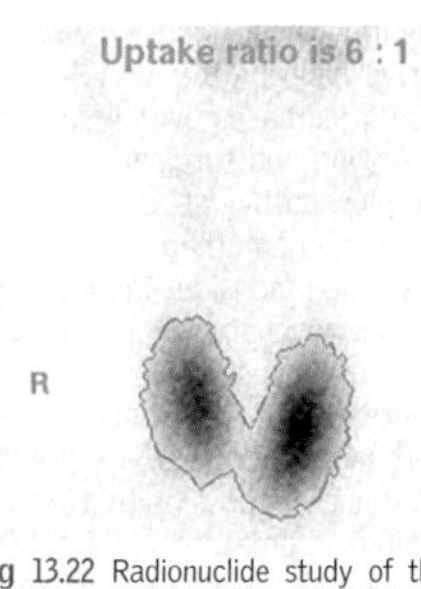

Fig 13.22 Radionuclide study of the thyroid showing changes consistent with Graves' disease (see also *hot and cold nodules* (p216) and *nuclear medicine*, p738). There is increased uptake of the radionuclide trace diffusely throughout both lobes of the gland.

Image courtesy of Norwich Radiology Department.

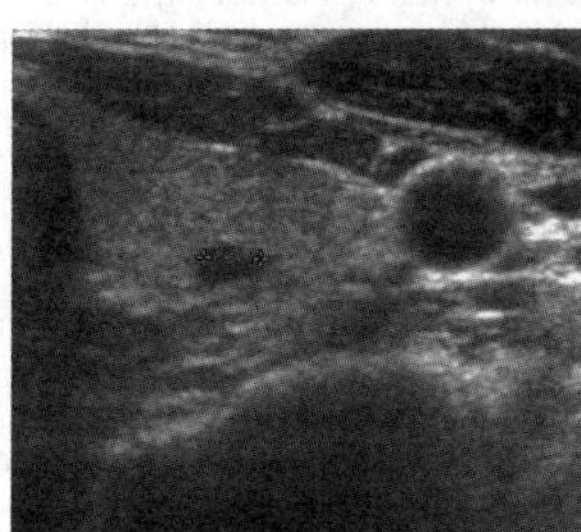

Fig 13.23 Transverse ultrasound of the left lobe of the thyroid showing a small low-reflectivity cyst within higher-reflectivity thyroid tissue. Note the proximity to the gland of the common carotid artery and internal jugular vein (the latter compressed slightly by pressure from the probe), both seen beneath the body of sternocleidomastoid muscle.

Image courtesy of Norwich Radiology Department.

Breast carcinoma

Epidemiology Affects 1 in 8 ♀; nearly 60 000 new cases per year in UK (incidence increasing). Rare in men (~1% of all breast cancers).

Risk factors Risk is related to family history, age, and uninterrupted oestrogen exposure, hence: nulliparity; 1st pregnancy >30yrs old, early menarche; late menopause; HRT; obesity; BRCA genes (p521); not breastfeeding; past breast cancer (metachronous rate ≈2%, synchronous rate ≈1%).

Pathology Non-invasive ductal carcinoma *in situ* (DCIS) is premalignant and seen as microcalcification on mammography (unifocal or widespread). Non-invasive lobular CIS is rarer and tends to be multifocal. Invasive ductal carcinoma is most common (~70%) whereas invasive lobular carcinoma accounts for 10-15% of breast cancers. Medullary cancers (~5%) tend to affect younger patients while colloid/mucoid (~2%) tend to affect the elderly. Others: papillary, tubular, adenoid-cystic and Paget's (p708). 60-70% of breast cancers are oestrogen receptor +ve, conveying better prognosis. ~30% over-express HER2 (growth factor receptor gene) associated with aggressive disease and poorer prognosis.

Investigations (See p82 for history and examination.) ►All lumps should undergo *'triple' assessment:* Clinical examination + histology/cytology + mammography/ultrasound; see fig 13.24.

Staging: *Stage 1:* Confined to breast, mobile. *Stage 2:* Growth confined to breast, mobile, lymph nodes in ipsilateral axilla. *Stage 3:* Tumour fixed to muscle (but not chest wall), ipsilateral lymph nodes matted and may be fixed, skin involvement larger than tumour. *Stage 4:* Complete fixation of tumour to chest wall, distant metastases. Also *TNM staging:* (p523) T1<2cm, T2, 2-5cm, T3 >5cm, T4, fixity to chest wall or *peau d'orange*; N1, mobile ipsilateral nodes; N2, fixed nodes; M1, distant metastases.

Treating local disease (Stage 1-2.)[7] •*Surgery:* Removal of tumour by wide local excision (WLE) or mastectomy ± breast reconstruction + axillary node sampling/surgical clearance or sentinel node biopsy (BOX 'Sentinel node biopsy'). •*Radiotherapy:* Recommended for all patients with invasive cancer after WLE. Risk of recurrence decreases from 30% to <10% at 10yrs and increases overall survival. Axillary radiotherapy used if lymph node +ve on sampling and surgical clearance not performed (↑risk of lymphoedema and brachial plexopathy). SE: pneumonitis, pericarditis, and rib fractures. •*Chemotherapy:* Adjuvant chemotherapy improves survival and reduces recurrence in most groups of women (consider in all except excellent prognosis patients), eg epirubicin + 'CMF' (cyclophosphamide + methotrexate + 5-FU). Neoadjuvant chemotherapy has shown no difference in survival but may facilitate breast-conserving surgery. •*Endocrine agents:* Aim to ↓oestrogen activity and are used in oestrogen receptor (ER) or progesterone receptor (PR) +ve disease. The ER blocker tamoxifen is widely used, eg 20mg/d PO for 5yrs post-op (may rarely cause uterine cancer so warn to report vaginal bleeding). Aromatase inhibitors (eg anastrozole) targeting peripheral oestrogen synthesis are also used (may be better tolerated). They are only used if post-menopausal. If pre-menopausal and an ER+ve tumour, ovarian ablation (via surgery or radiotherapy) or GnRH analogues (eg goserelin) ↓ recurrence and ↑ survival. •*Support:* Breastcare nurses •*Reconstruction options:* Eg tissue expanders/implants/nipple tattoos, latissimus dorsi flap, TRAM (transverse rectus abdominis myocutaneous) flap.

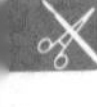

Treating distant disease (Stage 3-4.)[8] Long-term survival is possible and median survival is >2yrs. Staging investigations should include CXR, bone scan, liver USS, CT MRI or PET-CT (p739), + LFTs and Ca^{2+}. Radiotherapy (p526) to painful bony lesions (*bisphosphonates*, p677, may ↓ pain and fracture risk). Tamoxifen is often used in ER+ve if relapse after initial success, consider chemotherapy. Trastuzumab should be given for HER2 +ve tumours, in combination with chemotherapy. CNS surgery for solitary (or easily accessible) metastases may be possible; if not—radiotherapy. Get specialist help for arm lymphoedema (try decongestive methods first).

Preventing deaths •Promote awareness. •*Screening:* 2-view mammography every 3yrs for women aged 47-73 in UK has ↓breast cancer deaths by 30% in women >50yrs.

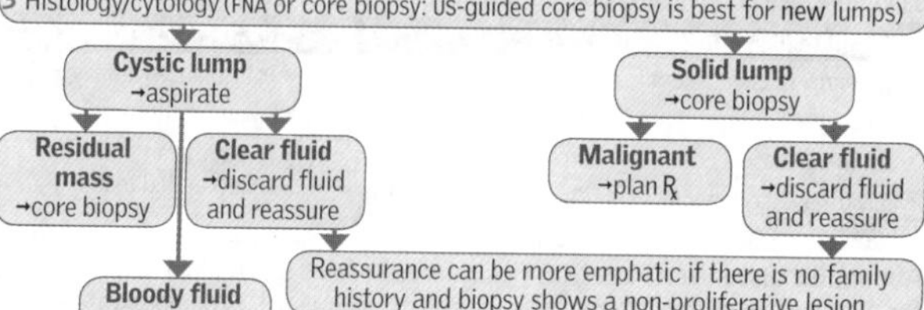

Fig 13.24 Triple assessment and investigation of a breast lump.
* US is more accurate at detecting invasive breast cancer, though mammography remains most accurate at detecting ductal carcinoma *in situ* (DCIS). MRI is used in the assessment of multifocal/bilateral disease and patients with cosmetic implants who are identified as high risk.

Sentinel node biopsy

Decreases needless axillary clearances in lymph node −ve patients.
- Patent blue dye and/or radiocolloid injected into periareolar area or tumour.
- A gamma probe/visual inspection is used to identify the sentinel node.
- The sentinel node is biopsied and sent for histology ± immunohistochemistry; further clearance only if sentinel node +ve.

Sentinel node identified in 90%. False −ve rates <5% for experienced surgeons.

Prognostic factors in breast cancer

Tumour size, grade, lymph node status, ER/PR status, presence of vascular invasion all help assess prognosis. Nottingham Prognostic Index (NPI) is widely used to predict survival and risk of relapse, and to help select appropriate adjuvant systemic therapy. NPI = *0.2 × tumour size (cm) + histological grade + nodal status*[6]
If treated with surgery alone, 10yr survival rates are: NPI <2.4: 95%; NPI 2.4–3.4: 85%; NPI 3.4–4.4: 70%; NPI 4.4–5.4: 50%; NPI >5.4: 20%.

Benign breast disease

Fibroadenoma: Usually presents <30yrs but can occur up to menopause. Benign overgrowth of collagenous mesenchyme of one breast lobule. Firm, smooth, mobile lump, the 'breast mouse'. Painless. May be multiple. ⅓ regress, ⅓ stay the same, ⅓ get bigger. Rx: observation and reassurance, but if in doubt refer for USS (usually conclusive) ± FNA. Surgical excision if large.

Breast cysts: Common >35yrs, esp. perimenopausal. Benign, fluid-filled rounded lump. Not fixed to surrounding tissue. Occasionally painful. Rx: diagnosis confirmed on aspiration (perform only if trained).

Infective mastitis/breast abscesses: Infection of mammary duct often associated with lactation (usually *Staph. aureus*). Abscess presents as painful, hot swelling of breast segment. Rx: antibiotics. Open incision or percutaneous drainage if abscess.

Duct ectasia: Typically around menopause. Ducts become blocked and secretions stagnate. Present with nipple discharge (green/brown/bloody) ± nipple retraction ± lump. Refer for confirmation of diagnosis. Usually no Rx needed. Advise to stop smoking.

Fat necrosis: Fibrosis and calcification after injury to breast tissue. Scarring results in a firm lump. Refer for triple assessment. No Rx once diagnosis confirmed.

6 Nodal status is scored 1-3: 1 = node -ve; 2 = 1-3 nodes +ve; 3 = >3 nodes +ve for breast cancer. Histological grade is also scored 1-3.

Abdominal masses

As with any mass (see p594), determine size, site, shape, and surface. Find out if it is pulsatile and if it is mobile. Examine supraclavicular and inguinal nodes. Is the lump ballotable (like bobbing an apple up and down in water)?

Right iliac fossa masses		
• Appendix mass/abscess • Caecal carcinoma • Crohn's disease • Pelvic mass (see later in topic)	• Intussusception • TB mass • Amoebic abscess • Actinomycosis (p389)	• Transplanted kidney • Kidney malformation • Tumour in an undescended testis.

Abdominal distension Flatus, fat, fluid, faeces, or fetus (p57)? Fluid may be outside the gut (ascites) or sequestered in bowel (obstruction; ileus). To demonstrate ascites elicit signs of a fluid thrill and/or shifting dullness (p61).

Causes of ascites		Ascites with portal hypertension	
• Malignancy • Infections—esp. TB • ↓Albumin (eg nephrosis)	• CCF; pericarditis • Pancreatitis • Myxoedema.	• Cirrhosis • Budd-Chiari syndrome (p696) • IVC or portal vein thrombosis.	• Portal nodes

Tests: Aspirate ascitic fluid (p764) for cytology, culture and albumin;[7] US.

Left upper quadrant mass Is it spleen, stomach, kidney, colon, pancreas, or a rare cause (eg neurofibroma)? Pancreatic cysts may be true (congenital; cystadenomas; retention cysts of chronic pancreatitis; cystic fibrosis) or pseudocysts (fluid in lesser sac from acute pancreatitis).

Splenomegaly Causes are often said to be infective, haematological, neoplastic, etc, but grouping by associated feature is more useful clinically:

Splenomegaly with fever	With lymphadenopathy	With purpura
• Infection[HS] (malaria, SBE/IE, hepatitis,[HS] EBV,[HS] TB, CMV, HIV) • Sarcoid; malignancy.[HS]	• Glandular fever[HS] • Leukaemias; lymphoma • Sjögren's syndrome.	• Septicaemia; typhus • DIC; amyloid[HS] • Meningococcaemia.
With arthritis	**With ascites**	**With a murmur**
• Sjögren's syndrome • Rheumatoid arthritis; SLE • Infection, eg Lyme (p422) • Vasculitis/Behçet's (p556).	• Carcinoma • Portal hypertension.[HS]	• SBE/IE • Rheumatic fever • Hypereosinophilia • Amyloid[HS] (p370).
With anaemia	**With ↓weight + *CNS* signs**	**Massive splenomegaly**
• Sickle-cell;[HS] thalassaemia[HS] • Leishmaniasis;[HS] leukaemia[HS] • Pernicious anaemia (p334) • POEMS syn. (p220).	• Cancer; lymphoma • TB; arsenic poisoning • Paraproteinaemia.[HS]	• Malaria (hyper-reactivity after chronic exposure) • Myelofibrosis; CML[HS] • Gaucher's syndrome[HS] • Leishmaniasis.

[HS] =causes of hepatosplenomegaly.

Smooth hepatomegaly Hepatitis, CCF, sarcoidosis, early alcoholic cirrhosis (a small liver is typical later); tricuspid incompetence (→ pulsatile liver).

Craggy hepatomegaly Secondaries or 1° hepatoma. (Nodular cirrhosis typically causes a small, shrunken liver, not an enlarged craggy one.)

Pelvic masses Fibroids, fetus, bladder, ovarian cysts or malignancies. *Is it truly pelvic?*—Yes, if by palpation you cannot get 'below it'.

Investigating lumps Check FBC (with film); CRP; U&E; LFT; Ca^{2+}; tumour markers only as appropriate. Imaging by CT or US (transvaginal approach may be useful); MRI also has a role, eg in assessment of liver masses (p286). *Others:* TB tests (p394). Biopsy to give a tissue diagnosis may be obtained using a fine needle guided by CT, US, or endoscopy.

Surgery

7 Subtract fluid albumin from serum albumin to obtain serum-ascites albumin gradient (SAAG). Gradient <11g/L suggests malignancy, infections, or pancreatitis.

The first successful laparotomy...

In 1809, an American surgeon by the name of Ephraim McDowell performed an astonishing operation: the first successful elective laparotomy for an abdominal tumour. It was an ovariotomy for an ovarian mass in a 44-year-old who, prior to physical examination by McDowell, was believed to be gravid. Not only was this feat performed in the age before anaesthesia and antisepsis, but it was also performed on a table in the front room of McDowell's Kentucky home, at that time on the frontier of the West in the United States. His account of the operation makes fascinating reading. While the strength of his diagnostic convictions combined with his speed and skill at operating is to be admired (the operation took 25 minutes), there is an even more laudable part played in this story. The patient, Mrs Jane Todd-Crawford, was fully willing to be involved with what can only be described as experimental surgery in the face of uncertainty. She defied pain simply by reciting psalms and hymns, and was back at home within 4 weeks with no complications, ultimately living another 33 years. We would be well served in remembering the exceptional commitment of Mrs Todd-Crawford. In the rush and hurry of our daily tasks perhaps it is all to easy to forget that the undertaking of surgery today may be no less fear-provoking for patients than it was 200 years ago.

The acute abdomen

Someone who becomes acutely ill and in whom symptoms and signs are chiefly related to the abdomen has an acute abdomen. Prompt laparotomy is sometimes essential: *repeated examination is the key to making the decision.*

Clinical syndromes that usually require laparotomy

1 *Rupture of an organ* (Spleen, aorta, ectopic pregnancy.) Shock is a leading sign—see table 13.10 for assessment of blood loss. Abdominal swelling may be seen. Any history of trauma: blunt trauma → spleen; penetrating trauma → liver? *Delayed* rupture of the spleen may occur weeks after trauma. Peritonism may be mild.

2 *Peritonitis* (Perforation of peptic ulcer/duodenal ulcer, diverticulum, appendix, bowel, or gallbladder.) Signs: prostration, shock, lying still, +ve cough test (p62), tenderness (± rebound/percussion pain, p62), board-like abdominal rigidity, guarding, and no bowel sounds. Erect CXR may show gas under the diaphragm (fig 13.26). NB: acute pancreatitis (p636) causes these signs, but does *not* require a laparotomy so don't be caught out and ►*always check serum amylase.*

Syndromes that may not require a laparotomy

Local peritonitis: Eg diverticulitis, cholecystitis, salpingitis, and appendicitis (the latter *will* need surgery). If abscess formation is suspected (swelling, swinging fever, and ↑WCC) do US or CT. Drainage can be percutaneous (US or CT-guided), or by laparotomy. Peritoneal inflammation can cause localized ileus with a 'sentinel loop' of intraluminal gas visible on plain AXR (p729).

Colic is a regularly waxing and waning pain, caused by muscular spasm in a hollow viscus, eg gut, ureter, salpinx, uterus, bile duct, or gallbladder (in the latter, pain is often dull and constant). Colic, unlike peritonitis, causes restlessness and the patient may well be pacing around when you go to review!

Obstruction of the bowel See p610.

Tests U&E; FBC; amylase; LFT; CRP; lactate (is there mesenteric ischaemia?); urinalysis. ►►Urine and serum hCG is vital to exclude ectopic pregnancy. Erect CXR (fig 13.26), AXR may show Rigler's sign (p728). Laparoscopy may avert open surgery. CT can be helpful provided it is readily available and causes no delay (pp732–3); US may identify perforation or free fluid (appropriate performer training is important).

Pre-op ►Don't rush to theatre. *Anaesthesia compounds shock*, so resuscitate properly first (p790) unless blood being lost faster than can be replaced, eg ruptured ectopic pregnancy, (*OHCS* p262), aneurysm leak (p654), trauma.

Plan Bed rest, keep NBM; assess volume status (BOX) and treat shock (p790); cross-match/group and save; analgesia (p574); arrange imaging; consider need for IVI, blood cultures, and antibiotics (eg piperacillin/tazobactam 4.5g/8h IV); ECG.

The medical acute abdomen Irritable bowel syndrome (p266) is the chief cause, so always ask about episodes of pain associated with loose stools, relieved by defecation, bloating, and urgency (but *not* blood—this may be UC). Other causes:

►►Myocardial infarction	Pneumonia (p166)	Sickle-cell crisis (p341)
Gastroenteritis or UTI	Thyroid storm (p834)	Phaeochromocytoma (p837)
Diabetes mellitus/DKA (p206)	Zoster (p404)	Malaria (p416)
Bornholm disease	Tuberculosis (p393)	Typhoid fever (p415)
Pneumococcal peritonitis	Porphyria (p692)	Cholera (p430)
Henoch-Schönlein (p702)	Narcotic addiction	*Yersinia enterocolitica* (p431)
Tabes dorsalis (p412)	PAN (p556)	Lead colic

Hidden diagnoses ►►Mesenteric ischaemia (p620), ►►acute pancreatitis (p636), and ►►leaking AAA (p654) are the *Unterseeboote* of the acute abdomen—unsuspected undetectable unless carefully looked for, and underestimatedly deadly. They may have non-specific symptoms and signs that are surprisingly mild, so always think of them when assessing the acute abdomen and hopefully you will 'spot' them ►Finally: *always exclude pregnancy (± ectopic?) in females.*

Acute cholecystitis
Duodenal ulcer
Hepatitis
Congestive hepatomegaly
Pyelonephritis
Appendicitis
(R) Pneumonia

Pancreatitis
Myocardial infarct
Peptic ulcer
Acute cholecystitis
Perforated oesophagus

Epigastrium

Ruptured spleen
Gastric ulcer
Aortic aneurysm
Perforated colon
Pyelonephritis
(L) Pneumonia

Intestinal obstruction
Acute pancreatitis
Early appendicitis
Mesenteric thrombosis
Aortic aneurysm
Diverticulitis

RUQ
LUQ
RLQ
LLQ

Appendicitis
Salpingitis
Tubo-ovarian abscess
Ruptured ectopic pregnancy
Renal/ureteric stone
Strangulated hernia
Mesenteric adenitis
Meckel's diverticulitis
Crohn's disease
Perforated caecum
Psoas abscess

Sigmoid diverticulitis
Salpingitis
Tubo-ovarian abscess
Ruptured ectopic pregnancy
Strangulated hernia
Perforated colon
Crohn's disease
Ulcerative colitis
Renal/ureteric stones

Fig 13.25 Causes of abdominal pain.

Assessing hypovolaemia from blood loss

►► Treat suspected shock rather than wait for BP to fall. The most likely cause of shock in a surgical patient is hypovolaemia. Check urine output, GCS, and capillary refill (CR) as measures of renal, brain, and skin perfusion.

When there is any blood loss, assess the status of the following:

Table 13.10 Estimating blood loss based on patient's initial presentation

Parameter	Class I	Class II	Class III	Class IV
Blood loss	<750mL	750–1500mL	1500–2000mL	>2000mL
	<15%	15–30%	30–40%	>40%
Pulse	<100bpm	>100bpm	>120bpm	>140bpm
BP	↔	↔	↓	↓
Pulse pressure	↔ or ↑	↓	↓	↓
Respirations	14–20/min	20–30/min	30–40/min	>35/min
Urine output	>30mL/h	20–30mL/h	5–15mL/h	Negligible
Mental state	Slightly anxious	Anxious	Confused →	→Lethargic
Fluid to give	Crystalloid	Crystalloid	Crystalloid + blood	

Assumes a body mass of 70kg.

An adaptation of 'Estimated blood loss based on initial presentation' table from the 9th edition of the *Advanced Trauma Life Support Manual*. Adapted with permission from the American College of Surgeons.

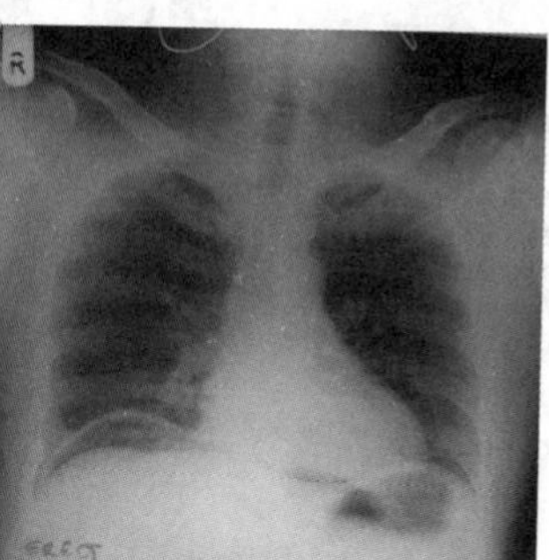

Fig 13.26 Erect CXR showing air beneath the right hemidiaphragm, indicating presence of a pneumoperitoneum. *Causes:*
- Bowel perforation (visible only in 75%) (fig 13.25).
- Gas-forming infection, eg *C. perfringens.*
- Iatrogenic, eg laparoscopic surgery (detectable on CXR up to 10d post-op).
- *Per vaginam* (eg sexual activity).
- Interposition of bowel between liver and diaphragm (Chilaiditi sign—not true free air).

Image courtesy of Mr P. Paraskeva.

Acute appendicitis

Incidence Most common surgical emergency (lifetime incidence = 6%). Can occur at any age, though highest incidence is between 10-20yrs.[8] It is rare before age 2 because the appendix is cone shaped with a larger lumen.

Pathogenesis Gut organisms invade the appendix wall after lumen obstruction by lymphoid hyperplasia, faecolith, or filarial worms. This leads to oedema, ischaemic necrosis, and perforation.

Presentation Classically periumbilical pain that moves to the RIF. Associated signs may include tachycardia, fever, peritonism with guarding and rebound or percussion tenderness in RIF. Pain on right during PR examination suggests an inflammed, low-lying pelvic appendix. Anorexia is an important feature; vomiting is rarely prominent—*pain normally precedes vomiting* in the surgical abdomen. Constipation is usual, though diarrhoea may occur. *Additional signs: Rovsing's sign* (pain > in RIF than LIF when the LIF is pressed). *Psoas sign* (pain on extending hip if retrocaecal appendix). *Cope sign* (pain on flexion and internal rotation of right hip if appendix in close relation to obturator internus).

Investigations Blood tests may reveal neutrophil leucocytosis and elevated CRP. US may help, but the appendix is not always visualized. CT has high diagnostic accuracy and is useful if diagnosis is unclear: it reduces –ve appendicectomy rate.

Variations in the clinical picture

- Inflammation in a retrocecal/retroperitoneal appendix (2.5%) may cause flank or RUQ pain; its only sign may be ↑tenderness on the right on PR.
- The child with vague abdominal pain who will not eat their favourite food.
- The shocked, confused octogenarian who is not in pain.
- Appendicitis occurs in ~1/1000 pregnancies. Mortality is higher, especially from 20wks' gestation. Perforation is more common, and increases fetal mortality. Pain is often less well localized (may be RUQ) and signs of peritonism less obvious.

Hints

- If a child is anxious, use their hand to press their tummy.
- Check for recent viral illnesses and lymphadenopathy—mesenteric adenitis?
- Don't *start* palpating in the RIF (makes it difficult to elicit pain elsewhere).
- Expect diagnosis to be wrong half the time. If diagnosis is uncertain, re-examine often. A normal appendix is removed in up to 20% of patients.

Treatment Prompt *appendicectomy* (fig 13.27). *Antibiotics:* piperacillin/tazobactam 4.5g/8h, 1 to 3 doses IV starting 1h pre-op, reduces wound infections. Give a longer course if perforated. *Laparoscopy:* Has diagnostic and therapeutic advantages (if surgeon experienced), especially in women and the obese. It is not recommended in cases of suspected gangrenous perforation as the rate of abscess formation may be higher.

Complications

- *Perforation* is commoner if a faecolith is present and in young children, as the diagnosis is more often delayed.
- *Appendix mass* may result when an inflamed appendix becomes covered with omentum. US/CT may help with diagnosis. Some advocate early surgery. Alternatively, initial conservative management—NBM and antibiotics. If the mass resolves, some perform an interval (ie delayed) appendicectomy. Exclude a colonic tumour (laparotomy or colonoscopy), which can present as early as the 4th decade.
- *Appendix abscess* May result if an appendix mass fails to resolve but enlarges and the patient gets more unwell. Treatment usually involves drainage (surgical or percutaneous under US/CT-guidance). Antibiotics alone may bring resolution.

8 There is a second peak between 60-70yrs; older adults may present later with atypical symptoms.

Explaining the patterns of abdominal pain

Internal organs and the visceral peritoneum have no somatic innervation, so the brain attributes the visceral (splanchnic) signals to a physical location whose dermatome corresponds to the same entry level in the spinal cord. Importantly, there is no laterality to the visceral unmyelinated C-fibre pain signals, which enter the cord bilaterally and at multiple levels. Division of the gut according to embryological origin is the important determinant here: see table 13.11.

Table 13.11 Somatic referral of abdominal pain

Gut	Division points	Somatic referral	Arterial supply
Fore	Proximal to 2nd part of duodenum	Epigastrium	Coeliac axis
Mid	Above to ⅔ along transverse colon	Periumbilical	Superior mesenteric
Hind	Distal to above	Suprapubic	Inferior mesenteric

Early inflammation irritates the structure and walls of the appendix, so a colicky pain is referred to the mid-abdomen—classically periumbilical. As the inflammation progresses and irritates the parietal peritoneum (especially on examination), the somatic, lateralized pain settles at McBurney's point, ⅔ of the way along from the umbilicus to the right anterior superior iliac spine.

These principles also help us understand patterns of *referred pain*. In pneumonia, the T9 dermatome is shared by the lung and the abdomen. Also, irritation of the underside of the diaphragm (sensory innervation is from above through the phrenic nerve, C3–5) by an inflamed gallbladder or a subphrenic abscess refers pain to the right shoulder: dermatomes C3–5.

ΔΔ

- Ectopic (►►do a pregnancy test!)
- UTI (test urine!)
- Mesenteric adenitis
- Cystitis.
- Cholecystitis
- Diverticulitis
- Salpingitis/PID
- Dysmenorrhoea
- Crohn's disease
- Perforated ulcer
- Food poisoning
- Meckel's diverticulum

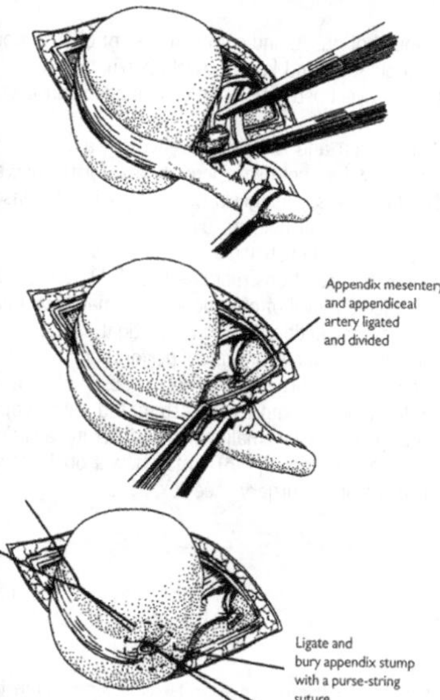
Appendix mesentery and appendiceal artery ligated and divided
Ligate and bury appendix stump with a purse-string suture

Fig 13.27 Appendicectomy.
Reproduced from McLatchie *et al.*, *Operative Surgery*, 2006, with permission from Oxford University Press.

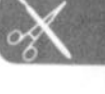

Obstruction of the bowel

Cardinal features of intestinal obstruction •*Vomiting*,[9] nausea and anorexia. •*Colic* occurs early (↓ in long-standing obstruction). •*Constipation* may be absolute (ie no faeces or flatus passed) in distal obstruction; less pronounced if obstruction is high. •*Abdominal distension* ↑ as the obstruction progresses with active, 'tinkling' bowel sounds.

The key decisions

1 *Is it obstruction of the small or large bowel?* In small bowel obstruction, vomiting occurs early, distension is less, and pain is higher in the abdomen; in large bowel obstruction, pain is more constant. The AXR plays a key role (fig 13.28 & p728).

2 *Is there an ileus or mechanical obstruction?* Ileus is functional obstruction from ↓bowel motility (see BOX 'Paralytic ileus or pseudo-obstruction?' & p728). Bowel sounds are absent; pain tends to be less.

3 *Is the obstructed bowel simple/closed loop/strangulated? Simple:* one obstructing point and no vascular compromise. *Closed loop:* obstruction at two points (eg sigmoid volvulus) forming a loop of grossly distended bowel at risk of perforation. *Strangulated:* blood supply is compromised and the patient is iller than you would expect. There is sharper, more constant, and *localized* pain. Peritonism is the cardinal sign. There may be fever + ↑WCC with other signs of mesenteric ischaemia (p620).

Causes See table 13.12.

Table 13.12 Causes of bowel obstruction

Causes: small bowel	Causes: large bowel	Rarer causes
• Adhesions (p581)	• Colon ca (p616)	• Crohn's stricture
• Hernias (p612)	• Constipation (p260)	• Gallstone ileus (p634)
	• Diverticular stricture	• Intussusception
	• Volvulus	• TB (developing world)
	• Sigmoid (see BOX 'Sigmoid volvulus')	• Foreign body
	• Caecal	

Management

- *General principles:* Cause, site, speed of onset, and completeness of obstruction determine definitive therapy: strangulation and large bowel obstruction require surgery; ileus and incomplete small bowel obstruction can be managed conservatively, at least initially.
- *Immediate action:* ►'Drip and suck'—NGT and IV fluids to rehydrate and correct electrolyte imbalance (p668). Being NBM does not give adequate rest for the bowel because it can produce up to 9L of fluid/d. Also: analgesia, blood tests (inc. amylase, FBC, U&E), AXR, erect CXR, catheterize to monitor fluid status.
- *Further imaging:* CT to establish the cause of obstruction (may show dilated, fluid-filled bowel and a transition zone at the site of obstruction—figs 13.29, 13.30). Oral Gastrografin® prior to CT can help identify level of obstruction and may have mild therapeutic action against mechanical obstruction. Consider investigating the cause of large bowel obstruction by colonoscopy but beware risk of perforation.
- *Surgery:* ►Strangulation needs emergency surgery. Closed loop obstruction may be managed with surgery or endoscopic decompression attempted. Endoscopic stenting may be used for obstructing large bowel malignancies either in palliation or as a bridge to surgery in acute obstruction (p616). Small bowel obstruction secondary to adhesions should rarely lead to surgery—see BOX, p581.

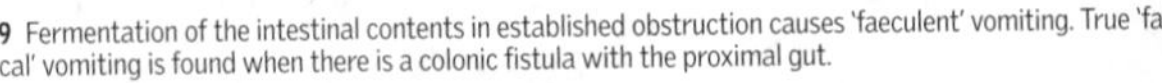

9 Fermentation of the intestinal contents in established obstruction causes 'faeculent' vomiting. True 'faecal' vomiting is found when there is a colonic fistula with the proximal gut.

Paralytic ileus or pseudo-obstruction?

Paralytic ileus is adynamic bowel due to the absence of normal peristaltic contractions. Contributing factors include abdominal surgery, pancreatitis (or any localized peritonitis), spinal injury, hypokalaemia, hyponatraemia, uraemia, peritoneal sepsis and drugs (eg tricyclic antidepressants).

Pseudo-obstruction resembles mechanical GI obstruction but with no obstructing lesion. *Acute* colonic pseudo-obstruction is called Ogilvie's syndrome (p706), and clinical features are similar to that of mechanical obstruction. Predisposing factors: puerperium; pelvic surgery; trauma; cardiorespiratory and neurological disorders. *Treatment:* Neostigmine or colonoscopic decompression are sometimes useful. In chronic pseudo-obstruction weight loss from malabsorption is a problem.

Sigmoid volvulus

Sigmoid volvulus occurs when the bowel twists on its mesentery, which can produce severe, rapid, strangulated obstruction (fig 13.28c). It tends to occur in the elderly, constipated, and comorbid patient, and is managed by insertion of a flatus tube or sigmoidoscopy. Sigmoid colectomy is sometimes required. ►If not treated successfully, it can progress to perforation and fatal peritonitis.

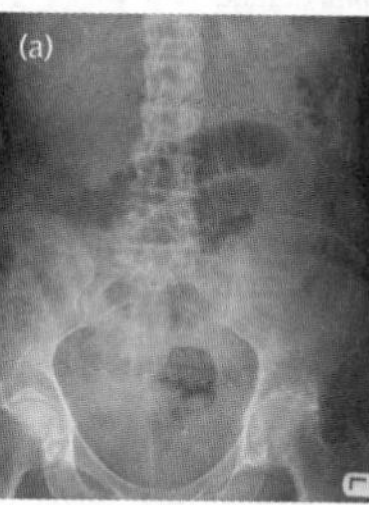

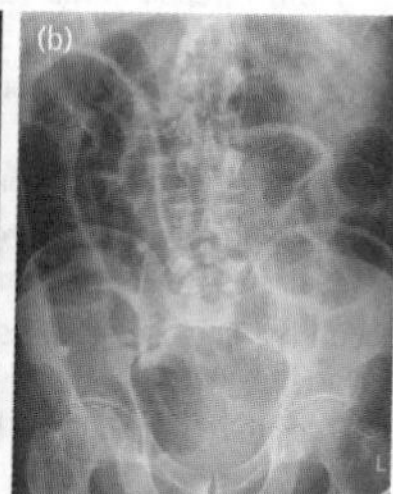

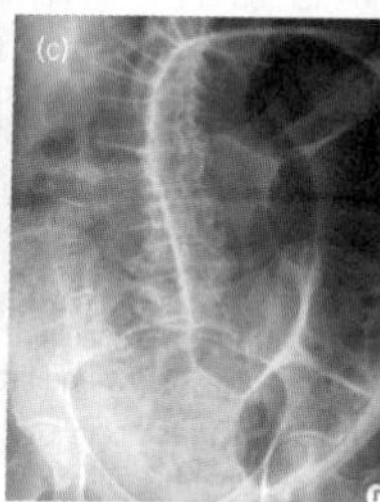

Fig 13.28 (a) Small bowel obstruction: AXR shows central gas shadows with *valvulae conniventes* that completely cross the lumen and no gas in the large bowel. (b) Large bowel obstruction: AXR shows peripheral gas shadows proximal to the blockage (eg in caecum) but not in the rectum. (c) Sigmoid volvulus: there is a characteristic AXR with an 'inverted U' loop of bowel that looks a bit like a coffee bean.

Images (a), (b), and (c) reproduced from Darby *et al.*, *Oxford Handbook of Medical Imaging*, 2011, with permission from Oxford University Press.

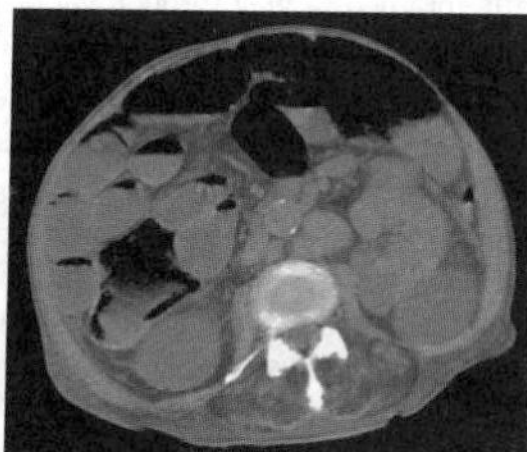

Fig 13.29 Unenhanced axial CT of the abdomen showing multiple loops of dilated, fluid-filled small bowel in a patient with small bowel obstruction.

Image courtesy of Norwich Radiology Dept.

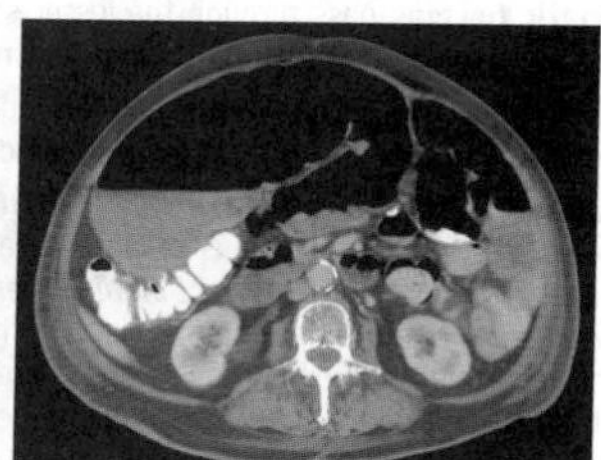

Fig 13.30 Axial CT of the abdomen post-oral contrast showing dilated loops of fluid and air-filled large bowel (contrast medium is in the small bowel).

Image courtesy of Norwich Radiology Dept.

Abdominal hernias

Definition The protrusion of a viscus or part of a viscus through a defect of the walls of its containing cavity into an abnormal position. See fig 13.31. *Terminology:*

- *Irreducible:* contents cannot be pushed back into place (see p614 for technique).
- *Obstructed:* bowel contents cannot pass—features of intestinal obstruction (p610).
- *Strangulated:* ischaemia occurs—the patient requires urgent surgery.
- *Incarceration:* contents of the hernial sac are stuck inside by adhesions.

Care must be taken with reduction as it is possible to push an incarcerated hernia back into the abdominal cavity, giving the initial appearance of successful reduction.

Inguinal hernia The commonest type in both ♂ & ♀ (but ♂>>♀), p614.

Femoral hernia Bowel enters the femoral canal, presenting as a mass in the upper medial thigh or above the inguinal ligament where it points down the leg, unlike an inguinal hernia which points to the groin. They occur more often in ♀ especially in middle age and the elderly. They are likely to be irreducible and to strangulate due to the rigidity of the canal's borders. *Anatomy:*See fig 13.32 *Differential diagnosis:* (See p651.) 1 Inguinal hernia. 2 Saphena varix. 3 An enlarged Cloquet's node (p615). 4 Lipoma. 5 Femoral aneurysm. 6 Psoas abscess. *Treatment:* Surgical repair is recommended. *Herniotomy* is ligation and excision of the sac, *herniorrhaphy* is repair of the hernial defect.

Paraumbilical hernias occur just above or below the umbilicus. Risk factors are obesity and ascites. Omentum or bowel herniates through the defect. Surgery involves repair of the rectus sheath (Mayo repair).

Epigastric hernias pass through linea alba above the umbilicus.

Incisional hernias follow breakdown of muscle closure after surgery (11-20%). If obese, repair is not easy. Mesh repair has ↓recurrence but ↑infection over sutures.

Spigelian hernias occur through the linea semilunaris at the lateral edge of the rectus sheath, below and lateral to the umbilicus.

Lumbar hernias occur through the inferior or superior lumbar triangles in the posterior abdominal wall.

Richter's hernias involve bowel wall only—not the whole lumen.

Maydl's hernias involve a herniating 'double loop' of bowel. The strangulated portion may reside as a single loop *inside* the abdominal cavity.

Littré's hernias are hernial sacs containing strangulated Meckel's diverticulum.

Obturator hernias occur through the obturator canal. Typically there is pain along the medial side of the thigh in a thin woman.

Sciatic hernias pass through the lesser sciatic foramen (a way through various pelvic ligaments). GI obstruction + a gluteal mass suggests this rare possibility.

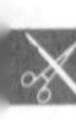

Sliding hernias contain a partially extraperitoneal structure (eg caecum on the right, sigmoid colon on the left). The sac does not completely surround the contents.

Paediatric hernias include *Umbilical hernias:* (3% of live births). Are a result of a persistent defect in the transversalis fascia. Surgical repair rarely needed as most resolve by the age of 3. *Indirect inguinal hernias* (~4% of all ♂ infants due to patent *processus vaginalis*—prematurity is a risk factor; uncommon in ♀ infants—consider testicular feminization.) Surgical repair is required. *Gastroschisis:* Protrusion of the abdominal contents through a defect in the anterior abdominal wall to the right of the umbilicus. Prompt surgical repair required. *Exomphalos:* Abdominal contents are found outside the abdomen, covered in a three-layer membrane consisting of peritoneum, Wharton's jelly, and amnion. Surgical repair less urgent because the bowel is protected by these membranes.

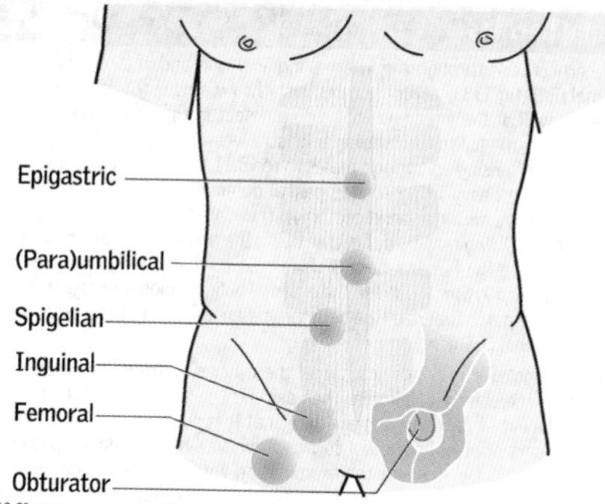

Fig 13.31 Some examples of hernias.

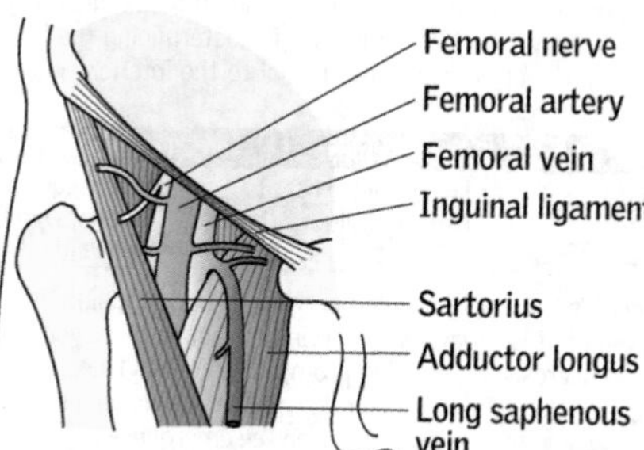

Fig 13.32 The boundaries of the femoral canal are anteriorly the inguinal ligament; medially the lacunar ligament (and pubic bone); laterally the femoral vein (and iliopsoas); and posteriorly the pectineal ligament and pectineus. The canal contains fat and Cloquet's node. The neck of the hernia is felt inferior and lateral to the pubic tubercle (inguinal hernias are superior and medial to this point).

Inguinal hernias

Indirect hernias pass through the internal inguinal ring and, if large, out through the external ring (fig. 13.33). *Direct* hernias push their way *directly* forward through the posterior wall of the inguinal canal, into a defect in the abdominal wall (Hesselbach's triangle; medial to the inferior epigastric vessels and lateral to the rectus abdominus). *Predisposing conditions:* males (♂:♀≈8:1), chronic cough, constipation, urinary obstruction, heavy lifting, ascites, past abdominal surgery (eg damage to the iliohypogastric nerve during appendicectomy). There are two landmarks to identify: *the deep (internal) ring* may be defined as being the mid-point of the inguinal ligament, ~1½cm above the femoral pulse (which crosses the mid-inguinal point); *the superficial (external) ring* is a split in the external oblique aponeurosis just superior and medial to the pubic tubercle (the bony prominence forming the medial attachment of the inguinal ligament).

Examination Look for previous scars; feel the other side (more common on the right); examine the external genitalia. Then ask: •Is the lump visible? If so, ask the patient to reduce it—if he cannot, make sure that it is not a scrotal lump. Ask him to cough. Appears *above and medial to the pubic tubercle*. •If no lump is visible, feel for a cough impulse. •Repeat the examination with the patient standing. *Distinguishing direct from indirect hernias:* This is loved by examiners but is of little clinical use—not least because repair is the same for both (see 'Repairs' later in topic). The best way is to reduce the hernia and occlude the deep (internal) ring with two fingers. Ask the patient to cough or stand—if the hernia is restrained, it is indirect; if not, it is direct. The 'gold standard' for determining the type of inguinal hernia is at surgery: direct hernias arise medial to the inferior epigastric vessels; indirect hernias are lateral.

Indirect hernias:	Direct hernias:	Femoral hernias:
• Common (80%) • Can strangulate.	• Less common (20%) • Reduce easily • Rarely strangulate.	• More frequent in females • Frequently irreducible • Frequently strangulate.

Irreducible hernias You may be called because a long-standing hernia is now irreducible and painful. It is always worth trying to reduce these yourself to prevent strangulation and necrosis (demanding prompt laparotomy). Learn how to do this from an expert, ie one of your patients who has been reducing his hernia for years. Then you will know how to act correctly when the emergency presents. Notice that such patients use the flat of the hand, directing the hernia from below, up towards the contralateral shoulder. Sometimes, as the hernia obstructs, reduction requires perseverance, which may be rewarded by a gurgle from the retreating bowel and a kiss from the attending spouse who had thought that surgery was inevitable.

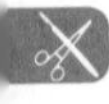

Repairs Weight loss (if over-weight) and stop smoking pre-op. Warn that hernias may recur and patients should be counselled about possibility of chronic pain post-operatively. Mesh techniques (eg Lichtenstein repair) have replaced older methods. In mesh repairs, a polypropylene mesh reinforces the posterior wall. Recurrence rate is less than with other methods (eg <2% vs 10%). (CI: strangulated hernias, contamination with pus/bowel contents.) Local anaesthetic techniques and day-case 'ambulatory' surgery may halve the price of surgery. This is important because this is one of the most common operations (>100 000 per year in the UK). *Laparoscopic repair* gives similar recurrence rates. Methods include *transabdominal pre-peritoneal* (TAPP) in which the peritoneum is entered and the hernia repaired, and *totally extraperitoneal* (TEP), which decreases the risk of visceral injury. For benefits of laparoscopic surgery see p592.

Return to work: Will depend upon surgical approach and patient—discuss this pre-operatively. Rest for 4wks and convalescence over 8wks with open approaches, but laparoscopic repairs may allow return to manual work (and driving) after ≤2wks if all is well.

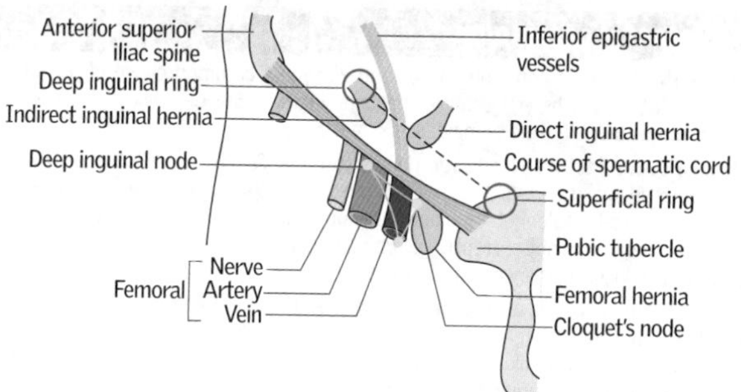

Fig 13.33 Anatomy of the inguinal canal. *Floor:* Inguinal ligament and lacunar ligament medially; *Roof:* Fibres of transversalis, internal oblique; *Anterior:* External oblique aponeurosis + internal oblique for the lateral ⅓; *Posterior:* Laterally, transversalis fascia; medially, conjoint tendon.

The contents of the inguinal canal in the male

- The external spermatic fascia (from external oblique), cremasteric fascia (from internal oblique and transverses abdominus), and internal spermatic fascia (from transversalis fascia) covering the cord.
- The spermatic cord:
  - Vas deferens, obliterated processus vaginalis, and lymphatics.
  - Arteries to the vas, cremaster, and testis.
  - The pampiniform plexus and the venous equivalent of the above.
  - The genital branch of the genitofemoral nerve and sympathetic nerves.
- The ilioinguinal nerve, which enters the inguinal canal via the anterior wall and runs anteriorly to the cord.

NB: in the female the round ligament of the uterus is in place of the male structures. A hydrocele of the canal of Nuck is the female equivalent of a hydrocele of the cord.

Colorectal carcinoma

This is the 3rd most common cancer and 2nd most common cause of UK cancer deaths (16 000 deaths/yr). Usually adenocarcinoma. 86% of presentations are in those >60yrs old. Lifetime UK incidence: ♂ = 1:15; ♀ = 1:19.

Predisposing factors Neoplastic polyps (see BOX & p520); IBD (UC and Crohn's); genetic predisposition (<8%), eg FAP and HNPCC (see p521); diet (low-fibre; ↑red and processed meat); ↑alcohol; smoking; previous cancer. *Prevention:* While routine chemoprevention is not currently recommended due to gastrointestinal SEs, aspirin ≥75mg/d reduces incidence and mortality.

Presentation depends on site: *Left-sided:* Bleeding/mucus PR; altered bowel habit or obstruction (25%); tenesmus; mass PR (60%). *Right:* ↓Weight; ↓Hb; abdominal pain; obstruction less likely. *Either:* Abdominal mass; perforation; haemorrhage; fistula. See p522 for a guide to urgent referral criteria. See fig 13.34 for distribution.

Tests FBC (microcytic anaemia); faecal occult blood (FOB, see BOX); sigmoidoscopy or colonoscopy (figs 6.7 & 6.8, p249), which can be done 'virtually' by CT (fig 16.31, p743); LFT; liver MRI/US. CEA (p531) may be used to monitor disease and effectiveness of treatment. If family history of FAP, refer for DNA test once >15yrs old.

Spread Local, lymphatic, by blood (liver, lung, bone) or transcoelomic. The TNM system (Tumour, Node, Metastases see table 13.13 and p523) is used to stage disease and is preferred to the older Dukes' classification (Dukes A: limited to muscularis mucosae; Dukes B: extension through muscularis mucosae; Dukes C: involvement of regional lymph nodes).

Surgery aims to cure and may ↑ survival times by up to 50%. In elective surgery, anastomosis is typically achieved at the 1st operation. *Laparoscopic surgery* has revolutionized surgery for colon cancer. It is as safe as open surgery and there is no difference in overall survival or disease recurrence. •Right hemicolectomy for caecal, ascending, or proximal transverse colon tumours. •Left hemicolectomy for tumours in distal transverse or descending colon. •Sigmoid colectomy for sigmoid tumours. •Anterior resection for low sigmoid or high rectal tumours. •Abdomino-perineal (AP) resection for tumours low in the rectum (≤8cm from anus): permanent colostomy and removal of rectum and anus. •Hartmann's procedure in emergency bowel obstruction, perforation, or palliation (p582). •Transanal endoscopic microsurgery allows local excision through a wide proctoscope for localized rectal disease. *Endoscopic stenting* should be considered for palliation in malignant obstruction and as a bridge to surgery in acute obstruction. Stenting ↓ need for colostomy, has less complications than emergency surgery, shortens intensive care and total hospital stays, and prevents unnecessary operations. Surgery with liver resection may be curative if single-lobe hepatic metastases and no extrahepatic spread.

Radiotherapy is mostly used in palliation for colonic cancer. It is occasionally used pre-op in rectal cancer to allow resection. Post-op radiotherapy is only used in patients with rectal tumours at high risk of local recurrence.

Chemotherapy Adjuvant chemotherapy for stage 3 disease has been shown to reduce disease recurrence by 30% and mortality by 25%. Benefits for stage 2 disease are more marginal and warrant an individualized approach. The FOLFOX regimen has become standard (fluorouracil, folinic acid and oxaliplatin). Chemotherapy is also used in palliation of metastatic disease. *Biological therapies:* Bevacizumab (anti-VEGF antibody) improves survival when added to combination therapy in advanced disease. Cetuximab and panitumumab (anti-EGFR agents) improve response rate and survival in KRAS wild-type metastatic colorectal cancer.

Prognosis Survival is dependent on age and stage; for stage 1 disease, 5yr survival is ~75% but this drops to just 5% with diagnosis at stage 4, hence the imperative for effective screening (BOX).

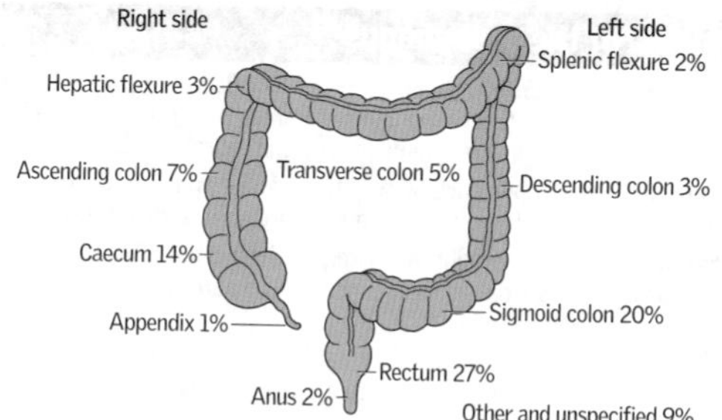

Fig 13.34 Distribution of colorectal carcinomas. These are averages: black females tend to have more proximal neoplasms. White men tend to have more distal neoplasms.

TNM staging in colorectal cancer

Table 13.13 Colorectal cancer: TNM staging

Tx	Primary tumour cannot be assessed	Nx	Nodes cannot be assessed
T_{is}	Carcinoma *in situ*	N0	No node spread
T1	Invading submucosa	N1	Metastases in 1–3 regional nodes
T2	Invading muscularis propria	N2	Metastases in >3 regional nodes
T3	Invading subserosa and beyond (not other organs)	M0	No distant spread
T4	Invasion of adjacent structures	M1	Distant metastasis

Reproduced with permission from Edge, SB *et al.* (Eds.), *AJCC Cancer Staging Manual*, 7th Edition. New York: Springer; 2010.

TNM status used to define overall stage. This is complex with several important subtypes, but in essence, stage 1 disease is T1 or T2/N0/M0; stage 2 is T3 or T4/N0/M0; stage 3 is characterized by N1 or N2 but still M0; stage 4 is M1.

Polyps, the challenges of screening, and the NHS

Polyps are growths that appear above the mucosa and can be inflammatory, hamartomatous, or neoplastic. Left *in situ*, polyps carry a risk of malignant transformation that will relate to size and histology (tubular or villous adenomas, esp. if >2cm). Patients with polyps may have no symptoms and thus a colonoscopy is required to detect and remove. Colonscopy allows the opportunity to detect colorectal cancer at an earlier stage when treatment may be more effective.

However, population-based colonoscopic screening is costly and some studies have suggested that the test does not impact on deaths from right-sided cancers which are rarer and harder to detect (fig 13.34). Therefore, the NHS has introduced a one-off screening flexible sigmoidoscopy offered to all people in their 55th year. Trial results have shown the incidence of colorectal cancer in the intervention (screening) group is reduced by 33% and mortality from colorectal cancer is reduced by 43%. Number needed to screen to prevent one diagnosis (=191); or death (=489).

In parallel, the NHS Bowel Cancer Screening Programme (introduced in 2006) offers colonoscopy to all men and women aged 60–75 who test positive for faecal occult blood (FOB) using a home testing kit performed every 2 years. This FOB-stratification targets screening to those in the highest risk groups, permitting detection of more advanced adenomas and early stage cancers. The relative risk of death from colorectal cancer in patients undergoing screening is reduced by 16%. A 11% increase in incidence rates since 2006 for people aged 60–69 is almost certainly due to earlier detection through the screening programme.

Carcinoma of the oesophagus

Incidence Australia <5/100 000/yr; UK <9; Iran >100. *Risk factors:* Diet, alcohol excess, smoking, achalasia, reflux oesophagitis ± Barrett's oesophagus (p695); obesity, hot drinks, nitrosamine exposure, Plummer-Vinson syndrome (p250). ♂:♀≈5:1.

Site 20% occur in the upper part, 50% in the middle, and 30% in the lower part. They may be squamous cell (proximal) or adenocarcinomas (distal; incidence rising).

Presentation Dysphagia; ↓weight; retrosternal chest pain. *Signs from the upper third of the oesophagus:* Hoarseness; cough (may be paroxysmal if aspiration pneumonia). *ΔΔ:* See 'Dysphagia', p250.

Tests Oesophagoscopy with biopsy is the investigation of choice ± EUS, CT/MRI for staging (fig 13.35), or laparoscopy if significant infra-diaphragmatic component. *Staging:* See table 13.14.

Treatment Survival rates are poor with or without treatment. If localized T1/T2 disease, radical curative oesophagectomy may be tried. Pre-op chemotherapy (cisplatin + fluorouracil) for localized disease may improve survival, but causes some morbidity. If surgery is *not* indicated, then chemoradiotherapy may be better than radiotherapy alone. Palliation in advanced disease aims to restore swallowing with chemo/radiotherapy, stenting, and laser use.

TNM staging in oesophageal cancer

Spread of oesophageal cancer is direct, by submucosal infiltration and local spread—or to nodes, or, later, via the blood.

Table 13.14 Oesophageal cancer: TNM staging

T_{is}	Carcinoma *in situ*	Nx	Nodes cannot be assessed
T1	Invading lamina propria/submucosa	N0	No node spread
T2	Invading muscularis propria	N1–N3	Regional node metastases
T3	Invading adventitia	M0	No distant spread
T4	Invasion of adjacent structures	M1	Distant metastasis

Reproduced with permission from Edge, SB *et al.* (Eds.), ***AJCC Cancer Staging Manual***, 7th Edition. New York: Springer; 2010.

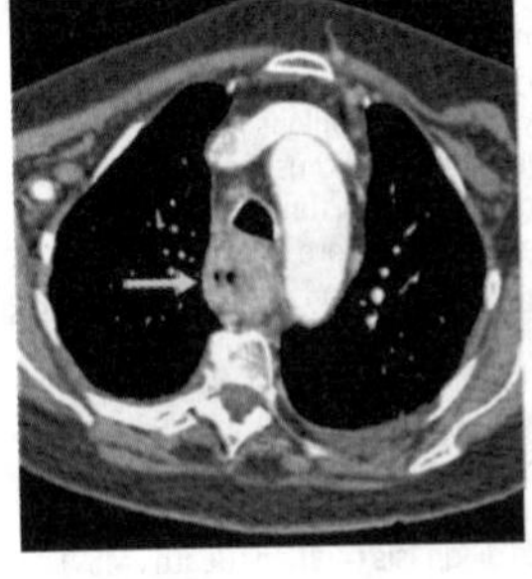

Fig 13.35 Axial CT of the chest after IV contrast medium showing concentric thickening of the oesophagus (arrow); the diagnosis here is oesophageal carcinoma. Loss of the fatty plane around the oesophagus suggests local invasion. Anterior to the oesophagus is the trachea and next to it is the arch of the aorta.

Image courtesy of Dr Stephen Golding.

Carcinoma of the stomach

Incidence of adenocarcinoma at the gastro-oesophageal junction is increasing in the West, though incidence of distal and gastric body carcinoma has fallen sharply. It remains a tumour notable for its gloomy prognosis and non-specific presentation.

Incidence 23/100 000/yr in the UK, but there are unexplained wide geographical variations; it is especially common in Japan, as well as Eastern Europe, China, and South America. ♂:♀≈2:1. *Risk factors:* Pernicious anaemia, blood group A, *H. pylori* (p252), atrophic gastritis, adenomatous polyps, lower social class, smoking, diet (high nitrate, high salt, pickling, low vitamin C), nitrosamine exposure.

Pathology A range of clinical and histological classifications are in use. Of note, 'early' gastric carcinoma (confined to mucosa and submucosa) carries a better prognosis with endoscopic resection often possible.

Presentation *Symptoms:* Often non-specific. Dyspepsia (p59; age ≥55yrs with treatment-refractory symptoms demands investigation), ↓weight, vomiting, dysphagia, anaemia. *Signs* suggesting incurable disease: epigastric mass, hepatomegaly; jaundice, ascites (p604); large left supraclavicular (Virchow's) node (=Troisier's sign); acanthosis nigricans (p562). Most patients in the West present with locally advanced (inoperable) or metastatic disease. *Spread* is local, lymphatic, blood-borne, and transcoelomic, eg to ovaries (Krukenberg tumour).

Tests Gastroscopy + multiple ulcer edge biopsies. ►*Aim to biopsy all gastric ulcers as even malignant ulcers may appear to heal on drug treatment.* Endoscopic ultrasound (EUS) can evaluate depth of invasion; CT/MRI helps staging. Staging laparoscopy is recommended for locally advanced tumours. Cytology of peritoneal washings can help identify peritoneal metastases.

Treatment See p622 for a description of surgical resections. Early gastric cancers may be resectable endoscopically (endoscopic mucosal resection). Partial gastrectomy may suffice for more advanced distal tumours. If proximal, total gastrectomy may be needed. Combination chemotherapy (eg epirubicin, cisplatin and fluorouracil) appears to increase survival in advanced disease. If given perioperatively in operable disease it improves survival compared to surgery alone. Surgical palliation is often needed for obstruction, pain, or haemorrhage. In locally advanced and metastatic disease, chemotherapy increases quality of life and survival. Targeted therapies are likely to have an increasing role, eg trastuzumab for HER-2-positive tumours.

5yr survival <10% overall, but nearly 20% for patients undergoing radical surgery. The prognosis is much better for 'early' gastric carcinoma.

Bile duct and gallbladder cancers

All are rare, have an overall poor prognosis, and are difficult to diagnose. They account for ~3% of all GI cancers worldwide, but there is geographical variation (↑ in north-east Thailand, Japan, Korea, and Eastern Europe). Most are adenocarcinomas. Primary sclerosing cholangitis (p282) is the commonest predisposing factor in the West. *Presentation:* Varies according to location and may include obstructive jaundice, pruritus, abdominal pain, weight loss, and anorexia. *Investigations:* US, CT, and ERCP. MRI has a role for determining extent of invasion in bile duct cancers.

Treatment:

- *Bile duct cancer:* surgical resection is the only potentially curative treatment yet ~80% present with inoperable disease. Palliation includes biliary stenting and chemotherapy.
- *Gallbladder cancer:* again, radical surgery is the only chance of cure. Patients with a calcified ('porcelain') gallbladder have an increased risk of cancer—prophylactic surgery should be considered. Palliative treatment of inoperable disease includes biliary stenting and chemotherapy.

Bowel ischaemia

There are three main types of bowel ischaemia: ►AF with abdominal pain should always prompt thoughts of mesenteric ischaemia.

1 **Acute mesenteric ischaemia** almost always involves the small bowel and may follow superior mesenteric artery (SMA; fig 13.36) thrombosis (~35%) or embolism (~35%), mesenteric vein thrombosis (~5%; younger patients with hypercoagulable states—tends to affect smaller lengths of bowel), or non-occlusive disease (~20%; occurs in low-flow states and usually reflects poor cardiac output, though there may be other factors such as recent cardiac surgery or renal failure). Other causes include trauma, vasculitis (p556), radiotherapy, or strangulation (volvulus or hernia, p612).

Presentation is a classical clinical triad: ►acute severe abdominal pain; no/minimal abdominal signs; rapid hypovolaemia→shock. Pain tends to be constant, central, or around the RIF. The degree of illness is often far out of proportion with clinical signs.

Tests: There may be ↑Hb (due to plasma loss), ↑WCC, modestly raised plasma amylase, and a persistent metabolic acidosis (high lactate). Early on, the abdominal x-ray shows a 'gasless' abdomen. CT/MR may show evidence of ischaemia with CT/MR angiography or formal arteriography if doubt remains. Often the diganosis is made on finding a nasty, necrotic bowel at laparotomy.

Treatment: The main life-threatening complications secondary to acute mesenteric ischaemia are 1 septic peritonitis and 2 progression of a systemic inflammatory response syndrome (SIRS) to multi-organ failure, mediated by bacterial translocation across the dying gut wall. Resuscitation with fluid, antibiotics (eg piperacillin/tazobactam, see table 9.3, p386), and, usually, LMWH/heparin are required. If arteriography is done, thrombolytics may be infused locally via the catheter. At surgery, dead bowel must be removed. Revascularization may be attempted on potentially viable bowel but it is a difficult process and often needs a 2nd laparotomy.

Prognosis: Poor for arterial thrombosis and non-occlusive disease (<40% survive), though not so bad for venous and embolic ischaemia.

2 **Chronic mesenteric ischaemia** (AKA intestinal angina.) The triad of severe, colicky post-prandial abdominal pain ('gut claudication'), ↓weight (eating hurts), and an upper abdominal bruit may be present ± PR bleeding, malabsoprtion, and N&V. Typically brought about through a combination of a low-flow state with atheroma (95% due to diffuse atherosclerotic disease in all three mesenteric arteries). It is rare and difficult to diagnose. *Tests:* CT angiography and contrast-enhanced MR angiography are replacing traditional angiography. *Treatment:* Once diagnosis is confirmed, surgery should be considered due to the ongoing risk of acute infarction. Percutaneous transluminal angioplasty and stent insertion has replaced open revascularization. It is associated with less post-operative morbidity and mortality, but has higher restenosis rates.

3 **Chronic colonic ischaemia** (AKA ischaemic colitis) usually follows low flow in the inferior mesenteric artery (IMA) territory and ranges from mild ischaemia to gangrenous colitis. *Presentation:* Lower left-sided abdominal pain ± bloody diarrhoea. *Tests:* CT may be helpful but lower GI endoscopy is 'gold-standard'. *Treatment:* Usually conservative with fluid replacement and antibiotics. Most recover but subsequent development of ischaemic strictures is common. Gangrenous ischaemic colitis (presenting with peritonitis and hypovolaemic shock) requires prompt resuscitation followed by resection of the affected bowel and stoma formation. Mortality is high.

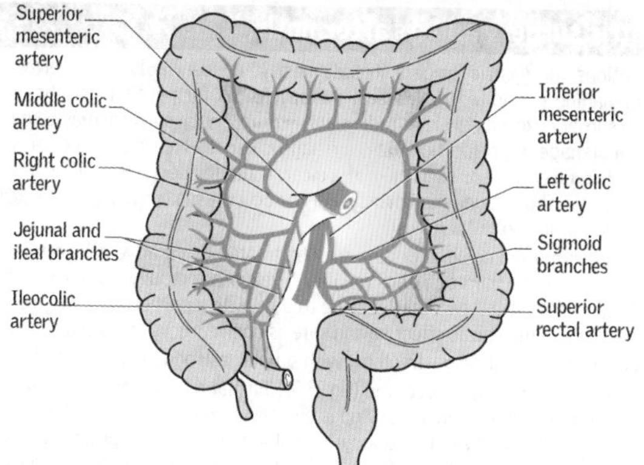

Fig 13.36 The arterial supply to the colon.

Gastric surgery and its aftermath

►Indications for gastric surgery include gastric cancer (p619) and perforated/haemorrhaging peptic ulcers. Medical therapy (p252) for peptic ulcers has made elective surgery exceedingly rare/redundant. ►►*Emergency surgery* may be needed for haemorrhage or perforation. Haemorrhage is usually treated by under-running the bleeding ulcer base or excision of the ulcer. If the former is done, then a biopsy should be taken to exclude malignancy. Perforation is usually managed by excision of the hole for histology, then closure.

Gastric carcinoma Localized disease may be treated by curative gastrectomy. Lesions in the proximal third or extensive infiltrative disease require total gastrectomy, while lesions in the distal two-thirds can be treated with a partial gastrectomy. Laparoscopic surgery may be as effective and safe as open surgery in specialist centres.

Surgery: *Billroth I:* Partial gastrectomy with simple gastroduodenal re-anastomosis. *Billroth II (AKA Polya) gastrectomy:* (fig 13.37) Partial gastrectomy with gastrojejunal anastomosis. The duodenal stump is oversewn (leaving a blind afferent loop), and anastomosis is achieved by a longitudinal incision into the proximal jejunum. *Roux-en-Y:* (fig 13.38) Following total or subtotal gastrectomy, the proximal duodenal stump is oversewn, the proximal jejunum is divided from the distal duodenum and connects with the oesophagus (or proximal stomach after subtotal gastrectomy), while the distal duodenum is connected to the distal jejunum.

Lymph node clearance is a controversial area. RCTs and meta-analyses suggest there may be limited benefit and increased morbidity associated with extended lymph node resections (D_2 or D_3) over resection limited to the perigastric nodes (D_1).

Physical complications of gastrectomy

- *Abdominal fullness:* Feeling of early satiety (± discomfort and distension) improving with time. Advise to take small, frequent meals.
- *Afferent loop syndrome:* Post-gastrectomy (eg Billroth II), the afferent loop may fill with bile after a meal, causing upper abdominal pain and bilious vomiting. This is difficult to treat—but often improves with time.
- *Diarrhoea:* May be disabling after vagotomy. Codeine phosphate may help.
- *Gastric tumour:* A rare complication of any surgery which ↓acid production.
- *↑Amylase:* If with abdominal pain, this may indicate afferent loop obstruction after Billroth II surgery and requires emergency surgery.

Metabolic complications

- *Dumping syndrome:* Fainting and sweating after eating due to food of high osmotic potential being dumped in the jejunum, causing oligaemia from rapid fluid shifts. 'Late dumping' is due to rebound hypoglycaemia and occurs 1-3h after meals. Both tend to improve with time but may be helped by eating less sugar, and more guar gum and pectin (slows glucose absorption). Acarbose may also help to reduce the early hyperglycaemic stimulus to insulin secretion.
- *Weight loss:* Often due to poor calorie intake.
- *Bacterial overgrowth ± malabsorption* (blind loop syndrome) may occur.
- *Anaemia:* Usually from lack of iron, hypochlorhydria, and stomach resection. B_{12} levels are frequently low but megaloblastic anaemia is rare.
- *Osteomalacia:* There may be pseudofractures which look like metastases.

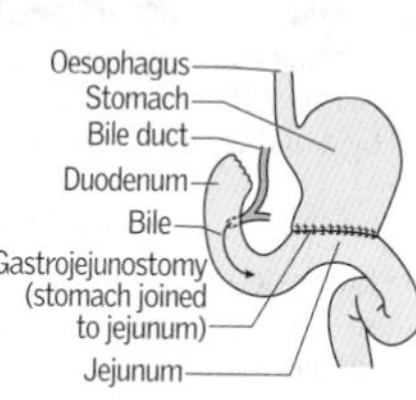

Fig 13.37 Billroth II.

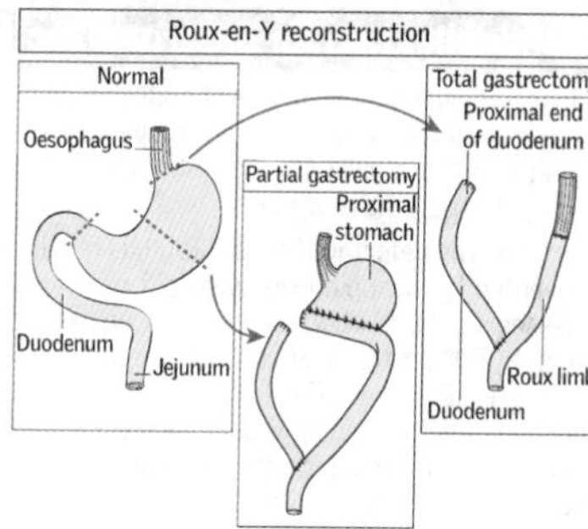

Fig 13.38 The Roux-en-Y reconstruction.

Theodor Billroth

Theodor Billroth was a surgeon of German-Austrian origin, whose name lives on as a set of operations on the stomach. He was a pioneer of abdominal surgery and the use of aseptic techniques, performing the first Billroth I procedure in 1881 for the resection of a pyloric gastric carcinoma. Among the many of his remarkable achievements is included the first laryngectomy. He was also a talented musician (a close friend of Brahms) and a dedicated educator with something of a realist's view of the world:

'*The pleasure of a physician is little, the gratitude of patients is rare, and even rarer is material reward, but these things will never deter the student who feels the call within him.*' Theodor Billroth (1829–94).

Fundoplication for gastro-oesophageal reflux

Laparoscopic fundoplication is the surgical procedure of choice when symptoms of GORD are refractory to medical therapy *and* there is severe reflux (confirmed by pH-monitoring)—see p254. Symptoms may be complicated by a hiatus hernia, which is repaired during the procedure.

Surgery The defect in the diaphragm is repaired by tightening the crura. Reflux is prevented by wrapping the gastric fundus around the lower oesophageal sphincter—see fig 13.39. There are various types of procedure, eg Nissen (360° wrap), Toupet (270° posterior wrap), Watson (anterior hemifundoplication). Laparoscopic surgery is at least as effective at controlling reflux as open surgery but with a lower mortality and morbidity. Wound infections and respiratory complications are also more common in open surgery, though the incidence of dysphagia is similar for the two procedures—but see p592.

Complications Dysphagia (if the wrap is too tight), 'gas-bloat syndrome' (inability to belch/vomit), and new-onset diarrhoea.

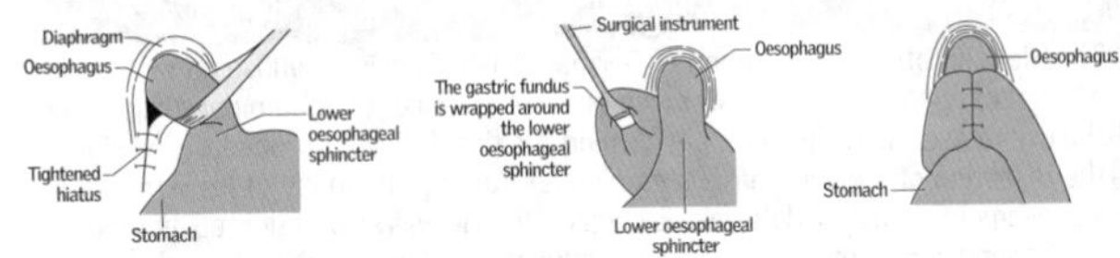

Fig 13.39 Laparoscopic Nissen fundoplication.

Oesophageal rupture

Causes •*Iatrogenic*, eg endoscopy/biopsy/dilatation (accounts for 85–90% of perforations). •*Trauma*, eg penetrating injury/ingestion of foreign body. •*Carcinoma* •*Boerhaave syndrome*—rupture due to violent vomiting. •*Corrosive ingestion*.

Clinical features Odynophagia, tachypnoea, dyspnoea, fever, shock, surgical emphysema (a crackling sensation felt on palpating the skin over the chest or neck caused by air tracking from the lungs. ΔΔ: Pneumothorax).

℞ Iatrogenic perforations are less prone to mediastinitis and sepsis and may be managed conservatively with NG tube, PPI, and antibiotics. Others require resuscitation, PPI, antibiotics, antifungals, and surgery (debridement of mediastinum and placement of T-tube for drainage and formation of a controlled oesophago-cutaneous fistula).

This page intentionally blank

Surgical management of obesity

Severe obesity is increasing in prevalence worldwide and is associated with type 2 diabetes mellitus (T2DM); hypertension; ischaemic heart disease; sleep apnoea; osteoarthritis; and depression. Bariatric surgery has become very successful at weight reduction, symptom improvement,and improving quality of life. Surgery increases life expectancy by around 3 years (but may not prolong survival in high-risk men).

Indications: According to NICE guidelines,[9] weight-loss surgery in adults should be considered if *all* the following criteria are met:

1. BMI ≥40 (or ≥35 with significant comorbidities that could improve with ↓weight).
2. Failure of non-surgical management to achieve and maintain clinically beneficial weight loss for 6 months.
3. Fitness for surgery and anaesthesia.
4. Intensive management in tier 3 service (provides guidance on diet, physical activity, and psychosocial concerns, as well as lifelong medical monitoring).
5. The patient must be well informed and motivated.

If BMI ≥50, or in newly diagnosed T2DM with BMI ≥30, surgery is recommended as first-line treatment.

Comparison with medical therapy Surgery is more effective in achieving weight loss than non-surgical management and weight loss is more likely to be maintained in the longer term. Adverse events are more common following surgery, and vary from one procedure to another.

Procedures There are two main mechanisms causing weight loss: 1 Restriction of calorie intake by reducing stomach capacity. 2 Malabsorption of nutrients by reducing the length of functional small bowel. NB: This also affects the levels of circulating gut peptides (eg PYY and GLP-1), which are thought to play a role in the mechanism of satiety and weight loss. Choose surgical intervention jointly with patient:

- *Laparoscopic adjustable gastric banding (LAGB):* This restrictive technique creates a pre-stomach pouch by placing a silicone band around the top of the stomach, which serves as a new smaller stomach. The band can be adjusted by addition or removal of saline through a subcutaneous port (see fig 13.40). LAGB is associated with improvements in comorbidities and quality of life. Weight loss is slower and less than with gastric bypass but there is lower mortality and fewer complications. Relatively non-invasive and band removal possible. *Complications:* pouch enlargement, band slip, band erosion, and port infection/breakage.
- *Sleeve gastrectomy:* (fig 13.41) Involves division of the stomach vertically, reducing it in size by about 75%. The pyloric valve at the bottom of the stomach is left intact so function and digestion are unaltered. The procedure is not reversible and may be a first stage for progression to Roux-en-Y gastric bypass or duodenal switch in very obese patients where a single-stage procedure would be technically difficult or unsafe.

- *Roux-en-Y gastric bypass:* (fig 13.42) Laparoscopic or open. A portion of the jejunum is attached to a small stomach pouch to allow food to bypass the distal stomach, duodenum, and proximal jejunum. It can be performed laparoscopically and works by both restriction and malabsorption. Mean excess weight loss at 5 years is 62.8%.Current evidence demonstrates greater weight loss, greater resolution of comorbidities, and lower reoperation rates compared to LAGB. *Complications:* micronutrient deficiency (requires vitamin supplementation and lifelong follow-up/ blood tests), dumping syndrome, wound infection, hernias, malabsorption, diarrhoea, and a mortality of <0.5% (at experienced centres).

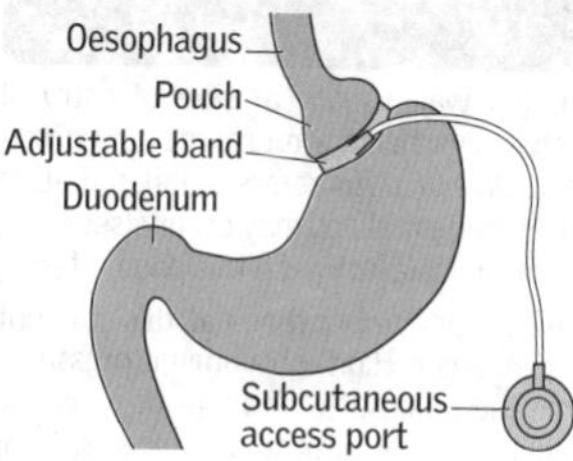

Fig 13.40 Adjustable gastric band.

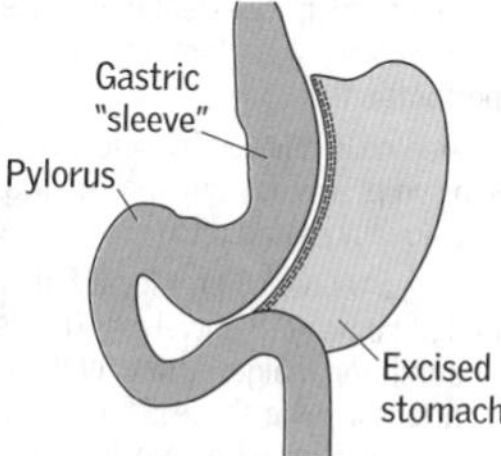

Fig 13.41 Vertical sleeve gastrectomy.

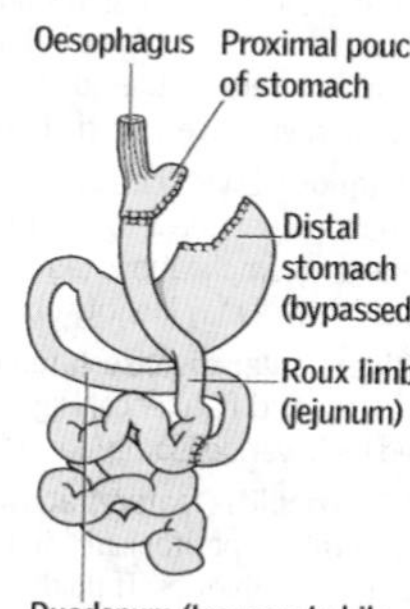

Fig 13.42 Gastric bypass.

Diverticular disease

A GI *diverticulum* is an outpouching of the gut wall, usually at sites of entry of perforating arteries. *Diverticulosis* means that diverticula are present, and *diverticular disease* implies they are symptomatic. *Diverticulitis* refers to inflammation of a diverticulum. Diverticula can be aquired or congenital and may occur elsewhere, but the most important are acquired colonic diverticula, to which this page refers.

Pathology Most within sigmoid colon with 95% of complications at this site, but right-sided and massive single diverticula can occur. High intraluminal pressures (due, perhaps, to lack of dietary fibre) force the mucosa to herniate through the muscle layers of the gut at weak points adjacent to penetrating vessels. 30% of Westerners have diverticulosis by age 60. The majority are asymptomatic.

Diagnosis Diverticula are a common incidental finding at colonoscopy (fig 6.11, p249). CT abdomen is best to confirm acute diverticulitis and can identify extent of disease and any complications (eg colovesical fistulae). Colonoscopy risk perforation in acute setting. AXR may identify obstruction or free air (perforation).

Diverticular disease Altered bowel habit ± left-sided colic relieved by defecation; nausea and flatulence. High-fibre diets do not help symptoms; try antispasmodics, eg mebeverine 135mg/8h PO. Surgical resection occasionally resorted to.

Diverticulitis features above + pyrexia, ↑WCC, ↑CRP/ESR, a tender colon ± localized or generalized peritonism. Mild attacks can be treated at home with bowel rest (fluids only) ± antibiotics. If fluids and pain not tolerated, admit for analgesia, NBM, IV fluids and IV antibiotics. Most attacks settle but complications include abscess formation (necessitating percutaneous CT-guided drainage), or perforation. ►Beware diverticulitis in immunocompromised patients (eg on steroids) who often have few symptoms and may present late.

Surgery The need for surgery is reflected by the degree of infective complications:

Stage 1	Pericolic or mesenteric abscess	Surgery rarely needed
Stage 2	Walled off or pelvic abscess	May resolve without surgery
Stage 3	Generalized purulent peritonitis	Surgery required
Stage 4	Generalized faecal peritonitis	Surgery required

Indications for elective surgery include stenosis, fistulae, or recurrent bleeding.

Complications ►►*Perforation:* There is ileus, peritonitis ± shock. Mortality: 40%. Manage as for an acute abdomen. At laparotomy a Hartmann's procedure may be performed (p582). Primary anastomosis is possible in selected patients. Emergency laparoscopic management is an emerging alternative.

- *Haemorrhage* is usually sudden and painless. It is a common cause of big rectal bleeds (p629). Embolization (at angiography) or colonic resection only necessary if ongoing massive bleeding and colonoscopic haemostasis has been unsuccessful.
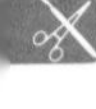
- *Fistulae:* Enterocolic, colovaginal, or colovesical (pneumaturia ± intractable UTIs). Treatment is surgical, eg colonic resection.
- *Abscesses*, eg with swinging fever, leucocytosis, and localizing signs, eg boggy rectal mass (pelvic abscess—drain rectally). If no localizing signs, remember the aphorism: *pus somewhere, pus nowhere = pus under the diaphragm*. A subphrenic abscess is a horrible way to die, so do an urgent ultrasound. Antibiotics ± ultrasound/CT-guided drainage may be needed.
- *Post-infective strictures* may form in the sigmoid colon.

Rectal bleeding—an acute management plan

Causes Diverticulitis, colorectal cancer, haemorrhoids, IBD, perianal disease, angiodyplasia (submucosal arteriovenous malformations, typically elderly). Rarities: trauma, ischaemia colitis, radiation proctitis, aorto-enteric fistula.

An acute management plan for this common surgical event:

- ►►*ABC* resuscitation, if necessary.
- ►►*History and examination.*
- ►►*Blood tests:* FBC, U&E, LFT, clotting, amylase (always thinking of pancreatitis), CRP, group and save—await Hb result before crossmatching unless unstable and bleeding.
- ►►*Imaging:* May only need plain AXR, but if there are signs of perforation (eg sepsis, peritonism) or if there is cardiorespiratory comorbidity, then request an erect CXR.
- ►►*Fluid management:* Insert 2 cannulae (≥18G) into the antecubital fossae. Insert a urinary catheter if there is a suspicion of haemodynamic compromise—there is no absolute indication, but remember that you are weighing up the risks and benefits. Give crystalloid as replacement and maintenance IVI. Blood transfusion only if significant blood loss (table 13.10, p607).
- ►►*Clotting:* Withold ± reverse anticoagulation and antiplatelet agents (p351).
- ►►*Antibiotics* may occasionally be required if there is evidence of sepsis or perforation, eg piperacillin/tazobactam 4.5g/8h IV.
- ►►*Keep bedbound:* The patient may feel the need to get out of bed to pass stool, but this could be another large bleed, resulting in collapse if they try to walk. ►Don't allow them to mobilize and inform the nursing staff of this.
- ►►*Start a stool chart* to monitor volume and frequency of motions. Send a sample for MC&S (x3 if known to have compromising comorbidity such as IBD).
- ►►*Diet:* Keep on clear fluids so that they can have something, yet the colon will be as clear as possible if colonoscopy required.
- ►►*Interventions* if bleeding not settling with conservative management: *Angiography* may allow localization of bleeding (eg sigmoid diverticulum or right sided angiodysplasia) as well as therapeutic embolization; *CT angiography* is a non-invasive alternative (without interventional options); *colonoscopy* may permit endoscopic haemostasis.
- ►►*Surgery:* The main indication for this is unremitting, massive bleeding that is not controlled by other means.

Perianal problems

Pruritus ani Itch occurs if the anus is moist/soiled; fissures, incontinence, poor hygiene, tight pants, threadworm, fistula, dermatoses, lichen sclerosis, anxiety, contact dermatitis (perfumed goods). Cause is often unknown. ℞: Avoid scratching, perianal hygiene, avoid foods which loosen stools. Soothing ointment, mild topical corticosteroid if perinanal inflammation (max 2wks), oral antihistamine for noctural itch.

Fissure-in-ano Painful tear in the squamous lining of the lower anal canal—often, if chronic, with a 'sentinel pile' or mucosal tag at the external aspect. 90% are posterior (anterior ones follow parturition). ♂>♀. *Causes:* Most are due to hard faeces. Spasm may constrict the inferior rectal artery, causing ischaemia, making healing difficult and perpetuating the problem. Rare causes (multiple ± lateral): syphilis; herpes; trauma; Crohn's; anal cancer; psoriasis. Groin nodes suggest a complicating factor (eg immunosuppression/HIV). ℞: 5% lidocaine ointment + GTN ointment (0.2–0.4%) *or* topical diltiazem (2%); dietary fibre, fluids, stool softener, and hygiene advice. Botulinum toxin injection (2nd line) and topical diltiazem (2%) are at least as effective as GTN with fewer side-effects. If conservative measures fail, surgical options include *lateral partial internal sphincterotomy.*

Surgery

Fistula-in-ano A track communicates between the skin and anal canal/rectum. Blockage of deep intramuscular gland ducts is thought to predispose to the formation of abscesses, which discharge to form the fistula. *Goodsall's rule* determines the path of the fistula track: if anterior, the track is in a straight line (radial); if posterior, the internal opening is *always* at the 6 o'clock position, taking a tortuous course. *Causes:* perianal sepsis, abscesses (see later in topic), Crohn's disease, TB, diverticular disease, rectal carcinoma, immunocompromise. *Tests:* MRI; endoanal US scan. ℞: Fistulotomy + excision. High fistulae (involving continence muscles of anus) require 'seton suture' tightened over time to maintain continence; low fistulae are 'laid open' to heal by secondary intention—division of sphincters poses no risk to continence.

Anorectal abscesses Usually caused by gut organisms (rarely staphs or TB). ♂:♀≈1:8. Perianal (~45%), ischiorectal (≲30%), intersphincteric (>20%), supralevator (~5%) (fig 13.43). ℞: Incise & drain under GA. *Associations:* DM, Crohn's, malignancy, fistulae.

Perianal haematoma (AKA thrombosed external pile—see p633). Strictly, it is actually a clotted venous saccule. It appears as a 2–4mm 'dark blueberry' under the skin at the anal margin. It may be evacuated under LA or left to resolve spontaneously.

Pilonidal sinus Obstruction of natal cleft hair follicles ~6cm above the anus. Ingrowing of hair excites a foreign body reaction and may cause secondary tracks to open laterally ± abscesses, with foul-smelling discharge. (Barbers get these between fingers.) ♂:♀≈10:1. Obese Caucasians and those from Asia, the Middle East, and Mediterranean at ↑risk. ℞: Excision of the sinus tract ± primary closure. Consider pre-op antibiotics. Complex tracks can be laid open and packed individually, or skin flaps can be used to cover the defect. Offer hygiene and hair removal advice.

Rectal prolapse The mucosa (partial/type 1), or all layers (complete/type 2—more common), may protrude through the anus. Incontinence in 75%. It is due to a lax sphincter, prolonged straining, and related to chronic neurological and psychological disorders. ℞: *Abdominal approach*: fix rectum to sacrum (rectopexy) ± mesh insertion ± rectosigmoidectomy. Laparoscopic rectoplexy is as effective as open repair. *Perineal approach*: Delorme's procedure (resect close to dentate line and suture mucosal boundaries), anal encirclement with a Thiersch wire.

Perianal warts Condylomata acuminata (viral warts) are treated with podophyllotoxin or imiquimod or cryotherapy/surgical excision. Giant condylomata acuminata of Buschke & Loewenstein may evolve into verrucous cancers (low-grade, non-metastasizing). Condylomata lata secondary to syphilis is treated with penicillin.

Proctalgia fugax Idiopathic, intense, brief, stabbing/crampy rectal pain, often worse at night. The mainstay of treatment is reassurance. Inhaled salbutamol or topical GTN (0.2–0.4%) or topical diltiazem (2%) may help.

Anal ulcers Consider Crohn's, anal cancer, lymphogranuloma venerum, TB, syphilis.

Skin tags Seldom cause trouble but are easily excised.

Anal cancer

Incidence: 1233 new cases of anal cancer in the UK (2013). *Risk factors:* Anoreceptive intercourse; HPV (HPV 16 associated with worse prognosis); HIV. *Histology:* Squamous cell (85%); rarely basaloid, melanoma, or adenocarcinoma. Anal margin tumours are usually well-differentiated, keratinizing lesions with a good prognosis. Anal canal tumours arise above dentate line, are poorly differentiated and non-keratinizing with a poorer prognosis. *Spread:* Tumours above the dentate line spread to pelvic lymph nodes; those below spread to the inguinal nodes. *Presentation:* Bleeding, pain, bowel habit change, pruritus ani, masses, stricture. *ΔΔ:* Perianal warts; leucoplakia; lichen sclerosis; Bowen's disease; Crohn's disease. *Treatment:* Chemo-irradiation (radiotherapy + fluorouracil + mitomycin/cisplatin) is usually preferred to anorectal excision & colostomy; 75% retain normal anal function.

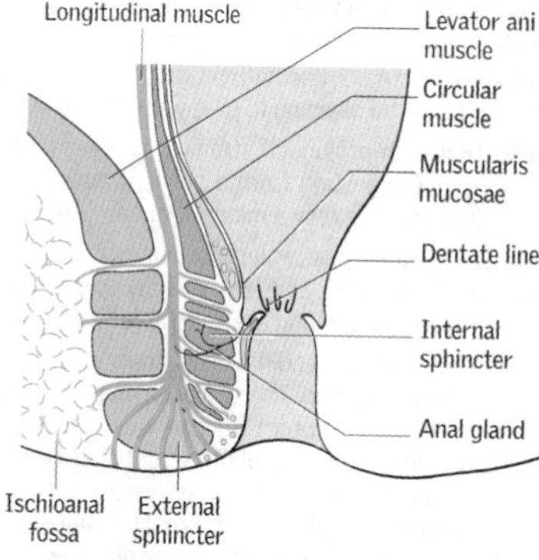

Fig 13.43 Anatomy of the anal canal. Perianal abscesses present as tender, inflamed, localized swellings at the anal verge. Ischiorectal abscesses are also tender but cause a diffuse, indurated swelling in the ischioanal fossa area. You will find your patient waiting anxiously for you, pacing about, or on the edge of their chair: avoiding all pressure is imperative. NB: above the dentate line = visceral nerve innervation (hence no pain sensation); below = somatic innervation (very sensitive to pain).

Haemorrhoids (piles)

Definition Haemorrhoids (≈*running blood* in Greek) are disrupted and dilated anal cushions. The anus is lined mainly by discontinuous masses of spongy vascular tissue—the anal cushions, which contribute to anal closure. Viewed from the lithotomy position, the three anal cushions are at 3, 7, and 11 o'clock (where the three major arteries that feed the vascular plexuses enter the anal canal). They are attached by smooth muscle and elastic tissue, but are prone to displacement and disruption, either singly or together. The effects of gravity (standing), increased anal tone (?stress), and the effects of straining at stool may make them become both bulky and loose, and so to protrude to form piles (Latin *pila*, meaning a ball). They are vulnerable to trauma (eg from hard stools) and bleed readily from the capillaries (bright red blood) of the underlying lamina propria. NB: piles are *not* varicose veins.

As there are no sensory fibres above the dentate line (squamomucosal junction), piles are not painful unless they thrombose when they protrude and are gripped by the anal sphincter, blocking venous return. See fig 13.44.

Differential diagnosis Perianal haematoma; anal fissure; abscess; tumour; proctalgia fugax. ►Never ascribe rectal bleeding to piles without examination or investigation.

Causes Constipation with prolonged straining is a key factor. In many the bowel habit may be normal. Congestion from a pelvic tumour, pregnancy, CCF, or portal hypertension are important in only a minority of cases. ►Elicit red flags in history.

Pathogenesis There is a vicious circle: vascular cushions protrude through a tight anus, become more congested, and hypertrophy to protrude again more readily. These protrusions may then strangulate. See table 13.15 for classification.

Symptoms Bright red rectal bleeding, often coating stools, on the tissue, or dripping into the pan after defecation. There may be mucous discharge and pruritus ani. Severe anaemia may occur. Symptoms such as weight loss, tenesmus, and change in bowel habit should prompt thoughts of other pathology. ►In all rectal bleeding do:

- An abdominal examination to rule out other diseases.
- PR exam: prolapsing piles are obvious. Internal haemorrhoids are not palpable.
- Colonoscopy/flexible sigmoidoscopy to exclude proximal pathology if ≳50 years old.

Treatment 1 *Medical:* (1st-degree.) ↑Fluid and fibre is key ± topical analgesics & stool softener (bulk forming). Topical steroids for short periods only.
2 *Non-operative:* (2nd & 3rd degree, or 1st degree if medical therapy failed.) •*Rubber band ligation.* Cheap, but needs skill. Banding produces an ulcer to anchor the mucosa (SE: bleeding, infection; pain). It has the lowest recurrence rate. •*Sclerosants.* (1st- or 2nd-degree.) 2mL of 5% phenol in oil is injected into the pile above the dentate line, inducing fibrotic reaction. Recurrence higher (SE: impotence; prostatitis). •*Infra-red coagulation.* Applied to localized areas of piles, it works by coagulating vessels and tethering mucosa to subcutaneous tissue. It is as successful as banding and may be less painful. •*Bipolar diathermy and direct current electrotherapy.* Causes coagulation and fibrosis after local application of heat. Success rates are similar to those of infrared coagulation, and complication rates are low.

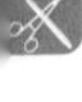

3 *Surgery:* •*Excisional haemorrhoidectomy* is the most effective treatment (excision of piles ± ligation of vascular pedicles, as day-case surgery, needing ~2wks off work). Scalpel, electrocautery, or laser may be used. •*Stapled haemorrhoidopexy* (procedure for prolapsing haemorrhoids) may result in less pain, a shorter hospital stay, and quicker return to normal activity than conventional surgery. It is used when there is a large internal component, but has a higher recurrence and prolapse rate than excisional. *Surgical complications* include constipation; infection; stricture; bleeding.

Prolapsed, thrombosed piles Analgesia, ice packs, and stool softeners. Pain usually resolves in 2-3wks. Some advocate early surgery.

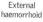

Table 13.15 Classification of haemorrhoids

1st degree	Remain in the rectum
2nd degree	Prolapse through the anus on defecation but spontaneously reduce
3rd degree	As for 2nd-degree but require digital reduction
4th degree	Remain persistently prolapsed

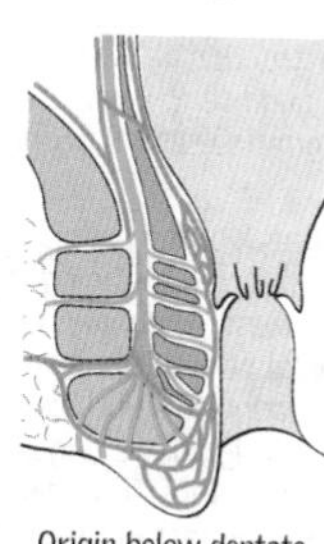

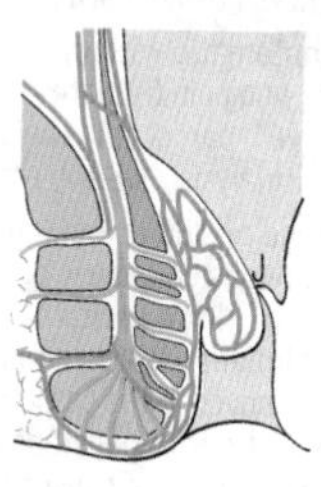

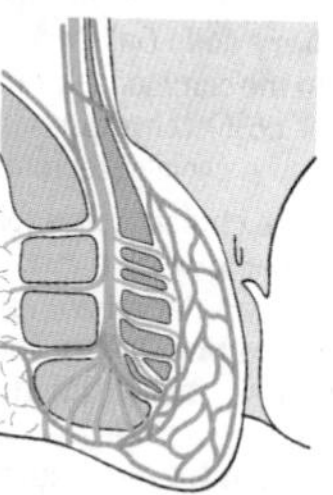

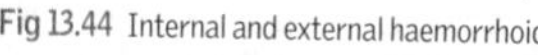
Fig 13.44 Internal and external haemorrhoids.

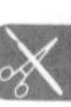

Gallstones

Bile contains cholesterol, bile pigments (from broken down Hb), and phospholipids. If the concentrations vary, different stones may form. *Pigment stones:* Small, friable, and irregular. *Causes:* haemolysis. *Cholesterol stones:* Large, often solitary. *Causes:* ♀, age, obesity (Admirand's triangle: ↑risk of stone if ↓lecithin, ↓bile salts, ↑cholesterol). *Mixed stones:* Faceted (calcium salts, pigment, and cholesterol). *Gallstone prevalence:* 8% of those over 40yrs. 90% remain asymptomatic. Risk factors for stones becoming symptomatic: smoking; parity.

Biliary colic Gallstones are symptomatic with cystic duct obstruction or if passed into the common bile duct (CBD[10]). RUQ pain (radiates → back) ± jaundice. ℞: Analgesia (see p636), rehydrate, NBM. Elective laparoscopic cholecystectomy (see BOX 'Early or delayed cholecystectomy?'). Do urinalysis, CXR, and ECG.

Acute cholecystitis follows stone or sludge impaction in the neck of the gallbladder (GB[10]), which may cause continuous epigastric or RUQ pain (referred to the right shoulder—see p609), vomiting, fever, local peritonism, or a GB mass. The main difference from *biliary colic* is the inflammatory component (local peritonism, fever, WCC↑; see table 13.16). If the stone moves to the CBD, obstructive jaundice and cholangitis may occur—see BOX 'Complications of gallstones'. *Murphy's sign:* lay 2 fingers over the RUQ; ask patient to breathe in. This causes pain & arrest of inspiration as an inflamed GB impinges on your fingers. It is only +ve if the same test in the LUQ does not cause pain. A *phlegmon* (RUQ mass of inflamed adherent omentum and bowel) may be palpable. *Tests:* ↑WCC, US—a thick-walled, shrunken GB (also seen in chronic disease), pericholecystic fluid, stones, CBD (dilated if >6mm). Plain AXR only shows ~10% of gallstones; it may identify a 'porcelain' GB (associated risk of cancer). *Treatment:* NBM, pain relief, IVI, and antibiotics, eg *co-amoxiclav* 625mg/8h IV. Laparoscopic cholecystectomy is the treatment of choice for all patients fit for GA. Open surgery is required if there is GB perforation. If elderly or high risk/unsuitable for surgery, consider percutaneous cholecystostomy; cholecystectomy can still be done later. Cholecystostomy is also the preferred treatment for acalculous cholecystitis.

Chronic cholecystitis Chronic inflammation ± colic. 'Flatulent dyspepsia': vague abdominal discomfort, distension, nausea, flatulence, and fat intolerance (fat stimulates cholecystokinin release and GB contraction). US to image stones and assess CBD diameter. MRCP (p742) is used to find CBD stones. ℞: Cholecystectomy. If US shows a dilated CBD with stones, ERCP (p742) + sphincterotomy before surgery. If symptoms persist post-surgery consider hiatus hernia/IBS/peptic ulcer/chronic pancreatitis/tumour.

Other presentations

- *Obstructive jaundice with CBD stones:* (See p272.) If LFT worsening, ERCP with sphincterotomy ± biliary trawl, then cholecystectomy may be needed, or open surgery with CBD exploration. If CBD stones are suspected pre-operatively, they should be identified by MRCP (p742).
- *Cholangitis:* (Bile duct infection.) Causing RUQ pain, jaundice, and rigors (Charcot's triad, BOX 'Complications of gallstones'). Treat with, eg piperacillin/tazobactam 4.5g/8h IV.
- *Gallstone ileus:* A stone erodes through the GB into the duodenum; it may then obstruct the terminal ileum. AXR shows: air in CBD (= pneumobilia), small bowel fluid levels, and a stone. Duodenal obstruction is rarer (Bouveret's syndrome).
- *Pancreatitis:* See p636.
- *Mucocoele/empyema:* Obstructed GB fills with mucus (secreted by GB wall)/pus.
- *Silent stones:* Do elective surgery on those with sickle cell, immunosuppression, (debatably diabetes) as well as all calcified/porcelain GBs.
- *Mirizzi's syndrome:* A stone in the GB presses on the bile duct causing jaundice.
- *Gallbladder necrosis:* Rare because of dual blood supply (hepatic artery via cystic artery, and from small branches of the hepatic artery in the GB fossa).
- *Other:* Causes of cholecystitis and biliary symptoms other than gallstones are rare Consider infection (typhoid, cryptosporidiosis, and brucellosis); cholecystokinin release; parenteral nutrition; anatomical abnormality; polyarteritis nodosa (p556).

10 Common abbreviations used in this section: CBD, common bile duct; GB, gallbladder.

Complications of gallstones

In the gallbladder & cystic duct:
- Biliary colic
- Acute and chronic cholecystitis
- Mucocoele
- Empyema
- Carcinoma
- Mirizzi's syndrome.

In the bile ducts:
- Obstructive jaundice
- Cholangitis
- Pancreatitis.

In the gut:
- Gallstone ileus.

Table 13.16 Biliary colic, cholecystitis, or cholangitis?

	RUQ pain	Fever/↑WCC	Jaundice
Biliary colic	✓	X	X
Acute cholecystitis	✓	✓	X
Cholangitis	✓	✓	✓

Early or delayed cholecystectomy?

For acute cholecystitis Laparoscopic cholecystectomy for acute cholecystitis has traditionally been performed 6–12wks after the acute episode due to anticipated increased mortality and conversion to open procedure. Early laparoscopic cholecystectomy, within 7d of symptom onset, is now the treatment of choice. Early surgery reduces the duration of hospital admission compared with delayed surgery, but does not reduce mortality or complications. Up to one-quarter of people scheduled for delayed surgery may require urgent operations because of recurrent or worsening symptoms.[10]

For biliary colic Patients with biliary colic due to gallstones waiting for an elective laparoscopic cholecystectomy may develop significant complications, such as acute pancreatitis (p636) during the waiting period. One high-bias trial found early laparoscopic cholecystectomy (within 24h of an acute episode) decreased potential complications that may develop during the wait for elective surgery.

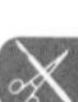

Acute pancreatitis

This unpredictable disease (mortality ~12%) is characterized by self-perpetuating pancreatic enzyme-mediated autodigestion; oedema and fluid shifts cause hypovolaemia, as extracellular fluid is trapped in the gut, peritoneum, and retroperitoneum (worsened by vomiting). Although pancreatitis is mild in 80% of cases; 20% develop severe complicated and life-threatening disease: progression may be rapid from mild oedema to necrotizing pancreatitis. ~50% of cases that advance to necrosis are further complicated by infection.

Causes The one mnemonic we can all agree on: 'GET SMASHED'. **G**allstones (~35%), **E**thanol (~35%), **T**rauma (~1.5%), **S**teroids, **M**umps, **A**utoimmune (PAN), **S**corpion venom, **H**yperlipidaemia, hypothermia, hypercalcaemia, **E**RCP (~5%) and emboli, **D**rugs. Also pregnancy and neoplasia or no cause found (~10–30%).

Symptoms Gradual or sudden severe epigastric or central abdominal pain (radiates to back, sitting forward may relieve); vomiting prominent.

Signs ►May be subtle in serious disease. ↑HR, fever, jaundice, shock, ileus, rigid abdomen ± local/general tenderness, periumbilical bruising (Cullen's sign) or flanks (Grey Turner's sign) from blood vessel autodigestion and retroperitoneal haemorrhage.

Tests Raised serum *amylase* (>1000U/mL or around 3-fold upper limit of normal). The degree of elevation is not related to severity of disease. ►Amylase may be normal even in severe pancreatitis (levels starts to fall within 24–48h). It is excreted renally so renal failure will ↑ levels. Cholecystitis, mesenteric infarction, and GI perforation can cause lesser rises. Serum *lipase* is more sensitive and specific for pancreatitis (especially when related to alcohol), and rises earlier and falls later. *ABG* to monitor oxygenation and acid-base status. *AXR:* No psoas shadow (↑retroperitoneal fluid), 'sentinel loop' of proximal jejunum from ileus (solitary air-filled dilatation). *Erect CXR* helps exclude other causes (eg perforation). *CT* is the standard choice of imaging to assess severity and for complications. *US* (if gallstones + ↑AST). *ERCP* if LFTs worsen. *CRP* >150mg/L at 36h after admission is a predictor of severe pancreatitis.

Management Severity assessment is essential (see BOX and table 13.17).

- Nil by mouth, consider NJ feeding (decrease pancreatic stimulation). Set up IVI and give lots of crystalloid, to counter third-space sequestration, until vital signs are satisfactory and urine flow stays at >30mL/h. Insert a urinary catheter and consider CVP monitoring.
- Analgesia: pethidine 75–100mg/4h IM, or morphine (may cause Oddi's sphincter to contract more, but it is a better analgesic and not contraindicated).
- Hourly pulse, BP, and urine output; daily FBC, U&E, Ca^{2+}, glucose, amylase, ABG.
- If worsening: ITU, O_2 if $\downarrow P_aO_2$. In suspected abscess formation or pancreatic necrosis (on CT), consider parenteral nutrition ± laparotomy & debridement ('necrosectomy'). Antibiotics may help in severe disease.
- ERCP + gallstone removal may be needed if there is progressive jaundice.
- Repeat imaging (usually CT) is performed in order to monitor progress.

ΔΔ Any acute abdomen (p606), myocardial infarct.

Early complications Shock, ARDS (p186), renal failure (►give lots of fluid!), DIC, sepsis, $\downarrow Ca^{2+}$, ↑glucose (transient; 5% need insulin).

Late complications (>1wk.) *Pancreatic necrosis* and *pseudocyst* (fluid in lesser sac, fig 13.45), with fever, a mass ± persistent ↑amylase/LFT; may resolve or need drainage. *Abscesses* need draining. *Bleeding* from elastase eroding a major vessel (eg splenic artery); embolization may be life-saving. *Thrombosis* may occur in the splenic/gastroduodenal arteries, or colic branches of the SMA, causing bowel necrosis. *Fistulae* normally close spontaneously. If purely pancreatic they do not irritate the skin. Some patients suffer *recurrent oedematous pancreatitis* so often that near-total pancreatectomy is contemplated. ►It can all be a miserable course.

Modified Glasgow criteria for predicting severity of pancreatitis

►Three or more positive factors detected within 48h of onset suggest severe pancreatitis, and should prompt transfer to ITU/HDU. Mnemonic: **PANCREAS.**

Table 13.17

P$_aO_2$	<8kPa
Age	>55yrs
Neutrophilia	WBC >15 x 10^9/L
Calcium	<2mmol/L
Renal function	Urea >16mmol/L
Enzymes	LDH >600iu/L; AST >200iu/L
Albumin	<32g/L (serum)
Sugar	Blood glucose >10mmol/L

These criteria have been validated for pancreatitis caused by gallstones and alcohol; Ranson's criteria are valid for alcohol-induced pancreatitis, and can only be fully applied after 48h, which does have its disadvantages. Other criteria for assessing severity include the Acute Physiology and Chronic Health Examination (APACHE)-II, and the Bedside Index for Severity in Acute Pancreatitis (BISAP).

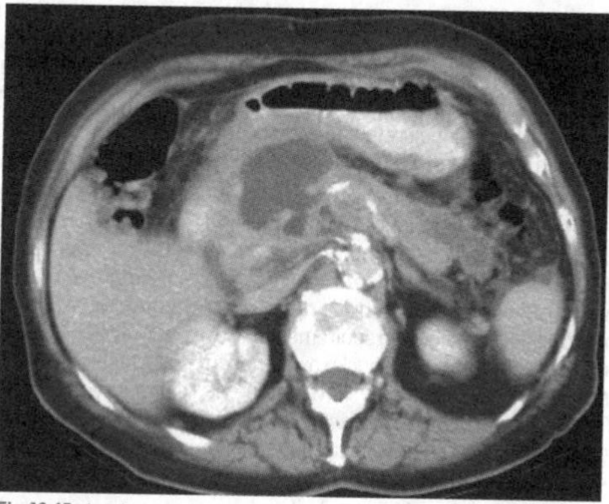

Fig 13.45 Axial CT of the abdomen (with IV and PO contrast media) showing a pancreatic pseudocyst occupying the lesser sac of the abdomen posterior to the stomach. It is called a 'pseudocyst' because it is not a true cyst, rather a collection of fluid in the lesser sac (ie not lined by epi/endothelium). It develops at ≥6wks. The cyst fluid is of low attenuation compared with the stomach contents because it has not been enhanced by the contrast media.

Image courtesy of Dr Stephen Golding.

Urinary tract calculi (nephrolithiasis)

Renal stones (calculi) consist of crystal aggregates. Stones form in collecting ducts and may be deposited anywhere from the renal pelvis to the urethra, though classically at: 1 Pelviureteric junction 2 Pelvic brim 3 Vesicoureteric junction.

Prevalence Common: lifetime incidence up to 15%. *Peak age:* 20–40yr. ♂:♀≈3:1.

Types •Calcium oxalate (75%). •Magnesium ammonium phosphate (struvite/triple phosphate; 15%). •Also: urate (5%), hydroxyapatite (5%), brushite, cystine (1%), mixed.

Presentation Asymptomatic or: 1 *Pain:* Excruciating spasms of renal colic 'loin to groin' (or genitals/inner thigh), with nausea/vomiting. Often cannot lie still (differentiates from peritonitis). *Obstruction of kidney:* felt in the loin, between rib 12 and lateral edge of lumbar muscles (like intercostal nerve irritation pain; the latter is not colicky, and is worsened by specific movements/pressure on a trigger spot). *Obstruction of mid-ureter:* may mimic appendicitis/diverticulitis. *Obstruction of lower ureter:* may lead to symptoms of bladder irritability and pain in scrotum, penile tip, or labia majora. *Obstruction in bladder or urethra:* causes pelvic pain, dysuria, strangury (desire but inability to void) ± interrupted flow. 2 *Infection:* Can coexist (↑risk if voiding impaired), eg UTI; pyelonephritis (fever, rigors, loin pain, nausea, vomiting); pyonephrosis (infected hydronephrosis) 3 *Haematuria.* 4 *Proteinuria.* 5 *Sterile pyuria.* 6 *Anuria.*

Examination Usually no tenderness on palpation. May be renal angle tenderness especially to percussion if there is retroperitoneal inflammation.

Tests FBC, U&E, Ca^{2+}, PO_4^{3-}, glucose, bicarbonate, urate. *Urine dipstick:* Usually +ve for blood (90%). *MSU:* MC&S. *Further tests for cause:* Urine pH; 24h urine for: calcium, oxalate, urate, citrate, sodium, creatinine; stone biochemistry (sieve urine & send stone).

Imaging: Non-contrast CT is investigation of choice for imaging stones (99% visible) & helps exclude differential causes of an acute abdomen. ►A ruptured abdominal aortic aneurysm may present similarly. 80% of stones are visible on KUB XR (kidneys + ureters + bladder). Look along ureters for calcification over the transverse processes of the vertebral bodies. US an alternative for hydronephrosis or hydroureter.

℞ *Initially:* Analgesia, eg diclofenac 75mg IV/IM, or 100mg PR. (If CI: *opioids*) + IV fluids if unable to tolerate PO; antibiotics (eg piperacillin/tazobactam 4.5g/8h IV, or gentamicin) if infection. *Stones <5mm in lower ureter:* ~90–95% pass spontaneously. ↑Fluid intake. *Stones >5mm/pain not resolving: Medical expulsive therapy:* ►start at presentation; nifedipine 10mg/8h PO or α-blockers (tamsulosin 0.4mg/d) promote expulsion and reduce analgesia requirements. Most pass within 48h (>80% after ~30d). If not, try extracorporeal shockwave lithotripsy (ESWL) (if <1cm), or ureteroscopy using a basket. ESWL: US waves shatter stone. SE: renal injury, may also cause ↑BP and DM. *Percutaneous nephrolithotomy (PCNL):* keyhole surgery to remove stones, when large, multiple, or complex. Open surgery is rare.

►*Indications for urgent intervention (delay kills glomeruli):* Presence of infection *and* obstruction—a percutaneous nephrostomy or ureteric stent may be needed to relieve obstruction (p640); urosepsis; intractable pain or vomiting; impending AKI; obstruction in a solitary kidney; bilateral obstructing stones.

Prevention *General:* Drink plenty. *Normal* dietary Ca^{2+} intake (low Ca^{2+} diets increase oxalate excretion). *Specifically:* •*Calcium stones:* in hypercalciuria, a thiazide diuretic is used to ↓Ca^{2+} excretion. •*Oxalate:* ↓oxalate intake; pyridoxine may be used (p295). •*Struvite (phosphate mineral):* treat infection promptly. •*Urate:* allopurinol (100–300mg/24h PO). Urine alkalinization may also help, as urate is more soluble at pH>6 (eg with potassium citrate or sodium bicarbonate). •*Cystine:* vigorous hydration to keep urine output >3L/d and urinary alkalinization (as above-mentioned). Penicillamine is used to chelate cystine, given with pyridoxine to prevent vitamin B_6 deficiency.

Questions to address when confronted by a stone

What is its composition? (See table 13.18.)

Table 13.18 Types, causes, and X-ray appearance of renal stones

Type	Causative factors	Appearance on X-ray
Calcium oxalate (fig 13.46)	Metabolic or idiopathic	Spiky, radio-opaque
Calcium phosphate	Metabolic or idiopathic	Smooth, may be large, radio-opaque
Magnesium ammonium phosphate (fig 13.47)	UTI (proteus causes alkaline urine and calcium precipitation and ammonium salt formation)	Large, horny, 'staghorn', radio-opaque
Urate (p680)	Hyperuricaemia	Smooth, brown, radiolucent
Cystine (fig 13.48)	Renal tubular defect	Yellow, crystalline, semi-opaque

Why has he or she got this stone now?

- *Diet:* chocolate, tea, rhubarb, strawberries, nuts, and spinach all ↑oxalate levels.
- *Season:* variations in calcium and oxalate levels are thought to be mediated by vitamin D synthesis via sunlight on skin.
- *Work:* can he/she drink freely at work? Is there dehydration?
- *Medications:* precipitating drugs include: diuretics, antacids, acetazolamide, corticosteroids, theophylline, aspirin, allopurinol, vitamin C and D, indinavir.

Are there any predisposing factors? For example:

- *Recurrent UTIs* (in magnesium ammonium phosphate calculi).
- *Metabolic abnormalities:*
  - Hypercalciuria/hypercalcaemia (p676): hyperparathyroidism, neoplasia, sarcoidosis, hyperthyroidism, Addison's, Cushing's, lithium, vitamin D excess.
  - Hyperuricosuria/↑plasma urate: on its own, or with gout.
  - Hyperoxaluria.
  - Cystinuria (p321).
  - Renal tubular acidosis (pp316-7).
- *Urinary tract abnormalities:* eg pelviureteric junction obstruction, hydronephrosis (renal pelvis or calyces), calyceal diverticulum, horseshoe kidney, ureterocele, vesicoureteric reflux, ureteral stricture, medullary sponge kidney.[11]
- *Foreign bodies:* eg stents, catheters.

Is there a family history? ↑Risk of stones 3-fold. Specific diseases include X-linked nephrolithiasis and Dent's disease (proteinuria, hypercalciuria, and nephrocalcinosis).

►*Is there infection above the stone?* Eg fever, loin tender, pyuria? This needs urgent intervention.

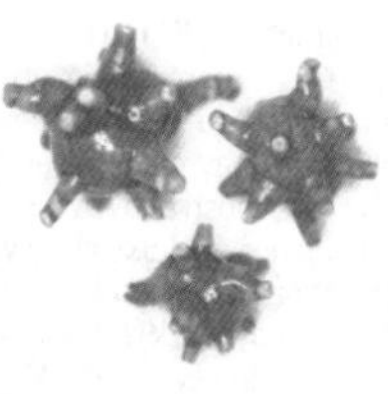

Fig 13.46 Calcium oxalate monohydrate.
Image courtesy of Dr Glen Austin.

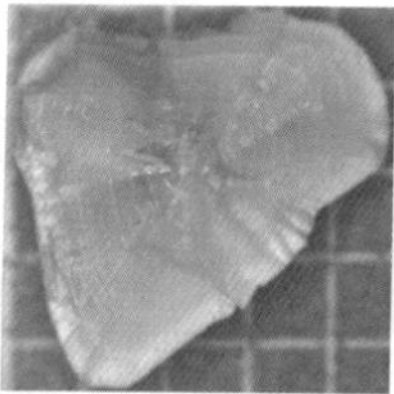

Fig 13.47 Struvite stone.
Image courtesy of Dr Glen Austin.

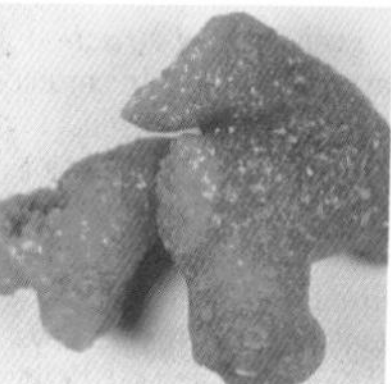

Fig 13.48 Cystine stone.
Image courtesy of Dr Glen Austin.

11 Medullary sponge kidney is a typically asymptomatic developmental anomaly of the kidney mostly seen in adult females, where there is dilatation of the collecting ducts, which if severe leads to a sponge-like appearance of the renal medulla. *Complications/associations:* UTIs, nephrolithiasis, haematuria and hypercalciuria, hyperparathyroidism (if present, look for genetic markers of MEN type 2A, see p223).

Urinary tract obstruction

►Urinary tract obstruction is common and should be considered in any patient with impaired renal function. ►►Damage can be permanent if the obstruction is not treated promptly. Obstruction may occur anywhere from the renal calyces to the urethral meatus, and may be *partial* or *complete, unilateral* or *bilateral*. Obstructing lesions are *luminal* (stones, blood clot, sloughed papilla, tumour: renal, ureteric, or bladder), *mural* (eg congenital or acquired stricture, neuromuscular dysfunction, schistosomiasis), or *extra-mural* (abdominal or pelvic mass/tumour, retroperitoneal fibrosis, or iatrogenic—eg post surgery). Unilateral obstruction may be clinically silent (normal urine output and U&E) if the other kidney is functioning. ►Bilateral obstruction or obstruction with infection requires urgent treatment. See p641.

Clinical features

- *Acute upper tract obstruction:* Loin pain radiating to the groin. There may be superimposed infection ± loin tenderness, or an enlarged kidney.
- *Chronic upper tract obstruction:* Flank pain, renal failure, superimposed infection. Polyuria may occur due to impaired urinary concentration.
- *Acute lower tract obstruction:* Acute urinary retention typically presents with severe suprapubic pain ± acute confusion (elderly); often acute on chronic (hence preceded by chronic symptoms , see next bullet point). Clinically: distended, palpable bladder containing ~600mL, dull to percussion. Causes include prostatic obstruction (usual cause in older ♂), urethral strictures, anticholinergics, blood clots eg from bladder lesion ('clot retention'), alcohol, constipation, post-op (pain/inflammation/anaesthetics), infection (p296), neurological (cauda equina syndrome, see p466).
- *Chronic lower tract obstruction: Symptoms:* urinary frequency, hesitancy, poor stream, terminal dribbling, overflow incontinence. *Signs:* distended, palpable bladder (capacity may be >1.5L) ± large prostate on PR. Complications: UTI, urinary retention, renal failure (eg bilateral obstructive uropathy—see BOX 'Obstructive uropathy'). Causes include prostatic enlargement (common); pelvic malignancy; rectal surgery; DM; CNS disease, eg transverse myelitis/MS; zoster (S2–S4).

Tests *Blood:* U&E, creatinine, FBC, and prostate-specific antigen (PSA, p530).[12] *Urine:* Dipstick and MC&S. *Ultrasound* (p744) is the imaging modality of choice for investigating upper tract obstruction: If there is hydronephrosis or hydroureter (distension of the renal pelvis and calyces or ureter), arrange a *CT scan.* This will determine the level of obstuction. NB: in ~5% of cases of obstruction, no distension is seen on US. *Radionuclide imaging* enables functional assessment of the kidneys.

Treatment *Upper tract obstruction:* Nephrostomy or ureteric stent. NB: stents may cause significant discomfort and patients should be warned of this and other risks (see BOX 'Problems of ureteric stenting'). α-blockers help reduce stent-related pain (↓ureteric spasm). Pyeloplasty, to widen the PUJ, may be performed for idiopathic PUJ obstruction.

Lower tract obstruction: Insert a urethral or suprapubic catheter (p762) to relieve acute retention. In chronic obstruction only catheterize patient if there is pain, urinary infection, or renal impairment; intermittent self-catheterization is sometimes required (p763). If in clot retention the patient will require a 3-way catheter and bladder washout. If >1L residual check U&E and monitor for post-obstructive diuresis (see BOX 'Obstructive uropathy'). Monitor weight, fluid balance, and U&E closely. Treat the underlying cause if possible, eg if prostatic obstruction, start an α-blocker (see p642). After 2–3 days, trial without catheter (TWOC, p763) may work (especially if <75yrs old and <1L drained or retention was triggered by a passing event, eg GA).

12 Do venepuncture for PSA **before** PR, as PR can ↑ total PSA by ~1ng/mL (free PSA ↑ by 10%). It's difficult to know if acute retention raises PSA, but relieving obstruction does cause it to drop.

Problems of ureteric stenting (depend on site)

Common:
- Stent-related pain
- Trigonal irritation
- Haematuria
- Fever
- Infection
- Tissue inflammation
- Encrustation
- Biofilm formation.

Rare:
- Obstruction
- Kinking
- Ureteric rupture
- Stent misplacement
- Stent migration (especially if made of silicone)
- Tissue hyperplasia
- Forgotton stents.

Obstructive uropathy

In chronic urinary retention, an episode of *acute* retention may go unnoticed for days and, because of their background symptoms, may only present when overflow incontinence becomes a nuisance—pain is not necessarily a feature. After diagnosing acute on chronic retention and placing a catheter, the bladder residual can be as much as 1.5L of urine. Don't be surprised to be called by the biochemistry lab to be told that the serum creatinine is 1000μmol/L! The good news is that renal function usually returns to baseline after a few days (there may be mild background impairment). Ask for an urgent renal us (fig 13.49) and consider the following in the acute plan to ensure a safe course:

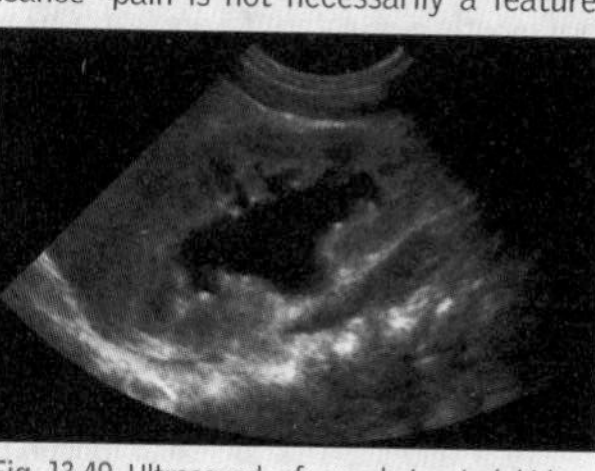

Fig 13.49 Ultrasound of an obstructed kidney showing hydronephrosis. Note dilatation of renal pelvis and ureter, and clubbed calyces.

Image courtesy of Norwich Radiology Department.

- **Hyperkalaemia** See p301.
- **Metabolic acidosis** On ABG there is likely to be a respiratory compensated metabolic acidosis. Concerns should prompt discussion with a renal specialist (a good idea anyway), in case haemodialysis is required (p306).
- **Post-obstructive diuresis** In the acute phase after relief of the obstruction, the kidneys produce *a lot* of urine—as much as a litre in the first hour. It is vital to provide resuscitation fluids and then match input with output. ►Fluid depletion rather than overload is the danger here.
- **Sodium- and bicarbonate-losing nephropathy** As the kidney undergoes diuresis, Na^+ and bicarbonate are lost in the urine in large quantities. Replace 'in for out' (as mentioned above) with isotonic 1.26% sodium bicarbonate solution—this should be available from ITU. Some advocate using 0.9% saline, though the chloride load may exacerbate acidosis. Withhold any nephrotoxic drugs.
- **Infection** Treat infection, bearing in mind that the ↑WCC and ↑CRP may be part of the stress response. Send a sample of urine for MC&S.

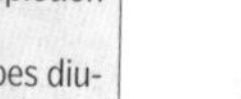

Benign prostatic hyperplasia

Benign prostatic hyperplasia (BPH) is common (24% if aged 40–64; 40% if older). *Pathology:* Benign nodular or diffuse proliferation of musculofibrous and glandular layers of the prostate. Inner (transitional) zone enlarges in contrast to peripheral layer expansion seen in prostate carcinoma. *Features: Lower urinary tract symptoms* (LUTS) = nocturia, frequency, urgency, post-micturition dribbling, poor stream/flow, hesitancy, overflow incontinence, haematuria, bladder stones, UTI. *Management:* Assess severity of symptoms and impact on life. PR exam. *Tests:* MSU; U&E; ultrasound (large residual volume, hydronephrosis—fig 13.49), PSA (prior to PR exam; see also BOX 'Advice to asymptomatic men', p645), transrectal US ± biopsy. Then consider:

- *Lifestyle:* Avoid caffeine, alcohol (to ↓urgency/nocturia). Relax when voiding. Void twice in a row to aid emptying. Control urgency by practising distraction methods (eg breathing exercises). Train the bladder by 'holding on' to ↑time between voiding.
- *Drugs* are useful in mild disease, and while awaiting surgery. • *α-blockers* are 1st line (eg tamsulosin 400mcg/d PO; also alfuzosin, doxazosin, terazosin). ↓Smooth muscle tone (prostate and bladder). SE: drowsiness; depression; dizziness; ↓BP; dry mouth; ejaculatory failure; extra-pyramidal signs; nasal congestion; ↑weight. • *5α-reductase inhibitors:* can be added, or used alone, eg finasteride 5mg/d PO (↓conversion of testosterone to the more potent androgen dihydrotestosterone). Excreted in semen, so use condoms; females should avoid handling. SE: impotence; ↓libido. ↓prostate size over 3–6mths and ↓ long-term retention risk.
- *Surgery:*
  - *Transurethral resection of prostate* (TURP) ≤14% become impotent (see BOX). Crossmatch 2U. Beware bleeding, clot retention, and post TURP syndrome: absorption of washout causing CNS & CVS disturbance. ~12% need redoing within 8yrs.
  - *Transurethral incision of the prostate* (TUIP) involves less destruction than TURP, and less risk to sexual function, gives similar benefit. Relieves pressure on the urethra. Maybe best surgical option for those with small glands <30g.
  - *Retropubic prostatectomy* is an open operation (if prostate very large).
  - *Transurethral laser-induced prostatectomy* (TULIP) may be as good as TURP.
  - *Robotic prostatectomy* is gaining popularity as a less traumatic and minimally invasive treatment option.

Advice for patients concerning transurethral prostatectomy (TURP)

Pre-op consent issues may centre on risks of the procedure, eg:

- Haematuria/haemorrhage
- Haematospermia
- Hypothermia
- Urethral trauma/stricture
- Post TURP syndrome (↓T°; ↓Na^+)
- Infection; prostatitis
- Erectile dysfunction ~10%
- Incontinence ≤10%
- Clot retention near strictures
- Retrograde ejaculation (common).

Post-operative advice

- Avoid driving for 2wks after the operation.
- Avoid sex for 2wks after surgery. Then get back to normal. The amount ejaculated may be reduced (as it flows backwards into the bladder—harmless, but may cloud the urine). It means you may be infertile. Erections may be a problem after TURP, but do not expect this: in some men, erections improve. Rarely, orgasmic sensations are reduced.
- Expect to pass blood in the urine for the first 2wks. A small amount of blood colours the urine bright red. Do not be alarmed.
- At first you may need to urinate *more* frequently than before. Do not be despondent. In 6wks things should be much better—but the operation cannot be guaranteed to work (8% fail, and lasting incontinence is a problem in 6%; 12% may need repeat TURPs within 8yrs, compared with 1.8% of men undergoing open prostatectomy).
- If feverish, or if urination hurts, take a sample of urine to your doctor.

Retroperitoneal fibrosis

Causes Idiopathic retroperitoneal fibrosis (RPF), inflammatory aneurysms of the abdominal aorta, and perianeurysmal RPF. With idiopathic RPF there is an associated inflammatory response resulting in fibrinoid necrosis of the vasa vasorum, affecting the aorta and small and medium retroperitoneal vessels. The ureters get embedded in dense, fibrous tissue resulting in progressive bilateral ureteric obstruction. Secondary causes of RPF include malignancy, typically lymphoma.

Associations Drugs (eg β-blockers, bromocriptine, methysergide, methyldopa), autoimmune disease (eg thyroiditis, SLE, ANCA+ve vasculitis), smoking, asbestos.

Typical patient Middle-aged ♂ with vague loin, back, or abdominal pain, ↑BP.

Tests *Blood:* ↑Urea and creatinine; ↑ESR; ↑CRP; anaemia. *Ultrasound:* Dilated ureters (hydronephrosis). *CT/MRI:* Periaortic mass (fig 13.50). Biopsy under imaging guidance is used to rule out malignancy.

Treatment Retrograde stent placement to relieve obstruction (removed after 12 months) ± ureterolysis (dissection of the ureters from the retroperitoneal tissue). Immunosuppression (in idiopathic RPF) with low-dose steroids has good long-term results.

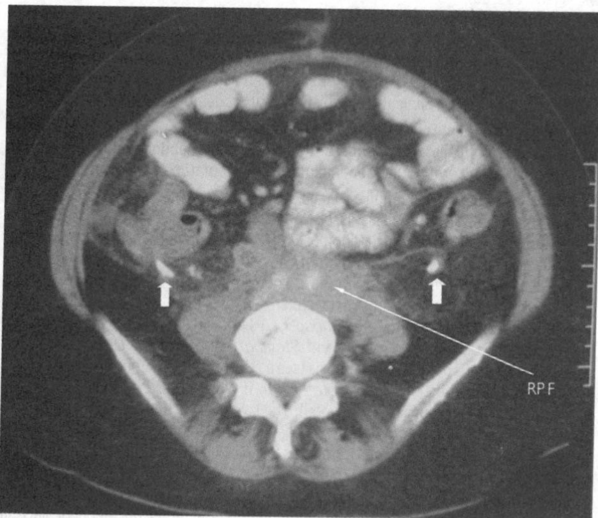

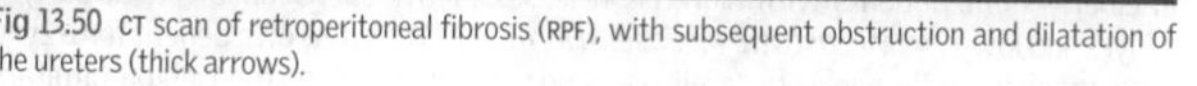

Fig 13.50 CT scan of retroperitoneal fibrosis (RPF), with subsequent obstruction and dilatation of the ureters (thick arrows).

Urinary tract malignancies

Renal cell carcinoma (RCC) arises from proximal renal tubular epithelium. *Epidemiology:* Accounts for 90% of renal cancers; mean age 55yrs. ♂:♀≈2:1. 15% of haemodialysis patients develop RCC. *Features:* 50% found incidentally. Haematuria, loin pain, abdominal mass, anorexia, malaise, weight loss, PUO—often in isolation. Rarely, invasion of left renal vein compresses left testicular vein causing a varicocele. Spread may be direct (renal vein), via lymph, or haematogenous (bone, liver, lung). 25% have metastases at presentation. *Tests:* BP: ↑from renin secretion. *Blood:* FBC (polycythaemia from erythropoietin secretion); ESR; U&E, ALP (bony mets?). *Urine:* RBCs; cytology. *Imaging:* US (p744); CT/MRI; CXR ('cannon ball' metastases). ℞: Radical nephrectomy (nephron-sparing surgery is as good for T1 tumours + preserves renal function). Cryotherapy and radiofrequency ablation is an option for patients unfit or unwilling to undergo surgery. RCC is generally radio- & chemoresistant. In those with unresectable or metastatic disease, options include: high-dose IL-2 and other T-cell activation therapies; anti-angiogenesis agents (eg pazopanib, sunitinib, axitinib, or bevacizumab); mTOR inhibitors, eg temsirolimus. The *Mayo prognostic risk score (SSIGN)* was developed to predict survival and uses information on tumour stage, size, grade, and necrosis. *Prognosis:* 10yr survival ranges from 96.5% (scores 0–1) to 19.2% (scores ≥ 10).

Transitional cell carcinoma (TCC) may arise in the bladder (50%), ureter, or renal pelvis. *Epidemiology:* Age >40yrs; ♂:♀≈4:1. *Risk factors:* p646. *Presentation:* Painless haematuria; frequency; urgency; dysuria; urinary tract obstruction. *Diagnosis:* Urine cytology; IVU; cystoscopy + biopsy; CT/MRI. ℞: See 'Bladder tumours', p646. *Prognosis:* Varies with clinical stage/histological grade: 10–80% 5yr survival.

Wilms' tumour (nephroblastoma) is a childhood tumour of primitive renal tubules and mesenchymal cells. *Prevalence:* 1:100 000—the chief abdominal malignancy in children. It presents with an abdominal mass and haematuria. ℞: *OHCS* p133.

Prostate cancer The commonest male malignancy. *Incidence:* ↑with age: 80% in men >80yrs (autopsy studies). *Associations:* +ve family history (x2–3 ↑risk, p521), ↑testosterone. Most are adenocarcinomas arising in peripheral prostate. Spread may be local (seminal vesicles, bladder, rectum) via lymph, or haematogenously (sclerotic bony lesions). *Symptoms:* Asymptomatic or nocturia, hesitancy, poor stream, terminal dribbling, or obstruction. ↓Weight ± bone pain suggests mets. *DRE exam of prostate:* may show hard, irregular prostate. *Diagnosis:* ↑PSA (normal in 30% of small cancers); transrectal US & biopsy; bone scan; CT/MRI. *Staging:* MRI. *Treatment: Disease confined to prostate:* options depend on prognosis (see BOX 'Prognostic factors'), patient preference, and comorbidities. •*Radical prostatectomy* if <70yrs gives excellent disease-free survival (laparoscopic surgery is as good). The role of adjuvant hormonal therapy is being explored. •*Radical radiotherapy* (± neoadjuvant & adjuvant hormonal therapy) is an alternative curative option that compares favourably with surgery (no RCTs). It may be delivered as external beam or brachytherapy. •*Hormone therapy alone* temporarily delays tumour progression but refractory disease eventually develops. Consider in elderly, unfit patients with high-risk disease. •*Active surveillance*—particularly if >70yrs and low-risk. *Metastatic disease:* •*Hormonal drugs* may give benefit for 1–2yrs. LHRH agonists, eg 12-weekly goserelin (10.8mg SC) first stimulate, then inhibit pituitary gonadotrophin. NB: risks tumour 'flare' when first used—start anti-androgen, eg cyproterone acetate, in susceptible patients. The LHRH antagonist degarelix is also used in advanced disease. *Symptomatic ℞:* Analgesia; treat hypercalcaemia; radiotherapy for bone mets/spinal cord compression. *Prognosis:* 10% die in 6 months, 10% live >10yrs. *Screening:* DRE of prostate; transrectal US; PSA (see BOX 'Advice to asymptomatic men').

Penile cancer *Epidemiology:* Rare in UK, more common in Far East and Africa, very rare in circumcised. Related to chronic irritation, viruses, smegma. *Presentation:* Chronic fungating ulcer, bloody/purulent discharge, 50% spread to lymph at presentation ℞: Radiotherapy & irridium wires if early; amputation & lymph node dissection if late.

Advice to asymptomatic men asking for a PSA blood test

- Many men over 50 consider a PSA test to detect prostatic cancer. *Is this wise?*
- The test is not very accurate, and we cannot say that those having the test will live longer—even if they turn out to have prostate cancer. Most men with prostate cancer die from an unrelated cause.
- If the test is falsely positive, you may needlessly have more tests, eg prostate sampling via the back passage (causes bleeding and infection in 1-5% of men).
- Only one in three of those with a high PSA level will have cancer.
- You may be worried needlessly if later tests put you in the clear.
- If a cancer is found, there's no way to tell *for sure* if it will impinge on health. You might end up having a bad effect from treatment that wasn't needed.
- There is much uncertainty on treating those who *do* turn out to have prostate cancer: options are radical surgery to remove the prostate (risks erectile dysfunction and incontinence), radiotherapy, or hormones.
- Screening via PSA has shown conflicting results. Some RCTs have shown no difference in the rate of death from prostate cancer, others have found reduced mortality, eg 1 death prevented per 1055 men invited for screening (if 37 cancers detected).

►Ultimately, you must decide for yourself what you want.

Prognostic factors in prostate cancer

A number of prognostic factors help determine if 'watchful waiting' or aggressive therapy should be advised: •Pre-treatment PSA level. •Tumour stage (as measured by the TNM system; p523). •Tumour grade—Gleason score. Gleason grading is from 1 to 5, with 5 being the highest grade, and carrying the poorest prognosis. Gleason grades are decided by analysing histology from two separate areas of tumour specimen, and adding them to get the total Gleason score for the tumour, from 2 to 10. Scores 8-10 suggest an aggressive tumour; 5-7: intermediate; 2-4: indolent.

Benign diseases of the penis

Balanitis Acute inflammation of the foreskin and glans. Associated with strep and staph infections. More common in diabetics. Often seen in young children with tight foreskins *Rx:* Antibiotics, circumcision, hygiene advice.

Phimosis The foreskin occludes the meatus. In young boys this causes recurrent balanitis and ballooning, but time (+ trials of gentle retraction) may obviate the need for circumcision. In adulthood presents with painful intercourse, infection, ulceration, and is associated with balanitis xerotica obliterans.

Paraphimosis Occurs when a tight foreskin is retracted and becomes irreplaceable, preventing venous return leading to oedema and even ischaemia of the glans. Can occur if the foreskin is not replaced after catheterization. ►►*Rx:* Ask patient to squeeze glans. Try applying a 50% glucose-soaked swab (oedema may follow osmotic gradient). Ice packs and lidocaine gel may also help. May require aspiration/dorsal slit/circumcision.

Prostatitis

May be acute or chronic. Usually those >35yrs. *Acute prostatitis* is caused mostly by *S. faecalis* and *E. coli*, also *Chlamydia* (and previously TB). *Features:* UTIs, retention, pain, haematospermia, swollen/boggy prostate on DRE. *Rx:* Analgesia; levofloxacin 500mg/24h PO for 28d. *Chronic prostatitis* may be bacterial or non-bacterial. Symptoms as for acute prostatitis, but present for >3 months. Non-bacterial chronic prostatitis does not respond to antibiotics. Anti-inflammatory drugs, α-blockers, and prostatic massage all have a place.

Bladder tumours

>90% are transitional cell carcinomas (TCCs) in the UK. Adenocarcinomas and squamous cell carcinomas are rare in the West (the latter may follow schistosomiasis). UK incidence ≈ 1:6000/yr. ♂:♀≈5:2. Histology is important for prognosis: *Grade 1*—differentiated; *Grade 2*—intermediate; *Grade 3*—poorly differentiated. 80% are confined to bladder mucosa, and only ~20% penetrate muscle (increasing mortality to 50% at 5yrs).

Presentation Painless haematuria; recurrent UTIs; voiding irritability.

Associations Smoking; aromatic amines (rubber industry); chronic cystitis; schistosomiasis (↑risk of squamous cell carcinoma); pelvic irradiation.

Tests

- Cystoscopy with biopsy is diagnostic.
- Urine: microscopy/cytology (cancers may cause sterile pyuria).
- CT urogram is both diagnostic and provides staging.
- Bimanual EUA helps assess spread.
- MRI or lymphangiography may show involved pelvic nodes.

Surgery

Staging See table 13.19.

Treating TCC of the bladder

- *Tis/Ta/T1:* (80% of all patients) Diathermy via transurethral cystoscopy/transurethral resection of bladder tumour (TURBT). Consider a regimen of intravesical *BCG* (which stimulates a non-specific immune response) for multiple small tumours or high-grade tumours. Alternative chemotherapeutic agents include mitomycin, epirubicin and gemcitabine. 5yr survival ≈ 95%.
- *T2–3:* Radical cystectomy is the 'gold standard'. Radiotherapy gives worse 5yr survival rates than surgery, but preserves the bladder. 'Salvage' cystectomy can be performed if radiotherapy fails, but yields worse results than primary surgery. Post-op chemotherapy (eg M-VAC: methotrexate, vinblastine, doxorubicin, and cisplatin) is toxic but effective. Neoadjuvant chemotherapy with M-VAC or GC (gemcitabine and cisplatin) has improved survival compared to cystectomy or radiotherapy alone. Methods to preserve the bladder with transurethral resection or partial cystectomy + systemic chemotherapy have been tried, but long-term results are disappointing. If the bladder neck is not involved, orthotopic reconstruction rather than forming a urostoma is an option (both using ~40cm of the patient's ileum), but adequate tumour clearance must not be compromised. ►The patient should have all these options explained by a urologist and an oncologist.
- *T4:* Usually palliative chemo/radiotherapy. Chronic catheterization and urinary diversions may help to relieve pain.

Follow-up History, examination, and regular cystoscopy: •*High-risk tumours:* Every 3 months for 2yrs, then every 6 months. •*Low-risk tumours:* First follow-up cystoscopy after 9 months, then yearly.

Tumour spread Local → to pelvic structures; lymphatic → to iliac and para-aortic nodes; haematogenous → to liver and lungs.

Survival This depends on age at surgery. For example, the 3yr survival after cystectomy for T2 and T3 tumours is 60% if 65–75yrs old, falling to 40% if 75–82yrs old (operative mortality is 4%). With unilateral pelvic node involvement, only 6% of patients survive 5yrs. The 3yr survival with bilateral or para-aortic node involvement is nil.

Complications Cystectomy can result in sexual and urinary malfunction. Massive bladder haemorrhage may complicate treatment or be a feature of disease treated palliatively. Determining the cause of bleeding is key. Consider alum solution bladder irrigation (if no renal failure) as 1st-line treatment for intractable haematuria in advanced malignancy: it is an inpatient procedure.

Table 13.19 TNM staging of bladder cancer (See also p523)

Tis	Carcinoma *in situ*
Ta	Tumour confined to epithelium
T1	Tumour in submucosa or lamina propria
T2	Invades muscle
T3	Extends into perivesical fat
T4	Invades adjacent organs
N0	No LN involved
N1–N3	Progressive LN involvement
M0	No metastases
M1	Distant metastasis

Reproduced with permission from Edge, SB *et al.* (Eds.), *AJCC Cancer Staging Manual*, 7th Edition. New York: Springer; 2010.

Is asymptomatic non-visible haematuria significant?

Dipstick tests are often done routinely for patients on admission. If non-visible (previously microscopic) haematuria is found, but the patient has no related symptoms, what does this mean? Before rushing into a barrage of investigations, consider:

- One study found that incidence of urogenital disease (eg bladder cancer) was no higher in those with asymptomatic microhaematuria than in those without.
- Asymptomatic non-visible haematuria is the sole presenting feature in only 4% of bladder cancers, and there is no evidence that these are less advanced than malignancies presenting with macroscopic haematuria.
- When monitoring those with treated bladder cancer for recurrence, non-visible-haematuria tests have a sensitivity of only 31% in those with superficial bladder malignancy, in whom detection would be most useful.
- Although 80% of those with flank pain due to a renal stone have microscopic haematuria, so do 50% of those with flank pain but no stone.

The conclusion is not that urine dipstick testing is useless, but that results should not be interpreted in isolation. ►Unexplained non-visible haematuria in those >50yrs should be referred under the 2-week rule. Smokers and those with +ve family history for urothelial cancer may also be investigated differently from those with no risk factors. It is worth considering, that in a young, fit athlete, the diagnosis is more likely to be exercise-induced haematuria. Wise doctors work collaboratively with their patients. 'Shall we let sleeping dogs lie?' is a reasonable question for *some* patients.

Urinary incontinence

►Think twice before inserting a urinary catheter.
►Carry out rectal examination to exclude faecal impaction.
►Is the bladder palpable after voiding (retention with overflow)?
►Is there neurological comorbidity: eg MS; Parkinson's disease; stroke; spinal trauma?

Incontinence in men Enlargement of the prostate is the major cause of incontinence: urge incontinence (see later in topic) or dribbling may result from partial retention of urine. TURP (p642) & other pelvic surgery may weaken the bladder sphincter and cause incontinence. Troublesome incontinence needs specialist assessment.

Incontinence in women Often under-reported with delays before seeking help.

- *Functional incontinence:* Ie when physiological factors are relatively unimportant. The patient is 'caught short' and too slow in finding the toilet because of (for example) immobility, or unfamiliar surroundings.
- *Stress incontinence:* Leakage from an incompetent sphincter, eg when intra-abdominal pressure rises (eg coughing, laughing). Increasing age and obesity are risk factors. The key to diagnosis is the loss of small (but often frequent) amounts of urine when coughing etc. Examine for pelvic floor weakness/prolapse/pelvic masses. Look for cough leak on standing and with full bladder. Stress incontinence is common in pregnancy and following birth. It occurs to some degree in ~50% of post-menopausal women. In elderly women, pelvic floor weakness, eg with uterine prolapse or urethrocele (*OHCS* p290), is a very common association.
- *Urge incontinence/overactive bladder syndrome:* The urge to urinate is quickly followed by uncontrollable and sometimes complete emptying of the bladder as the detrusor muscle contracts. Urgency/leaking is precipitated by: arriving home (latchkey incontinence, a conditioned reflex); cold; the sound of running water; caffeine; and obesity. *Δ:* urodynamic studies. *Cause:* detrusor overactivity (see table 13.20), eg from central inhibitory pathway malfunction or sensitization of peripheral afferent terminals in the bladder; or a bladder muscle problem. Check for organic brain damage (eg stroke; Parkinson's; dementia). *Other causes:* urinary infection; diabetes; diuretics; atrophic vaginitis; urethritis.

In both sexes incontinence may result from confusion or sedation. Occasionally it may be purposeful (eg preventing admission to an old people's home) or due to anger.

Management ►Effective treatment can have a huge impact on quality of life.

Check for: UTI; DM; diuretic use; faecal impaction; palpable bladder; GFR.

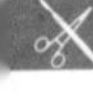

- *Stress incontinence:* Pelvic floor exercises are 1st line (8 contractions ×3/d for 3 months). Intravaginal electrical stimulation may also be effective, but is not acceptable to many women. A ring pessary may help uterine prolapse, eg while awaiting surgical repair. *Surgical options* (eg tension-free vaginal tape) aim to stabilize the mid-urethra. Urethral bulking also available. Medical options: duloxetine 40mg/12h PO (50% have ≥50% ↓ in incontinence episodes). SE = nausea.
- *Urge incontinence:* The patient (or carer) should complete an 'incontinence' chart for 3d to define the pattern of incontinence. Examine for spinal cord and CNS signs (including cognitive test, p64); and for vaginitis (if postmenopausal). Vaginitis can be treated with topical oestrogen therapy for a limited period. Bladder training (may include pelvic floor exercises) and weight loss are important. Drugs may help reduce night-time incontinence (see BOX) but can be disappointing. Consider aids eg absorbent pad. If ♂ consider a condom catheter.

►Do urodynamic assessment (cystometry & urine flow rate measurement) before any surgical intervention to exclude detrusor overactivity or sphincter dyssynergia.

Table 13.20 Managing detrusor overactivity in urge incontinence

Agents for detrusor overactivity	Notes
Antimuscarinics: eg tolterodine *SR* 4mg/24h; SE: dry mouth, eyes/skin, drowsiness, constipation, tachycardia, abdominal pain, urinary retention, sinusitis, oedema, ↑weight, glaucoma precipitation. Up to 4mg/12h may be needed (unlicensed).	Improves frequency & urgency. Alternatives: solifenacin 5mg/24h (max 10mg); oxybutynin, but more SE unless transdermal route or modified release used; trospium or fesoterodine (prefers M3 receptors). Avoid in myasthenia, and if glaucoma or UC are uncontrolled.
Topical oestrogens	Post-menopausal urgency, frequency + nocturia may occasionally be improved by raising the bladder's sensory threshold. Systemic therapy worsens incontinence.
β3 adrenergic agonist: mirabegron 50mg/24h; SE tachycardia; CI: severe HTN; Caution if renal/hepatic impairment.	Consider if antimuscarinics are contraindicated or clinically ineffective, or if SE unacceptable.
Intravesical botulinum toxin (Botox®)	Consider if above medications ineffective.
Percutaneous posterior tibial nerve stimulation (PTNS). (A typical treatment consists of ×12 weekly 30 min sessions.)	Consider if drug treatment ineffective and Botox® not wanted. PTNS delivers neuromodulation to the S2–S4 junction of the sacral nerve plexus.
Neuromodulation via transcutaneous electrical stimulation	Sacral nerve stimulation inhibits the reflex behaviour of involuntary detrusor contractions.
Modulation of afferent input from bladder	Gabapentin (unlicensed).
Hypnosis, psychotherapy, bladder training*	(These all require good motivation.)
Surgery (eg clam ileocystoplasty)	Reserved for troublesome or intractable symptoms. The bladder is bisected, opened like a clam, and 25cm of ileum is sewn in.

NB: desmopressin nasal spray 20mcg nocte reduces urine production and ∴ nocturia in overactive bladder. Unsuitable if elderly (SE: fluid retention, heart failure, ↓Na^+).

*Mind over bladder: •Void when you DON'T have urge; DON'T go to the bathroom when you do have urge. •Gradually extend the time between voiding. •Schedule your trips to toilet. •Stretch your bladder to normal capacity. • When urge comes, calm down and make it go using mind over bladder tricks.

Not all male urinary symptoms are prostate-related!

Detrusor overactivity Men get this as well as women. Pressure-flow studies help diagnose this (as does detrusor thickness ≥2.9mm on US).

Primary bladder neck obstruction A condition in which the bladder neck does not open properly during voiding. Studies in men and women with voiding dysfunction show that it is common. The cause may be muscular or neurological dysfunction or fibrosis. *Diagnosis:* Video-urodynamics, with simultaneous pressure-flow measurement, and visualization of the bladder neck during voiding. *Treatment:* Watchful waiting; α-blockers (p642); surgery.

Urethral stricture This may follow trauma or infection (eg gonorrhoea)—and frequently leads to voiding symptoms, UTI, or retention. Malignancy is a rare cause. *Imaging:* Retrograde urethrogram or antegrade cystourethrogram if the patient has an existing suprapubic catheter. ***Internal urethrotomy*** involves incising the stricture transurethrally using endoscopic equipment—to release scar tissue. *Stents* incorporate themselves into the wall of the urethra and keep the lumen open. They work best for short strictures in the bulbar urethra (anterior urethral anatomy, from proximal to distal: prostatic urethra→posterior or membranous urethra→bulbar urethra→penile or pendulous urethra→fossa navicularis→meatus).

Lumps in the groin and scrotum

►Testicular lump = cancer until proved otherwise.
►Acute, tender enlargement of testis = torsion (p652) until proved otherwise.

Diagnosing scrotal masses (fig 13.51)

1 *Can you get above it?* 2 *Is it separate from the testis?* 3 *Cystic or solid?*

- Cannot get above: inguinoscrotal hernia (p614) or hydrocele extending proximally.
- Separate and cystic: epididymal cyst.
- Separate and solid: epididymitis/varicocele.
- Testicular and cystic: hydrocele.

►Testicular and solid—*tumour*, haematocele, granuloma (p196), orchitis, gumma (p412). US may help.

Epididymal cysts Usually develop in adulthood and contain clear or milky (spermatocele) fluid. They lie above and behind the testis. Remove if symptomatic.

Hydroceles (Fluid within the tunica vaginalis.) *Primary* (associated with a patent processus vaginalis, which typically resolves during the 1st year of life) or *secondary* to testis tumour/trauma/infection. Primary hydroceles are more common, larger, and usually in younger men. Can resolve spontaneously. *℞:* Aspiration (may need repeating) or surgery: plicating the tunica vaginalis (Lord's repair)/inverting the sac (Jaboulay's repair). ►Is the testis normal after aspiration? If any doubt, do US.

Epididymo-orchitis *Causes: Chlamydia* (eg if <35yrs); *E. coli*; mumps; *N. gonorrhoeae*; TB. *Features:* Sudden-onset tender swelling, dysuria, sweats/fever. Take '1st catch' urine sample; look for urethral discharge. Consider STI screen. Warn of possible infertility and symptoms worsening before improving. *℞:* If <35yrs; doxycycline 100mg/12h (covers chlamydia; treat sexual partners). If gonorrhoea suspected add ceftriaxone 500mg IM stat. If >35yrs (mostly non-STI), associated UTI is common so try ciprofloxacin 500mg/12h or ofloxacin 200mg/12h. Antibiotics should be used for 2-4wks. Also: analgesia, scrotal support, drainage of any abscess.

Varicocele Dilated veins of pampiniform plexus. Left side more commonly affected. Often visible as distended scrotal blood vessels that feel like 'a bag of worms'. Patient may complain of dull ache. Associated with subfertility, but repair (via surgery or embolization) seems to have little effect on subsequent pregnancy rates.

Haematocele Blood in tunica vaginalis, follows trauma, may need drainage/excision.

Testicular tumours The commonest malignancy in ♂ aged 15–44; 10% occur in undescended testes, even after orchidopexy. A contralateral tumour is found in 5%. *Types:* Seminoma, 55% (30–65yrs); non-seminomatous germ cell tumour, 33% (NSGCT; previously teratoma; 20–30yrs); mixed germ cell tumour, 12%; lymphoma.

Signs: Typically painless testis lump, found after trauma/infection ± haemospermia, secondary hydrocele, pain, dyspnoea (lung mets), abdominal mass (enlarged nodes), or effects of secreted hormones. 25% of seminomas & 50% of NSGCTs present with metastases. *Risk factors:* Undescended testis; infant hernia; infertility.

Staging: **1** No evidence of metastasis. **2** Infradiaphragmatic node involvement (spread via the para-aortic nodes *not* inguinal nodes). **3** Supradiaphragmatic node involvement. **4** Lung involvement (haematogenous).

Tests: (Allow staging.) CXR, CT, excision biopsy. α-FP (eg >3IU/mL)[13] and β-hCG are useful tumour markers and help monitor treatment (p531); check *before & during* ℞.

℞: Radical orchidectomy (inguinal incision; occlude the spermatic cord before mobilization to ↓risk of intra-operative spread). Options are constantly updated (surgery, radiotherapy, chemotherapy). Seminomas are exquisitely radiosensitive. Stage 1 seminomas: orchidectomy + radiotherapy cures ~95%. Do close follow-up to detect relapse. Cure of NSGCT, even if metastases are present, is achieved by 3 cycles of bleomycin + etoposide + cisplatin. 5yr survival >90% in all groups.
►Encourage regular self-examination (prevents late presentation).

13 αFP is *not* ↑ in pure seminoma; may also be ↑ in: hepatitis, cirrhosis, liver cancer, open neural tube defect.

Surgery

Diagnosing groin lumps: lateral to medial thinking

- Psoas abscess—may present with back pain, limp, and swinging pyrexia.
- Neuroma of the femoral nerve.
- Femoral artery aneurysm.
- Saphena varix—like a hernia, it has a cough impulse.
- Lymph node.
- Femoral hernia.
- Inguinal hernia.
- Hydrocele or varicocele.
- Also consider an undescended testis (cryptorchidism).

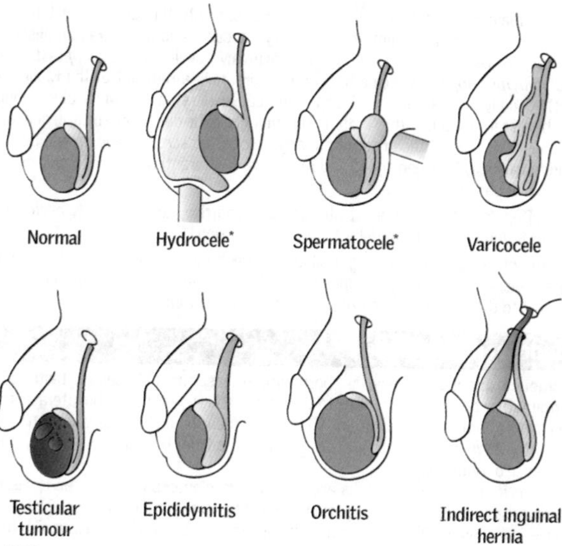

Fig 13.51 Diagnosis of scrotal masses. (*=transilluminates: position of pen torch shown in image).

►►Torsion of the testis

The aim is to recognize this condition before the cardinal signs and symptoms are fully manifest, as prompt surgery saves testes. If surgery is performed in <6h the salvage rate is 90–100%; if >24h it is 0–10%.

►*If in any doubt, surgery is required. If suspected refer immediately to urology.*

Symptoms: Sudden onset of pain in one testis, which makes walking uncomfortable. Pain in the abdomen, nausea, and vomiting are common.

Signs: Inflammation of one testis—it is very tender, hot, and swollen. The testis may lie high and transversely. Torsion may occur at any age but is most common at 11-30yrs. With *intermittent torsion* the pain may have passed on presentation, but if it was severe, and the lie is horizontal, prophylactic fixing may be wise.

ΔΔ: The main one is epididymo-orchitis (p650) but with this the patient tends to be older, there may be symptoms of urinary infection, and more gradual onset of pain. Also consider tumour, trauma, and an acute hydrocele. NB: *torsion of testicular or epididymal appendage* (the hydatid of Morgagni—a remnant of the Müllerian duct)—usually occurs between 7-12yrs, and causes less pain. Its tiny blue nodule may be discernible under the scrotum. It is thought to be due to the surge in gonadotrophins which signal the onset of puberty. *Idiopathic scrotal oedema* is a benign condition usually between ages 2 and 10yrs, and is differentiated from torsion by the absence of pain and tenderness.

Tests: Doppler US may demonstrate lack of blood flow to testis. Only perform if diagnosis equivocal—do not delay surgical exploration.

Treatment: ►Ask consent for possible orchidectomy + *bilateral* fixation (orchidopexy)—see p568. At surgery expose and untwist the testis. If its colour looks good, return it to the scrotum and fix *both* testes to the scrotum.

Undescended testes

Incidence About 3% of boys are born with at least one undescended testis (30% of premature boys) but this drops to 1% after the first year of life. Unilateral is four times more common than bilateral. (If bilateral then should have genetic testing.)

- *Cryptorchidism:* Complete absence of the testis from the scrotum (anorchism is absence of both testes).
- *Retractile testis:* The genitalia are normally developed but there is an excessive cremasteric reflex. The testis is often found at the external inguinal ring. ℞: reassurance (examining while in a warm bath, for example, may help to distinguish from maldescended/ectopic testes).
- *Maldescended testis:* May be found anywhere along the normal path of descent from abdomen to groin.
- *Ectopic testis:* Most commonly found in the superior inguinal pouch (anterior to the external oblique aponeurosis) but may also be abdominal, perineal, penile, and in the femoral triangle.

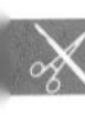

Complications of maldescended and ectopic testis Infertility; ×40 increased risk of testicular cancer (risk remains after surgery but in cryptorchidism may be ↓ if orchidopexy performed before aged 10), increased risk of testicular trauma, increased risk of testicular torsion. Also associated with hernias (due to patent processus vaginalis in >90%, p613) and other urinary tract anomalies.

Treatment of maldescended and ectopic testis restores (potential for) spermatogenesis; the increased risk of malignancy remains but becomes easier to diagnose.

Surgery: Orchidopexy, usually dartos pouch procedure, is performed in infancy testis and cord are mobilized following a groin incision, any processus vaginalis or hernial sac is removed and the testis is brought through a hole made in the dartos muscle into the resultant subcutaneous pouch where the muscle prevents retraction.

Hormonal: Hormonal therapy, most commonly human chorionic gonadotrophin (hCG), is sometimes attempted if an undescended testis is in the inguinal canal.

▸▸Aneurysms of arteries

An artery with a dilatation >50% of its original diameter has an aneurysm; remember this is an ongoing process. True aneurysms are abnormal dilatations that involve all layers of the arterial wall. False aneurysms (pseudoaneurysms) involve a collection of blood in the outer layer only (adventitia) which communicates with the lumen (eg after trauma). Aneurysms may be fusiform (eg most AAAs) or sac-like (eg Berry aneurysms; fig 10.17 p479).

Causes Atheroma, trauma, infection (eg mycotic aneurysm in endocarditis; tertiary syphilis—especially thoracic aneurysms), connective tissue disorders (eg Marfan's, Ehlers-Danlos), inflammatory (eg Takayasu's aortitis, p712).

Common sites Aorta (infrarenal most common), iliac, femoral, and popliteal arteries.

Complications Rupture; thrombosis; embolism; fistulae; pressure on other structures.

Screening All ♂ at age 65yr are invited for screening in UK, decreases mortality from ruptured AAA.

Ruptured abdominal aortic aneurysm (AAA) Death rates/year from ruptured AAAs rise with age: 125 per million in those aged 55–59; 2728 per million if over 85yrs. *Symptoms & signs:* Intermittent or continuous abdominal pain (radiates to back, iliac fossae, or groins; ▸don't dismiss this as renal colic), collapse, an *expansile* abdominal mass (it expands and contracts, unlike swellings that are purely pulsatile, eg nodes overlying arteries), and shock. If in doubt, assume a ruptured aneurysm.

Unruptured AAA *Definition:* >3cm across. *Prevalence:* 3% of those >50yrs. ♂:♀ >3:1. Less common in diabetics. *Cause:* Degeneration of elastic lamellae and smooth muscle loss. There is a genetic component. *Symptoms:* Often none, they *may* cause abdominal/back pain, often discovered incidentally on abdominal examination (see BOX). *Monitoring:* RCTs have failed to demonstrate benefit from early endovascular repair (EVAR, see later in paragraph) of aneurysms <5.5cm (where rupture rates are low). Risk of rupture below this size is <1%/yr, compared to ~25%/yr for aneurysms >6cm across. ~75% of aneurysms under monitoring will eventually need repair. Rupture is more likely if: •↑BP •Smoker •♀ •Positive family history. Modify risk factors if possible at diagnosis. *Elective surgery:* Reserve for aneurysms ≥5.5cm or expanding at >1cm/yr, or symptomatic aneurysms. Operative mortality: ~5%; complications include spinal or visceral ischaemia and distal emboli from dislodged thrombus debris. Studies show that age >80yrs should not, in itself, preclude surgery. *Stenting (EVAR):* Major surgery can be avoided by inserting an endovascular stent via the femoral artery. EVAR has less early mortality but higher graft complications, eg failure of stent-graft to totally exclude blood flow to the aneurysm—'endoleak'. See fig 13.52.

Emergency management of a ruptured abdominal aneurysm

Mortality—treated: 41% and improving; untreated: ~100%.

- ▸▸Summon a vascular surgeon and an experienced anaesthetist; warn theatre.
- ▸▸Do an ECG, and take blood for amylase, Hb, crossmatch (10–40U may eventually be needed). Catheterize the bladder.
- ▸▸Gain IV access with 2 large-bore cannulae. Treat shock with O Rh−ve blood (if not cross matched), but keep systolic BP ≤100mmHg to avoid rupturing a contained leak (NB: *raised* BP is common early on).
- ▸▸Take the patient straight to theatre. Don't waste time on X-rays: fatal delay may result, though CT can help in a stable patient with an uncertain diagnosis.
- ▸▸Give prophylactic antibiotics, eg co-amoxiclav 625mg IV.
- ▸▸Surgery involves clamping the aorta above the leak, and inserting a Dacron® graft (eg 'tube graft' or, if significant iliac aneurysm also, a 'trouser graft' with each 'leg' attached to an iliac artery).

▶▶Thoracic aortic dissection

Blood splits the aortic media with sudden tearing chest pain (± radiation to back). As the dissection extends, branches of the aorta occlude sequentially leading to hemiplegia (carotid artery), unequal arm pulses and BP, or acute limb ischaemia, paraplegia (anterior spinal artery), and anuria (renal arteries). Aortic valve incompetence, inferior MI, and cardiac arrest may develop if dissection moves proximally. *Type A* (70%) dissections involve the ascending aorta, irrespective of site of the tear, while if the ascending aorta is not involved it is called *type B* (30%). ▶▶All patients with type A thoracic dissection should be considered for surgery: *get urgent cardiothoracic advice*. Definitive treatment for type B is less clear and may be managed medically, with surgery reserved for distal dissections that are leaking, ruptured, or compromising vital organs. *Management:* •Crossmatch 10U blood. •ECG & CXR (expanded mediastinum is rare). •CT or transoesophageal echocardiography (TOE). Take to ITU; hypotensives: keep systolic at ~100-110mmHg: labetalol (p140) or esmolol ($t½$ is ultra-short) by IVI is helpful here (calcium-channel blockers may be used if β-blockers contraindicated). Acute operative mortality: <25%.

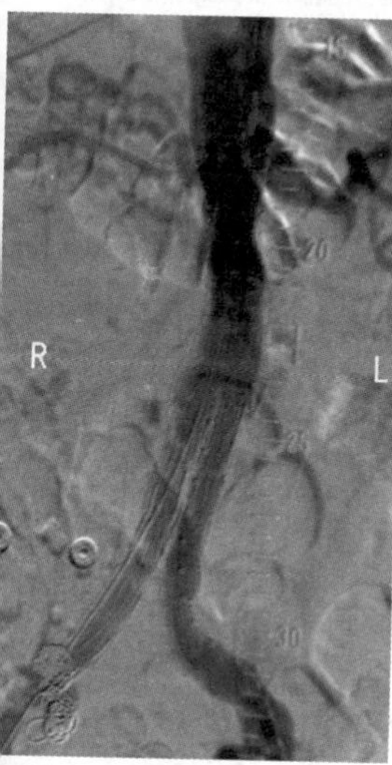

Fig 13.52 Stenting: not an open or closed case ... this is a digital subtraction angiogram showing correct positioning of an endovascular stent at the end of the procedure. Although less invasive than open repair, some are unsuited to this method, owing to the anatomy of their aneurysm. Lifelong monitoring is needed: stents may leak and the aneurysm progress (the risk can be reduced by coiling the internal iliac arteries, as shown).

Image courtesy of Norwich Radiology Dept.

Peripheral arterial disease (PAD)

Occurs due to atherosclerosis causing stenosis of arteries (fig 13.53) via a multi-factorial process involving modifiable and non-modifiable risk factors. 65% have coexisting clinically relevant cerebral or coronary artery disease. ►Cardiovascular risk factors should be identified and treated aggressively. The chief feature of PAD is intermittent claudication (= *to limp*). Prevalence = 10%.

Symptoms Cramping pain in the calf, thigh, or buttock after walking for a given distance (the claudication distance) and relieved by rest (calf claudication suggests femoral disease while buttock claudication suggests iliac disease). Ulceration, gangrene (p660), and foot pain at rest—eg burning pain at night relieved by hanging legs over side of bed—are the cardinal features of *critical ischaemia*. Buttock claudication ± impotence imply Leriche's syndrome (p704). Young, heavy smokers are at risk from Buerger's disease (thromboangiitis obliterans, p696).

Fontaine classification for PAD: **1** Asymptomatic. **2** Intermittent claudication. **3** Ischaemic rest pain. **4** Ulceration/gangrene (critical ischaemia).

Signs Absent femoral, popliteal, or foot pulses; cold, white leg(s); atrophic skin; punched out ulcers (often painful); postural/dependent colour change; Buerger's angle (angle that leg goes pale when raised off the couch) of <20° and capillary filling time >15s are found in severe ischaemia.

Tests Exclude DM, arteritis (ESR/CRP). FBC (anaemia, polycythaemia); U&E (renal disease); lipids (dyslipidaemia); ECG (cardiac ischaemia). Do thrombophilia screen and serum homocysteine if <50 years. *Ankle-brachial pressure index (ABPI):* Normal = 1–1.2; PAD = 0.5–0.9; critical limb ischaemia <0.5 or ankle systolic pressure <50mmHg. Beware falsely high results from incompressible calcified vessels in severe atherosclerosis, eg DM.

Imaging *Colour duplex US* 1st line. If considering intervention *MR/CT angiography* (fig 13.54) for extent and location of stenoses and quality of distal vessels ('run-off').

℞ 1 *Risk factor modification:* Quit smoking (vital). Treat hypertension and high cholesterol. Prescribe an antiplatelet agent (unless contraindicated), to prevent progression and to reduce cardiovascular risk. *Clopidogrel* is recommended as 1st-line.

2 *Management of claudication:* •*Supervised exercise programmes* reduce symptoms by improving collateral blood flow (2h per wk for 3 months). Encourage patients to excercise to the point of maximal pain. •*Vasoactive drugs*, eg naftidrofuryl oxalate, offer modest benefit and are recommended only in those who do not wish to undergo revascularization and if exercise fails to improve symptoms.

If conservative measures have failed and PAD is severely affecting a patient's lifestyle or becoming limb-threatening, intervention is required.

- *Percutaneous transluminal angioplasty (PTA)* is used for disease limited to a single arterial segment (a balloon is inflated in the narrowed segment). 5-year patency is 79% (iliac) and 55% (femoral). Stents can be used to maintain artery patency.
- *Surgical reconstruction:* If atheromatous disease is extensive but distal run-off is good (ie distal arteries filled by collateral vessels), consider arterial reconstruction with a bypass graft (fig 13.54). Procedures include femoral–popliteal bypass, femoral-femoral crossover, and aorto-bifemoral bypass grafts. Autologous vein grafts are superior to prosthetic grafts (eg Dacron® or PTFE) when the knee joint is crossed.
- *Amputation* <3% of patients with intermittent claudication require major amputation within 5 years (↑ in diabetes, p212). Amputation may relieve intractable pain and death from sepsis and gangrene. A decision to amputate must be made by the patient, usually against a background of failed alternative strategies. The knee should be preserved where possible as it improves mobility and rehabilitation potential (this must be balanced with the need to ensure wound healing). Rehabilitation should be started early with a view to limb fitting. Gabapentin (regimen p504) can be used to treat the gruelling complication of phantom limb pain.
- *Future therapies:* Early-phase clinical trials have demonstrated the safety and benefit of gene therapy (eg hepatocyte growth factor) in critical limb ischaemia

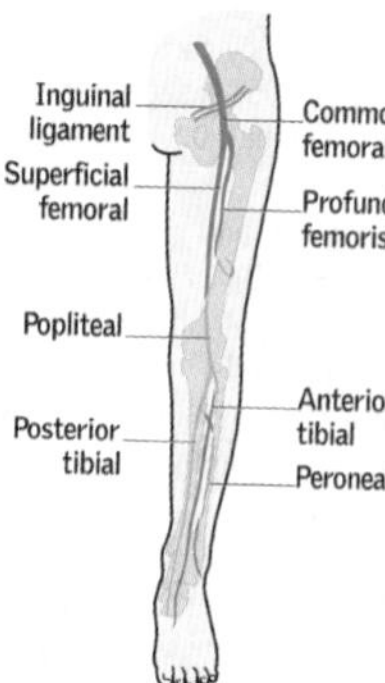

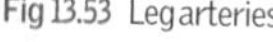
Fig 13.53 Leg arteries.

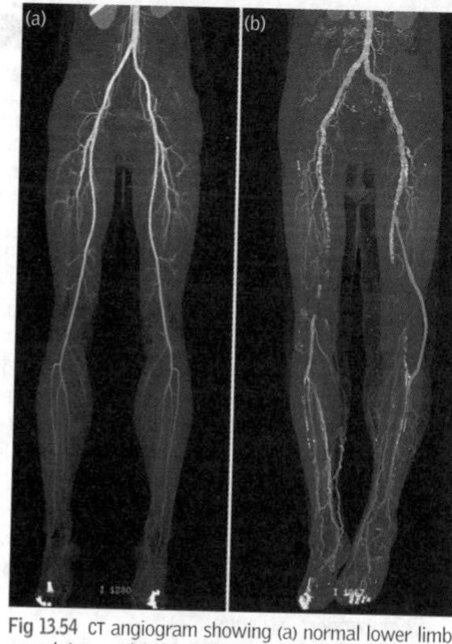

Fig 13.54 CT angiogram showing (a) normal lower limb vasculature and (b) heavily diseased arteries with previous left femoral anterior tibial bypass.

Reproduced from 'Diagnosis and management of peripheral arterial disease', *BMJ*, Peach *et al.*, 345:e5208, 2012, with permission from BMJ Publishing Group Ltd.

Acute limb ischaemia

►►Surgical emergency requiring revascularization within 4–6h to save the limb. May be due to thrombosis *in situ* (~40%), emboli (38%), graft/angioplasty occlusion (15%), or trauma. Thrombosis more likely in known 'vasculopaths'; emboli are sudden, eg in those without previous vessel disease; they can affect multiple sites, and there may be a bruit. Mortality: 22%. Amputation rate: 16%.

- *Symptoms and signs:* The 6 'P's of acute ischaemia: **p**ale, **p**ulseless, **p**ainful, **p**aralysed, **p**araesthetic, and '**p**erishingly cold'. Onset of fixed mottling implies irreversibility. Emboli commonly arise from the heart (AF; mural thrombus) or aneurysms. ►In patients with *known* PAD, sudden deterioration of symptoms with deep duskiness of the limb may indicate acute arterial occlusion. This appearance is due to extensive pre-existing collaterals and must not be misdiagnosed as gout/cellulitis.
- *Management:* ►This is an emergency and may require urgent open surgery or angioplasty. If diagnosis is in doubt, do urgent arteriography. If the occlusion is embolic, the options are surgical embolectomy (Fogarty catheter) or local thrombolysis, eg tissue plasminogen activator (t-PA, p345), balancing the risks of surgery with the haemorrhagic complications of thrombolysis.
- Anticoagulate with heparin after either procedure and look for the source of emboli. ►Be aware of possible post-op reperfusion injury and subsequent compartment syndrome.

Varicose veins (VVs)

Long, tortuous, & dilated veins of the superficial venous system (see fig 13.55).

Pathology Blood from superficial veins of the leg passes into deep veins via perforator veins (perforate deep fascia) and at the saphenofemoral and saphenopopliteal junctions. Valves prevent blood from passing from deep to superficial veins. If they become incompetent there is venous hypertension and dilatation of the superficial veins occurs. *Risk factors:* Prolonged standing, obesity, pregnancy, family history, and contraceptive pill. *Causes:* Primary mechanical factors (in ~95%); secondary to obstruction (eg DVT, fetus, pelvic tumour), arteriovenous malformations, overactive muscle pumps (eg cyclists); rarely congenital valve absence.

Symptoms 'My legs are ugly.' Pain, cramps, tingling, heaviness, and restless legs. But studies show these symptoms are only slightly commoner in those with VVs.

Signs Oedema; eczema; ulcers; haemosiderin; haemorrhage; phlebitis; *atrophie blanche* (white scarring at the site of a previous, healed ulcer); lipodermatosclerosis (skin hardness from subcutaneous fibrosis caused by chronic inflammation and fat necrosis). On their own VVs don't cause DVTs (except possibly ***proximally spreading thrombophlebitis*** of the long saphenous vein).

Examination See p78.

Treatment ►NICE guidelines[11] suggest that the criteria for specialist referral of patients with VVs should be: bleeding, pain, ulceration, superficial thrombophlebitis, or 'a severe impact on quality of life' (ie not for cosmetic reasons alone).

- ***Treat any underlying cause.***
- ***Education***—avoid prolonged standing and elevate leg(s) whenever possible; support stockings (compliance is a problem); lose weight; regular walks (calf muscle action aids venous return).
- ***Endovascular treatment*** (less pain and earlier return to activity than surgery.)
  - ***Radiofrequency ablation (VNUS Closure®)***—a catheter is inserted into the vein and heated to 120°C destroying the endothelium and 'closing' the vein. Results are as good as conventional surgery at 3 months.
  - ***Endovenous laser ablation (EVLA)*** is similar but uses a laser. Outcomes are similar to surgical repair after 2yrs (in terms of quality of life and recurrence).
  - ***Injection sclerotherapy***—either liquid or foam can be used. Liquid sclerosant is indicated for varicosities below the knee if there is no gross saphenofemoral incompetence. It is injected at multiple sites and the vein compressed for a few weeks to avoid thrombosis (intravascular granulation tissue obliterates the lumen). Alternatively foam sclerosant is injected under ultrasound guidance at a single site and spreads rapidly throughout the veins, damaging the endothelium. Ultrasound monitoring prevents inadvertent spread of foam into the femoral vein. It achieves ~80% complete occlusion but is not more effective than liquid sclerotherapy or surgery.

  - ***Surgery***—there are several choices, depending on vein anatomy and surgical preference, eg saphenofemoral ligation (Trendelenburg procedure); multiple avulsions; stripping from groin to upper calf (stripping to the ankle is not needed, and may damage the saphenous nerve). *Post-op:* bandage legs tightly and elevate for 24h. Surgery is more effective than sclerotherapy in the long term. ►Before surgery and after venous mapping, ensure that all varicosities are indelibly marked *to either side* (to avoid tattooing if the incision is made through inked skin).

Saphena varix Dilatation in the saphenous vein at its confluence with the femoral vein (the SFJ). It transmits a cough impulse and may be mistaken for an inguinal or femoral hernia, but on closer inspection it may have a bluish tinge.

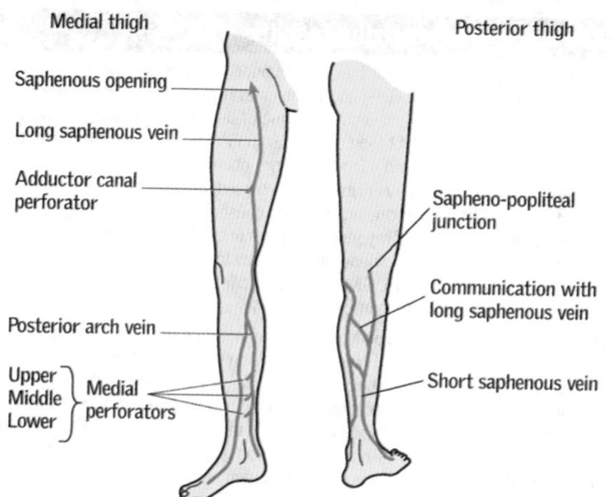

Fig 13.55 The superficial veins of the leg.

When do varicose veins become an illness?

Perhaps when they hurt? Or is this too simple? 'Certain illnesses are desirable: they provide a compensation for a functional disorder...' (Albert Camus); *this is known to be common with VVs.* Perhaps many opt for surgery as a displacement activity to confronting deeper problems. We adopt the sickness role when we want sympathy. Somatization is hard to manage; here is one approach to consider:

- Give time; don't dismiss these patients as 'just the "worried well"'.
- Explore factors perpetuating illness behaviour (misinformation, social stressors).
- Agree a plan that makes sense to the patient's holistic view of themself.
- Treat any underlying depression (drugs and cognitive therapy, *OHCS* p344).

Gangrene and necrotizing fasciitis

Definitions Gangrene is death of tissue from poor vascular supply and is a sign of critical ischaemia (see p656). Tissues are black and may slough. *Dry gangrene* is necrosis in the absence of infection. Note a line of demarcation between living and dead tissue.[14] ℞: restoration of blood supply ± amputation. *Wet gangrene* is tissue death and infection (associated with discharge) occurring together (p213, fig 5.10). ℞: analgesia; broad-spectrum IV antibiotics; surgical debridement ± amputation. *Gas gangrene* is a subset of necrotizing myositis caused by spore-forming clostridial species. There is rapid onset of myonecrosis, muscle swelling, gas production, sepsis, and severe pain. Risk factors include diabetes, trauma, and malignancy. ℞: remove all dead tissue (eg amputation). Give benzylpenicillin ± clindamycin. *Hyperbaric O_2* can improve survival and ↓ the number of debridements.

►►**Necrotizing fasciitis** is a rapidly progressive infection of the deep fascia causing necrosis of subcutaneous tissue. Prompt recognition (difficult in the early stages) and aggressive treatment is required. ►*In any atypical cellulitis, get early surgical help.* There is intense pain over affected skin and underlying muscle. Group A β-haemolytic streptococci is a major cause, although infection is often polymicrobial. Fournier's gangrene is necrotizing fasciitis localized to the scrotum and perineum. ℞: Radical debridement ± amputation; IV antibiotics, eg benzylpenicillin and clindamycin.

Skin ulcers

Ulcers are abnormal breaks in an epithelial surface. Leg ulcers affect ~2% in developed countries.

Causes May be multiple. For leg ulcers, venous disease accounts for 70%, mixed arterial and venous disease for 15%, and arterial disease alone for 2%. Other contributory factors include neuropathy (eg in DM), lymphoedema, vasculitis, malignancy (p596), infection (eg TB, syphilis), trauma (eg pressure sores: see fig 10.16, p473), pyoderma gangrenosum, drugs (eg nicorandil, hydroxyurea).

History Ask about number, pain, trauma. Explore comorbidities—eg VVs, peripheral arterial disease, diabetes, vasculitis. Length of history? Is the patient taking steroids? Are self-induced ulcers, *dermatitis artefacta,* a possibility? Has a biopsy been taken?

Examination Note features such as site, number, surface area, depth, edge, base, discharge, lymphadenopathy, sensation, and healing (see BOX). If in the legs, note features of venous insufficiency or arterial disease and, if possible, apply a BP cuff to perform ankle-brachial pressure index (ABPI).

Tests Skin and ulcer biopsy may be necessary—eg to assess for vasculitis (will need immunohistopathology) or malignant change in an established ulcer (Marjolin's ulcer = SCC presenting in chronic wound). If ulceration is the first sign of a suspected systemic disorder then further screening tests will be required.

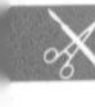

Management Managing ulcers is often difficult and expensive. Treat the cause(s) and focus on prevention. Optimize nutrition. Are there adverse risk factors (drug addiction, or risk factors for arteriopathy, eg smoking)? Get expert nursing care. Consider referral to specialist community nurse or leg ulcer/tissue viability clinic:

- 'Charing-Cross' 4-layer compression bandaging is better than standard bandages (use only if arterial pulses OK: ABPI (p656) should be >0.8). Honey dressings can improve healing in mild-moderate burns, but as an adjuvant to compression bandaging for leg ulcers they do not significantly improve healing rate.Negative pressure wound therapy (eg VAC®) helps heal diabetic ulcers.
- Surgery, larval therapy, and hydrogels are used to debride sloughy necrotic tissue (avoid hydrogels in diabetic ulcers due to ↑risk of wet gangrene).

►Routine use of antibiotics does not improve healing. Only use if there is infection (not colonization).

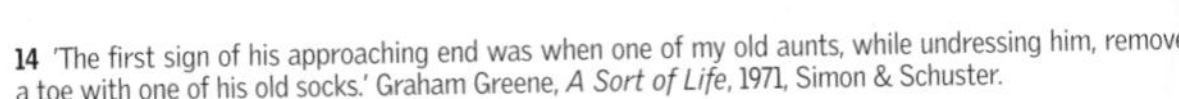

14 'The first sign of his approaching end was when one of my old aunts, while undressing him, removed a toe with one of his old socks.' Graham Greene, *A Sort of Life*, 1971, Simon & Schuster.

Features of skin ulceration to note on examination

Site Above the medial malleolus ('gaiter' area) is the favourite place for *venous ulcers* (fig 13.56; mostly related to superficial venous disease, but may reflect venous hypertension via damage to the valves of the deep venous system, eg 2° to DVT). Venous hypertension leads to the development of superficial varicosities and skin changes (*lipodermatosclerosis* = induration, pigmentation, and inflammation of the skin). Minimal trauma to the leg leads to ulceration which often takes many months to heal. Ulcers on the sacrum, greater trochanter, or heel suggest *pressure sores* (*OHCS* p604), particularly if the patient is bed-bound with suboptimal nutrition.

Temperature The ulcer and surrounding tissues are cold in an ischaemic ulcer. If the skin is warm and well perfused then local factors are more likely.

Surface area Draw a map of the area to quantify and time any healing (a wound >4wks old is a chronic ulcer as distinguished from an acute wound).

Shape Oval, circular (cigarette burns), serpiginous (*Klebsiella granulomatis*, p412); unusual morphology can be secondary to mycobacterial infection, eg cutaneous tuberculosis or scrofuloderma (*tuberculosis colliquativa cutis*, where an infected lymph node ulcerates through to the skin).

Edge Shelved/sloping ≈ healing; punched-out ≈ ischaemic or syphilis; rolled/everted ≈ malignant; undermined ≈ TB.

Base Any muscle, bone, or tendon destruction (malignancy; pressure sores; ischaemia)? There may be a grey-yellow slough, beneath which is a pale pink base. *Slough* is a mixture of fibrin, cell breakdown products, serous exudate, leucocytes, and bacteria—it need not imply infection, and can be part of the normal wound healing process. *Granulation tissue* is a deep pink gel-like matrix contained within a fibrous collagen network and is evidence of a healing wound.

Depth If not uncomfortable for the patient (eg in neuropathic ulceration), a probe can be used to gauge how deep the ulceration extends.

Discharge Culture before starting any antibiotics (which usually don't work). A watery discharge is said to favour TB; ►bleeding can ≈ malignancy.

Associated lymphadenopathy Suggests infection or malignancy.

Sensation Decreased sensation around the ulcer implies neuropathy.

Position in phases of extension/healing Healing is heralded by granulation, scar formation, and epithelialization. Inflamed margins ≈ extension.

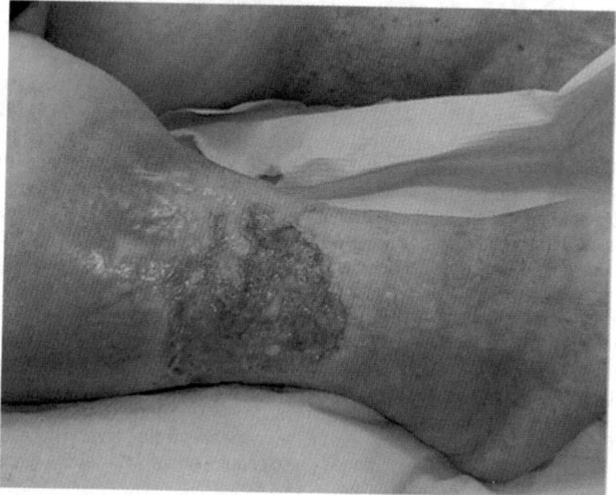

Fig 13.56 Venous ulcer in the gaiter area in an obese woman.

Reproduced from Burge *et al.*, *Oxford Handbook of Medical Dermatology*, 2016, with permission from Oxford University Press.

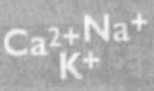

Contents

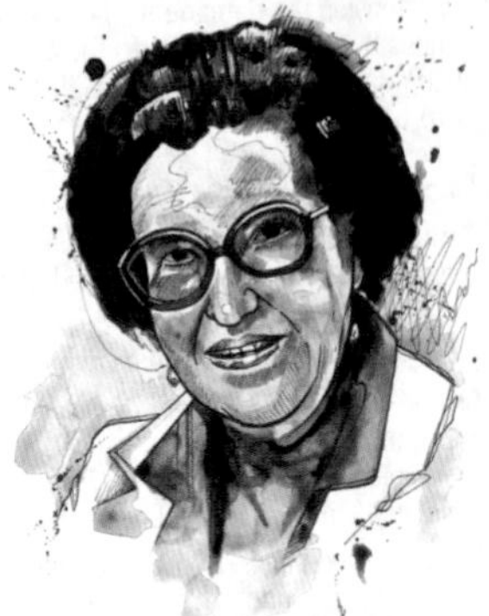

Fig 14.1 Rosalyn Yalow (1921-2011). Trained in nuclear physics, and made good use of this when she developed the radioimmunoassay technique to allow trace amounts of peptides to be measured in serum using antibodies. This revolutionized laboratory medicine, making reliable assays for hormones widely available, and underpinned the development of endocrinology. It was also employed to screen blood against a range of pathogens, and the technique is still commonly used today. She was awarded the Nobel prize for her work in 1977, and commented to a group of children that: 'Initially, new ideas are rejected...Later they become dogma, if you're right. And if you're really lucky you can publish your rejections as part of your Nobel presentation.'

On being normal in the society of numbers

Laboratory medicine reduces our patients to a few easy-to-handle numbers: this is the discipline's great attraction—and its greatest danger. The normal range (reference interval) is usually that which includes 95% of a given population (given a normal distribution, see p750). If variation is randomly distributed, 2.5% of our results will be 'too high', and 2.5% 'too low' on an average day, when dealing with apparently normal people. This statistical definition of normality is the simplest. Other definitions may be *normative*—ie stating what an upper or lower limit *should* be. The upper end of the reference interval for plasma cholesterol may be given as 6mmol/L because this is what biochemists state to be the *desired* maximum. 40% of people in some populations will have a plasma cholesterol greater than 6mmol/L and thus may be at increased risk. The WHO definition of anaemia in pregnancy is an Hb of <110g/L, which makes 20% of mothers anaemic. This 'lax' criterion has the presumed benefit of triggering actions that result in fewer deaths from haemorrhage. So do not just ask 'What is the normal range?'—also enquire about who set the range, for what population, and for what reason.

We thank Dr Petra Sulentic, our Specialist Reader, for her contribution to this chapter.

The essence of laboratory medicine

General principles

- Laboratory testing may contribute to four aspects of medicine:
  - diagnosis (eg TSH in hypothyrodism)
  - prognosis (eg clotting in liver failure)
  - monitoring disease activity or progression (eg creatinine in chronic kidney disease)
  - screening (eg phenylketonuria in newborn babies).
- Only do a test if the result will influence management. Make sure you look at the result.
- ►Always interpret laboratory results in the context of the patient's clinical picture.
- If a result does not fit with the clinical picture, trust clinical judgement and repeat the test. Could it be an artefact? The 'normal' range for a test (reference interval) is usually defined as the interval, symmetrical about the mean, containing 95% of results in a given population (p751). The more tests you run, the greater the probability of an 'abnormal' result of no significance (see p751).
- Laboratory staff like to have contact with you. They are an excellent source of help and information for both requests and results.
- ►Involve the patient. Don't forget to explain to them where the test fits into their overall management plan.

Getting the best out of the lab—a laboratory decalogue

1. Interest someone from the laboratory in your patient's problem.
2. Fill in the request form fully.
3. Give clinical details, not your preferred diagnosis.
4. Ensure that the lab knows who to contact.
5. Label specimens as well as the request form.
6. Follow the hospital labelling routine for crossmatching.
7. Find out when analysers run, especially batched assays.
8. Talk with the lab before requesting an unusual test.
9. Be thoughtful: at 16:30h the routine results are being sorted.
10. Plot results graphically: abnormalities show sooner.

Artefacts and pitfalls in laboratory tests

- Do not take blood samples from an arm that has IV fluid running into it.
- Repeat any unexpected and inconsistent result before acting on it.
- For clotting time do not sample from a heparinized IV catheter.
- Serum K^+ is overestimated if the sample is old or haemolysed (this occurs if venepuncture is difficult).
- If using Vacutainers, fill *plain* tubes first—otherwise, anticoagulant contamination from previous tubes can cause errors.
- Total calcium results are affected by albumin concentration (p676).
- INR may be overestimated if citrate bottles are underfilled.
- Drugs may cause *analytic* errors (eg prednisolone cross-reacts with cortisol). Be suspicious if results are unexpected.
- Food may affect result, eg bananas raise urinary HIAA (p271).

Ford Madox Ford 1915 '*The Good Soldier*'

Normal values can have hidden historical, social, and political desiderata—just like the normal values novelists ascribe to their characters: '*Conventions and traditions I suppose work blindly but surely for the preservation of the normal type; for the extinction of proud, resolute and unusual individuals... Society must go on, I suppose, and society can only exist if the normal, if the virtuous, and the slightly-deceitful flourish, and if the passionate, the headstrong, and the too-truthful are condemned to suicide and to madness. Yes, society must go on; it must breed, like rabbits. That is what we are here for ... But, at any rate, there is always Leonora to cheer you up; I don't want to sadden you. Her husband is quite an economical person of so normal a figure that he can get quite a large proportion of his clothes ready-made. That is the great desideratum of life.*'

Oxford World's Classics, pp181–92

Biochemistry—some major disease patterns

Dehydration ↑Urea (disproportionate relative to smaller ↑ in creatinine),[1] ↑albumin (also useful to plot change in a patient's condition), ↑haematocrit (PCV); also ↓urine volume and ↓skin turgor.

Abnormal kidney function There are two major biochemical pictures (table 14.1): *Low GFR:* Usually oliguric. *Causes:* early acute oliguric renal failure (p298), chronic kidney disease (p302). In chronic kidney disease also ↓Hb, ↑PTH, and renal bone disease. *Tubular dysfunction:* Results from damage to tubules. Diagnosis is made by testing renal concentrating ability (p241). May be polyuric with ↑urinary glucose, amino acids, proteins (lysozyme, β_2-microglobulin), or phosphate. *Causes:* recovery from acute kidney injury, hypercalcaemia, hyperuricaemia, myeloma, pyelonephritis, hypokalaemia, Wilson's disease, galactosaemia, and heavy metal poisoning.

Table 14.1 Biochemical profile in abnormal kidney function

	Low GFR	Tubular dysfunction
Urea & creatinine	↑	Normal
K^+ & urate	↑	↓
H^+	↑	↑
HCO_3^-	↓	↓
PO_4^{3-}	↑	↓
Ca^{2+}	↓	Normal

Thiazide and loop diuretics ↓Na^+, ↓K^+, ↑HCO_3^-, ↑urea.

Bone disease See table 14.2 for typical biochemical patterns.

Table 14.2 Serum biomarkers in common diseases of bone

	Ca^{2+}	PO_4^{3-}	ALP
Osteoporosis (p682)	Normal	Normal	Normal
Osteomalacia (p684)	↓	↓	↑
Paget's	Normal	Normal	↑↑
Myeloma	↑	↑, normal	Normal
Bone metastases	↑	↑, normal	↑
1° Hyperparathyroidism	↑	↓, normal	Normal, ↑
Hypoparathyroidism	↓	↑	Normal
Renal failure (low GFR)	↓	↑	Normal, ↑

Hepatocellular disease ↑Bilirubin, ↑↑AST, ALP ↑ slightly, ↓albumin. Also ↑clotting times. For details of the differences between AST and ALT, see p291.

Cholestasis ↑Bilirubin, ↑↑γGT, ↑↑ALP, ↑AST.

Excess alcohol intake Evidence of hepatocellular disease. Early evidence if ↑γGT ↑MCV, and ethanol in blood before lunch.

Myocardial infarction ↑Troponin, ↑CK, ↑AST, ↑LDH (p118).

Addison's disease ↑K^+, ↓Na^+, ↑urea.

Cushing's syndrome May show ↓K^+, ↑HCO_3^-, ↑Na^+.

Conn's syndrome May show ↓K^+, ↑HCO_3^-. Na^+ normal or ↑. (Also hypertension.)

Diabetes mellitus ↑Glucose, (↓HCO_3^- if acidotic).

Diabetes insipidus ↑Na^+, ↑plasma osmolality, ↓urine osmolality. (Both hypercalcaemia and hypokalaemia may cause nephrogenic diabetes insipidus.)

Inappropriate ADH secretion (SIADH) (See p673.) ↓Na^+ with ↓↔ urea and creatinine ↓plasma osmolality. ↑Urine osmolality (>plasma osmolality), ↑urine Na^+ (>20mmol/L

Some immunodeficiency states Normal serum albumin but *low* total prote (because immunoglobulins are missing. Also makes crossmatching difficult becau expected haemagglutinins are absent; *OHCS* p198).

1 Dehydration affects urea more than creatinine because in dehydration a greater proportion of filter urea is reabsorbed by the kidney. Creatinine is hardly reabsorbed at all.

Laboratory results: ▸▸ when to take action NOW

- On receiving a dangerous result, first check the name and date.
- Go to the bedside. If the patient is conscious, turn off any IVI (until fluid is checked: a mistake may have been made) and ask the patient how he or she is. *Any fits, faints, collapses, or unexpected symptoms?*
- Be sceptical of an unexpectedly, wildly abnormal result with a well patient. Compare with previous values. Could the specimens have got muddled up; whose is it? Is there an artefact? Was the sample taken from the 'drip' arm? Is a low calcium due to a low albumin (p676)? Perhaps the lab is using a new analyser with a faulty wash cycle? ►*When in doubt, seek help and repeat the test.*

The following values are somewhat arbitrary and must be taken as a guide only. Many results less extreme than those listed will be just as dangerous if the patient is old, immunosuppressed, or has some other pathology such as pneumonia.

Plasma biochemistry:

►►The main risks when plasma electrolytes are dangerously abnormal (table 14.3) are of cardiac arrhythmias and CNS events such as seizures.

Table 14.3 Dangerous levels of the common serum elecrolytes

Electrolyte	Lower limit	Upper limit	Relevant pages
Na^+	<120mmol/L	>155mmol/L	p672
K^+	<2.5mmol/L	>6.5mmol/L	p674, p301
Corrected Ca^{2+}	<2.0mmol/L	>3.5mmol/L	p676, p678
Glucose	<2.0mmol/L	>20mmol/L	p832, p834

Blood gases:

- P_aO_2 <8.0kPa = *Severe hypoxia. Give* O_2. See p188.
- pH <7.1 = *Dangerous acidosis. See* p670 *to determine the cause.*

Haematology results:

- Hb <70g/L with low mean cell volume (<75fL) or history of bleeding. This patient may need urgent transfusion (no spare capacity)—ask about symptoms, co-morbidities, and baseline Hb. Check haematinics before transfusion. See p324.
- Platelets <40×10⁹/L. May need a platelet transfusion; call a haematologist.
- *Plasmodium falciparum* seen on blood film. *Start antimalarials now*. See p418.
- ESR >30mm/h + headache. *Could there be giant cell arteritis?* See p556.

CSF results:

►►Never delay treatment when bacterial meningitis is suspected.

- >1 neutrophil/mm³. *Is there meningitis: usually >1000 neutrophils?* See p822.
- Positive Gram stain. *Talk to a microbiologist; urgent blind therapy*. See p822.

Conflicting, equivocal, or inexplicable results: ►Get prompt help.

Fluid balance and IV fluid therapy

Fluid requirement Roughly 2–2.5L in a normal person (~70kg) over 24h. Normal daily losses are through urine (1500mL), stool (200mL), and insensible losses (800mL). This requirement is normally met through food (1000mL) and drink (1500mL).

Intravenous fluids Given if sufficient fluids cannot be given orally. About 2–2.5L of fluid containing roughly 70mmol Na^+ and 70mmol K^+ per 24h are required.[1] Thus, a good regimen is 2–2.5L of 0.18% glucose with sodium chloride with 20–30mmol of K^+ per litre of fluid. Alternative routes are via a central venous line or subcutaneously. However, remember that all cannulae carry a risk of MRSA infection: femoral > jugular > subclavian > peripheral, so always resume oral fluid intake as soon as possible.

►In a sick patient, don't forget to include additional sources of fluid loss when calculating daily fluid requirements, such as drains, fevers, or diarrhoea (see BOX 'Special cases'). Daily weighing helps to monitor overall fluid balance, as will fluid balance charts.

►Examine patients regularly to assess fluid balance (see BOX 'Assessing fluid balance').

Fluid compartments and types of IV fluid

For a 70kg man, *total bodily fluid* is ~42L (60% body weight). Of this, ⅔ is intracellular (28L) and ⅓ is extracellular (14L). Of the extracellular compartment, ⅓ is intravascular, ie blood (5L). Different types of IV fluid will equilibrate with the different fluid compartments depending on the osmotic content of the given fluid.

5% glucose: (=Dextrose.) Isotonic, but contains only a small amount of glucose (50g/L) and so provides little energy (~10% daily energy per litre). The liver rapidly metabolizes all the glucose leaving only water, which rapidly equilibrates throughout all fluid compartments. It is, therefore, useless for fluid resuscitation (only 1/9 will remain in the intravascular space), but suitable for maintaining hydration. Excess 5% glucose IV may lead to water overload and hyponatraemia (p672).

0.9% saline: ('Normal saline.') Has about the same Na^+ content as plasma (150mmol/L) and is isotonic with plasma. 0.9% saline will equilibrate rapidly throughout the extracellular compartment only, and takes longer to reach the intracellular compartment than 5% glucose. It is, therefore, appropriate for fluid resuscitation, as it will remain predominantly in the extracellular space (and thus ⅓ of the given volume in the intravascular space), as well as for maintaining hydration. Hypertonic and hypotonic saline solutions are also available, but are for specialist use only.

Colloids: (eg Gelofusine®.) Have a high osmotic content similar to that of plasma and therefore remain in the intravascular space for longer than other fluids, making them appropriate for fluid resuscitation, but not for general hydration. Colloids are expensive, and may cause anaphylactic reactions. In reality, effective fluid resuscitation will use a combination of colloid and 0.9% saline.

Hypertonic glucose (10% or 50%): May be used in the treatment of hypoglycaemia It is irritant to veins, so care in its use is needed. Infusion sites should be inspectec regularly, and flushed with 0.9% saline after use.

Glucose with sodium chloride: (One-fifth 'normal saline.') Isotonic, containing 0.18% saline (30mmol/L of Na^+) and 4% glucose (222mmol/L). It has roughly the quantity o Na^+ required for normal fluid maintenance, when given 10-hourly in adults, but is now most commonly used in a paediatric setting.

Hartmann's solution: Contains Na^+ 131mmol, Cl^- 111mmol, lactate 29mmol, K 5mmol, HCO_3^- 29mmol, and Ca^{2+} 2mmol per litre of fluid. It is an alternative to 0.9% saline, and some consider it more physiological.

Assessing fluid balance

Underfilled:

- Tachycardia
- Postural drop in BP (low BP is a late sign of hypovolaemia)
- ↓capillary refill time
- ↓urine output
- Cool peripheries
- Dry mucous membranes
- ↓skin turgor
- Sunken eyes.

Overfilled:

- ↑JVP (p43)
- Pitting oedema of the sacrum, ankles, or even legs and abdomen
- Tachypnoea
- Bibasal crepitations
- Pulmonary oedema on CXR (fig 16.3, p723).

See also p134 for signs of heart failure.

The JVP is a substitute marker of central venous pressure, and when assessing fluid balance is difficult, a CVP line may help to guide fluid management.

Special cases

Acute blood loss: Resuscitate with colloid or 0.9% saline via large-bore cannulae until blood is available.
Children: Use glucose with sodium chloride for fluid maintenance: 100mL/kg for the first 10kg, 50mL/kg for the next 10kg, and 20mL/kg thereafter—all per 24h.
Elderly: May be more prone to fluid overload, so use IV fluids with care (smaller fluid bolus).
GI losses: (Diarrhoea, vomiting, NG tubes, etc.) Replace lost K^+ as well as lost fluid volume.
Heart failure: Use IV fluids with care to avoid fluid overload (p134).
Liver failure: Patients often have a raised total body sodium, so use salt-poor albumin or blood for resuscitation, and avoid 0.9% saline for maintenance.
Acute pancreatitis: Aggressive fluid resuscitation is required due to large amounts of sequestered 'third-space' fluid (p636).
Poor urine output: Aim for >1 mL/kg/h; the minimum is >0.5mL/kg/h. Give a fluid challenge, eg 500mL 0.9% saline over 1h (or half this volume in heart failure or the elderly), and recheck the urine output. If not catheterized, exclude retention; if catheterized, ensure the catheter is not blocked!
Post-operative: Check the operation notes for intraoperative losses, and ensure you chart and replace added losses from drains, etc.
Shock: Resuscitate with colloid or 0.9% saline via large-bore cannulae. Identify the type of shock (p790).
Transpiration losses: (Fever, burns.) Beware the large amounts of fluid that can be lost unseen through transpiration. Severe burns in particular may require aggressive fluid resuscitation (p846).

Potassium in IV fluids

- Potassium ions can be given with 5% glucose or 0.9% saline, usually 20mmol/L or 40mmol/L.
- K^+ may be retained in renal failure, so beware giving too much IV.
- Gastrointestinal fluids are rich in K^+, so increased fluid loss from the gut (eg diarrhoea, vomiting, high-output stoma, intestinal fistula) will need increased K^+ replacement.

►The maximum concentration of K^+ that is safe to infuse via a peripheral line is 40mmol/L, at a maximum rate of 20mmol/h in a cardiac monitored patient. Fluid-restricted patients may require higher concentrations or rates in life-threatening hypokalaemia. Faster rates risk cardiac dysrhythmias and asystole, and higher concentrations thrombophlebitis, depending on the size of the vein, so give concentrated solutions >40mmol/L via a central venous catheter, and use ECG monitoring for rates >10mmol/h. For symptoms and signs of hyper- and hypokalaemia see p674.

Electrolyte physiology and the kidney

The kidney Controls the homeostasis of a number of serum electrolytes (including Na^+, K^+, Ca^{2+}, and PO_4^{3-}), helps to maintain acid-base balance, and is responsible for the excretion of many substances. It also makes erythropoietin and renin, and hydroxylates 25-hydroxyvitamin D to 1,25-dihydroxyvitamin D (see p676 for Ca^{2+} and PO_4^{3-} physiology). All of these functions can be affected in chronic kidney disease (p302), but it is the biochemical effects of kidney failure that are used to monitor disease progression.

The renin-angiotensin-aldosterone system Plasma is filtered by the glomeruli, and Na^+, K^+, H^+, and water are reabsorbed from this filtrate under the control of the renin-angiotensin-aldosterone system. *Renin* is released from the juxtaglomerular apparatus (fig 7.13, p316) in response to low renal flow and raised sympathetic tone, and catalyses the conversion of *angiotensinogen* (a peptide made by the liver) to *angiotensin I*. This is then converted by angiotensin-converting enzyme (ACE), which is located throughout the vascular tree, to *angiotensin II*. The latter has several important actions including efferent renal arteriolar constriction (thus ↑perfusion pressure), peripheral vasoconstriction, and stimulation of the adrenal cortex to produce *aldosterone*, which activates the Na^+/K^+ pump in the distal renal tubule leading to reabsorption of Na^+ and water from the urine, in exchange for K^+ and H^+. Glucose spills over into the urine when the plasma concentration > renal threshold for reabsorption (≈10mmol/L, but this varies between people, and is ↓ in pregnancy).

Control of sodium Control is through the action of aldosterone on the distal convoluted tubule (DCT) and collecting duct to increase Na^+ reabsorption from the urine. The natriuretic peptides ANP, BNP, and CNP (p137) contribute to Na^+ homeostasis by reducing Na^+ reabsorption from the DCT and inhibiting renin. A *high GFR* (see later in this topic) results in increased Na^+ loss, and *high renal tubular flow* and haemodilution decrease Na^+ reabsorption in the proximal tubule.

Control of potassium Most K^+ is intracellular, and thus serum K^+ levels are a poor reflection of total body potassium. The concentrations of K^+ and H^+ in extracellular fluid tend to vary together. This is because these ions compete with each other in the exchange with Na^+ that occurs across most cell membranes and in the distal convoluted tubule of the kidney, where Na^+ is reabsorbed from the urine. Thus, if the H^+ concentration is high, less K^+ will be excreted into the urine. Similarly, K^+ will compete with H^+ for exchange across cell membranes and extracellular K^+ will accumulate. Insulin and catecholamines both stimulate K^+ uptake into cells by stimulating the Na^+/K^+ pump.

Serum osmolality A laboratory measurement of the number of osmoles per *kilogram* of solvent. It is approximated by *serum osmolarity* (the number of osmoles per *litre* of solution) using the equation $2(Na^+ + K^+)$ + Urea + Glucose, since these are the predominant serum electrolytes. Normal serum osmolarity is 280–300mmol/L which will always be a little less than the laboratory-measured osmolality—the *osmolar gap*. However, if the osmolar gap is greater than 10mmol/L, this indicates the presence of additional solutes: consider diabetes mellitus or high blood ethanol, methanol, mannitol, or ethylene glycol.

Control of water Control is mainly via serum Na^+ concentration, since water intake and loss are regulated to hold the extracellular concentration of Na^+ constant. Raised plasma osmolality (eg dehydration or ↑glucose in diabetes mellitus) causes thirst through the hypothalamic thirst centre and the release of antidiuretic hormone (ADH) from the posterior pituitary. ADH increases the passive water reabsorption from the renal collecting duct by opening water channels to allow water to flow from the hypotonic luminal fluid into the hypertonic renal interstitium. Low plasma osmolality inhibits ADH secretion, thus reducing renal water reabsorption.

Glomerular filtration rate (GFR) Defined as the volume of fluid filtered by the glomeruli per minute (units mL/min), and is one of the primary measures of disease progression in chronic kidney disease. It can be estimated in a number of different ways (see BOX).

Estimating GFR

Calculating GFR is useful because it is a more sensitive indication of the degree of renal impairment than serum creatinine. Subjects with low muscle mass (eg the elderly, women) can have a 'normal' serum creatinine, despite a significant reduction in GFR. This can be important when prescribing nephrotoxic drugs, or drugs that are renally excreted, which may therefore accumulate to toxic levels in the serum.

A number of methods for estimating GFR exist, all relying on a calculation of the clearance of a substance that is renally filtered and then not reabsorbed in the renal tubule. For example, the rate of clearance of creatinine can be used as a marker for the rate of filtration of fluid and solutes in the glomerulus because it is only slightly reabsorbed from the renal tubule. The more of the filtered substance that is reabsorbed, however, the less accurate the estimate of GFR.

MDRD (Modification of Diet in Renal Disease Study Group): This provides an estimate of GFR from four simple parameters: *serum creatinine, age, gender*, and *race (black/non-black)*. It is one of the best validated for monitoring patients with established moderately severe renal impairment,[2] and most labs now routinely report estimated GFR (eGFR) using the MDRD equation on all U&E reports:

$$\text{eGFR} = 32788 \times \text{serum creatinine}^{-1.154} \times \text{age}^{-0.203} \times [1.212 \textit{ if black}] \times [0.742 \textit{ if female}]$$

However, a number of caveats exist, so that it is best used in monitoring declining renal function rather than labelling elderly patients with mild renal impairment:

- It is not validated for mild renal impairment, and therefore its use for screening *general* populations is questionable.
- Inter-individual variations (and thus confidence intervals) are wide, although for each individual variations are small so that a decline in eGFR over a number of serum samples is always significant.
- Single results may be affected by variations in serum creatinine, such as after a protein-rich meal.

Cockcroft-Gault equation: This provides an estimate of creatinine clearance. It is an improvement on the MDRD equation because it also takes into account the patient's weight. However, 10% of creatinine is actively excreted in the tubules, and therefore creatinine clearance overestimates true GFR and underestimates renal impairment. Moreover, the equation assumes ideal body weight and is thus unreliable in the obese or oedematous. Also unreliable in unstable renal function.

$$\text{Creatinine clearance} = \frac{(140 - \text{age}) \times \text{weight (kg)} \times [0.85 \textit{ if female}] \times [1.212 \textit{ if black}]}{0.813 \times \text{serum creatinine } (\mu\text{mol/L})}$$

Creatinine clearance can also be calculated by measuring the excreted creatinine in a ***24h urine collection*** and comparing it with the serum creatinine concentration. However, the accuracy of collection is vital but often poor, making this an unreliable and inconvenient method.

GFR can also be measured by injection of a radioisotope followed by sequential blood sampling (*^{51}Cr-EDTA*) or by an isotope scan (eg DTPA ^{99}Tc, p190). These methods allow a more accurate estimate of GFR than creatinine clearance, since smaller proportions of these substances are reabsorbed in the tubules. They also have the advantage of being able to provide split renal function.

Inulin clearance: The gold standard for calculating GFR, because 100% of filtered inulin (not insulin) is retained in the luminal fluid and therefore reflects exactly the rate of filtration of water and solutes in the glomerulus. However, measuring inulin clearance again requires urine collection over several hours, and also a constant IV infusion of inulin, and is therefore inconvenient to perform.

Acid-base balance

Arterial blood pH is closely regulated in health to 7.40 ± 0.05 by various mechanisms including bicarbonate, other plasma buffers such as deoxygenated haemoglobin, and the kidney. Acid-base disorders needlessly confuse many people, but if a few simple rules are applied, then interpretation and diagnosis are easy. The key principle is that primary changes in HCO_3^- are *metabolic* and in CO_2 *respiratory*. See fig 14.2.

A simple method

1 *Look at the pH*, is there an acidosis or alkalosis?
- pH <7.35 is an acidosis; pH >7.45 is an alkalosis.

2 *Is the CO_2 abnormal?* (Normal range 4.7-6.0kPa.)
If so, is the change in keeping with the pH?
- CO_2 is an acidic gas—is CO_2 raised with an acidosis, lowered with an alkalosis? If so, it is in keeping with the pH and thus caused by a *respiratory* problem. If there is no change, or an opposite one, then the change is compensatory.

3 *Is the HCO_3^- abnormal?* (Normal concentration 22-28mmol/L.)
If so, is the change in keeping with the pH?
- HCO_3^- is alkaline—is HCO_3^- raised with an alkalosis, lowered with an acidosis? If so, the problem is a *metabolic* one.

4 *Is the P_aO_2 abnormal?* Interpret in the context of the FiO_2.

An example Your patient's blood gas shows: pH 7.05, CO_2 2.0kPa, HCO_3^- 8.0mmol/L. There is an *acidosis*. The CO_2 is low, and thus it is a compensatory change. The HCO_3^- is low and is thus the primary change, ie a *metabolic* acidosis.

The anion gap Estimates unmeasured plasma anions ('fixed' or organic acids such as phosphate, ketones, and lactate—hard to measure directly). It is calculated as the difference between plasma cations (Na^+ and K^+) and anions (Cl^- and HCO_3^-). Normal range: 10-18mmol/L. It is helpful in determining the cause of a metabolic acidosis.

Metabolic acidosis ↓pH, ↓HCO_3^-

Causes of metabolic acidosis and an increased anion gap:

Due to increased production, or reduced excretion, of fixed/organic acids. HCO_3^- falls and unmeasured anions associated with the acids accumulate.
- Lactic acid (shock, infection, tissue ischaemia).
- Urate (renal failure).
- Ketones (diabetes mellitus, alcohol).
- Drugs/toxins (salicylates, biguanides, ethylene glycol, methanol).

Causes of metabolic acidosis and a normal anion gap:

Due to loss of bicarbonate or ingestion of H^+ ions (Cl^- is retained).
- Renal tubular acidosis.
- Diarrhoea.
- Drugs (acetazolamide).
- Addison's disease.
- Pancreatic fistula.
- Ammonium chloride ingestion.

Metabolic alkalosis ↑pH, ↑HCO_3^-
- Vomiting.
- K^+ depletion (diuretics).
- Burns.
- Ingestion of base.

Respiratory acidosis ↓pH, ↑CO_2
- Type 2 respiratory failure due to any lung, neuromuscular, or physical cause (p188)
- Most commonly chronic obstructive pulmonary disease (COPD). Look at the P_aO_2. It will probably be low. Is oxygen therapy required? Use controlled O_2 (Venturi connector) if COPD is the underlying cause, as too much oxygen may make matters worse (p189).

►► Beware exhaustion in asthma, pneumonia, and pulmonary oedema, which can present with this picture when close to respiratory arrest. A normal or high P_aCO_2 is worrying. These patients require urgent ITU review for ventilatory support.

Respiratory alkalosis ↑pH, ↓CO_2
A result of hyperventilation of any cause. *CNS causes:* Stroke; subarachnoid bleed; meningitis. *Others:* Mild/moderate asthma; anxiety; altitude; ↑T°; pregnancy; pulmonary emboli (reflex hyperventilation); drugs, eg salicylates.

Terminology To aid understanding, we have used the terms acidosis and alkalosis, where a purist would sometimes have used acidaemia and alkalaemia. Technically acidaemia is the state of having a low blood pH, whereas acidosis refers to the processes which generate H^+, leading to the acidaemia.

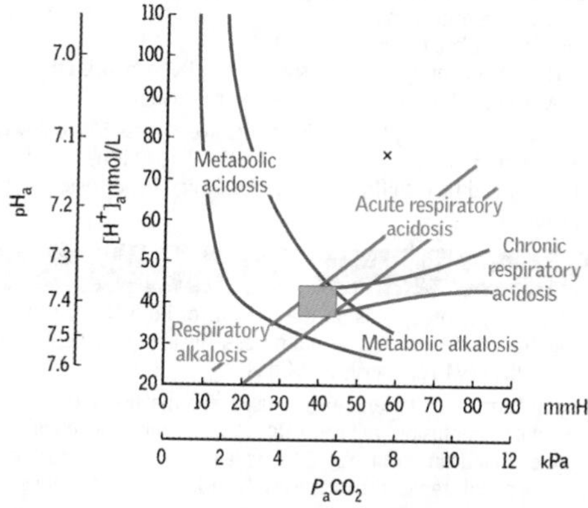

Fig 14.2 The shaded area represents normality. This method is very powerful. The result represented by point ×, for example, indicates that the acidosis is in part respiratory and in part metabolic. Seek a cause for each.

Hypernatraemia

Signs and symptoms Lethargy, thirst, weakness, irritability, confusion, coma, and fits, along with signs of dehydration (p666). *Laboratory features:* ↑Na^+, ↑PCV, ↑alb, ↑urea.

Causes

Usually due to water loss in excess of Na^+ loss:

- Fluid loss without water replacement (eg diarrhoea, vomit, burns).
- Diabetes insipidus (p240). Suspect if large urine volume. This may follow head injury, or CNS surgery, especially pituitary.
- Osmotic diuresis (for diabetic coma, see p832).
- Primary aldosteronism: rarely severe, suspect if ↑BP, ↓K^+, alkalosis (↑HCO_3^-).
- Iatrogenic: incorrect IV fluid replacement (excessive saline).

Management Give water orally if possible. If not, give glucose 5% IV slowly (1L/6h) guided by urine output and plasma Na^+. Use 0.9% saline IV if hypovolaemic, since this causes less marked fluid shifts and is hypotonic in a hypertonic patient. Avoid hypertonic solutions.

Hyponatraemia

Plasma Na^+ concentration depends on the amount of both Na^+ and water in the plasma. Hyponatraemia therefore does not necessarily imply Na^+ depletion. Assessing fluid status is the key to diagnosis (see fig 14.3).

Signs and symptoms Look for anorexia, nausea, and malaise initially, followed by headache, irritability, confusion, weakness, ↓GCS, and seizures, depending on the severity and rate of change in serum Na^+. Cardiac failure or oedema may help to indicate the cause. Hyponatraemia also increases the risk of falls in the elderly.[3]

Causes See fig 14.3. Artefactual causes include: •blood sample was from a drip arm •high serum lipid/protein content causing ↑serum volume, with ↓Na^+ concentration but normal plasma osmolality •if hyperglycaemic (≳20mmol/L) add ~4.3mmol/L to plasma Na^+ for every 10mmol/L rise in glucose above normal.

Iatrogenic hyponatraemia If 5% glucose is infused continuously without adding 0.9% saline, the glucose is quickly used, rendering the fluid hypotonic and causing hyponatraemia, esp. in those on thiazide diuretics, women (esp. pre-menopausal), and those undergoing physiological stress (eg post-operative, septic). In some patients, only marginally low plasma Na^+ levels cause serious effects (eg ~128mmol/L)—don't attribute odd CNS signs to non-existent strokes/TIAs if ↓Na^+.

Management

- Correct the underlying cause; never base treatment on Na^+ concentration alone. The presence of symptoms, the chronicity of the hyponatraemia, and state of hydration are all important. Replace Na^+ and water at the same rate they were lost.
- *Asymptomatic chronic hyponatraemia*, fluid restriction is often sufficient if asymptomatic, although demeclocycline (ADH antagonist) may be required. If hypervolaemic (cirrhosis, CCF), treat the underlying disorder first.
- *Acute or symptomatic hyponatraemia*, or if *dehydrated*, cautious rehydration with 0.9% saline may be given, but do not correct changes rapidly as *central pontine myelinolysis*[2] may result. Maximum rise in serum Na^+ 15mmol/L per day if chronic, or 1mmol/L per hour if acute. Consider using furosemide when not hypovolaemic to avoid fluid overload.
- *Vasopressor receptor antagonists* ('vaptans', eg tolvaptan) promote water excretion without loss of electrolytes, and appear to be effective in treating hypervolaemic and euvolaemic hyponatraemia but are expensive.[4]

►►*In emergency:* (Seizures, coma) seek expert help. Consider hypertonic saline (eg 1.8% saline) at 70mmol Na^+/h ± furosemide. Aim for a gradual increase in plasma Na^+ to ≈125mmol/L. Beware heart failure and central pontine myelinolysis.[2]

2 Central pontine myelinolysis: irreversible and often fatal pontine demyelination seen in malnourished alcoholics or rapid correction of ↓Na^+. There is subacute onset of lethargy, confusion, pseudobulbar palsy, para- or quadriparesis, 'locked-in' syndrome, or coma.

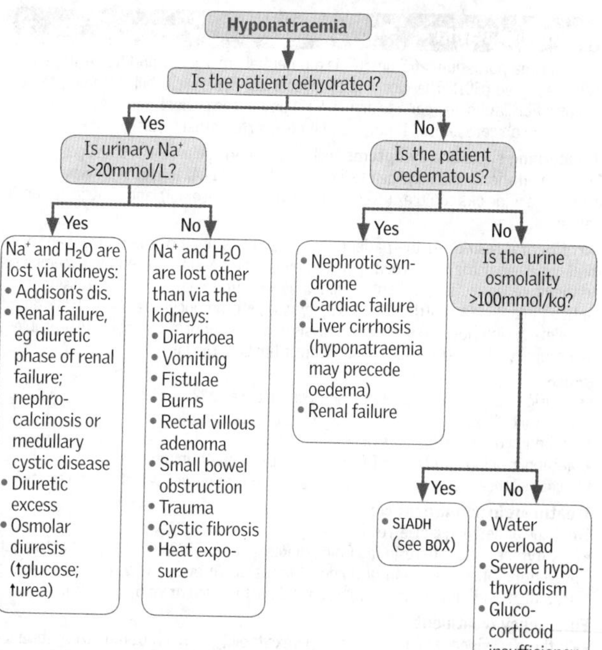

Fig 14.3 Hyponatraemia.

Syndrome of inappropriate ADH secretion (SIADH)

An important, but over-diagnosed, cause of hyponatraemia. The diagnosis requires concentrated urine (Na^+ > 20mmol/L and osmolality > 100mosmol/kg) in the presence of hyponatraemia (plasma Na^+ < 125mmol/L) and low plasma osmolality (< 260mosmol/kg), in the absence of hypovolaemia, oedema, or diuretics.

Causes:
- *Malignancy:* lung small-cell, pancreas, prostate, thymus, or lymphoma.
- *CNS disorders:* meningoencephalitis, abscess, stroke, subarachnoid or subdural haemorrhage, head injury, neurosurgery, Guillain-Barré, vasculitis, or SLE.
- *Chest disease:* TB, pneumonia, abscess, aspergillosis, small-cell lung cancer.
- *Endocrine disease:* hypothyroidism (not true SIADH, but perhaps due to excess ADH release from carotid sinus baroreceptors triggered by ↓ cardiac output).
- *Drugs:* opiates, psychotropics, SSRIs, cytotoxics.
- *Other:* acute intermittent porphyria, trauma, major abdominal or thoracic surgery, symptomatic HIV.

Treatment: Treat the cause and restrict fluid. Consider salt ± loop diuretic if severe. Demeclocycline is used rarely. Vasopressin receptor antagonists ('vaptans', p672) are an emerging class of drug used in SIADH and other types of hyponatraemia.

Hyperkalaemia

▶▶A plasma potassium >6.5mmol/L is a potential emergency and needs urgent assessment (see p301). The worry is of myocardial hyperexcitability leading to ventricular fibrillation and cardiac arrest. First assess the patient—do they look unwell, is there an obvious cause? If not, could it be an artefactual result?

Concerning signs and symptoms Include a fast irregular pulse, chest pain, weakness, palpitations, and light-headedness. ECG: (see fig 14.4) tall tented T waves, small P waves, a wide QRS complex (eventually becoming sinusoidal), and ventricular fibrillation.

Artefactual results: If the patient is well, and has none of the above-mentioned findings, repeat the test urgently as it may be artefactual, caused by: •haemolysis (difficult venepuncture; patient clenched fist) •contamination with potassium EDTA anticoagulant in FBC bottles (do FBCs *after* U&Es) •thrombocythaemia (K^+ leaks out of platelets during clotting) •delayed analysis (K^+ leaks out of RBCs; a particular problem in a primary care setting due to long transit times to the lab).[5]

Causes

- Oliguric renal failure.
- K^+-sparing diuretics.
- Rhabdomyolysis (p319).
- Metabolic acidosis (DM).
- Excess K^+ therapy.
- Addison's disease (see p226).
- Massive blood transfusion.
- Burns.
- Drugs, eg ACE-i, suxamethonium.
- Artefactual result (see earlier 'Artefactual results').

Treatment in non-urgent cases

Treat the underlying cause; review medications.

- Polystyrene sulfonate resin (eg Calcium Resonium® 15g/8h PO) binds K^+ in the gut, preventing absorption and bringing K^+ levels down over a few days. If vomiting prevents PO administration, give a 30g enema, followed at 9h by colonic irrigation.

Emergency treatment

▶▶If there is evidence of myocardial hyperexcitability, or K^+ is >6.5mmol/L, get senior assistance, and treat as an emergency (see p301).

Hypokalaemia

If K^+ <2.5mmol/L, urgent treatment is required. Note that hypokalaemia exacerbates digoxin toxicity.

Signs and symptoms Muscle weakness, hypotonia, hyporeflexia, cramps, tetany, palpitations, light-headedness (arrhythmias), constipation.

ECG Small or inverted T waves, prominent U waves (after T wave), a long PR interval, and depressed ST segments.

Causes

- Diuretics.
- Vomiting and diarrhoea.
- Pyloric stenosis.
- Rectal villous adenoma.
- Intestinal fistula.
- Cushing's syndrome/steroids/ACTH.
- Conn's syndrome.
- Alkalosis.
- Purgative and liquorice abuse.
- Renal tubular failure (p316 & p664).

If on diuretics, ↑HCO_3^- is the best indication that hypokalaemia is likely to have been long-standing. Mg^{2+} may be low, and hypokalaemia is often difficult to correct until Mg^{2+} levels are normalized. Suspect Conn's syndrome if hypertensive, hypokalaemic alkalosis in someone not taking diuretics (p228).

In *hypokalaemic periodic paralysis*, intermittent weakness lasting up to 72h appears to be caused by K^+ shifting from extra- to intracellular fluid. See *OHCS* p652.

Treatment *If mild:* (>2.5mmol/L, no symptoms.) Give oral K^+ supplement (≥80mmol/24h, eg Sando-K® 2 tabs/8h). Review K^+ after 3 days. If taking a thiazide diuretic, and K^+ >3.0 consider repeating and/or K^+-sparing diuretic. *If severe:* (<2.5mmol/L, and/or dangerous symptoms.) Give IV potassium cautiously, not more than 20mmol/h, and not more concentrated than 40mmol/L. Do not give K^+ if oliguric. ▶▶*Never* give K^+ as a fast stat bolus dose.

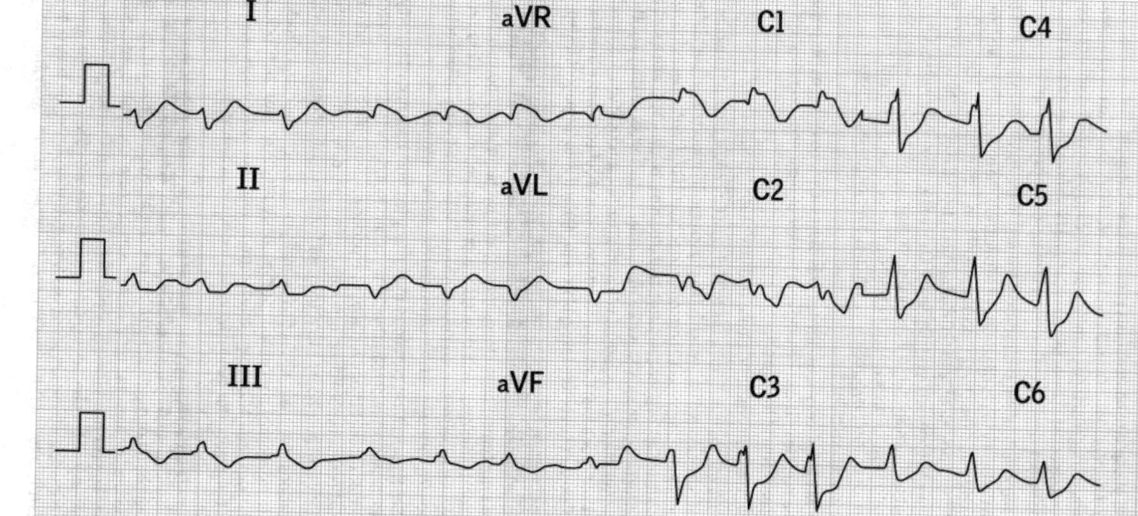

Fig 14.4 Hyperkalaemia—note the flattening of the P waves, prominent T waves, and widening of the QRS complex.

Calcium and phosphate physiology

Calcium and phosphate homeostasis is maintained through:

Parathyroid hormone (PTH): Overall effect is ↑Ca^{2+} & ↓PO_4^{3-}. Secretion by four parathyroid glands is triggered by ↓serum ionized Ca^{2+}; controlled by −ve feedback loop. Actions are: •↑osteoclast activity releasing Ca^{2+} and PO_4^{3-} from bones •↑Ca^{2+} & ↓PO_4^{3-} reabsorption in the kidney •↑renal production of 1,25-dihydroxy-vitamin D_3.

Vitamin D and calcitriol: Vit D is hydroxylated first in the liver to 25-hydroxy-vit D, and again in the kidney to 1,25-dihydroxy-vit D (calcitriol), the biologically active form, and 24,25-hydroxy-vit D (inactive). Calcitriol production is stimulated by ↓Ca^{2+}, ↓PO_4^{3-}, and ↑PTH. *Actions are:* •↑Ca^{2+} and ↑PO_4^{3-} absorption from the gut •inhibition of PTH release •enhanced bone turnover •↑Ca^{2+} and ↑PO_4^{3-} reabsorption in the kidney. Cholecalciferol (vit D_3—from animal sources) and ergocalciferol (vit D_2—from vegetables) are biologically identical in their activity. Disordered regulation of calcitriol underlies familial normocalcaemic hypercalciuria, which is a major cause of calcium oxalate renal stone formation (p638).

Calcitonin: Made in C-cells of the thyroid, this causes ↓Ca^{2+} and ↓PO_4^{3-}, but its physiological role is unclear. It can be used as a marker of recurrence or metastasis in medullary carcinoma of the thyroid.

Magnesium: ↓Mg^{2+} prevents PTH release, and may cause hypocalcaemia.

Plasma binding: Labs usually measure total plasma Ca^{2+}. ~40% is bound to albumin, and the rest is free ionized Ca^{2+} which is the physiologically important amount (often available on blood gas analyser). Therefore, *correct total Ca^{2+} for albumin* as follows: add 0.1mmol/L to Ca^{2+} level for every 4g/L that albumin is below 40g/L, and a similar subtraction for raised albumin. However, many other factors affect binding (eg other proteins in myeloma, cirrhosis, individual variation) so be cautious in your interpretation. If in doubt over a high Ca^{2+}, take blood specimens uncuffed (remove tourniquet after needle in vein, but before taking blood sample), and with the patient fasted.

Hypercalcaemia

Signs and symptoms 'Bones, stones, groans, and psychic moans.' Abdominal pain; vomiting; constipation; polyuria; polydipsia; depression; anorexia; weight loss; tiredness; weakness; hypertension, confusion; pyrexia; renal stones; renal failure; ectopic calcification (eg cornea—see BOX); cardiac arrest. *ECG:* ↓QT interval.

Causes (See fig 14.5.) Most commonly malignancy (eg from bone metastases, myeloma, PTHrP) or primary hyperparathyroidism. Others include sarcoidosis, vit D intoxication, thyrotoxicosis, lithium, tertiary hyperparathyroidism, milk-alkali syndrome, and familial benign hypocalciuric hypercalcaemia (rare; defect in calcium-sensing receptor). HIV can cause both ↑ & ↓Ca^{2+} (perhaps from PTH-related bone remodelling).[6]

Investigations The main distinction is malignancy vs 1° hyperparathyroidism. Pointers to malignancy are ↓albumin, ↓Cl^-, alkalosis, ↓K^+, ↑PO_4^{3-}, ↑ALP. ↑PTH indicates hyperparathyroidism. Also FBC, protein electrophoresis, CXR, isotope bone scan, 24h urinary Ca^{2+} excretion (for familial hypocalciuric hypercalcaemia).

Causes of metastatic (ectopic) calcification 'PARATHORMONE'

Parathormone (PTH)↑ (p222) and other causes of ↑Ca^{2+}, eg sarcoidosis; **A**myloidosis; **R**enal failure (relates to ↑PO_4^{3-}); **A**ddison's disease (adrenal calcification); **T**B nodes; **T**oxoplasmosis (CNS); **H**istoplasmosis (eg in lung); **O**verdose of vitamin D; **R**aynaud's-associated diseases (eg SLE; systemic sclerosis p552; dermatomyositis); **M**uscle primaries/leiomyosarcomas); **O**ssifying metastases (**o**steosarcoma) or **o**varian mets (to peritoneum); **N**ephrocalcinosis; **E**ndocrine tumours (eg gastrinoma).

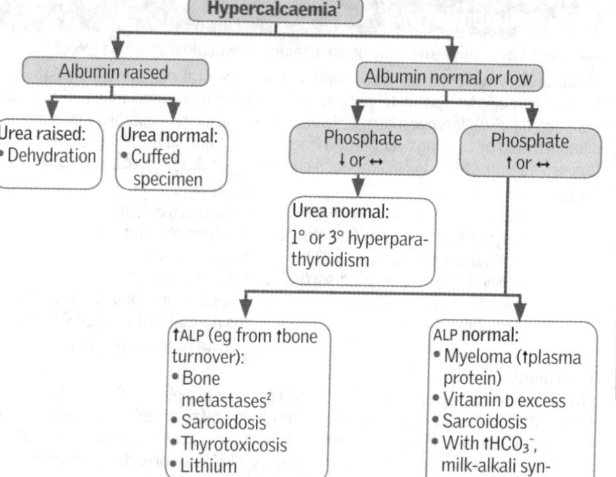

Fig 14.5 Hypercalcaemia.

1 This diagram is only a guide: use in conjunction with the clinical picture.

2 Most common primary: breast, kidney, lung, thyroid, prostate, ovary, colon.

3 Ingesting too much calcium and alkali (eg in milk) can cause hypercalcaemia with metastatic calcification and renal failure. Thyrotoxicosis causes alkalaemia because of hyperventilation.[7]

Treating acute hypercalcaemia

Diagnose and treat the underlying cause. If Ca^{2+} >3.5mmol/L and symptomatic:

1 *Correct dehydration:* If dehydrated give IV 0.9% saline.

2 *Bisphosphonates:* These prevent bone resorption by inhibiting osteoclast activity. A single dose of pamidronate lowers Ca^{2+} over 2-3d; maximum effect is at 1wk. *Infuse slowly*, eg 30mg in 300mL 0.9% saline over 3h via a largish vein. Max dose 90mg (see table 14.4). Zoledronic acid is significantly more effective in reducing serum Ca^{2+} than previously used bisphosphonates.[8] Usually, a single dose of 4mg IV (diluted to 100mL, over 15min) will normalize plasma Ca^{2+} within a week. *SE*, flu symptoms, ↓PO_4^{3-}, bone pain, myalgia, nausea, vomiting, headache, lymphocytopenia, ↓Mg^{2+}, ↓Ca^{2+}, seizures.

3 *Further management:* Chemotherapy may help in malignancy. Steroids are used in sarcoidosis, eg prednisolone 40–60mg/d. Salmon calcitonin acts similarly to bisphosphonates, and has a quicker onset of action, but is now rarely used. NB: the use of furosemide is contentious, as supporting RCT evidence is scant.[9,10] It helps to promote renal excretion of Ca^{2+}, but can exacerbate hypercalcaemia by worsening dehydration. Thus it should only be used once fully rehydrated, and with concomitant IV fluids (eg 0.9% saline 1L/4–6h). Avoid thiazides.

Table 14.4 Disodium pamidronate doses

Calcium (mmol/L; corrected)	Single-dose pamidronate (mg)
<3	15–30
3–3.5	30–60
3.5–4	60–90
>4	90

Hypocalcaemia

►Apparent hypocalcaemia may be an artefact of hypoalbuminaemia (p676).

Signs and symptoms See BOX.[11] *Mild:* cramps, perioral numbness/paraesthesiae. *Severe:* carpopedal spasm (especially if brachial artery compressed, *Trousseau's sign*; see fig 14.6), laryngospasm, seizures. Neuromuscular excitability may also be demonstrated by tapping over parotid (facial nerve) causing facial muscles to twitch (*Chvostek's sign*; see fig 14.7). Cataract if chronic hypocalcaemia. *ECG:* Long QT interval.

Causes *With ↑PO_4^{3-}*
- Chronic kidney disease (p302).
- Hypoparathyroidism (incl thyroid or parathyroid surgery, p222).
- Pseudohypoparathyroidism (p222).
- Acute rhabdomyolysis.
- Hypomagnesaemia.

With ↔ or ↓PO_4^{3-}
- Vitamin D deficiency.
- Osteomalacia (↑ALP).
- Acute pancreatitis.
- Over-hydration.
- Respiratory alkalosis (total Ca^{2+} is normal, but ↓ionized Ca^{2+} due to ↑pH ∴ symptomatic).

Treatment
- *Mild symptoms:* Give calcium 5mmol/6h PO, with daily plasma Ca^{2+} levels.
- *In chronic kidney disease:* See p302. May require **alfacalcidol**, eg 0.5–1mcg/24h PO.
- *Severe symptoms:* Give 10mL of 10% **calcium gluconate** (2.25mmol) IV over 30min, and repeat as necessary. If due to respiratory alkalosis, correct the alkalosis.

Features of hypocalcaemia 'SPASMODIC'

Spasms (carpopedal spasms = Trousseau's sign)
Perioral paraesthesiae
Anxious, irritable, irrational
Seizures
Muscle tone ↑ in smooth muscle—hence colic, wheeze, and dysphagia
Orientation impaired (time, place, and person) and confusion
Dermatitis (eg atopic/exfoliative)
Impetigo herpetiformis (↓Ca^{2+} and pustules in pregnancy—rare and serious)
Chvostek's sign; **c**horeoathetosis; **c**ataract; **c**ardiomyopathy (long QT interval on ECG).

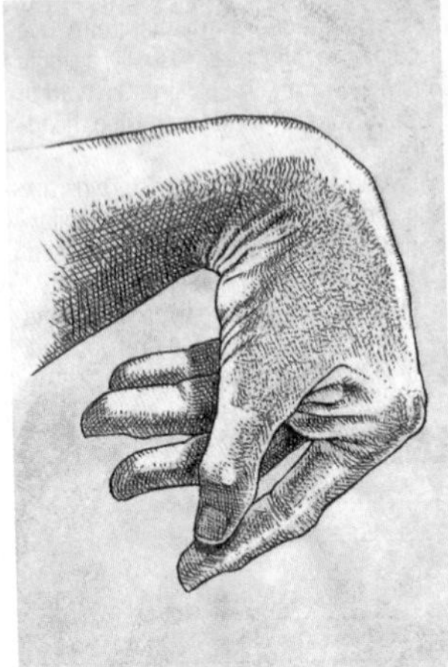

Fig 14.6 Trousseau's sign: on inflating the cuff, the wrist and fingers flex and draw together (carpopedal spasm).

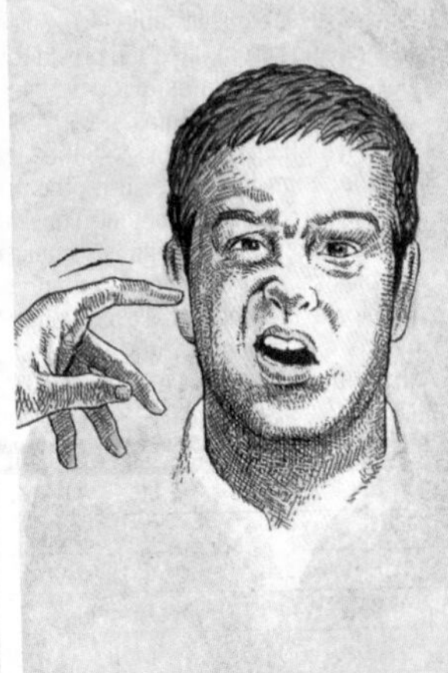

Fig 14.7 Chvostek's sign: the corner of the mouth twitches when the facial nerve is tapped over the parotid.

Phosphate

Hypophosphataemia Common and of little significance unless severe (<0.4mmol/L). *Causes:* Vitamin D deficiency, alcohol withdrawal, refeeding syndrome (p587), inadequate oral intake, severe diabetic ketoacidosis, renal tubular dysfunction and 1° hyperparathyroidism. *Signs and symptoms:* Muscle weakness or rhabdomyolysis, red cell, white cell and platelet dysfunction, and cardiac arrest or arrhythmias. *Treatment:* Oral or parenteral phosphate supplementation, eg Phosphate Polyfusor® IVI (100mmol PO_4^{3-} in 500mL). Never give IV phosphate to a patient who is hypercalcaemic or oliguric.

Hyperphosphataemia Most commonly due to chronic kidney disease, when it is treated with phosphate binders, eg sevelamer 800mg/8h PO during meals. Also catabolic states such as tumour lysis syndrome (p529).

Magnesium

Magnesium is distributed 65% in bone and 35% in cells; plasma concentration tends to follow that of Ca^{2+} and K^+.

Hypomagnesaemia Causes paraesthesiae, ataxia, seizures, tetany, arrhythmias. Digitalis toxicity may be exacerbated. *Causes:* Diuretics, severe diarrhoea, ketoacidosis, alcohol abuse, total parenteral nutrition (monitor weekly), ↓Ca^{2+}, ↓K^+, and ↓PO_4^{3-}. *Treatment:* If needed, give magnesium salts, PO or IV (eg 8mmol $MgSO_4$ IV over 3min to 2h, depending on severity, with frequent Mg^{2+} levels).

Hypermagnesaemia Rarely requires treatment unless severe (>7.5mmol/L). *Causes:* Renal failure or iatrogenic (eg excessive antacids). *Signs:* If severe: neuromuscular depression, ↓BP, ↓pulse, hyporeflexia, CNS & respiratory depression, coma.

Zinc

Zinc deficiency This may occur in parenteral nutrition or, rarely, from a poor diet (too few cereals and dairy products; anorexia nervosa; alcoholism). Rarely it is due to a genetic defect. *Symptoms:* Alopecia, dermatitis (look for red, crusted skin lesions especially around nostrils and corners of mouth), night blindness, diarrhoea. *Diagnosis:* Therapeutic trial of zinc (plasma levels are unreliable as they may be low, eg in infection or trauma, without deficiency).

Selenium

An essential element present in cereals, nuts, and meat. Low soil levels in some parts of Europe and China cause deficiency states. Required for the antioxidant glutathione peroxidase, which ↓ harmful free radicals. Selenium is also antithrombogenic, and is required for sperm motility proteins. Deficiency may increase risk of neoplasia and atheroma, and may lead to a cardiomyopathy or arthritis. Serum levels are a poor guide. Toxic symptoms may also be found with over-energetic replacement.

Urate and the kidney

Causes of hyperuricaemia High levels of urate in the blood (hyperuricaemia) may result from increased turnover (15%) or reduced excretion of urate (85%). Either may be drug induced.

- *Drugs:* Cytotoxics, thiazides, loop diuretics, pyrazinamide.
- *Increased cell turnover:* Lymphoma, leukaemia, psoriasis, haemolysis, muscle death (rhabdomyolysis, p319; tumour lysis syndrome, p529).
- *Reduced excretion:* Primary gout (p548), chronic kidney disease, lead nephropathy, hyperparathyroidism, pre-eclampsia (*OHCS* p48).
- *Other:* Hyperuricaemia may be associated with hypertension and hyperlipidaemia. Urate may be raised in disorders of purine synthesis such as the *Lesch-Nyhan syndrome* (*OHCS* p648).

Hyperuricaemia and renal failure Severe renal failure from any cause may be associated with hyperuricaemia, and rarely this may give rise to gout. Sometimes the relationship of cause and effect is reversed so that it is the hyperuricaemia that causes the renal failure. This can occur following cytotoxic treatment (tumour lysis syndrome, p529), and in muscle necrosis.

How urate causes renal failure: Urate is poorly soluble in water, so over-excretion can lead to crystal precipitation. Renal failure occurs most commonly because urate precipitates in the renal tubules. This may occur at plasma levels ≥1.19mmol/L. In some instances, ureteric obstruction from urate crystals may occur. This responds to retrograde ureteric catheterization and lavage.

Prevention of renal failure: Before starting chemotherapy, ensure good hydration and initiate **allopurinol** (xanthine oxidase inhibitor) or **rasburicase** (recombinant urate oxidase), which prevent a sharp rise in urate following chemotherapy (see p528). There is a remote risk of inducing xanthine nephropathy.

Treatment of hyperuricaemic acute kidney injury: Exclude bilateral ureteric obstruction, then give prompt rehydration ± loop diuretic to wash uric acid crystals out of the renal tubules, and correct electrolyte abnormalities. Once oliguria is established, haemodialysis is required (in preference to peritoneal dialysis). There is no evidence for either preventing (see previous paragraph) or treating hyperuricaemic renal failure.

Gout See p548.

Urate renal stones Urate stones (fig 14.8) comprise 5-10% of all renal stones and are radiolucent.

Incidence: ~5-10% in temperate climates (double if confirmed gout),[12] but up to 40% in hot, arid climates. ♂:♀≈4:1. But most urate stone formers have no detectable abnormalities in urate metabolism.

Risk factors: Acidic or strongly concentrated urine; ↑urinary excretion of urate; chronic diarrhoea; distal small bowel disease or resection (regional enteritis); ileostomy; obesity; diabetes mellitus; chemotherapy for myeloproliferative disorders; inadequate caloric or fluid intake.

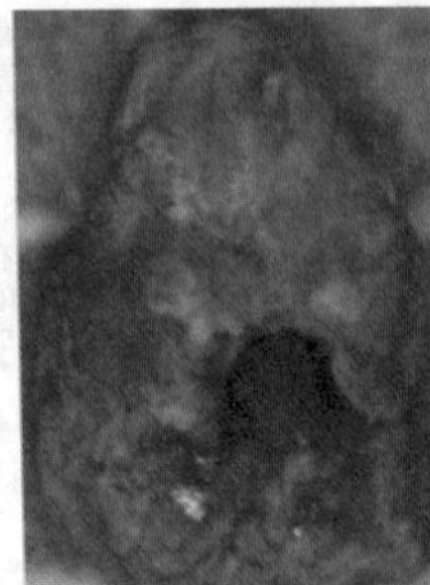

Fig 14.8 Urate stone.

©Dr G. Austin

Treatment: Hydration to increase urine volume (aim >2L/d). Unlike most other renal calculi, existing uric acid stones can often be dissolved with either systemic or topical alkalinizing agents. Potassium citrate or potassium bicarbonate at a dose titrated to alkalinize the urine to a pH of 6-7 dissolves some urate stones. If hyperuricosuria, consider dietary management ± allopurinol (xanthine oxidase inhibitor).

This page intentionally blank

Metabolic bone diseases: osteoporosis

Osteoporosis implies reduced bone mass. It may be 1° (age-related) or 2° to another condition or drugs. If trabecular bone is affected, crush fractures of vertebrae are common (hence the 'littleness' of little old ladies and their dowager's hump); if cortical bone is affected, long bone fractures are more likely, eg femoral neck: the big cause of death and orthopaedic expense (80% hip fractures in the UK occur in women >50yrs).

Prevalence (In those >50yrs): ♂ 6%, ♀ 18%. Women lose trabeculae with age, but in men, although there is reduced bone formation, numbers of trabeculae are stable and their lifetime risk of fracture is less.

Risk factors Age-independent risk factors for 1° osteoporosis: parental history, alcohol >4 units daily, rheumatoid arthritis, BMI <19, prolonged immobility, and untreated menopause. See BOX 'Osteoporosis risk factors' for other risk factors, including for 2° osteoporosis.

Investigations *X-ray* (low sensitivity/specificity, often with hindsight after a fracture). Bone densitometry (DEXA—see BOX 'DEXA bone densitometry'; table 14.5). *Bloods:* Ca^{2+}, PO_4^{3-}, and ALP normal. Consider specific investigations for 2° causes if suggestive history. *Biopsy* is unreliable and unnecessary with non-invasive techniques available.

Management Loss of bone mineral density may not be entirely irreversible. Age, number of risk factors, and bone mineral density (DEXA scan; see BOX 'DEXA bone densitometry') guide the pharmacological approach (eg FRAX, which is a WHO risk assessment tool for estimating 10-yr risk of osteoporotic fracture in untreated patients; see www.shef.ac.uk/frax),[13,14] although DEXA is not necessary if age >75yrs. Lifestyle measures should apply to all (including those at risk but not yet osteoporotic).

Lifestyle measures:
- Quit smoking and reduce alcohol consumption.
- Weight-bearing exercise may increase bone mineral density.[15]
- Balance exercises such as tai chi reduce risk of falls.
- Calcium and vitamin D-rich diet (use supplements if diet is insufficient—see 'Pharmacological measures' later in this topic).
- Home-based fall-prevention programme, with visual assessment and a home visit. NB: hip-protectors are unreliable for preventing fractures.[16]

Pharmacological measures:
- *Bisphosphonates:* alendronic acid is 1st line (10mg/d or 70mg/wk; not if eGFR <35). Use also for prevention in long-term steroid use. If intolerant, try etidronate or risedronate. Tell patient to swallow pills with *plenty* of water while remaining upright for >30min and wait 30min before eating or other drugs. (SE: photosensitivity; GI upset; oesophageal ulcers—stop if dysphagia or abdo pain; rarely, jaw osteonecrosis).
- *Calcium and vitamin D:* rarely used alone for prophylaxis, as questionable efficacy and some evidence of a small ↑CV risk. Offer if evidence of deficiency, eg calcium 1g/d + vit D 800u/d. Target serum 25-hydroxy-vitamin D level ≥75nmol/L.
- *Strontium ranelate:* due to an increased risk of cardiac problems it should only be used in those with severe intolerance of other agents and without cardiovascular disease.
- *Hormone replacement therapy (HRT)* can prevent (not treat) osteoporosis in postmenopausal women. Relative risk of breast cancer is 1.4 if used >10yrs; ↑CV risk.
- *Raloxifene* is a selective oestrogen receptor modulator (SERM) that acts similarly to HRT, but with ↓ breast cancer risk.
- *Teriparatide* (recombinant PTH) is useful in those who suffer further fractures despite treatment with other agents. There is a potential ↑ risk of renal malignancy.
- *Calcitonin* may reduce pain after a vertebral fracture.
- *Testosterone* may help in hypogonadal men by promoting trabecular connectivity.
- *Denosumab*, a monoclonal Ab to RANK ligand, given SC twice yearly ↓ reabsorption.

DEXA bone densitometry: WHO osteoporosis criteria

It is better to scan the hip than the lumbar spine. Bone mineral density (g/cm^2) is compared with that of a young healthy adult. The 'T-score' is the number of standard deviations (SD, p751) the bone mineral density (BMD) is from the youthful average. Each decrease of 1 SD in BMD ≈ 2.6-fold ↑ in risk of hip fracture.

Table 14.5 Interpreting DEXA bone scan results

T-score >0	BMD is better than the reference.
0 to −1	BMD is in the top 84%: no evidence of osteoporosis.
−1 to −2.5	Osteopenia. Risk of later osteoporotic fracture. Offer lifestyle advice.
−2.5 or worse	Osteoporosis. Offer lifestyle advice and treatment (p682). Repeat DEXA in 2yrs.

Some indications for DEXA:

- NICE suggests DEXA if previous low-trauma fracture, or for women ≥ 65yrs with one or more risk factors for osteoporosis, or younger if two or more. The benefits of universal screening for osteoporosis remain unproven, but some authorities recommend this for men and women over 70—and earlier if risk factors are present.[17]
- DEXA is not needed pre-treatment for women over 75yrs if previous low-trauma fracture, or ≥ 2 present of rheumatoid arthritis, alcohol excess, or positive family history.
- Prior to giving long-term prednisolone (eg ≳3 months at >5mg/d). Steroids cause osteoporosis by promoting osteoclast bone resorption, ↓muscle mass, and ↓Ca^{2+} absorption from the gut.
- Men or women with osteopenia if low-trauma, non-vertebral fracture.
- Bone and bone-remodelling disorders (eg parathyroid disorders, myeloma, HIV, esp. if on protease inhibitors).

Osteoporosis risk factors: 'SHATTERED'

Steroid use of >5mg/d of prednisolone.
Hyperthyroidism, hyperparathyroidism, hypercalciuria.
Alcohol and tobacco use ↑.
Thin (BMI <18.5).
Testosterone ↓ (eg antiandrogen ca prostate ℞).
Early menopause.
Renal or liver failure.
Erosive/inflammatory bone disease (eg myeloma or rheumatoid arthritis).
Dietary ↓Ca^{2+}/malabsorption; diabetes mellitus type 1.

Metabolic bone diseases: osteomalacia

In osteomalacia, there is a normal amount of bone but its mineral content is low (there is excess uncalcified osteoid and cartilage). This is the reverse of osteoporosis in which mineralization is unchanged, but there is overall bone loss. Rickets is the result if this process occurs during the period of bone growth; osteomalacia is the result if it occurs after fusion of the epiphyses.

Signs and symptoms

Rickets: Growth retardation, hypotonia, apathy in infants. Once walking: knock-kneed, bow-legged, and deformities of the metaphyseal-epiphyseal junction (eg the rachitic rosary). Features of ↓Ca^{2+}—often mild (p678). Children with rickets are ill.

Osteomalacia: Bone pain and tenderness; fractures (esp. femoral neck); proximal myopathy (waddling gait), due to ↓PO_4^{3-} and vitamin D deficiency per se.

Causes

Vitamin D deficiency: Due to malabsorption (p266), poor diet, or lack of sunlight.

Renal osteodystrophy: Renal failure leads to 1,25-dihydroxy-cholecalciferol deficiency [1,25(OH)$_2$-vitamin D deficiency]. See also *renal bone disease* (p312).

Drug-induced: Anticonvulsants may induce liver enzymes, leading to an increased breakdown of 25-hydroxy-vitamin D.

Vitamin D resistance: A number of mainly inherited conditions in which the osteomalacia responds to high doses of vitamin D (see 'Treatment' later in this topic).

Liver disease: Due to reduced hydroxylation of vitamin D to 25-hydroxy-cholecalciferol and malabsorption of vitamin D, eg in cirrhosis (p276).

Tumour-induced osteomalacia: (Oncogenic hypophosphataemia.) Mediated by raised tumour production of phosphatonin fibroblast growth factor 23 (FGF-23) which causes hyperphosphaturia. ↓serum PO_4^{3-} often causes myalgia and weakness.[18]

Investigations

Plasma: Mildly ↓Ca^{2+} (but may be severe); ↓PO_4^{3-}; ↑ALP; PTH high; ↓25(OH)-vitamin D, except in vitamin D resistance. In renal failure, ↓1,25(OH)$_2$-vitamin D (p312).

Biopsy: Bone biopsy shows incomplete mineralization. Muscle biopsy (if proximal myopathy) is normal.

X-ray: In osteomalacia, there is a loss of cortical bone; also, apparent partial fractures without displacement may be seen especially on the lateral border of the scapula, inferior femoral neck, and medial femoral shaft (Looser's zones; see fig 14.9). Cupped, ragged metaphyseal surfaces are seen in rickets (fig 14.10).

Treatment

- In dietary insufficiency, give vitamin D, eg as one calcium D_3 forte tablet/12h PO.
- In malabsorption or hepatic disease, give vitamin D_2 (ergocalciferol), up to 40 000U (=1mg) daily, or parenteral calcitriol, eg 7.5mg monthly.
- If due to renal disease or vitamin D resistance, give alfacalcidol (1α-hydroxy-vitamin D_3) 250ng–1mcg daily, or calcitriol (1,25-dihydroxy-vitamin D_3) 250ng–1mcg daily, and adjust dose according to plasma Ca^{2+}. ►►Alfacalcidol and calcitriol can cause dangerous hypercalcaemia.
- Monitor plasma Ca^{2+}, initially weekly, and if nausea/vomiting.

Vitamin D-resistant rickets Exists in two forms. Type I has low renal 1α-hydroxylase activity, and type II has end-organ resistance to 1,25-dihydroxy-vitamin D_3, due to a point mutation in the receptor. Both are treated with large doses of calcitriol.

X-linked hypophosphataemic rickets Dominantly inherited—due to a defect in renal phosphate handling (due to mutations in the PEX or PHEX genes which encode an endopeptidase). Rickets develops in early childhood and is associated with poor growth. Plasma PO_4^{3-} is low, ALP is high, and there is phosphaturia. Treatment is with high doses of oral phosphate, and calcitriol.

Metabolic bone diseases: Paget's disease of bone

Also called *osteitis deformans*, there is increased bone turnover associated with increased numbers of osteoblasts and osteoclasts with resultant remodelling, bone enlargement, deformity, and weakness. Rare in the under-40s. Incidence rises with age (3% over 55yrs old). Commoner in temperate climates, and in Anglo-Saxons.

Clinical features Asymptomatic in ~70%. Deep, boring pain, and bony deformity and enlargement—typically of the pelvis, lumbar spine, skull, femur, and tibia (classically a bowed sabre tibia; fig 14.11). *Complications* include pathological fractures, osteoarthritis, ↑Ca^{2+}, nerve compression due to bone overgrowth (eg deafness, root compression), high-output CCF (if >40% of skeleton involved), and osteosarcoma (<1% of those affected for >10yrs—suspect if sudden onset or worsening of bone pain).[19]

Radiology X-ray Localized enlargement of bone. Patchy cortical thickening with sclerosis, osteolysis, and deformity (eg *osteoporosis circumscripta* of the skull). Affinity for axial skeleton, long bones, and skull. Bone scan may reveal 'hot spots'.

Blood chemistry Ca^{2+} and PO_4^{3-} normal; ALP markedly raised.

Treatment If analgesia fails, alendronic acid may be tried to reduce pain and/or deformity. It is more effective than etidronate or calcitonin, and as effective as IV pamidronate. Follow expert advice.

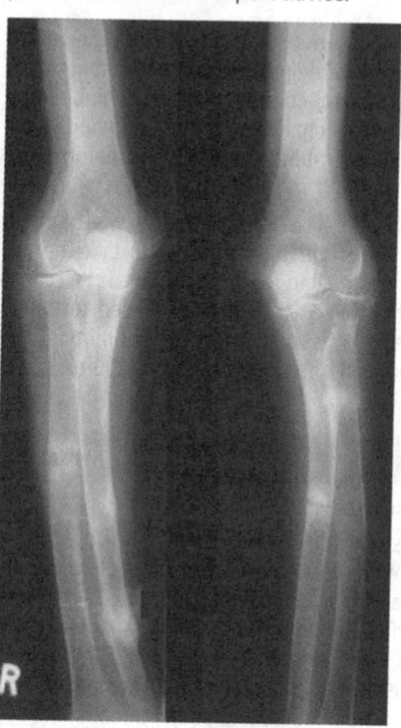

Fig 14.9 Osteomalacia. Cortical bone lucency and Looser's zones are seen in both forearms of a patient with osteomalacia.
Image courtesy of Dr Ian Maddison.

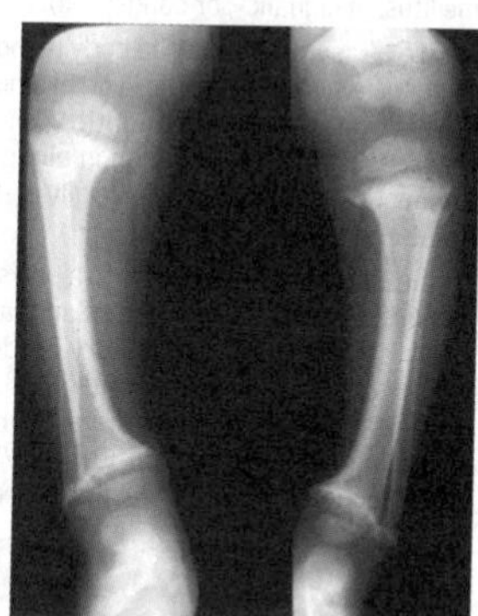

Fig 14.10 Rickets. Typical ragged metaphyseal surfaces are seen in the knee and ankle joints of a child with rickets, with bowing of the long bones.
Image courtesy of Dr Ian Maddison.

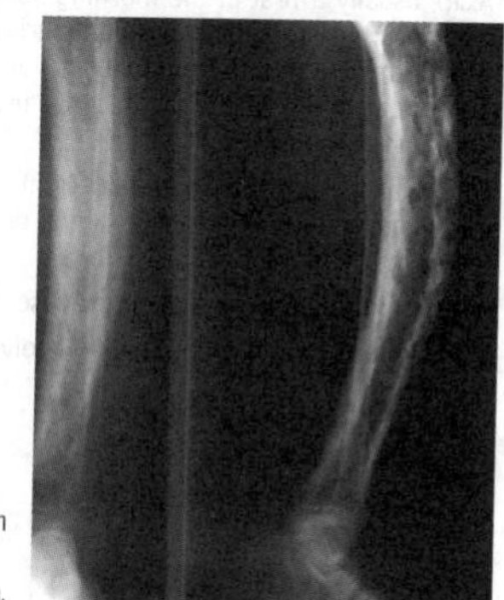

Fig 14.11 Paget's disease. The 'sabre tibia' seen in Paget's disease, with multiple sclerotic lesions.
Image courtesy of Dr Ian Maddison.

Plasma proteins

The plasma contains a number of proteins including albumin, immunoglobulins, α_1-antitrypsin, α_2-macroglobulin, caeruloplasmin, transferrin, low-density lipoprotein (LDL), fibrinogen, complement, and factor VIII. The most abundant is albumin (see fig 14.12).

Albumin Synthesized in the liver; $t\frac{1}{2}\approx 20$d. It binds bilirubin, free fatty acids, Ca^{2+}, and some drugs. *Low albumin:* Results in oedema, and is caused by: •↓*synthesis:* liver disease, acute phase response (due to ↑vascular permeability—eg sepsis, trauma, surgery), malabsorption, malnutrition, malignancy •↑*loss:* nephrotic syndrome, protein-losing enteropathy, burns •*haemodilution:* late pregnancy, artefact (eg from 'drip' arm). Also posture (↑5g/L if upright) and genetic variations. *High albumin:* Causes are dehydration; artefact (eg stasis).

Immunoglobulins (Antibodies) are synthesized by B cells. Five isoforms Ig A,D,E,G,M exist in humans, and IgG is the most abundant circulating form. *Specific monoclonal band* in paraproteinaemia (see p370). *Diffusely raised* in chronic infections, TB, bronchiectasis, liver cirrhosis, sarcoidosis, SLE, RA, Crohn's disease, 1° biliary cirrhosis, hepatitis, and parasitaemia. *Low* in nephrotic syndrome, malabsorption, malnutrition, and immune deficiency states (eg severe illness, renal failure, diabetes mellitus, malignancy, or congenital).

Acute phase response The body responds to a variety of insults with, among other things, the synthesis, by the liver, of a number of proteins (normally present in serum in small quantities)—eg α_1-antitrypsin, fibrinogen, complement, haptoglobin, and CRP. A concomitant reduction in albumin level, is characteristic of conditions such as infection, malignancy (especially α_2-fraction), trauma, surgery, and inflammatory disease.

CRP So called because it binds to a polysaccharide (fraction C) in the cell wall of pneumococci. Levels help monitor inflammation/infection (normal <8mg/L). Like the ESR, it is raised in many inflammatory conditions, but changes more rapidly. It increases in hours and begins to fall within 2-3d of recovery; thus it can be used to follow disease activity (eg Crohn's disease) or the response to therapy (eg antibiotics). CRP values in mild inflammation 10-50mg/L; active bacterial infection 50-200mg/L; severe infection or trauma >200mg/L; see table 14.6.

Urinary proteins

Urinary protein loss >150mg/d is pathological (p294).

Albuminuria Usually caused by renal disease (p294). *Microalbuminuria:* Urinary protein loss between 30 and 300mg/d (so not visible on normal dipstick) and may be seen with diabetes mellitus, ↑BP, SLE, and glomerulonephritis (see p314 for role in DM). Can also be quantified by measuring the urinary *albumin:creatinine ratio* (A:CR), usually a first-in-the-morning spot urine sample. A level >30mg/mmol indicates albuminuria, and microalbuminuria is defined as >2.5mg/mmol in men and >3.5 in women. This is a useful screening test in diabetics, and subjects with reduced eGFR. Note some labs measure total urinary protein not albumin—a P:CR of 50, is equivalent to an A:CR of 30.[20]

Bence Jones protein Consists of light chains excreted in excess by some patients with myeloma (p368). They are not detected by dipsticks and may occur with normal serum electrophoresis.

Haemoglobinuria Caused by intravascular haemolysis (p336).

Myoglobinuria Caused by rhabdomyolysis (p319).

Table 14.6 C-reactive protein (CRP)

Marked elevation	Normal-to-slight elevation
Bacterial infection	Viral infection
Abscess	Steroids/oestrogens
Crohn's disease	Ulcerative colitis
Connective tissue diseases (except SLE)	SLE
Neoplasia	Morbid obesity
Trauma	Atherosclerosis
Necrosis (eg MI)	

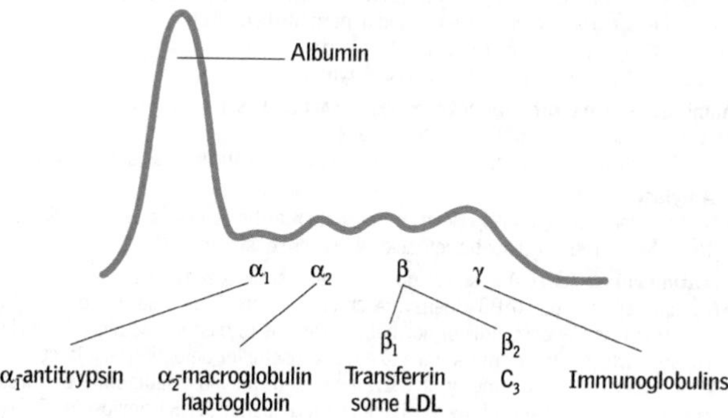

Fig 14.12 A normal electrophoretic scan.

Plasma enzymes

►Reference intervals vary between laboratories. See p752 for a guide to normal values.

Raised levels of specific enzymes can be a useful indicator of a disease. However, remember that most can be raised for other reasons too. Levels may be raised due to cellular damage, ↑cell turnover, cellular proliferation (malignancy), enzyme induction, and ↓clearance. The major causes of *raised enzymes:*

Alkaline phosphatase (Several distinguishable isoforms exist, eg liver and bone.)
- Liver disease (suggests cholestasis; also cirrhosis, abscess, hepatitis, or malignancy).
- Bone disease (isoenzyme distinguishable, reflects osteoblast activity) especially Paget's, growing children, healing fractures, bone metastases, osteomalacia, osteomyelitis, chronic kidney disease, and hyperparathyroidism.
- Congestive cardiac failure (moderately raised).
- Pregnancy (placenta makes its own isoenzyme).

Alanine and aspartate aminotransferase (ALT and AST)
- Liver disease (suggests hepatocyte damage).
- AST also ↑ in MI, skeletal muscle damage (especially crush injuries), and haemolysis.

α-Amylase
- Acute pancreatitis (smaller rise in chronic pancreatitis as less tissue remaining).
- *Also:* severe uraemia, diabetic ketoacidosis, severe gastroenteritis, and peptic ulcer.

Creatine kinase (CK) ►A raised CK does not necessarily mean an MI.
- Myocardial infarction (p118; isoenzyme 'CK-MB'. Diagnostic if CK-MB >6% of total CK, or CK-MB mass >99 percentile of normal). CK returns to baseline within 48h (unlike troponin, which remains raised for ~10 days), ∴ useful for detecting re-infarction.
- Muscle damage (rhabdomyolysis, p319; prolonged running; haematoma; seizures; IM injection; defibrillation; bowel ischaemia; myxoedema; dermatomyositis, p552)—and *drugs* (eg statins).

Gamma-glutamyl transferase (GGT, γGT)
- Liver disease (particularly alcohol-induced damage, cholestasis, drugs).

Lactate dehydrogenase (LDH)
- Myocardial infarction (p118).
- Liver disease (suggests hepatocyte damage).
- Haemolysis (esp. sickle cell crisis), pulmonary embolism, and tumour necrosis.

Troponin
- Subtypes troponin T and troponin I are used clinically.
- Cardiac damage or strain (MI—p118, pericarditis, myocarditis, PE, sepsis, CPR).
- Chronic kidney disease (troponin T only; elevation less marked; aetiology unknown).

Enzyme inducers and inhibitors

Hepatic drug metabolism is mainly by conjugation or oxidation. The oxidative pathways are catalysed by the family of cytochrome P450 isoenzymes, the most important of which is the CYP 3A4 isoenzyme. The cytochrome P450 pathway may be either induced or inhibited by a range of commonly used drugs and foods (table 14.7).

This can lead to important interactions or side-effects. For example, phenytoin reduces the effectiveness of the contraceptive pill due to more rapid oestrogen metabolism, and ciprofloxacin retards the metabolism of methylxanthines (aminophylline) which leads to higher plasma levels and potentially more side-effects. The *BNF* contains a list of the major interactions between drugs.

Table 14.7 Common inhibitors and inducers of cytochrome P450 isoenzymes

Enzyme inducers	Enzyme inhibitors	
Phenytoin	SSRIs	Amiodarone
Rifampicin	Ciprofloxacin	Diltiazem
Carbamazepine	Isoniazid	Verapamil
Alcohol	Macrolides	Omeprazole
St John's wort	HIV protease inhibitors	Grapefruit juice
Barbiturates	Imidazole and triazole antifungal agents	

Hyperlipidaemia

Lipids travel in blood packaged with proteins as lipoproteins. There are four classes: chylomicrons and VLDL (mainly triglyceride), LDL (mainly cholesterol), and HDL (mainly phospholipid) (for abbreviations see footnote[3]). The evidence that cholesterol is a major risk factor for cardiovascular disease (CVD) is undisputed ('4S' STUDY,[21] WOSCOPS,[22] CARE STUDY,[23] HEART PROTECTION STUDY[24]) and indeed it may even be the 'green light' that allows other risk factors to act.[25] Half the UK population have a serum cholesterol putting them at significant risk of CVD. HDL appears to correlate inversely with CVD.

Who to screen for hyperlipidaemia

►NB: full screening requires a fasting lipid profile.

Those at risk of hyperlipidaemia: •Family history of hyperlipidaemia. •Corneal arcus <50yrs old. •Xanthomata or xanthelasmata (fig 14.13).

Those at risk of CVD: •Known CVD. •Family history of CVD <60yrs old. •DM or impaired glucose tolerance. •Hypertension. •Smoker. •↑BMI. •Low socioeconomic or Indian Asian background.

Types of hyperlipidaemia

Common primary hyperlipidaemia: Accounts for 70% of hyperlipidaemia. ↑LDL only.

Familial primary hyperlipidaemias: Multiple phenotypes exist (see table 14.8). *Risk of ↑↑CVD*, although evidence suggests protection from CVD is achieved with lower doses of statin than for common primary hyperlipidaemia.[26] Refer to specialist.

Secondary hyperlipidaemia: Causes include: Cushing's syndrome, hypothyroidism, nephrotic syndrome, or cholestasis. ↑LDL. Treat the cause first.

Mixed hyperlipidaemia: Results in ↑ in both LDL and triglycerides. Caused by type 2 diabetes mellitus, metabolic syndrome, alcohol abuse, and chronic renal failure.

Management

Identify familial or 2° hyperlipidaemias, as ℞ may differ. Give lifestyle advice; aim for BMI of 20–25; encourage a Mediterranean-style diet—↑fruit, vegetables, fish, unsaturated fats; and ↓red meat; ↑exercise. Top ℞ priority are those with known CVD (there is no need to calculate their risk: *ipso facto* they already have high risk). Second ℞ priority is primary prevention in patients with chronic kidney disease or type-1 diabetes, and those with a 10-yr risk of CVD >10%, *irrespective of baseline lipid levels*.

- *1st-line therapy:* Atorvastatin 20mg PO at night, for primary prevention, and 80mg for secondary prevention and primary prevention in those with kidney disease.[27] Simvastatin 40mg, is an alternative. ↓cholesterol synthesis in the liver by inhibiting HMGCOA reductase. CI: porphyria, cholestasis, pregnancy. SE: myalgia ± myositis (stop if ↑CK ≥10-fold; if any myalgia, check CK; risk is 1 per 100 000 treatment-years),[28] abdominal pain, and ↑LFTs (stop if AST ≥100U/L). Cytochrome P450 inhibitors (p689) ↑serum concentrations (200mL of grapefruit juice ↑simvastatin concentration by 300%, and atorvastatin ↑80%, but pravastatin is almost unchanged).Current guidelines suggest a target plasma cholesterol reduction of ≥40 % in those with CVD.
- *2nd-line therapy:* Ezetimibe—a cholesterol absorption inhibitor, may be used in statin intolerance or combination with statins to achive target reduction.
- *3rd-line therapy:* Alirocumab—a monoclonal antibody against PCSK9 (acts to reduce hepatocyte LDL receptor expression). Very effective in reducing LDL,[29] but expensive and needs to be given by injection every 2 weeks. Others: fibrates, eg bezafibrate (useful in mixed hyperlipidaemias); anion exchange resins, eg colestyramine; nicotinic acid (↑HDL; ↓LDL; SE: severe flushes; aspirin 300mg ½h pre-dose helps this).
- *Hypertriglyceridaemia:* Responds best to fibrates, nicotinic acid, or fish oil.

Xanthomata These yellow lipid deposits may be: *eruptive* (itchy nodules in crops in hypertriglyceridaemia); *tuberous* (plaques on elbows and knees); or *planar*—also called palmar (orange streaks in palmar creases), 'diagnostic' of remnant hyperlipidaemia; or in tendons (p38), eyelids (*xanthelasma*, see fig 14.13), or cornea (*arcus*, p39)

3 Abbreviations: (V)LDL = (very) low-density lipoprotein; IDL = intermediate-density lipoprotein; HDL = high-density lipoprotein; chol = cholesterol; trig = trigylcerides.

Primary hyperlipidaemias

Table 14.8 Classification of primary hyperlipidaemias

Familial hyperchylomicronaemia (lipoprotein lipase deficiency or apoCII deficiency)[I]	Chol <6.5 Trig 10–30 Chylomicrons ↑		Eruptive xanthomata; lipaemia retinalis; hepatosplenomegaly
Familial hypercholesterolaemia[II] (LDL receptor defects)	Chol 7.5–16 Trig <2.3	↑LDL	Tendon xanthoma; corneal arcus; xanthelasma
Familial defective apolipoprotein B-100[IIa]	Chol 7.5–16 Trig <2.3	↑LDL	Tendon xanthoma; arcus; xanthelasma
Common hypercholesterolaemia[IIa]	Chol 6.5–9 Trig <2.3	↑LDL	*The commonest 1° lipidaemia*; may have xanthelasma or arcus
Familial combined hyperlipidaemia[IIb, IV, OR V]	Chol 6.5–10 Trig 2.3–12	↑LDL ↑VLDL ↓HDL	*Next commonest 1° lipidaemia*; xanthelasma; arcus
Dysbetalipoproteinaemia (remnant particle disease)[III]	Chol 9–14 Trig 9–14	↑IDL ↓HDL ↓LDL	Palmar striae; tubero-eruptive xanthoma
Familial hypertriglyceridaemia[IV]	Chol 6.5–12 Trig 3.0–6.0	↑VLDL	
Type V hyperlipoproteinaemia	Trig 10–30; chylomicrons found		Eruptive xanthomata; lipaemia retinalis; hepatosplenomegaly

Blue superscript numbers = WHO phenotype; chol/trig levels given in mmol/L.

Primary HDL abnormalities:

- Hyperalphalipoproteinaemia: ↑HDL, chol >2.
- Hypoalphalipoproteinaemia (Tangier disease): ↓HDL, chol <0.92.

Primary LDL abnormalities:

- Abetalipoproteinaemia (ABL): trig <0.3, chol <1.3, missing LDL, VLDL, and chylomicrons. Autosomal recessive disorder of fat malabsorption causing vitamin A & E deficiency, with retinitis pigmentosa, sensory neuropathy, ataxia, pes cavus, and acanthocytosis.
- Hypobetalipoproteinaemia: chol <1.5, ↓LDL, ↓HDL. Autosomal codominant disorder of apolipoprotein B metabolism. ↑longevity in heterozygotes. Homozygotes present with a similar clinical picture to ABL.

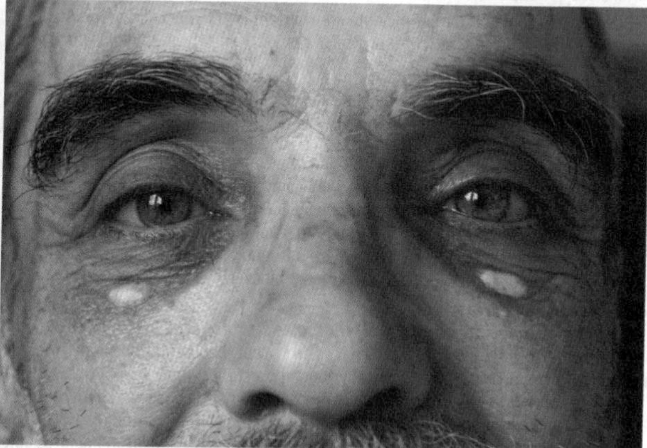

Fig 14.13 Xanthelasma. *Xanthos* is Greek for yellow, and *elasma* means plate. Xanthelasmata are lipid-laden yellow plaques, typically a few millimetres wide. They congregate around the lids, or just below the eyes, and signify hyperlipidaemia.

The porphyrias

The porphyrias are a heterogenous group of rare diseases caused by various errors of haem biosynthesis (produced when iron is chelated into protoporphyrin IXα), which may be genetic or acquired. Depending on the stage in haem biosynthesis that is faulty, there is accumulation of either porphyrinogens, which are unstable and oxidize to porphyrins, or their precursors, porphobilinogen and δ-aminolaevulinic acid. Porphyrin precursors are neurotoxic, while porphyrins themselves induce photosensitivity and the formation of toxic free radicals.

- Alcohol, lead, and iron deficiency cause abnormal porphyrin metabolism.
- Genetic counselling (*OHCS* p154) should be offered to all patients and their families.

Acute porphyrias Occur when the accumulation of porphyrinogen precursors predominates, and are characterized by acute neurovisceral crises, though some forms have additional photosensitive cutaneous manifestations.

Acute intermittent porphyria: ('*The Madness of King George*.') A low-penetrant autosomal dominant condition (porphobilinogen deaminase gene); 28% have no family history (*de novo* mutations). ~10% of those with the defective gene have neurovisceral symptoms. Attacks are intermittent, more common in women and those aged 18–40, and may be precipitated by drugs. Urine porphobilinogens are raised during attacks (the urine may go deep red on standing) and also, in ~50%, between attacks. Faecal porphyrin levels are normal. There is never cutaneous photosensitivity. It is the commonest form of porphyria—prevalence in UK: 1-2/100 000.

Variegate porphyria and hereditary coproporphyria: Autosomal dominant, characterized by photosensitive blistering skin lesions and/or acute attacks. The former is prevalent in Afrikaners in South Africa. Porphobilinogen is high only during an attack, and other metabolites may be detected in faeces.

Triggers of an acute attack: Include infection, starvation (including pre-operative 'nil-by-mouth'), reproductive hormones (pregnancy, premenstrual), smoking, anaesthesia, and cytochrome P450 enzyme inducers (alcohol, and other drugs—see BOX).

Features of an acute attack:

- *Gastrointestinal:* abdominal pain, vomiting, constipation.
- *Neuropsychiatric:* peripheral neuropathy (weakness, hypotonia, pain, numbness), seizures (often associated with severe ↓Na^+), psychosis (or other odd behaviour).[4]
- *Cardiovascular:* hypertension, tachycardia, shock (due to sympathetic overactivity).
- *Other:* fever, ↓Na^+, ↓K^+, proteinuria, urinary porphobilinogens, discoloured urine. Rare but serious complications include bulbar and respiratory paralysis.

►►Beware the 'acute abdomen' in acute intermittent porphyria: colic, vomiting, fever, and ↑WCC—so mimicking an acute surgical abdomen. Anaesthesia could be disastrous.

Treatment of an acute attack:

- Remove precipitants (review medications; treat intercurrent illness/infection).
- IV fluids to correct electrolyte imbalance.
- High carbohydrate intake (eg Hycal®) by NG tube, or IV if necessary.
- IV haematin is 1st-line (inhibits production of porphyrinogen precursors).
- Nausea controlled with prochlorperazine 12.5mg IM.
- Sedate if necessary with chlorpromazine 50–100mg PO/IM.
- Pain control with opiate or opioid analgesia (avoid oxycodone).
- Seizures can be controlled with diazepam (although this will prolong the attack).
- Treat tachycardia and hypertension with a β-blocker.

Non-acute porphyrias

Porphyria cutanea tarda (PCT), *erythropoietic protoporphyria,* and *congenital erythropoietic porphyria* are characterized by cutaneous photosensitivity alone, as there is no overproduction of porphyrinogen precursors, only porphyrins. PCT presents in adults with blistering skin lesions ± facial hypertrichosis and hyperpigmentation. Total plasma porphyrins and LFTs are ↑. Screen for associated disorders: hep C, HIV, iron overload, hepatocellular ca. ℞: phlebotomy, iron chelators, chloroquine, sunscreens.

Drugs to avoid in acute intermittent porphyria

There are many, many drugs that may precipitate an acute attack ± quadriplegia, and this is by no means an exhaustive list (see *BNF/Oxford Textbook of Medicine*).

►► For an up-to-date list of drugs considered safe in acute porphyria see www.wmic.wales.nhs.uk/porphyria-safe-list-may-2016/

- Diclofenac
- Alcohol
- Oral contraceptive pill & HRT
- Tricyclic antidepressants
- Benzodiazepines
- Anaesthetic agents (barbiturates, halothane)
- Antibiotics (cephalosporins, sulfonamides, macrolides, tetracyclines, rifampicin, trimethoprim, chloramphenicol, metronidazole)
- Metoclopramide
- ACE-inhibitors
- Ca^{2+}-channel blockers
- Statins
- Anticonvulsants
- Furosemide
- Sulfonylureas
- Lidocaine
- Gold salts
- Antihistamines
- Amphetamines.

4 Be sure I looked at her eyes
Happy and proud; at last I knew
Porphyria worshipped me; surprise
Made my heart swell, and still it grew
While I debated what to do.
That moment she was mine, mine, fair,
Perfectly pure and good: I found
A thing to do, and all her hair
In one long yellow string I wound
Three times her little throat around,
And strangled her ...

From *Porphyria's Lover* by Robert Browning.

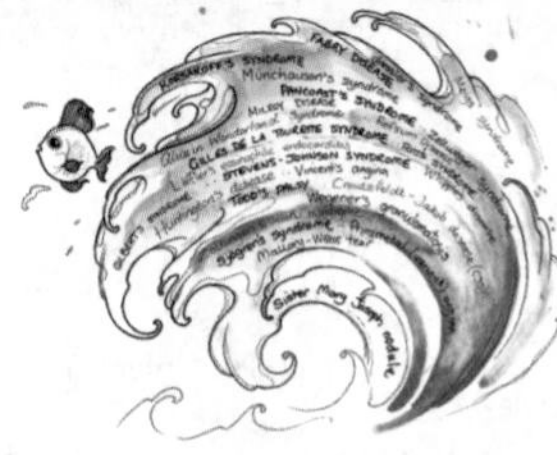

Fig 15.1 'No scientific discovery is named after its original discoverer', asserts Professor Stephen Stigler in '*Stigler's Law of Eponymy*', and in doing so, names the sociologist RK Merton as its discoverer—deliberately making Stigler's law exemplify itself. Is the same true in medicine? At least six others described Alzheimer's disease before Alois Alzheimer in 1906, and Tetralogy of Fallot (named after Étienne-Louis Fallot in 1888) was first described in 1672 by Niels Stenson. Not all medical eponyms obey Stigler's law. Forty years after it was first described, the French neurologist Jean-Marie Charcot (himself associated with at least 15 medical eponyms) attributed the name 'Parkinson's Disease' to the illness outlined in James Parkinson's 1817 essay '*The Shaking Palsy*'. Monochromatic doctors may try to abolish eponyms by regimenting them to histologically driven disease titles. But classifications vary as facts emerge, and as a result the renaming of non-eponyms becomes essential. Eponyms, however, carry on forever, because they imply nothing about causes.

Alice in Wonderland syndrome Altered perception in size and shape of body parts or objects ± an impaired sense of passing time—as experienced by *Alice* in Lewis Carroll's novel. Seen in epilepsy, migraine, and cerebral lesions.[1,2] *Alice Pleasance Liddell, 1865–1934*

Arnold-Chiari malformation Malformed cerebellar tonsils and medulla herniate through the foramen magnum. This may cause infantile hydrocephalus with mental retardation, optic atrophy, ocular palsies, and spastic paresis of the limbs. Spina bifida, syringomyelia (p516), or focal cerebellar and brainstem signs may occur (p499). There may be bony abnormalities of the base of the skull. Often presents in early adulthood. MRI aids diagnosis. *Julius Arnold, 1835–1915 (German pathologist); Hans Chiari, 1851–1916 (Austrian pathologist)*

Baker's cyst Fluid from a knee effusion escapes to form a popliteal cyst (often swollen and painful) in a sub-gastrocnemius bursa.[3] Usually secondary to degeneration. *ΔΔ:* DVT (exclude if calf swelling); sarcoma. *Imaging:* USS; MRI. *℞:* None if asymptomatic. NSAIDs/ice if painful. Spontaneous resolution may take 10–20 months. Arthroscopy + cystectomy may be needed. *William M Baker, 1838–1896 (British surgeon)*

Bazin's disease (*Erythema induratum.*) Localized areas of fat necrosis that produce painful, firm nodules ± ulceration and an indurated rash, characteristically on adolescent girls' calves. It is associated with TB. *Nodular vasculitis* is a variant unrelated to TB.[4] *Pierre-Antoine-Ernest Bazin, 1807–1878 (French dermatologist)*

Behçet's disease A systemic inflammatory disorder of unknown cause, associated with HLA-B5. It is most common along the old Silk Road, from the Mediterranean to China. *Features:* Recurrent oral and genital ulceration, uveitis, skin lesions (eg erythema nodosum, papulopustular lesions); arthritis (non-erosive large joint oligoarthropathy); thrombophlebitis; vasculitis; myo/pericarditis; CNS involvement (pyramidal signs); and colitis. *Diagnosis:* Mainly clinical. *Pathergy test:* needle prick leads to papule formation within 48hrs. *℞:* Colchicine for orogenital ulceration; steroids, azathioprine/cyclophosphamide for systemic disease. Infliximab has a role in ocular disease unresponsive to topical steroids.[5] *Hulusi Behçet, 1889–1948 (Turkish dermatologist)*

Berger's disease (*IgA nephropathy*, p311.) Ranges from invisible haematuria to rapidly progressive glomerulonephritis. Biopsy shows mesangial IgA deposition. Usually indolent disease, but progression to end-stage renal failure occurs. *℞:* ACE-i/ARB if ↑BP or proteinuria. Immunosuppression considered for progressive disease.[6] *Jean Berger, 1930–2011 (French nephrologist)*

Bickerstaff's brainstem encephalitis Ophthalmoplegia, ataxia, areflexia, and extensor plantars ± tetraplegia ± coma, and a *reversible* brain death picture (but there is *no* structural damage). *MRI:* hyperintense brainstem signals. GQ1b antibodies +ve.[7] Plasmapheresis may help. *Edwin R Bickerstaff, 1920–2008 (British physician)*

We thank Dr Simon Eyre, our Specialist Reader, for his contribution to this chapter.

Barrett's oesophagus

Barrett's oesophagus is metaplasia of the normal stratified squamous epithelium of the distal oesophagus to a columnar epithelium, as a result of chronic GORD (p254). Estimates of prevalence vary widely, but in patients with a history of symptomatic GORD, rates of ≈8% have been reported. Importantly, screening studies in *asymptomatic* individuals have reported rates of ≈6%. General population-based screening is not recommended, although screening endoscopy may be considered in individuals with chronic GORD symptoms and *multiple* risk factors (>50 years old, obesity, ♂, white race, family history of Barrett's or oesophageal adenocarcinoma). *Diagnosis:* Biopsy of endoscopically visible columnarization allows histological corroboration. The length should be recorded (using the Prague classification). *Management:* ►Focus on detecting and preventing the most significant associated morbidity: oesophageal adenocarcinoma. The risk of progression is low (0.1–0.4% per patient per year, much lower than previously suggested). Risk factors for malignant transformation include ↑age, ♂, long segment of oesophagus involved, and evidence of dysplasia. Endoscopic surveillence for dysplasia is controversial and the evidence base is lacking. Current guidelines suggest that patients without dysplasia and in whom the length of involved oesophagus is <3cm should be considered for discharge from surveillance programmes, depending on the precise histology.[8] For those with more extensive disease, endoscopic assessment every 2–3 years is appropriate. If high-grade dysplasia or intramural carcinoma is detected, ***endoscopic resection*** or mucosal radiofrequency ablation (RFA) is recommended. If low-grade dysplasia is detected, it should be confirmed by repeat examination after 6 months and by an independent pathologist, prior to RFA.[9]

Norman Rupert Barrett, 1903–1979 (British surgeon)

Brugada syndrome

Note right bundle branch block and the unusual morphology of the raised ST segments in V_1–V_3 (fig 15.2; there are three ECG variants of this pattern). This predominently autosomal dominant condition causing faulty sodium channels predisposes to fatal arrhythmias (eg ventricular fibrillation), typically in young males (eg triggered by a fever).[10] It is preventable by implanting a defibrillator. ►*Consider primary electrical cardiac disease in all with unexplained syncope.* Programmed electrical stimulation may be needed. Relatives of those with sudden unexplained death may undergo unmasking of arrhythmias by IV ajmaline tests—but some results are false +ve. Use judgement in subjecting those with ST abnormalities but no symptoms to electrophysiological tests, right ventricular myocardial biopsy, and MRI. Mutations in the SCN5A gene (encodes the cardiac voltage-gated $Na_v1.5$ channel) are found in 15–20%. Other mutations have also been described.[11]

Pedro & Josep Brugada, described 1992 (Spanish cardiologists).

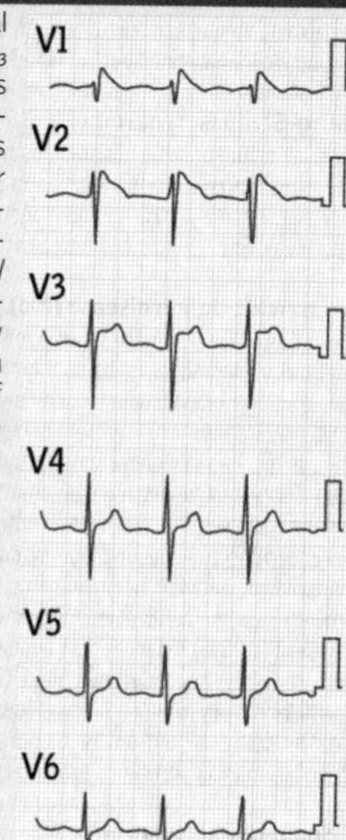

Fig 15.2 Note right bundle branch block and ST morphology in leads V_{1-3}.

Courtesy of Dr Shayashi.

Brown-Séquard syndrome A lesion in one half of the spinal cord (due to hemisection or unilateral cord lesion) causes: •Ipsilateral UMN weakness below the lesion (severed corticospinal tract, causing spastic paraparesis, brisk reflexes, extensor plantars). •Ipsilateral loss of proprioception and vibration (dorsal column severed). •Contralateral loss of pain and temperature sensation (severed spinothalamic tract which has crossed over; fig 10.35 p516). *Causes:* Bullet, stab, tumour, disc hernia, myelitis,[12] septic emboli. *Imaging:* MRI. *Charles-Édouard Brown-Séquard, 1817-1894 (Mauritian neurologist)*

Budd-Chiari syndrome Hepatic vein obstruction by thrombosis or tumour causes congestive ischaemia and hepatocyte damage. Abdominal pain, hepatomegaly, ascites, and ↑ALT occur. Portal hypertension occurs in chronic forms. *Causes:* Include hypercoagulable states (combined OCP, pregnancy, malignancy, paroxysmal nocturnal haemoglobinuria, polycythaemia, thrombophilia), TB, liver, renal, or adrenal tumour. *Tests:* USS + Dopplers, CT, or MRI. Angioplasty or a transjugular intrahepatic portosystemic shunt (TIPSS) may be needed. Anticoagulate (lifelong) unless there are varices. Consider liver transplant in fulminant hepatic necrosis or cirrhosis.[13]

George Budd, 1808-1882 (British physician); Hans Chiari, 1851-1916 (Austrian pathologist)

Buerger's disease (*Thromboangiitis obliterans.*) Non-atherosclerotic smoking-related inflammation and thrombosis of veins and middle-sized arteries causing thrombophlebitis and ischaemia (→ulcers, gangrene). *Cause:* Unknown. Stopping smoking is vital. Most patients are men aged 20-45yrs (see BOX 'Poisoning your boss'). *Leo Buerger, 1879-1943 (US physician)*

Caplan's syndrome Multiple lung nodules in coal workers with RA, caused by an inflammatory reaction to anthracite (also associated with silica or asbestos exposure). CXR: bilateral peripheral nodules (0.5-5cm). ΔΔ: TB. *Anthony Caplan, 1907-1976 (British physician)*

Charcot-Marie-Tooth syndrome (*Peroneal muscular atrophy.*) This inherited neuropathy starts in puberty with weak legs and foot drop + variable loss of sensation and reflexes. The peroneal muscles atrophy, leading to an inverted champagne bottle appearance. Atrophy of hand and arm muscles also occurs. The most common form, CMT1A (PMP22 myelin gene mutation on chr. 17), has AD inheritance. Quality of life is good; *total* incapacity rare. Hand pain/paraesthesiae may respond to nerve release.

Jean-Marie Charcot, 1825-1893; Pierre Marie, 1853-1940 (French neurologists); Howard H Tooth, 1856-1926 (British physician)

Churg-Strauss syndrome *(Eosinophilic granulomatosis with polyangiitis.)* A triad of adult-onset asthma, eosinophilia, and vasculitis (± vasospasm ± MI ± DVT), affecting lungs, nerves, heart, and skin. A septic-shock picture/systemic inflammatory response syndrome may occur (with glomerulonephritis/renal failure, esp. if ANCA +ve). ℞: Steroids; biological agents if refractory disease, eg rituximab.[14]

Jacob Churg, 1910-2005; Lotte Strauss, 1913-1985 (US pathologists)

Creutzfeldt-Jakob disease (CJD) The cause is a prion (PrPSc), a misfolded form of a normal protein (PrPc), that can transform other proteins into prion proteins (hence its infectivity). ↑PrPSc leads to spongiform changes (tiny cavities ± tubulovesicular structures) in the brain.[15] Most cases are *sporadic* (incidence: 1-3/million/yr). *Variant* CJD (vCJD; ≈225 cases worldwide)[16] is transmitted via contaminated CNS tissue affected by bovine spongiform encephalopathy (BSE) (see BOX 'Signs that may distinguish variant CJD'). *Inherited forms:* (eg Gerstmann-Sträussler-Scheinker syndrome, P102L mutation in PRNP gene with ataxia ± self-mutilation), the 'normal' protein is too unstable, readily transforming to PrPSc. *Iatrogenic causes:* Contaminated surgical instruments, corneal transplants, growth hormone from human pituitaries, and blood (vCJD only).[17] Prion protein resists sterilization. *Signs:* Progressive dementia, focal CNS signs, myoclonus (present in 95%),[18] depression, eye signs (diplopia, supranuclear palsies, complex visual disturbances, homonymous field defects, hallucinations, cortical blindness).[19] *Tests:* Tonsil/olfactory mucosa biopsy;[20] CSF gel electrophoresis; MRI. *Treatment:* None proven. Death occurs in ~6 months in sporadic CJD (a little slower in variant CJD). *Prevention:* Regulations to ↓spread of BSE and transmission to humans + ↓iatrogenic transmission.

Hans G Creutzfeldt, 1885-1964 (German pathologist); Alfons M Jakob 1884-1931 (German neurologist)

ABC

Crigler-Najjar syndrome Two rare syndromes of inherited unconjugated hyperbilirubinaemia presenting in the 1st days of life with jaundice ± CNS signs. *Cause:* Mutation in UGT enzyme activity causing absent (type 1) or impaired (type 2; mild) ability to excrete bilirubin. ℞: T1: phototherapy and plasmapheresis to control jaundice; liver transplant before irreversible kernicterus (*OHCS* p115) develops.[21] T2: usually no ℞ needed. *John F Crigler 1919-2002; Victor A Najjar b1914 (US paediatricians)*

Signs that may distinguish variant CJD from sporadic CJD (sCJD)

- An earlier age at presentation (median 29yrs vs 60yrs in sporadic CJD).
- Longer survival and later dementia (median 14 months vs 4 for sporadic CJD).
- Psychiatric features are an early sign (anxiety, withdrawal, apathy, agitation, a permanent look of fear in the eyes, depression, personality change, insomnia). Hallucinations and delusions may occur—before akinetic mutism.
- Painful sensory symptoms are commoner (eg foot pain hyperaesthesia).
- More normal EEG (sporadic CJD has a characteristic spike and wave pattern).
- Mean CSF tau-pT181/tau protein ratio is 10-fold higher in vCJD than in sCJD.[22]
- Homozygosity for methionine at codon 129 of the PRP gene is typical.

Fame and infamy in the search for lost youth

After his neurological experiments, Brown-Séquard, the most visionary of all neuroanatomists and the grandfather of HRT, proclaimed he had found the secret of perpetual youth after injecting himself with a concoction of testicular blood, semen, and testicular extracts from dogs and guinea pigs. In the 1880s, over 12 000 doctors were queuing up to use his special extracts on patients, which he gave away free, provided results were reported back to him. 314 out of 405 cases of spinal syphilis improved, and his own urinary flow rate rose by 25%. Endocrinologists never forgave him for bringing their science into disrepute. To this day, no one really knows if his (literally) seminal work has given us anything of any practical value. But he might be pleased to know that testosterone is now known to have the urodynamic benefits he anticipated, at least in men with hypogonadism.[23]

Like many brilliant men, he had a cruel streak, backing clitoridectomy for preventing blindness and other imaginary complications of 'masturbatory melancholia'. Had he not been blinded by 19th-century ideas about female sexuality, could he have found a marvellous use for his concoctions, for 21st-century 'hypoactive sexual desire disorder'? Possibly, but only if he relied on placebo responses.[24,25]

Poisoning your boss

In 1931, Buerger's disease caused gangrene in the toes of Harvey Cushing (p224)—the most cantankerous (and greatest) neurosurgeon ever. He had to be wheeled to the operating theatre to carry on his brilliant art (and to continue terrifying his assistants).[26] He had to retire partially, whereupon his colleagues presented him with a magnificent silver cigarette box, containing 2000 cigarettes (to which he was addicted)—one for each brain tumour he had removed during his long career, so verifying the truth that although we owe everything to our teachers, we must eventually kill them to move out from under their shadow.[1]

Why bother studying rare diseases? The Liberski imperative...

For centuries, kuru was no bigger than a man's hand; a cloud barely visible on our horizon; a rare disease in cannibals beyond the Pacific. But meticulous work on kuru led to knowledge of prion diseases *before* the 1990s epidemic of vCJD. If in the 1950s, Gajdusek and Zigas had not been intrigued as to why kuru affected women and children more than men (their strange neural diet was the culprit), the discovery of vCJD would have been delayed, as no surveillance would have been in place. Neural tissue might still be in our food chain, with dreadful consequences. But further than this, the notion of 'protein-misfolding diseases'[2] would have been delayed by decades. So this is the lesson: ►*let curiosity flourish*. This is Liberski's imperative.[27] So now let's scan our horizon for other intriguing clouds.

ABC

1 *Der Vogel kämpft sich aus dem Ei. Das Ei ist die Welt. Wer geboren werden will, muss eine Welt zerstören*. The bird struggles out of the egg. The egg is the world. Whoever will be born, must first destroy a world. (Hermann Hesse. *Demian*; 1917.)

2 Cystic fibrosis (misfolded CFTR protein), Marfan's (misfolded fibrillin),[28] Fabry (misfolded α-galactosidase), Gaucher's (misfolded β-glucocerebrosidase), retinitis pigmentosa 3 (misfolded rhodopsin); some cancers may be caused by misfolding of tumour suppressor proteins (von Hippel–Lindau protein).

Devic's syndrome (*Neuromyelitis optica*; NMO.) Inflammatory demyelination causes attacks of optic neuritis ± myelitis.[29] Abnormal CSF (may mimic bacterial meningitis) and serum anti-AQP4 antibody (in 65%) help distinguish it from MS[30] (**table 15.1**). *R*: IV steroids; plasma exchange. Azathioprine and rituximab[31] help prevent relapses. ***Prognosis:*** Variable; complete remission may occur. *Eugène Devic, 1858-1930 (French neurologist)*

Dressler's syndrome This develops 2-10wks after an MI, heart surgery (or even pacemaker insertion). It is thought that myocardial injury stimulates formation of autoantibodies against heart muscle. ***Symptoms:*** Recurrent fever and chest pain ± pleural or pericardial rub (from serositis). Cardiac tamponade may occur, so avoid anticoagulants. *R*: Aspirin, NSAIDs, or steroids. *William Dressler, 1890-1969 (US cardiologist)*

Dubin-Johnson syndrome There is defective hepatocyte excretion of conjugated bilirubin. Typically presents in late teens with intermittent jaundice ± hepatosplenomegaly (autosomal recessive). ***Tests:*** ↑Bilirubin; ALT and AST are normal; bilirubinuria on dipstick; ↑ratio of urinary coproporphyrin I to III. Liver biopsy: diagnostic pigment granules.[32] *R*: Usually none needed. *Isadore N Dubin, 1913-1981; Frank B Johnson, b1919 (US pathologists)*

Dupuytren's contracture (fig 15.3) Progressive shortening and thickening of the palmar fascia causing finger contracture and loss of extension (often 5th finger). ***Prevalence:*** ~10% of ♂ >65yrs (↑ if +ve family history). ***Associations:*** Smoking, alcohol use, heavy manual labour, trauma, DM, phenytoin, HIV. Peyronie's may coexist (p708). It is thought to be caused by local hypoxia. *R*: Collagenase injections.[33] Surgery may be needed. *Baron Guillaume Dupuytren, 1777-1835 (French surgeon, famed also for treating Napoleon's haemorrhoids)*

Ekbom's syndrome (*Restless legs*.) Criteria: **1** Compelling desire to move legs. **2** Worse at night. **3** Relieved by movement. **4** Unpleasant leg sensations (eg shootings or tinglings) worse at rest. ***Mechanism:*** Endogenous opioid system fault causes altered central processing of pain. ***Prevalence:*** 1-3%. ♀:♂≈2:1. ***Associations:*** Iron deficiency, uraemia, pregnancy, DM, polyneuropathy, RA, COPD. ***Exclude:*** Cramps, positional discomfort, and local leg pathology. *R*: Dopamine agonists are commonly used; also, anticonvulsants, opioids, and benzodiazepines.[34]

Karl Axel Ekbom, 1907-1977 (Swedish neurologist)

Fabry disease X-linked lysosomal storage disorder caused by abnormalities in the GLA gene, leading to a deficiency in α-galactosidase A. There is accumulation of glycosphingolipids in skin (angiokeratoma classically in a 'swimming trunk' distribution), eyes (corneal verticillata), heart (hypertrophy, mitral valve prolapse, dilated aortic root, arrhythmias, angina), kidneys (renal failure, p320), CNS (stroke) and nerves (neuropathy/acroparaesthesia). Prior to enzyme replacement, premature death in the 6th decade was due to CV and renal disease. *R*: Enzyme replacement therapy with α or β human agalsidase.[35] *Johannes Fabry, 1860-1930 (German dermatologist)*

Fanconi anaemia Autosomal recessive, defective stem cell repair & chromosomal fragility leads to aplastic anaemia, ↑risk of AML and breast ca (BRCA2), skin pigmentation, absent radii, short stature, microcephaly, syndactyly, deafness, ↓IQ, hypopituitarism, and cryptorchidism. *R*: Stem-cell transplant. *Guido Fanconi, 1892-1979 (Swiss paediatrician)*

Felty's syndrome A triad of rheumatoid arthritis + ↓WCC + splenomegaly (±hypersplenism, causing anaemia and ↓platelets), recurrent infections, skin ulcers, and lymphadenopathy. 95% are Rh factor +ve. Splenectomy may raise the WCC. *R*: DMARDs (p547) ± *rituximab* if refractory.[36] *Augustus Roi Felty, 1895-1964 (US physician)*

ABC

Fitz-Hugh-Curtis syndrome Liver capsule inflammation causing RUQ pain due to transabdominal spread of chlamydial or gonococcal infection, often with PID ± 'violin-string' adhesions. *R*: Antibiotics for PID (+ treat sexual partners) ± laparoscopic division of adhesions. *Thomas Fitz-Hugh, 1894-1963 (US physician); Arthur H Curtis, 1881-1955 (US gynaecologist)*

Foster Kennedy syndrome Optic atrophy of one eye due to optic nerve compression (most commonly from an olfactory groove meningioma), with papilloedema of the other eye secondary to ↑ICP. There is also central scotoma and anosmia.

Robert Foster Kennedy, 1884-1952 (British neurologist)

Friedreich's ataxia Expansions of the trinucleotide repeat GAA in the frataxin gene (recessive) causes degeneration of many nerve tracts: spinocerebellar tracts degenerate causing cerebellar ataxia, dysarthria, nystagmus, and dysdiadochokinesis. Loss of corticospinal tracts occurs (weakness and extensor plantar response) with peripheral

Devic's syndrome and multiple sclerosis

Table 15.1 Distinguishing Devic's syndrome from multiple sclerosis

	Devic's syndrome	Multiple sclerosis
Course	Monophasic or relapsing	Relapsing usually; see p496
Attack severity	Usually severe	Often mild
Respiratory failure	~30%, from cervical myelitis	Rare
MRI head	Usually normal	Many periventricular white-matter lesions
MRI cord lesions	Longitudinal, central	Multiple, small, peripheral
CSF oligoclonal bands	Absent	Present
Permanent disability	Unusual, and attack-related	In late progressive disease
Other autoimmunities	In ≤50% (eg Sjögren's)	Uncommon

Diagnostic criteria for Devic's Optic neuritis, myelitis, and ≥2 out of 3 of: •MRI evidence of a continuous cord lesion for ≥3 segments. •Brain MRI at onset non-diagnostic for MS. •NMO-IgG (anti-AQP4) serum or CSF positivity (poorer prognosis). NB: CNS involvement beyond the optic nerves and cord is compatible with NMO.

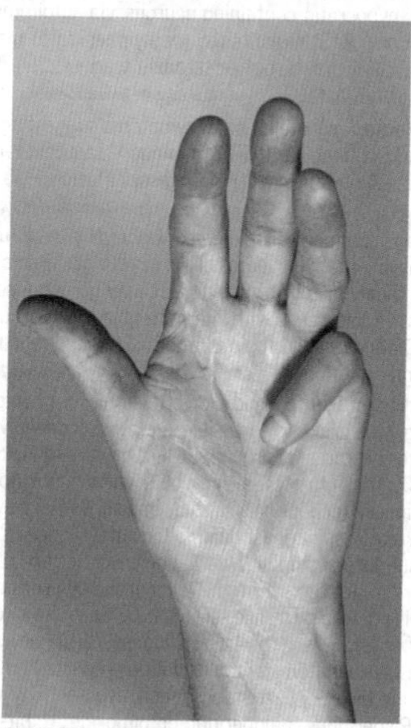

Fig 15.3 Dupuytren's contracture of the 5th finger. Note scar from previous surgery to the index finger.

nerve damage, so tendon reflexes are paradoxically depressed (differential diagnosis p446). There is also dorsal column degeneration, with loss of positional and vibration sense. Pes cavus and scoliosis occur. Cardiomyopathy may cause CCF. Typical age at death: ~50yrs. ℞: There is no cure. Treat CCF, arrhythmias, and DM.

Nikolaus Friedreich, 1825–1882 (German neurologist)

Froin's syndrome ↑ CSF protein + xanthochromia with normal cell count—a sign of blockage in spinal CSF flow (eg from a spinal tumour). *Georges Froin, 1874–1932 (French physician)*

Gardner's syndrome A dominant variant of familial adenomatous polyposis, caused by mutations in the APC gene (5q21). There are multiple colon polyps (which inevitably become malignant; p520),[37] benign bone osteomas, epidermal cysts, dermoid tumours, fibromas, and neurofibromas. *Fundoscopy* reveals black spots (congenital hypertrophy of retinal pigment epithelium); this helps pre-symptomatic detection. *Presentation:* Can present from 2–70yrs with colonic (eg bloody diarrhoea) or extracolonic symptoms. Prophylactic surgery (eg proctocolectomy) is the only curative treatment. Endoscopic polypectomy with long-term celecoxib therapy has been used to postpone prophylactic colectomy.[38] *Eldon J Gardner, 1909–1989 (US physician)*

Gélineau's syndrome (*Narcolepsy.*) The patient, usually a young man, succumbs to irresistible attacks of inappropriate sleep ± vivid hypnogogic hallucinations, cataplexy (sudden hypotonia), and sleep paralysis (paralysis of speech and movement, while fully alert, at sleep onset or on waking). *Hypothesis:* Mutations lead to loss of hypothalamic hypocretin-containing neurons, via autoimmune destruction.[39] 95% are +ve for HLA DR2. ℞: Stimulants (eg methylphenidate) may cause dependence ± psychosis. Modafinil may be better. SE: anxiety, aggression, dry mouth, euphoria, insomnia, ↑BP, dyskinesia, ↑ALP. *Jean-Baptiste-Édouard Gélineau, 1828–1906 (French physician)*

Gerstmann's syndrome A constellation of symptoms suggesting a dominant parietal lesion: finger agnosia (inability to identify fingers), agraphia (inability to write), acalculia (inability to calculate), and left-right disorientation.

Josef Gerstmann, 1887–1969 (Austrian neurologist)

Gilbert's syndrome A common cause of *unconjugated* hyperbilirubinaemia due to ↓ UGT-1 activity (the enzyme that conjugates bilirubin with glucuronic acid). *Prevalence:* 1–2%; 5–15% have a family history of jaundice. It may go unnoticed for many years and usually presents in adolescence with intermittent jaundice occuring during illness, exercise or fasting. *Diagnosis:* Mild ↑bilirubin; normal FBC and reticulocytes (ie no haemolysis). It is a benign condition. *Nicolas Augustin Gilbert, 1858–1927 (French physician)*

Gilles de la Tourette syndrome Tonic, clonic, dystonic, or phonic tics: jerks, blinks, sniffs, nods, spitting, stuttering, irrepressible explosive obscene verbal ejaculations (coprolalia, in 20%) or gestures (coprophilia, 6%),[40] grunts, squeaks, burps, twirlings, and nipping others ± tantrums. There may be a witty, innovatory, phantasmagoric picture, with mimicry (echopraxia), antics, impishness, extravagance, audacity, dramatizations, surreal associations, uninhibited affect, speed, 'go', vivid imagery and memory, and hunger for stimuli. *The tic paradox:* Tics are *voluntary*, but often *unwanted*: the desire to tic stems from the relief of the odd sensation that builds up prior to the tic and is relieved by it, 'like scratching a mosquito bite, tics lead to more tics'.[41] *Mean age of onset:* 6yrs. ♂:♀≈4:1. *Pathogenesis:* Unknown; multiple genetic loci implicated and neuroanatomical abnormalities reported on MRI. *Associations:* Obsessive-compulsive disorder; attention deficit hyperactivity disorder. ℞: (None may be wanted.) Risperidone, haloperidol, or pimozide. Habit-reversal training.[42] Deep brain stimulation is rarely indicated, but may help.

ABC

Marquis Georges Albert Édouard Brutus Gilles de la Tourette, 1857–1904 (French neurologist)

Goodpasture's disease *(A pulmonary-renal syndrome.)* Acute glomerulonephritis + lung symptoms (haemoptysis/diffuse pulmonary haemorrhage) caused by antiglomerular basement membrane antibodies (binding kidney's basement membrane and alveolar membrane). *Tests:* CXR: infiltrates due to pulmonary haemorrhage, often in lower zones. Kidney biopsy: crescentic glomerulonephritis. ℞: ►►Treat shock. Vigorous immunosuppressive treatment and plasmapheresis.

Ernest William Goodpasture, 1886–1960 (US pathologist)

Cataplexy is highly specific for narcolepsy/Gélineau's syndrome

Daytime sleepiness has many causes, but if it occurs with cataplexy the diagnosis 'must' be narcolepsy. Cataplexy is bilateral loss of tone in antigravity muscles provoked by emotions such as laughter, startle, excitement, or anger. Associated phenomena include: falls, mouth opening, dysarthria, mutism, and phasic muscle jerking around the mouth. Most attacks are brief, but injury can occur (eg if several attacks per day). It is comparable to the atonia of rapid eye movement sleep *but without loss of awareness*. ΔΔ: bradycardia, migraine, atonic/akinetic epilepsy, delayed sleep phase syndrome, conversion disorder, malingering, and psychosis.

Don't confuse cata*plexy* with cata*lepsy*—a waxy flexibility where involuntary statue-like postures are effortlessly maintained (frozen) despite looking most uncomfortable.

Guillain-Barré syndrome (*Acute inflammatory demyelinating polyneuropathy.*)[43,44] (table 15.2) *Incidence:* 1-2/100 000/yr. *Signs:* A few weeks after an infection a symmetrical ascending muscle weakness starts. *Triggers: Campylobacter jejuni*, CMV, mycoplasma, zoster, HIV, EBV, vaccinations. The trigger causes antibodies which attack nerves. In 40%, no cause is found. It may advance quickly, affecting all limbs at once, and can lead to paralysis. There is a progressive phase of up to 4 weeks, followed by recovery. Unlike other neuropathies, *proximal* muscles are more affected, eg trunk, respiratory, and cranial nerves (esp. VII). Pain is common (eg back, limb) but sensory signs may be absent. *Autonomic dysfunction:* Sweating, ↑pulse, BP changes, arrhythmias. *Nerve conduction studies:* Slow conduction. *CSF:* ↑Protein (eg >5.5g/L), normal CSF white cell count. Respiratory involvement (the big danger) requires transfer to ITU. Do forced vital capacity (FVC) 4-hourly. ►*Ventilate sooner rather than later*, eg if FVC <1.5L, P_aO_2 <10kPa, P_aCO_2 >6kPa. ℞: IV immunoglobulin 0.4g/kg/24h for 5d. Plasma exchange is good too (?more SE).[45] Steroids have no role. *Prognosis:* Good; ~85% make a complete or near-complete recovery. 10% are unable to walk alone at 1yr. *Complete paralysis is compatible with complete recovery. Mortality:* 10%.

George C Guillain, 1876–1961; Jean-Alexandre Barré, 1880–1967 (French neurologists)

Henoch-Schönlein purpura (HSP) (fig 15.5) A small vessel vasculitis, presenting with purpura (non-blanching purple papules due to intradermal bleeding), often over buttocks and extensor surfaces, typically affecting young ♂. There may be glomerulonephritis (p310), arthritis, and abdominal pain (± intussusception), which may mimic an 'acute abdomen'. ℞: Mostly supportive.

Eduard H Henoch, 1820–1910 (German paediatrician); Johann L Schönlein, 1793–1864 (German physician)

Horner's syndrome A triad of **1** *miosis* (pupil constriction, fig 15.4) **2** partial *ptosis* (drooping upper eyelid) + *apparent enophthalmos* (sunken eye) **3** *anhidrosis* (ipsilateral loss of sweating). Due to interruption of the face's sympathetic supply, eg at the brainstem (demyelination, vascular disease), cord (syringomyelia), thoracic outlet (Pancoast's tumour, p708), or on the sympathetic's trip on the internal carotid artery into the skull (fig 15.6), and orbit. *Johann Friedrich Horner, 1831–1886 (Swiss ophthalmologist)*

Huntington's disease Incurable, progressive, autosomal dominant, neurodegenerative disorder presenting in middle age, often with prodromal phase of mild symptoms (irritability, depression, incoordination). Progresses to chorea, dementia ± fits & death (within ~15yrs of diagnosis). *Pathology:* Atrophy and neuronal loss of striatum and cortex. *Genetic basis:* Expansion of CAG repeat on Chr. 4. ℞: (p87.) No treatment prevents progression. Counselling for patient and family.[46]

George Huntington, 1850–1916 (US physician)

Jervell and Lange-Nielsen syndrome Congenital, bilateral, autosomal recessive, sensorineural deafness, and long QT interval (p96, hence syncope, VT, *torsades*, ± sudden death—50% by age 15 if untreated). KCNQ1 or KCNE1 gene mutation causes K^+ channelopathy. ℞: β-blocker, pacemaker, ICD, cochlear implants.[47]

Anton Jervell, 1901–1987; Fred Lange-Nielsen, 1919–1989 (Norwegian physicians)

Kaposi's sarcoma (KS) A spindle-cell tumour derived from capillary endothelial cells, caused by human herpes virus 8 (=Kaposi's sarcoma-associated herpes virus KSHV). It presents as purple papules (½–1cm) or plaques on skin (fig 15.7) and mucosa (look in mouth, but any organ). It metastasizes to nodes. There are four types: **1** Classic, a rare disease of the elderly. **2** Endemic, a disease of children documented prior to HIV. **3** Iatrogenic KS due to immunosuppression, eg organ transplant recipients. **4** AIDS-associated KS. Usually presents with low CD4 count and can indicate failure of HAART (p402). However ⅓ presents in HIV with near normal CD4 counts and an undetectable viral load. Initiation of HAART with rapid immune system constitution can precipitate KS. Lung KS may present in HIV +ve men and women as dyspnoea and haemoptysis. Bowel KS may cause nausea, abdominal pain. *Rare sites:* CNS, larynx, eye, glands, heart, breast, wounds, or biopsy sites. Δ: Biopsy. ℞: Optimize HAART, local radiotherapy, surgical excision, intralesional therapy (vincristine, bleomycin), topical retinoids, interferon alfa, interleukin-12. Current research includes thalidomide, VEGF monoclonal antibodies, and sirolimus. *Moricz Kaposi, 1837–1902 (Hungarian dermatologist)*

ABC

Guillain-Barré polyneuritis

Table 15.2 Diagnostic criteria

Features required for	Features supporting diagnosis
Progressive weakness of >1 limb Areflexia	• Progression over days, up to 4wks • Near symmetry of sytoms
Features making diagnosis doubtful • Sensory level • Marked, persistent asymmetry of weakness • Severe bowel and bladder dysfunction • CSF WCC >50	• Sensory symptoms/signs only mild • CN involvement (eg bilateral facial weakness) • Recovery starts ~2wks after the period of progression has finished • Autonomic dysfunction • Absence of fever at onset • CSF protein ↑ with CSF WCC $<10\times10^6$/L • Typical electrophysiological tests

Variants of Guillain-Barré syndrome include:

Chronic inflammatory demyelinating polyradiculopathy (CIDP): Characterized by a slower onset and recovery.

Miller Fisher syndrome: Comprises of ophthalmoplegia, ataxia, and areflexia. Associated with anti-GQ1b antibodies in the serum.

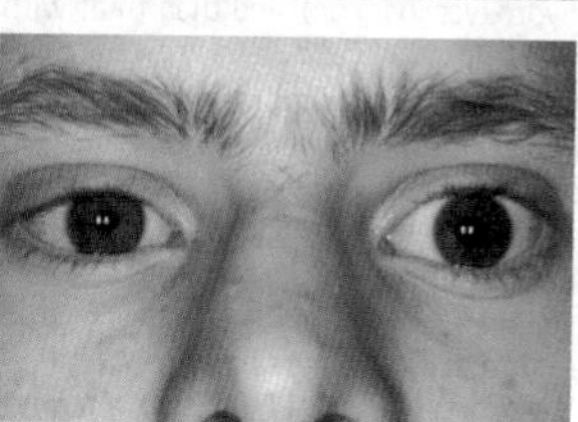

Fig 15.4 Right Horner's: everything reduces: pupil, eye, sweating, etc.

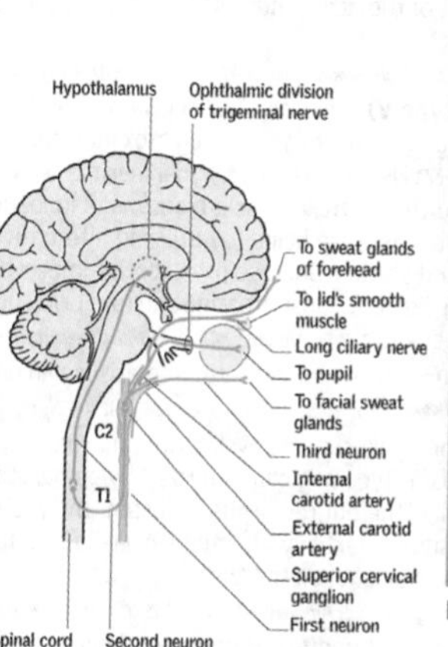

Fig 15.6 Pathways in Horner's syndrome.

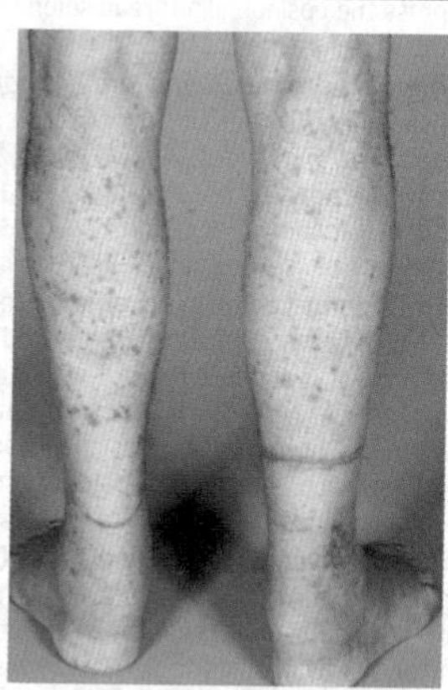

Fig 15.5 Henoch-Schönlein vasculitis.

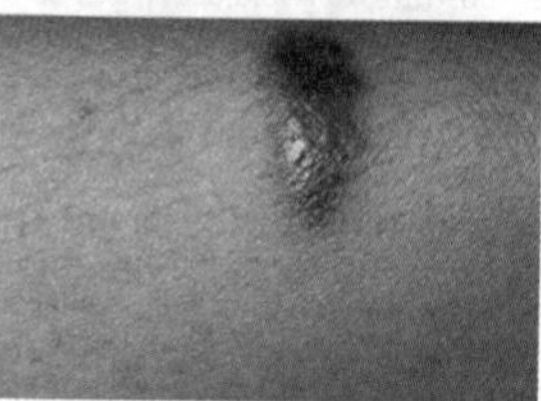

Fig 15.7 Kaposi's sarcoma.

Reproduced from *Oxford Handbook of Medical Dermatology*, 2010, with permission from Oxford University Press.

Klippel-Trénaunay syndrome A triad of port wine stain, varicose veins, and limb hypertrophy, due to vascular malformation. Usually sporadic (although AD inheritance has been reported).[48] *Maurice Klippel, 1858–1942; Paul Trénaunay, 1875–1938 (French physicians)*

Korsakoff's syndrome Hypothalamic damage & cerebral atrophy due to thiamine (vitamin B_1) deficiency (eg in alcoholics). May accompany Wernicke's encephalopathy. There is ↓ability to acquire new memories, confabulation (invented memory, owing to retrograde amnesia), lack of insight & apathy. ℞: See *Wernicke's*, p714; patients rarely recover. *Sergei Sergeievich Korsakoff, 1853–1900 (Russian neuropsychiatrist)*

Langerhans cell histiocytosis (*Histiocytosis X.*) A group of single- (73%, eg bone) or multisystem (27%) disorders, with infiltrating granulomas containing dendritic (Langerhans) cells. ♂:♀ ≈1.5:1; at-risk organs are liver, lung, spleen, marrow. Pulmonary disease presents with pneumothorax or pulmonary hypertension. CXR/CT: nodules and cysts + honeycombing in upper and middle zones. Δ: Biopsy (skin, lung). ℞: Local excision, steroids, vinblastine ± etoposide if severe.[49] *OHCS* p644. *Paul Langerhans, 1847–1888 (German pathologist)*

Leriche's syndrome Absent femoral pulse, claudication/wasting of the buttock, a pale cold leg, and erectile dysfunction from aorto-iliac occlusive disease, eg a saddle embolus at the aortic bifurcation. Surgery may help. *René Leriche, 1879–1955 (French surgeon)*

Löffler's eosinophilic endocarditis Restrictive cardiomyopathy + eosinophilia (eg 120 × 10^9/L). It may be an early stage of tropical endomyocardial fibrosis (and overlaps with hypereosinophilic syndrome, p330) but is distinct from eosinophilic leukaemia. *Signs:* Heart failure (75%) ± mitral regurgitation (49%) ± heart block. ℞: Suppress the eosinophilia (prednisolone ± hydroxycarbamide), and then treat with anti-heart failure medication. *Wilhelm Löffler, 1887–1972 (Swiss physician)*

Löffler's syndrome (*Pulmonary eosinophilia.*) An allergic infiltration of the lungs by eosinophils. Allergens include: *Ascaris lumbricoides, Trichinella spiralis, Fasciola hepatica, Strongyloides, Ankylostoma, Toxocara, Clonorchis sinensis*, sulfonamides, hydralazine, and nitrofurantoin. Often symptomless with incidental CXR (diffuse fan-shaped shadows), or cough, fever, eosinophilia (in ~20%) & larval migrans (p433). ℞: Eradicate cause. Steroids (if idiopathic). *Wilhelm Löffler, 1887–1972 (Swiss physician)*

Lown-Ganong-Levine syndrome A pre-excitation syndrome, similar to Wolf-Parkinson-White (WPW, p133), characterized by a short PR interval (<0.12sec), a normal QRS complex (as opposed to the δ-waves of WPW), and risk of supraventricular tachycardia (but not AF/flutter). The cause is not completely understood, but may be due to paranodal fibres that bypass all or part of the atrioventricular node. The patient may complain of intermittent palpitations.[50]
Bernard Lown, b1921 (US cardiologist); William F Ganong, 1924–2007 (US physiologist); Samuel A Levine, 1891–1966 (US cardiologist)

McArdle's glycogen storage disease (type V) Absence of muscle phosphorylase enzyme with resulting inability to convert glycogen into glucose (eg R50X mutation of PYGM gene; autosomal recessive). Fatigue & crises of cramps ± hyperthermia. Rhabdomyolysis/myoglobinuria follow exercise. *Tests:* ↑↑CK. Muscle biopsy is diagnostic (necrosis and atrophy). ℞: Moderate aerobic exercise helps (by utilizing alternative fuel substrates).[51] Avoid heavy exertion and statins. Sucrose pre-exercise improves performance, as does a carbohydrate-rich diet. Low-dose creatine and ramipril (only if D/D ACE phenotype) may be of minimal benefit.[52] *Brian McArdle, 1911–2002 (British paediatrician)*

ABC

Mallory-Weiss tear Persistent vomiting/retching *causes* haematemesis via an oesophageal mucosal tear. *George K Mallory, 1900–1986 (US pathologist); Soma Weiss, 1898–1942 (US physician)*

Marchiafava-Bignami syndrome Corpus callosum demyelination and necrosis, most often secondary to chronic alcoholism. Type A is characterized by coma, stupor, and pyramidal tract features involving the entire corpus callosum. In type B, symptoms are mild and the corpus callosum is partially affected.[53] Δ: MRI. ℞: As for Wernicke's, p714 (see BOX 'Adverse effects of alcohol on the CNS').
Ettore Marchiafava, 1847–1935; Amico Bignami, 1862–1929 (Italian pathologists)

Marchiafava-Micheli syndrome (*Paroxysmal nocturnal haemoglobinuria*, PNH.) An acquired clonal expansion of a multipotent stem cell manifesting with haemolytic anaemia (from complement-mediated intravascular haemolysis), large vessel thromboses and deficient haematopoiesis (ranging from mild to pancytopenia). See BOX 'Paroxysmal nocturnal haemoglobulinuria' fig 15.8, and p338.
Ettore Marchiafava, 1847–1935 (Italian pathologist); Ferdinando Micheli, 1872–1936 (Italian physician)

Paroxysmal nocturnal haemoglobinuria: the darkest hour

In paroxysmal nocturnal haemoglobinuria (PNH), surface proteins are missing in all blood cells due to a somatic mutation in the X-linked PIG-A gene. Cells lack the glycosyl-phosphatidylinositol (GPI) anchor that binds the surface proteins to cell membranes. This causes uncontrolled amplification of the complement system and leads to destruction of the RBC membrane and release of haemoglobin into the circulation (fig 15.8). NB: the phenomenom of haemoglobinuria[3] is not all that reliable. A much better test even than a marrow biopsy (right-hand panel, showing a clone of PNH cells) is flow cytometric analysis of GPI-anchored proteins on peripheral blood cells. This can determine the size of the PNH clone and type of GPI deficiency (complete or partial). ℞: Most benefit from supportive measures—but allogeneic stem cell transplantation is the only cure. Eculizumab is a monoclonal antibody that targets the C5 protein of the complement system. Blockade prevents activation of the complement distal pathway, reducing haemolysis, stabilizing haemoglobin, and reducing transfusion requirements.[54]

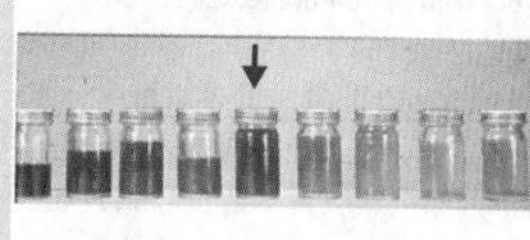

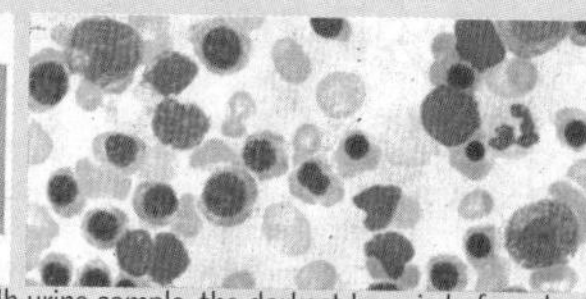

Fig 15.8 Urine and blood in PNH. In this 24h urine sample, the darkest hour is before dawn. Haemolysis occurs throughout the day and night, but the urine concentrated overnight produces the dramatic change in colour.

Courtesy of the Crookston Collection.

Adverse effects of alcohol on the CNS

- ↓Inhibitions (risk taking; ↑unsafe sex)
- Wernicke's encephalopathy
- Korsakoff's syndrome
- Hepatic encephalopathy
- Cerebral atrophy (dementia)
- Central pontine myelinolysis
- Cerebellar atrophy (eg falls)
- Stroke (ischaemic and haemorrhagic)
- Seizures
- Marchiafava-Bignami syndrome.

ABC

3 In haemoglobinuria, urine dipstick will be positive for blood but microscopy of urine does not show RBCs (thus differentiating it from haematuria, but not myoglobinuria—where CK ± AST will be high).

Marfan's syndrome (table 15.3) Autosomal dominant disorder (fibrillin-1) with ↓extracellular microfibril formation; but ~25% have no family history. *Major criteria:* (Diagnostic if >2): lens dislocation (*ectopia lentis*; fig 15.9); aortic dissection/dilatation; dural ectasia; *skeletal features:* arachnodactyly (long spidery fingers), armspan > height, pectus deformity, scoliosis, pes planus. *Minor signs:* Mitral valve prolapse, high-arched palate, joint hypermobility. Diagnosis is clinical; MRI for dural ectasia. *℞:* The danger is aortic dissection: β-blockers slow dilatation of the aortic root. Annual echos, surgical repair when aortic diameter is >5cm. In pregnancy ↑risk of dissection. Homocystinuria has similar skeletal deformities.

Antoine Bernard-Jean Marfan, 1858–1942 (French paediatrician)

Table 15.3 Comparing Marfan's and homocystinuria

Marfan's	vs	Homocystinuria
Upwards lens dislocation		Downwards lens dislocation
Aortic valve incompetence		Heart rarely affected
Normal intelligence		Mental retardation
Scoliosis, flat feet, herniae		Recurrent thromboses, osteoporosis
Life expectancy is lower due to cardiovascular risks		Positive urine cyanide-nitroprusside test Response to treatment with pyridoxine

Meckel's diverticulum The distal ileum contains embryonic remnants of gastric and pancreatic tissue. There may be gastric acid secretion, causing GI pain & occult bleeding. Δ: Radionucleotide scan; laparotomy. *Johann Friedrich Meckel, 1781–1833 (German anatomist)*

Meigs' syndrome A triad of **1** benign ovarian tumour (fibroma) **2** pleural effusion (R>L) & **3** ascites. It resolves on tumour resection. *Joe Vincent Meigs, 1892–1963 (US gynaecologist)*

Ménétrier's disease Giant gastric mucosal folds up to 4cm high, in the fundus, with atrophy of the glands + ↑mucosal thickness + hypochlorhydria + protein-losing gastropathy (hence hypoalbuminaemia ± oedema). *Causes:* CMV, *strep*, *H. pylori*. There may be epigastric pain, vomiting, ± ↓weight. It is pre-malignant. *℞:* Treat *H. pylori* or CMV if present; give high-dose PPI; if this fails, consider epidermal growth factor blockade with cetuximab or gastrectomy (eg if intractable symptoms or malignant change). Epidermal growth factor receptor blockade with cetuximab is 1st-line treatment.[55] Surgery if intractable symptoms or malignant change. *Pierre Eugène Ménétrier, 1859–1935 (French pathologist)*

Meyer-Betz syndrome (*Paroxysmal myoglobinuria.*) Rare idiopathic condition causing necrosis of exercising muscles. There is muscle pain, weakness, and discoloured urine: pink→brown (as ↑myoglobin is excreted). Acute kidney injury can result from myoglobinuria (p319). DIC is associated. *Tests:* ↑WCC, ↑LFT, ↑LDH, ↑CPK, ↑urine myoglobin. *Diagnosis:* Muscle biopsy, ↑CPK, and ↑serum myoglobin. Exertion should be avoided. *Friedrich Meyer-Betz, described 1910 (German physician)*

Mikulicz's syndrome Benign persistent swelling of lacrimal and parotid (or submandibular) glands due to lymphocytic infiltration. Exclude other causes (sarcoidosis, TB, viral infection, lymphoproliferative disorders). It is thought to be an IgG4-related plasmacytic systemic disease.[56] *Johann Freiherr von Mikulicz-Radecki, 1850–1905 (Polish-Austrian surgeon)*

ABC

Milroy disease 1° congenital lymphoedema. Mutations in the VEGFR3 gene (dominant) cause lymphatic malfunction with lower leg swelling from birth (fig 15.10). Δ: Lymphoscintigraphy; genetic testing. *℞:* •Compression hosiery/bandages. •Encourage exercise. •Good skin hygiene. •Treat cellulitis actively. *William Forsyth Milroy, 1855–1942 (US physician)*

Münchausen's syndrome Vivid liars, who are addicted to institutions, flit from hospital to hospital, feigning illness, eg hoping for a laparotomy or mastectomy, or they complain of awful bleeding, odd eye movements, curious fits, sexual assaults, throat closings, false asthma, or heart attacks. Münchausen-by-proxy entails injury to a dependent person by a carer (eg mother) to gain medical attention.

Karl Friedrich Hieronymus, Freiherr von Münchausen, 1720–1797 (German aristocrat). Described by RAJ Asher in 1951[57]

Ogilvie's syndrome *(Acute colonic pseudo-obstruction.)* Colonic obstruction in the absence of a mechanical cause, associated with recent severe illness or surgery. *℞:* Correct U&E. Colonoscopy allows decompression, and excludes mechanical causes. Neostigmine is also effective, suggesting parasympathetic suppression is to blame.[58] Surgery is rarely needed (eg if perforation). *William Heneage Ogilvie, 1887–1971 (British surgeon)*

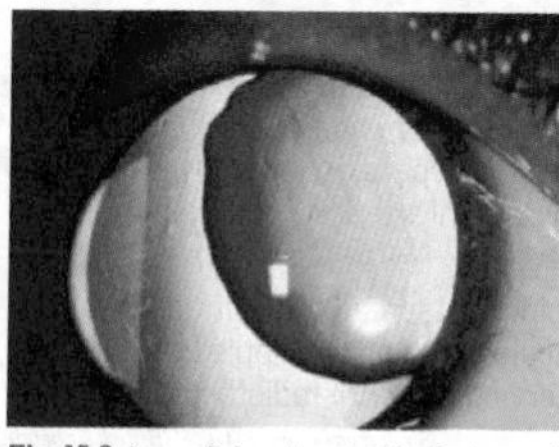

Fig 15.9 Lens dislocation in Marfan's syndrome: here the lens is dislocated superiorly and medially.

Courtesy of Prof Jonathan Trobe.

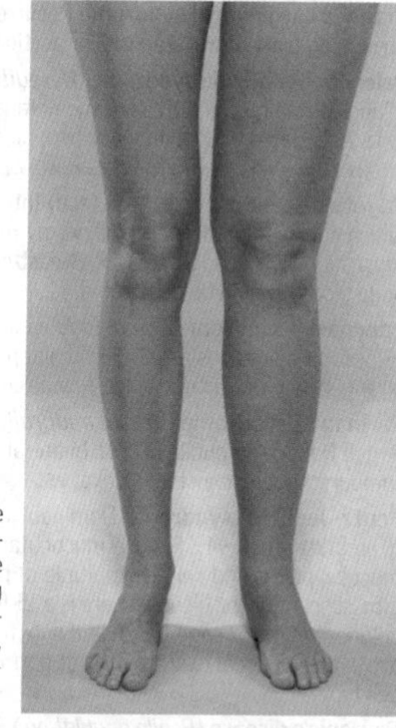

Fig 15.10 Milroy disease. Lymphoedema may be primary, as in Milroy or Meige disease, and is a feature in both Turner and Noonan syndromes. More commonly it is secondary to other conditions, eg cancer (after surgery, lymph node dissection, radiotherapy, or from direct tumour effect), cellulitis, varicose veins, or immobility/dependency. Filariasis (p421) is a common cause in tropical regions.

Who was Baron Münchausen?

Baron Karl Münchausen was an 18th-century German aristocrat and fabulist, whose tall tales became first a popular book, then a byword for circular logic, and finally a medical syndrome of self-delusion. He is famous for riding cannonballs, travelling to the moon, and pulling himself out of a swamp by his own hair. ►►In emergencies (we've all had that sinking feeling...), this method may save your life, for example in your final exams (fig 15.11):

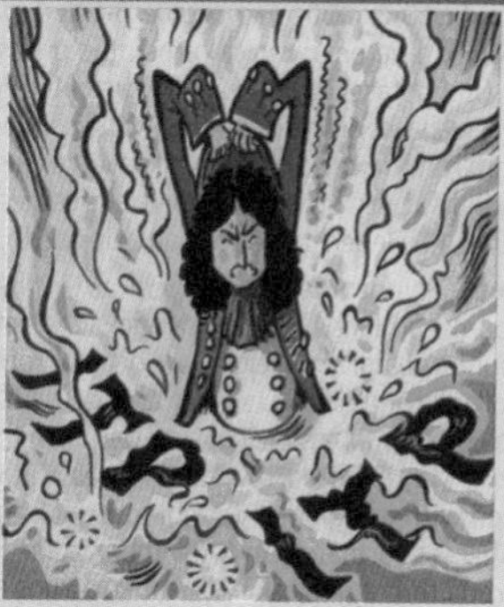

Examiner: 'What is ITP?'

You: 'ITP is idiopathic thrombocytopenic purpura.' (you have scored 50% already).

Examiner: 'And what is idiopathic thrombocytopenic purpura?'

You: 'It's when a cryptogenic cause of a low platelet count leads to purpura.'

Fig 15.11 Münchausen during his finals.

You have deployed your skills with logical brilliance, without adding a single insight. For this Münchausen circularity you may be awarded 100%—unless your examiner is a philosopher, when the right answer would be 'What is ITP? I don't know—and nor do you'—but don't try this too often. You see, you must never forget that medicine is marvellously scientific, and no one is popular who dares cast doubt on this article of faith.

Ortner's cardiovocal syndrome Recurrent laryngeal nerve palsy from a large left atrium (eg from mitral stenosis) or aortic dissection. *Norbert Ortner, 1865–1935 (Austrian physician)*

Osler-Weber-Rendu syndrome (*Hereditary telangiectasia.*) Autosomal dominant telangiectasia of skin & mucous membranes (causing epistaxis and GI bleeds), see fig 15.12. Associated with pulmonary, hepatic, and cerebral arteriovenous malformations.

William Osler, 1849–1919 (Canadian); Frederick Weber, 1863–1962 (British); Henri Rendu, 1844–1902 (French)—physicians

Paget's disease of the breast (PDB) Intra-epidermal spread of an intraduct cancer, which can look just like eczema. ►Any red, scaly lesion at the nipple (see fig 15.13) *must* suggest PDB: do a biopsy. ℞: Breast-conserving surgery + radiotherapy. Sentinel node biopsy should be performed. *Sir James Paget, 1814–1899 (British surgeon)*

Pancoast's syndrome Apical lung ca invades the sympathetic plexus in the neck (→ipsilateral Horner's, p702) ± brachial plexus (→arm pain ± weakness) ± recurrent laryngeal nerve (→hoarse voice/bovine cough). *Henry Pancoast, 1875–1939 (US radiologist)*

Parinaud's syndrome (*Dorsal midbrain syndrome.*) Upward gaze palsy + pseudo-Argyll Robertson pupils (p72) ± bilateral papilloedema. *Causes:* Pineal or midbrain tumours; upper brainstem stroke; MS. *Henry Parinaud, 1844–1905 (French neuro-ophthalmologist)*

Peutz-Jeghers' syndrome Dominant germline mutations of tumour suppressor gene STK11 (in 66–94%) cause mucocutaneous dark freckles on lips (fig 15.14), oral mucosa, palms and soles, + multiple GI polyps (hamartomas), causing obstruction, intussusception, or bleeds. There is a 15-fold ↑risk of developing GI cancer∴ perform colonoscopy (from age 18yrs) and OGD (from age 25yrs) every 3yrs. NB: hamartomas are excessive focal overgrowths of normal cells in an organ composed of the same cell type. *Johannes LA Peutz, 1886–1957 (Dutch physician); Harold J Jeghers, 1904–1990 (US physician)*

Peyronie's disease (*Penile angulation.*) *Pathogenesis:* A poorly understood connective tissue disorder most commonly attributed to repetitive microvascular trauma during sexual intercourse, resulting in penile curvature and painful erectile dysfunction (in 50%; p230). *Prevalence:* 3–9%. *Typical age:* >40yrs. *Associations:* Dupuytren's (p698); atheroma; radical prostatectomy. *ΔΔ:* Haemangioma. *Tests:* Ultrasound/MRI. ℞: Oral potassium para-aminobenzoate (Potaba®), intralesional verapamil, clostridial collagenase, or interferon α2B; topical verapamil 15% gel; iontophoresis with verapamil and dexamethasone. All have various success.[59] *Surgery:* (If disease stable for >3 months) tunica plication ± penile prostheses. Manage associated depression (seen in 48%). Penile rehabilitation can help (p230).[60] *Francois Gigot de la Peyronie, 1678–1747 (French surgeon)*

Pott's syndrome *(Spinal TB.)* Rare in the West, this is usually from an extra-spinal source, eg lungs. *Features:* Backache, and stiffness of *all* back movements. Fever, night sweats, and weight loss occur. Progressive bone destruction leads to vertebral collapse and gibbus (sharply angled spinal curvature). Abscess formation may lead to cord compression, causing paraplegia, and bowel/bladder dysfunction (p466). *X-rays:* (fig 15.15) Narrow disc spaces and vertebral osteoporosis, leading to destruction with wedging of vertebrae. Lesions in the thoracic spine often lead to kyphosis. Abscess formation in the lumbar spine may track down to the psoas muscle, and erode through the skin. ℞: Anti-TB drugs (p394). *Sir Percival Pott, 1714–1788 (British surgeon)*

ABC

Prinzmetal (variant) angina Angina from coronary artery spasm, which may lead to MI, ventricular arrhythmias or sudden death. Severe chest pain occurs *without* physical exertion. Triggers include hyperventilation, cocaine and tobacco use. *ECG:* ST elevation. ℞: Establish the diagnosis. GTN treats angina. Use Ca^{2+}-channel blockers (p114) and long-acting nitrates as prophylaxis. *Myron Prinzmetal, 1908–1987 (US cardiologist)*

Raynaud's syndrome This is peripheral digital ischaemia due to paroxysmal vasospasm, precipitated by cold or emotion. Fingers or toes ache and change colour: pale (ischaemia) →blue (deoxygenation) →red (reactive hyperaemia). It may be idiopathic (Raynaud's *disease*—prevalence: 3–20%; ♀:♂ >1:1) or have an underlying cause (Raynaud's *phenomenon*; fig 15.16). *Tests:* Exclude an underlying cause (see BOX 'Conditions in which Raynaud's phenomenon may be exhibited'). ℞: Keep warm (eg hand warmers); stop smoking.[4] Nifedipine 5–20mg/8h PO helps, as may evening primrose oil, sildenafil, and epoprostenol (for severe attacks/digital gangrene). Relapse is common. Chemical or surgical (lumbar or digital) sympathectomy may help in those with severe disease. *AG Maurice Raynaud, 1834–1881 (French physician)*

Prinzmetal angina and vascular hyperreactivity

Coronary spasm causes Prinzmetal angina and also contributes to coronary heart disease in general, eg acute coronary syndrome (esp. in Japan). Coronary spasm can be induced by ergonovine, acetylcholine, and methacholine (the former is used diagnostically).[5] These cause vasodilation by endothelium-derived nitric oxide when vascular endothelium is functioning normally, whereas they cause vasoconstriction if the endothelium is damaged. In the light of these facts, patients with coronary spasm are thought to have a disturbance in endothelial function as well as local hyperreactivity of the coronary arteries.

If full anti-anginal therapy does not reduce symptoms, stenting or intracoronary radiation (20Gy brachytherapy) to vasospastic segments may be tried. Prognosis is good (especially if non-smoker, no past MI, and no diabetes; progress to infarction is quite rare);[61] β-blockers and large doses of aspirin are contraindicated.

Prinzmetal angina is associated with vascular hyperreactivity/vasospastic disorders such as Raynaud's phenomenon and migraine. It is also associated with circle of Willis occlusion from intimal thickening (moyamoya disease).

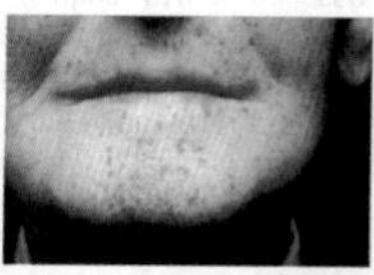

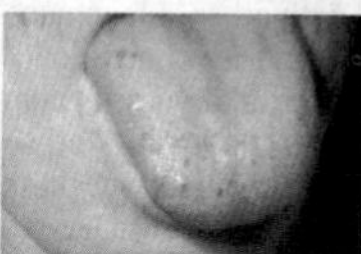

Fig 15.12 Telangiectasia in Osler-Weber-Rendu syndrome.

Reproduced from Cox and Roper, *Clinical Skills*, 2005, with permission from Oxford University Press.

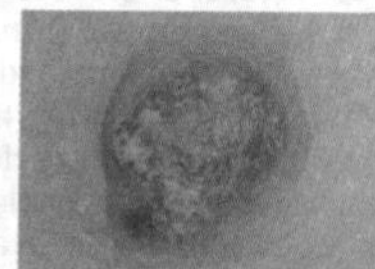

Fig 15.13 Paget's disease of the breast.

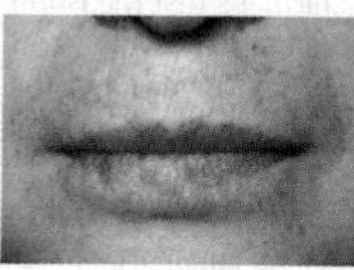

Fig 15.14 Perioral pigmentation, seen in Peutz-Jeghers' syndrome.

Reproduced from Cox and Roper, *Clinical Skills*, 2005, with permission from Oxford University Press.

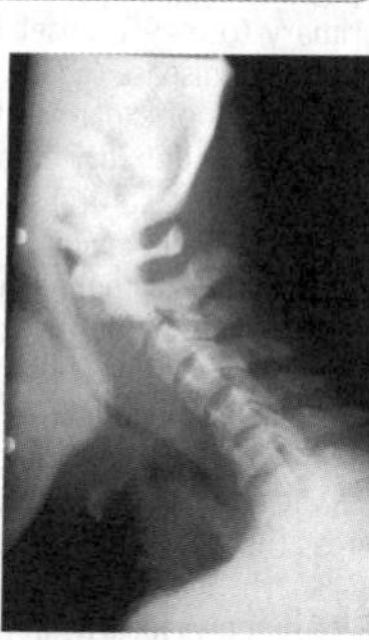

Fig 15.15 TB of axis: soft tissue swelling displaces the retropharyngeal air-tissue boundary forwards. There is an anterior defect in the vertebra, below the axis peg.

Courtesy of Dr Ian Maddison, myweb.lsbu.ac.uk.

Conditions in which Raynaud's phenomenon may be exhibited

Connective tissue disorders: Systemic sclerosis, SLE, rheumatoid arthritis, dermatomyositis/polymyositis.

Occupational: Using vibrating tools.

Obstructive: Thoracic outlet obstruction, Buerger's disease, atheroma.

Blood: Thrombocytosis, cold agglutinin disease, polycythaemia rubra vera (p366), monoclonal gammopathies.

Drugs: β-blockers.

Others: Hypothyroidism.

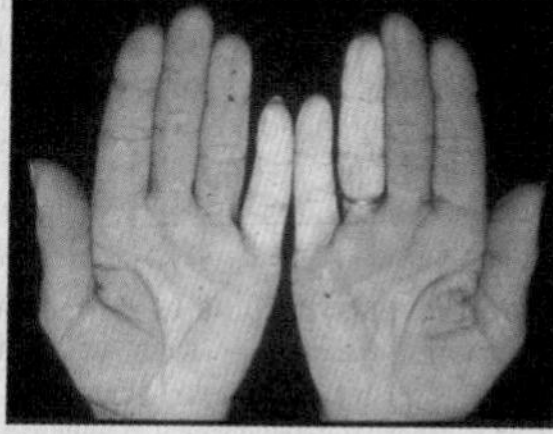

Fig 15.16 Raynaud's phenomenon in SLE.

Courtesy of the Crookston Collection.

4 Patient information on Raynaud's is available from www.raynauds.org.uk.

5 Since Prinzmetal angina is not a 'demand-induced' symptom, but a supply (vasospastic) abnormality, exercise tolerance tests don't help. The most sensitive and specific test is IV ergonovine; 50mcg at 5min intervals in a specialist lab until a +ve result or 400mcg is given. When positive, the symptoms and ↑ST should be present. Nitroglycerin rapidly reverses the effects of ergonovine if refractory spasm occurs.[62]

Refsum disease Phytanic acid accumulates in tissues and serum, due to PHYH or PEX7 gene mutation (recessive). This leads to anosmia (a universal finding) and early-onset retinitis pigmentosa, with variable combinations of neuropathy, deafness, ataxia, ichthyosis, and cardiomyopathy. *Tests:* ↑Plasma phytanic acid. ℞: Restrict foods containing phytanic acid (animal fats, dairy products, green leafy vegetables); plasmapheresis is used for severe symptoms.[63] *Sigvald Bernhard Refsum, 1907–1991 (Norwegian physician)*

Romano-Ward syndrome A dominant mutation in a K^+ channel subunit causes long QT syndrome ± episodic VT, VF, *torsades*, ± sudden death. (Jervell and Lange-Nielsen syn is similar, p702.) *Cesarino Romano, 1924–2008 (Italian paediatrician); Owen C Ward, b1923 (Irish paediatrician)*

Rotor syndrome A rare, benign, autosomal recessive disorder. Primary non-haemolytic conjugated hyperbilirubinaemia, with almost normal hepatic histology (no pigmentation, in contrast to DJS, p698). Typically presents in childhood with mild jaundice. Cholescintigraphy reveals an 'absent' liver. *Arturo Belleza Rotor, 1907–1988 (Filipino physician)*

Sister Mary Joseph nodule An umbilical metastatic nodule from an intra-abdominal malignancy (fig 15.17). *Sister Mary Joseph Dempsey, 1856–1939 (US catholic nun & Dr William Mayo's surgical assistant)*

Sjögren's syndrome A chronic inflammatory autoimmune disorder, which may be primary (♀:♂≈9:1, onset 4th–5th decade) or secondary, associated with connective tissue disease (eg RA, SLE, systemic sclerosis). There is lymphocytic infiltration and fibrosis of exocrine glands, especially lacrimal and salivary glands. *Features:* ↓Tear production (dry eyes, keratoconjunctivitis sicca), ↓salivation (xerostomia—dry mouth, caries), parotid swelling. Other glands are affected causing vaginal dryness, dyspareunia, dry cough, and dysphagia. Systemic signs include polyarthritis/arthralgia, Raynaud's, lymphadenopathy, vasculitis, lung, liver, and kidney involvement, peripheral neuropathy, myositis, and fatigue. It is associated with other autoimmune diseases (eg thyroid disease, autoimmune hepatitis, PBC) and an ↑risk of non-Hodgkin's B-cell lymphoma. *Tests:* Schirmer's test measures conjunctival dryness (<5mm in 5min is +ve). Rose Bengal staining may show keratitis (use a slit-lamp). Anti-Ro (SSA; in 40%) & anti-La (SSB; in 26%) antibodies may be present (in pregnancy, these cross the placenta and cause fetal congenital heart block in 5%). ANA is usually +ve (74%); rheumatoid factor is +ve in 38%. There may be hypergammaglobulinaemia. Biopsy shows focal lymphocytic aggregation. ℞: Treat sicca symptoms: eg hypromellose (artificial tears), frequent drinks, sugar-free pastilles/gum. NSAIDs and hydroxychloroquine are used for arthralgia. Immunosuppressants may be indicated in severe systemic disease.[64] *Henrik Conrad Samuel Sjögren, 1899–1986 (Swedish ophthalmologist)*

Stevens-Johnson syndrome A severe form of erythema multiforme (p562), and a variant of toxic epidermal necrolysis. It is caused by a hypersensitivity reaction, usually to drugs (eg salicylates, sulfonamides, penicillin, barbiturates, carbamazepine, phenytoin), but is also seen with infections or cancer. There is ulceration of the skin and mucosal surfaces (see fig 15.18). Typical target lesions develop, often on the palms or soles with blistering in the centre. There may be a prodromal phase with fever, malaise, arthralgia, myalgia ± vomiting and diarrhoea. ℞: Mild disease is usually self-limiting—remove any precipitant and give supportive care (eg calamine lotion for the skin). Steroid use is controversial—trials have been variable, so ask a dermatologist and ophthalmologist. IV immunoglobulin has shown benefit. Plasmapheresis and immunosuppressive agents may have a role.[65] *Prognosis:* Mortality ~5%. May be severe for the first 10d before resolving over 30d. Damage to the eyes may persist and blindness can result. *Albert M Stevens 1884–1945; Frank C Johnson, 1894–1934 (US paediatricians)*

Sturge-Weber syndrome (SWS) Essential features: **1** Facial cutaneous capillary malformation (port wine stain; PWS) in the ophthalmic dermatome (V1 ± V2/V3). **2** Clinical signs or radiologic evidence of a leptomeningeal vascular malformation. 75% of patients with unilateral involvement develop seizures by age 1yr (95% if bilateral)—due (in part) to the increased metabolic demand of a developing brain in the setting of vascular compromise. Early management of seizures is critical to minimize brain injury. Some patients have severe cognitive and neurologic deficits beyond simple seizure activity. Screen early for glaucoma (50%). EEG and MRI help establish early diagnosis and treatment in patients at risk for SWS. Treat the PWS early with pulsed dye laser. *William A Sturge, 1850–1919; Frederick P Weber, 1863–1962 (British physicians)*

Causes of a long QT interval

Many conditions and drugs (check *BNF*) cause a long QT interval. Brugada syndrome (p695) is similar, predisposing to sudden cardiac death.

Congenital: Romano-Ward syndrome (autosomal dominant). Jervell and Lange-Nielsen syndrome (autosomal recessive) with associated deafness (p702).

Cardiac: Myocardial infarction or ischaemia; mitral valve prolapse.

HIV: May be a direct effect of the virus or from protease inhibitors.

Metabolic: ↓K^+; ↓Mg^{2+}; ↓Ca^{2+}; starvation; hypothyroidism; hypothermia.

Toxic: Organophosphates.

Anti-arrhythmic drugs: Quinidine; amiodarone; procainamide; sotalol.

Antimicrobials: Erythromycin; levofloxacin; pentamidine; halofantrine.

Antihistamines: Terfenadine; astemizole.

Motility drugs: Domperidone.

Psychoactive drugs: Haloperidol; risperidone; tricyclics; SSRIs.

Connective tissue diseases: Anti-Ro/SSA antibodies (p552).

Herbalism: Ask about Chinese folk remedies (may contain unknown amounts of arsenic). Cocaine, quinine, and artemisinins (and other antimalarials) are examples of herbalism-derived products that can prolong the QT interval.

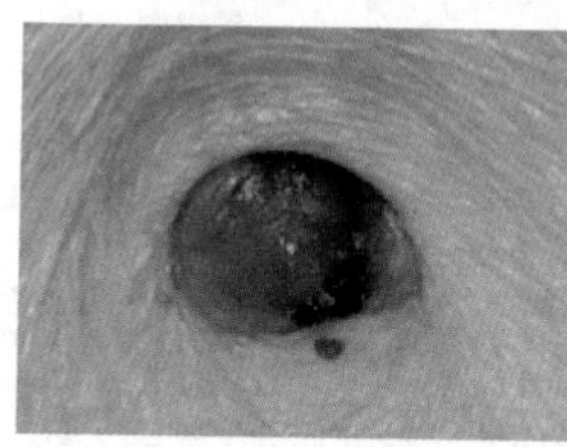

Fig 15.17 Sister Mary Joseph nodule.
Reproduced from *Postgraduate Medical Journal*, 'Sister Joseph nodule', J E Clague, 78(917), 174, 2002 with permission from BMJ Publishing Group Ltd.

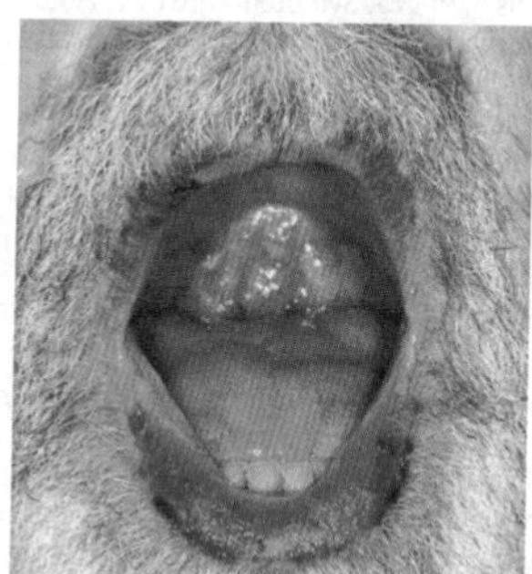

Fig 15.18 Stevens-Johnson syndrome.
Reproduced from Emberger *et al*, Stevens-Johnson syndrome associated with anti-malarial prophylaxis. *Clinical Infectious Diseases* (2003) 37:1, with permission from Oxford University Press.

Takayasu's arteritis (*Aortic arch syndrome; pulseless disease.*) Rare outside of Japan, this systemic vasculitis affects the aorta and its major branches. Granulomatous inflammation causes stenosis, thrombosis, and aneurysms. It often affects women aged 20–40yrs. Symptoms depend on the arteries involved. The aortic arch is often affected, with cerebral, ophthalmological, and upper limb symptoms, eg dizziness, visual changes, weak arm pulses. Systemic features are common—eg fever, weight loss, and malaise. ↑BP is often a feature, due to renal artery stenosis. Complications include aortic valve regurgitation, aortic aneurysm and dissection; ischaemic stroke (↑BP and thrombus); and ischaemic heart disease. ***Diagnosis:*** ↑ESR and CRP; MRI/PET allows earlier diagnosis than standard angiography. ℞: Prednisolone (1mg/kg/d PO). Methotrexate or cyclophosphamide have been used in resistant cases. BP control is essential to ↓risk of stroke. Angioplasty ± stenting, or bypass surgery is performed for critical stenosis. ***Prognosis:*** ~95% survival at 15 years.

Mikito Takayasu, 1860–1938 (Japanese ophthalmologist)

Tietze's syndrome (*Idiopathic costochondritis.*) Localized pain/tenderness at the costosternal junction, enhanced by motion, coughing, or sneezing. The 2nd rib is most often affected. The diagnostic key is *localized* tenderness which is marked (flinches on prodding). ***Treatment:*** Simple analgesia, eg NSAIDs. Its importance is that it is a benign cause of what at first seems to be alarming, eg cardiac pain. In lengthy illness, local steroid injections may be used. *Alexander Tietze, 1864–1927 (German surgeon)*

Todd's palsy Transient neurological deficit (paresis) after a seizure. There may be face, arm, or leg weakness, aphasia, or gaze palsy, lasting from ~30min–36h. The aetiology is unclear. *Robert Bentley Todd, 1809–1860 (Irish-born physician)*

Vincent's angina (*Necrotizing ulcerative gingivitis.*) Mouth infection with ulcerative gingivitis from *Borrelia vincentii* (a spirochaete) + fusiform bacilli, often affecting young ♂ smokers with poor oral hygiene. Try amoxicillin 500mg/8h and metronidazole 400mg/8h PO, + chlorhexidine mouthwash. *Jean Hyacinthe Vincent, 1862–1950 (French physician)*

Von Hippel-Lindau syndrome A dominant germline mutation of a tumour suppressor gene. It predisposes to bilateral renal cysts and clear cell renal carcinoma (p320), retinal & cerebellar haemangioblastoma, and phaeochromocytoma. See figs 15.19, 15.20. It may present with visual impairment or cerebellar signs (eg unilateral ataxia). *Eugen von Hippel, 1867–1939 (German ophthalmologist); Arvid Lindau, 1892–1958 (Swedish pathologist)*

Von Willebrand's disease (VWD) Von Willebrand's factor (VWF) has three roles in clotting: **1** To bring platelets into contact with exposed subendothelium. **2** To make platelets bind to each other. **3** To bind to factor VIII, protecting it from destruction in the circulation. There are >22 types of VWD; the commonest are:
Type I: (60–80%) ↓Levels of of VWF. Symptoms are mild. Autosomal dominant.
Type II: (20–30%) Abnormal VWF, with lack of high-molecular-weight multimers. Usually autosomal dominant inheritance. Bleeding tendency varies. There are 4 subtypes.
Type III: (1–5%) Undetectable VWF levels (autosomal recessive with gene deletions). VWF antigen is lacking and there is ↓factor VIII. Symptoms can be severe.
Signs are of a platelet-type disorder (p344): bruising, epistaxis, menorrhagia, ↑bleeding post-tooth extraction. ***Tests:*** ↑APTT, ↑bleeding time, ↓factor VIIIC (clotting activity), VWF ↓Ag; ↔INR and platelets. ℞: Get expert help. Desmopressin is used in mild bleeding, VWF-containing factor VIII concentrate for surgery or major bleeds. Avoid NSAIDs. *Erik Adolf von Willebrand, 1870–1949 (Finnish physician)*

ABC

Wallenberg's lateral medullary syndrome This relatively common syndrome comprises lesions to multiple CNS nuclei, caused by posterior or inferior cerebellar artery occlusion leading to brainstem infarction (fig 15.21). ***Features:*** • Dysphagia dysarthria (IX and X nuclei). • Vertigo, nausea, vomiting, nystagmus (vestibular nucleus). • Ipsilateral ataxia (inferior cerebellar peduncle). • Ipsilateral Horner's syndrome (descending sympathetic fibres). • Loss of pain and temperature sensation on the ipsilateral face (V nucleus) and contralateral limbs (spinothalamic tract). There is no limb weakness as the pyramidal tracts are unaffected.

In the rarer ***medial medullary syndrome***, vertebral or anterior spinal artery occlusion causes ipsilateral tongue paralysis (XII nucleus) with contralateral limb weakness (pyramidal tract, sparing the face) and loss of position sense.

Adolf Wallenberg, 1862–1949 (German neurologist)

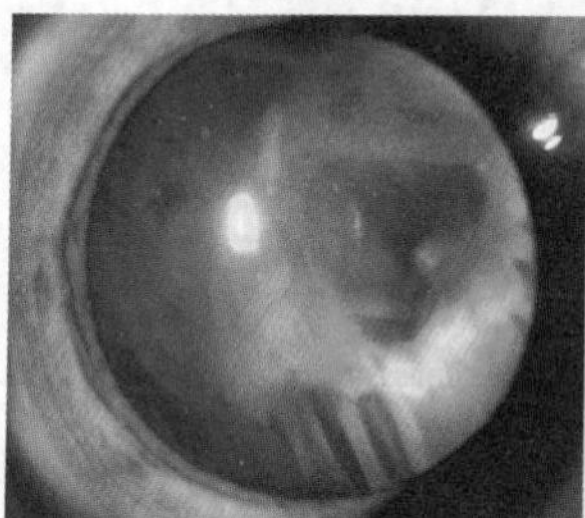

Fig 15.19 Von Hippel-Lindau syndrome showing retinal detachment.

Reproduced with permission from the National Eye Institute, National Institutes of Health.

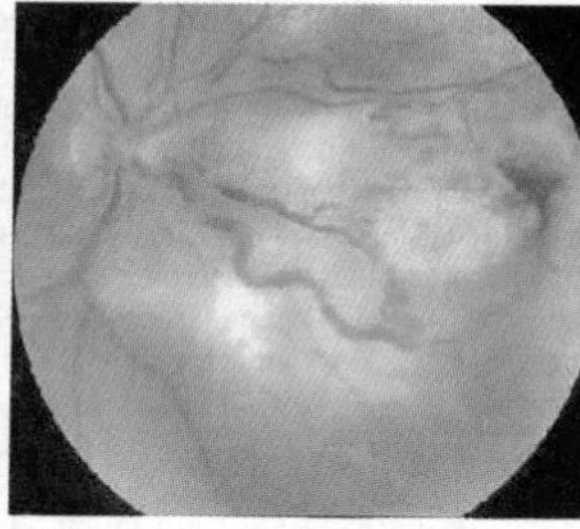

Fig 15.20 Von Hippel-Lindau syndrome showing a retinal tumour.

Reproduced with permission from the National Eye Institute, National Institutes of Health.

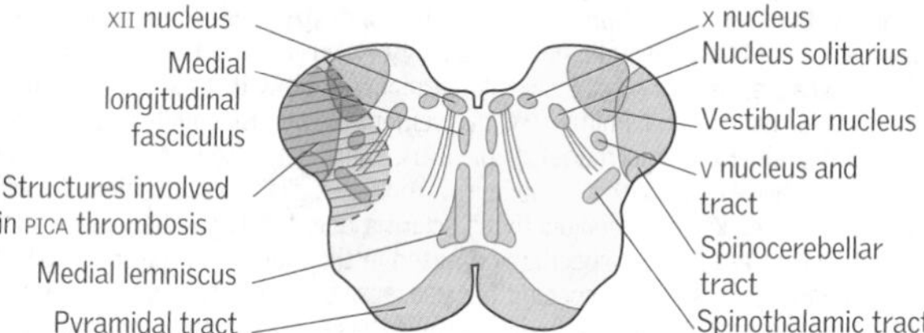

Fig 15.21 Cross section of the medulla showing structures involved in Wallenberg's lateral medullary syndrome (posterior inferior cerebellar artery thrombosis).

Waterhouse-Friderichsen's (WhF) syndrome Bilateral adrenal cortex haemorrhage, often occurring in rapidly deteriorating meningococcal sepsis, alongside widespread purpura, meningitis, coma, and DIC (fig 15.22). The meningococcal endotoxin acts as a potent initiator of inflammatory and coagulation cascades. Other causes include *H. influenzae*, pneumococcal, streptococcal, and staphylococcal sepsis. Adrenal failure causes shock, as normal vascular tone requires cortisol to set activity of α- and β-adrenergic receptors, and aldosterone is needed to maintain extracellular fluid volume. *Treatment:* ▸▸Antibiotics, eg ceftriaxone (p822) and hydrocortisone 200mg/4h IV for adrenal support. ICU admission.

Rupert Waterhouse, 1873–1958 (British physician); Carl Friderichsen, 1886–1979 (Danish paediatrician)

Weber's syndrome (*Superior alternating hemiplegia.*) Ipsilateral oculomotor nerve palsy with contralateral hemiplegia, due to infarction of one-half of the midbrain, after occlusion of the paramedian branches of the basilar or posterior cerebral arteries. *Herman David Weber, 1823–1918 (German-born physician whose son described Sturge–Weber syndrome)*

Wegener's granulomatosis This has been renamed ***granulomatosis with polyangiitis (GPA)***, in part because of concerns over the suitability of Friedrich Wegener, a member of the Nazi party during WWII, to be the source of an eponym. GPA is a multisystem disorder of unknown cause characterized by necrotizing granulomatous inflammation and vasculitis of small and medium vessels. It has a predilection for the upper respiratory tract, lungs, and kidneys. *Features:* Upper airways disease is common, with nasal obstruction, ulcers, epistaxis, or destruction of the nasal septum causing a characteristic 'saddle-nose' deformity.[6] Sinusitis is often a feature. Renal disease causes rapidly progressive glomerulonephritis with crescent formation, proteinuria, or haematuria. Pulmonary involvement may cause cough, haemoptysis (severe if pulmonary haemorrhage), or pleuritis. There may also be skin purpura or nodules, peripheral neuropathy, mononeuritis multiplex, arthritis/arthralgia, or ocular involvement, eg keratitis, conjunctivitis, scleritis, episcleritis, uveitis. *Tests:* cANCA directed against PR3 is most specific and raised in the majority of patients (p553). Some patients express pANCA specific for MPO. ↑ESR/CRP. Urinalysis should be performed to look for proteinuria or haematuria. If these are present, consider a renal biopsy. CXR may show nodules ± fluffy infiltrates of pulmonary haemorrhage. CT may reveal diffuse alveolar haemorrhage. Atypical cells from cytology of sputum/BAL can be confused with bronchial carcinoma.[66] *Treatment:* Depends on the extent of disease. Severe disease (eg biopsy-proven renal disease) should be treated with corticosteroids and cyclophosphamide (or rituximab) to induce remission. Azathioprine and methotrexate are usually used as maintenance. Indications for plasma exchange include patients presenting with severe renal disease (eg creatinine >500µmol/L) and those with pulmonary haemorrhage. Co-trimoxazole should be given as prophylaxis against *Pneumocystis jirovecii* and staphylococcal colonization.

Friedrich Wegener, 1907–1990 (German pathologist)

Wernicke's encephalopathy Thiamine (vitamin B_1) deficiency with a classical triad of **1** confusion **2** ataxia and **3** ophthalmoplegia (nystagmus, lateral rectus, or conjugate gaze palsies). There is inadequate dietary intake, ↓GI absorption, and impaired utilization of thiamine resulting in focal areas of brain damage, including periaqueductal punctate haemorrhages (mechanism unclear). Always consider this diagnosis in alcoholics: it may also present with memory disturbance, hypotension, hypothermia, or reduced consciousness.[67] *Recognized causes:* Chronic alcoholism, eating disorders, malnutrition, prolonged vomiting, eg with chemotherapy, GI malignancy, or hyperemesis gravidarum. *Diagnosis:* Primarily clinical. Red cell transketolase activity is decreased (rarely done). *Treatment: Urgent* replacement to prevent irreversible Korsakoff's syndrome (p704). Give thiamine (Pabrinex®), 2 pairs of high-potency ampoules IV/IM/8h over 30min for 2d, then 1 pair OD for a further 5d. Oral supplementation (100mg OD) should continue until no longer 'at risk' (+ give other B vitamins). Anaphylaxis is rare. If there is coexisting hypoglycaemia (often the case in this group of patients), make sure thiamine is given before glucose, as Wernicke's can be precipitated by glucose administration to a thiamine-deficient patient. *Prognosis:* Untreated, death occurs in 20%, and Korsakoff's psychosis occurs in 85%—a quarter of whom will require long-term institutional care. *Karl Wernicke, 1848–1905 (German neurologist)*

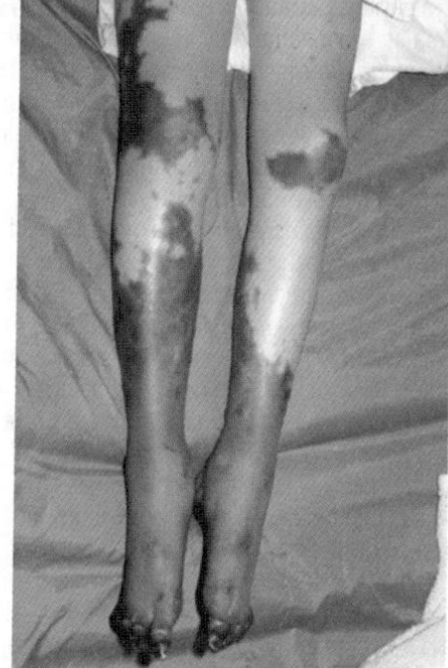

Fig 15.22 Meningococcal sepsis with purpura.

6 Common causes of a 'saddle-nose' deformity are trauma and iatrogenic (eg post-rhinoplasty). Rarer causes (popular with some finals examiners): GPA, relapsing polychondritis, syphilis, and leprosy.

Whipple's disease A rare disease[68] featuring GI malabsorption which usually occurs in middle-aged white males, most commonly in Europe. It is fatal if untreated and is caused by *Tropheryma whippelii*, which, combined with defective cell-mediated immunity, produces a systemic disease. *Features:* Often starts insidiously with arthralgia (chronic, migratory, seronegative arthropathy affecting mainly peripheral joints). GI symptoms commonly include colicky abdominal pain, weight loss, steatorrhea/diarrhoea, which leads to malabsorption (p266). Systemic symptoms such as chronic cough, fever, sweats, lymphadenopathy, and skin hyperpigmentation also occur. Cardiac involvement may lead to endocarditis, which is typically blood culture negative. CNS features include a reversible dementia, ophthalmoplegia, and facial myoclonus (if all together, they are highly suggestive)—also hypothalamic syndrome (hyperphagia, polydipsia, insomnia). NB: CNS involvement may occur without GI involvement. *Tests:* Diagnosis requires a high level of clinical suspicion. Jejunal biopsy shows stunted villi. There is deposition of macrophages in the lamina propria-containing granules which stain positive for periodic acid-Schiff (PAS). Similar cells may be found in affected samples, eg CSF, cardiac valve tissue, lymph nodes, synovial fluid. The bacteria may be seen within macrophages on electron microscopy. PCR of bacterial RNA can be performed on serum or tissue. MRI may demonstrate CNS involvement. ℞: Should include antibiotics which cross the blood-brain barrier. Current recommendations: IV ceftriaxone (or penicillin+streptomycin) for 2wks then oral co-trimoxazole for 1 year. Shorter courses risk relapse. A rapid improvement in symptoms usually occurs.

George Hoyt Whipple, 1878–1976 (US pathologist)

Zellweger syndrome (*Cerebrohepatorenal syndrome.*) A rare recessive disorder characterized by absent peroxisomes (intracellular organelles required for many cellular activities including lipid metabolism). The syndrome has a similar molecular basis to infantile Refsum's syndrome, and although more severe, exhibits comparable biochemical abnormalities (p710). Clinical features include craniofacial abnormalities, severe hypotonia and mental retardation, glaucoma, cataracts, hepatomegaly, and renal cysts. A number of causative PEX gene mutations have been identified. Life expectancy is usually a few months only. *Hans Zellweger, 1909–1990 (US paediatrician)*

Zollinger-Ellison syndrome This is the association of peptic ulcers with a gastrin-secreting adenoma (gastrinoma). Gastrin excites excessive gastric acid production, which may produce multiple ulcers in the duodenum and stomach. The adenoma is usually found in the pancreas, although it may arise in the stomach or duodenum. Most cases are sporadic; 20% are associated with multiple endocrine neoplasia, type 1 (MEN1, p223). 60% are malignant; metastases are found in local lymph nodes and the liver. *Symptoms:* Include abdominal pain and dyspepsia, from the ulcer(s), and chronic diarrhoea due to inactivation of pancreatic enzymes (also causes steatorrhoea) and damage to intestinal mucosa. *Incidence:* ~0.1% of patients with peptic ulcer disease. Suspect in those with multiple peptic ulcers, ulcers distal to the duodenum, or a family history of peptic ulcers (or of islet cell, pituitary, or parathyroid adenomas). *Tests:* (fig 15.23) ↑Fasting serum gastrin level (>1000pg/mL). Measure three fasting levels on different days. Hypochlorhydria (reduced acid production, eg in chronic atrophic gastritis) should be excluded as this also causes a raised gastrin level: gastric pH should be <2. The secretin stimulation test is useful in suspected cases with only mildly raised gastrin levels (100–1000pg/mL). The adenoma is often small and difficult to image; a combination of somatostatin receptor scintigraphy, endoscopic ultrasound, and CT is used to localize and stage the adenoma. OGD evaluates gastric/duodenal ulceration. ℞: High-dose proton pump inhibitors, eg omeprazole: start with 60mg/d and adjust according to response. Measuring intragastric pH helps determine the best dose (aim to keep pH at 2-7). All gastrinomas have malignant potential—and surgery is better sooner than later (with lymph node clearance generally recommended if >2cm in size). Surgery may be avoided in MEN1, as adenomas are often multiple, and metastatic disease is rare. If well-differentiated (G1 and G2) somatostatin analogues may be 1st-line and chemotherapy with streptozotocin (if available) + doxorubicin/*5-FU* is 2nd-line. In G3, etoposide + cisplatin is possible.[69] Selective embolization may be done for hepatic metastases. *Prognosis:* 5yr survival: 80% if single resectable lesion, ~20% with hepatic metastases. Screen all patients for MEN1. *Robert M Zollinger, 1903–1992; Edwin H Ellison, 1918–1970 (US surgeons)*

ABC

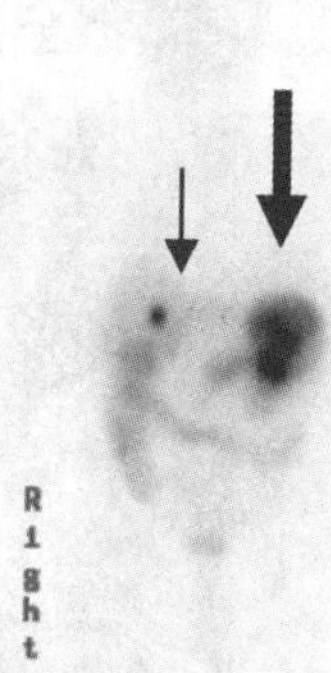

Fig 15.23 OctreoScan in patient with metastatic MEN 1 gastrinoma. Solitary hepatic metastatic deposit (thin arrow), gastric neuroendocrine tumour (thick arrow).

Epilogue

25% of patients with rare diseases have to wait from 5-30 years for a diagnosis. 40% are misdiagnosed resulting in inappropriate drugs or psychological treatments—eg 20% of people with Ehlers-Danlos syndrome (p149) had to consult over 20 doctors before the diagnosis was made,[70] causing understandable loss of confidence in our profession. Lack of appropriate referral and rejection because of disease complexity are common problems. Let us cultivate our networks with each other and approach 'unexplained symptoms' with an open mind.

16 Radiology

Contents

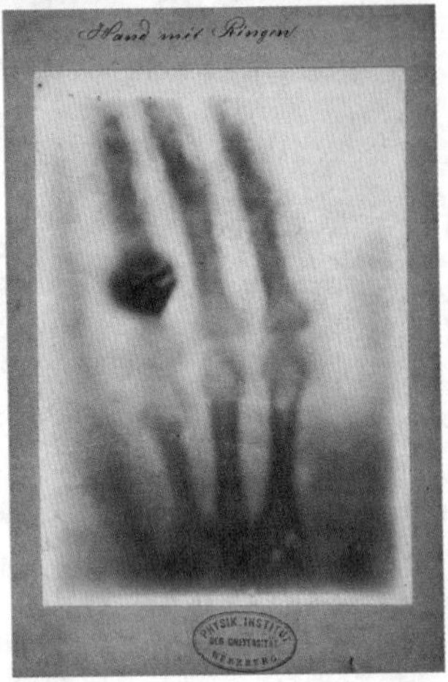

Fig 16.1 The first X-ray, taken by Wilhelm Röntgen of his wife's hand (for which he won the first Nobel Prize in Physics in 1901). Upon seeing the ghostly image she cried 'I have seen my death!' Could this exclamation have prophesized the radiation-induced malignancies that have plagued the recipients (and administrators) of X-rays since their conception (see BOX)? Despite the obvious commercial potential, Röntgen declined to take out any patents on his new technology, preferring to see it developed for the benefit of humanity. Fate did not repay this generosity: his personal wealth depreciated away in the German hyperinflation of the 1920s, and he spent his later years in bankruptcy.

We thank Professor Peter Scally, Dr Dean McCoombe, and Dr Paul Thomas, our Specialist Readers for this chapter.

Typical effective doses

The effective dose of an examination is calculated as the weighted sum of the doses to different body tissues. The weighting factor for each tissue depends on its sensitivity. The effective dose thus provides a single dose estimate related to the total radiation risk, no matter how the radiation dose is distributed around the body. This table is certainly not to be learnt; rather it serves as a reminder of the relative exposures to radiation that we prescribe in practice. ►Remember that US and MRI involve no radiation, would they provide the answer?

Table 16.1 Radiation doses in common radiological investigations

Procedure	Typical effective dose (mSv)	CXR equivalents	Approx. equivalent period of background radiation
X-ray examinations			
Limbs and joints	<0.01	<1	<2 days
Chest (PA)	0.015	1	2.5 days
Abdomen	0.4	30	2 months
Lumbar spine	0.6	40	3 months
CT head	1.4	90	7.5 months
CT chest	6.6	440	3 years
CT abdo/pelvis	6.7	450	3 years
Radionuclide studies			
Lung ventilation	0.4	30	9 weeks
Lung perfusion	1	70	6 months
Bone	3	200	1.4 years
PET head	7	460	3.2 years
PET-CT	18	1200	8.1 years

Reproduced from iRefer *Making the Best Use of Clinical Radiology*, 7th edition, ©Royal College of Radiologists, 2012.

Justifying exposure to ionizing radiation

The very nature of ionizing radiation that gives us vision into the human body also gives it lethal properties. In considering the decision to expose patients to radiation, the clinical benefits should outweigh the risks of genetic mutation and cancer induction. These risks can be hard to quantify (and estimates vary wildly—extrapolation of effects from doses associated with nuclear explosions are likely unreliable) but even with strict guidelines we still have a tendency to over-exposure in medical practice. Perhaps the best advice is to be certain of the importance of every dose of radiation that you sanction, and mindful of the comparative doses involved (see table 16.1).

The responsibility lies with us not to rely too heavily on radiology. ►Don't request examinations to comfort patients (or appease their consultants), to replace images already acquired elsewhere (or lost) simply to avoid medico-legal issues, or when the result will not affect management. To give an idea of relative doses, a CT of the abdomen and pelvis gives a typical effective dose of 500 times as much radiation as a CXR. This important factor also tells us about the preference of ultrasound over CT when investigating abdominal and pelvic complaints such as acute appendicitis, especially given the youthful demographics of this diagnosis.

►Unwitting exposure of the unborn fetus to radiation is inexcusable at any stage of gestation—unless the mother's life is in immediate danger—and it is the responsibility of the referring clinician, as well as the radiographer and the radiologist, to ensure that this is avoided.

The art of the request

One of the most nerve-wracking moments that you can encounter as a recently qualified doctor is having to request an investigation from a seasoned consultant radiologist. What information do you need to give? How much? Who do you ask? Put yourself on the other side: what does the radiologist need to know to decide who needs what imaging and when? Keep the following in mind when requesting (never ordering!) an investigation:

Patient details Get the patient's name right! Include hospital number and date of birth on all requests.

Clinical details Think of your clinical question, what answer are you hoping radiology will provide? It can:

- *Confirm* a suspected diagnosis.
- *'Exclude'* something important (though remember that exclusion is never 100%).
- *Define* the extent of a disease.
- *Monitor* the progress of a disease.

► Don't forget to mention pertinent facts that may change the way the investigation is carried out: an agitated or confused patient may need sedation prior to an MRI of their head. A CT scan on a patient with an acutely raised creatinine may need to be done without contrast medium. Insertion of a drain on a patient with deranged clotting may need to wait while this is corrected. Include recent creatinine, Hb, and clotting on the form if appropriate. Don't forget to mention anticoagulants, eg warfarin, LMWH, and aspirin for intervention requests.

Investigation details What scan do you think is required, and how soon do you need it? Different clinical questions require different procedures. If you think the patient has a collection, would you like them to drain it? Always state whether intervention is required (eg US abdo ± drain insertion). Remember that the radiologist ultimately decides what imaging or procedure they undertake based on the information you have provided.

Tips

- Know your patient well, but keep your request brief and accurate.
- Know the clinical question and how the answer will change your management.
- Look up previous imaging before you go; asking for a CT on a patient who had one yesterday makes you look foolish and will not go down well.
- If in doubt, or if the investigation is very urgent, go down to the department in person. Regard this as an important opportunity: involving a radiologist will result in the best selection of imaging technique for your clinical question, will help expedite urgent requests, and should be of educational value for you.

If your request is turned down Don't be afraid to (politely) ask why. If you or your team still feel it is warranted, look back at the request; did you miss a relevant piece of information that would change the mind of the radiologist? If you still draw a blank, try speaking to a radiologist who specializes in that particular technique. Many teams have clinical radiology meetings; think about approaching someone who appreciates why you are asking that particular question. Alternatively, go back to your team; speak to your senior, who may have a better understanding of why the investigation is needed and be able to convey this to the radiologist.

►Remember that there is a patient at the heart of this, and you are their advocate. If the results of an investigation will change their management then explain this to the radiologist. Moreover, don't forget to explain it to your patient. Being whisked off to the department for investigation and intervention can be particularly terrifying if you aren't expecting it.

Interpreting an image

You won't always be able to get an immediate radiologist's interpretation so it is important to know how to review an image. ►First make sure the image you are looking at is of your patient. Check its date. And remember:

- *Practice makes perfect*—always look at the image before checking the report, learning how to distinguish normal from abnormal.
- *Understand how the scan is done*—this makes interpretation easier and helps you appreciate which scan will give the answer you need. It also gives practical clues to the result—eg a routine CXR is performed in the postero-anterior (PA) direction (the source posterior to the patient to minimize the cardiac shadow).
- *Use a systematic approach*—so that you don't miss subtleties.
- *Understand your anatomy*—virtually all investigations yield a 2D image from a 3D structure. An understanding of anatomical relationships of the area in question will help reconstruct the images in your mind.
- *Orientation*—for axial cross-sectional imaging this is as if you are looking up at the supine patient ►*from the feet*. For images with non-conventional orientations (eg MRCP) look on the image for clue markings, or rely on your knowledge of anatomy—it can be tricky to visualize oblique sections!
- *Remember the patient*—an investigation is only one part of the clinical work-up, don't rely solely on the investigation result for your management decisions. Go back to see the patient after looking at the investigation and reading the radiologist's report: you might notice something that you didn't before.

Presenting an image

Everyone has their own method for presenting, and the right way is *your own way*. As long as you cover everything systematically—because we all get 'hot-seat amnesia' at some point—the particulars will take care of themselves. Continue to polish your own method and remember a few extra tips for when an image is presented expectantly by your consultant/examiner and the floor is yours. A brief silence with a thoughtful expression as you analyse the image is fine, then:

- State the written details: name, date of birth, where and how the imaging was taken. Look for clues: weighting of an MRI, a '+ c' indicating that contrast medium has been used, the phase of the investigation (arterial/venous/portal), or even the name of the organ printed on an ultrasound.
- State the type, mode, and technical quality of investigation—not always easy!

Going through this list also gives you a bit of thinking time. Then:

- Start with life-threatening or very obvious abnormalities. *Then be systematic:*
- Is the patient's position adequate? Any lines, leads, or tubes? Note their position.
- Just like the bedside clues in a physical examination, there are clues in radiology examinations. Note oxygen masks, ECG leads, venous access, infusion apparatus, and invasive devices. Identifying what they are also helps you to look through what may otherwise appear to be a cluttered mess.
- Note any abnormalities and try to contextualize these with whatever you already know of the patient. The abnormality may be hiding in plain sight, but if struggling, step back and note any asymmetry or areas that just 'look different'.
- With cross-sectional imaging, scan through adjacent sections noting the anatomy of one organ system or structure at a time (this may mean going up and down through a CT abdomen multiple times).
- Giving a differential diagnosis is good practice, as not all findings are diagnostic.
- If there is additional clinical information that would help you to make a diagnosis, don't be afraid to ask. After all, we treat patients and not images!

Remember: •X-ray=*radiodensity* (lucency/opacity). •CT=*attenuation*. •US=*echogenicity*. •MRI=*signal intensity*.

Chest x-ray—part 1

Images are usually taken on inspiration with the x-ray source behind the patient (postero-anterior, PA). Mobile images may be antero-posterior (AP, fig 16.6), magnifying heart size. If supine, distribution of air and fluid in lungs and pleural cavities is altered and the diaphragm is elevated.

Acclimatize yourself to the four cardinal elements of the chest radiograph, memorably (albeit slightly inaccurately) termed bone, air, fat, and 'water'/soft tissue. Each has its own radiographic density. ►*A border is only seen at an interface of two densities,* eg heart (soft tissue) and lung (air); this 'silhouette' is lost if air in the lung is replaced by consolidation ('water'). The silhouette sign localizes pathology (eg middle lobe pneumonia or collapse causing loss of clarity of the right heart border, fig 16.2). When interpreting a CXR use a systematic approach that works for you, eg:

Technical quality

- *Rotation:* The sternal ends of the clavicles should symmetrically overlie the transverse processes of the 4th or 5th thoracic vertebrae. A rotated image can alter the position of structures, eg rotation to the right projects the aortic arch vessels over the right upper zone, appearing as though there is a mass.
- *Inspiration:* There should be 5 to 7 ribs visible anteriorly (or 10 posteriorly). Hyperinflation can be abnormal, eg COPD. Poor inspiration can mimic cardiomegaly, as the heart is usually pulled down (hence elongated) with inspiration, and crowding of vessels at the lung bases can mimic consolidation or collapse. This is common in patients who are acutely unwell, particularly those in pain or unconscious. Take care in interpreting these images.
- *Exposure:* An under-exposed image will be too white and an over-exposed image will be too black. Both cause a loss of definition and quality although some compensation can be made with standard viewing software.
- *Position:* The entire lung margin should be visible.

Trachea Normally central or just to the right. Deviated by collapse (towards the lesion), expansion (away from the lesion), or patient rotation.

Mediastinum May be: *Widened* by mediastinal fat; retrosternal thyroid; aortic aneurysm/unfolding; lymph node enlargement (sarcoidosis, lymphoma, metastases, TB); tumour (thymoma, teratoma); cysts (bronchogenic, pericardial); paravertebral mass (TB). *Shifted* towards a collapsed lung or away from processes that add volume (eg a large mass or a tension pneumothorax).

There are three bulges normally visible on the left border of the mediastinum that help identify pathology if abnormal. From superior to inferior they are: **1** Aortic knuckle. **2** Pulmonary outflow tract. **3** Left ventricle.

Hila The left hilum is higher than the right or at the same level (not lower); they should be the same size and density. The hila may be: *Pulled up or down* by fibrosis or collapse. *Enlarged* by: pulmonary arterial hypertension; bronchogenic ca; lymph nodes. ►Sarcoidosis, TB, and lymphoma can give *bilateral* hilar lymphadenopathy. *Calcified* due to: sarcoid, past TB; silicosis; histoplasmosis (p408).

Heart Normally less than half of the width of the thorax (cardiothoracic ratio <0.5). ⅓ should lie to the right of the vertebral column, ⅔ to the left. It may appear elongated if the chest is hyperinflated (COPD); or enlarged if the image is AP or if there is LV failure (fig 16.3), or a pericardial effusion. Are there calcified valves?

Diaphragm The right side is often slightly higher (due to the liver). *Causes of raised hemidiaphragm:* Trouble above the diaphragm—lung volume loss or inflammation. Trouble with the diaphragm—stroke; phrenic nerve palsy (causes, p504; any mediastinal mass?). Trouble below the diaphragm—hepatomegaly; subphrenic abscess. NB subpulmonic effusion (effusions having a similar contour to the diaphragm without a characteristic meniscus) and diaphragm rupture give apparent elevation. NB: bilateral palsies (polio, muscular dystrophy) cause hypoxia.

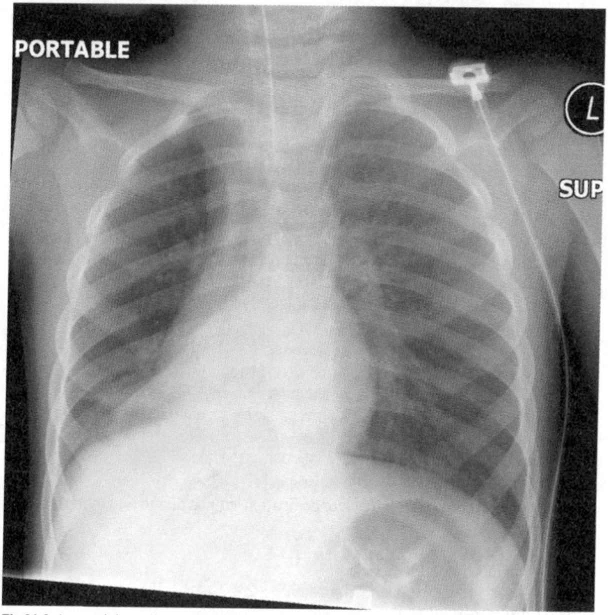

Fig 16.2 Lower lobe collapse (right lung). The right heart border is obscured. Volume loss in the right lower zone results in a hyper-expanded right upper lobe that is more radiolucent than the left upper lobe.

Courtesy of Dr Edmund Godfrey.

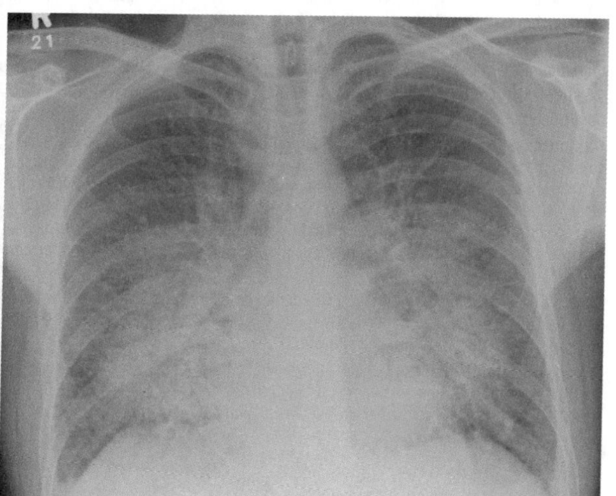

Fig 16.3 'Bat's wing', peri-hilar pulmonary oedema indicating heart failure and fluid overload.

Courtesy of Dr Edmund Godfrey.

Chest x-ray—part 2: the lungs

The apex of the lower lobe rises up to the 4th rib posteriorly, so it is difficult to ascribe the true location of a lobe on a PA image without additional information from a lateral view. It may therefore be better to use the term 'zone' rather than lobe when localizing a lesion.

Opacification Lung opacities are described as nodular, reticular (network of fine lines, interstitial), or alveolar (fluffy). A single nodule may be called a space-occupying lesion (SOL).

Nodules: (If >3cm across, the term pulmonary mass is used instead.)
- Neoplasia: metastases (often missed if small), lung cancer, hamartoma, adenoma.
- Infections: varicella pneumonia, septic emboli, abscess (eg as an SOL), hydatid.
- Granulomas: miliary TB, sarcoidosis (see GPA, p714), histoplasmosis.
- Pneumoconioses (except asbestosis), Caplan's syndrome (p696).

Reticular opacification: =Lung parenchymal changes.
- Acute interstitial oedema.
- Infection: acute (viral, bacterial), chronic (TB, histoplasmosis).
- Fibrosis: usual interstitial pneumonia (UIP), non-specific interstitial pneumonia (NSIP), drugs (eg methotrexate, bleomycin, crack cocaine), connective tissue disorders (rheumatoid arthritis—p546, GPA—p714, SLE, PAN, systemic sclerosis—p552, sarcoidosis), industrial lung diseases (silicosis, asbestosis).
- Malignancy (lymphangitis carcinomatosa).

Alveolar opacification: = Airspace opacification, can be due to any material filling the alveoli:
- Pus—pneumonia.
- Blood—haemorrhage, DIC (p352).
- Water—heart, renal, or liver failure (p302, p274), ARDS (p186), smoke inhalation (p847), drugs (heroin), O_2 toxicity, near drowning (*OHCS* p768).
- Cells—lymphoma, adenocarcinoma.
- Protein—alveolar proteinosis, ARDS, fat emboli (~7d post fracture).

'Ring' opacities: Either airways seen end-on (bronchitis; bronchiectasis) or cavitating lesions, eg abscess (bacterial, fungal, amoebic), tumour, or pulmonary infarct (wedge-shaped with a pleural base).

Linear opacities: Septal lines (Kerley B lines, ie interlobular lymphatics seen with fluid, tumour, or dusts); atelectasis; pleural plaques (asbestos exposure).

White-out of whole hemithorax: (fig 16.4) Pneumonia, large pleural effusion, ARDS, post-pneumonectomy.

Gas outside the lungs Check for a pneumothorax (hard to spot if apical or in a supine image, can you see vascular markings right out to the periphery?), surgical emphysema (trauma, iatrogenic), and gas under the diaphragm (surgery, perforated viscus, trauma). *Pneumomediastinum:* Air tracks along mediastinum, into the neck. Due to rupture of alveolar wall (eg asthma or pulmonary barotrauma) or bronchial or oesophageal trauma (can be iatrogenic, eg from endoscope). *Pneumopericardium:* Rare (usually iatrogenic).

Bones Check the *clavicles* for fracture, *ribs* for fractures and lesions (eg metastases), *vertebral column* for degenerative disease, collapse, or destruction, and *shoulders* for dislocation, fracture, and arthritis.

An apparently normal CXR? Check for tracheal compression, absent breast shadow (mastectomy), double left heart border (left lower lobe collapse, fig 16.5), fluid level behind the heart (hiatus hernia, achalasia), and paravertebral abscess (TB).

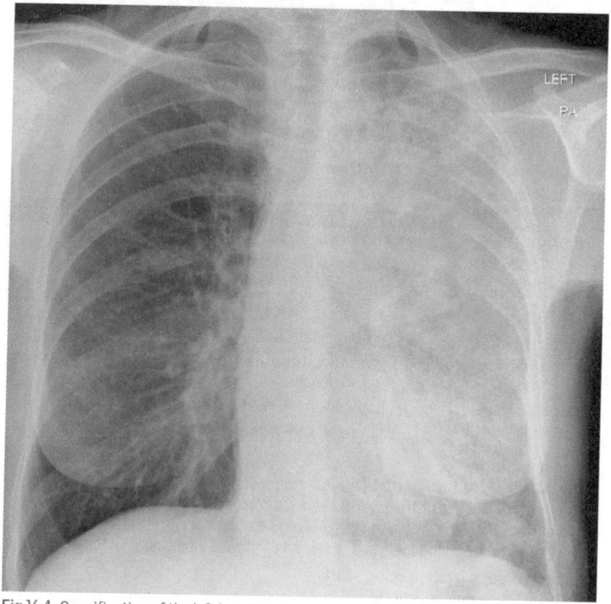

Fig 16.4 Opacification of the left hemithorax from consolidation.

Courtesy of Dr Edmund Godfrey.

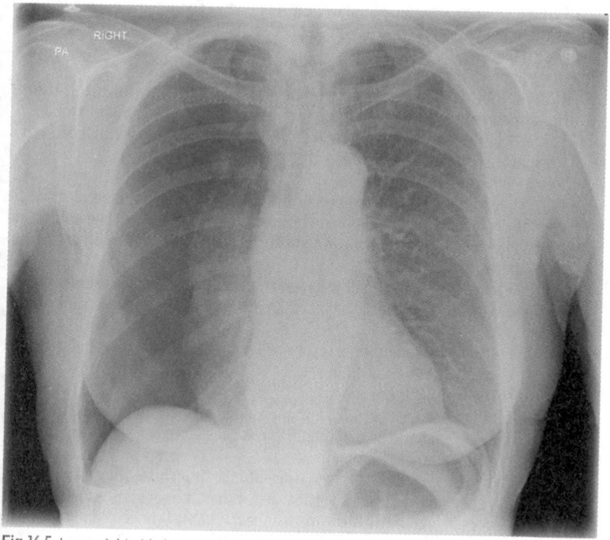

Fig 16.5 Large right-sided pneumothorax; note the trachea remains central, suggesting this is a simple pneumothorax, not a tension pneumothorax.

Courtesy of Dr Edmund Godfrey.

Chest x-ray—part 3

Confirming the position of various tubes, lines, and leads on a CXR can be a daunting task, as incorrect positioning can have deadly consequences: an NG tube which is misplaced can cause aspiration pneumonia, or a poorly positioned CVC can lead to fatal arrhythmias. However, this can be a straightforward task if you recall some basic anatomy (figs 16.6, 16.7; table 16.2).

►If you are unsure, always ask a senior.

Table 16.2 Radiological confirmation of device placement

Line/tube/lead	Correct position for tip(s)
CVC (p774)	In the SVC or brachiocephalic vein
PICC	In the SVC or brachiocephalic vein
Tunnelled line, eg Hickman	At the junction of the SVC and right atrium
Endotracheal	3-7 cm above the carina (in adult)
Nasogastric (p759)	10cm beyond the gastro-oesophageal junction
Chest drain (p766)	In the pleural space tracking either up (for pneumothorax) or down (for effusion)
Cardiac pacemaker/temporary pacing wire (p776)	Atrial lead—in the right appendage Ventricular lead—in the apex of the right ventricle

Normal anatomy

- The SVC begins at the right 1st anterior intercostal space.
- The right atrium lies at the level of the 3rd intercostal space.
- The carina should be visible at the level of T5–T7 thoracic vertebrae.
- The right atrial appendage sits at the level of the 3rd intercostal space.

Common bleeps from nursing staff

1 *Central line not aspirating:*
   - Is the tip in the right place (see earlier in topic) or has it gone up into the internal jugular, too far in (sitting against the tricuspid valve, does the patient have an arrhythmia?) or not far enough in (sitting against a venous valve)?
   - Is the tip kinked, suggesting it may be in a side vessel or against the vessel wall?
   - If the line looks appropriately positioned, consider flushing gently, could the line be blocked?

2 *Patient not ventilating well:*
   - Is the ET tube down the right main bronchus (causes left lung collapse, or rarely right pneumothorax)? Retract tube to correct position (see earlier in topic).
   - Is the ET tube blocked? Most have a secondary port allowing ventilation even if the main hole is blocked, get anaesthetic assistance!

3 *Chest drain not bubbling/swinging:*
   - Is it correctly positioned (see earlier in topic)—if not in the pleural space, it cannot drain the air/fluid. Common problems include sitting in the soft tissue of the chest wall, or sitting above the effusion, below the pneumothorax, or in the oblique fissure.
   - Is it blocked? If draining an effusion and correctly positioned, consider gently flushing with 10mL of sterile saline, then aspirating. If not successful, obtain senior advice.
   - Has the effusion/pneumothorax resolved? Pneumothoraces can rapidly resolve with a correctly positioned drain.

4 *Unable to aspirate from NG tube:*
   - Is NG tube not far enough in/coiled in oesophagus? Tip is radio-opaque and should be visible below the diaphragm, if it is coiled it may lie in the pharynx or anywhere along the mediastinum.
   - Is NG tube passing down the trachea and into the bronchus? The oesophagus is (generally speaking) a straight vertical line, if the tube veers off to left or right before it goes below the diaphragm, assume it is in the bronchus and replace it.

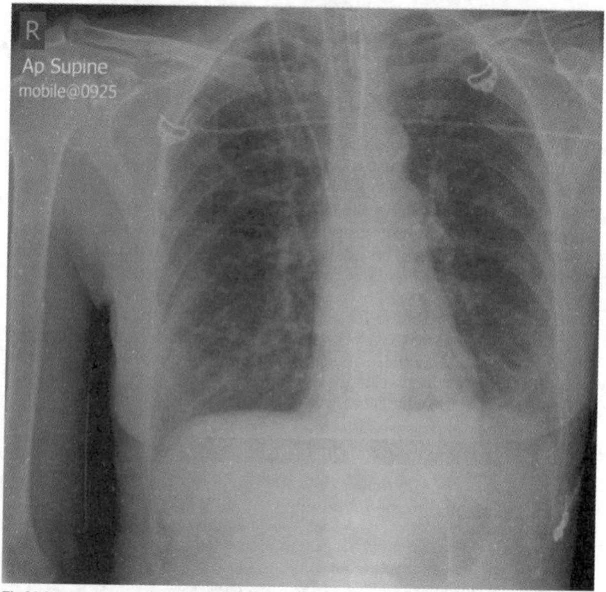

Fig 16.6 Image from ICU showing ET tube, CVC, and NG tube *in situ* with ECG leads placed across the chest.
Image courtesy of Dr Elen Thomson, Leeds Teaching Hospitals.

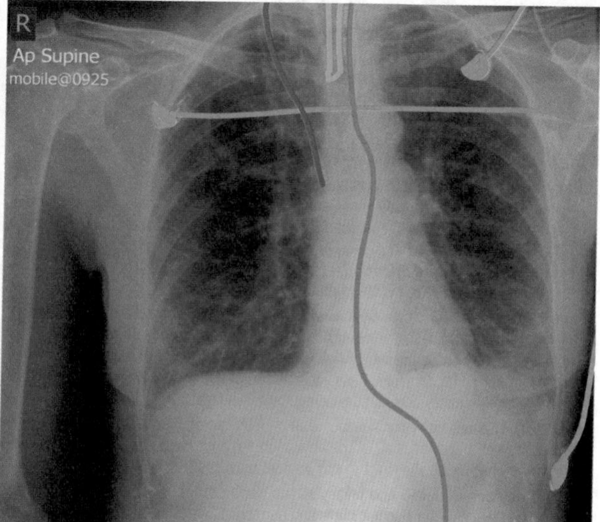

Fig 16.7 Knowing where lines and tubes should be placed is an essential skill. An ET tube (orange) should sit 3–7cm above the carina; this one is slightly high. The tip of the CVC (red, here a right internal jugular line) should lie in the SVC, as seen here, or just in the right atrium. The tip of the NG tube (green) must be seen below the diaphragm to ensure it is placed in the oesophagus, not the trachea. Do not confuse external leads (blue) with internal lines.

Plain abdominal x-ray

These are rarely diagnostic and involve a radiation dose equivalent to 50 CXRs. Indications for AXR with acute abdominal symptoms:

- Suspicion of obstruction (or intussusception, eg in paediatrics).
- Acute flare of inflammatory bowel disease (eg to confirm/exclude megacolon).
- Renal colic with known renal stones (if first presentation, CT KUB is better).
- Ingestion of a sharp or poisonous foreign body (eg lithium battery).

Bowel gas pattern is best assessed on supine images and free intraperitoneal gas (signifying perforation) is best seen on an erect CXR (fig 13.26, p607).

Gas patterns Look for: an abnormal quantity of gas in the stomach, small intestine, or colon. Decide whether you are looking at small or large bowel (fig 16.8; table 16.3).

Small bowel diameter is normally ~2.5cm, the colon ~5cm, the caecum up to 10cm. Dilated small bowel is seen in obstruction and paralytic ileus. Dilated large bowel (≳6cm) is seen in both these, and also in 'toxic dilatation', and, in the elderly, in benign hypotonicity. Grossly dilated segments of bowel (coffee bean sign) are seen in sigmoid and caecal volvulae—fig 13.28c, p611. Loss of normal mucosal folds and bowel wall thickening are seen in inflammatory colitis (eg IBD)—fig 16.9. 'Thumb-printing' is protrusion of thickened mural folds into the lumen, seen in large bowel ischaemia and colitis.

Table 16.3 Radiological gas patterns in the bowel

Small bowel	Large bowel	Ileus
• Smaller calibre • Central; multiple loops • *Valvuli conniventes:* folds that go from wall to wall, all the way across the lumen; more regular and finer than haustra • Grey (contains air and fluid)	• Larger calibre • Peripheral • *Semi-lunar folds:** don't go all the way across the lumen, but may appear to do so if viewed from an angle • Blacker (contains gas)†	• Both small and large bowel visible • There is no clear transition point that corresponds to an obstructing lesion

*Semi-lunar folds (plicae semilunares) lie in between adjacent haustra.
†The ascending colon contains liquid faeces, but the descending colon contains faecal pellets (*scybala*).

Gas outside the lumen You must explain any gas outside the lumen of the gut. It could be: **1** Pneumoperitoneum; signs on the supine AXR include: gas on both sides of the bowel wall (Rigler's sign), a triangle of gas in the RUQ trapped beneath the falciform ligament, and a circle of gas beneath the anterior abdominal wall. Seen with bowel perforation but also after laparoscopic surgery. **2** Gas in the urinary tract—eg in the bladder from a fistula. **3** Gas in the biliary tree (see next paragraph), or rarely **4** Intramural gas, found in bowel necrosis.

Biliary tree *Any stones:* ~10% visible on plain AXR. *Any gas:* (Pneumobilia.) Caused by: •post-ERCP/sphincterotomy •post-surgery (eg Whipple's) •recent stone passage •anaerobic cholangitis (rare) •gallbladder-bowel fistula: gallstone migrates directly into the bowel (Rigler's triad is seen in 25%: pneumobilia, small bowel obstruction, an ectopic gallstone). ***Calcification:*** ('Porcelain gallbladder'.) Chronic inflammation from gallstones (associated with gallbladder cancer).

Urinary tract Check for calculi (visible in 90% of cases)[1] and normal anatomy: ***Kidneys:*** Length equivalent to 2½–3½ vertebral bodies, slope inferolaterally. Right is lower than the left ('pushed down' by the liver). Their outline can usually be seen due to surrounding layer of perinephric fat. ***Ureters:*** Pass near the tips of the lumbar transverse processes, cross the sacroiliac joints, down to the ischial spines, and turn medially to join the bladder.

Other soft tissues Look for size/position of: liver, spleen, and bladder. A big liver will push bowel to the left side of the abdomen. An enlarged spleen displaces bowel and stomach bubble to the right. A big bladder elevates these.

Medical devices Double-J and biliary stents, nephrostomy and gastrostomy tubes, intrauterine devices, laparoscopic clips, and peritoneal dialysis catheters can be seen.

Bones and joints Plain AXR is not ideal, but there may be important abnormalities. In the lumbar spine, look for scoliosis and degeneration (osteophytes, joint space narrowing) as well as bone metastases or sacroiliitis.

1 Don't get confused by other calcifications—eg phleboliths: harmless calcifications found in the perivesical veins (rounded with a radiolucent centre).

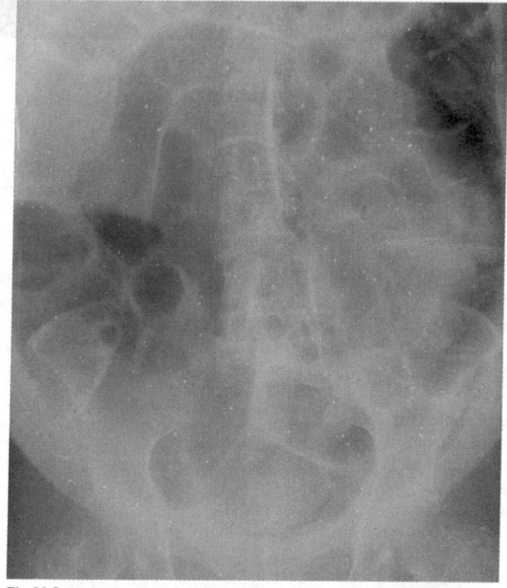

Fig 16.8 Multiple dilated air-filled loops of large and small bowel. This pattern is seen in ileus. Courtesy of Norwich Radiology Department.

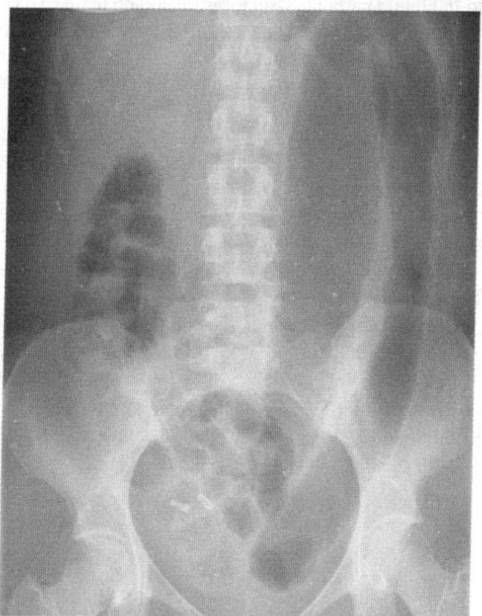

Fig 16.9 Abdominal image showing toxic megacolon associated with ulcerative colitis, note colon wall thickening and loss of mucosal folds. Courtesy of Dr Edmund Godfrey.

Computed tomography (CT)

Can give whole-body images in under one breath (thanks to continuous, helical data acquisition). Within a single slice (eg 0.5 or 5mm thick), CT records the attenuation (=loss of energy from, eg absorption or reflection) of different tissues to ionizing radiation and calculates a mean value for a given volume of tissue (a 'voxel'). This value is represented in greyscale as a single point, called a pixel, in the final 2D image (or 3D 'reconstruction'—fig 16.13). The greyscale of the pixel is measured on the Hounsfield scale (see fig 16.10) relative to the attenuation of water, 0 Hounsfield units (HU), and air, −1000HU. The human eye and display systems have a limited greyscale range, so different settings (levels and 'windows') are used to focus on differences in attenuation in ranges typical for tissues of different density, eg bone or lung (fig 16.11).

►CTs are responsible for up to 40% of iatrogenic radiation in high-use settings, which could account for ~1% of all cancers: always balance benefits of CT vs other modalities with less or no radiation (ultrasound; MRI), particularly in the young or in those with chronic disease likely to undergo multiple imaging investigations. Discuss with a radiologist—there are several technical aspects of imaging that can limit radiation dose whilst still providing clinically useful information.

Imaging of choice for

- Staging and monitoring most malignant disease.
- Intracranial pathology, eg stroke, trauma, ↑ICP, and space-occupying lesions.
- Trauma.
- Pre-operative assessment of complex masses.
- Assessment of acute abdomen (figs 16.15, 16.16). NB ultrasound increasingly used (p736).
- Following abdominal surgery.

Contrast medium (p748) Enhance anatomical detail by use of a high- or low (water)-attenuating medium to fill the lumen of a structure. *Give IV* to image vascular anatomy (fig 16.12) and vascular structures (including highly perfused tumours). Images acquired at different times ('phases') after injection will show the agent in arterial or venous structures or during 'washout' (=clearing). *Perfusion CT* maps cerebral blood flow by acquiring serial images after contrast administration then combines these into a colour-coded image of perfusion times (fig 16.14). Ensure IV cannulae secure and sufficient gauge to allow for rapid injection of agent as bolus—extravasation of contrast can cause significant tissue damage. *Give PO* eg 1–12h before imaging bowel. *Give PR* for examining distal colonic lumen.

Contrast-enhanced CTs may include a pre-contrast series. Unenhanced imaging alone reduces radiation exposure and may be adequate for images of the brain, spine, lung, and musculoskeletal system or necessary in those with renal failure (contrast is nephrotoxic).

Streak artefact Remember that the CT slice image is a matrix representation of the attenuation produced by rotating around the patient. High-attenuation items such as metal fillings, clips, and prostheses (and even bone) can cause interference.

CT combined with PET (See p739.) Combines the anatomical detail of CT with the metabolic information of PET, to aid assessment of, eg neoplastic lesions. Radiation doses are much higher than CT alone.

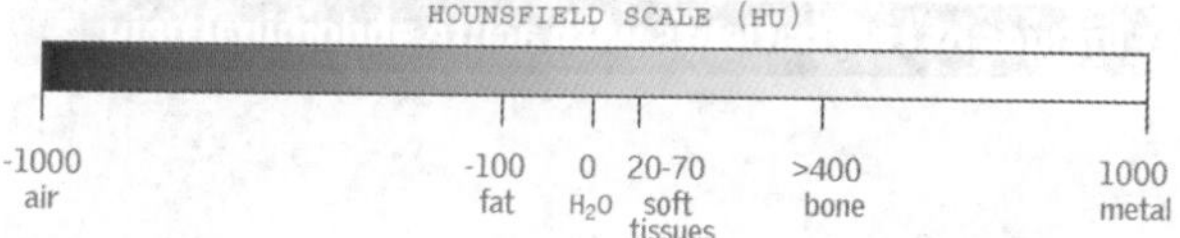

Fig 16.10 The Hounsfield scale.

Courtesy of Dr T Turmezei.

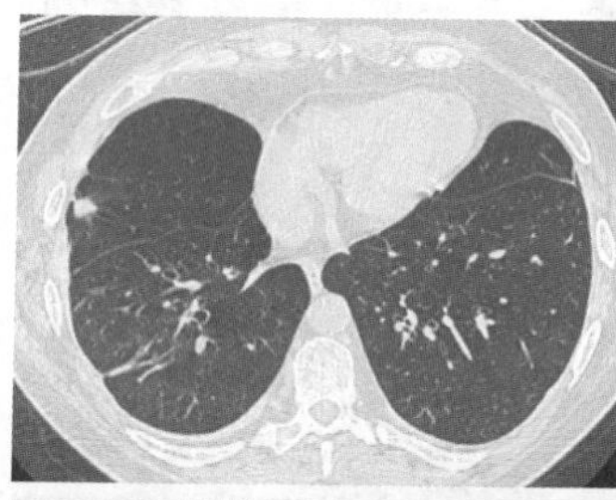

Fig 16.11 Axial high-resolution CT chest on a lung window algorithm; note solitary lesion in the right lung (in this case, from GPA).

Courtesy of Norwich Radiology Dept.

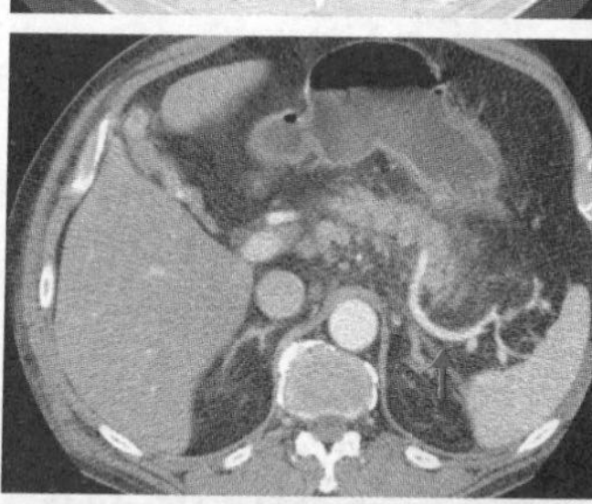

Fig 16.12 Axial CT of the abdomen after IV contrast (arterial phase). The tortuous splenic artery is enhanced (arrow)—so is the aorta, but not the inferior vena cava (compare to water in the stomach).

Courtesy of Norwich Radiology Dept.

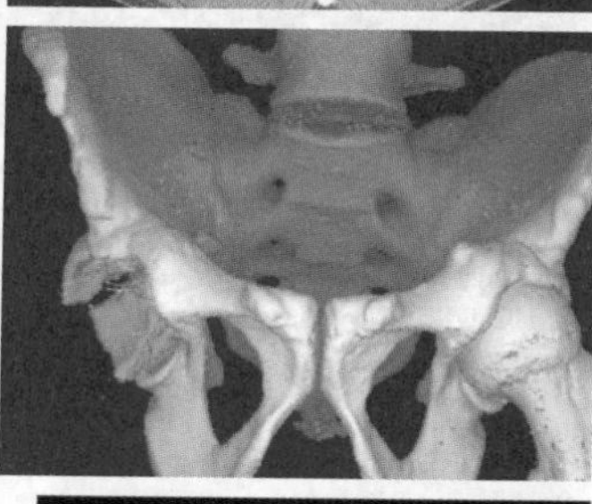

Fig 16.13 Surface rendered 3D CT reconstruction of the pelvis. The posterior aspect of the right acetabulum is fractured. The right femur has been digitally removed for better viewing.

Courtesy of Norwich Radiology Dept.

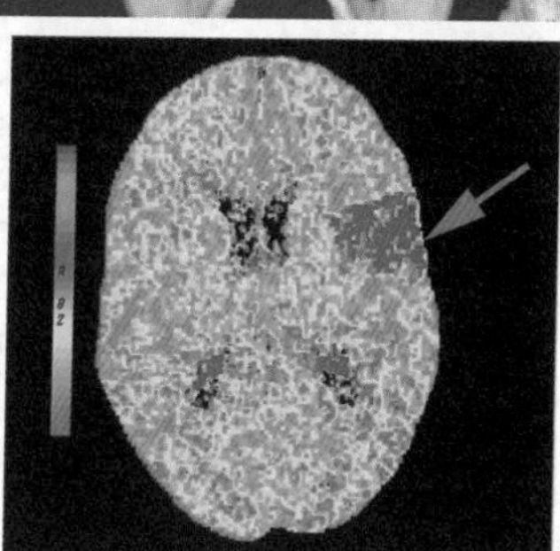

Fig 16.14 Cerebral perfusion CT showing ischaemia around the Sylvian fissure (arrow).

Courtesy of Dr C Cousens.

CT images of two patients with acute abdominal pain

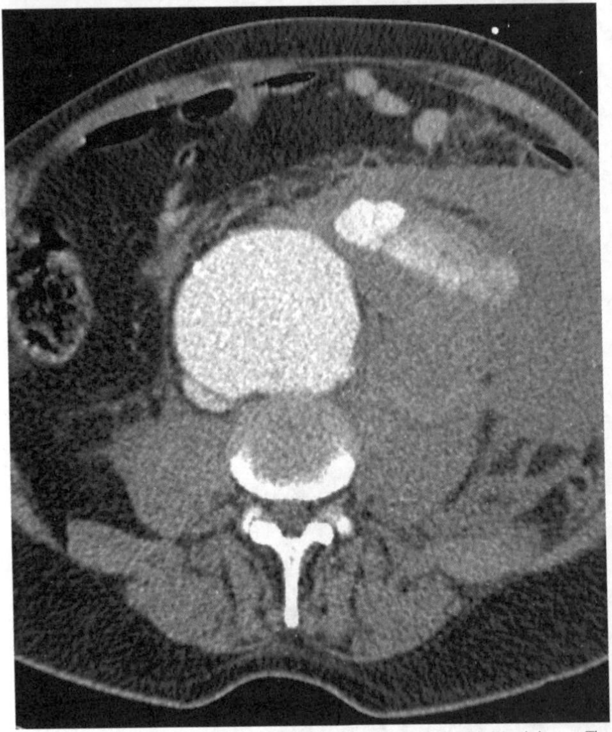

Fig 16.15 The history was of central abdominal pain with a non-peritonitic abdomen. The CT shows a leaking AAA. Under fluoroscopic screening, this can be repaired using stents, inserted via femoral arterial puncture and deployed in the aneurysm (p654). This kind of endovascular aneurysm repair (EVAR) is commonly used in the treatment of leaking AAA as well as elective repair of intact but enlarging aneurysms.

The changing roles of surgeons and CT in the acutely unwell

In the days when general surgeons did their rounds towards the end of an on-call day, there would be wards of patients with undiagnosed abdominal pain having 'drip-and-suck' regimens (IVI and NGT) while awaiting improvement or a change in their clinical condition that revealed the need for surgery. On opening up, the surgeon would try to deal with whatever pathology was found. With increased subspecialization and accurate emergency imaging (CT and US), patients are now matched to a team best equipped to deal with their condition. In this context, drip-and-suck is on the ebb, giving way to imaging, early intervention, rapid discharge, or onward referral. With increasing pressures to safeguard surgical beds for elective cases and on junior surgeons to polish their surgical logbooks in decreased training hours, can come attempts to deflect away from surgical teams the care of patients in whom imaging or clinical circumstances suggest no current requirement for an operation. But is this always appropriate? Do we expect on-call surgeons to be practitioners of medicine, assessing and managing patients with surgical pathology, even if a trip to the operating theatre is not currently called for, or simply technicians restricted to cutting?

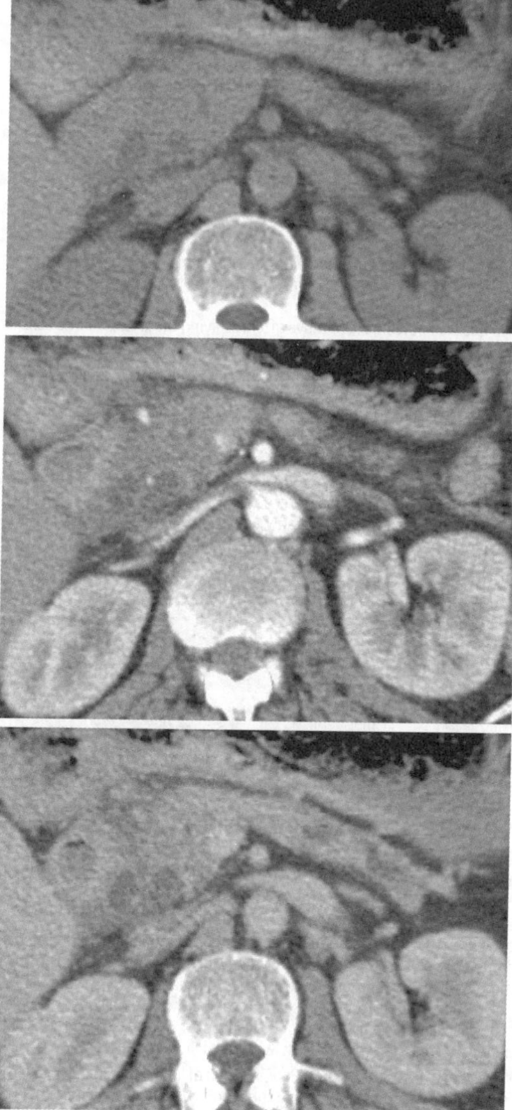

Fig 16.16 Triple-phase CT abdomen, cropped to show the pancreas. Top panel—unenhanced image, middle panel—arterial phase of contrast medium to look for pseudocysts and parenchymal enhancement, bottom panel—portal venous phase to look at veins. The history here was also central abdominal pain with a non-peritonitic abdomen. The CT shows an enlarged pancreatic head with fat stranding around the duodenopancreatic groove ('groove pancreatitis'), and two small areas of fluid attenuation posteriorly, likely to be pseudocysts.

Top panel courtesy of Dr Edmund Godfrey.

Magnetic resonance imaging (MRI)

1 A large proportion of the human body is fat or water (~80%).
2 Fat and water contain a large number of hydrogen nuclei (unpaired protons).
3 The spin of a positively charged hydrogen nucleus gives it magnetic polarity.

Thus...

- Placing the human body in a magnetic field aligns its hydrogen nuclei either with (parallel) or against (anti-parallel) the field.
- A radiofrequency (RF) pulse at the resonant frequency flips a few nuclei away from their original alignment by an angle depending on the amount of energy they absorb.
- When the RF pulse stops, the nuclei flip back (or *relax*) into their original alignment, emitting the energy (called an *echo*) that was absorbed from the RF pulse.
- Measuring and plotting the energy of the returning signal according to location (provided the nuclei haven't moved) gives a picture of fat, tissue, and water as distributed throughout the body.
- The hydrogen nuclei in flowing blood move after receiving the RF pulses. The echo is not detected, and so the vessel lumen appears black (flow void).

Rather than radiodensity or attenuation, the correct descriptive terminology for the greyscale seen in MRI is signal intensity: high signal appears white and low signal black (see table 16.4). Weighting is a quality of MRI that is dependent on the time between the RF pulses (repetition time, TR) and the time between an RF pulse and the echo (echo time, TE). MR images are most commonly T1-weighted (good for visualizing anatomy) or T2-weighted (good for visualizing disease) but can also be a mixture of both, called proton density (PD) weighting. FLAIR sequences produce heavily T2-weighted images. A good way to determine the weighting of an MR image is to look for water—eg in the aqueous humour of the eye, CSF, or synovial fluid (see table 16.4; fig 16.17).

Table 16.4 MRI sequence characteristics

	T1-weighted	T2-weighted
TR	Short (<1000ms)	Long (>2000ms)
TE	Short (<30ms)	Long (>80ms)
Low signal ■	Water Flowing Hb Fresh Hb Haemosiderin	Bone Flowing Hb DeoxyHb Haemosiderin Melanin
High signal □	Bone marrow Fat Cholesterol Gadolinium (p762) MetHb	Water Cholesterol Fresh Hb MetHb

Fig 16.17 T1-weighted MRI of the hips. Normal adult bone marrow is high signal due to fat; note also low signal from urine in the bladder.

Courtesy of Norwich Radiology Department

Advantages MRI's great bonus is that it does not involve ionizing radiation. It has no known long-term adverse effects. It is *excellent for imaging soft tissues* (water- and hence proton-dense) and is preferred over CT for musculoskeletal disorders and for many intracranial, head, and neck pathologies (figs 16.18–16.20). Multiplanar acquisition of images can provide multiple views and 3D reconstruction from one scan. MR angiography is also excellent for reconstructing vascular anatomy. This avoids the need for invasive angiography with femoral puncture or CT contrast in patients with renal impairment.

Disadvantages Long acquisition times. Poor imaging of lung parenchyma. Claustrophobic. Incompatible with some metal implants. High cost and specialized interpretation (=limited availability).

Contraindications *Absolute:* •Pacemakers; other implanted electrical devices. •Metallic foreign bodies, eg intra-ocular (consider orbital X-ray to exclude), shrapnel. •Non-compatible surgical clips/coils/heart valves. *Relative:* •If unable to complete the pre-scan questionnaire. •Cochlear implants. NB: orthopaedic prostheses and extracranial metallic clips are generally safe. ►If uncertain, ask a radiologist. *Contrast.* •Renal impairment (gadolinium can cause systemic fibrosis). •Allergy. •Pregnancy.

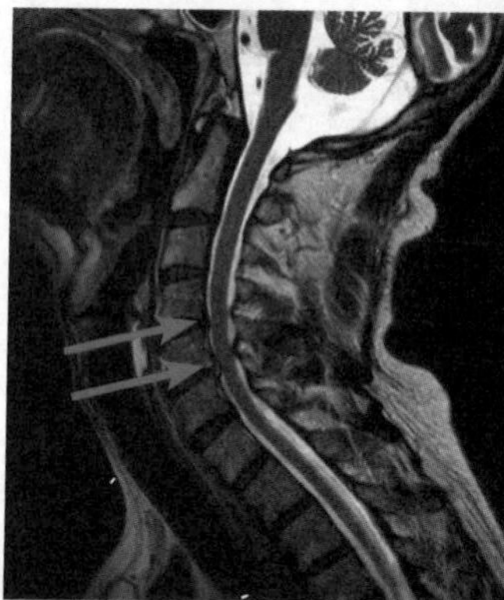

Fig 16.18 T2-weighted sagittal MRI of the cervical spine. There is impingement of the spinal cord at the C4/5 and C5/6 levels caused by degenerative disease. C2 (axis) is identifiable from the odontoid peg, which is embryologically derived from the body of C1 (atlas).
Courtesy of Norwich Radiology Department.

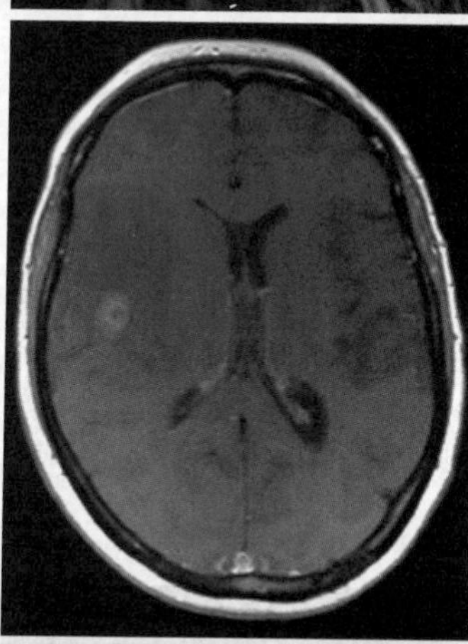

Fig 16.19 Axial T1-weighted MRI of the brain post-IV gadolinium. In the right temporo-parietal region there is a small area of high signal enhancement with a more central area of low signal, surrounded by a region of low signal (presumably vasogenic cerebral oedema) in comparison to the normal brain tissue. This is all causing mass effect with effacement of the sulci and adjacent right frontal horn of the lateral ventricle. There is very subtle midline shift.
Courtesy of Norwich Radiology Department.

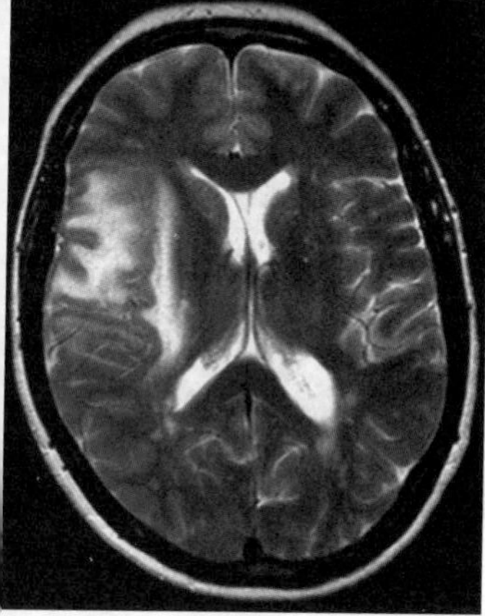

Fig 16.20 Axial T2-weighted MRI of the same patient at the same level as fig 16.19. The high signal in the temporo-parietal region is the oedema causing mass effect. The diagnosis was of a solitary metastasis. In this T2-weighted image the oedema and the cerebrospinal fluid are of high signal due to their water content.
Courtesy of Norwich Radiology Department.

Ultrasound (US)

Unlike the other methods of imaging, US doesn't use electromagnetic radiation. Instead, it relies on properties of longitudinal sound waves. This has made it a popular and safe form of imaging with increasingly widespread applications. High-frequency sound waves (3–15MHz) are generated in the transducer (transmitter and receiver) by the vibrations of a piezo-electric quartz crystal as a voltage is applied. Passage of sound waves through tissue is affected by *attenuation* and *reflection*. Attenuation disperses waves out of the receiver's range, but it is the waves reflected back to the transducer that determine the image. Its quality depends on the difference in *acoustic impedance* between adjacent soft tissues.

Processing With the help of software a real-time 2D image is made. During processing, an average attenuation value is assumed throughout the tissue examined, so if a higher-than-average attenuation structure is in the superficial tissues (eg fibrous tissue, calcification, or gas), then everything deep to it will be in a low intensity (black) acoustic shadow. If a lower-than-average attenuation object (eg fluid-filled/cystic structure) is in the superficial tissues then everything deep to it will be high intensity (white) or enhanced. If a tissue interface is strongly disparate, eg gas in the intestine, then all the waves are reflected back, making it impossible to image beyond it. See also figs 16.21–16.24.

Modes *B:* (Brightness) is the most common, giving 2D slices that map the different magnitudes of echo in greyscale. *M:* (Movement) traces the movement of structures within the line of the sound beam. It is used in imaging, eg heart valves (p110).

Duplex ultrasonography (flow and morphology) By combining Doppler effects (shifts in wavelength caused by movement of a source or reflecting surface) with B-mode ultrasound technology, flow characteristics of blood can be inferred (fig 16.21). This is extremely useful in arterial and venous studies, and echocardiography.

Advantages Portable; fast; non-ionizing; cheap; real-time; can be used with intervention; can enter organs, eg rectum, vagina, bowel. *Endoscopic US* can be used to stage and biopsy lung and GI tract cancers, eg stomach, pancreas, and also image the heart = transoesophageal echocardiogram or TOE, p110.

Disadvantages Operator dependent—interoperator variability high; poor quality if patient is obese; interference from bone, bowel gas, calculi, or superimposed organs can limit depth and quality of imaging.

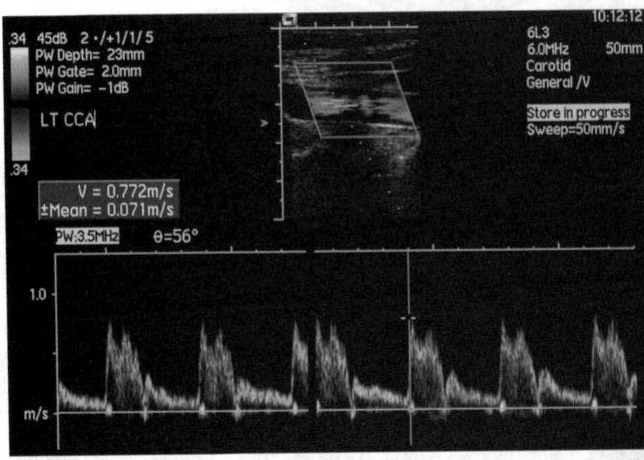

Fig 16.21 A normal Duplex US of the right common carotid artery with a flow rate=77cm/s. The Doppler trace (orange) is displayed below the main image.

Courtesy of Norwich Radiology Department.

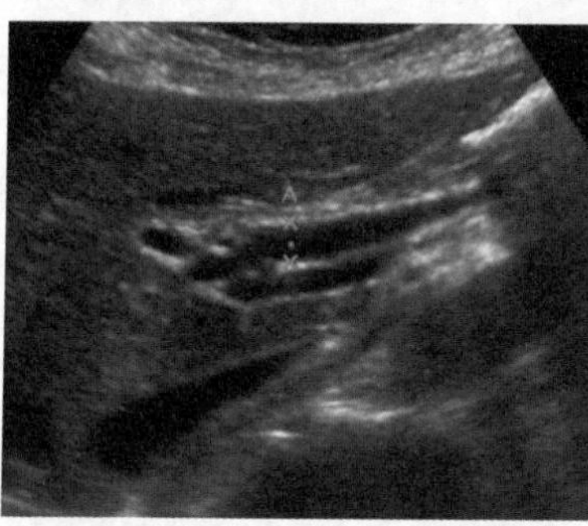

Fig 16.22 Ultrasound of the liver shows the common bile duct (CBD) to be dilated. Distal obstruction of the CBD causes proximal dilatation of the duct. It is important to correlate the width of the CBD with the ALP, as the normal diameter varies with age and previous interventions. Also check that the distal CBD tapers as it enters the duodenum. NB: the portal vein lies posterior to the duct (along with the hepatic artery) in the free edge of the lesser omentum. Next, ask 'What is causing the obstruction?' and 'Where can I get that information?'

Courtesy of Norwich Radiology Department.

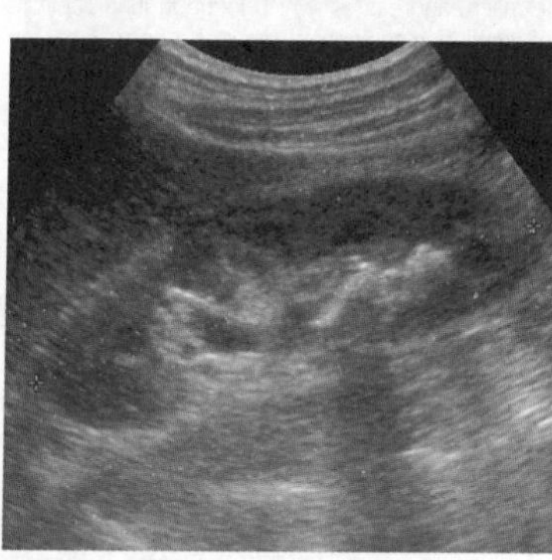

Fig 16.23 Ultrasound of the kidney. At first the image may seem normal but there is a wedge of posterior acoustic shadow cast by the object which is causing increased echogenicity in the lower pole calyces. Acoustic shadows in the kidney suggest stones—as here—or nephrocalcinosis.

Courtesy of Norwich Radiology Department.

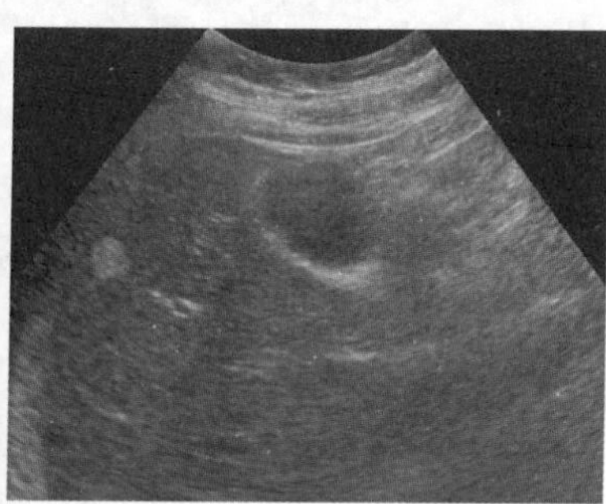

Fig 16.24 Longitudinal ultrasound of the right lobe of the liver showing a well-defined small area of echogenicity. This is the typical appearance of a liver haemangioma, a common benign liver lesion.

Courtesy of Norwich Radiology Department.

The majority of medical imaging is concerned with passing external waves (eg radiation) through the patient to a detector, and measuring scatter, slowing, or other alterations by various tissues. Nuclear medicine is the opposite; it measures emitted radiation from an internal source, introduced into the patient via injection, inhalation, or ingestion. It can be diagnostic (eg PET scanning) or therapeutic (eg radioiodine (I^{131}) ablation in thyrotoxicosis).

Because molecules labelled with radioisotopes are introduced into the patient, there is exposure to ionizing radiation, though doses are usually less than those from CT (see table 16.1, p719). The selection of molecule for labelling depends on the tissue of interest, as it should be something that will be readily taken up by that tissue, eg bisphosphonates for bone, glucose for fast-turnover tissue. Examples include:

Ventilation/perfusion (VQ) scan Uses inhaled technetium (Tc) or, less commonly, xenon-133 (^{133}Xe) plus injected ^{99m}Tc macro-aggregates, which lodge in lung capillaries. Normal perfusion excludes PE but ventilation component requires a normal CXR for comparison (figs 16.25, 16.26). Due to the large number of 'indeterminate' scans VQ is considered inferior to CTPA for the investigation of PE except in pregnancy (see p192).

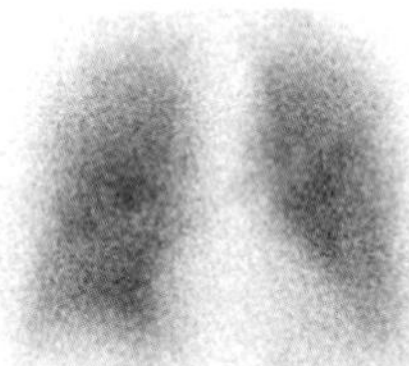

Fig 16.25 Ventilation scintigram. Courtesy of Norwich Radiology Department.

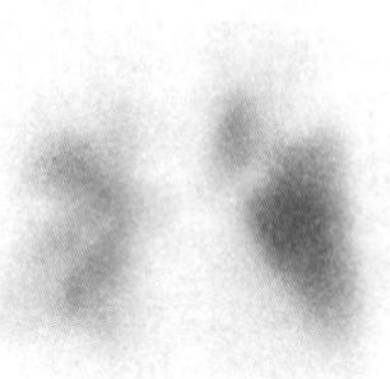

Fig 16.26 Perfusion scintigram showing mismatches with **fig 16.25**. Courtesy of Norwich Radiology Department.

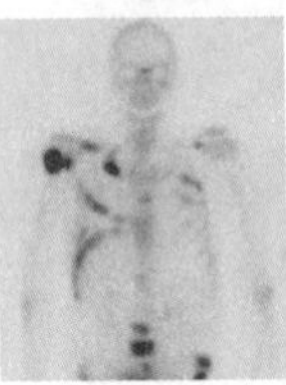

Fig 16.27 Bone scintigram showing metastases. Courtesy of Norwich Radiology Department.

Bone scintigraphy ^{99m}Tc-labelled bisphosphonates are readily taken up by bone, and concentrate in areas of pathology, eg tumours, fractures. It is much more sensitive in identifying metastases than X-ray, where lesions may not appear until >50% of bone matrix has been destroyed (**fig** 16.27).

Thyroid disease TcO_4 is used for differentiating Graves', toxic multinodular goitre, and subacute thyroiditis (fig 13.22, p601) as well as identifying ectopic tissue, functioning nodules, and residual/recurrent thyroid tissue after surgery. ~15% of cold (non-functioning) nodules are malignant. Hot nodules are often toxic adenomas.

Phaeochromocytoma Iodine-123 (^{123}I) meta-iodobenzylguanidine (MIBG) is taken up by sympathetic tissues, and indicates functioning, ectopic, and metastatic adrenal medullary (+other neural crest) tumours. ^{131}I-MIBG is also used for treatment.

Hyperparathyroidism ^{99m}Tc-methoxyisobutyl isonitrile (MIBI) scans can detect parathyroid adenomas.

Haemorrhage Red cells are removed from the patient and labelled with ^{99m}Tc, then re-injected to allow identification of a bleeding point. Used in both acute (after endoscopy and CT) and chronic GI bleeding, red cell scans are more sensitive than CT angiography and useful in intermittent bleeding, although localization can be challenging.

Renal function Chromium-51 (^{51}Cr) EDTA or DTPA (^{99m}Tc, p669) is used to assess GFR. ^{99m}Tc-mercapto-acetyltriglycine (MAG3) technique assesses relative (left-right) renal function and renal transit time (eg in renovascular disease). ^{99m}Tc-dimercaptosuccinic acid (DMSA) scanning (fig 16.28) is the gold standard for evaluation of renal scarring that occurs, eg in reflux nephropathy.

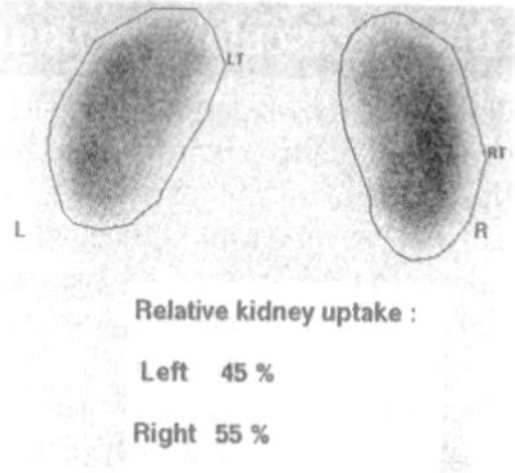

Fig 16.28 DMS showing relative renal function of each kidney.

Courtesy of Norwich Radiology Department.

Positron emission tomography (PET) One of the key investigations in malignancy, but also has a wide range of other uses. If the tracer chosen is ^{18}F-fluorodeoxyglucose (FDG), a short half-life glucose analogue, it becomes concentrated in metabolically active tissues. FDG decays rapidly to produce a positron that, after travelling a few millimetres through tissue, annihilates with an electron to produce a pair of high-energy photons (gamma rays), which PET detects. Normal high uptake of FDG occurs in brain, liver, kidney, bladder, larynx, and lymphoid tissue of pharynx and must be considered when assessing images. *Neoplasms* have high uptake of FDG with hotspots suggesting primary disease or metastases. Since inflammatory lesions will also show high uptake, there is a risk of false-positive results (eg sarcoid, TB); diagnosis must be confirmed with histology of suspicious lesions. PET allows *staging* of many solid organ malignancies (lung, melanoma, oesophageal) as well as lymphomas, and is particularly useful for *planning* of radiotherapy and surgery for both primary disease and metastases. PET can also be used to image occult sources of infection. PET can be combined with CT or MRI to provide high-quality images combining anatomy with physiology. A range of alternative tracers are now entering clinical use with radiotracers conjugated to other tissue-specific substrates (eg ^{11}C-labelled metomidate to detect tumors of adrenocortical origin, somatostatin tracers in neuroendocrine tumours, and amyloid tracers in Alzheimer's disease).

Single photon emission computed tomography (SPECT) Similar to PET but rather than using positron emission, it uses a radioisotope-labelled molecule as per conventional nuclear imaging, but with two gamma cameras for detection. The images produced are of lower resolution than PET but the isotopes used are longer lived and more easily available. Examples include myocardial perfusion scanning (p741).

CT *Cardiac CT:* Modern CT scanners can acquire images with sufficient speed and resolution to image coronary arteries and exclude significant disease with a negative predictive value of 97–99%. It can also visualize CABG patency, provide coronary artery Ca^{2+} scoring (a risk factor for coronary artery disease, p117), demonstrate cardiac anatomy including congenital anomalies, and estimate ventricular function. *Vascular CT:* Has become routine in emergency assessment of suspected dissections, ruptured aneurysms, and arterial and venous thromboses (fig 16.29). CT angiography has overtaken invasive angiography in the assessment of many conditions such as stable angina and renal artery stenosis.

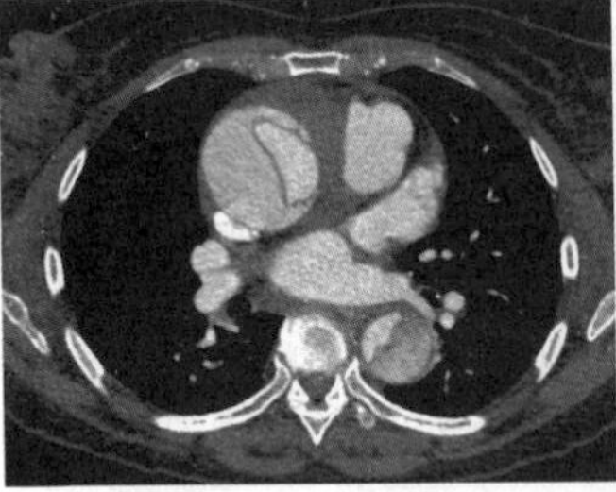

Fig 16.29 CT angiogram showing type A (ascending) aortic dissection with haemopericardium.

Courtesy of Dr C Cousins.

Catheter angiography Wherever intervention may be required, contrast studies such as angiography provide both image clarity and the possibility of proceeding to intervention, eg angioplasty or stenting of vessels, endovascular repair of aneurysms, clipping/coiling of aneurysms (see p746). Remember that these have a high burden of both radiation and contrast medium, so check renal function before requesting. *Complications* include those of arterial puncture (bleeding, infection, thrombosis, dissection, pseudoaneurysm formation) plus cholesterol emboli, thromboemboli, and vasospasm.

MRI *Cardiac MRI* using ECG-gating to acquire the imaging data and relate it to the position in the cardiac cycle (best when the patient is in sinus rhythm) can reduce movement artefact and lead to excellent resolution images for functional assessment. This, coupled with a lack of radiation, makes it ideal for the assessment of a wide range of structural and functional heart diseases. Flow velocities can be measured and, because the flow is proportional to the pressure differences, degrees of stenosis and regurgitation across heart valves can be calculated. Myocardial infarction, perfusion, and viability can also be imaged with the use of IV gadolinium contrast (p748). *Vascular MRI* is used to limit radiation exposure where multiple investigations may be required over a long time period, eg follow-up of intracranial aneurysm coiling, aortic root size in a young patient with Marfan's syndrome (p706), or Takayasu's arteritis (p712).

Ultrasound Non-invasive, relatively low cost, and with no radiation, US is excellent for assessing the heart and vasculature particularly in acute settings where the test can be performed at the bedside. *Cardiac US* (=echocardiography) evaluates myocardial and valvular anatomy and function (p110). The use of exercise or pharmacological agents for 'stress echocardiography' can permit more detailed functional assessment. *Vascular US* Doppler ultrasonography is widely used for detection of thrombotic disease (eg DVT p578, portal vein thrombosis p276) and carotid atherosclerosis (p472).

Multiple gated acquisition (MUGA) scanning is a non-invasive way to measure left ventricle ejection fraction. After injection of ^{99m}Tc-labelled RBCs, a dynamic image of the left ventricle is obtained for a few hundred heartbeats by gamma camera. Since estimates of LVEF show less inter-operator variation than with echocardiograpy, uses include the detailed serial assessment of LVEF in patients undergoing cardiotoxic chemotherapy (eg anthracyclines, trastuzumab).

Myocardial perfusion imaging A non-invasive method of assessing regional myocardial blood flow and the cellular integrity of myocytes. The technique uses radionuclide tracers which cross the myocyte membrane and are trapped intracellularly. Thallium-201 (^{201}Tl), a K^+ analogue, is distributed via regional myocardial blood flow and requires cellular integrity for uptake. Newer technetium-99 (^{99}Tc)-based agents are similar to ^{201}Tl but have improved imaging characteristics, and can be used to assess myocardial perfusion and LV performance in the same study (fig 16.30). Myocardial territories supplied by unobstructed coronary vessels have normal perfusion whereas regions supplied by stenosed coronary vessels have poorer relative perfusion, a difference that is accentuated by exercise. For this reason, exercise tests are used in conjunction with radionuclide imaging to identify areas at risk of ischaemia/infarction. Exercise scans are compared with resting views: *reversible* (ischaemia) or *fixed defects* (infarct) can be seen and the coronary artery involved reliably predicted. Drugs (eg adenosine, dobutamine, and dipyridamole) can also be used to induce perfusion differences between normal and underperfused tissues.

Myocardial perfusion imaging adds information in patients presenting with acute MI (to determine the amount of myocardium salvaged by thrombolysis) and in diagnosing acute chest pain in those without classical ECG changes (to define the presence of significant perfusion defects).

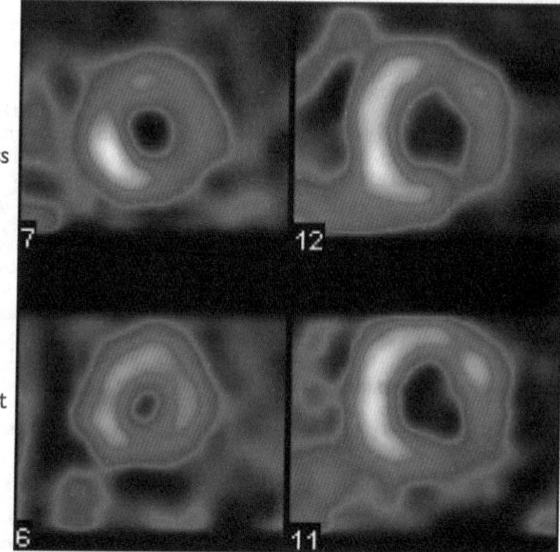

Fig 16.30 ^{99}Tc perfusion study showing perfusion defect in the left ventricle anterior and lateral walls at stress which is partially reversible (difference between stress and rest images). This study is good for small vessel disease such as in diabetes; CT and coronary angiography do not show small vessel disease well.

Courtesy of Dr C Cousins.

Gastrointestinal imaging

Ultrasound Widely used for imaging all intra-abdominal organs, including an emerging role in small bowel imaging (though overlying bowel gas can cast acoustic shadows). US is the 1st-line imaging choice for abnormal LFTs, jaundice, hepatomegaly, renal dysfunction, and abdominal masses. Ensure the patient is 'nil by mouth' for 4 hours beforehand (aids gallbladder filling). Pelvic US needs a full bladder (consider clamping the catheter if appropriate). US may also guide diagnostic biopsy and therapeutic aspiration of cysts or collections.

CT plays an important role in the investigation of acute abdominal pain (see pp730–3). It is unparalleled in the detection of free gas and intra-abdominal collections, and allows good visualization of the colon and retroperitoneal areas. Oral or IV contrast medium enhances definition (p730). The big disadvantage is the radiation dose. *CT colonography* (*CTC*; fig 16.31) uses rectal air or CO_2 insufflation, usually coupled with an oral 'stool tagging' agent to visualize the colonic mucosa in those unfit for endoscopic evaluation or in whom endoscopic evaluation has failed (eg in a stenosing tumour, where it can be used to assess the proximal colon and allow assessment of liver and nodal metastases at the same time). A negative test can be regarded as definitive but if polyps or masses are seen then patients will usually require a colonoscopy.

Wireless capsule endoscopy: See p248.

Magnetic resonance imaging (MRI) This gives excellent soft tissue imaging, giving it an important role in imaging the liver, biliary system, pancreas, and pancreatic duct (MRCP—magnetic resonance cholangiopancreatography; fig 16.32). As well as assessing potential malignant disease, MRCP is the imaging modality of choice for detection of common bile duct stones that can be missed on US. MRI performed after fluid loading of the small bowel (fluid delivered orally=MRI enterography; fluid delivered via nasoduodenal tube=MRI enteroclysis) permits assessment of small bowel inflammation (eg Crohn's) and lesions that can be challenging to reach with conventional endoscopy.

Endoscopic retrograde cholangiopancreatography (ERCP; fig 16.33) *Indications:* No longer routinely used for diagnosis, it still has a significant therapeutic role: sphincterotomy for common bile duct stones; stenting of benign or malignant strictures and obtaining brushings to diagnose the nature of a stricture. *Method:* A catheter is advanced from a side-viewing duodenoscope via the ampulla into the common bile duct. Contrast medium is injected and images taken to show lesions in the biliary tree and pancreatic ducts. *Complications:* Pancreatitis; bleeding; cholangitis; perforation. Mortality <0.2% overall; 0.4% if performing stone removal.

Endoscopic ultrasound (EUS; see p736.) Commonly used in diagnosis of upper GI abnormalities, and is excellent for diagnosis of oesophageal, gastric, and pancreatic cancers. It allows staging by assessing depth of invasion, as well as histological diagnosis by biopsy of lesions.

Contrast studies (fig 16.34) These can help in dysphagia (p250) and assessing integrity of anastomoses post-op. Real-time fluoroscopic imaging studies assess swallowing function. Barium gives better contrast but iodine-based water-soluble contrast medium is used if there is a concern of perforation. *Contrast enemas* are increasingly obsolete and now used to exclude a leak following a low anterior resection, for proctograms, and not much else.

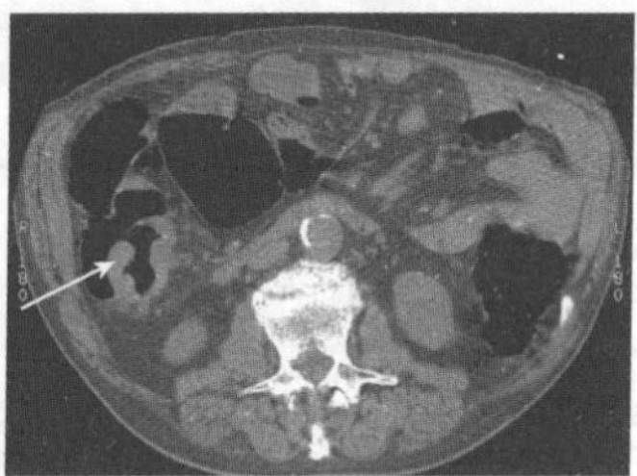

Fig 16.31 Axial CT colonogram: mural thickening (?ascending colon tumour).
Courtesy of Norwich Radiology Department.

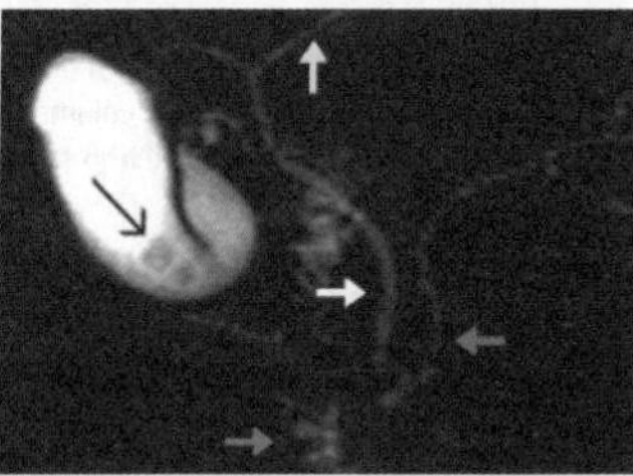

Fig 16.32 MRCP of the biliary system showing: left hepatic duct (yellow arrow); multiple gallstones in the gallbladder (black arrow); common bile duct (white arrow); pancreatic duct (red arrow); duodenum (green arrow).
Courtesy of Norwich Radiology Department.

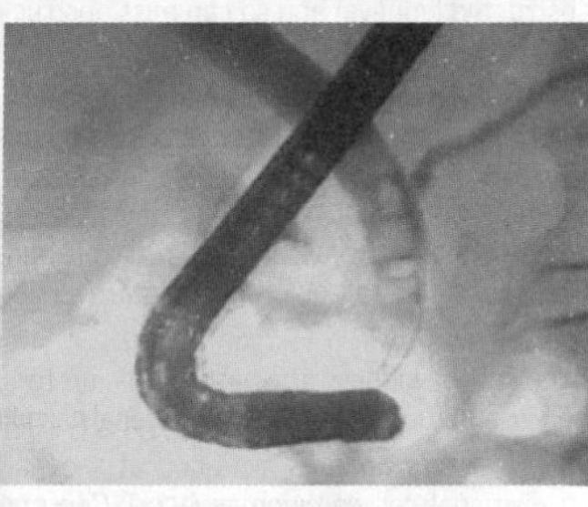

Fig 16.33 The ERCP shows a dilated common bile duct. The multiple filling defects are calculi within and obstructing the duct.
Courtesy of Norwich Radiology Department.

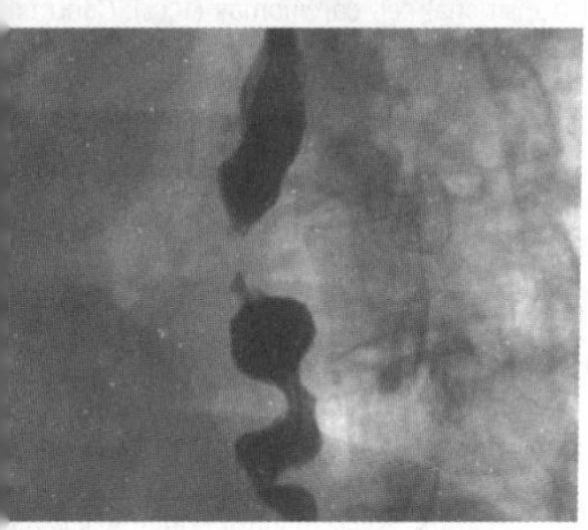

Fig 16.34 Barium swallow: note 'corkscrew' appearance of the oesophagus found in some motility disorders.
Courtesy of Norwich Radiology Department.

Ultrasound
Imaging modality of choice for genitourinary problems. Can be used to assess:
Kidneys:
- Renal size—small in chronic kidney disease, large in renal masses, cysts, hypertrophy if other kidney missing, polycystic kidney disease (fig 16.35), and rarities (eg amyloidosis, p370).
- Hydronephrosis, which may indicate ureteric obstruction or reflux (fig 13.49, p641).
- Perinephric collections (trauma, post-biopsy).
- Renal perfusion (assessment of renovascular disease: Doppler US of renal arteries).
- Transplanted kidneys (collections, obstruction, perfusion).

Lower urinary tract:
- Bladder volume: useful in assessment of the need to catheterize (see p640) or for assessment of adequacy of bladder emptying (post-micturition residual volume).
- Prostate: transrectal ultrasound enables US-guided biopsy of focal lesions. NB: prostate size does not correlate with symptoms.

Other:
- Ovarian cysts, size, infections (pyosalpinx), uterine fibroids and other masses.
- Testicular masses, hydrocele, varicocele.

Advantages: Fast; cheap; independent of renal function; no IV contrast or radiation risk. *Disadvantages:* Intraluminal masses (transitional cell ca) in the upper tracts may not be seen; not a functional study; only suggests obstruction if there is dilatation of the collecting system (95% of obstructed kidneys) and so can miss obstruction from, eg retroperitoneal fibrosis.

CT (fig 16.36) First choice in renal colic. Performed without intravenous contrast so safe in renal impairment; such unenhanced images miss <2% of stones, but can show other pathologies. With IV contrast, CT can delineate masses (cystic or solid, contrast enhancement, calcification, local/distant extension, renal vein involvement); assess renal trauma (presence of two kidneys; haemorrhage; devascularization; laceration; urine leak); and show retroperitoneal lesions. CT has all but replaced intravenous urography and the radiation dose is similar.

Plain abdominal X-ray Can be used to look at the kidneys, the paths of the ureters, and bladder. However, in practice it is only useful for monitoring known renal calculi.

Contrast studies *Retrograde pyelography/ureterograms* are good at showing pelvi-calyceal, ureteric anatomy, and transitional cell carcinomas (TCCs). Contrast medium is injected via a ureteric catheter. With the advent of cystoscopy, allowing immediate intervention, these are rarely done in isolation. However, contrast medium is routinely used in cystoscopic placement of retrograde stents for obstruction

Percutaneous nephrostomy. Used in obstruction to decompress the renal pelvis which is punctured under local anaesthetic with imaging guidance. Images are obtained following contrast injection (antegrade pyelogram). A nephrostomy tube is then placed to allow decompression, sometimes followed by an antegrade stent if there is no easily treatable cause of obstruction.

Renal arteriography (fig 16.37) Therapeutic indications: angioplasty; stenting; embolization (bleeding tumour, trauma, AV malformation).

Magnetic resonance imaging (MRI) Soft tissue resolution can help clarify equivocal CT findings. Magnetic resonance angiography (MRA) helps image renal artery anatomy/stenosis (fig 16.38) and is also used in the assessment of potential live donors for kidney transplant, as well as to monitor patients following embolization of tumours, arteriovenous malformations, and aneurysms.

Radionuclide imaging See p738.

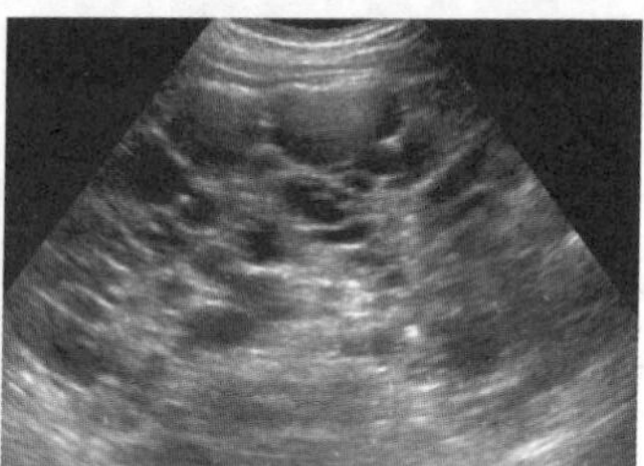

Fig 16.35 Ultrasound of the kidney showing multiple simple cysts.

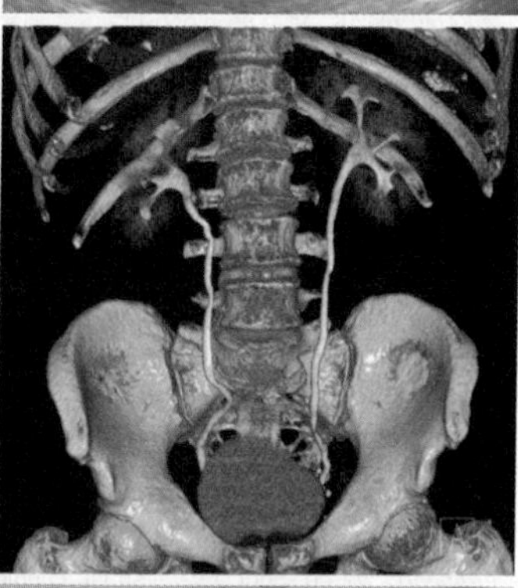

Fig 16.36 3D reconstruction of CT urogram showing normal appearances of both kidneys, ureters, and bladder.

Courtesy of Dr Edmund Godfrey.

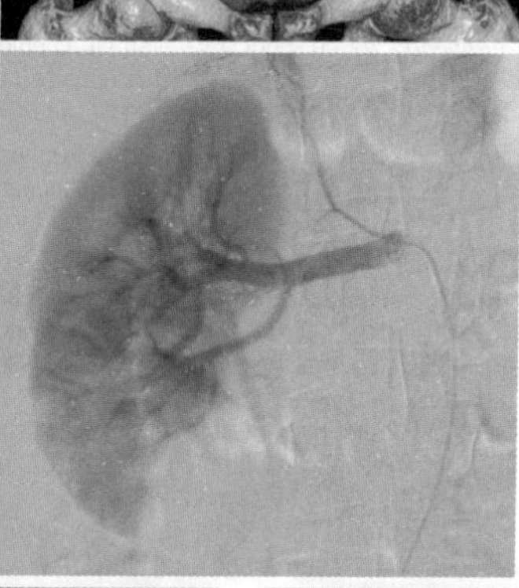

Fig 16.37 Renal artery digital subtraction angiogram (DSA; DSA is the final arbiter of renal artery stenosis). It is possible to tell that this is a DSA as no other structure has any definition or contrast in the image. There is, however, some interference from overlying bowel gas, which is not an uncommon problem. GI tract peristalsis can be diminished during the examination by using IV buscopan.

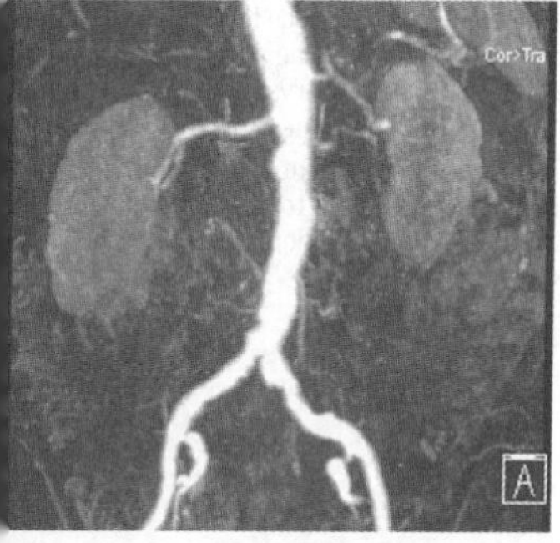

Fig 16.38 Coronal 3D MRA of the kidneys showing two renal arteries supplying the left kidney. This is important information pre-transplant. Anomalous renal arteries are common and, like the normal renal arteries, are end arteries, hence the consequence of infarction if tied at surgery.

CT (fig 16.39) Imaging modality of choice for patients presenting with acute neurological symptoms suggestive of a stroke. It is better than MRI at showing *acute haemorrhage* and *fractures*, and is much easier to do in ill or anaesthetized patients, and so is good in emergencies. The attenuation of biological soft tissues is in a narrow range from about +80 for blood and muscle, to 0 for CSF, and down to −100 for fat (Hounsfield units, p730). IV contrast medium initially gives an angiographic effect, whitening the vessels. Later, if there is a defect in the blood-brain barrier (eg tumours or infection), contrast medium will opacify a lesion's margins, giving enhancing white areas.

- Some CNS areas, eg pituitary gland, choroid plexus, have no blood-brain barrier and enhance normally.
- Fresh blood is of higher attenuation (ie whiter) than brain tissue.
- In old haematomas, Hb breaks down and loses attenuation, so a subacute subdural haematoma at 2wks may be of the same attenuation as adjacent brain.
- A chronic subdural haematoma will be of relatively low attenuation.

CT is often used in *acute stroke* to exclude haemorrhage (eg pre-antiplatelets) and with perfusion scanning (fig 16.14) to aid management decisions regarding thrombolysis. The actual area of infarction/ischaemia may not show up for a day or so, and will be low-attenuation cytotoxic oedema (affecting both white and grey matter—look for loss of grey matter definition).

Tumours and abscesses appear similar, eg a ring-enhancing mass, surrounding vasogenic oedema, and mass effect. Vasogenic oedema (from leaky capillaries) is extracellular and spreads through the white matter (grey matter spared). Mass effect causes compression of the sulci and ipsilateral ventricles, and may also cause herniation (subfalcine, transtentorial, or tonsillar). ►See p483 (and also fig 16.40).

Another indication for CT is acute, *severe headache*, eg suggestive of subarachnoid haemorrhage (p478). An unenhanced CT may show fresh blood, hydrocephalus or ↑ICP, any of which could make LP unsafe.

CT angiography gives excellent mapping of the cerebral circulation (fig 16.41), and can be done directly after unenhanced CT, looking for an aneurysm if the unenhanced CT shows subarachnoid haemorrhage.

MRI (MRI in stroke: fig 10.19, p481) The chief image sequences are:

- *T1-weighted images:* Give good anatomical detail to which the T2 image can be compared. Fat is brightest (↑signal intensity); other tissues are darker to varying degrees. Flowing blood is low signal. Gadolinium contrast (p748) usually results in an increase in signal intensity. See table 16.4.
- *T2-weighted images:* These provide the best detection of most lesions as they usually contain some oedema or fluid and therefore appear white (eg fig 16.20, p735). Fat and fluid appear brightest. Flowing blood is again low signal.

Magnetic resonance angiography maps carotid, vertebrobasilar, and cerebral arterial circulations (and sinuses, veins). Functional MRI can image local blood flow.

Catheter angiography (fig 16.42) Less commonly used since the advent of MRA and CT angiography and perfusion techniques, though it has the advantage of allowing immediate therapy—eg coil embolization of saccular aneurysms.

Radionuclide imaging (p738) PET is mostly used as a research tool in dementia but perfusion scintigraphy scan be used in the assessment of Alzheimer's disease, other dementias, and localizing epileptogenic foci. SPECT to visualize uptake of ^{123}I FP-CIT (DaTSCAN™) can be used to assess reduced striatal dopaminergic transport in Parkinson's disease.

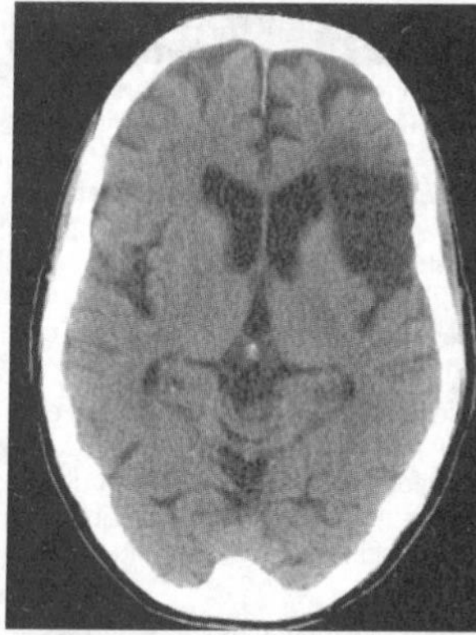

Fig 16.39 Unenhanced axial CT head: note the old infarct in the left middle cerebral artery territory.

Courtesy of Norwich Radiology Department.

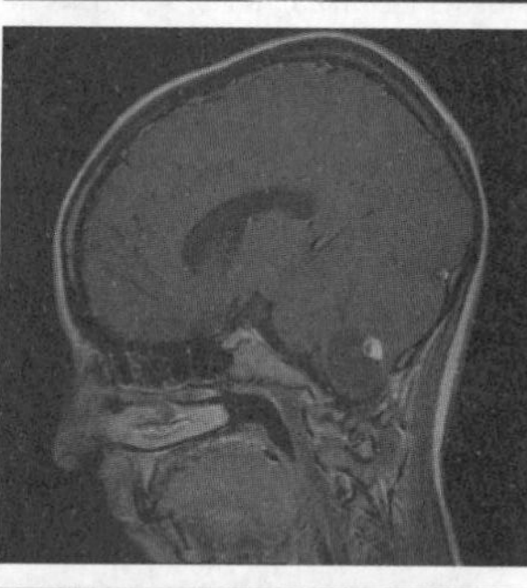

Fig 16.40 T1-weighted MRI of the brain showing a haemangioblastoma in a patient with Von Hippel-Lindau syndrome (p712). Note enhancement with contrast medium.

Courtesy of Dr Edmund Godfrey.

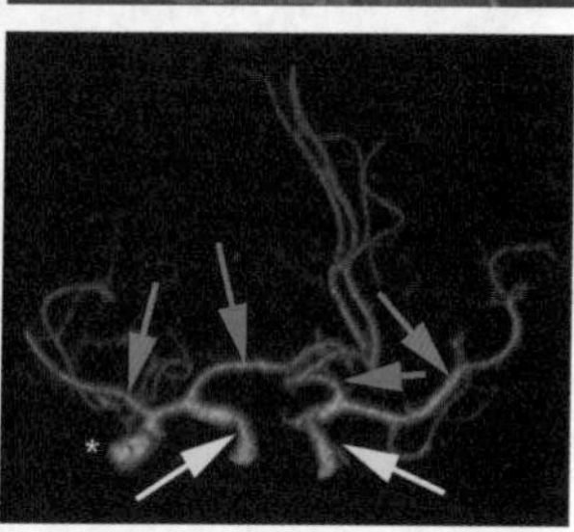

Fig 16.41 A 3D reconstruction of a CT angiogram of the paired internal carotid arteries (yellow arrows) and their branches (anterior cerebral arteries—green arrows, middle cerebral arteries—red arrows), seen from the front and slightly to the right. There is an aneurysm of the right middle cerebral artery (*).

Courtesy of Norwich Radiology Department.

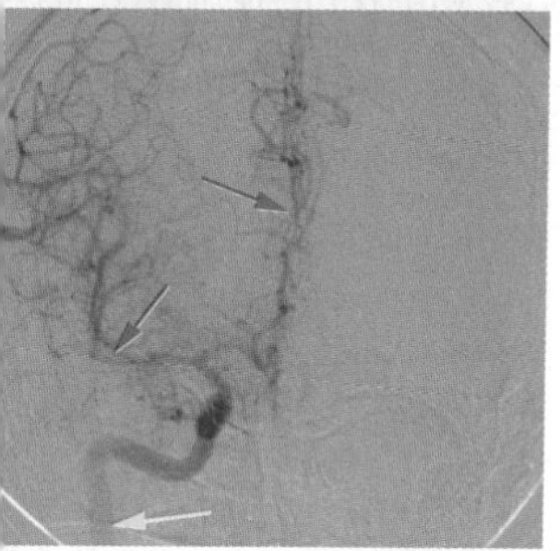

Fig 16.42 Digital subtraction angiogram (DSA). The right internal carotid artery (yellow arrow), anterior cerebral artery (green arrow), and middle cerebral artery (red arrow) are shown.

Courtesy of Norwich Radiology Department.

Contrast media in imaging

The use of a contrast medium can alter the electron density of two previously similar tissues, thus allowing them to be distinguished. Contrast medium is usually administered by the following routes:

- *PO:* Barium- or iodine-based agents for, eg swallow or enhancing visualization of bowel lumen on CT.
- *Inhaled:* Technetium or xenon used in ventilation scintigraphy.
- *IV:* (Most widespread clinical application.) Iodine or gadolinium.
- *PR:* Air or CO_2 can be introduced to the colon for CT colonography, iodinated contrast medium is used for water-soluble enemas.

Iodine-based contrast agents Iodine is used because of its relatively high electron density and good physiological tolerance. When used with CT, the examination is said to be contrast enhanced—look for '+ c' amongst the scan details. *Exercise caution in:* renal or cardiac impairment; myeloma; diabetes; sickle cell disease; elderly; infants; the acutely unwell. ►Avoid iodine-based agents in active hyperthyroidism.

►Have renal function to hand in these patients (see p315). Minor reactions include nausea, vomiting, and a sensation of warmth. More severe reactions include urticaria, bronchospasm, angioedema, and low BP (1:250); theoretical risk of death for 1:150 000.

►Metformin should be withheld for 48h after IV contrast administration because of the risk of lactic acidosis.

Barium sulfate Used in examination of the GI tract. Water-insoluble particles of 0.6–1.4μm diameter are mixed with large organic molecules such as pectin and gum to promote good flow, mucosal adherence, and high density in thin layers. *Complications:* Chemical pneumonitis or peritonitis. Never administer if you suspect perforated viscus.

Water-soluble, non-ionic, iodine-based contrast agents Used instead of barium where there is a risk of peritoneal contamination (eg fistula, megacolon, ulceration, diverticulitis, bowel anastomosis, acute intestinal haemorrhage). Gastrograffin should not be used.

►Contains iodine so establish allergy history and thyroid status.

Air In CT colonography, air (or CO_2) is insufflated as a negative contrast medium after barium administration to enhance mucosal definition. Water can also be used PO and PR to outline the lumen of the gut.

Gadolinium A lanthanide series element with paramagnetic qualities that is administered intravenously (as gadolinium-DTPA) to enhance the contrast of certain structures in MRI. It works by reducing the time to relaxation (TR) of hydrogen nuclei in its proximity and appears as high signal on T1-weighted scans. It does not cross the blood-brain barrier so is useful in enhancing isointense extra-axial tumours such as meningiomas. It can also highlight areas where the blood-brain barrier has broken down secondary to inflammatory or neoplastic processes. It is renally excreted: ►check eGFR: if significantly reduced, gadolinium is contraindicated, as up to 30% may develop progressive nephrogenic systemic fibrosis/nephrogenic fibrosing dermopathy which causes generalized fibrosis which impairs movement and breathing—and which may be fatal. Aberrations in calcium-phosphate metabolism and erythropoietin treatment seem to increase risk. Other adverse reactions include headache, nausea, and local irritation at the site of injection, with idiosyncratic reaction reported in less than 1%.

Imaging the acutely unwell patient

Asking yourself '*Does this investigation need to be done right now?*' will often yield the answer '*No!*', yet there are a few occasions when early imaging can provide vital diagnostic information and influence the prognosis for a patient:

- Acute cauda equina syndrome (p466): ►►MRI lumbar spine.
- Suspected thoracic aorta dissection (p655): ►►CT thorax + IV contrast, MRI or transoesophageal echo (TOE). The mediastinum is rarely widened on CXR.
- Suspected leaking abdominal aortic aneurysm (p654): ►►CT aorta.
- Acute kidney injury (p298): ►►US of renal tract to exclude obstruction.
- Acute pulmonary oedema: ►►portable CXR: don't delay to get an ideal film.
- Acute abdomen with signs of peritonism: ►►erect CXR to find intraperitoneal free gas (fig 13.26, p607; ≈GI perforation). Remember: post-op there will be detectable gas (air/CO_2) in the abdomen for ~10 days. ►►CT if suspicion of intra-abdominal source for sepsis or pathology requiring prompt surgery (eg appendicitis). US for ectopic pregnancy.
- Any patient with post-traumatic midline cervical spine tenderness—not just for the emergency department! ►►Collar and backboard immobilization followed by a CT. All the vertebrae down to the top of T1 must be visualized and cleared before it is safe to take the collar off.
- Sudden-onset focal neurology, worst-ever headache, deteriorating GCS: ►►CT head, then LP if no evidence of ↑ICP.

Remember that imaging—or re-imaging for a poor quality film—should never delay the definitive treatment of an emergency condition, eg:

- Tension pneumothorax (p814 and fig 16.43): ►►decompression *not* CXR.
- Intra-abdominal haemorrhage or viscus rupture (p606): ►►laparotomy.
- High clinical suspicion of torsion of testis (p652): ►►surgery *not* Doppler US.

Prior to the advent of interventional radiology, a collapsed, shocked patient with an acute abdomen would have skipped CT and gone straight for a laparotomy. However, you should bear in mind that ruptured aneurysms are increasingly being managed by endovascular repair under fluoroscopic guidance (p654) so this is one area where rapid imaging may be preferable to immediate intervention.

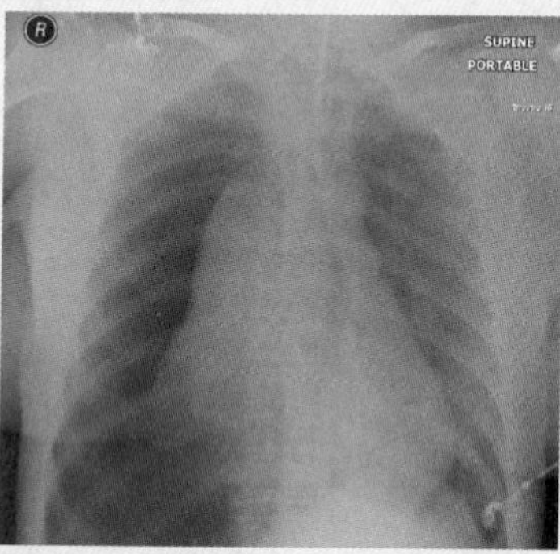

Fig 16.43 This is a great educational image from ICU. The inexperienced doctor could be distracted by the poor quality image, missing the lung bases: technicians do their best under difficult conditions. To ask for a new CXR here would be a mistake ►►note the large right-sided tension pneumothorax needing immediate decompression! *Lungs:* The right lung field is too black compared to the left, the right hemidiaphragm is depressed, and the right lung is seen collapsed against the mediastinum. *Mediastinum:* Left-shifted, obstructing venous return—so ↓cardiac output, and a threat to life. Is it being pushed or pulled? Check hila, bones, and soft tissues. Since the right lung is collapsed and mediastinum shifted to left this suggests ►►right tension pneumothorax. Needle thoracocentesis decompression and a chest drain are needed now.

Courtesy of Dr Edmund Godfrey.

Contents

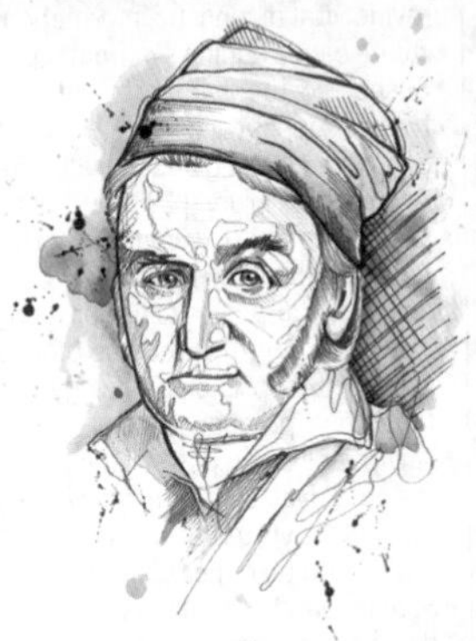

Fig 17.1 Carl Friedrich Gauss (1777–1855) was a German astronomer and mathematician who made many contributions to science, not least of which was establishing the normal (Gaussian) distribution (see p751). After his death, Gauss's brain was examined by anatomist Rudolph Wagner, to test the popular theory that intellectual ability correlated with physical properties of the brain such as weight and surface markings. While his brain was noted to display an unusually intricate pattern of sulci, lack of similarly patterned sulci among the brains of other intellectuals cast doubts on the theory. Further lack of evidence to support Wagner's hypothesis came when Gauss' brain was weighed: it would perhaps have amused Gauss to learn that the weight of his brain, whilst slightly above average, lay very much within the central region of a Gaussian distribution. After some rather sloppy housekeeping, Gauss' brain was stored in a mislabelled pot at the University in Göttingen, accidentally switched with that of his contemporary, the physician Conrad Fuchs. Over 150 years later, some careful searching of the archives and a MRI scanner revealed the switch.

- *The normal (Gaussian) distribution curve.* This bell-shaped graph (fig 17.2) is the theoretical basis of reference intervals, and explains 'lab error'—why some tests repeated at close intervals may reveal slightly different values. Hb for example, has a lab error of ~5g/L. This emphasizes the importance of the *clinical picture* in decision-making, rather than treating the numbers alone: don't subject anaemic patients to blood transfusions unless they have a clinical need. See p324.
- *Range* is the lowest and highest value of all observations in the set being studied.
- *Arithmetic mean* is the sum of all observations ÷ by the number of observations.
- *Median* is the middle value (eg 9 data points are higher and 9 are lower). If their distribution is Normal, then the median coincides with the mean.
- *Standard deviation (SD)* is the square root of the variance (the average of the square of the distance of each data point from the mean). When the distribution of the observations is Normal, 95% of observations are located in the interval 'mean ± 1.96 SD'. This is the basis of the reference interval.
- *Standard error of the mean* gives an estimate of the reliability of the mean of a sample representing the mean of the population from which the sample was taken, and is the SD of the sample ÷ by the square root of the number of observations in the sample. Thus the larger the sample size, the smaller the standard error of the mean—the basis of ensuring that clinical trial evidence is based upon enough observations to be confident that differences seen between groups do not occur by chance alone.

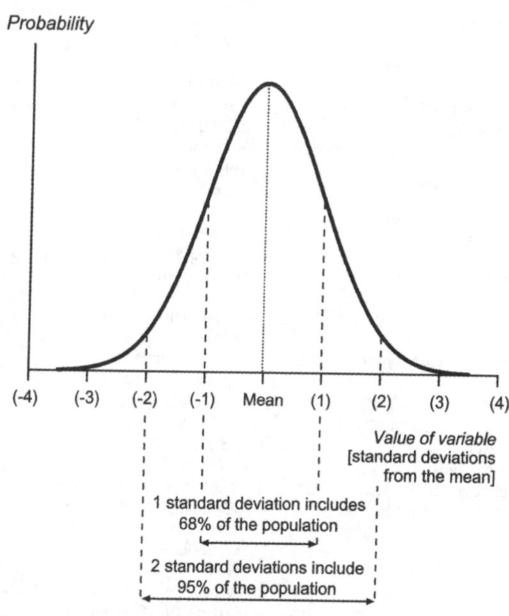

g 17.2 Normal (Gaussian) distribution curve.

Reproduced from Bhopal, *Concepts of Epidemiology*, 2008, with permission from Oxford University Press.

Biochemistry reference intervals

See p662 for the *philosophy of the normal range*; see OHCS p220 for *children*.

Drugs (and other substances) may interfere with any chemical method; as these effects may be method dependent, it is difficult for the clinician to be aware of all the possibilities. If in doubt, discuss with the lab.

Table 17.1

Substance	Specimen	Reference interval (*labs vary, so a guide only*)	Your hospital
Adrenocorticotrophic hormone	P	<80ng/L	
Alanine aminotransferase (ALT)	P	5–35U/L	
Albumin[1]	P	35–50g/L	
Aldosterone[2]	P	100–500pmol/L	
Alkaline phosphatase[1]	P	30–130U/L (adults)	
α-amylase	P	0–180IU/dL	
α-fetoprotein	S	<10kU/L	
Angiotensin II[2]	P	5–35pmol/L	
Antidiuretic hormone (ADH)	P	0.9–4.6pmol/L	
Aspartate transaminase	P	5–35U/L	
Bicarbonate[1]	P	24–30mmol/L	
Bilirubin	P	3–17μmol/L	
BNP (see p137)	P	<50ng/L	
C-reactive protein	P	<10mg/L	
Calcitonin	P	<0.1mcg/L	
Calcium (ionized)	P	1.0–1.25mmol/L	
Calcium[1] (total) See p676 to correct for albumin	P	2.12–2.60mmol/L	
Chloride	P	95–105mmol/L	
Cholesterol[3] (see p690)	P	<5.0mmol/L	
VLDL (see p690)	P	0.128–0.645mmol/L	
LDL	P	<2.0mmol/L	
HDL	P	0.9–1.93mmol/L	
Cortisol	P	AM 450–700nmol/L Midnight 80–280nmol/L	
Creatine kinase (CK)	P	♂ 25–195U/L ♀ 25–170U/L	
Creatinine[1] (proportional to lean body mass)	P	70–100μmol/L	
Ferritin	P	12–200mcg/L	
Folate	S	2.1mcg/L	
Follicle-stimulating hormone (FSH)	P/S	2–8U/L in ♀ (luteal); >25U/L in menopause	
Gamma-glutamyl transpeptidase	P	♂ 11–51U/L ♀ 7–33U/L	
Glucose (fasting)	P	3.5–5.5mmol/L	
Growth hormone	P	<20mu/L	
HbA1c = glycosylated Hb (DCCT)	B	4–6%. 7% ≈ good DM control	
HbA1c IFCC (more specific than DCCT)	B	20–42mmol/mol; 53 ≈ good DM control	
Iron	S	♂ 14–31μmol/L ♀ 11–30μmol/L	
Lactate	P ABG	Venous 0.6–2.4mmol/L Arterial 0.6–1.8mmol/L	
Lactate dehydrogenase (LDH)	P	70–250U/L	
Lead	B	<1.8mmol/L	
Luteinizing hormone (LH) (premenopausal)	P	3–16U/L (luteal)	
Magnesium	P	0.75–1.05mmol/L	
Osmolality	P	278–305mosmol/kg	

Parathyroid hormone (PTH)	P	<0.8–8.5pmol/L
Potassium	P	3.5–5.3mmol/L
Prolactin	P	♂ <450U/L ♀ <600U/L
Prostate-specific antigen (PSA)	P	0–4mcg/mL, age specific, see p530
Protein (total)	P	60–80g/L
Red cell folate	B	0.36–1.44µmol/L (160–640mcg/L)
Renin[2] (erect/recumbent)	P	2.8–4.5/ 1.1–2.7pmol/mL/h
Sodium[1]	P	135–145mmol/L
Thyroid-binding globulin (TBG)	P	7–17mg/L
Thyroid-stimulating hormone (TSH)	P	0.5–4.2mU/L widens with age, p216 assays vary; 4–5 is a grey area
Thyroxine (T_4)	P	70–140nmol/L
Thyroxine (free)	P	9–22pmol/L
Total iron-binding capacity	S	54–75µmol/L
Triglycerides (fasting)	P	0.50–2.3mmol/L
Triiodothyronine (T_3)	P	1.2–3.0nmol/L
Troponin T (see p119)	P	<0.1mcg/L
Urate[1]	P	♂ 210–480µmol/L ♀ 150–390µmol/L
Urea[1]	P	2.5–6.7mmol/L
Vitamin B_{12}	S	0.13–0.68nmol/L (>150ng/L)
Vitamin D	S	50nmol/L (total)

P=plasma (eg citrate bottle); S=serum (clotted; no anticoagulant); B=whole blood (EDTA bottle); ABG=arterial blood gas).

1 See *OHCS* p9 for reference intervals in pregnancy.

2 The sample requires special handling: contact the laboratory.

3 Desired upper limit of cholesterol would be <6mmol/L. In some populations, 7.8mmol/L is the top end of the distribution.

Table 17.2

Arterial blood gases reference intervals	
pH: 7.35–7.45	P_aCO_2: 4.7–6.0kPa
P_aO_2: >10.6kPa	Base excess: ±2mmol/L

Note: 7.6mmHg = 1kPa (atmospheric pressure ≈ 100kPa)

Table 17.3

Urine reference intervals	Reference interval	Your hospital
Cortisol (free)	<280nmol/24h	
Hydroxyindole acetic acid	16–73µmol/24h	
Hydroxymethylmandelic acid	16–48µmol/24h	
Metanephrines	0.03–0.69µmol/mmol creatinine (or <5.5µmol/day)	
Osmolality†	350–1000mosmol/kg	
17-oxogenic steroids	♂ 28–30µmol/24h ♀ 21–66µmol/24h	
17-oxosteroids (neutral)	♂ 17–76µmol/24h ♀ 14–59µmol/24h	
Phosphate (inorganic)	15–50mmol/24h	
Potassium	14–120mmol/24h	
Protein	<150mg/24h	
Protein	creatinine ratio <3mg/mmol	
Sodium†	100–250mmol/24h	

† Interpret based upon plasma values.

Haematology reference intervals

Table 17.4 (For B_{12}, folate, Fe, and TIBC, see pp752-3.)

Measurement	Reference interval	Your hospital
White cell count (WCC)	4.0-11.0 × 10^9/L	
Red cell count	♂ 4.5-6.5 × 10^{12}/L	
	♀ 3.9-5.6 × 10^{12}/L	
Haemoglobin	♂ 130-180g/L	
	♀ 115-160g/L	
Packed red cell volume (PCV) or haematocrit	♂ 0.4-0.54L/L ♀ 0.37-0.47L/L	
Mean cell volume (MCV)	76-96fL	
Mean cell haemoglobin (MCH)	27-32pg	
Mean cell haemoglobin concentration (MCHC)	300-360g/L	
Red cell distribution width (RCDW, RDW)	11.6-14.6% (p325)	
Neutrophils	2.0-7.5 × 10^9/L	
	40-75% WCC	
Lymphocytes	1.0-4.5 × 10^9/L	
	20-45% WCC	
Eosinophils	0.04-0.44 × 10^9/L	
	1-6% WCC	
Basophils	0.0-0.10 × 10^9/L	
	0-1% WCC	
Monocytes	0.2-0.8 × 10^9/L	
	2-10% WCC	
Platelet count	150-400 × 10^9/L	
Reticulocyte count	0.8-2.0%[1] 25-100 × 10^9/L	
Erythrocyte sedimentation rate	Depends on age (p372)	
Prothrombin time (citrated bottle) (factors I, II, VII, X)	10-14s	
Activated partial thromboplastin time (VIII, IX, XI, XII)	35-45s	

Therapeutic ranges for INR: see p351.

1 Only use percentages as reference interval if red cell count is normal; otherwise, use the absolute value.

This page intentionally blank

Drug therapeutic ranges in plasma

►Ranges should only be used as a guide to treatment. A drug in an apparently too low concentration may still be clinically useful, while some patients require (and tolerate) levels in the 'toxic' range.

►The time since the last dose should be specified on the request form.

Amikacin.[1] Peak (1h post IV dose): 20-30mg/L. Trough: <10mg/L.

Carbamazepine.[1] Optimal concentration: 20-50μmol/L (4-12mg/L).

Digoxin[1] (6-12h post dose) 1-2.6nmol/L (0.8-2mcg/L). <1.3nmol/L may be toxic if there is hypokalaemia. *Signs of toxicity*—CVS: arrhythmias, heart block. CNS: confusion, insomnia, agitation, seeing too much yellow (xanthopsia), delirium. GI: nausea.

Gentamicin[1,2] (p387) and *tobramycin.*[1,2] The potential for oto- and nephrotoxicity is high if aminoglycosides are used inappropriately, so only prescribe for short therapeutic courses and follow local expert advice/guidelines. *CI* in severe renal or liver failure, ascites, burns, high cardiac output states (eg anaemia, Paget's disease), children, and pregnancy. *Signs of toxicity:* tinnitus, deafness, nystagmus, vertigo, renal failure. *Once-daily dosing* with dose adjustment is prefered as this has fewer SEs and better bactericidal activity (eg gentamicin 5mg/kg/d or tobramycin 4mg/kg/d; check with pharmacist in obese patients or when using tobramycin in cystic fibrosis). An exception to this dosing is endocarditis: split dosing (eg gentamicin 1mg/kg/8h or 12-hourly in renal failure) increases the synergistic bactericidal effect of other agents. Trough (just before dose) levels and renal function should initially be monitored daily (can be twice weekly in stable patients with normal renal function)—aim for *trough:* <1mg/L for both gentamicin and tobramycin. If the trough level is out of range, withold the next dose until level <1mg/L (recheck after 12-24h).

Lithium[2] (12h post dose). Guidelines vary: 0.4-0.8mmol/L is reasonable. *Early* signs of toxicity (Li^+ >1.5mmol/L): tremor. *Intermediate:* lethargy. *Late:* (Li^+ >2mmol/L) spasms, coma, fits, arrhythmias, renal failure (haemodialysis may be needed). See *OHCS* p349.

Phenytoin.[1,2] Trough: 40-80μmol/L (10-20mg/L). Beware if ↑↓albumin, as the assay is for bound phenytoin, while it is free phenytoin that is pharmacologically important. *Signs of toxicity:* ataxia, diplopia, nystagmus, sedation, dysarthria.

Theophylline 10-20mg/mL (55-110μmol/L). (►See p810.) Take sample 4-6h after starting an infusion (which should be stopped for ~15min just before the specimen is taken). *Signs of toxicity:* arrhythmias, anxiety, tremor, convulsions.

Vancomycin.[1,2] Renally excreted; dosing guided by age and renal function but typically 500mg-1g/12h. Check trough levels prior to 3rd dose, aiming for: 5-10 mg/L (10-15mg/L in SBE/IE and less-sensitive MRSA infections). If levels too low check drug being given then cautiously increase dose; if levels high then confirm timing of dose/levels, omit next dose, recheck levels, and consider decreasing dose or frequency.

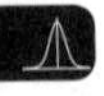

1 Trough levels should be taken just before the next dose. If values abnormally high, check that sample was indeed a trough level and not taken post-dose.
2 Drugs for which *routine* monitoring is indicated.

Some important drug interactions

►See *BNF*.

►See p689 for a list of cytochrome P450 inducers and inhibitors. Note: '↑' = effect of drug increased; '↓' = effect decreased.

Drugs

Adenosine: ↓ by: aminophylline. ↑ by: dipyridamole.
Aminoglycosides: ↑ by: loop diuretics.
Antidiabetic drugs: (All) ↑ by: alcohol, β-blockers, bezafibrate, monoamine oxidase inhibitors. ↓ by: contraceptive steroids, corticosteroids, diazoxide, diuretics, (possibly also lithium).
- *Metformin* ↑ by: cimetidine. With alcohol: lactic acidosis risk.
- *Sulfonylureas* ↑ by: azapropazone, chloramphenicol, bezafibrate, co-trimoxazole, miconazole, sulfinpyrazone. ↓ by: rifampicin (nifedipine occasionally).

Antiretroviral agents (HIV): See p402.
Angiotensin-converting enzyme (ACE) inhibitors: ↓ by: NSAIDs, oestrogens.
Antihistamines: Avoid anything that ↑concentrations and risk of arrhythmias, eg anti-arrhythmics, antifungals, antipsychotics, β-blockers, diuretics, halofantrine, macrolide antibiotics (erythromycin, azithromycin, etc), protease inhibitors (p402), SSRIs (p448), tricyclics.
Azathioprine: ↑ by: allopurinol.
β-blockers: Avoid verapamil. ↓ by: NSAIDs. Lipophilic β-blockers (eg propranolol) are metabolized by the liver, and concentrations are ↑ by cimetidine. This does not happen with hydrophilic β-blockers (eg atenolol).
Carbamazepine: ↑ by: erythromycin, isoniazid, verapamil.
Ciclosporin: ↑ by: erythromycin, grapefruit juice, nifedipine. ↓ by: phenytoin.
Cimetidine: ↑ the effect of: amitriptyline, lidocaine, metronidazole, pethidine, phenytoin, propranolol, quinine, theophylline, warfarin.
Contraceptive steroids: ↓ by: antibiotics, barbiturates, carbamazepine, phenytoin, rifampicin.
Digoxin: ↑ by: amiodarone, carbenoxolone and diuretics (due to ↓K^+), quinine, verapamil.
Diuretics: ↓ by: NSAIDs—particularly indometacin.
Ergotamine: ↑ by: erythromycin (ergotism may occur).
Fluconazole: Avoid concurrent astemizole.
Lithium: ↑ by: thiazide diuretics.
Methotrexate: ↑ by: aspirin, NSAIDs. Many antibiotics (check *BNF*).
Phenytoin: ↑ by: chloramphenicol, cimetidine, disulfiram, isoniazid, sulfonamides. ↓ by: carbamazepine.
Potassium-sparing diuretics with ACE-inhibitors: Hyperkalaemia.
Theophyllines: ↑ by: cimetidine, ciprofloxacin, erythromycin, contraceptive steroids, propranolol. ↓ by: barbiturates, carbamazepine, phenytoin, rifampicin. See p810.
Valproate: ↓ by: carbamazepine, phenobarbital, phenytoin.
Warfarin and nicoumalone: (Nicoumalone=acenocoumarol) ↑ by: alcohol, allopurinol, amiodarone, aspirin, chloramphenicol, cimetidine, ciprofloxacin, co-trimoxazole, danazol, dipyridamole, disulfiram, erythromycin (and broad-spectrum antibiotics), gemfibrozil, glucagon, ketoconazole, metronidazole, miconazole, nalidixic acid, neomycin, NSAIDs, phenytoin, quinidine, simvastatin (but not pravastatin), sulfinpyrazone, sulfonamides, tetracyclines, levothyroxine.
Warfarin and nicoumalone: ↓ by: aminoglutethimide, barbiturates, carbamazepine, contraceptive steroids, dichloralphenazone, griseofulvin, rifampicin, phenytoin, vitamin K.
Zidovudine (AZT): ↑ by: paracetamol (↑marrow toxicity).

IVI solutions to avoid

Glucose: Avoid furosemide, ampicillin, hydralazine, insulin, melphalan, phenytoin, and quinine.
0.9% saline: Avoid amphotericin, lidocaine, nitroprusside.

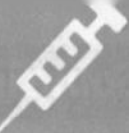

Contents

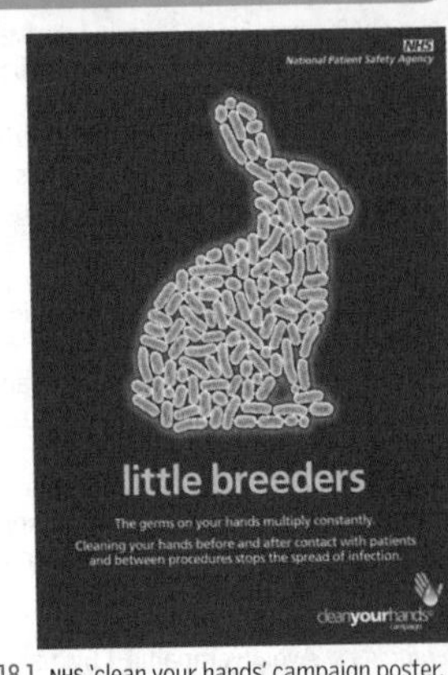
NHS
National Patient Safety Agency
little breeders
The germs on your hands multiply constantly.
Cleaning your hands before and after contact with patients and between procedures stops the spread of infection.
cleanyourhands

Fig 18.1 NHS 'clean your hands' campaign poster.
 https://www.whatdotheyknow.com/request/21861/response/56086/attach/3/04072%20Hand%20Hygiene%205%201.1.pdf

Hungarian obstetrician Ignaz Semmelweis demonstrated the benefits of handwashing in the 1840s: he observed that maternal mortality was nearly three times as high on a doctor-run maternity ward compared to a midwife-run ward. The explanation remained elusive until Semmelweis' friend Jakob Kolletschka died after receiving an accidental scalpel cut from a student during a post-mortem demonstration. Semmelweis recognized in Kolletschka's death many of the features of the dying mothers. The explanation: the maternity ward doctors' day started with post-mortem examinations, from which they would procede to perform vaginal examinations on the living without washing their hands. Noticing this, Semmelweis introduced the practice of washing hands with chloride of lime and cut death rates to that of the midwives' patients. Despite the evidence he amassed, Semmelweis's theory was rejected by his contemporaries, a rejection which undoubtedly contributed to his psychiatric distress, eventual commitment to an asylum, and ultimate death from the blows of his guards. It would take another 20 years and countless deaths before Lister published his landmark work on the use of carbolic acid in surgery.

Take a minute to wash your hands thoroughly before undertaking any procedure. This prerequisite will not only reduce infection risk for your patients, but give you a moment for mindfulness: focus on the hot water running over your hands, breathe deeply, and for a while forget about your list of jobs. Perhaps spare Dr Kolletschka a thought. You may find that the subsequent procedure goes more smoothly than anticipated.

Training and the business of medicine

As medical training has evolved in an environment where patient safety is paramount, the old adage of 'see one, do one, teach one' is no longer relevant. 'Just having a go' when you aren't confident can have devastating consequences for the patient, and also for you and your future. This creates tensions for training, but these are not insurmountable. Seek out opportunities to learn practical procedures, ideally in a controlled, elective setting, so that your first attempt isn't a life-or-death emergency attempt—time spent in theatres or ICU will pay dividends in this regard. Many seniors will be happy to make time to teach if you contact them in advance—let them know you are interested and leave your bleep. ►Even in an emergency setting, it is still wiser to seek help rather than attempting an urgent procedure for the first time.

We thank our Specialist Reader, Dr Andrew Johnston, for his contribution to this chapter.

Nasogastric tubes

These tubes are passed into the stomach via the nose. Large (eg 16F) are good for drainage but can be uncomfortable for patients. Small (eg 10F) are more comfortable for feeding but can be difficult to aspirate and are poor for drainage. Used:

- To decompress the stomach/gastrointestinal tract especially when there is obstruction, eg gastric outflow obstruction, ileus, intestinal obstruction.
- For gastric lavage.
- To administer feed/drugs, especially in critically ill patients or those with dysphagia, eg motor neuron disease, post CVA.

Passing the tube Nurses are experts and will ask you (who may never have passed one) to do so only when they fail—so the first question to ask is: 'Have you asked the charge-nurse from the ward next door?'

- Wear non-sterile gloves and an apron to protect both you and the patient.
- Explain the procedure. Take a new, cool (hence less flexible) tube. Have a cup of water to hand. Lubricate well with aqueous gel.
- Use the tube, by holding it against the patient's head, to estimate the length required to get from the nostril to the back of the throat.
- Place lubricated tube in nostril with its natural curve promoting passage down, rather than up. The right nostril is often easier than the left but, if feasible, ask the patient for their preference. Advance directly backwards (not upwards).
- When the tip is estimated to be entering the throat, rotate the tube by ~180° to discourage passage into the mouth.
- Ask the patient to swallow a sip of water, and advance as they do, timing each push with a swallow. *If this fails:* Try the other nostril.
- The tube has distance markings along it: the stomach is at ~35–40cm in adults, so advance > this distance, preferably 10–20cm beyond. Tape securely to the nose.

Confirming position This is vital prior to commencing any treatment through the tube. Misplaced nasogastric tubes have led to a number of preventable deaths, and feeding via a misplaced tube is considered an NHS Never Event (a serious, largely preventable patient safety incident that should *never* occur if the available preventative measures have been implemented).

- Use pH paper to test that you are in the stomach: aspirated gastric contents are acid (pH ≤5.5) although antacids or PPIs may increase the pH. Small tubes can be difficult to aspirate, try withdrawing or advancing a few cm or turning the patient on the left side to help dip the tube in gastric contents. Aspirates should be >0.5mL and tested directly on unhandled pH paper. Allow 10s for colour change to occur.
- If the pH is >5.5 and the NGT is needed for drug or feed administration then the position must be checked radiologically. Request a CXR/abdo X-ray (tell the radiologist why you need it). Look for the radio-opaque line/tip (this can be hard to see, look below the diaphragm, but if in doubt, ask for help from the radiologist).
- *The 'whoosh' test is NOT an accepted method of testing for tube position.*
- Either spigot the tube, or allow to drain into a dependent catheter bag secured to clothing (zinc oxide tape around tube to form a flap, safety pin through flap).

►Do not pass a tube nasally if there is any suspicion of a facial fracture.

►Get senior help if the patient has recently had upper GI surgery—it is not good practice to push the tube through a fresh anastomosis.

Complications •Pain, or, rarely: •Loss of electrolytes •Oesophagitis •Tracheal or duodenal intubation •Necrosis: retro- or nasopharyngeal •Stomach perforation.

Weaning When planning removal of an NGT *in situ* for decompression or relief of obstruction, it is wise to wean it so that the patient manages well without it. Drainage should be <750mL/24 hours for successful weaning.

- First it should be on free drainage with, eg, 4hrly aspirations.
- Then spigot with 4hrly aspirations.
- Then spigot only. If this is tolerated along with oral intake then it is probably safe to remove the tube; if not, then take a step backwards.

Placing IV cannulae

►Much of what we do is not evidence based; however, in more recent years, particularly in intensive care units, the rise of hospital-acquired infections and multidrug-resistant organisms has prompted a review of standard practice and a series of evidence-based interventions put together as a 'care bundle' to reduce hospital-acquired infections. The technique for placing a cannula is best shown at the bedside by an expert, but following these simple rules will significantly reduce the risk of infection from the cannula.

Preparation is key, remember the following before you start

1 *Equipment:* Set up a tray with cleaning swabs, gauze, cannulae (swallow your pride and take at least three of different sizes, see table 18.1), dressings, 0.9% saline, 10mL syringe, needle-free adaptor (eg octopus with bionector), blood tubes if required, portable sharps bin → needlestick injuries do happen.
2 *Patient:* Have them lying down, explain procedure, obtain verbal consent, place tourniquet around arm, rest the arm below the heart to aid venous filling.
3 *Site:* Look for the best vein—it should be palpable; some of the best veins are not easily visible, some of the most visible collapse on insertion. Tapping gently helps. ►*Never cannulate:* AV fistulae arms, limbs with lymphoedema. ►*Avoid:* Sites crossing a joint (if possible), the cephalic vein in a renal patient.
4 *Consider:* EMLA® cream, cold spray, or 1% lidocaine for children or those with needle phobia. EMLA® takes 45min to work, but can save you hassle later.

Insertion care bundle

1 Aseptic technique. 2 Hand hygiene. 3 Apron + non-sterile gloves. 4 Skin preparation—2% chorhexidine in 70% isopropyl alcohol (allow to dry for 30 seconds). Do not repalpate vein after cleaning unless wearing sterile gloves. 5 Dressing—sterile and transparent so that insertion site can be observed.

After insertion

1 Take blood with syringe or adaptor. 2 Remove tourniquet. 3 Attach needle-free device (if appropriate) and flush with 10mL 0.9% saline. 4 Apply dressing. 5 Let nursing staff know that cannula is in place and ready for use. 6 Document insertion according to local policy. 7 Write up appropriate fluids or parenteral medication.

When seeing your patient on the daily ward round (and to avoid being called to review or replace cannulae at 6pm) do a RAID[1] assessment: consider if the drip is:

Required—can the patient manage with oral medication/fluids?

Appropriate—should you consider a PICC, central line, long-term line, etc?

Infected—any signs of inflammation or infection? Remove if yes. Peripheral cannulae should be replaced every 72–96 hours.

Dressed properly—many drips are replaced early because they have 'fallen out', or are kinked from poor dressings.

Tissued or infected cannulae need replacing, either with another peripheral cannula, or with a longer-term access device, such as a PICC line.

If you fail after three attempts ►Shocked patients need fluid quickly: if you are having trouble putting in a drip, call your senior. The following advice assumes that the drip is not immediately life-saving. ►►If it is, see BOX.

- Ask for help—from colleagues or seniors—do not be ashamed, everyone has to learn and even senior doctors have bad days; a fresh pair of eyes can be all it takes. As a house officer, one of us was asked to place a drip when a very shame-faced consultant had 'had a go' to prove he still could, and found out that he couldn't!
- Help yourself—try putting the hand in warm water, using a small amount of GTN paste over the vein, or using ultrasound if available to help you identify the vein.
- If there is no one else to help, take a break and come back in half an hour. Veins come and go, and coming back with fresh eyes can make all the difference.

Table 18.1 Intravenous cannulae sizes and UK colour conventions

Gauge	Colour	Diameter (mm)	Length (mm)	Flow rate (mL/min)
14G	ORANGE/BROWN	2.0	45	250
16G	GREY	1.7	42	170
18G	GREEN	1.2	40	90
20G	PINK	1.0	32	55
22G	BLUE	0.28	25	25
24G	YELLOW	0.07	19	24

Flow rate is given as maximum flow rate under gravity; faster rates may be achievable with rapid infusion devices. According to Poiseuille's law[1] the flow rate (Q) of a fluid through a tubular structure is inversely proportional to viscosity (η) and length (l) and proportional to the pressure difference across it ($P_i - P_o$) and the radius *to the power of* 4(r^4). Hence:

$$Q \propto \frac{(P_i - P_o)r^4}{\eta l}$$

A last throw of the dice

Just once it may come down to you. For some, this is one of the challenges and thrills in medicine. There may be no one else available to help when there is an absolute and urgent indication for IV drugs/fluids/blood—and all of the previously discussed measures have been tried, and have failed. Think of lonesome night shifts, over-run emergency departments, a disaster scene, war, or medicine in the field. The following measures are not recommended for non-life-threatening scenarios:

- ▸▸Don't worry. Have a good look again. Feet (avoid in diabetics)? Inside of the forearm? Upper arm?
- ▸▸Have you really exhausted all of your options for help from a colleague? Maybe the anaesthetist or ICU registrar is approachable—they do have remarkable skills.
- ▸▸Is the patient familiar with his/her own veins (eg previous IV drug abuser)?
- ▸▸If there is only a small amount of IV medication required and a small, short vein, you may be able to gain access with a carefully placed butterfly needle that is taped down. Some drugs cannot be passed this way (eg amiodarone, K^+).
- ▸▸The external jugular vein may become prominent when the patient is head down (Trendelenburg) by 5–10° (►not in situations of fluid overload, LVF, ↑ICP). Only attempt cannulation of this vein if you are not going to jeopardize future central line insertion, and if you can clearly determine the surrounding anatomy.
- ▸▸In an arrest situation, the 2015 Advanced Life Support Guidelines recommend the intraosseous route in both adults and children if venous access is not possible; access devices should be available within resuscitation settings (eg emergency department).

Only do the following if you have had the appropriate training/experience:

- ▸▸In children, consider cannulating a scalp vein.
- ▸▸Central venous catheterization (p775). This may be just as hard in a profoundly hypovolaemic arrest patient, and a good knowledge of local anatomy and of the procedure (± ultrasound guidance) will be invaluable.

If you don't have an intraosseous access device, a cut down to the long saphenous vein may be attempted, *in extremis, even if you have no prior experience* (at this site you won't kill by being ham-fisted). ▸▸Make a transverse incision 1-2cm anterior and superior to the medial malleolus. ▸▸Free vein with forceps. ▸▸Cannulate it under direct vision. ►*Here, 'first do no harm' is trumped by 'nothing ventured, nothing gained'.*

Hopefully, it shouldn't ever have to come to these measures, but one day...

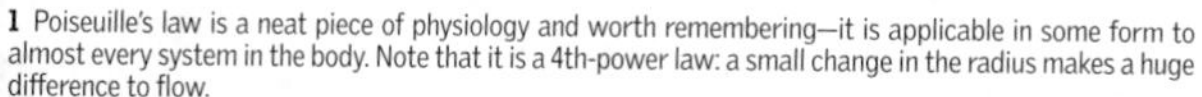

1 Poiseuille's law is a neat piece of physiology and worth remembering—it is applicable in some form to almost every system in the body. Note that it is a 4th-power law: a small change in the radius makes a huge difference to flow.

Catheterizing bladders

Urinary tract infections are the second commonest health care-associated infection, and urinary catheters are frequently to blame. Think, does the patient really need a catheter? If so, use the smallest you can and take out as soon as possible.

Size (in French gauge): 12=small; 16=large; 20=very large (eg 3-way). **Material** Coated latex catheters are soft and a good short-term option ►but unsuitable in true latex allergy. Silastic (silicone) catheters may be used long term, but cost more. Silver alloy coating reduces infections. **Shape** Foley is typical (fig 18.2); coudé (elbow) catheters have an angled tip to ease around prostates but are more risky; 3-way catheters are used in clot or debris retention and have an extra lumen for irrigation fluid, attached to the irrigation set via an extra port on the distal end (fig 18.3). Get urology advice before starting irrigation. Condom catheters are often preferred by patients (less discomfort) even though they may leak and fall off.

Catheter problems • *Infection:* ~5% develop bacteraemia (most will have bacterial colonization, antibiotics may not be required unless systemically unwell—discuss with microbiology). A stat dose of, eg gentamicin 80mg is sometimes given pre-insertion despite a lack of evidence for benefit. Check your local policy. • *Bladder spasm:* May be painful—try reducing the water in the balloon or an anticholinergic drug, eg oxybutynin.

Per urethram Aseptic technique required.

Indications • Relieve urinary retention. • Monitor urine output in critically ill patients. • Collect uncontaminated urine for diagnosis. ► It is contraindicated in urethral injury (eg pelvic fracture) and acute prostatitis.

- Explain the procedure, and obtain verbal consent. Prepare a catheterization trolley: gloves, catheter, lidocaine jelly, cleaning solution, drape, kidney dish, gauze swabs, drainage bag, 10mL water and syringe, specimen container.
- Lie the patient supine: women with knees flexed and hips abducted with heels together. Use a gloved hand to clean urethral meatus in a pubis-to-anus direction, holding the labia apart with the other hand. With uncircumcised men, retract the foreskin to clean the glans; use a gloved hand to hold the penis still. The hand used to hold the penis or labia should not touch the catheter. Place a sterile drape with a hole in the middle to help you maintain asepsis. Remember: left hand dirty, right hand clean.
- Put sterile lidocaine 1-2% gel on the catheter tip and ≤10mL into the urethra (≤5mL if ♀). In men, lift and gently stretch the penis upwards to eliminate any urethral folds that may lead to false passage formation.
- Use steady gentle pressure to advance the catheter, rotating slightly can help it slide in. ►Never force the catheter. Tilting the penis up towards the umbilicus while inserting may help negotiate the prostate. Insert to the hilt; wait until urine emerges before inflating the balloon. Remember to check the balloon's capacity before inflation (written on the outer end). Collect a sterile specimen and attach a drainage bag. Pull the catheter back so that the balloon comes to rest at the bladder neck.
- If you are having trouble getting past the prostate, try: more lubrication, a gentle twisting motion; a larger catheter; or call the urologists, who may use a guidewire.

►Remember to reposition the foreskin in uncircumcised men after the catheter is inserted to prevent oedema of the glans and paraphimos.

Documentation: In the notes be sure to document the indication for catheterization, size of catheter, whether insertion was difficult or straightforward, any complications, residual volume and colour of urine. It is good practice to document that the foreskin has been replaced. Sign with your name, date, and designation.

Suprapubic catheterization: Sterile technique required ►Absolutely contraindicated unless there is a large bladder palpable or visible on ultrasound, because of the risk of bowel perforation. Be wary, particularly if there is a history of abdominal or pelvic surgery. Suprapubic catheter insertion is high risk and you should be trained before attempting it, speak to the urologists first.

Self-catheterization

This is a good, safe way of managing chronic retention from a neuropathic bladder (eg in multiple sclerosis, diabetic neuropathy, spinal tumour, or trauma). Never consider a patient in difficulties from a big residual volume to be too old, young, or disabled to learn. 5-yr-old children can learn the technique, and can have their lives transformed—so motivation may be excellent. There may be fewer UTIs as there is no residual urine—and less reflux obstructive uropathy. Assessing suitability entails testing sacral dermatomes: a 'numb bum' implies ↓sensation of a full bladder; higher sensory loss may mean catheterization will be painless. Get help from your continence adviser who will be in a position to teach the patient or carer that catheterizations must be gentle (the catheter is of a much smaller calibre), particularly if sensation is lacking, and must number >4/d ('always keep your catheter with you; don't wait for an urge before catheterizing'). See fig 18.4.

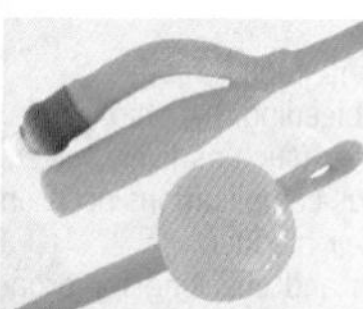
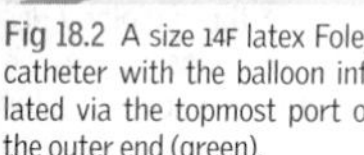

Fig 18.2 A size 14F latex Foley catheter with the balloon inflated via the topmost port of the outer end (green).

© Dr Tom Turmezei (not to scale).

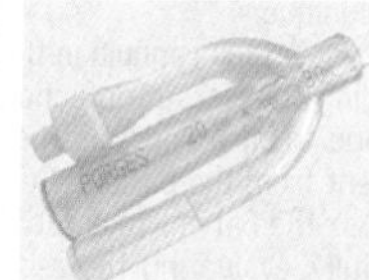

Fig 18.3 The external end of a size 20F 3-way catheter. The lowest port is for the bladder irrigation fluid and the uppermost port (yellow) is for balloon inflation.

© Dr Tom Turmezei (not to scale).

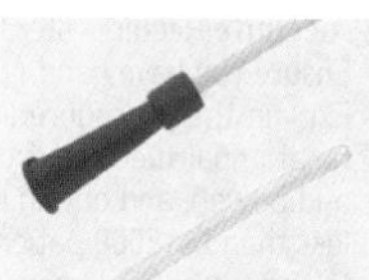

Fig 18.4 A size 10F catheter for self-catheterization. They are usually smaller than indwelling catheters, eg 10F compared to 14F. Note that this catheter also has no balloon.

© Dr Tom Turmezei (not to scale).

'The catheter is not draining...'

You will be asked to check catheters that are not draining. Check the fluid chart and the patient:

- *Previously good output, now anuric:* Blocked catheter until proven otherwise. Was the urine clear previously or bloodstained? Consider flushing the catheter: with aseptic technique flush and withdraw 20mL of sterile 0.9% saline with a bladder syringe. This may get the flow going again. A 3-way catheter may be needed if there is clot or debris retention. If it blocks again, replace it. Repeated flushes lead to infection.
- *Slow decline in urine output over several hours:* In a dehydrated/post-op patient a fluid challenge of 500mL STAT (250mL if cardiac comorbidity) may help, come back and check the response in 30min. Check all other parameters (eg pulse, BP, CVP) and increase rate of background IV fluids if appropriate.
  ▸▸Acute kidney injury (p298): if urine output has tailed off and now stopped, the cause is often renal hypoperfusion (ie pre-renal failure), but consider other factors, eg nephrotoxic drugs.
- *Catheter is bypassing:* A condom catheter may be more appropriate.
- *Catheter has dislodged into the proximal (prostatic) urethra:* Possible even if the balloon is fully inflated. Consider this if a flush enters but cannot be withdrawn. If the patient still needs a catheter then replace it, consider a larger size.
- *The catheter has perforated the lower urinary tract on insertion and is not lying in the bladder or urethra:* ▸▸If suspected, call the urologists immediately.

Remember: urine output should be >400mL in 24h or >0.5mL/kg/h (see p576).

Trial without catheter (TWOC)

When it is time to remove a catheter, the possibility of urinary retention must be considered. Remove the catheter first thing one morning. If retention does occur, insert a long-term catheter (eg silicone), consider an α-blocker (p642), and arrange urology TWOC clinic follow-up.

Draining ascites

For patients with refractory or recurrent ascites that is symptomatic, it is possible to drain the ascites using a long pig-tail catheter. Paracentesis in such patients even in the presence of spontaneous bacterial peritonitis may be safe. Learn at the bedside from an expert.

Contraindications (these are relative, not absolute) End-stage cirrhosis; coagulopathy; hyponatraemia (≤126mmol/L); sepsis. The main complication of the procedure is severe hypovolaemia secondary to reaccumulation of the ascites, so intravascular replenishment with a plasma expander is required. For smaller volumes, eg less than 5L, 500mL of 5% human albumin or Gelofusine® would be sufficient. For volumes over 5L, reasonable replacement would be 100mL 20% human albumin IV for each 1-3 litres of ascites drained (check your local policy). You may need to call the haematology lab to request this in advance.

Procedure Requires sterile technique.

- Ensure you have good IV access—eg 18G cannula in the antecubital fossa.
- Explain the procedure including the risks of infection, bleeding, hyponatraemia, renal impairment, and damage to surrounding structures (such as liver, spleen, and bowel), and obtain consent from the patient. Serious complications occur in less than 1 in 1000 patients. Ask the patient to empty their bladder.
- Examine the abdomen carefully, evaluating the ascites and checking for organomegaly. Mark where you are going to enter. If in doubt, ask the radiology department to ultrasound the abdomen and mark a spot for drainage. Approach from the left side unless previous local surgery/stoma prevents this—call a senior for support and advice if this is the case.
- Prepare a tray with 2% chlorhexidine solution, sterile drapes, 1% lidocaine, syringes, needles, sample bottles, and your drain. Clean the abdomen thoroughly and place sterile drapes, ensure you maintain sterile technique throughout. Infiltrate the local anaesthetic.
- Perform an ascitic tap (see p765) first so that you know you are in the correct place: remove 20mL fluid for MC&S.
- Away from the patient, carefully thread the catheter over the (large and long) needle using the guide so that the pig-tail has been straightened out. Remove the guide.
- With the left hand hold the needle ~2.5cm (1 inch) from the tip—this will stop it from advancing too far (and from performing an aortic biopsy). With the right hand, hold the other end.
- Gently insert the needle perpendicular to the skin at the site of the ascitic tap up to your hold with your left hand—ascites should now drain easily. If necessary, advance the needle and catheter a short distance until good flow is achieved.
- Advance the catheter over the needle with your left hand, keeping the needle in exactly the same place with your right hand. ►Do not re-advance the needle because it will go through the curled pig-tail and do not withdraw it because you won't be able to thread in the catheter.
- When fully inserted, remove the needle, connect the catheter to a drainage bag (keep it below the level of the abdomen), and tape it down securely to the skin.
- The patient should stay in bed as the ascites drains.
- Document clearly in the notes the indication for the procedure, that consent was obtained, clotting and U&Es checked pre-procedure, how much lidocaine was required, how much fluid was removed for investigations, and whether there were any complications to the procedure.
- Replenish intravascular volume with human albumin (see 'Contraindications' earlier in topic).
- Ask the nursing staff to remove the catheter after 6h or after a pre-determined volume has been drained (up to 20L can come off in 6h) and document this clearly in the medical notes. Drains are removed after 4-6h to prevent infection.
- Check U&Es after the procedure and re-examine the patient.

Diagnostic taps

If you are unsure whether a drain is needed, a diagnostic tap can be helpful. Whatever fluid you are sampling, a green needle carries far less risk than a formal drain. It also allows you to decide whether a drain is required.

Ascites may be sampled to give a cytological or bacterial diagnosis, eg to exclude spontaneous bacterial peritonitis (SBP; p276). Before starting, know the patient's platelets + clotting times. If they are abnormal, seek help before proceeding.

- Place the patient flat and tap out the ascites, marking a point where fluid has been identified, avoiding vessels, stomas, and scars (adhesions to the anterior abdominal wall). The left side may be safer—less chance of nicking liver (fig 18.5).
- Clean the skin. Infiltrate some local anaesthetic, eg 1% lidocaine (see p573).
- Insert a 21G needle on a 20mL syringe into the skin and advance while aspirating until fluid is withdrawn, try to obtain 60mL of fluid.
- Remove the needle, apply a sterile dressing.
- Send fluid to microbiology (15mL) for microscopy and culture, biochemistry (5mL for protein, see p192), and cytology (40mL). Call microbiology to forewarn them if urgent analysis of the specimen is required.

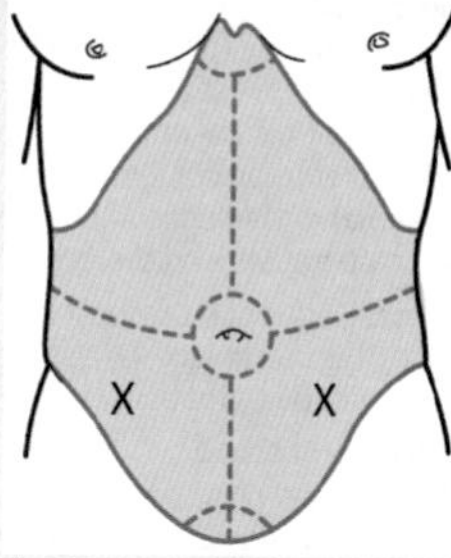

Fig 18.5 Always tap out the ascites, but aim approximately for 5cm medial to and superior to the anterior superior iliac spine. If in doubt, ask for an ultrasound to mark the spot.

Diagnostic aspiration of a pleural effusion

- If not yet done, a CXR may help evaluate the side and size of the effusion.
- Ideally use US guidance at the bedside (↑ chance of successful aspirate and ↓ chance of organ puncture). If this is unavailable, ask an ultrasonographer to mark a spot, or percuss the upper border of the pleural effusion and choose a site 1 or 2 intercostal spaces below it (usually posteriorly or laterally).
- Clean the area around the marked spot with 2% chlorhexidine solution.
- Infiltrate down to the pleura with 5-10mL of 1% lidocaine.
- Attach a 21G needle to a syringe and insert it just above the upper border of the rib below the mark to avoid the neurovascular bundle (fig 18.6). Aspirate whilst advancing the needle. Draw off 10-30mL of pleural fluid. Send fluid to the lab for chemistry (protein, glucose, pH, LDH); bacteriology (microscopy and culture, auramine stain, TB culture); cytology, and, if indicated, amylase and immunology (rheumatoid factor, antinuclear antibodies, complement).

►►If you cannot obtain fluid with a 21G needle, seek help.

- If any cause for concern, arrange a repeat CXR.

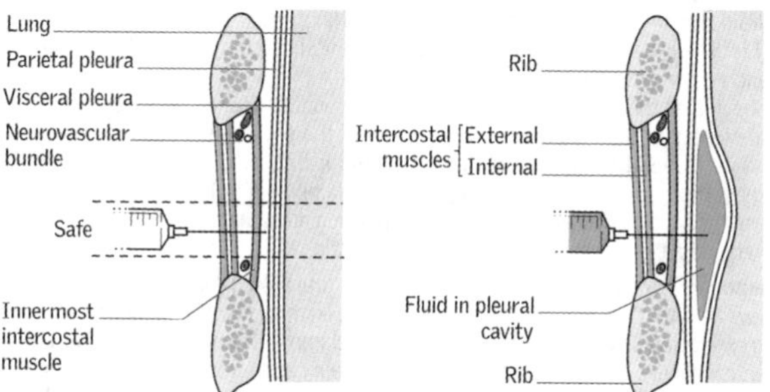

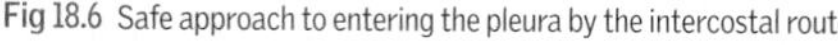
Fig 18.6 Safe approach to entering the pleura by the intercostal route.

Inserting a chest drain

Indications

- Pneumothorax (p814): ventilated; tension; persistent/recurrent despite aspiration (eg <24h after 1st aspiration); large 2nd spontaneous pneumothorax if >50yrs old.
- Malignant pleural effusion, empyema, or complicated parapneumonic effusion.
- Pleural effusion compromising ventilation, eg in ICU patients.
- Traumatic haemopneumothorax.
- Post-operatively: eg thoracotomy; oesophagectomy; cardiothoracic surgery.

►Pleural effusions are best drained under US guidance using a Seldinger technique. This technique is also used for pneumathoraces (except in traumatic or post-operative situations) without US guidance; for this reason it is detailed here.

Sterile procedure

- Identify the point for drainage. In effusions, this should be done with US, ideally under direct guidance or with a marked spot. For pneumothoraces, check the drainage point from CXR/CT/examination.
- Preparation: trolley with dressing pack; 2% chlorhexidine; needles; 10mL syringes; 1% lidocaine; scalpel; suture; Seldinger chest drain kit; underwater drainage bottle; connection tubes; sterile H_2O; dressings. Incontinence pad under patient.
- Choose insertion site: 4-6th intercostal space, anterior- to mid-axillary line—the 'safe triangle' (see BOX 'The "safe triangle" for insertion' and fig 18.7). A more posterior approach, eg the 7th space posteriorly, may be required to drain a loculated effusion (under direct US visualization) and occasionally the 2nd intercostal space in the mid-clavicular line may be used for apical pneumothoraces—however, both approaches tend to be less comfortable.
- Maintain sterile technique—clean and place sterile drapes. Scrub for insertion.
- Prepare your underwater drain by filling the bottle to the marked line with sterile water. Ensure this is kept sterile until you need it.
- Infiltrate down to pleura with 10mL of 1% lidocaine and a 21G needle. Check that air/fluid can be aspirated from the proposed insertion site; if not, do not proceed.
- Attach the Seldinger needle to the syringe containing 1-2mL of sterile saline. The needle is bevelled and will direct the guidewire; in general advance bevel up for pneumothoraces, bevel down for effusions.
- Insert the needle gently, aspirating constantly. When fluid/air is obtained in the syringe, stop, note insertion depth from the markings on the Seldinger needle. Remove syringe, thread the guidewire through the needle. Remove the needle and clamp the guidewire to the sterile drapes to ensure it does not move. Using the markings on the Seldinger needle, move the rubber stops on the dilators to the depth noted earlier, to prevent the dilator slipping in further than intended.
- Make a nick in the skin where the wire enters, and slide the dilators over the wire sequentially from smallest to largest to enlarge the hole, keep gauze on hand. Slide the Seldinger drain over the wire into the pleural cavity. Remove the wire and attach a 3-way tap to the drain, then connect to the underwater drainage bottle.
- Suture the drain in place using a drain stitch—make a stitch in the skin close to the drain site, tie this fairly loosely with a double knot. Then tie the suture to the drain. It is usually best to be shown this before attempting it for yourself. Dress the drain, and ensure it is well taped down.
- Check that the drain is swinging (effusion) or bubbling (pneumothorax) and ensure the water bottle remains below the level of the patient at all times. If the drain needs to be lifted above the patient, clamp it briefly. ►You should never clamp chest drains inserted for pneumothoraces. Clamping for pleural effusions can control the rate of drainage and prevent expansion pulmonary oedema.
- Request a CXR to check the position of the drain.

Removal *In pneumothorax:* Consider when drain is no longer bubbling and CXR shows re-inflation. Give analgesia beforehand, eg morphine. Smartly withdraw during expiration or Valsalva. There is no need to clamp the drain beforehand as reinsertion is unlikely. *In effusions:* Generally the drain can be removed when drainage is <200mL/24h, but for cirrhotic hydrothoraces the chest drain is treated similarly to the ascitic drain (see p764) with HAS supplementation and removal at 4-6 hours.

The 'safe triangle' for insertion of a chest drain

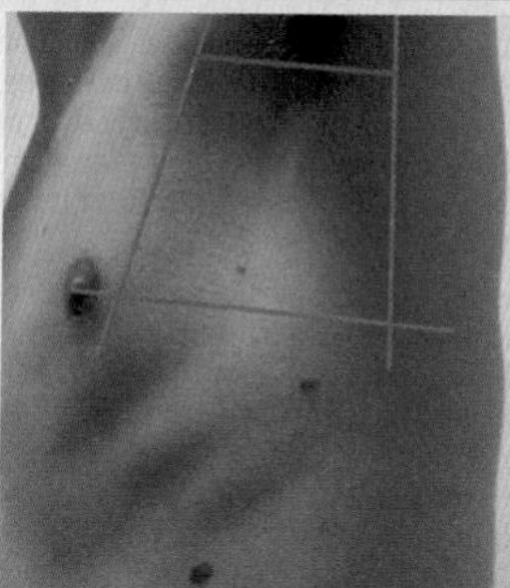

Fig 18.7 The safe 'triangle' is not really a triangle, as the axilla cuts off the point of the triangle. Draw a line along the lateral border of pectoralis major, a line along the anterior border of latissimus dorsi, and a line superior to the horizontal level of the nipple. The apex of the triangle is the axilla. Often chest drains are inserted directly under ultrasound guidance, or with a pre-marked spot; however, in an emergency or for aspiration, the landmarks of the safe triangle are important to know.

Complications

- Thoracic or abdominal organ injury. • Lymphatic damage ∴ chylothorax.
- Damage to long thoracic nerve of Bell ∴ wing scapula. • Rarely, arrhythmia.

Watch out for:

- Retrograde flow back into the chest.
- Persistent bubbling—there may be a continual leak from the lung.
- Blockage of the tube from clots or kinking—no swinging or bubbling.
- Malposition—check position with CXR.

Relieving a tension pneumothorax

Symptoms Acute respiratory distress, chest pain, ►►respiratory arrest.

Signs Hypotension; distended neck veins; asymmetrical lung expansion; trachea and apex deviated away from side of reduced air entry and hyperresonance to percussion. ►►There is no time for a CXR (but see fig 16.43, p749).

Aim To release air from the pleural space. In a tension pneumothorax, air is drawn into the intrapleural space with each breath, but cannot escape due to a valve-like effect of the tiny flap in the parietal pleura. The increasing pressure progressively embarrasses the heart and the other lung.

►►100% oxygen.

Prodedure

- Insert a large-bore IV cannula (eg Venflon®) usually through the 2nd intercostal space in the midclavicular line or the 'safe triangle' for chest drain insertion (see BOX 'The "safe triangle" for insertion'). Remove the stylet, allowing the trapped air to escape, usually with an audible hiss. This converts the tension pneumothorax to an open pneumothorax. Tape securely. • Don't recover the cannula as tensioning will recur.
- Proceed to formal chest drain insertion (see p766).

Aspiration of a pneumothorax

Identify the 2nd intercostal space in the midclavicular line (or 4-6th intercostal space in the midaxillary line) and infiltrate with 1% lidocaine down to the pleura overlying the pneumothorax.

- Insert a 16G cannula into the pleural space. Remove the needle and connect the cannula to a 3-way tap and a 50mL syringe. Aspirate up to 2.5L of air (50mL×50). Stop if resistance is felt, or if the patient coughs excessively.
- Request a CXR to confirm resolution of the pneumothorax. If successful, consider discharging the patient and repeating the CXR after 24h to exclude recurrence, and again after 7-10d. Advise to avoid air travel for 6 weeks after a normal CXR. Diving should be permanently avoided.
- If aspiration is unsuccessful (in a significant, symptomatic pneumothorax), insert an intercostal drain (see p766).

Lumbar puncture (LP)

Contraindications •Bleeding diathesis. •Cardiorespiratory compromise. •Infection at site of needle insertion. Most importantly: ►► ↑ICP (suspect if very severe headache, ↓level of consciousness with falling pulse, rising BP, vomiting, focal neurology, or papilloedema)—LP in these patients will cause coning, so unless it is a routine procedure, eg for known idiopathic intracranial hypertension, obtain a CT prior to LP. CT is not infallible, so be sure your indication for LP is strong.

Method Explain to the patient what sampling CSF entails, why it is needed, that co-operation is vital, and that they can communicate with you at all stages.

- Place the patient on his or her left side, with the back on the edge of the bed, fully flexed (knees to chin). A pillow under the head and another between the knees may keep them more stable.
- Landmarks: plane of iliac crests through the level of L3/4 (see fig 18.8). In adults, the spinal cord ends at the L1/2 disc (fig 18.9). Mark L3/4 intervertebral space (or one space below, L4/5), eg by a gentle indentation of a needle cap on the overlying skin (better than a ballpoint pen mark, which might be erased by the sterilizing fluid).
- Use aseptic technique (hat, mask, gloves, gown) and 2% chlorhexidine in 70% alcohol to clean the skin, allow to dry and then place sterile drapes.
- Open the spinal pack. Assemble the manometer and 3-way tap. Have three plain sterile tubes and one fluoride tube (for glucose) ready.
- Using a 25G (orange) needle, raise a bleb of local anaesthetic, then use a 21G (green) needle to infiltrate deeper.
- Wait 1min, then insert spinal needle (22G, stilette in place) perpendicular to the body, through your mark, aiming slightly up towards the umbilicus. Feel resistance of spinal ligaments, and then the dura, then a 'give' as the needle enters the subarachnoid space. NB: keep the bevel of the needle facing up, parallel with dural fibres.
- Withdraw stilette. Check CSF fills needle and attach manometer (3-way tap turned off towards you) to measure 'opening' pressure.
- Catch fluid in three sequentially numbered bottles (10 drops per tube).
- Reinsert stilette then remove needle and apply dressing. Document the procedure clearly in the notes including CSF appearance and opening pressure.
- Send CSF promptly for *microscopy, culture, protein, lactate, and glucose* (do plasma glucose too)—call the lab to let them know. If applicable, also send for: cytology, fungal studies, TB culture, virology (± herpes and other PCR), syphilis serology, oligoclonal bands (+serum sample for comparison) if multiple sclerosis suspected. Is there xanthochromia (p478)?
- If you fail; ask for help—try with the patient sitting or with radiological guidance.

CSF composition *Normal values:* Lymphocytes <5/mm^3; no polymorphs; protein <0.4g/L; glucose >2.2mmol/L (or ≥50% plasma level); pressure <200mm CSF. *In meningitis:* See p822. *In multiple sclerosis:* See p496.

Bloody tap: This is an artefact due to piercing a blood vessel, which is indicated (unreliably) by fewer red cells in successive bottles, and no yellowing of CSF (xanthochromia). To estimate how many white cells (*W*) were in the CSF before the blood was added, use the following:

$$W = \text{CSF WCC} - [(\text{blood WCC} \times \text{CSF RBC}) \div \text{blood RBC}].$$

If the blood count is normal, the rule of thumb is to subtract from the total CSF WCC (per μL) one white cell for every 1000 RBCs. To estimate the true protein level, subtract 10mg/L for every 1000 RBCs/mm^3 (be sure to do the count and protein estimation on the same bottle). NB: high protein levels in CSF make it appear yellow. *Subarachnoid haemorrhage:* Xanthochromia (yellow supernatant on spun CSF). Red cells in equal numbers in all bottles (unreliable). RBCs will excite an inflammatory response (eg CSF WCC raised), most marked after 48h. *Raised protein:* Meningitis; MS; Guillain-Barré syndrome. *Very raised CSF protein:* Spinal block; TB; or severe bacterial meningitis.

Complications

• Post-dural puncture headache. • Infection. • Bleeding. • Cerebral herniation (rare, check for signs of ↑ICP before proceeding). • Minor/transient neurological symptoms, eg paraesthesia, radiculopathy.

Any change in lower body neurology after an LP (pain, weakness, sensory changes, bladder/bowel disturbance) should be treated as cauda equina compression (haematoma/abscess) until proven otherwise. Obtain an urgent MRI spine.

Post-LP brain MRI scans often show diffuse meningeal enhancement with gadolinium. This is thought to be a reflection of increased blood flow secondary to intracranial hypotension. Interpret these scans with caution and in the context of the patient's clinical situation. Ensure the reason for the scan and current neurological examination are discussed with the radiologist pre procedure.

Post-LP headache

Risk 10–30%, typically occurring within 24h of LP, resolution over hours to 2wks (mean: 3–4d). Patients describe a constant, dull ache, more frontal than occipital. The most characteristic symptom is of positional exacerbation—worse when upright. There may be mild meningism or nausea. The pathology is thought to be continued leakage of CSF from the puncture site and intracranial *hypo*tension, though there may be other mechanisms involved.

Prevention Use the smallest spinal needle that is practical (22G) and keep the bevel aligned as described on p768. Blunt needles (more expensive) can reduce risk and are recommended (ask an anaesthetist about supply); however, collection of CSF takes too long (>6min) if needles smaller than 22G are used. Before withdrawing the needle, reinsert the stilette.

Treatment Despite years of anecdotal advice to the contrary, none of the following has ever been shown to be a risk factor: position during or after the procedure; hydration status before, during, or after; amount of CSF removed; immediate activity or rest post-LP. Time is a consistent healer. For severe or prolonged headaches, ask an anaesthetist about a blood patch. This is a careful injection of 20mL of autologous venous blood into the adjacent epidural space (said to 'clog up the hole'). Immediate relief occurs in 95%.

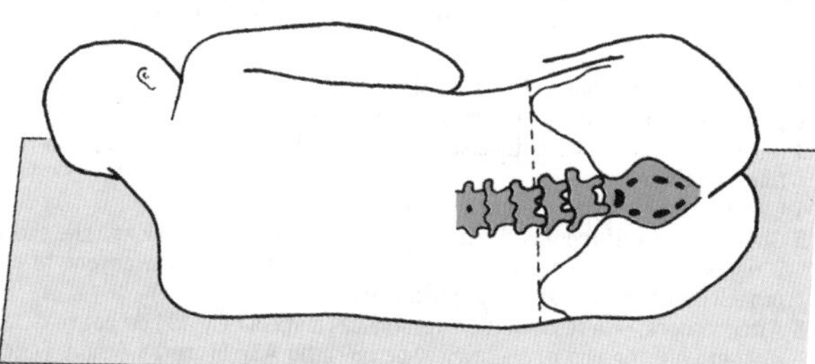

Fig 18.8 Defining the 3rd–4th lumbar vertebral interspace.

Adapted with permission from Vakil *et al.*, *Diagnosis and Management of Medical Emergencies*, 1977 Oxford University Press.

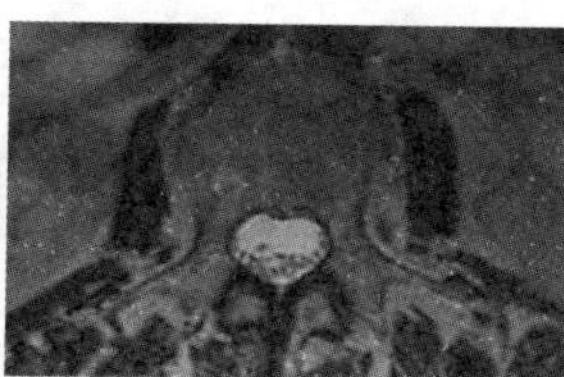

Fig 18.9 Axial T2-weighted MRI of the lumbar spine. The conus ends at the L1/L2 level with continuation of the cauda equina. Lumbar puncture below the L2 level will not damage the cauda equina as the nerve roots will part around an LP needle.

Image courtesy of Norwich Radiology Dept.

Cardioversion/defibrillation

►Do not wait for a crisis before familiarizing yourself with the defibrillator, as there are several types. All hospitals should include this information in your induction but check how the machine on your ward works.

Indications To restore sinus rhythm if VF/VT; AF, flutter, or supraventricular tachycardias if other treatments (p126) have failed, or there is haemodynamic compromise (p130 & p806). This may be done as an emergency, eg VF/VT, or electively, eg AF.

Aim To completely depolarize the heart using a direct current.

Procedure ►►*For VF/pulseless VT follow the ALS algorithm on p894 and call the arrest team!*

- Unless critically unwell, conscious patients require a general anaesthetic or monitored heavy sedation.
- If elective cardioversion of AF ensure adequate anticoagulation beforehand.
- Almost all defibrillators are now paddle-free and use 'hands-free' pads instead (less chance of skin arc than jelly). Place the pads on chest, one over apex (p39) and one below right clavicle. The positions are often given by a diagram on the reverse of the pad.

Fig 18.10 The dampened sine monophasic waveform.

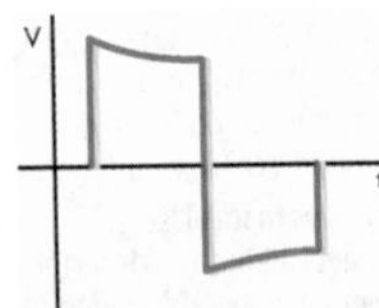

Fig 18.11 Rectilinear biphasic waveform with truncated exponential decay. Most new external defibrillators use this waveform.

Cardioversion: Synchronize the shock with the rhythm by pressing the 'SYNC' button on the machine. This ensures the shock does not initiate a ventricular arrhythmia. However, this only works for cardioversion; if the sync mode is engaged in *VF*, the defibrillator will not discharge.

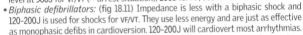

- *Monophasic defibrillators:* (fig 18.10) Set the energy level at 360J for VF/VT (►►arrest situation); 200J for AF; 50J for atrial flutter.
- *Biphasic defibrillators:* (fig 18.11) Impedance is less with a biphasic shock and 120–200J is used for shocks for VF/VT. They use less energy and are just as effective as monophasic defibs in cardioversion. 120–200J will cardiovert most arrhythmias.
- *Automatic external defibrillators:* (AEDs) Can be used by anyone who can turn them on and apply the pads. Follow the instructions given by the AED.

Shocking

1. Consider anticoagulation in AF (see p130).
2. Clearly state that you are charging the defibrillator.
3. Make sure no one else is touching the patient, the bed, or anything is in turn touching these.
4. Clearly state that you are about to shock the patient.
5. Give the shock. If there is a change in rhythm before you shock and the shock is no longer required, turn the dial to 'discharge'. Do not allow anyone to approach until the reading has dropped to 0J.
6. After a shock: ►►in resuscitation, resume CPR immediately and do not reassess rhythm until the end of the cycle (see p894, fig A3); in cardioversion, watch ECG; consider need to repeat the shock. Up to three are usual for AF/flutter.
7. Get an up-to-date 12-lead ECG.

►In children, use 4J/kg in VF/VT; see *OHCS* p239.

Taking arterial blood gas (ABG) samples

Having an artery sampled is more unpleasant for the patient than venepuncture: explain that it is going to feel different and is for a different purpose (p162 for indications and analysis). The usual site is the radial artery at the wrist. ►*Check with the patient that they do not have an arteriovenous fistula for haemodialysis. Never, ever sample from a fistula.*

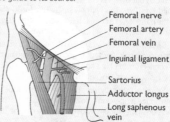

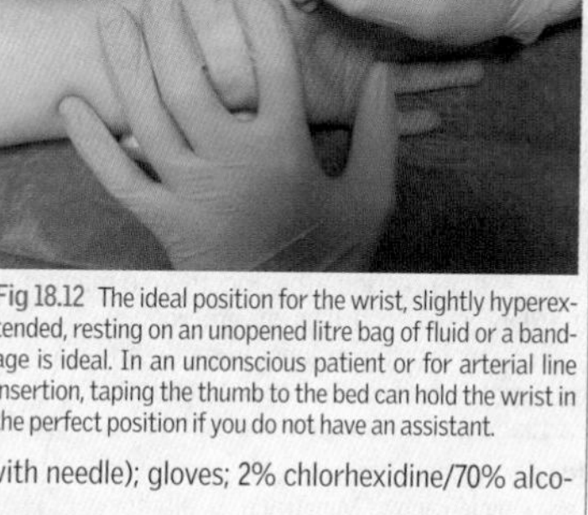

Fig 18.12 The ideal position for the wrist, slightly hyperextended, resting on an unopened litre bag of fluid or a bandage is ideal. In an unconscious patient or for arterial line insertion, taping the thumb to the bed can hold the wrist in the perfect position if you do not have an assistant.

Procedure:

- Get kit ready; include: portable sharps bin; pre-heparinized syringe; needle (blue size (23G) is good, although many syringes now come pre-made with needle); gloves; 2% chlorhexidine/70% alcohol swab; gauze; tape.
- Feel thoroughly for the best site. Look at both sides.
- Wipe with cleaning swab. Let the area dry. Get yourself comfortable.
- If the patient is drowsy or unconscious, ask an assistant to hold the hand and arm with the wrist slightly extended (fig 18.12).
- Before sampling, expel any excess heparin in the syringe. Infiltration over the artery with a small amount of 1% lidocaine (p573) through a 25G (orange) needle makes the procedure painless.
- Hold the syringe like a pen, with the needle bevel up. Let the patient know you are about to take the sample. Feel for the pulse with your other hand and enter at 45°, aiming beneath the finger you are feeling with.
- In most syringes, the plunger will move up on its own in a pulsatile manner if you are in the artery; rarely, entry into a vein next to the artery will give a similar result. Colour of the blood is little guide to its source.
- Allow the syringe to fill with 1-2mL, then remove the needle and apply firm pressure for 5 minutes (10 if anticoagulated).
- Expel any air from the syringe as this will alter the oxygenation of the blood. Cap and label the sample, check the patient's temperature and FiO_2 (0.21 if on air). Take the sample to the nearest analysis machine or send it by express delivery to the lab (which may be by your own feet, get someone else to apply pressure) as it should be analysed within 15 minutes of sampling.
- Syringes and analysis machines differ, so get familiar with the local nuances.

Femoral nerve
Femoral artery
Femoral vein
Inguinal ligament
Sartorius
Adductor longus
Long saphenous vein

Fig 18.13 The femoral artery is amenable to ABG sampling.

The other site that is amenable to ABG sampling is the femoral artery (fig 18.13). Surprisingly this may be less uncomfortable as it is a relatively less sensitive area and because, when supine, the patient cannot see the needle and thus may feel less apprehensive. The brachial artery can also be used, but be aware that the median nerve sits closely on its medial side and it is an end-artery. Normal values: p753.

Cricothyroidotomy Thsi is an emergency procedure to overcome airway obstruction above the level of the larynx. It should only be done in absolute 'can't intubate, can't ventilate' situations, ie where ventilation is impossible with a bag and mask (± airway adjuncts) and where there is an immediate threat to life. If not, call anaesthetics or ENT for immediate help.

Indications Upper airway obstruction when endotracheal intubation not possible, eg irretrievable foreign body; facial oedema (burns, angio-oedema); maxillofacial trauma; infection (epiglottitis).

Procedure Lie the patient supine with neck extended (eg pillow under shoulders) unless there is suspected cervical-spine instability. Run your index finger down the neck anteriorly in the midline to find the notch in the upper border of the thyroid cartilage (the Adam's apple): just below this, between the thyroid and cricoid cartilages, is a depression—the cricothyroid membrane (see fig 18.14). If you cannot feel the depression and it is an emergency, you can access the trachea directly approximately halfway between the cricoid cartilage and the suprasternal notch.

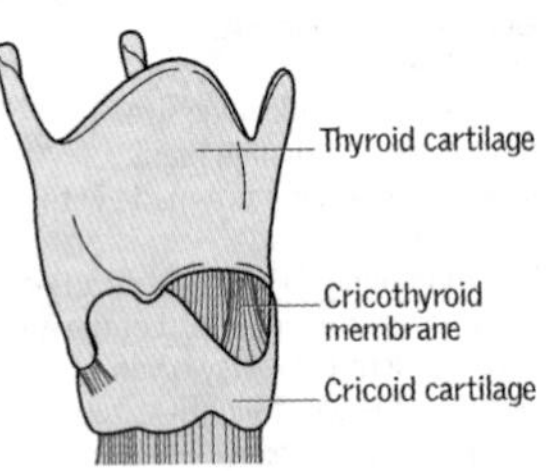

Fig 18.14 The cricothyroid membrane.

Ideally use a purpose-designed kit (eg QuickTrach®, MiniTrach®), all hospitals will stock one version. If no kit is available then a cannula (needle cricothyroidotomy) can buy time, and in out-of-hospital situations a blade and empty biro case have saved lives. ►►Needle and kit cricothyroidotomies are temporary measures pending formal tracheostomy.

1 *Needle cricothyroidotomy:* Pierce the membrane perpendicular to the skin with large-bore cannula (14G) attached to syringe: withdrawal of air confirms position; lidocaine may or may not be required. Slide cannula over needle at 45° to the skin superiorly in the sagittal plane. Use a Y-connector (see fig 18.16) or improvise connection to O_2 supply at 15L/min: use thumb on Y-connector to allow O_2 in over 1s and CO_2 out over 4s ('transtracheal jet insufflation'). This is the preferred method in children <12yrs. This will only sustain life for 30–45min before CO_2 builds up. However, if the patient has a completely obstructed airway then they will not be able to exhale through this, and it will lead to cardiovascular compromise and pneumothoraces.

2 *Cricothyroidotomy kit:* Most contain a guarded blade, and a large (4–6mm) shaped cannula (cuffed or uncuffed depending on brand) over an introducer, plus a connector and binding tape. The patient will have to be ventilated via a bag, as the resistance is too high to breathe spontaneously. This will sustain for 30–45min.

3 *Surgical cricothyroidotomy:* Smallest tube for prolonged ventilation is 6mm. Introduce high-volume, low-pressure cuff tracheostomy tube through a horizontal incision in membrane. Take care not to cut the thyroid or cricoid cartilages.

Complications Local haemorrhage ± aspiration; posterior perforation of trachea ± oesophagus; subglottic stenosis; laryngeal stenosis if membrane over-incised in childhood; tube blockage; subcutaneous tunnelling; vocal cord paralysis or hoarseness (the recurrent laryngeal nerve runs superiorly in the tracheo-oesophageal groove).

Emergency needle pericardiocentesis

Fig 18.15 Emergency needle pericardiocentesis.

- Get your senior's help (for whom this page may serve as an *aide-memoire*).
- Equipment: 20mL syringe, long 18G cannula, 3-way tap, ECG monitor, skin cleanser. Use ECHO guidance if there is time.
- If time allows, use full aseptic technique, at a minimum clean skin with 2% chlorhexidine in 70% alcohol and wear sterile gloves, and, if conscious, use local anaesthesia and sedation, eg with slow IV midazolam: titrate up to 3.5-5mg—start with 2mg over 1min, 0.5-1mg in elderly (in whom the maximum dose is 3.5mg; inject at the rate of 2mg/min)—antidote: flumazenil 0.2mg IV over 15s, then 0.1mg every 60s, up to 1mg in total.
  ►*Ensure you have IV access and full resuscitation equipment to hand.*
- Introduce needle at 45° to skin just below and to left of xiphisternum, aiming for tip of left scapula (fig 18.15). Aspirate continuously and watch ECG. Frequent ventricular ectopics or an injury pattern (↓ST segment) on ECG imply that the myocardium has been breached—withdraw slightly. As soon as fluid is obtained through the needle, slide the cannula into place.
- Evacuate pericardial contents through the syringe and 3-way tap. Removal of only a small amount of fluid (eg 20mL) can produce marked clinical improvement. If you are not sure whether the fluid you are aspirating is pure blood (eg on entering a ventricle), see if it clots (heavily bloodstained pericardial fluid does not clot), or measure its PCV (though this may be difficult in the acute setting but some blood gas analysers may give this).
- You can leave the cannula *in situ* temporarily, for repeated aspiration. If there is reaccumulation, insert a drain but pericardiectomy may be needed.
- Send fluid for microscopy and culture, as needed, including tests for TB.

Complications: Laceration of ventricle or coronary artery (± subsequent haemopericardium); aspiration of ventricular blood; arrhythmias (ventricular fibrillation); pneumothorax; puncture of aorta, oesophagus (± mediastinitis), or peritoneum (± peritonitis).

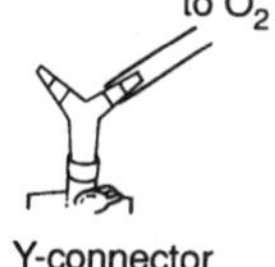

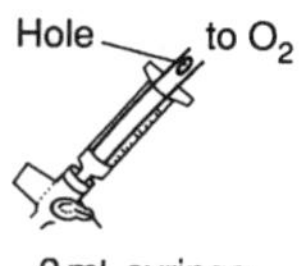

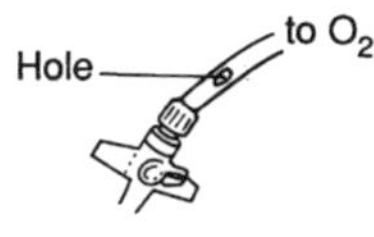

Fig 18.16 Methods of providing oxygen.

Central venous cannulation

Central venous cannulae may be inserted to measure central venous pressure (CVP), to administer certain drugs (eg amiodarone, chemotherapy), or for intravenous access (fluid, parenteral nutrition). In an emergency, the procedure can be done using the landmark method (see p775), though NICE recommends that all routine internal jugular catheters should be placed with US guidance. Even if the line is not placed under direct US visualization, a look to check vessel size, position in relation to artery, and patency (no thrombus or stenosis) is extremely useful. For contraindications, see table 18.2.

Table 18.2 Contraindications to central venous cannulation

Absolute	Relative
Infection at insertion site	Coagulopathy
	Ipsilateral carotid endarterectomy
	Newly inserted cardiac pacemaker leads
	Thrombus within the vein
	Venous stenosis
	Ipsilateral abnormal anatomy

Sites of insertion These include the internal jugular vein (see p775 and p43), subclavian vein, and the femoral vein. The choice depends largely on operator experience, but evidence suggests that the femoral approach is associated with a higher rate of line infection and thrombosis. Overall, the internal jugular approach (with ultrasound guidance) is most commonly used and risks fewer complications than the subclavian. If possible, get written consent (p568). Check clotting and platelets. The technique for internal jugular (routine) and femoral (emergency) are given here.

Complications (~20%.) Insertion is not without hazard, so decide whether the patient requires a line first, and then ask for help if you are inexperienced.
►Bleeding; arterial puncture/cannulation; AV fistula formation; air embolism; pneumothorax; haemothorax; chylothorax (lymph); phrenic nerve palsy (the right phrenic nerve passes over the brachiocephalic artery, posterior to the subclavian vein—hiccups may be a sign of injury); phlebitis; thrombus formation on tip or in vein (if high risk for thromboembolism, eg malignancy, consider anticoagulation, eg LMWH); bacterial colonization; cellulitis; sepsis (can be reduced by adherence to a strict aseptic technique; if taking blood cultures in a febrile patient with a central venous line, remember to take samples from the central line and from a peripheral vein).

Peripherally inserted central cannulas (PICC lines) These are a good alternative to central lines, as they can stay *in situ* for up to 6 months, and provide access for blood sampling, fluids, antibiotics (allowing home IV therapy). They are placed using a Seldinger technique, puncturing the brachial or basilic vein then threading the line into the subclavian or superior vena cava. Because of the insertion site there is a much lower risk of pneumo- or haemothorax, but they are tricky to insert in an emergency.

Removing central lines Should be done carefully with aseptic technique. Position the patient slightly head down, remove dressings, clean and drape the area, remove sutures. Ask the patient to inhale and hold their breath, then ►breathe out smoothly while you are pulling the line out. This helps to prevent air emboli. Ask the patient to rehearse this sequence with you to ensure they have understood their role. Apply pressure for 5 minutes (longer if coagulopathic).

Internal jugular catheterization

Internal jugular Should be the approach of choice in a non-emergency situation. Ideally the right side as it offers a direct route to the heart and there is less chance of misplacement of the line compared to the left. The subclavian approach is trickier and best taught by an expert. Use US guidance if at all possible, ideally to insert the line under direct vision, but at least to define the anatomy. If possible, have the patient attached to a cardiac monitor in case of arrhythmias.

- Position the patient slightly head down to avoid air embolism and fill the veins to improve your chances of success. ►This can compromise cardiac function and precipitate acute LVF so check if your patient has a cardiac history. Minimize the time the patient is head down; if they are unable to lie flat, consider a femoral approach. Turn their head slightly to the left.
- This should be a sterile procedure so use full aseptic technique (hat, mask, gloves, gown) and clean with 2% chlorhexidine in 70% isopropyl alcohol before draping. Ensure your equipment is prepared, flush the catheter lumens with saline.
- If US is unavailable, the *landmark procedure* can be used to identify insertion point—approximately at the junction of the two heads of sternocleidomastoid at about the level of the thyroid cartilage (fig 18.17). Feel gently for the carotid pulse, then infiltrate with 1% lidocaine just lateral to this. The vein is usually superficial (fig 18.18).
- Insert the introducer needle with a 5mL syringe attached, advance gently at a 45° angle, aiming for the ipsilateral nipple and aspirating continuously. If you are using US, watch the needle tip enter the vein, if the landmark approach keep your fingers on the carotid pulse.
- As soon as blood is aspirated, lay down the US probe and hold the introducer needle in position, remove the syringe and thread the guidewire through the needle. It should pass easily, if there is resistance try lowering the angle of the needle and gently advancing the wire. If the wire will not pass do not remove it alone, the tip can shear off and embolize; remove the needle with the wire, apply pressure and attempt a second puncture.

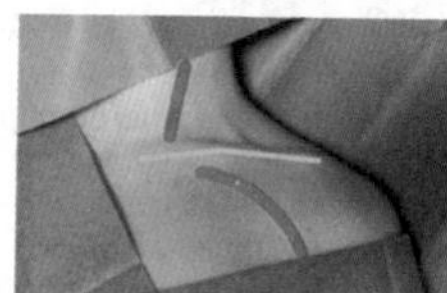

Fig 18.17 Position of internal jugular and subclavian veins (red) compared to the clavicle (yellow).

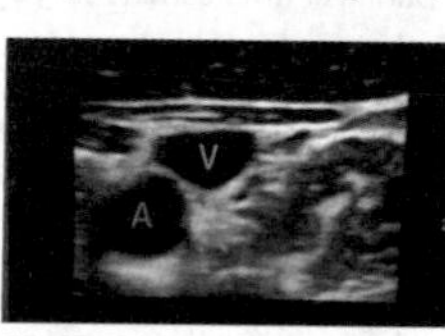

Fig 18.18 Vessels seen on ultrasound. The compressible vein is above the artery.

- If the wire threads easily, insert to 30cm (see markings on the wire), remove the needle keeping hold of the wire at all times. Make a nick in the skin with a scalpel at the insertion point, and gently thread the dilator over the wire. You do not need to insert the dilator far, only as far as the vein (you often feel a loss of resistance as the dilator enters the vein, so insert gently: a pneumothorax can result from enthusiastic dilating).
- Remove the dilator, keeping hold of the wire, thread the flushed catheter over the wire, then remove the wire. The line should sit at about 13cm on the right side (17cm on the left). Check you can aspirate blood from each lumen, then flush them.
- Suture the catheter in place (many have little 'wings' for suturing) and dress. Request a CXR to confirm position and exclude pneumothorax. The tip of the catheter should sit vertically in the SVC.

Femoral vein In an emergency situation where ultrasound is not easily accessible, if the patient is unable to lie flat, or where speed is of the essence, the femoral approach is often the safest, as there is no risk of pneumothorax or haemothorax and a much reduced risk of arrhythmia. The technique is similar to internal jugular, except the insertion point is just medial to the femoral artery at the groin crease.

Subclavian vein Should be taught by an expert and should ideally be carried out under US guidance. Some physicians prefer this approach, but even in experienced hands there is a ↑risk of complications compared to US-guided internal jugular lines.

Inserting a temporary cardiac pacemaker

Often it is wiser to liaise with a specialist pacing centre to arrange prompt, definitive pacing than to try temporary transvenous pacing, which often has complications (see later in topic) and therefore may delay a definitive procedure.

Possible indications in the acute phase of myocardial infarction

- *Complete AV block:*
  - With inferior MI (right coronary artery occlusion) pacing may only be needed if symptomatic; spontaneous recovery may occur.
  - With anterior MI (representing massive septal infarction).
- *Second-degree block:*
  - Wenckebach (p99; implies decremental AV node conduction; may respond to atropine in an inferior MI; pace if anterior MI).
  - Mobitz type 2 block is usually associated with distal fascicular disease and carries high risk of complete heart block, so pace in both types of MI.
- *First-degree block:* Observe carefully: 40% develop higher degrees of block.
- *Bundle branch block:* Pace prophylactically if evidence of trifascicular disease (p100) or non-adjacent bifascicular disease.
- *Sino-atrial disease + serious symptoms:* Pace unless responds to atropine.

Other indications where temporary pacing may be needed

- Pre-op: if surgery is required in patients with type 2 or complete heart block (whether or not MI has occurred); do 24h ECG; liaise with the anaesthetist.
- Drug poisoning, eg with β-blockers, digoxin, or verapamil.
- Symptomatic bradycardia, uncontrolled by atropine or isoprenaline.
- Suppression of drug-resistant VT and SVT (overdrive pacing; do on ICU).
- Asystolic cardiac arrest with P-wave activity (ventricular standstill).
- During or after cardiac surgery—eg around the AV node or bundle of His.

Technique for temporary transvenous pacing Learn from an expert.

- *Preparation:* Monitor ECG; have a defibrillator to hand, ensure the patient has peripheral access; check that a radiographer with screening equipment is present. If you are screening, wear a protective lead apron.
- *Insertion:* Using an aseptic technique, place the introducer into the (ideally right) internal jugular vein (p775) or subclavian. If this is difficult, access to the right atrium can be achieved via the femoral vein. Pass the pacing wire through the introducer into the right atrium, ideally under radiological screening. It will either pass easily through the tricuspid valve or loop within the atrium. If the latter occurs, it is usually possible to flip the wire across the valve with a combined twisting and withdrawing movement (fig 18.19). Advance the wire slightly. At this stage the wire may try to exit the ventricle through the pulmonary outflow tract. A further withdrawing and rotation of the wire will aim the tip at the apex of the right ventricle. Advance slightly again to place the wire in contact with the endocardium. Remove any slack to ↓risk of subsequent displacement.
- *Checking the threshold:* Connect the wire to the pacing box and set the 'demand' rate slightly higher than the patient's own heart rate and the output to 3V. A paced rhythm should be seen. Find the pacing threshold by slowly reducing the voltage until the pacemaker fails to stimulate the tissue (pacing spikes are no longer followed by paced beats). The threshold should be less than 1V, but a slightly higher value may be acceptable if it is stable—eg after a large infarction.
- *Setting the pacemaker:* Set the output to 3V or over 3 times the threshold value (whichever is higher) in 'demand' mode. Set the rate as required. Suture the wire to the skin, and fix with a sterile dressing.
- Check the position of the wire (and exclude pneumothorax) with a CXR.
- Recurrent checks of the pacing threshold are required over the next few days. The formation of endocardial oedema can raise the threshold by a factor of 2-3.

Complications Pneumothorax; sepsis; cardiac perforation; pacing failure: from loss of capture, loss of electrical continuity in pacing circuit, or electrode displacement.

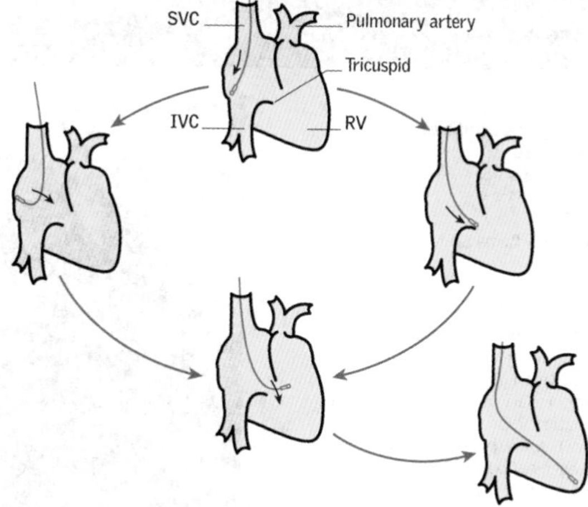

Fig 18.19 Siting a temporary cardiac pacemaker.

Non-invasive transcutaneous cardiac pacing

This method (performed through a defibrillator with external pacing facility) has the advantages of being quicker, less risky than the transvenous route, and easier to perform. Its main disadvantage is the pain caused by skeletal muscle contraction in the non-sedated patient. Indications for pacing via the transcutaneous route are as p776, *plus* if transvenous pacing (or someone able to perform it) is unavailable or will be delayed in an emergency situation.

- Give sedation and analgesia, eg midazolam + morphine IV titrated to effect.
- Clipping chest hair may help improve electrical contact; ►don't shave the skin, as nicks can predispose to electrical burns. Ensure the skin is dry.
- Almost all modern transcutaneous devices can function through defibrillation 'hands-free' pads, and so these can be applied as for defibrillation (see p770). If necessary, the pads can be placed in an AP position: anteriorly over the V2–V3 electrode position and posteriorly at the same level, just below the scapula.
- Select 'demand' mode, (which synchronizes the stimulus with the R wave, so avoiding pacing on the T wave—which can provoke VF or VT) and adjust the ECG gain so that QRS complexes can be seen.
- Select an appropriate pacing rate: eg 60–90bpm in an adult.
- Set the pacing current at the lowest setting and turn on the pacemaker.
- Increase the pacing current until electrical capture occurs (normally from 50–100mA), which can be confirmed by seeing a wide QRS complex and a T wave on the trace (ventricular electrical capture).
- There will be some interference from skeletal muscle contraction on the ECG trace, as well as possible artefact, which could be mistaken for a QRS complex. The absence of a T wave in the former is an important discriminator between the two.
- CPR can continue with the pads in place, though only when the pacing unit is *off*.
- Once adequate cardiac output has been maintained, seek expert help and arrange transvenous pacing.

19 Emergencies

Contents

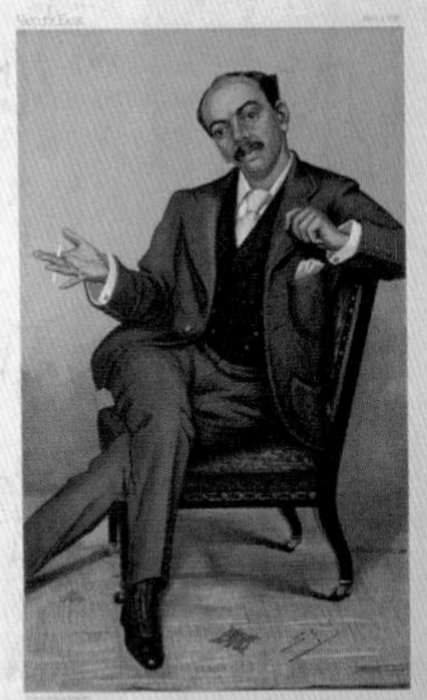

Fig 19.1 Dr Leander Starr Jameson (1853–1917) was a Victorian physician barely known to the history of our profession and yet immortalized by the idealization of his character in Rudyard Kipling's poem '*If*'. Kipling's words contain much that might guide the doctor faced with a sudden and unexpected emergency. Beyond the oft quoted exhortation to '*keep your head when all about you are losing theirs*', Kipling also endorsed an appropriate degree of self-confidence ('*trust yourself when all men doubt you, But make allowance for their doubting too*'), encouraged realism ('*meet with Triumph and Disaster And treat those two impostors just the same*'), and a large measure of courage ('*force your heart and nerve and sinew To serve your turn long after they are gone, And so hold on when there is nothing in you Except the Will which says to them: "Hold on!"*'). But what of Dr James? As a house officer in London, he broke down from overwork and moved to take up what would become a distinguished practice in South Africa. A foray into the military ill-suited him and he ended up in jail for leading a botched raid that was so out-of-character that it seems he allowed himself to become a scapegoat for others higher in government. He died in November 1917, outliving Kipling's son John, who was killed in the trenches in 1915 at the age of 18, and to whom '*If*' was addressed: '*Yours is the Earth and everything that's in it, And—which is more—you'll be a Man, my son.*'

We thank Dr Andrew Johnston and Bernard Ho, our Junior Reader, for their contribution.

Introduction to emergencies

Some doctors enjoy the adrenaline rush of seeing an emergency case and pulling someone back from the edge of death. Some fear the emergency take, worried as to what they will miss, how many will die. There is no right approach; the emergency room needs both thought and practicality to manage patients. A patient who comes in flat and can be resuscitated gives the whole team a boost, as right there in front of us is the proof that we can make a difference. However, a patient who comes in well and collapses, dying before we can even decide what is wrong, can bring the whole team down. There are nights where we save life after life, and nights where we can't; sometimes a death is inevitable, despite our best efforts. You are a doctor, but you are a human being as well, and losing a patient can feel like a personal failure. However, remember that when we lose a patient it is the disease that has killed them, not us. Try to take a few minutes and reflect on what happened; ask if you could have done anything differently. Should you have sought help sooner? Discussing with a senior can be helpful, as can writing down your reflection, not in a portfolio for discussion at your appraisal, but in anonymous format for your own education. Watch the team at an arrest, the best leaders are the ones who have learned to stand back, assess the whole situation, and take enough time to see where the critical intervention is needed. There is no substitute for experience, nobody becomes a consultant overnight, but watch the best clinicians at work and you will learn both practical and life skills.

Most important in an emergency situation is communication. Wherever you can, involve the relatives and the whole team in discussions, but remember that at the heart of this is a patient. What do they want? Never be afraid to ask the patient directly, they may hold very strong views. However, it is up to us as physicians to be honest with them about their prognosis—do not offer a treatment you know is not in the best interests of the patient, and this includes resuscitation. When faced with death, many patients are afraid—our role is to try to relieve that fear, whether by intervening to delay death, or by easing their passing. But we cannot ever prevent death, we simply delay it. As Shakespeare has *Julius Caesar* say:

'Of all the wonders that I have yet heard, it seems to me most strange that men should fear, seeing that death, a necessary end, will come when it will come.'

ABCDE preliminary assessment (primary survey)

Airway — Protect cervical spine, if injury possible.
Assessment: any signs of obstruction? Ascertain patency.
Management: establish a patent airway.

Breathing — *Assessment:* determine respiratory rate, check bilateral chest movement, percuss, and auscultate.
Management: if no respiratory effort, treat as arrest (see p894, fig A3), intubate and ventilate. If breathing compromised, give high-concentration O_2, manage according to findings, eg relieve tension pneumothorax.

Circulation — *Assessment:* check pulse and BP; check if peripherally shut down; check capillary refill; look for evidence of haemorrhage.
Management: if shocked, treat as on p790.
If no cardiac output, treat as arrest (see p894, fig A3).

Disability — Assess 'level of consciousness' with **AVPU** score (**a**lert? responds to **v**oice? to **p**ain? **u**nresponsive?); check pupils: size, equality, reactions. *Glasgow Coma Scale*, if time allows.

Exposure — Undress patient, but cover to avoid hypothermia.

Quick history from relatives assists diagnosis: *Events* surrounding onset of illness, evidence of overdose/suicide attempt, any suggestion of trauma? *Past medical history,* especially diabetes, asthma, COPD, alcohol, opiate or street drug abuse, epilepsy or recent head injury, recent travel. *Medication,* current drugs. *Allergies*.

Once ventilation and circulation are adequate, proceed to carry out history, examination, investigations, and management in the usual way.

Headache: differential diagnosis

The vast majority of headaches are benign, but when taking a history do not forget to ask about the following[1] (early diagnosis can save lives):

Worrying features or 'red flags'

- First and worst headache—*subarachnoid haemorrhage* (p478).
- Thunderclap headache—*subarachnoid haemorrhage* (p478: p480 for other causes).
- Unilateral headache and eye pain—*cluster headache, acute glaucoma* (p456).
- Unilateral headache and ipsilateral symptoms—*migraine, tumour, vascular* (p458).
- Cough-initiated headache—*↑ICP/venous thrombosis* (p480).
- Worse in the morning or bending forward—*↑ICP/venous thrombosis* (p480).
- Persisting headache ± scalp tenderness in over-50s—*giant cell arteritis* (p556).
- Headache with fever or neck stiffness—*meningitis* (p822).
- Change in the pattern of 'usual headaches' (p456).
- Decreased level of consciousness (p456).

Two other vital questions:

- Where have you been? (Malaria, p416).
- Might you be pregnant? (Pre-eclampsia; especially if proteinuria and ↑BP, p458.)

Always examine a patient presenting with a severe headache; if nothing about history or examination is concerning, both you and the patient will be reassured, but subtle abnormalities are important not to miss.

No signs on examination

- Tension headache (p456).
- Migraine (p458).
- Cluster headache (p457).
- Post-traumatic (p456).
- Drugs (nitrates, calcium-channel antagonists) (p114).
- Carbon monoxide poisoning or anoxia. (p842)
- Subarachnoid haemorrhage (p478).

Signs of meningism?

- Meningitis (may not have fever or rash—p822).
- Subarachnoid haemorrhage (p478—examination may be normal).

Decreased conscious level or localizing signs?

- Stroke (p470).
- Encephalitis/meningitis (p822).
- Cerebral abscess (p824).
- Subarachnoid haemorrhage (pp478-9, figs 10.17, 10.18).
- Venous sinus occlusion (p480—focal neurological deficits).
- Tumour (p498).
- Subdural haematoma (p482).
- TB meningitis (p393).

Papilloedema?

- Tumour (p498).
- Venous sinus occlusion (p480—focal neurological deficits).
- Malignant (accelerated phase) hypertension (p138).
- Idiopathic intracranial hypertension (p498).
- Any CNS infection, if prolonged (eg >2wks)—eg TB meningitis (p393).

Others

- Giant cell arteritis (p556—↑ESR and tender scalp over temporal arteries).
- Acute glaucoma (p456—painful red eye—get pressures checked urgently).
- Vertebral artery dissection (p470—neck pain and cerebellar/medullary signs).
- Cervical spondylosis (p508).
- Sinusitis.
- Paget's disease (p685—↑ALP).
- Altitude sickness (*OHCS* p770).

This page intentionally blank

Breathlessness: emergency presentations

There may not be time to ask or the patient may not be able to give you a history in acute breathlessness, this in itself can be a helpful sign (inability to complete sentences in one breath = severe breathlessness, inability to speak/impaired conscious level = life-threatening). Collateral history of known respiratory disease, anaphylaxis, or other history can be extremely helpful but do not delay. Assess the patient for the following:

Wheezing?
- Asthma (p810).
- COPD (p812).
- Heart failure (p800).
- Anaphylaxis (p794).

Stridor? (Upper airway obstruction.)
- Foreign body or tumour.
- Acute epiglottitis (younger patients).
- Anaphylaxis (p794).
- Trauma, eg laryngeal fracture.

Crepitations?
- Heart failure (p800).
- Pneumonia (p816).
- Bronchiectasis (p172).
- Fibrosis (p198).

Chest clear?
- Pulmonary embolism (p818).
- Hyperventilation.
- Metabolic acidosis, eg diabetic ketoacidosis (p832).
- Anaemia (p324).
- Drugs, eg salicylates.
- Shock (may cause 'air hunger', p790).
- *Pneumocystis jirovecii* pneumonia (p400).
- CNS causes.

Others
- Pneumothorax (p814—pain, increased resonance, tracheal deviation if tension pneumothorax).
- Pleural effusion (p192—'stony dullness').

Key investigations
- Baseline observations—O_2 sats, pulse, temperature, peak flow.
- ABG if saturations <94% or concern about acidosis/drugs/sepsis.
- ECG (signs of PE, LVH, MI?).
- CXR.
- Baseline blood: glucose, FBC, U&E, consider drug screen.

This page intentionally blank

Chest pain: differential diagnosis

First exclude any potentially life-threatening causes, by virtue of history, brief examination, and limited investigations. Then consider other potential causes. For the full assessment of cardiac pain, see pp94, 118.

Life-threatening

- Acute myocardial infarction (pp796–9).
- Angina/acute coronary syndrome (pp796–9).
- Aortic dissection (p655).
- Tension pneumothorax (p814).
- Pulmonary embolism (p818).
- Oesophageal rupture (p820).

Others

- Pneumonia (p816).
- Chest wall pain:
  - Muscular.
  - Rib fractures.
  - Bony metastases.
  - Costochondritis.
- Gastro-oesophageal reflux (p254).
- Pleurisy (p166).
- Empyema (p170).
- Pericarditis (p154).
- Oesophageal spasm (p250).
- Herpes zoster (p404).
- Cervical spondylosis (p508).
- Intra-abdominal:
  - Cholecystitis (p634).
  - Peptic ulceration (p252).
  - Pancreatitis (p270).
- Sickle-cell crisis (p340).

Before discharging patients with undiagnosed chest pain, be sure in your own mind that the pain is not cardiac (this pain is usually dull, may radiate to jaw, arm, or epigastrium, and is usually associated with exertion). Carry out key investigations and discuss options with a colleague, and the patient. *Safety-net*, telling the patient to return or seek advice if they develop worrying features (specify these) or the pain does not settle.

Key investigations

- CXR.
- ECG.
- FBC, U&E, and troponin (p118). Consider D-dimer only if low probability of venous thromboembolism. See 'Modified Wells' score for PE, p191.

►Just because the patient's chest wall is tender to palpation, this doesn't mean the cause of the chest pain is musculoskeletal. Even if palpation reproduces the same type of pain, ensure that you exclude all potential life-threatening causes. Although chest wall tenderness has discriminatory value against cardiac pain, it may be a feature of a pulmonary embolism.

⚠

This page intentionally blank

Coma

Definition *Unrousable unresponsiveness*. Quantify using *Glasgow Coma Scale* (GCS).

Causes of impaired conscious level/coma

Metabolic:

- Drugs, poisoning, eg carbon monoxide, alcohol, tricyclics.
- Hypoglycaemia, hyperglycaemia (ketoacidotic, or HONK, pp832–4).
- Hypoxia, CO_2 narcosis (COPD).
- Septicaemia (p792).
- Hypothermia.
- Myxoedema (p834), Addisonian crisis (p836).
- Hepatic/uraemic encephalopathy (pp275, 298).

Neurological:

- Trauma.
- Infection: meningitis (p822); encephalitis (eg herpes simplex—p404), *tropical*: malaria (p416; do thick films), typhoid, typhus, rabies, trypanosomiasis.
- Tumour: 1° or 2° (p528).
- Vascular: stroke (p470), subdural (p482), subarachnoid (p478), hypertensive encephalopathy (p140).
- Epilepsy: non-convulsive status (p484) or post-ictal state.

Immediate management See fig 19.2 (and coma CNS exam, p789).

- Assess Airway, Breathing, and Circulation. Consider intubation if GCS <8 (p788). Support the circulation if required (ie IV fluids). Give O_2 and treat any seizures. Protect the cervical spine unless trauma is known not to be the cause.
- Check blood glucose; give eg 200mL 10% glucose IV stat if hypoglycaemia possible.
- IV thiamine if any suggestion of Wernicke's encephalopathy; see later in topic.
- IV naloxone (0.4–2mg IV) for opiate intoxication (may also be given IM or via ET tube); IV flumazenil (p842) for benzodiazepine intoxication only if airway compromised as risk of seizures especially if concomitant tricyclic intoxication.

Examination ►*Vital signs are vital—obtain full set, including temperature.*

- Signs of trauma—haematoma, laceration, bruising, CSF/blood in nose or ears, fracture 'step' deformity of skull, subcutaneous emphysema, 'panda eyes'.
- Stigmata of other illnesses: liver disease, alcoholism, diabetes, myxoedema.
- Skin for needle marks, cyanosis, pallor, rash (meningitis; typhus), poor turgor.
- Smell the breath (alcohol, hepatic fetor, ketosis, uraemia).
- Opisthotonus (fig 9.45, p436) ≈meningitis or tetanus. Decerebrate/decorticate (p788)?
- Meningism (pp456, 822) ►but do *not* move neck unless cervical spine is cleared.
- Pupils (p789) size, reactivity, gaze.
- Heart/lung exam for BP, murmurs, rubs, wheeze, consolidation, collapse.
- Abdomen/rectal for organomegaly, ascites, bruising, peritonism, melaena.
- Are there any foci of infection (abscesses, bites, middle ear infection)?
- Any features of meningitis: neck stiffness, rash, focal neurology?
- Note the *absence* of signs, eg *no* pin-point pupils in a known heroin addict.

Quick history From family, ambulance staff, bystanders: abrupt or gradual onset? How found—suicide note, seizure? If injured, suspect cervical spinal injury and do not move spine (*OHCS* p782). Recent complaints—headache, fever, vertigo, depression? Recent medical history—sinusitis, otitis, neurosurgery, ENT procedure? Past medical history—diabetes, asthma, ↑BP, cancer, epilepsy, psychiatric illness? Drug or toxin exposure (especially alcohol or other recreational drugs)? Any travel?

If the diagnosis is unclear:

- Treat the treatable: O_2; naloxone as above; glucose (eg 200mL of 10% IV); Pabrinex IV for Wernicke's encephalopathy, p714; septic specifics: cefotaxime 2g/12h IV (meningitis, p822), artemether/quinine (malaria, p418), aciclovir (encephalitis, p824).
- Do routine biochemistry, haematology, thick films, blood cultures, blood ethanol, drug screen, etc.
- Arrange urgent CT head, if normal, and no CI, proceed to LP.

The diagnosis should now be clear, eg hypo/hyperglycaemia; alcohol excess; poisoning; uraemia; pneumonia; subarachnoid; hypertensive/hepatic encephalopathy.

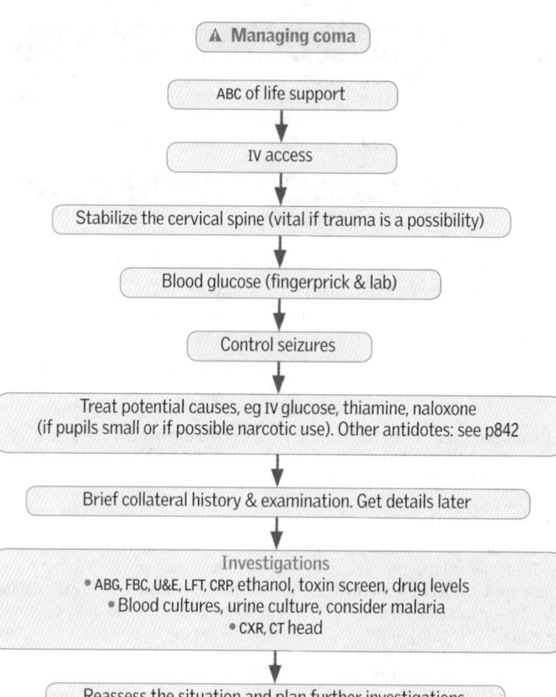

Fig 19.2 Managing coma. NB: check pupils every few minutes during the early stages, particularly if trauma is the likely cause. Doing so is the quickest way to find a localizing sign (so helpful in diagnosis, but remember that false localizing signs do occur)—and observing changes in pupil behaviour (eg becoming fixed and dilated) is the quickest way of finding out just how bad things are.

The Glasgow Coma Scale (GCS)

This gives a reliable, objective way of recording the conscious state of a person. It can be used by medical and nursing staff for initial and continuing assessment. It has value in predicting ultimate outcome. Three types of response are assessed, note in each case the best response (or best of any limb) which should be recorded (table 19.1).

Table 19.1 The Glasgow Coma Scale

⚠ Best motor response	Best verbal response	Eye opening
6 Obeying commands	**5** Oriented (time, place, person)	**4** Spontaneous
5 Localizing to pain	**4** Confused conversation	**3** In response to speech
4 Withdrawing to pain	**3** Inappropriate speech	**2** In response to pain
3 Flexor response to pain	**2** Incomprehensible sounds	**1** None
2 Extensor response to pain	**1** None	
1 No response to pain		

Adapted from 'Assessment of coma and impaired consciousness: a practical scale', Graham Teasdale and Bryan Jennett, *The Lancet*, Vol 304, No. 7872, 81–84 (1974), Elsevier.

An overall score is made by summing the score in the three areas assessed.
- No response to pain + no verbalization + no eye opening = 3.
- Severe injury, GCS ≤8—consider airway protection.
- Moderate injury, GCS 9–12.
- Minor injury, GCS 13–15.

Causing pain is not a pleasant thing, there are acceptable and unacceptable methods. Try fingernail bed pressure with a pen/pencil, sternal pressure (not a rub), or suprascapular squeeze. Abnormal responses to pain can help to localize the damage:
- *Flexion* = decorticate posture (arms bent inwards on chest, thumbs tucked in a clenched fist, legs extended) implies damage above the level of the red nucleus in the midbrain.[1]
- *Extension* = decerebrate posture (adduction and internal rotation of shoulder, pronation of forearm) indicates midbrain damage below the level of the red nucleus.

NB: an abbreviated coma scale, **AVPU**, is sometimes used in the initial assessment ('primary survey') of the critically ill:

A = **a**lert

V = responds to **v**ocal stimuli

P = responds to **p**ain

U = **u**nresponsive

NB: GCS scoring is different in young children; see *OHCS* p201.

1 Red nucleus output reinforces upper limb antigravity flexion. When its output is damaged, the unregulated reticulospinal and vestibulospinal tracts reinforce extension tone of upper and lower limbs.

The neurological examination in coma

This is aimed at locating the pathology in one of two places. Altered level of consciousness implies either:

1. A diffuse, bilateral, cortical dysfunction (usually producing loss of awareness with normal arousal), or
2. Damage to the ascending reticular activating system (ARAS) located throughout the brainstem from the medulla to the thalami (usually producing loss of arousal with unassessable awareness). The brainstem can be affected directly (eg pontine haemorrhage) or indirectly (eg compression from transtentorial or cerebellar herniation secondary to a mass or oedema).

Systematic examination:

- Level of consciousness; describe using *objective* words/AVPU.
- Respiratory pattern (p53)—Cheyne-Stokes (brainstem lesions or compression) hyperventilation (acidosis, hypoxia, or, rarely, neurogenic), ataxic or apneustic (breath-holding) breathing (brainstem damage with grave prognosis).
- Eyes—almost all patients with ARAS pathology will have eye findings:
  1. *Visual fields*—in light coma, test fields with visual threat. No blink in one field suggests hemianopia and contralateral hemisphere lesion.
  2. *Pupils—normal direct and consensual reflexes present* = intact midbrain. *Midposition (3-5mm) non-reactive ± irregular* = midbrain lesion. *Unilateral dilated and unreactive* ('fixed') = 3rd nerve compression. *Small, reactive* = pontine lesion ('pin-point pontine pupils') or drugs. *Horner's syndrome* (p702, fig 15.4) = ipsilateral lateral medulla or hypothalamus lesion, may precede uncal herniation. Beware patients with false eyes or who use eye drops for glaucoma.
  3. *Extraocular movements (EOMS)*—observe resting position and spontaneous movement; then test the vestibulo-ocular reflex (VOR) with either the *doll's-head manoeuvre* (normal if the eyes keep looking at the same point in space when the head is quickly moved laterally or vertically) or *ice water calorics* (normal if eyes deviate towards the cold ear with nystagmus to the other side). If present, the VOR exonerates most of the brainstem from the VIIth nerve nucleus (medulla) to the IIIrd (midbrain). *Don't move the head unless the cervical spine is cleared.*
  4. *Fundi*—papilloedema, subhyaloid haemorrhage, hypertensive retinopathy, signs of other disease (eg diabetic retinopathy).
- Examine for CNS asymmetry (tone, spontaneous movements, reflexes). One way to test for hemiplegia in coma is to raise both arms together and compare how they fall under gravity. If one descends fast, like a lead weight, but the other descends more gracefully, you have found a valuable focal sign of cortical dysfunction. The same applies to the legs.

Reproduced from 'Assessment of coma and impaired consciousness: a practical scale', Graham Teasdale and Bryan Jennett, *The Lancet*, Vol 304, No. 7872, 81–84 (1974), Elsevier.

Emergencies

⚠

►►Shock

Circulatory failure resulting in inadequate organ perfusion. Often defined by ↓BP—systolic <90mmHg—or mean arterial pressure (MAP) <65mmHg—with evidence of tissue hypoperfusion, eg mottled skin, urine output (UO) of <0.5mL/kg/h, serum lactate >2mmol/L. *Signs:* ↓GCS/agitation, pallor, cool peripheries, tachycardia, slow capillary refill, tachypnoea, oliguria.

MAP = cardiac output (CO) × systemic vascular resistance (SVR).
CO = stroke volume × heart rate.
► ∴ shock can result from inadequate CO or a loss of SVR, or both.

Inadequate cardiac output

- *Hypovolaemia:*
  - Bleeding: trauma, ruptured aortic aneurysm, GI bleed.
  - Fluid loss: vomiting, burns, 'third-space' losses, eg pancreatitis, heat exhaustion.
- *Pump failure:*
  - Cardiogenic shock, eg ACS, arrhythmias, aortic dissection, acute valve failure.
  - Secondary causes, eg PE, tension pneumothorax, cardiac tamponade.

Peripheral circulatory failure (loss of SVR)

- *Sepsis:* (p792) Infection with any organism can cause acute vasodilation from inflammatory cytokines. Gram -ves can produce endotoxin, causing sudden and severe shock but without signs of infection (fever, ↑WCC). Classically patients with sepsis are warm & vasodilated, but may be cold & shut down. Other diseases, eg pancreatitis, can give a similar picture associated with the inflammatory cascade.
- *Anaphylaxis:* p794.
- *Neurogenic:* Eg spinal cord injury, epidural or spinal anaesthesia.
- *Endocrine failure:* Addison's disease, p836 or hypothyroidism; see p834.
- *Other:* Drugs, eg anaesthetics, antihypertensives, cyanide poisoning.

Assessment ►►ABCDE (p779). With shock we are dealing primarily with 'C' so get large-bore IV access ×2 and check ECG for rate, rhythm (very fast or very slow will compromise cardiac output), and signs of ischaemia.

- *General review:* Cold and clammy suggests cardiogenic shock or fluid loss. Look for signs of anaemia or dehydration, eg skin turgor, postural hypotension? Warm and well perfused, with bounding pulse points to septic shock. Any features suggestive of anaphylaxis—history, urticaria, angioedema, wheeze?
- *CVS:* Usually tachycardic (unless on β-blocker, or in spinal shock—*OHCS* p757) and hypotensive. But in the young and fit, or pregnant women, the systolic BP may remain normal, although the pulse pressure will narrow, with up to 30% blood volume depletion. Difference between arms (>20mmHg)—aortic dissection (p655)?
- *JVP or central venous pressure:* If raised, cardiogenic shock likely.
- *Check abdomen:* Any signs of trauma, or aneurysm? Any evidence of GI bleed?

Management ►If BP unrecordable, call the cardiac arrest team.

- *Septic shock:* See p792.
- *Anaphylaxis:* See p794.
- *Cardiogenic shock:* See p802.
- *Hypovolaemic shock:* Identify and treat underlying cause. Raise the legs.
  - Give fluid bolus 10–15mL/kg crystalloid via large peripheral line, if shock improves repeat, titrate to HR (aim <100), BP (aim SBP >90) and UO (aim >0.5mL/kg/h).
  - If no improvement after 2 boluses, consider referral to ICU.
- *Haemorrhagic shock:* Stop bleeding if possible. See table 19.2 for grading.
  - If still shocked despite 2L crystalloid or present with class III/IV shock then crossmatch blood (request O Rh-ve in an emergency, see p348).
  - Give FFP with red cells (1:1 ratio); aim for platelets >100 and fibrinogen >1 (guided by results, but eg 1 pool of platelets and 2 pools of cryoprecipitate per 6–8 units of red cells). Consider tranexamic acid 2g IV. Discuss with haematology early.

- *Heat exposure (heat exhaustion):*
  - Tepid sponging + fanning; avoid ice and immersion. Resuscitate with IVI, eg 0.9% saline ± hydrocortisone 100mg IV. Lorazepam 1–2mg IV or chlorpromazine 25mg IM/IV may be used to stop shivering. Stop cooling when core temperature <39°C.

Table 19.2 Categorizing shock

⚠ Class of shock	1	2	3	4
Blood loss (estimated mL or % of circulating vol)	<750mL or <15%	750-1500mL 15-30%	1500-2000mL 30-40%	>2000mL >40%
Heart rate	<100bpm	>100bpm	120-140bpm	>140bpm
Systolic BP	Normal	Normal	Low	Unrecordable
Pulse pressure	Normal	Narrow	Narrow	V narrow/ absent
Capillary refill	Normal	>2 seconds	>2 seconds	Absent
Respiratory rate	14-20/min	20-30/min	>30/min	>35/min
Urine output	>30mL/h	20-30mL/h	5-20mL/h	Negligible
Cerebral function	Normal/ anxious	Anxious/ hostile	Anxious/ confused	Confused/unre-sponsive

Sepsis

Sepsis is a major killer. There are >150 000 cases of sepsis in the UK each year resulting in >44 000 deaths, and much morbidity.

Sepsis Life-threatening organ dysfunction caused by a dysregulated host response to infection.

Septic shock Sepsis in combination with:
- EITHER lactate >2mmol/L despite adequate fluid resuscitation
- OR the patient is requiring vasopressors to maintain MAP ≥65mmHg.

⚠ Sepsis recognition

Many sepsis-related deaths could be prevented with earlier treatment. Often, the key failure in sepsis management is not recognizing sepsis in time. Early warning scores (p892, fig A1) help identify inpatients who are becoming septic.

Have a low threshold for assessing for sepsis if:
- the patient has communication difficulties: limited English; limited verbal communication; cognitive impairment
- the patient is immunosuppressed, on chemotherapy, or an IV drug user
- the patient recently had surgery or is pregnant/recently gave birth
- the patient has indwelling lines/other foreign material.

⚠ Assessing risk in sepsis

Table 19.3 Risk criteria in sepsis

⚠ Moderate- to high-risk criteria	High-risk criteria
Reports of altered mental state or acute deterioration in functional status	Objective evidence of altered mental state
Respiratory rate (RR) 21-24	RR>24; new requirement for FiO_2 >40% to keep sats >92% (>88% in COPD)
Systolic blood pressure (SBP) 91-100mmHg	SBP <90 or >40mmHg less than baseline
Heart rate 91-130bpm or new arrhythmia	Heart rate >130bpm
Urine output: nil for 12-18h; 0.5-1.0mL/kg/h if catheterized	Urine output: nil for 18h; <0.5mL/kg/h if catheterized
Local signs of infection, incl. redness, swelling, or discharge around wound	Mottled, ashen, or cyanotic skin. Non-blanching rash (p822)
Rigors, or temperature <36°C	
Impaired immunity (illness or drugs)	
Recent surgery/trauma/invasive procedure	

When there is a suspicion of sepsis, the criteria in table 19.3 are used to assess the patient's risk of death or serious illness from sepsis as follows:
High risk: At least one high-risk criterion OR at least two moderate- to high-risk criteria with AKI or LACTATE >2.
Moderate to high risk: At least one moderate- to high-risk criterion.
Low risk: No moderate- or high-risk criteria.

Acute management in sepsis ►Early recognition and treatment is key. See fig 19.3.[2]
Antibiotics: These should be broad spectrum and start within 1h. Consider covering for non-bacterial microbes, eg give aciclovir if HSV encephalitis is suspected.
Fluids: Give within 1h if high risk with SBP <90, AKI, or lactate >2 (consider if <2).
- Give 500mL boluses of crystalloids with 130-154mmol/L sodium (eg 0.9% saline) over 15mins. Caution in heart failure.

- If no improvement after two boluses, speak with a senior.

Oxygen: Give oxygen as required for target saturations. These will be 94-98% (or 88-92% if the patient is at risk of CO_2 retention, eg in severe COPD).
Critical care review: Speak with critical care early if intensive care support (eg inotropes, ventilation, haemofiltration, intensive monitoring) may be required.
Surgical involvement: Eg emergency wound debridement.
Manage acute complications: Shock (p790), AKI (p298), DIC (p352), ARDS (p186), arrhythmias (may spontaneously resolve when sepsis improves).

⚠ Acute management of sepsis in adults

Recognize the need to assess for sepsis

- Consider possibility of sepsis in any patient with signs or symptoms that are suggestive of infection (eg productive cough or offensive oozing wound)
- Consider non-specific signs (patient/carer concern; altered mental state; feeling generally unwell), particularly when there is reason to have low threshold for sepsis assessment (see BOX)

↓

Gather information

History: Full medical history: take time to clarify the time course of symptoms and any travel history

Examination:

- General: capillary refill time, mottled/ashen skin, conscious level
- Localize source of infection: don't forget to assess wounds/ulcers which may be hidden by dressings

Bedside tests: Blood gas for lactate, observations incl. HR, BP, RR, sats, temperature; ECG; urine dip and urine output monitoring

↓

Assess risk (see BOX)

High risk	**Moderate to high risk**	**Low risk**
Request immediate senior review	Clinician review within 1h. Senior review within 3h if cause not identified	Manage according to clinical judgement

↓

Investigations

Blood tests: Serial ABGs, or VBGs for lactate; blood cultures; U&E, CRP, FBC, LFT, clotting screen

Micro samples: Sputum and urine for MC&S; swab any wounds; consider LP; send fluid from drains and lines; joint aspirates; ascitic tap

Imaging: CXR, consider CT/USS/MRI/echo of suspected source

↓

Treatment

Antibiotics ± other antimicrobials

Fluids

Oxygen

Liaise with other teams

- Critical care, surgeons, medical specialties

Manage acute complications

↓

Review

Immediately alert a consultant if, after 1h of antibiotics and fluids:

- SBP <90 • RR >30 • Reduced GCS
- Raised lactate not reduced by >20%

►►Consider critical care referral.

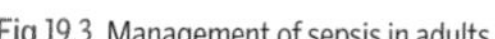

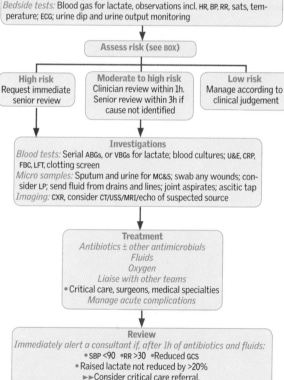

Fig 19.3 Management of sepsis in adults.

►►Anaphylactic shock

Type I IgE-mediated hypersensitivity reaction. Release of histamine and other agents causes: capillary leak; wheeze; cyanosis; oedema (larynx, lids, tongue, lips); urticaria. More common in atopic individuals. An *anaphylactoid reaction* results from direct release of mediators from inflammatory cells, without involving antibodies, usually in response to a drug, eg acetylcysteine.

Examples of precipitants

- Drugs, eg penicillin, and contrast media in radiology.
- Latex.
- Stings, eggs, fish, peanuts, strawberries, semen (rare).

Signs and symptoms

- Itching, sweating, diarrhoea and vomiting, erythema, urticaria, oedema.
- Wheeze, laryngeal obstruction, cyanosis.
- Tachycardia, hypotension.

Mimics of anaphylaxis

- Carcinoid (p271).
- Phaeochromocytoma (p228, p837).
- Systemic mastocytosis.
- Hereditary angioedema.

Management ►See fig 19.4.

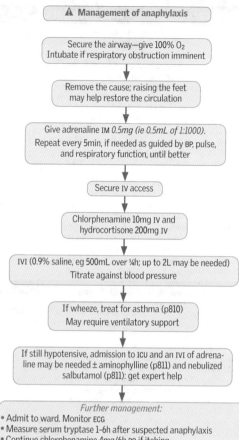

⚠ Management of anaphylaxis

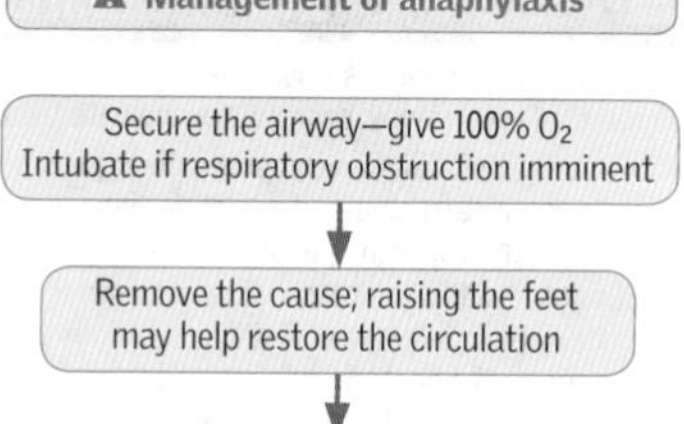

Secure the airway—give 100% O_2
Intubate if respiratory obstruction imminent

↓

Remove the cause; raising the feet may help restore the circulation

↓

Give adrenaline IM *0.5mg (ie 0.5mL of 1:1000)*.
Repeat every 5min, if needed as guided by BP, pulse, and respiratory function, until better

↓

Secure IV access

↓

Chlorphenamine 10mg IV and hydrocortisone 200mg IV

↓

IVI (0.9% saline, eg 500mL over ¼h; up to 2L may be needed)
Titrate against blood pressure

↓

If wheeze, treat for asthma (p810)
May require ventilatory support

↓

If still hypotensive, admission to ICU and an IVI of adrenaline may be needed ± aminophylline (p811) and nebulized salbutamol (p811): get expert help

↓

Further management:
- Admit to ward. Monitor ECG
- Measure serum tryptase 1-6h after suspected anaphylaxis
- Continue chlorphenamine 4mg/6h PO if itching
- Suggest a 'MedicAlert' bracelet naming the culprit allergen
- Teach about self-injected adrenaline (eg 0.3mg, Epipen®) to prevent a fatal attack
- Skin-prick tests showing specific IgE help identify allergens to avoid

ig 19.4 Management of anaphylaxis.

►Adrenaline (=epinephrine) is given IM and NOT IV unless the patient is severely ill, r has no pulse. The IV dose is *different*: 100mcg/min—titrating with the response. his is 0.5mL of *1:10 000 solution* IV per minute. Stop as soon as a response has been btained.

f on a β-blocker, consider salbutamol IV in place of adrenaline.

Acute coronary syndrome—with ST-elevation

Acute coronary syndrome (ACS) includes unstable angina, STEMI, and NSTEMI (p798). STEMI is a common medical emergency; prompt appropriate treatment saves lives.[3]

Initial treatment ►See fig 19.5. Take brief history, do a quick physical examination and a 12-lead ECG. Observe on cardiac monitor or telemetry in case of dysrhythmia. Other tests on admission: U&E, troponin, glucose, cholesterol, FBC, CXR.

- *Aspirin:* 300mg PO (if not already given); consider ticagrelor (180mg PO) or prasugrel (60mg PO if no history of stroke/TIA and <75yrs) as newer alternatives to clopidogrel (300mg PO) as they have been shown to be superior in outcome studies.
- *Morphine:* 5–10mg IV (repeat after 5min if necessary). Give anti-emetic with the 1st dose of morphine: metoclopramide 10mg IV (1st line), or cyclizine 50mg IV (2nd line).
- *GTN:* routine use now not recommended in the acute setting unless patient is hypertensive or in acute LVF. Useful as anti-anginal in chronic/stable patients.
- *Oxygen* is recommended if patients have SaO_2 <95%, are breathless or in acute LVF.
- *Restore coronary perfusion* in those presenting <12h after symptom onset (see BOX).
- *Anticoagulation:* An injectable anticoagulant must be used in primary PCI. Bivalirudin is preferred, if not available use enoxaparin ± a GP IIb/IIIa blocker.
- *β-blockers* provide additional benefit when started early, eg bisoprolol 2.5mg PO OD. Ensure no evidence of cardiogenic shock, heart failure, asthma/COPD, or heart block.

Right ventricular infarction Confirm by demonstrating ST elevation in $rV_{3/4}$ and/or echo. NB: rV_4 means that V_4 is placed in the right 5th intercostal space in the midclavicular line. Treat hypotension and oliguria with fluids (avoid nitrates and diuretics). Monitor BP carefully, and assess early signs of pulmonary oedema. Intensive monitoring and inotropes may be useful in some patients.

⚠ Reperfusion therapy

Early coronary reperfusion saves lives; decisions must be taken quickly so seek senior advice early. Look for typical clinical symptoms of MI plus ECG criteria:

- ST elevation >1mm in ≥2 adjacent limb leads or >2mm in ≥2 adjacent chest leads.
- LBBB (unless known to have LBBB previously).
- Posterior changes: deep ST depression and tall R waves in leads V_1 to V_3.

Therapy may be percutaneous intervention (PCI—with angiographic identification of the culprit blockage(s) and revascularization via deployment of an expandable metal stent) or thrombolysis (with systemically administered clot-dissolving enzymes):

- *Primary PCI:* ►►Should be offered to all patients presenting within 12h of symptom onset with a STEMI who either are at or can be transferred to a primary PCI centre within 120min of first medical contact. If this is not possible, patients should receive thrombolysis and be transferred to a primary PCI centre after the infusion for either rescue PCI (if residual ST elevation) or angiography (if successful). Use beyond 12h if evidence of ongoing ischaemia or in stable patients presenting after 12–24h may be appropriate—seek specialist advice.
- *Thrombolysis:* ►►Benefit reduces steadily from onset of pain, target time is <30min from admission; use >12h from symptom onset requires specialist advice. ►Do not thrombolyse ST depression alone, T-wave inversion alone, or normal ECG. Thrombolysis is best achieved with tissue plasminogen activators (eg tenecteplase as a single IV bolus). *CI:* •Previous intracranial haemorrhage. •Ischaemic stroke <6months. •Cerebral malignancy or AVM. •Recent major trauma/surgery/head injury (<3wks). •GI bleeding (<1 month). •Known bleeding disorder. •Aortic dissection. •Non-compressible punctures <24h, eg liver biopsy, lumbar puncture. *Relative CI:* •TIA <6 months. •Anticoagulant therapy. •Pregnancy/<1wk post partum. •Refractory hypertension (>180mmHg/110mmHg). •Advanced liver disease. •Infective endocarditis. •Active peptic ulcer. •Prolonged/traumatic resuscitation

►Patients with STEMI who do not receive reperfusion (eg presenting >12h after symptom onset) should be treated with fondaparinux, or enoxaparin/unfractionated heparin if not available.

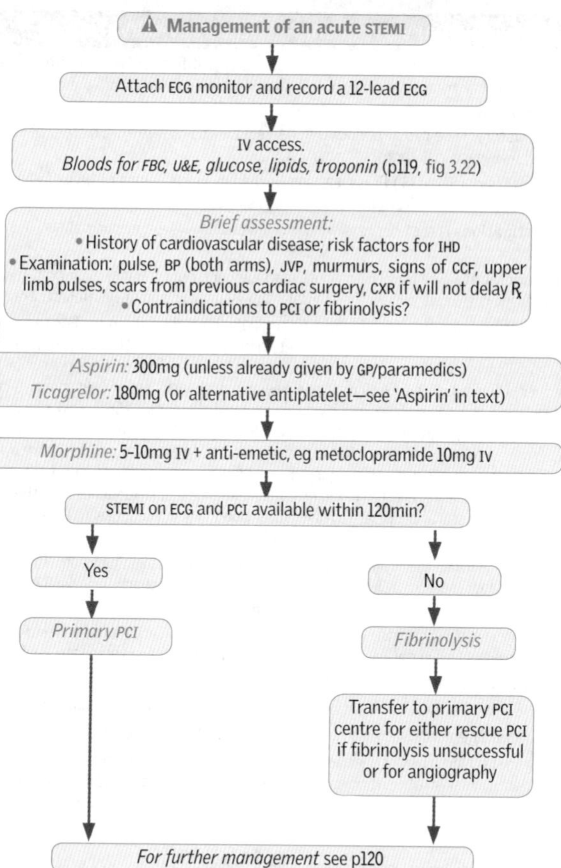

⚠ Management of an acute STEMI
Attach ECG monitor and record a 12-lead ECG
IV access.
Bloods for FBC, U&E, glucose, lipids, troponin (p119, fig 3.22)
Brief assessment:
• History of cardiovascular disease; risk factors for IHD
• Examination: pulse, BP (both arms), JVP, murmurs, signs of CCF, upper limb pulses, scars from previous cardiac surgery, CXR if will not delay Rx
• Contraindications to PCI or fibrinolysis?
Aspirin: 300mg (unless already given by GP/paramedics)
Ticagrelor: 180mg (or alternative antiplatelet—see 'Aspirin' in text)
Morphine: 5–10mg IV + anti-emetic, eg metoclopramide 10mg IV
STEMI on ECG and PCI available within 120min?
Yes
Primary PCI
No
Fibrinolysis
Transfer to primary PCI centre for either rescue PCI if fibrinolysis unsuccessful or for angiography
For further management see p120

Fig 19.5 Management of an acute STEMI.

Acute coronary syndrome—without ST-elevation

First stabilize with medical therapy; early risk stratification will identify those in need of further treatment and prompt angiography (involve cardiologists).[4]

Assessment

Brief history: (See p36.) Previous angina, relief with rest/nitrates, history of cardiovascular disease, risk factors for IHD.

Examination: (See p38.) Pulse, BP, JVP, cardiac murmurs, signs of heart failure, peripheral pulses, scars from previous cardiac surgery.

Investigations ECG: ST depression; flat or inverted T-waves; or normal; FBC, U&E, troponin, glucose, random cholesterol; CXR.

Management ►See fig 19.6 for acute management, but p796 if ST elevation. The aim of therapy is to control pain then initiate anti-ischaemic and antiplatelet therapy.

Oral antiplatelet therapy: Aspirin 300mg PO, followed by 75mg OD. For those with confirmed ACS give a second antiplatelet agent, eg clopidogrel (300mg PO then 75mg OD PO). Ticagrelor (180mg then 90mg/12h PO) is a prefered alternative, particularly in higher risk groups[5] (eg • ≥60yrs age •previous stroke, TIA, MI, or CABG •known coronary artery stenosis ≥50% in ≥2 vessels or carotid stenosis ≥50% •DM •peripheral arterial disease •chronic kidney disease). Prasugrel (60mg then 10mg/d PO) is an alternative to clopidogrel for those undergoing PCI. In practice, if the history is typical but ECG changes are non-diagnostic and troponin results are awaited, treatment with eg clopridogrel is often given on clinical suspicion; if troponin testing then confirms ACS, it is still appropriate to give either ticagrelor or prasugrel to those patients in whom it is indicated, even if clopidogrel has already been given.

Anticoagulation: Ideally fondaparinux (factor Xa inhibitor) 2.5mg OD; if not available, use low-molecular-weight heparin (LMWH, eg enoxaparin 1mg/kg/12h) or unfractionated heparin (aim APTT 50–70s) until discharge.

β-blockers: In higher-risk patients with no contraindications (consider diltiazem as alternative). ►Do not use β-blockers with verapamil—can precipitate asystole.

Nitrates (PO or IV): For recurrent chest pain.

ACE-i: Should be given to all patients unless there are CI (monitor renal function).

Lipid management: Start early, eg atorvastatin 80mg OD (see p120).

Prognosis Overall risk of death ~1–2%, but ~15% for refractory angina despite medical therapy. Risk stratification can help predict those most at risk and allow intervention to be targeted at those individuals: calculate using GRACE score.[2] The following are associated with an increased risk:

- History of unstable angina.
- ST depression or widespread T-wave inversion.
- Raised troponin (except patients with ST elevation MI).
- Age >70 years.
- General comorbidity, previous MI, poor LV function or DM.

►High-risk patients should be considered for inpatient coronary angiography. Symptomatic lesions may be addressed by coronary stenting or CABG (see p123).

Further measures

- Wean off *glyceryl trinitrate* (GTN) infusion when stabilized on oral drugs.
- Continue fondaparinux (or LMWH or heparin) until discharge.
- Observe on cardiac monitor or telemetry in case of dysrhythmia. Check serial ECGs and troponin >12h after pain.
- Address modifiable risk factors: smoking, hypertension, hyperlipidaemia, diabetes
- Gentle mobilization.
- Ensure patient on dual antiplatelet therapy, β-blocker, ACE inhibitor, and statin.

►*If symptoms recur, refer to cardiologist for urgent angiography & PCI or CABG.*

2 GRACE = Global Registry of Acute Coronary Events. Risk is scored based on age, heart rate, BP, renal function, Killip class of heart failure, and other events, eg raised troponin. Very complicated to calculate so recommendation by European Society of Cardiology is to use an online calculator eg http://www.outcomes-umassmed.org/grace/.

⚠ Acute management of cardiac chest pain

Monitor closely; record ECG while in pain

↓

If SaO_2 <90% or breathless, low-flow O_2

↓

Analgesia: Eg morphine 5–10mg IV + metoclopramide 10mg IV

↓

Nitrates: GTN spray or sublingual tablets as required

↓

Aspirin: 300mg PO.
Consider need for second antiplatelet agent (see 'Oral antiplatelet therapy' in text)

↓

Measure troponin and clinical parameters to risk assess, eg GRACE score[2]

↓

Invasive strategy (high-risk pt):
- *Rise in troponin OR:*
- *Dynamic ST or T-wave changes*
- *Secondary criteria—diabetes, CKD, LVEF <40%, early angina post MI, recent PCI, prior CABG, intermediate to high-risk GRACE score*

Conservative strategy (low-risk pt):
- *No recurrence of chest pain*
- *No signs of heart failure*
- *Normal ECG*
- *—ve baseline (± repeat) troponin*

May be discharged (check troponin interval required with your laboratory and retest after delay if necessary). Arrange further outpatient investigation, eg stress test.

↓ (from invasive strategy)

Fondaparinux: 2.5mg OD SC or LMWH 1mg/kg/12h SC

↓

Second antiplatelet agent (see text), eg *ticagrelor* 180mg PO (or *clopidogrel* 300mg PO in lower risk, or *prasugrel* 60mg OD if proceeding to PCI)

↓

IV *nitrate* if pain continues
(eg GTN 50mg in 50mL 0.9% saline at 2–10mL/h)
titrate to pain, and maintain systolic BP >100mmHg

↓

Oral *β-blocker*, eg bisoprolol 2.5mg OD
CI: cardiogenic shock, heart failure, asthma/COPD or heart block; consider rate-limiting calcium antagonist (eg verapamil 80–120mg/8h PO, or diltiazem 60–120mg/8h PO)

↓

Prompt cardiologist review for angiography
1. Urgent (<120min after presentation) if ongoing angina and evolving ST changes, signs of cardiogenic shock or life-threatening arrhythmias
2. Early (<24h) if GRACE score >140 and high-risk patient
3. Within 72h if lower-risk patient

Fig 19.6 Acute management of chest pain and ACS without ST-segment elevation.

►►Severe pulmonary oedema

Causes

- Cardiovascular, usually left ventricular failure (post-MI or ischaemic heart disease). Also valvular heart disease, arrhythmias, and malignant hypertension.
- ARDS (p186) from any cause, eg trauma, malaria, drugs. Look for predisposing factors, eg trauma, post-op, sepsis. *Is aspirin overdose or glue-sniffing/drug abuse likely*? Ask friends/relatives.
- Fluid overload.
- Neurogenic, eg head injury.

Differential diagnosis Asthma/COPD, pneumonia, and pulmonary oedema are often hard to distinguish, especially in the elderly, where they may coexist. If the patient is extremely unwell and you are not sure, consider treating all three (eg with salbutamol nebulizer, furosemide IV, diamorphine, amoxicillin—p386).

Symptoms Dyspnoea, orthopnoea (eg paroxysmal), pink frothy sputum. NB: note drugs recently given and other illnesses (recent MI/COPD or pneumonia).

Signs Distressed, pale, sweaty, ↑pulse, tachypnoea, pink frothy sputum, pulsus alternans, ↑JVP, fine lung crackles, triple/gallop rhythm (p44), wheeze (cardiac asthma). Usually sitting up and leaning forward. Quickly examine for possible causes.

Investigations

- CXR (p135, pp722–4): cardiomegaly, signs of pulmonary oedema: look for shadowing (usually bilateral), small effusions at costophrenic angles, fluid in the lung fissures, and Kerley B lines (septal linear opacities).
- ECG: signs of MI, dysrhythmias.
- U&E, troponin, ABG.
- Consider echo.
- BNP (p137) may be helpful if diagnosis in question (high negative predictive value).

Management ►See fig 19.7. ►►Begin treatment before investigations.

Monitoring progress: BP; pulse; cyanosis; respiratory rate; JVP; urine output; ABG. Observe on cardiac monitor or telemetry in case of dysrhythmia.

Once stable and improving:

- Daily weights, aim reduction of 0.5kg/day, check obs at least QDS.
- Repeat CXR.
- Change to oral furosemide or bumetanide.
- If on large doses of loop diuretic, consider the addition of a thiazide (eg bendroflumethiazide or metolazone 2.5-5mg daily PO).
- ACE-i if LVEF <40%. If ACE-i contraindicated, consider hydralazine and nitrate (may also be more effective in African-Caribbeans).
- Also consider β-blocker and spironolactone (if LVEF <35%).
- Is the patient suitable for biventricular pacing or cardiac transplantation?
- Optimize management of AF if present (p130); consider anticoagulation.

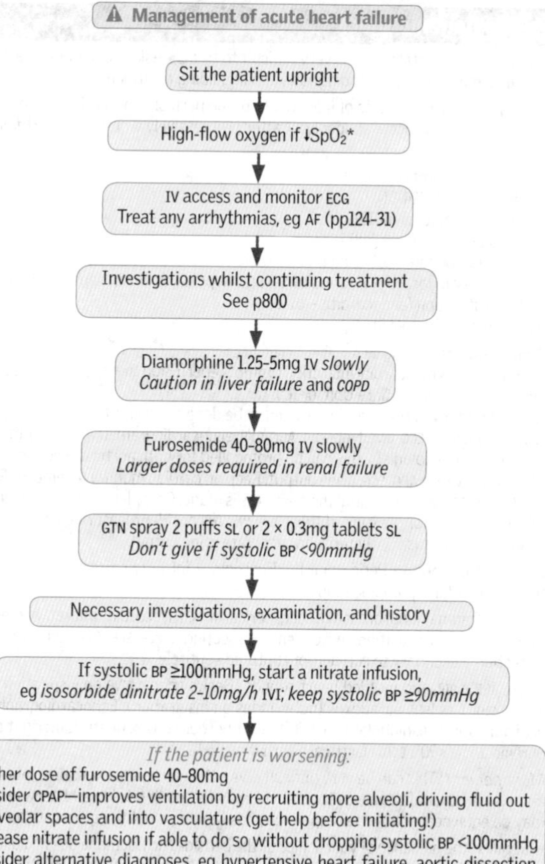

⚠ Management of acute heart failure
Sit the patient upright
High-flow oxygen if ↓SpO_2*
IV access and monitor ECG
Treat any arrhythmias, eg AF (pp124–31)
Investigations whilst continuing treatment
See p800
Diamorphine 1.25–5mg IV *slowly*
Caution in liver failure and COPD
Furosemide 40–80mg IV slowly
Larger doses required in renal failure
GTN spray 2 puffs SL or 2 × 0.3mg tablets SL
Don't give if systolic BP *<90mmHg*
Necessary investigations, examination, and history
If systolic BP ≥100mmHg, start a nitrate infusion,
eg *isosorbide dinitrate 2–10mg/h* IVI; *keep systolic* BP *≥90mmHg*
If the patient is worsening:
• Further dose of furosemide 40–80mg
• Consider CPAP—improves ventilation by recruiting more alveoli, driving fluid out of alveolar spaces and into vasculature (get help before initiating!)
• Increase nitrate infusion if able to do so without dropping systolic BP <100mmHg
• Consider alternative diagnoses, eg hypertensive heart failure, aortic dissection, pulmonary embolism, pneumonia
If systolic BP <100mmHg, treat as cardiogenic shock (p802) and refer to ICU

*Avoid supplemental oxygen if not hypoxaemic since may cause vasoconstriction and reduce cardiac output. If known COPD, hypoxaemia still needs correcting; give high-flow oxygen but monitor closely for CO_2 retention (check serial ABG if needed) and reduce flow as soon as possible.

Fig 19.7 Management of heart failure.

►►Cardiogenic shock

This has a high mortality and is very difficult to treat. ►Ask a senior physician's help both in formulating an *exact* diagnosis and in guiding treatment.

Cardiogenic shock is a state of inadequate tissue perfusion primarily due to cardiac dysfunction. It may occur suddenly, or after progressively worsening heart failure.

Causes

- Myocardial infarction (pp796–9).
- Arrhythmias (pp124–31).
- Pulmonary embolus (p818).
- Tension pneumothorax (p814).
- Cardiac tamponade (p154 and later in topic).
- Myocarditis; myocardial depression (drugs, hypoxia, acidosis, sepsis) (p152).
- Valve destruction (endocarditis—p150).
- Aortic dissection (p655).

Management ►See fig 19.8.

►►If the cause is myocardial infarction prompt reperfusion therapy is vital (see p796).

- Manage in Coronary Care Unit, or ICU.
- Investigation and treatment may need to be done concurrently.
- *Investigations:* ECG, U&E, troponin, ABG, CXR, echocardiogram. If indicated, CT thorax (speak with radiologists, this can be protocolled for both aortic dissection and PE).
- *Monitor:* CVP, BP, ABG, ECG, urine output. Keep on cardiac monitor/telemetry. Record a 12-lead ECG every hour until the diagnosis is made. Consider a CVP line and an arterial line to monitor pressure, if these are *in situ* consider measuring cardiac output and volume status.[3] Catheterize for accurate urine output.

Cardiac tamponade Pericardial fluid collects → intrapericardial pressure rises → heart cannot fill → pumping stops.

Causes: Trauma, lung/breast cancer, pericarditis, myocardial infarct, bacteria, eg TB. *Rarely:* ↑urea, radiation, myxoedema, dissecting aorta, SLE. Also coronary artery dissection (secondary to PCI) and/or ruptured ventricle.

Signs: ↓BP, ↑JVP, and muffled heart sounds (Beck's triad); ↑JVP on inspiration (Kussmaul's sign); pulsus paradoxus (pulse fades on inspiration). Echocardiography may be diagnostic. CXR: globular heart; left heart border convex or straight; right cardiophrenic angle <90°. ECG: electrical alternans (p154).

Management: This can be very difficult. Everything is against you: time, physiology, and your own confidence, as the patient may be too ill to give a history, and signs may be equivocal—but bitter experience has taught us not to equivocate for long.

►►Request the presence of your senior at the bedside (do not make do with telephone advice). With luck, prompt pericardiocentesis (p773) brings swift relief. While awaiting this, give O_2, monitor ECG, and set up IVI. Take blood for group & save. NB: there may be a role for cardiothoracic surgery (eg CABG, ventricular repair, or pericardial window) as a definitive solution to some causes.

3 Eg Pulse contour cardiac output (PICCO) or lithium dilution cardiac output (LIDCO). Both use injection (PICCO = cold water, LIDCO = lithium) to estimate filling pressure, extravascular water (ie pulmonary oedema) and cardiac output. The time from injection via a central vein to detection via an arterial line, plus dilution gives estimates of cardiac output and volume status and can guide fluid and inotrope therapy.

⚠ Management of cardiogenic shock

Oxygen
Titrate to maintain arterial saturations of 94–98% (88–92% if COPD)

↓

Diamorphine 1.25–5mg IV for pain and anxiety

↓

Investigations and *close monitoring* (see p802)

↓

Correct arrhythmias (pp124–31), U&E abnormalities, or acid-base disturbance

↓

Optimize filling pressure with clinical assessment of pulse, BP, JVP/CVP (if in ICU consider using PICCO, LIDCO, transoesophageal doppler or Swan-Gantz catheter to estimate cardiac output and fluid balance)

↓

Underfilled?
Give a plasma expander 100mL every 15min IV
Aim MAP 70mmHg, CVP 8–10mmHg

Well/over-filled?
Inotropic support, eg dobutamine 2.5–10mcg/kg/min IVI. Aim MAP 70mmHg

↓

Look for and treat any reversible cause:
MI or PE—consider thrombolysis;
surgery for: acute VSD, mitral, or aortic incompetence

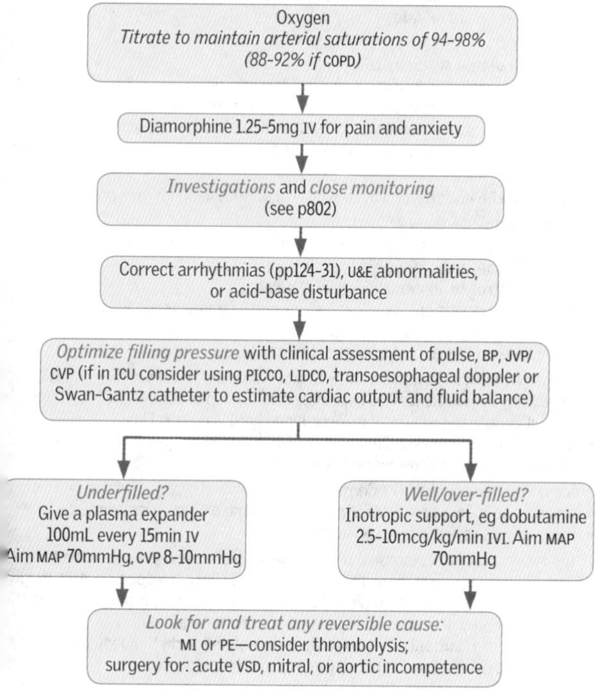

Fig 19.8 Management of cardiogenic shock. MAP = mean arterial pressure.

▶▶Broad complex tachycardia

ECG shows rate of >100bpm and QRS complexes >120ms (>3 small squares on ECGs done at the standard UK rate of 25mm/s). Identify the underlying rhythm and treat accordingly.[6]

Differential diagnosis (See p128.)
- *Ventricular tachycardia (VT) including torsade de pointes.* Single ventricular ectopics should not cause confusion; if >3 together at a rate >100, this is VT.
- SVT (p806) with aberrant conduction, eg AF or atrial flutter, with bundle branch block.
- Pre-excited tachycardias, eg AF, atrial flutter, or AV re-entry tachycardia, with underlying WPW (p133).

Identifying the underlying rhythm (See p128.) ▶▶If in doubt, treat as VT.

Management ▶See fig 19.9.[6]
- Connect patient to a cardiac monitor and have a defibrillator to hand.
- Monitor O_2 sats and if <90% give supplemental oxygen.
- Correct electrolyte abnormalities, esp K^+ and Mg^{2+}.
- Check for adverse signs. Low cardiac output (clammy, ↓consciousness, BP <90); oliguria; angina; pulmonary oedema.
- Obtain 12-lead ECG (request CXR) and obtain IV access.

If haemodynamically unstable VT: ▶▶Synchronized DC shock (see p894, fig A3).
- Correct any hypokalaemia and hypomagnesaemia: up to 60mmol KCl at 30mmol/h and 4mL 50% magnesium sulfate over 30min both via central line.
- Follow with amiodarone 300mg IV over 10–20min (peripherally only in emergency).
- For refractory cases consider procainamide or sotalol.

If haemodynamically stable VT: Correct hypokalaemia and hypomagnesaemia: as above
- Amiodarone 300mg IV over 20–60min (avoid if long QT) via central line.
- If this fails, use synchronized DC shock.

After correction of VT: Establish the cause (via the history and tests described above).
- Maintenance anti-arrhythmic therapy may be required. If VT occurs after MI, give IV amiodarone infusion for 12–24h; if 24h after MI, also start oral anti-arrhythmic sotalol (if good LV function) or amiodarone (if poor LV function).
- Prevention of recurrent VT: surgical isolation of the arrhythmogenic area or an implantable cardioverter defibrillator (ICD) may help.

Ventricular fibrillation: (ECG p129, fig 3.29) Use non-synchronized DC shock (there is no R wave to trigger defibrillation, p770): see p894, fig A3.

If SVT with aberrant conduction: Manage as SVT with eg adenosine (see p806).

Ventricular extrasystoles (ectopics): These are the commonest post-MI arrhythmia but they are also seen in healthy people (often >10/h). Patients with frequent ectopics post-MI have a worse prognosis, but there is no evidence that antidysrhythmic drugs improve outcome, indeed they may increase mortality.

Torsade de pointes: A form of VT, with a constantly varying axis, often in the setting of long QT syndromes (ECG p129, fig 3.31). Causes (p711): congenital or from drugs (eg some antidysrhythmics, tricyclics, antimalarials, antipsychotics). Torsade in the setting of congenital long-QT syndromes can be treated with high doses of β-blockers.

In acquired long-QT syndromes (p711), stop all predisposing drugs, correct hypokalaemia, and give magnesium sulfate (2g IV over 10min). Alternatives include: overdrive pacing (pace at a faster rate, then slow reduce) or isoprenaline IVI to increase heart rate.

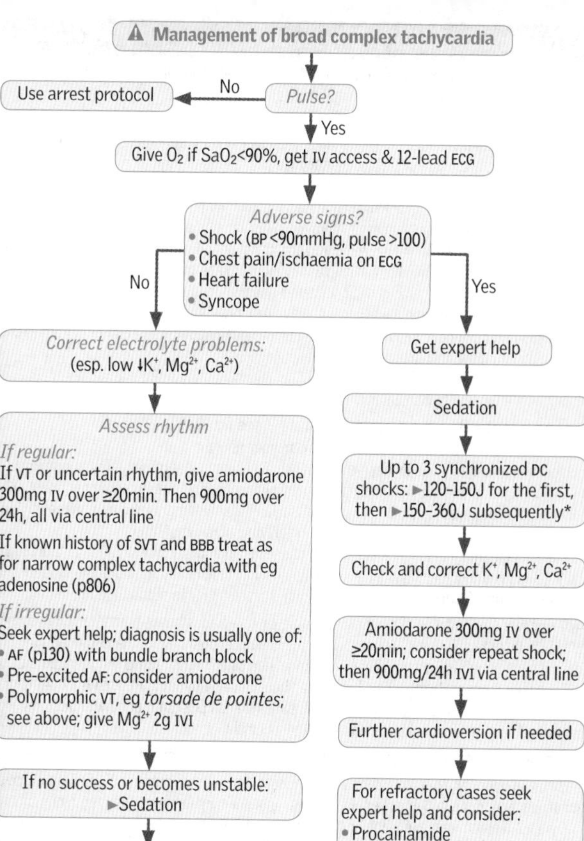

*Check your defibrillator: energies given are for a typical biphasic defibrillator (preferred); if a monophasic shock used, higher energies will be required.

Fig 19.9 Management of broad complex tachycardia.

►►Narrow complex tachycardia

ECG shows rate of >100bpm and QRS complex duration of <120ms (<3 small squares on ECGs done at the standard UK rate of 25mm/s).

Differential diagnosis (See p126.)

- *Sinus tachycardia:* Normal P wave followed by normal QRS—not an arrhythmia! Do not attempt to cardiovert; if necessary (ie not a physiological response to fever/hypovolaemia) rate control with β-blockers.
- *Atrial tachyarrhythmias:* Rhythm arises in atria, AV node is a bystander.
  - Atrial fibrillation (AF): absent P wave, irregular QRS complexes.
  - Atrial flutter: atrial rate ~260–340bpm. Sawtooth baseline, due to a re-entrant circuit usually in the right atrium. Ventricular rate often 150bpm (2:1 block).
  - Atrial tachycardia: abnormally shaped P waves, may outnumber QRS.
  - Multifocal atrial tachycardia: ≥3 P-wave morphologies, irregular QRS complexes.
- *Junctional tachycardia:* AV node is part of the pathway. P wave either buried in QRS complex or occurring after QRS complex.
  - AV nodal re-entry tachycardia.
  - AV re-entry tachycardia, includes an accessory pathway, eg WPW (p133).

Management ►Be guided by patient status,[6] see fig 19.10.[6]

►►If the patient is compromised, use DC cardioversion.

- Otherwise, identify the underlying rhythm and treat accordingly. The most important thing is to decide whether the rhythm is regular or not (irregular is likely AF).
- Vagal manoeuvres (carotid sinus massage, Valsalva manoeuvre) transiently increase AV block, and may unmask an underlying atrial rhythm.
- If unsuccessful, give adenosine, which causes transient AV block. It has a short half-life (10–15s) and works by: **1** transiently slowing ventricles to show the underlying atrial rhythm; **2** cardioverting a junctional tachycardia to sinus rhythm.

Adenosine: Consult *BNF* if on dipyridamole or has had a heart transplant. Give 6mg IV bolus into a large vein, followed by 0.9% saline flush, while recording a rhythm strip. If unsuccessful, after 2min give 12mg, then one further 12mg bolus. Warn about SE: transient chest tightness, dyspnoea, headache, flushing. *Relative CI:* Asthma 2nd/3rd-degree AV block or sinoatrial disease (unless pacemaker). *Interactions:* Potentiated by dipyridamole; antagonized by theophylline.

Specifics *Sinus tachycardia:* Identify and treat underlying cause.

Supraventricular tachycardia: If adenosine fails, use verapamil 2.5–5mg IV over 2min. NB: NOT if on a β-blocker. If no response, a further 5mg IV over 3min (if age <60yrs). Alternatives: atenolol 2.5mg IV repeated at 5min intervals until 10mg given or amiodarone. If unsuccessful, use DC cardioversion.

Atrial fibrillation/flutter: Manage with rate control; seek help if resistant (p130).

Atrial tachycardia: Rare; may be due to digoxin toxicity: withdraw digoxin, consider digoxin-specific antibody fragments. Maintain K^+ at 4–5mmol/L.

Multifocal atrial tachycardia: Most commonly occurs in COPD. Correct hypoxia and hypercapnia. Consider verapamil if rate remains >110bpm.

Junctional tachycardia: Where anterograde conduction through the AV node occurs, vagal manoeuvres are worth trying. Adenosine will usually cardiovert a junctional rhythm to sinus rhythm. If it fails or recurs, β-blockers (or verapamil—*not* with β-blockers, digoxin, or class I agents such as quinidine). If this does not control symptoms, consider radiofrequency ablation.

►Seek specialist advice if resistant junction tachycardia, or accessory pathway.

⚠ **Wolff-Parkinson-White (WPW) syndrome** (*ECG* p133, fig 3.37.) Caused by congenital accessory conduction pathway between atria and ventricles. Resting ECG shows short PR interval and widened QRS complex due to slurred upstroke or 'delta wave'. Two types: WPW type A (+ve δ wave in V_1), WPW type B (–ve δ wave in V_1). Present with SVT which may be due to an AVRT (p126), pre-excited AF, or pre-excited atrial flutter. Risk of degeneration to VF and sudden death. ℞: Flecainide, propafenone, sotalol, or amiodarone. Refer to cardiologist for electrophysiology and ablation of the accessory pathway.

⚠ Management of narrow complex tachycardia (supraventricular tachycardia)

Give O_2 if SaO_2 <90%, get IV access & 12-lead ECG

Adverse signs?
- Shock
- Chest pain/ischaemia on ECG
- Heart failure
- Syncope

No → Is the rhythm regular?

- **Yes →** Start continuous ECG trace. Perform vagal manoeuvres (caution if possible digoxin toxicity, acute ischaemia or carotid bruit)
  - If vagal manoeuvres fail, give adenosine 6mg bolus IV, then 12mg, and further 12mg if necessary (verapamil 2.5–5mg over 2min is an alternative if adenosine contraindicated or does not succeed)
  - Sinus rhythm achieved?
    - **Yes →** *Probable paroxysmal re-entrant SVT* Assess ECG for eg WPW. If recurrent consider referral for electrophysiology/prophylaxis
    - **No →** *Possible atrial flutter* Seek expert help. Control rate with, eg β-blocker
- **No →** *Probable AF* See BOX

Yes → Get expert help
- Sedation
- Up to 3 synchronized DC shocks: ►70–120J for the first (120–150J for AF), then ►120–360J subsequently*
- Check and correct K^+, Mg^{2+}, Ca^{2+}
- Amiodarone 300mg IV over ≥20min; consider repeat shock; then 900mg/24h IVI via central line

*Check your defibrillator: energies given are for a typical biphasic defibrillator (preferred); if a monophasic shock used, higher energies will be required.

Fig 19.10 Management of narrow complex tachycardia (supraventricular tachycardia).

⚠ Irregular narrow complex tachycardia

- Treat as AF—by far the most likely diagnosis.
- Control rate with:
  - β-blocker: eg metoprolol 1–10mg IV, give small increments to slow rate
  - rate-limiting Ca^{2+}-channel blocker eg verapamil 5–10mg IV
  - digoxin is an alternative in heart failure (load with eg 500mcg PO then 500mcg PO after 8h and further 250mcg PO after 8h)
  - amiodarine (may also control rhythm—see last bullet point in this box).
- Consider anticoagulation with warfarin or NOAC to ↓ risk of stroke.
- If onset definitely <48h, or if effectively anticoagulated for >3wk, consider cardioversion with synchronized DC cardioversion under sedation (see p770). Chemical cardioversion may be achieved with flecanide 300mg PO (only if definitely no structural heart damage) or amiodarone, 300mg IVI over 20–60min, then 900mg over 24h.

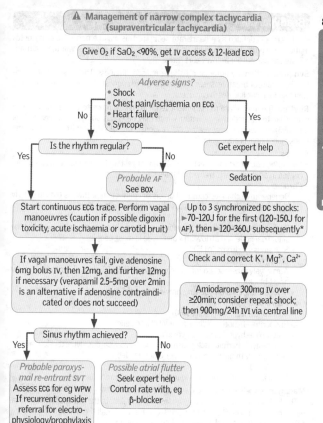

Bradycardia

Bradycardia is defined as a heart rate <60bpm. This may be normal and asymptomatic in very fit, young individuals whose high stroke volumes will maintain adequate cardiac output at low heart rates.

Symptoms Often asymptomatic. Fatigue, nausea, dizziness. The presence of syncope, chest pain, or breathlessness is concerning and suggests the presence of adverse signs; sudden cardiac death can occur.

Rhythm The immediate management tends to relate more to cause and adverse signs than to the underlying rhythm, which may be •sinus bradycardia •heart block (see p98) •AF with a slow ventricular response •atrial flutter with a high-degree block •junctional bradycardia.

Causes

- *Physiological:* Heart rates as low as 40bpm at rest and 30bpm in sleep can be accepted in asymptomatic trained athletes.
- *Cardiac:*
  - Degenerative changes causing fibrosis of conduction pathways (risk in elderly patients; may have previous ECGs showing bundle branch block or 1st- or 2nd-degree heart block).
  - Post-MI—particularly after an inferior MI (the right coronary artery supplies the sinoatrial node and atrioventricular node in most people).
  - Sick sinus syndrome (p125).
  - Iatrogenic—ablation, surgery.
  - Aortic valve disease, eg infective endocarditis (p150; do daily ECGs looking for heart block).
  - Myocarditis, cardiomyopathy, amyloid, sarcoid, SLE.
- *Non-cardiac origin:*
  - Vasovagal—very common (p460).
  - Endocrine—hypothyroidism, adrenal insufficiency.
  - Metabolic—hyperkalaemia, hypoxia.
  - Other—hypothermia, ↑ICP (Cushing's triad: bradycardia, hypertension, and irregular breathing: ►► urgent senior input needed).
- *Drug-induced:*
  - β-blockers, amiodarone, verapamil, diltiazem, digoxin.

Management ►Follow a logical approach,[6] see fig 19.11.[6]

►►Think ahead. If you may need an anaesthetist to sedate the patient for transcutaneous pacing, or a cardiologist for transvenous pacing, call them now.

- Perform a 12-lead ECG, check electrolytes (including K^+, Ca^{2+}, Mg^{2+}), do digoxin levels.
- Connect patient to cardiac monitor/telemetry.
- Address the cause: correct metabolic defects; if the patient has adverse signs or is deteriorating, give antidotes to medicines likely to have caused the bradycardia (eg glucagon if β-blocker overdose).
- If the patient has adverse signs or risk of asystole, give atropine (not to be given if patient has a transplanted heart).
- If atropine is insufficient and adverse signs persist, transcutaneous pacing should be considered (p777). If this cannot be initiated immediately (eg waiting for an anaesthetist), consider other medications such as isoprenaline infusion.
- Remember electrical 'capture' with transcutaneous pacing does not guarantee mechanical 'capture'. Once pacing is established, check the patient's pulse.

►It is possible to have two patients sat next to each other with identical bradycardic ECG tracings, one of whom is peri-arrest, the other is sat comfortably and cannot understand your concern. The clinical state is more important than the numbers on the screen.

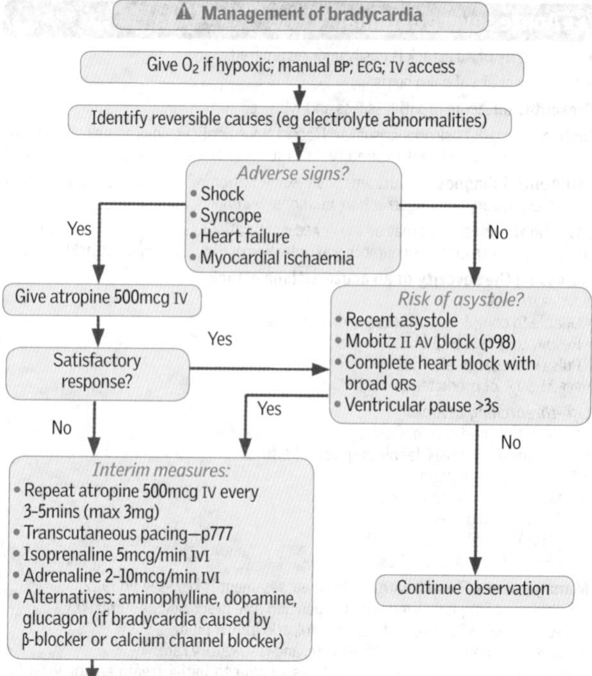

Fig 19.11 Management of bradycardia.

►►Acute severe asthma

►The severity of an attack is easily underestimated.

►An atmosphere of calm helps.

Presentation Acute breathlessness and wheeze.

History (See p48.) Ask about usual and recent treatment; previous acute episodes and their severity and best peak expiratory flow rate (PEF). Have they been admitted to ICU?

Differential diagnosis Acute infective exacerbation of COPD, pulmonary oedema, upper respiratory tract obstruction, pulmonary embolus, anaphylaxis.

Investigations PEF—but may be too ill; ABG if saturations <92% or life-threatening features; CXR (if suspicion of pneumothorax, infection or life-threatening attack); FBC; U&E.

Assessing the severity of an acute asthma attack

Severe attack:

- Unable to complete sentences in one breath.
- Respiratory rate ≥25/min.
- Pulse rate ≥110 beats/min.
- PEF 33–50% of predicted or best.

Life-threatening attack:

- PEF <33% of predicted or best.
- Silent chest, cyanosis, feeble respiratory effort.
- Arrhythmia or hypotension.
- Exhaustion, confusion, or coma.
- Arterial blood gases:
  - Normal/high P_aCO_2 >4.6kPa.
  - P_aO_2 <8kPa, or S_aO_2 <92%.

Management ►Rapid treatment and reassessment is key,[7] see fig 19.12.

- Salbutamol 5mg nebulized with oxygen and give prednisolone 30mg PO.
- If PEF remains <75%, repeat salbutamol; add ipratropium.
- Monitor oxygen saturation, heart rate, and respiratory rate.
- Admit all with severe features not responding to initial treatment or with life-threatening features.

NB: the routine use of antibiotics is not recommended in exacerbations of asthma.

Discharge Patients with PEF >75% within 1h of initial treatment can be discharged if no other reason to admit. Otherwise, before discharge patients must have:

- been stable on discharge medication for 24h
- had inhaler technique checked
- peak flow rate >75% predicted or best with diurnal variability <25%
- steroid (inhaled *and* oral) and bronchodilator therapy
- their own PEF meter and have written management plan
- GP appointment within 2d
- respiratory clinic appointment within 4wks.

Drugs used in acute asthma

Salbutamol (β_2-agonist). SE: tachycardia, arrhythmias, tremor, ↓K^+.

Hydrocortisone and *prednisolone* (steroid; reduces inflammation).

Aminophylline is used much less frequently and is not routinely recommended in current *BTS* guidelines, but may be initiated by respiratory team or ICU. It inhibits phosphodiesterase; ↑[cAMP]. *SE:* ↑pulse, arrhythmias, nausea, seizures. The amount of IVI aminophylline may need altering according to the individual patient: always check the *BNF*. Monitor ECG. ►Aim for plasma concentration of 10–20mcg/mL (55–110μmol/L). Serious toxicity (↓BP arrhythmias, cardiac arrest) can occur at concentrations ≥25mcg/mL. Measure plasma K^+: theophyllines may cause ↓K^+. Don't load patients already on oral preparations. Stick with one brand (bioavailability varies).

⚠ Management of acute asthma

Assess severity of attack:
PEF, ability to speak, RR, pulse rate, O_2 sats
Warn ICU if severe or life-threatening attack

↓

Immediate treatment:
Supplemental O_2 to maintain sats 94–98%
Salbutamol 5mg (or terbutaline 10mg) nebulized with O_2
If severe/life-threatening add in ipratropium 0.5mg/6h to nebulizers
Hydrocortisone 100mg IV or prednisolone 40–50mg PO

↓

Reassess every 15min:
- If PEF <75% repeat salbutamol nebulizers every 15–30min, or 10mg/h continuously. Add ipratropium if not already given
- Monitor ECG; watch for arrhythmias
- Consider single dose of magnesium sulfate ($MgSO_4$) 1.2–2g IV over 20min in those with severe/life-threatening features without good initial response to therapy

↓

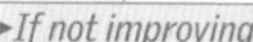

►►If not improving:
Refer to ICU for consideration of ventilatory support and intensification of medical therapy, eg aminophylline, IV salbutamol if any of the following signs are present:
- Deteriorating PEF
- Persistent/worsening hypoxia
- Hypercapnia
- ABG showing low pH or high H^+
- Exhaustion, feeble respiration
- Drowsiness, confusion, altered conscious level
- Respiratory arrest

If improving within 15–30min:
- Continue nebulized salbutamol every 4–6h (+ ipratropium if started in previous step)
- Prednisolone 40–50mg PO OD for 5–7 days
- Monitor peak flow and O_2 sats, aim 94–98% with supplemental if needed
- If PEF >75% 1h after initial treatment, consider discharge with outpatient follow-up

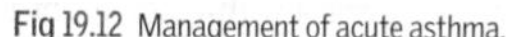

Fig 19.12 Management of acute asthma.

Acute exacerbations of COPD

A common medical emergency especially in winter. May be triggered by viral or bacterial infections.

Presentation Increasing cough, breathlessness, or wheeze. Decreased exercise capacity.

History (See p48.) Ask about usual/recent treatments (especially home oxygen), smoking status, and exercise capacity (may influence a decision to ventilate the patient).

Differential diagnosis Asthma, pulmonary oedema, upper respiratory tract obstruction, pulmonary embolus, anaphylaxis.

Investigations
- ABG (p771).
- CXR to exclude pneumothorax and infection.
- FBC; U&E; CRP. Theophylline level if patient on therapy at home.
- ECG.
- Send sputum for culture if purulent.
- Blood cultures if pyrexial.

Management ►Ensure oxygenation then treat the reversible,[8] see fig 19.13.
- Look for a cause, eg infection, pneumothorax.
- Prior to discharge, liaise with GP regarding steroid reduction, domiciliary oxygen (p184), smoking cessation, and pneumococcal and flu vaccinations (p166).

Treatment of stable COPD and more advanced disease: See pp184–5.

Consider the ceiling of care: What is in the best interests of the patient? Invasive ventilation for exacerbations of COPD may not be appropriate: it can be difficult to wean patients off ventilatory support, and brings with it the risk of ventilator-associated pneumonias and pneumothoraces from ruptured bullae. If possible, speak to the patient early, before deterioration, try to ascertain their wishes. Patients who have previously been ventilated may not wish to repeat the experience. Consider comorbidities, FEV_1, functional status, whether the patient requires home oxygen, and whether the patient has previously been admitted to ICU (and if so, whether they were easily weaned from invasive ventilation). Involve the patient, the family, your seniors, and ICU early in making a decision.

Oxygen therapy

- The greatest danger is hypoxia, which probably accounts for more deaths than hypercapnia. *Don't leave patients severely hypoxic.*
- However, in some patients, who rely on their hypoxic drive to breathe, too much oxygen may lead to a reduced respiratory rate and hypercapnia, with a consequent fall in conscious level. Always prescribe O_2 as if it were a drug.
- Care is always required with O_2, especially if there is evidence of CO_2 retention. Start with 24–28% O_2 in such patients.
- ►► Whenever you initiate or change oxygen therapy, do consider an ABG within 1h.
- Monitor the patient carefully. Aim to raise the P_aO_2 above 8.0kPa with a rise in P_aCO_2 <1.5kPa.
- In patients without evidence of retention at baseline use 28–40% O_2, but still monitor and repeat ABG.

⚠ Management of acute COPD

Nebulized bronchodilators:
Salbutamol 5mg/4h and ipratropium 500mcg/6h
Investigate: CXR, ABG

↓

Controlled oxygen therapy if S_aO_2 <88% or P_aO_2 <7 kPa:
Start at 24–28%, aim sats 88–92%
Adjust according to ABG, aim P_aO_2 >8.0kPa with a rise in P_aCO_2 <1.5kPa

↓

Steroids:
IV hydrocortisone 200mg and oral prednisolone 30mg OD (continue for 7–14d)

↓

Antibiotics:
Use if evidence of infection, eg amoxicillin 500mg/8h PO, alternatively clarithromycin or doxycycline (p387)

↓

Physiotherapy to aid sputum expectoration

↓

If no response to nebulizers and steroids:
Consider IV aminophylline*

↓

If no response:

1. Consider non-invasive positive pressure ventilation† (NIPPV) if respiratory rate >30 or pH <7.35, or P_aCO_2 rising despite best medical treatment. *OR*:
2. Consider a respiratory stimulant drug, eg doxapram 1.5–4mg/min IV in patients who are not suitable for mechanical ventilation. *SE*: *agitation, confusion, tachycardia, nausea*. It is a short-term measure, used only if NIV is not available

↓

Consider intubation and ventilation if pH <7.26 and P_aCO_2 is rising despite non-invasive ventilation only where appropriate (see 'Consider the ceiling of care' in text)

*Load with 250mg over 20min, then infuse at a rate of ~500mcg/kg/h (300mcg/kg/h if elderly), where kg is ideal body weight. Do not give a loading dose to patients on maintenance methylxanthines (theophyllines/aminophylline; see p811). Check plasma levels if given for >24h. ECG monitoring is required.

†This may alone serve as a rescue therapy, be an intermittent step before ventilation, or be considered as a 'ceiling of therapy' for those deemed not suitable for mechanical ventilation.

Fig 19.13 Management of acute COPD.

►►Pneumothorax

Causes

- *Spontaneous:* (Especially in young thin men) due to rupture of a subpleural bulla.
- *Chronic lung disease:* Asthma; COPD; cystic fibrosis; lung fibrosis; sarcoidosis.
- *Infection:* TB; pneumonia; lung abscess.
- *Traumatic:* Including iatrogenic (CVP line insertion, pleural aspiration or biopsy, percutaneous liver biopsy, positive pressure ventilation).
- *Carcinoma.*
- *Connective tissue disorders:* Marfan's syndrome, Ehlers-Danlos syndrome.

Clinical features

Symptoms: Can be asymptomatic (especially in fit young people with small pneumothoraces) or sudden onset of dyspnoea and/or pleuritic chest pain. Patients with asthma or COPD may present with a sudden deterioration. Mechanically ventilated patients can suddenly develop hypoxia or an increase in ventilation pressures.

Signs: Reduced expansion, hyper-resonance to percussion, and diminished breath sounds on the affected side. With a *tension pneumothorax*, the trachea will be deviated away from the affected side and the patient will be very unwell.

Tests ►*A CXR should not be performed if a tension pneumothorax is suspected, as it will delay immediate necessary treatment.* Otherwise, request an expiratory film, and look for an area devoid of lung markings, peripheral to the edge of the collapsed lung (see p725). Ensure the suspected *pneumothorax is not a large emphysematous bulla*. Check *ABG* in dyspnoeic/hypoxic patients and those with chronic lung disease.

Management ►See fig 19.14. Depends on whether it is a primary pneumothorax or secondary (=underlying lung disease or smoker >50yrs old), size, and symptoms.[9]

- Size is measured from the visible lung margin to chest wall *at level of the hilum*.
- Pneumothorax due to trauma or mechanical ventilation requires a chest drain.
- Aspiration of a pneumothorax, see p767.
- Insertion and management of a chest drain, see p766. Use a small tube (10–14F) unless blood/pus is also present. Tubes may be removed 24h after the lung has re-expanded and air leak has stopped (ie the tube stops bubbling). This is done during expiration or a Valsalva manoeuvre.

Surgical advice: Arrange if: bilateral pneumothoraces; lung fails to expand within 48h of intercostal drain insertion; persistent air leak; two or more previous pneumothoraces on the same side; or history of pneumothorax on the opposite side.

►►Tension pneumothorax

►► This is a medical emergency. (See fig 16.43, p749.)

Essence Air drawn into the pleural space with each inspiration has no route of escape during expiration. The mediastinum is pushed over into the contralateral hemithorax, kinking and compressing the great veins. Unless the air is rapidly removed, cardiorespiratory arrest will occur.

Signs Respiratory distress, tachycardia, hypotension, distended neck veins, trachea deviated away from side of pneumothorax. Increased percussion note, reduced air entry/breath sounds on the affected side.

Treatment

To remove the air, insert a large-bore (14–16G) needle with a syringe, partially filled with 0.9% saline, into the 2nd intercostal interspace in the midclavicular line on the side of the suspected pneumothorax. Remove plunger to allow the trapped air to bubble through the syringe (with saline as a water seal) until a chest tube can be placed. Alternatively, insert a large-bore Venflon in the same location.

►► Do this *before* requesting a CXR.

►► Then insert a chest drain. See p766.

⚠ Acute management of pneumothorax

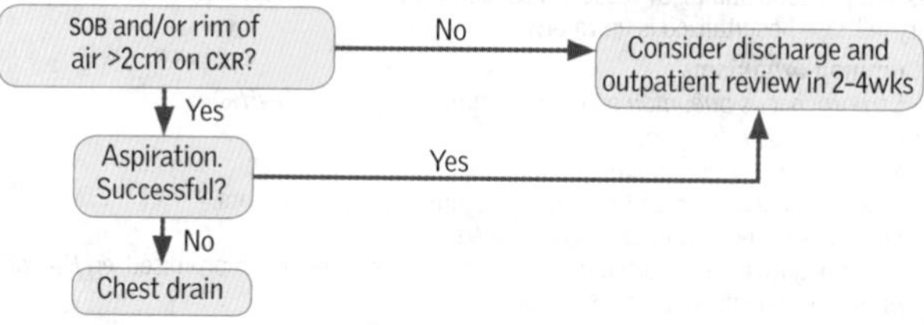

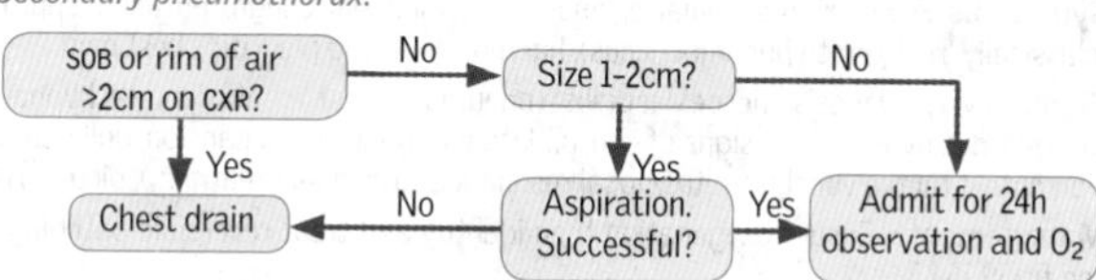

Fig 19.14 Acute management of pneumothorax.

Pneumonia

An infection of the lung parenchyma. Incidence of community-acquired pneumonia is 5-11 per 1000 adults. Of these, 1-3 per 1000 will require hospitalization, and mortality in those hospitalized is up to 14%.

Common organisms

- *Streptococcus pneumoniae* is the commonest cause (60-75%).
- *Haemophilus influenzae.*
- *Mycoplasma pneumoniae.*
- *Staphylococcus aureus* found more commonly in ICU patients.
- *Legionella* species and *Chlamydia psittaci.*
- Gram-negative bacilli, often hospital-acquired or immunocompromised, eg *Pseudomonas*, especially in those with COPD.
- Viruses including influenza account for up to 15%.

Symptoms Fever, rigors, malaise, anorexia, dyspnoea, cough, purulent sputum (classically 'rusty' with pneumococcus), haemoptysis, and pleuritic chest pain.

Signs Fever, cyanosis, herpes labialis (pneumococcus), confusion, tachypnoea, tachycardia, hypotension, signs of consolidation (diminished expansion, dull percussion note, ↑ tactile vocal fremitus/vocal resonance, bronchial breathing), pleural rub.

Management ►Ensure oxygenation then identify and treat reversible pathology,[10] see fig 19.15.

Investigations: Assess severity—this will guide both investigation and treatment.

- CXR (X-ray images, fig 16.4 on p725).
- Oxygen saturation and ABG if S_aO_2 <92% or severe pneumonia.
- FBC, U&E, LFT, CRP.
- Blood cultures (if CURB-65 ≥2).
- Sputum cultures (if CURB-65 ≥3 or if CURB-65 =2 and not had antibiotics yet).
- Urine pneumococcal antigen (if CURB-65 ≥2); *Legionella* antigen (if CURB-65 ≥3 or if clinical suspicion).
- Consider need for viral throat swabs and mycoplasma PCR/serology.
- Pleural fluid may be aspirated for culture (if CURB-65 ≥2).
- Consider bronchoscopy and bronchoalveolar lavage if the patient is immunocompromised or on ICU.

Severity: Calculate the core adverse features 'CURB-65' score: •**C**onfusion (abbreviated mental test ≤8). •**U**rea >7mmol/L. •**R**espiratory rate ≥30/min. •**B**P <90/60mmHg. •Age ≥**65**. *Score:* 0-1: home treatment if possible; ≥2: hospital therapy; ≥3: indicates severe pneumonia and should consider ICU referral.

Other features increasing the risk of death are: coexisting disease; bilateral/multilobar involvement; P_aO_2 <8kPa or S_aO_2 <92%.

Treatment: See antibiotic guidance (table 4.2 on p167). Most patients who require IV antibiotics can safely be switched to PO therapy by day 3.

Complications (Of infection or treatment.) Pleural effusion, empyema, lung abscess, respiratory failure, septicaemia, pericarditis, myocarditis, cholestatic jaundice, acute kidney injury.

Management of pneumonia

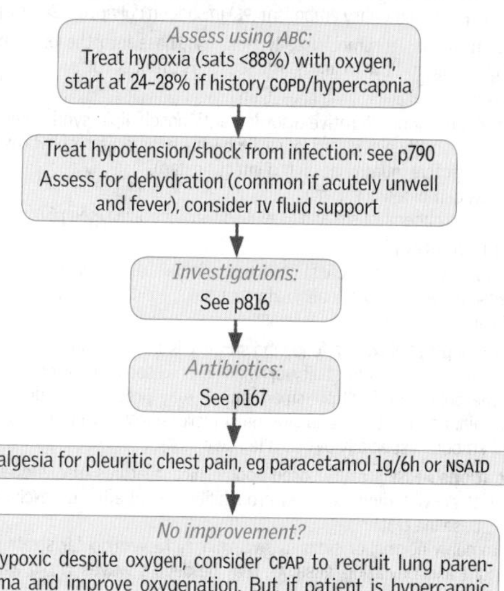

Fig 19.15 Management of pneumonia.

Pulmonary embolism (PE)

►Always suspect pulmonary embolism (PE) in sudden collapse 1-2wks after surgery.

Mechanism Venous thrombi, usually from DVT, pass into the pulmonary circulation and block blood flow to lungs. The source is often occult.

Risk factors
- Malignancy; myeloproliferative disorder; antiphospholipid syndrome.
- Surgery—especially pelvic and lower limb (much lower if prophylaxis used).
- Immobility; active inflammation (eg infection, IBD).
- Pregnancy; combined OCP; HRT.
- Previous thromboembolism and inherited thrombophilia, see p374.

Signs and symptoms
- Acute dyspnoea, pleuritic chest pain, haemoptysis, and syncope.
- Hypotension, tachycardia, gallop rhythm, ↑JVP, loud P_2, right ventricular heave, pleural rub, tachypnoea, cyanosis, AF.

With thromboprophylaxis, PE following surgery is far less common, but PE may occur after any period of immobility, or with no predisposing factors. Breathlessness may be the only sign. Multiple small emboli may present less dramatically with pleuritic pain, haemoptysis, and gradually increasing breathlessness. ►Look for a source of emboli—especially DVT (is a leg swollen?).

Investigations ►Risk stratify based upon clinical features (use 2-level Wells' score for PE—p191). A −ve D-dimer in a low-probability patient effective excludes PE.[11]
- U&E, FBC, baseline clotting.
- *ECG:* commonly normal or sinus tachycardia; right ventricular strain pattern V_1–V_3 (p98), right axis deviation, RBBB, AF, may be deep S waves in I, Q waves in III, inverted T waves in III ('$S_I Q_{III} T_{III}$').
- *CXR:* often normal; decreased vascular markings, small pleural effusion. Wedge-shaped area of infarction. Atelectasis.
- *ABG:* hyperventilation + poor gas exchange: ↓P_aO_2, ↓P_aCO_2, ↑pH.
- *Serum D-dimer:* low specificity (↑ if thrombosis, inflammation, post-op, infection, malignancy) ∴ check only in patients with low pre-test probability (p191).
- *CT pulmonary angiography* (CTPA) is sensitive and specific and is the test of choice for high-risk patients or low-risk patients with a +ve D-dimer. If unavailable, a *ventilation-perfusion (V/Q) scan* can aid diagnosis but frequently produces equivocal results

Management ►See fig 19.16 for immediate management.[11]

►If good story and signs, make the diagnosis. Start treatment (fig 19.16) before definitive investigations: most PE deaths occur within 1h.
- Commence LMWH or fondaparinux.
- If there is haemodynamic instability, consider thromolysis.
- Long-term anticoagulation: either DOAC (p350—switch directly from LMWH) or warfarin (continue LMWH until INR >2).
- Is there an underlying cause, eg thrombophilia (p374), SLE, or polycythaemia? Consider malignancy (take a careful history and perform a full physical examination; check CXR, FBC, LFT, Ca^{2+}; urinalysis; consider CT abdomen/pelvis and mammogram).
- If obvious remedial cause, 3 months of anticoagulation (p351) may be enough; otherwise, continue for ≥3-6 months (long term if recurrent emboli, or underlying malignancy).

Prevention See p190.

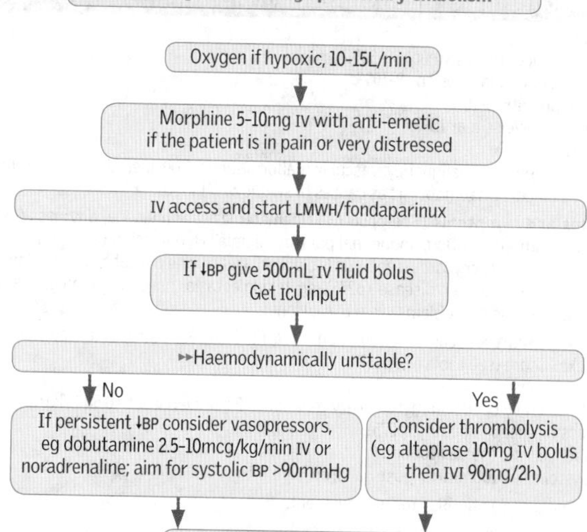

Fig 19.16 Management of large pulmonary embolism.

►►Acute upper gastrointestinal bleeding

Causes
- Peptic ulcer disease (PUD) 35–50%.
- Gastroduodenal erosions 8–15%.
- Oesophagitis 5–15%.
- Mallory–Weiss tear 15%.
- Varices 5–10%.
- Other: upper GI malignancy, vascular malformations. Consider also facial trauma, nose bleed, or haemoptysis as causes of *swallowed* blood.

Signs and symptoms (See pp56–63.) Haematemesis, or melaena, dizziness (especially postural), fainting, abdominal pain, dysphagia? Hypotension (in young may be postural only), tachycardia (not if on β-blocker), ↓JVP, ↓urine output, cool and clammy, signs of chronic liver disease (p276), eg telangiectasia, purpura, jaundice. NB: ask about previous GI problems, drug use, alcohol.

Management ►Focus on circulation,[12] see fig 19.17. Risk stratify based upon, eg Rockall score (see table 6.6, p257).

Is the patient shocked?
- Peripherally cool/clammy; capillary refill time >2s; urine output <0.5mL/kg/h.
- ↓GCS or encephalopathy (p275).
- Tachycardic (pulse >100bpm).
- Systolic BP <100mmHg; postural drop >20mmHg.

If shocked: See fig 19.17 for management.

If haemodynamically stable:
- Insert two large-bore (14–16G) IV cannulae and take blood for FBC, U&E, LFT, clotting, and group & save.
- Give IV fluids (p821) to restore intravascular volume; avoid saline if cirrhotic/varices; consider a CVP line to monitor and guide fluid replacement.
- Organize a CXR, ECG, and check ABG.
- Consider a urinary catheter and monitor hourly urine output.
- Transfuse if significant Hb drop (<70g/L).
- Correct clotting abnormalities (vitamin K (p274), FFP, platelets).
- If suspicion of varices (eg known history of liver disease or alcohol excess) then give terlipressin IV (1–2mg/6h for ≤3d) and initiate broad-spectrum IV antibiotics (eg piperacillin/tazobactam IV 4.5g/8h).
- Monitor pulse, BP, and CVP (keep >5cmH_2O) at least hourly until stable.
- Arrange an urgent *endoscopy* (p248).
- If endoscopic control fails, surgery or emergency mesenteric angiography/embolization may be needed. For uncontrolled oesophageal variceal bleeding, a Sengstaken–Blakemore tube may compress the varices, but should only be placed by someone with experience.

Acute drug therapy: There is no role for routine administration of PPI pre-endoscopy (provided endoscopy can be arranged in a timely manner). In patients undergoing successful endoscopic haemostasis, give PPI (eg omeprazole 40mg/12h IV/PO). Treat if positive for *H. pylori* (p253).

Rebleeds Serious event: 40% of patients who rebleed will die. If 'at risk' maintain a high index of suspicion. If a rebleed occurs, check vital signs every 15min and call senior cover for repeat endoscopy and/or surgical intervention.

Signs of a rebleed:

- Rising pulse rate.
- Falling JVP ± decreasing hourly urine output.
- Haematemesis or 'fresh' melaena (NB: it is normal to pass decreasing amounts of melaena for 24h post-haemostasis, as blood makes its way through the GI tract).
- Fall in BP (a late and sinister finding) and decreased conscious level.

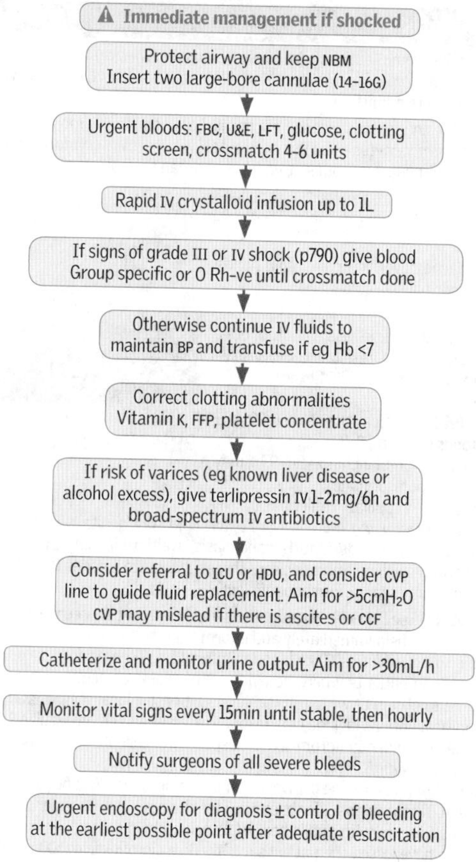

⚠ Immediate management if shocked

Protect airway and keep NBM
Insert two large-bore cannulae (14–16G)

↓

Urgent bloods: FBC, U&E, LFT, glucose, clotting screen, crossmatch 4–6 units

↓

Rapid IV crystalloid infusion up to 1L

↓

If signs of grade III or IV shock (p790) give blood
Group specific or O Rh-ve until crossmatch done

↓

Otherwise continue IV fluids to maintain BP and transfuse if eg Hb <7

↓

Correct clotting abnormalities
Vitamin K, FFP, platelet concentrate

↓

If risk of varices (eg known liver disease or alcohol excess), give terlipressin IV 1–2mg/6h and broad-spectrum IV antibiotics

↓

Consider referral to ICU or HDU, and consider CVP line to guide fluid replacement. Aim for >5cmH_2O
CVP may mislead if there is ascites or CCF

↓

Catheterize and monitor urine output. Aim for >30mL/h

↓

Monitor vital signs every 15min until stable, then hourly

↓

Notify surgeons of all severe bleeds

↓

Urgent endoscopy for diagnosis ± control of bleeding at the earliest possible point after adequate resuscitation

Fig 19.17 Immediate management of suspected upper GI bleed with shock.

▸▸Meningitis

▸**Primary care** Prompt actions save lives. ▸▸*If suspect meningitis arrange urgent transfer to secondary care. If a non-blanching rash is present,* give benzylpenicillin 1.2g IM/IV before admitting.

Organisms Meningococcus or pneumococcus. Less commonly *Haemophilus influenzae; Listeria monocytogenes*. HSV, VZV, enteroviruses. CMV, cryptococcus (p400), or TB (p393) if immunocompromised, eg HIV +ve, organ transplant, malignancy.

Differential Malaria, encephalitis, septicaemia, subarachnoid, dengue, tetanus.

Features

Early: Headache, fever, leg pains, cold hands and feet, abnormal skin colour.

Later:

- Meningism: neck stiffness, photophobia, Kernig's sign (pain + resistance on passive knee extension with hip fully flexed).
- ↓GCS, coma.
- Seizures (~20%) ± focal CNS signs (~20%) ± opisthotonus (p436, fig 9.46).
- Petechial rash (non-blanching—fig 19.18; may only be 1 or 2 spots, or none).
- Shock: prolonged capillary refill time; DIC; ↓BP.

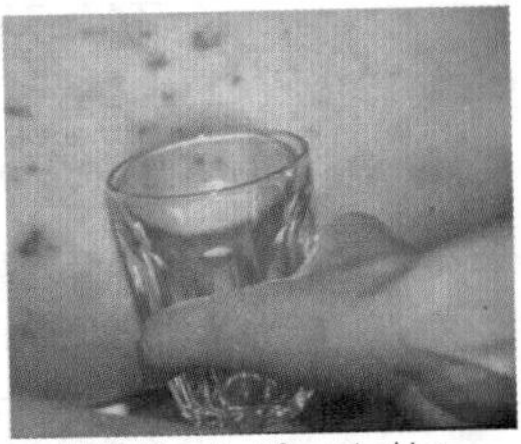

Fig 19.18 Glass test for petechiae.
Courtesy of Meningitis Research Foundation.

Signs of disease causing meningitis: Zoster; cold sore/genital vesicles (HSV); HIV signs (lymphadenopathy, dermatitis, candidiasis, uveitis); bleeding ± red eye (leptospirosis); parotid swelling (mumps); sore throat ± jaundice ± nodes (glandular fever, p405); splenectomy scar (∴ immunodeficient).

Management ▸See fig 19.19; investigations and treatment proceed in parallel.[13]

- *If ↑ICP*, summon help immediately and inform ICU.
- *Initiate early antibiotics.* Take blood cultures first. Then perform LP prior to antibiotics only in patients where no evidence of shock, petechial rash or ↑ICP and where able to obtain LP within 1h (table 19.4). Consult local policies and seek advice. Empirical options include ceftriaxone 2g/12h IV; add eg amoxicillin 2g/4h IV if >60yrs age or immunocompromised. If suspect viral encephalitis see p824.
- *If features of menigism* give dexamethasone 10mg/6h IV
- *Other investigations,* U&E, FBC (↓WBC≈immunocompromise: get help), LFT, glucose, coagulation. Throat swabs (1 for bacteria, 1 for virology). CXR. Consider HIV, TB tests.
- *Prophylaxis* (discuss with public health/ID): •Household contacts in droplet range. •Those who have kissed the patient's mouth. Give ciprofloxacin (500mg PO, 1 dose; child 5–12yrs: 250mg; child <5yrs: 30mg/kg to max 125mg).

⚠ Lumbar puncture in meningitis

Table 19.4 CSF analysis in meningitis

CSF in meningitis	Bacterial	Tuberculous (p393)	Viral ('aseptic')
Appearance	Often turbid	Often fibrin web	Usually clear
Predominant cell	Polymorphs*	Mononuclear*	Mononuclear
Cell count/mm³	Eg 90–1000 or more	10–1000	50–1000
Glucose	<½ plasma	<½ plasma	>½ plasma
Protein (g/L)	>1.5	1–5	<1
Bacteria	In smear & culture	Often none in smear	None seen or cultured

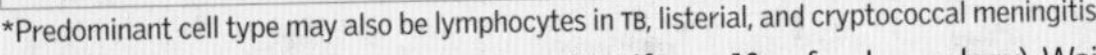

*Predominant cell type may also be lymphocytes in TB, listerial, and cryptococcal meningitis.

Perform LP (p768) without waiting for CT (not if GCS≤12 or focal neurology). Wait for clotting screen only if suspect coagulopathy. Record opening pressure—7–18cm CSF normal but ↑ in meningitis. Send CSF for MC&S, protein, lactate, glucose, virology/PCR. *Normal values:* ≤5 lymphocytes/mm³ with no neutrophils is normal. Protein: 0.15–0.45g/L. CSF glucose: 2.8–4.2mmol/L.

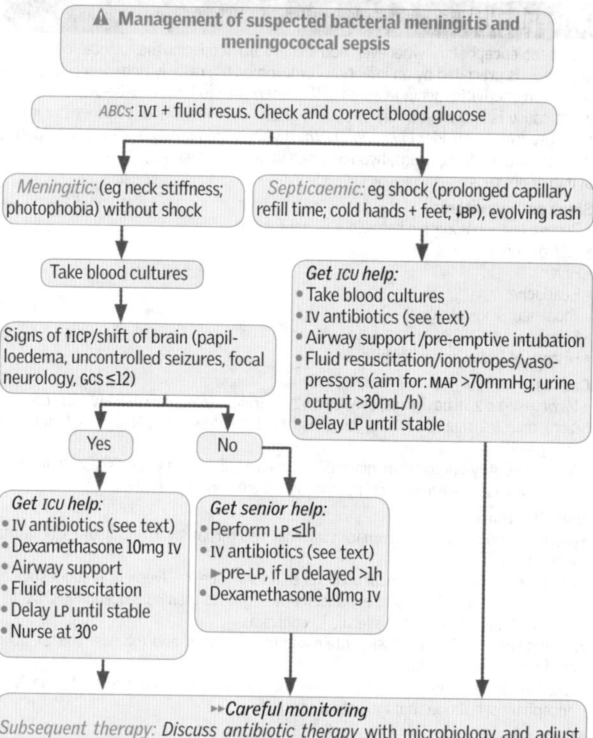

Fig 19.19 Management of suspected bacterial meningitis and meningococcal sepsis in immunocompetent adults.

Encephalitis

►Suspect encephalitis whenever odd behaviour, ↓consciousness, focal neurology or seizure is preceded by an infectious prodrome (↑T°, rash, lymphadenopathy, cold sores, conjunctivitis, meningeal signs). It is often wise to treat (see below) before the exact cause is known—usually viral, and often never identified. Without the infectious prodrome consider *encephalopathy:* hypoglycaemia, hepatic encephalopathy, diabetic ketoacidosis, drugs, hypoxic brain injury, uraemia, SLE, Wernicke's (give vit B_1 if in doubt p714).

Signs and symptoms
- Bizarre encephalopathic behaviour or confusion.
- ↓GCS or coma.
- Fever.
- Headache.
- Focal neurological signs.
- Seizures.
- History of travel or animal bite.

Causes
- *Viral:* HSV-1 & 2, arboviruses, CMV, EBV, VZV (varicella-zoster virus), HIV (seroconversion), measles, mumps, rabies, Japanese B encephalitis, West Nile virus, tick-borne encephalitis.
- *Non-viral:* Any bacterial meningitis, TB, malaria, listeria, Lyme disease, legionella, leptospirosis, aspergillosis, cryptococcus, schistosomiasis, typhus.

Investigations
- *Bloods:* Blood cultures; serum for viral PCR (also throat swab and MSU); toxoplasma IgM titre; malaria film.
- *Contrast-enhanced CT:* Focal bilateral temporal lobe involvement is suggestive of HSV encephalitis. Meningeal enhancement suggests meningoencephalitis. Do before LP. MRI is alternative if allergic to contrast.
- *LP:* Typically moderately ↑CSF protein and lymphocytes, and ↓glucose (p822). Send CSF for viral PCR including HSV.
- *EEG:* Urgent EEG showing diffuse abnormalities may help confirm a diagnosis of encephalitis, but does not indicate a cause.

Management
- ►Mortality in untreated viral encephalitis is ~70%. ►►Aim to start aciclovir within 30min of the patient arriving (10mg/kg/8h IV over 1h) for 14d as empirical treatment for HSV (21d if immunosuppressed). Specific therapies also exist for CMV and toxoplasmosis (p425).
- Supportive therapy, in high-dependency unit or ICU environment if necessary.
- Symptomatic treatment: eg phenytoin for seizures (p826).

Cerebral abscess

Suspect this in any patient with ↑ICP, especially if there is fever or ↑WCC. It may follow ear, sinus, dental, or periodontal infection; skull fracture; congenital heart disease; endocarditis; bronchiectasis. It may also occur in the absence of systemic signs of inflammation.

Signs Seizures, fever, localizing signs, or signs of ↑ICP. Coma. Signs of sepsis elsewhere (eg teeth, ears, lungs, endocarditis).

Investigations CT/MRI p746 (eg 'ring-enhancing' lesion); ↑WCC, ↑ESR; biopsy.

⚠ **Treatment** Urgent neurosurgical referral; treat ↑ICP (p830). If frontal sinuses or teeth are the source, the likely organism will be *Strep. milleri* (microaerophilic), or oropharyngeal anaerobes. In ear abscesses, *B. fragilis* or other anaerobes are most common. Bacterial abscesses are often peripheral; toxoplasma lesions (p425) are deeper (eg basal ganglia). NB: ask yourself: is the patient immunocompromised? Discuss with infectious diseases/microbiology.

This page intentionally blank

▸▸Status epilepticus

This means seizures lasting for >30min, or repeated seizures without intervening consciousness. Mortality and the risk of permanent brain damage increase with the length of attack. Aim to terminate seizures lasting more than a few minutes as soon as possible (<20min).

Status usually occurs in patients with known epilepsy. If it is the 1st presentation, the chance of a structural brain lesion is high (>50%). Diagnosis of tonic-clonic status is usually clear. Non-convulsive status (eg absence status or continuous partial seizures with preservation of consciousness) may be more difficult: look for subtle eye or lid movement. For other signs, see pp484, 490-3. An EEG can be very helpful. ▸*Could the patient be pregnant* (any pelvic mass)? If so, eclampsia (*OHCS* p48) is the likely diagnosis, check the urine and BP: call a senior obstetrician—immediate delivery may be needed.

Investigations

- Bedside glucose, the following tests can be done once ℞ has started: lab glucose, ABG, U&E, Ca^{2+}, FBC, ECG.
- Consider anticonvulsant levels, toxicology screen, LP, culture blood and urine, EEG, CT, carbon monoxide level.
- Pulse oximetry, cardiac monitor.

Management ▸See fig 19.20. Basic life support—and these agents:[14]

1. *Lorazepam:* 0.1mg/kg (usually 4mg) as a slow bolus into a large vein. If no response after 10-20min give a second dose. Beware respiratory arrest during the last part of the injection. Have full resuscitation facilities to hand for all IV benzodiazepine use. The rectal route is an alternative for diazepam if IV access is difficult. *Buccal midazolam* is an easier to use oral alternative where no IV access (eg in a community setting); dose for those 10yrs old and older 10mg; if 1-5yrs 5mg, if 5-10yrs 7.5mg; squirt half the volume between the lower gum and the cheek on each side. While waiting for this to work, prepare other drugs. If fits continue ...
2. *Phenytoin infusion:* 15-18mg/kg IVI (roughly 1g if 60kg, and 1.5g if 80kg; max 2g), at a maximum rate of 50mg/min (don't put diazepam in same line: they don't mix). Beware ↓BP and do not use if bradycardic or heart block. Requires BP and ECG monitoring. 100mg/6-8h is a maintenance dose (check levels). If fits continue ...
3. *Seek ICU help:* Paralysis and anaesthesia with eg propofol is required. Close monitoring, especially respiratory function, is vital. Consider whether this could be pseudoseizures (p490), particularly if there are odd features (pelvic thrusts; resisting attempts to open lids and your attempts to do passive movements; arms and legs flailing around).
4. *Dexamethasone:* 10mg IV if vasculitis/cerebral oedema (tumour) possible.

As soon as seizures are controlled, start oral drugs (p492). Ask what the cause was, eg hypoglycaemia, pregnancy, alcohol, drugs, CNS lesion or infection, hypertensive encephalopathy, inadequate anticonvulsant dose/compliance (p490).

⚠

⚠ Management of convulsive status epilepticus

Open and secure the airway (adjuncts as necessary)
Remove false teeth if poorly fitting

↓

Oxygen, 100% + suction (as required)

↓

IV access and take blood:
U&E, LFT, FBC, glucose, Ca^{2+}
Toxicology screen if indicated
Anticonvulsant levels

↓

IV bolus—to stop seizures: eg lorazepam 4mg
Give 2nd dose of lorazepam if no response after 10–20min

↓

Thiamine 250mg IV over 30min if alcoholism or malnourishment suspected
Glucose 50mL 50% IV, unless glucose known to be normal
Treat acidosis if severe (contact ICU)

↓

Correct hypotension with fluids

↓

IV infusion: If seizures continue, start phenytoin, 15–18mg/kg IVI, at a rate of 50mg/min. Monitor ECG and BP. 100mg/6–8h is a maintenance dose (check levels)

↓

General anaesthesia: Continuing seizures after 60–90mins of above therapies require expert help with paralysis (eg propofol infusion) and ventilation with continuous EEG monitoring in ICU. NB: ►*never* spend longer than 20min on someone with status epilepticus without having help at the bedside from an anaesthetist

Fig 19.20 Management of status epilepticus.

►►Head injury

►If the pupils are unequal, diagnose rising intracranial pressure (ICP), eg from extradural haemorrhage, and summon urgent neurosurgical help (p482). Retinal vein pulsation at fundoscopy helps exclude ↑ICP.

Initial management ►See fig 19.21. Write full notes. Record times.

►►Stabilization of airway, breathing, and circulation (ABC) remains the 1st priority. If GCS ≤8 then seek urgent anaesthetic and ICU help to protect airway.[15]

- Involve neurosurgeons early, especially if ↓GCS, or if ↑ICP suspected.
- Examine the CNS. Chart pulse, BP, T°, respirations + pupils every 15min.
- Assess anterograde amnesia (loss from the time of injury, ie post-traumatic) and retrograde amnesia (for events prior to injury)—extent of retrograde loss correlates with severity of injury, and never occurs without anterograde amnesia.
- Nurse semi-prone if no spinal injury; meticulous care to airway and bladder.

Perform a CT head <1h if:

- GCS <13 on initial assessment, or GCS <15 at 2h following injury.
- Focal neurological deficit.
- Suspected open or depressed skull fracture, or signs of basal skull fracture: periobital ecchymoses ('panda' eyes/racoon sign), postauricular ecchymosis (Battle's sign), CSF leak through nose/ears, haemotympanum.
- Post-traumatic seizure.
- Vomiting more than once.

Perform a CT head <8h if: Any loss of consciousness or amnesia *AND* any of: •age ≥65 •coagulopathy •high-impact injury, eg struck by or ejected from motor vehicle; fall >1m or >5 stairs •retrograde amnesia of >30min.

Suspected cervical spine injuries: Perform a CT cervical spine <1h if:

- GCS <13 on initial assessment.
- The patient has been intubated.
- Definitive diagnosis of cervical spine injury is needed urgently (eg before surgery).
- The patient is having other body areas scanned, eg multi-region trauma.
- Clinical suspicion of cervical spine injury *AND ANY OF:* •age 65 years or older •high-impact injury •focal neurological deficit •paraesthesia in the upper or lower limbs.

►If above-listed criteria are *NOT* met *AND IF ANY OF* the following low-risk features are present, then assess neck movement: •simple rear-end motor vehicle collision •comfortable in a sitting position •ambulatory since injury •no midline cervical spine tenderness •delayed onset of neck pain. If patient unable actively to rotate neck 45° to left and right or if a low-risk feature not present, then obtain plain X-rays of cervical spine <1h. If X-rays technically inadequate, suspicious, or definitely abnormal, proceed to CT.

Admit if: •new, clinically significant abnormalities on CT •GCS<15 after CT, regardless of result or continuing worrying signs (eg vomiting) •when CT indications met but CT unavailable •other concerns (eg drugs or alcohol, other injuries, CSF leak, shock, suspected non-accidental injury, meningism).

►Do not attribute ↓GCS to alcohol until a significant head injury has been excluded. Alcohol is an unlikely cause of coma if plasma alcohol <44mmol/L. If unavailable, estimate blood alcohol level from the osmolar gap (p668). If blood alcohol ≈ 40mmol/L, osmolar gap ≈ 40mmol/L.

Discuss with neurosurgical unit all with significant abnormalities on CT or with eg persistent GCS ≤8 or deteriorating GCS (especially motor component), persistent confusion, progressive focal neurology, seizure without full recovery, penetrating injuries, or CSF leak. If transfer is required, ensure skilled medical escort and consider need for intubation prior to transfer.

Complications *Early:* Extradural/subdural haemorrhage, seizures. *Late:* Subdural (p482), seizures, diabetes insipidus, parkinsonism, dementia.

Indicators of a bad prognosis Old age, decerebrate rigidity, extensor spasms, prolonged coma, ↑BP, ↓P_aO_2 (on blood gases), T° >39°C. 60% of those with loss of consciousness of >1 month will survive 3–25yrs, but may need daily nursing care.

▲ Immediate management plan for head injury

ABC

↓

Oxygen if saturations <92% or hypoxic on ABG
Intubate and hyperventilate if necessary
Immobilize neck until injury to cervical spine excluded

↓

Stop blood loss and support circulation
Treat for shock if required (p790)

↓

Treat seizures with lorazepam ± phenytoin (p826)

↓

Assess level of consciousness (GCS):
►►If GCS ≤8 ICU involvement to manage airway
Assess for anterograde and retrograde amnesia

↓

Rapid examination survey

↓

Investigations:
U&Es, glucose, FBC, blood alcohol,
toxicology screen, ABGs, and clotting

↓

Neurological examination

↓

Brief history:
When? Where? How? Had a fit? Lucid interval? Alcohol?

↓

Evaluate lacerations of face or scalp:
Palpate deep wounds with sterile glove to check for
step deformity. Note obvious skull/facial fractures

↓

Check for CSF leak, from nose (rhinorrhoea) or ear (otorrhoea)
Any blood behind the ear drum?
If either is present, suspect basilar skull fracture: do CT
Give tetanus toxoid, and refer at once to neurosurgeons

↓

Palpate the neck posteriorly for tenderness and deformity:
If detected, or if the patient has other indicators for neck imaging, immobilize the neck and get cervical spine x-ray or CT neck (see text)

↓

Radiology:
As indicated: CT of head/neck (see text)
Consider need for trauma series (eg CT chest/abdo/pelvis)

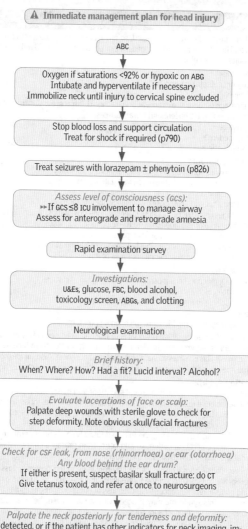

Fig 19.21 Immediate management plan for head injury.

►►Raised intracranial pressure (ICP)

The volume inside the cranium is fixed, so any increase in the contents can lead to raised ICP. This can be mass effect, oedema, or obstruction to fluid outflow. Normal ICP in adults is <15mmHg.

Causes
- Primary or metastatic tumours.
- Head injury.
- Haemorrhage (subdural, extradural, subarachnoid, intracerebral, intraventricular).
- Infection: meningitis, encephalitis, brain abscess.
- Hydrocephalus.
- Cerebral oedema.
- Status epilepticus.

Signs and symptoms
- Headache (worse on coughing, leaning forwards), vomiting.
- Altered GCS: drowsiness, listlessness, irritability, coma.
- History of trauma.
- ↓HR and ↑BP (Cushing's response); Cheyne–Stokes respiration.
- Pupil changes (constriction at first, later dilation—do not mask these signs by using agents such as tropicamide to dilate the pupil to aid fundoscopy).
- ↓Visual acuity; peripheral visual field loss.
- Papilloedema is an unreliable sign, but venous pulsation at the disc may be absent (absent in ~50% of normal people, but *loss* of it is a useful sign).

Investigations
- U&E, FBC, LFT, glucose, serum osmolality, clotting, blood culture.
- Consider toxicology screen.
- CXR—any source of infection that might indicate abscess?
- CT head.
- Then consider LP if safe. Measure the opening pressure!

Management ►See fig 19.22. The goal is to ↓ICP and avert secondary injury. Urgent neurosurgery is required for the definitive treatment of ↑ICP from focal causes (eg haematomas). This is achieved via a craniotomy or burr hole. Also, an ICP monitor (or bolt) may be placed to monitor pressure. *Holding measures* are listed in fig 19.22.

Herniation syndromes

Uncal herniation is caused by a lateral supratentorial mass, which pushes the ipsilateral inferomedial temporal lobe (uncus) through the temporal incisura and against the midbrain. The IIIrd nerve, travelling in this space, gets compressed, causing a dilated ipsilateral pupil, then ophthalmoplegia (a fixed pupil localizes a lesion poorly but is 'ipsilateralizing'). This may be followed (quickly) by contralateral hemiparesis (pressure on the cerebral peduncle) and coma from pressure on the ascending reticular activating system (ARAS) in the midbrain.

Cerebellar tonsil herniation is caused by ↑pressure in the posterior fossa forcing the cerebellar tonsils through the foramen magnum. Ataxia, VIth nerve palsies, and upgoing plantar reflexes occur first, then loss of consciousness, irregular breathing, and apnoea. This syndrome may proceed very rapidly given the small size of, and poor compliance in, the posterior fossa.

Subfalcian (cingulate) herniation is caused by a frontal mass. The cingulate gyrus (medial frontal lobe) is forced under the rigid falx cerebri. It may be silent unless the anterior cerebral artery is compressed and causes a stroke—eg contralateral leg weakness ± abulia (lack of decision-making).

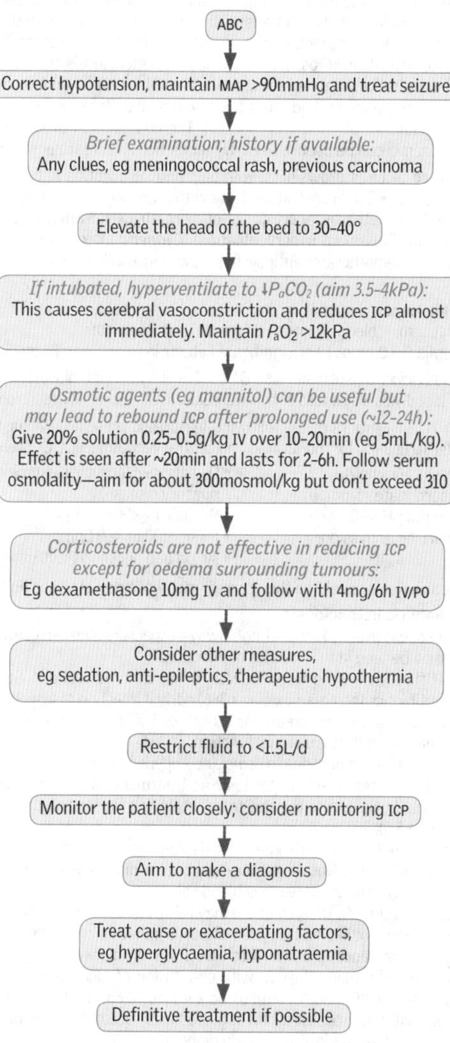

⚠ Immediate management plan for raised intracranial pressure
ABC
Correct hypotension, maintain MAP >90mmHg and treat seizures
Brief examination; history if available:
Any clues, eg meningococcal rash, previous carcinoma
Elevate the head of the bed to 30–40°
If intubated, hyperventilate to ↓P_aCO_2 (aim 3.5–4kPa):
This causes cerebral vasoconstriction and reduces ICP almost immediately. Maintain P_aO_2 >12kPa
Osmotic agents (eg mannitol) can be useful but may lead to rebound ICP after prolonged use (~12–24h):
Give 20% solution 0.25–0.5g/kg IV over 10–20min (eg 5mL/kg). Effect is seen after ~20min and lasts for 2–6h. Follow serum osmolality—aim for about 300mosmol/kg but don't exceed 310
Corticosteroids are not effective in reducing ICP except for oedema surrounding tumours:
Eg dexamethasone 10mg IV and follow with 4mg/6h IV/PO
Consider other measures, eg sedation, anti-epileptics, therapeutic hypothermia
Restrict fluid to <1.5L/d
Monitor the patient closely; consider monitoring ICP
Aim to make a diagnosis
Treat cause or exacerbating factors, eg hyperglycaemia, hyponatraemia
Definitive treatment if possible

Fig 19.22 Immediate management plan for raised intracranial pressure.

Diabetic ketoacidosis (DKA)

Mechanism Normally the body metabolizes carbohydrates, leading to efficient energy production. Ketoacidosis is an alternative metabolic pathway used in starvation states; it is far less efficient, and produces acetone as a byproduct (hence the fruity breath of patients in ketosis). In acute diabetic ketoacidosis, there is excessive glucose, but because of a lack of insulin, this cannot be taken up into cells to be metabolized, so pushing the body into a starvation-like state where ketoacidosis is the only mechanism of energy production. The combination of severe acidosis and hyperglycaemia can be deadly, so early recognition and treatment is important.

Typical picture Gradual drowsiness, vomiting, and dehydration in type 1 diabetic (very rarely type 2). ►Do glucose in *all* those with unexplained vomiting, abdo pain, polyuria, polydipsia, lethargy, anorexia, ketotic breath, dehydration, coma, or deep breathing (sighing 'Kussmaul' hyperventilation). *Triggers:* Infection, eg UTI; surgery; MI; pancreatitis; chemotherapy; antipsychotics; wrong insulin dose/non-compliance.

Diagnosis

1. Acidaemia (venous blood pH <7.3 or HCO_3^- < 15.0mmol/L).
2. Hyperglycaemia (blood glucose >11.0mmol/L) or known DM.
3. Ketonaemia (≥3.0mmol/L) or significant ketonuria (more than 2+ on dipstick).

Tests: ECG, CXR. *Urine:* Dipstick and MSU. *Blood:* Capillary and lab glucose, ketones, pH (use venous blood; ABG only if ↓GCS or hypoxia), U&E, HCO_3^-, osmolality, FBC, blood culture.

Severe DKA If one or more of the following features is present on admission, consider transfer to HDU/ICU for monitoring and central venous access. Get senior help!

- Blood ketones >6mmol/L.
- Venous bicarbonate <5mmol/L.
- Venous/arterial pH <7.0.
- K <3.5mmol/L on admission.
- GCS <12.
- O_2 sats <92% on air (assuming no respiratory disease).
- Systolic BP <90mmHg.
- Pulse >100 or <60 bpm.
- Anion gap above 16 (p670).

Management ►Replace volume then correct metabolic defects,[16] see fig 19.23.

Pitfalls in diabetic ketoacidosis

- *Plasma glucose* is usually high, but not always, especially if insulin continued.
- *High WCC* may be seen in the absence of infection.
- *Infection.* Often there is no fever. Do MSU, blood cultures, and CXR. Start broad-spectrum antibiotics (eg co-amoxiclav, p386) early if infection is suspected.
- *Creatinine.* Some assays for creatinine cross-react with ketone bodies, so plasma creatinine may not reflect true renal function.
- *Hyponatraemia* is common, due to osmolar compensation for the hyperglycaemia. ↑ or ↔ [Na^+] indicates severe water loss. As treatment commences Na^+ rises as water enters cells. Na^+ is also low due to an artefact; corrected plasma [Na^+] = Na^+ + 2.4[(glucose −5.5)/5.5].
- *Ketonuria* does not equate with ketoacidosis. Anyone may have up to ++ketonuria after an overnight fast. Not all ketones are due to diabetes—consider alcohol if glucose normal. Always check venous blood ketones.
- *Recurrent ketoacidosis.* Blood glucose may return to normal long before ketones are removed from the blood, and premature termination of insulin infusion may lead to lack of clearance and return to DKA. This may be avoided by maintaining a constant rate of insulin infusion (with co-infusion of glucose 10% to maintain plasma glucose at 6-10mmol/L) until blood ketones <0.6mmol/L and pH >7.3.
- *Acidosis* but without gross elevation of glucose may occur, but consider overdose (eg aspirin) and lactic acidosis (in elderly diabetics).

- *Serum amylase* is often raised (up to ×10) and non-specific abdominal pain is common, even in the absence of pancreatitis.

Complications ►Cerebral oedema (get help if sudden CNS decline), aspiration pneumonia, hypokalaemia, hypomagnesaemia, hypophosphataemia, thromboembolism.

Prevention ►Talk to the patient: evaluate compliance and educate about triggers.

⚠ Management plan for diabetic ketoacidosis

ABC approach, 2 large-bore cannulae:
Start fluid: 1L 0.9% saline over 1h (if systolic BP <90mmHg then give 500mL bolus over 15mins and reassess—if systolic BP still <90mmHg then seek senior review and give further 500mL bolus; if BP remains <90mmHg then involve ICU)

↓

Tests: Venous blood gas for pH, bicarbonate; bedside and lab glucose and ketones; U&Es, FBC, CRP; CXR, ECG

↓

Insulin: Add 50 units human soluble insulin to 50mL 0.9% saline. Infuse continuously at 0.1 unit/kg/h. Continue patient's regular long-acting insulin at usual doses and times; consider initiating long-acting insulin in newly diagnosed T1DM. ►Aim for a fall in blood ketones of 0.5mmol/L/h, or a rise in venous bicarbonate of 3mmol/L/h with a fall in glucose of 3mmol/L/h. If not achieving this, increase insulin infusion by 1 unit/h until target rates achieved

↓

Check capillary blood glucose and ketones hourly
Check VBG (pH, HCO_3^-, K^+) at 2h, 4h, 8h, 12h, and 24h (or more frequent)

↓

Continue fluids and assess need for K^+ (see below)

↓

Consider catheter if not passed urine by 1h, aim for urine output 0.5mL/kg/h. Consider NG tube if vomiting or drowsy
Start all patients on LMWH

↓

Avoid hypoglycaemia! When glucose <14mmol/L start 10% glucose at 125mL/h to run alongside saline and prevent hypoglycaemia

↓

Continue fixed-rate insulin until ketones <0.6mmol/L, venous pH >7.3, and venous bicarb >15mmol/L. Do not rely on urinary ketones to indicate resolution—they stay positive after DKA resolved
Find and treat infection/cause for DKA

Fig 19.23 Management plan for diabetic ketoacidosis.

⚠ Fluid replacement

- 0.9% saline is the replacement fluid of choice.
- Typical fluid deficit is 100mL/kg, so for an average 70kg man = 7 litres.
- Give eg 1L in 1h (faster if systolic BP <90mmHg) then: 1L over 2h, 1L over 2h, 1L over 4h, 1L over 4 h, 1L over 8h. This regimen may not be appropriate for all: reassess frequently, especially if young, elderly, pregnant, or comorbidities.
- Bicarbonate may increase risk of cerebral oedema and is not recommended.

⚠ Potassium replacement

- Typical deficit = 3-5mmol/kg, plasma K^+ falls with treatment as K^+ enters cells.
- Don't add K^+ to the 1st bag. Thereafter add K^+ according to most recent VBG result (table 19.5).

Table 19.5 Potassium replacement in DKA

Serum K^+ (mmol/L)	Amount of KCl to add per litre of IV fluid
>5.5	Nil
3.5–5.5	40mmol
<3.5	Seek help from HDU/ICU for higher doses

Other diabetic emergencies

Hypoglycaemia Usually *rapid* onset; may be accompanied by odd behaviour (eg aggression), sweating, ↑pulse, seizures. *Management:* ▸▸If conscious, orientated, and able to swallow, give 15–20g of quick-acting carbohydrate snack (eg 200mL orange juice) and recheck blood glucose after 10–15mins (repeat snack up to 3 times). If conscious but uncooperative, squirt glucose gel between teeth and gums. In unconscious patients, or those not responding to these measures, start glucose IVI (eg 10% at 200mL/h if conscious; 10% at 200mL/15mins if unconscious), or give glucagon 1mg IV/IM (will not work in malnourished patients). Expect prompt recovery. Once blood glucose >4.0mmol/L and patient has recovered, give long-acting carbohydrate (eg slice of toast).

Hyperglycaemic hyperosmolar state (HHS) Seen in unwell patients with type 2 DM.[17] The history is longer (eg 1wk), with marked dehydration and glucose >30mmol/L. There is no switch to ketone metabolism, so ketonaemia stays <3mmol/L and pH >7.3. Osmolality is typically >320mosmol/kg: ▸*Occlusive events are a danger* (focal CNS signs, chorea, DIC, leg ischaemia/rhabdomyolysis)—give LMWH prophylaxis to all unless contraindication (p350). Rehydrate slowly with 0.9% saline IVI over 48h, typical deficits are 110–220mL/kg, ie 8–15L for a 70kg adult. Replace K^+ when urine starts to flow (see DKA BOX, p833). ▸Only use insulin if blood glucose not falling by 5mmol/L/h with rehydration or if ketonaemia—start slowly 0.05u/kg/h. Keep blood glucose at least 10–15mmol/L for first 24 hours to avoid cerebral oedema. Look for the cause, eg MI, drugs, sepsis, or bowel infarct.

Lactic acidosis A rare but serious complication of DM with metformin use or septicaemia. Blood lactate: >5mmol/L. Seek expert help. Treat sepsis vigorously, maintain blood pressure and hence tissue perfusion. Stop metformin.

Thyroid emergencies

Myxoedema coma The ultimate hypothyroid state before death.

Signs and symptoms: Looks hypothyroid (p220, p221, fig 5.16); often >65yrs; hypothermia; hyporeflexia; ↓glucose; bradycardia; coma; seizures. May have had radioiodine, thyroidectomy, or pituitary surgery (signs of hypopituitarism, p232). Psychosis (myxoedema madness) may precede coma. *Precipitants:* infection, MI, stroke, or trauma.

Examination: Goitre; cyanosis; ↓BP (cardiogenic); heart failure; signs of precipitants.

Treatment: Preferably on ICU.

- Blood for: T_3, T_4, TSH, FBC, U&E (often ↓Na^+), cultures, cortisol, glucose.
- ABG for P_aO_2. High-flow O_2 if cyanosed. Ventilation may be needed.
- Correct any hypoglycaemia.
- Give T_3 (liothyronine) 5–20mcg/12h IV slowly. Be cautious: you may precipitate manifestations of ischaemic heart disease. Alternative regimens involve levothyroxine.
- Give hydrocortisone 100mg/8h IV—vital if pituitary hypothyroidism is suspected (ie no goitre, no previous radioiodine, and no previous thyroid surgery).
- If infection suspected, give antibiotic, eg co-amoxiclav 1.2g/8h IV.
- Caution with fluid, rehydrate as needed but watch for cardiac dysfunction; BP may not respond to fluid and inotropes may be needed.
- Active warming (blankets, fluids) may be needed for *hypothermia*. Beware complications (hypoglycaemia, pancreatitis, arrhythmias). See p848.

Further ℞: T_3 5–20mcg/4–12h IV until sustained improvement (~2–3d) then levothyroxine 50mcg/24h PO. Hydrocortisone + IV fluids as needed (hyponatraemia is dilutional).

Hyperthyroid crisis (thyrotoxic storm) *Signs and symptoms:* ♀:♂≈4:1. Severe hyperthyroidism (see p218): ↑T°, agitation, confusion, coma, tachycardia, AF, D&V, goitre, thyroid bruit, acute abdomen (exclude surgical causes), heart failure.

Precipitants: Recent thyroid surgery or radioiodine; infection; MI; trauma.

Diagnosis: Do not wait for test results if urgent treatment is needed. Do TSH, free T_4, and free T_3. Confirm with technetium uptake if possible.

Treatment: ▸See fig 19.24. Seek endocrinology advice and aim to: **1** Counteract peripheral effects of thyroid hormones. **2** Inhibit thyroid hormone synthesis. **3** Treat systemic complications. If you are not making headway in 24h, thyroidectomy may be an option.

⚠ Management plan for thyrotoxic storm

IV access, fluids if dehydrated. NG tube if vomiting

↓

Take blood for: T_3, T_4, TSH, cultures (if infection suspected)

↓

Sedate if necessary (eg chlorpromazine 50mg PO/IM). Monitor BP

↓

If no contraindication, and cardiac output OK, give propranolol 60mg/4–6h PO; max IV dose: 1mg over 10min; may need repeating every few hours. In asthma/poor cardiac output, propranolol has caused cardiac arrest in thyroid storm, so ultra-short-acting β-blockers have a role, eg IV esmolol. Consider diltiazem if β-blockers contraindicated. ►*Get help*

↓

High-dose digoxin may be needed to slow the heart, but ensure adequately β-blocked, give with cardiac monitoring

↓

Antithyroid drugs: carbimazole 15–25mg/6h PO (or via NGT); after 4h give Lugol's solution (aqueous iodine oral solution) 0.3mL/8h PO well diluted in water for 7-10d to block thyroid

↓

Hydrocortisone 100mg/6h IV or dexamethasone 2mg/6h PO to prevent peripheral conversion T_4 to T_3

↓

Treat suspected infection, eg with co-amoxiclav 1.2g/8h IV

↓

Adjust IV fluids as necessary; cool with tepid sponging ± paracetamol

↓

Continuing treatment: After 5d reduce carbimazole to 15mg/8h PO. After 10d stop propranolol and iodine. Adjust carbimazole (p218)

Fig 19.24 Management plan for thyrotoxic storm.

Addisonian crisis

Signs and symptoms Patients may present in shock (↑HR; vasoconstriction; postural hypotension; oliguria; weak; confused; comatose)—often (but not always) in a patient with known Addison's (eg when oral steroid has not been increased to cover stress such as pneumonia), or someone on long-term steroids who has forgotten their tablets. Remember bilateral adrenal haemorrhage (eg meningococcaemia) as a cause. An alternative presentation is with hypoglycaemia.

Precipitating factors Infection, trauma, surgery, missed medication.

Management If suspected, treat before biochemical results.

- Bloods for cortisol and ACTH (this needs to go straight to laboratory, call ahead!), U&Es—can have ↑K^+ (check ECG and give calcium gluconate if needed, see p301) and ↓Na^+ (salt depletion, should resolve with rehydration and steroids).
- Hydrocortisone 100mg IV stat.
- IV fluid bolus eg 500mL 0.9% saline to support BP, repeated as necessary.
- Monitor blood glucose: the danger is hypoglycaemia.
- Blood, urine, sputum for culture, then antibiotics if concern about infection.

Continuing treatment

- Glucose IV may be needed if hypoglycaemic.
- Give IV fluids as guided by clinical state and to correct U&E imbalance.
- Continue hydrocortisone, eg 100mg/8h IV or IM.
- Change to oral steroids after 72h if patient's condition good.
- Fludrocortisone may well be needed if the cause is adrenal disease: ask an expert.
- Search for (and vigorously treat) the underlying cause. Get endocrinological help.

Hypopituitary coma

Think of decompensated chronic hypophyseal failure whenever hypothermia, refractory hypotension ± septic signs *without* fever occur with short stature or loss of axillary/pubic hair ± gonadal atrophy. ►Waiting for lab confirmation may be fatal. It *usually* develops gradually in a person with known hypopituitarism. If rapid onset due to pituitary infarction (eg postpartum, Sheehan's, p232), subarachnoid haemorrhage is often misdiagnosed as symptoms include headache and meningism.

Presentation Headache; ophthalmoplegia; ↓consciousness; hypotension; hypothermia; hypoglycaemia; signs of hypopituitarism (p232).

Tests Cortisol; T_4; TSH; ACTH; glucose. Pituitary fossa CT/MRI.

Treatment ►Hydrocortisone, eg 100mg IV/6h.

- Only after hydrocortisone begun: liothyronine (L-tri-iodothyronine sodium), eg 10mcg/12h PO or by slow IV: 5–20mcg/12h (4-hourly may be needed).
- Prompt surgery is needed if the cause is pituitary apoplexy (p234).

Phaeochromocytoma emergencies

Patients with phaeochromocytoma may have had undiagnosed symptoms for some time, but stress, abdominal palpation, parturition, general anaesthetic, or contrast media used in imaging can cause acute *hypertensive crises*.

Signs and symptoms Pallor, pulsating headache, hypertension, feels 'about to die', pyrexial. *ECG*: signs of LVF, ↑ST segment, VT, and cardiogenic shock.

Treatment ►Get help. Take to ICU.

Principle is combined α- and β-adrenoreceptor blockade, but α must be started first, as unopposed β-blockade can worsen hypertension.

- Start with short-acting, IV α-blocker, eg phentolamine 2-5mg IV. Repeat to maintain safe BP.
- When BP controlled, give long-acting α-blocker, eg phenoxybenzamine 10mg/24h PO (increase by 10mg/d as needed, up to 30mg/12h PO); SE: postural hypotension; dizziness; tachycardia; nasal congestion; miosis; idiosyncratic marked BP drop after 1st dose. The idea is to ↑ the dose until BP is controlled and there is no significant postural hypotension. Alternative α_1-selective blockers, eg doxazosin, are preferred in some centres, particularly if surgery is not an option, eg metastatic tumour.
- A β_1-blocker may also be given at this stage to control any tachycardia or myocardial ischaemia/dysrhythmias (p114).
- Surgery is usually done electively after 4-6wks to allow full α-blockade and volume expansion. When admitted for surgery the phenoxybenzamine dose is increased until significant postural hypotension occurs.

Acute poisoning—general measures

Diagnosis Mainly from the history. The patient may not tell the truth about what has been taken. If there are any tablets with the patient, use *MIMS Colour Index*, *EMIMS* images, *BNF* descriptions, or the computerized system 'TICTAC' (ask pharmacy) to identify tablets and plan specific treatment.

TOXBASE The best resource for managing acute poisoning: www.toxbase.org—check with your Emergency Department about log-in details for your hospital.

Clues May become apparent from examination:
- *Fast or irregular pulse:* Salbutamol, antimuscarinics, tricyclics, quinine, or phenothiazine poisoning.
- *Respiratory depression:* Opiate (p842) or benzodiazepine (p842) toxicity.
- *Hypothermia:* Phenothiazines (p843), barbiturates.
- *Hyperthermia:* Amphetamines, MAOIs, cocaine, or ecstasy (p843).
- *Coma:* Benzodiazepines, alcohol, opiates, tricyclics, or barbiturates.
- *Seizures:* Recreational drugs, hypoglycaemic agents, tricyclics, phenothiazines, or theophyllines.
- *Constricted pupils:* Opiates (p842) or insecticides (organophosphates, p843).
- *Dilated pupils:* Amphetamines, cocaine, quinine, or tricyclics.
- *Hyperglycaemia:* Organophosphates, theophyllines, or MAOIs.
- *Hypoglycaemia:* (p834) Insulin, oral hypoglycaemics, alcohol, or salicylates.
- *Renal impairment:* Salicylate (p844), paracetamol (p844), or ethylene glycol.
- *Metabolic acidosis:* Alcohol, ethylene glycol, methanol, paracetamol, or carbon monoxide poisoning (p842).
- ↑*Osmolality:* Alcohols (ethyl or methyl); ethylene glycol. See p668.

Management ►See fig 19.25.
- *Take blood* as appropriate (p840). Always check paracetamol and salicylate levels.
- *Empty stomach* if appropriate (p840).
- *Consider specific antidote* (p842) or oral activated charcoal (p840).
- *If you are not familiar with the poison* get more information. *Toxbase* (www.toxbase.org) should be your first thought. If no information here or in doubt how best to act, phone the Poisons Information Service: in the UK phone 0844 892 0111.

Continuing care Measure temperature, pulse, BP, and blood glucose regularly. Keep on cardiac monitor. If unconscious, nurse semi-prone, turn regularly. Catherize if the bladder is distended, or acute kidney injury (p298) is suspected, or forced diuresis undertaken. Consider ICU, eg if ↓respiration.

Psychiatric assessment Be sympathetic despite the hour! Interview relatives and friends if possible. Aim to establish:
- *Intentions at time.* Was this a suicide attempt, if so was the act planned? What precautions against being found? Did the patient seek help afterwards? Does the patient think the method was dangerous? Was there a final act (eg suicide note)?
- *Present intentions.* Do they still feel suicidal? Do they wish it had worked?
- *What problems* led to the act: do they still exist?
- Is there a *psychiatric disorder* (depression, alcoholism, personality disorder, schizophrenia, dementia)?
- What are the patient's *resources* (friends, family, work, personality)?

The assessment of suicide risk: The following ↑ chance of future suicide: original intention was to die; present intention is to die; presence of psychiatric disorder; poor resources; previous suicide attempts; socially isolated; unemployed; male; >50yrs old. See *OHCS* p358. There is ↑risk of death in the first year following initial presentation.

Referral to psychiatrist: This depends partly on local resources. Refer all with presence of psychiatric disorder or high suicide risk. Consider discussing all presentations with deliberate self-poisoning.

Mental Capacity Act or the Mental Health Act: (In England and Wales) may provide for the detention of the patient against his or her will: see *OHCS* p406.

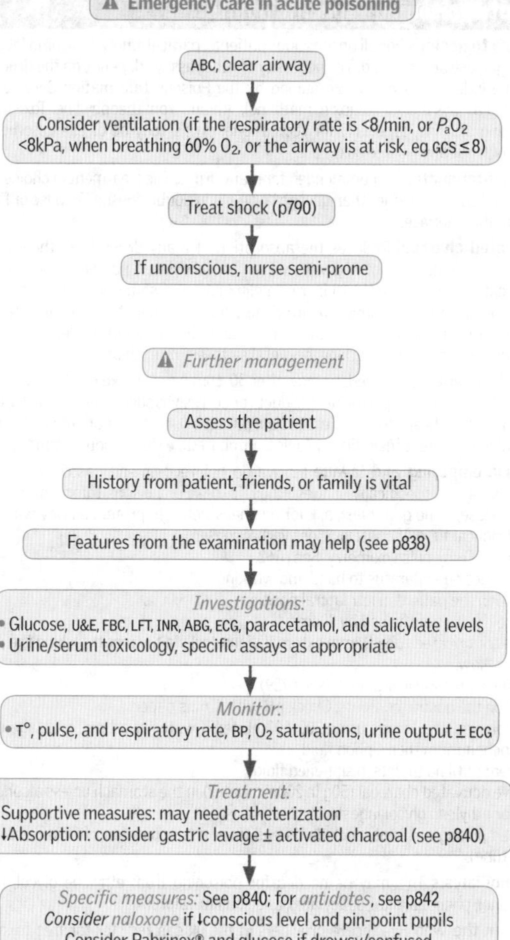

Emergency care in acute poisoning
ABC, clear airway
Consider ventilation (if the respiratory rate is <8/min, or P_aO_2 <8kPa, when breathing 60% O_2, or the airway is at risk, eg GCS ≤8)
Treat shock (p790)
If unconscious, nurse semi-prone
Further management
Assess the patient
History from patient, friends, or family is vital
Features from the examination may help (see p838)
Investigations:
• Glucose, U&E, FBC, LFT, INR, ABG, ECG, paracetamol, and salicylate levels
• Urine/serum toxicology, specific assays as appropriate
Monitor:
• T°, pulse, and respiratory rate, BP, O_2 saturations, urine output ± ECG
Treatment:
• Supportive measures: may need catheterization
• ↓Absorption: consider gastric lavage ± activated charcoal (see p840)
Specific measures: See p840; for antidotes, see p842
Consider naloxone if ↓conscious level and pin-point pupils
Consider Pabrinex® and glucose if drowsy/confused

Fig 19.25 Emergency care in acute poisoning.

Acute poisoning—specific points

Plasma toxicology For all unconscious patients, paracetamol and aspirin levels and blood glucose are required. The necessity of other assays depends on the drug taken and the index of suspicion. Be guided by the Poisons Information Service. More common assays include: digoxin; methanol; lithium; iron; theophylline. Toxicological screening of urine, especially for recreational drugs, may be of use in some cases (although not always, see BOX).

GI decontamination Recommended for many drugs. The treatment of choice is now activated charcoal rather than gastric lavage. If in doubt, consult Toxbase or Poisons Information Service.

Activated charcoal Reduces the absorption of many drugs from the gut when given as a single dose of 50g with water, eg salicylates, paracetamol. It is given in repeated doses (50g/4h) to increase elimination of some drugs from the blood, eg carbamazepine, dapsone, theophyllines, quinine, phenobarbital, and paraquat. Lower doses are used in children. Do not use with petroleum products, corrosives, alcohols, clofenotane, malathion, or metal salts (eg iron, lithium).

Gastric lavage Rarely used. Lavage after 30-60min may make matters worse. ►*Do not empty stomach* if petroleum products or corrosives such as acids, alkalis, bleach, descalers have been ingested (*exception:* paraquat), or if the patient is unconscious or unable to protect their airway (unless intubated). ►Never induce vomiting.

Gastric emptying and lavage NB: we do not recommend gastric lavage is attempted unless specifically suggested by Toxbase or Poisons Information Service. If comatose, or no gag reflex, ask for an anaesthetist to protect airway with cuffed endotracheal tube. If conscious, get verbal consent.

- Monitor O_2 by pulse oximetry. See p162.
- Have suction apparatus to hand and working.
- Position the patient in left lateral position.
- Raise the foot of the bed by 20cm.
- Pass a lubricated tube (14mm external diameter) via the mouth, asking the patient to swallow.
- Confirm position in stomach (see p759).
- Siphon the gastric contents. Check pH with litmus paper.
- Perform gastric lavage using 300-600mL tepid water at a time. Massage the left hypochondrium then siphon fluid.
- Repeat until no tablets in siphoned fluid.
- Leave activated charcoal (50g in 200mL water) in the stomach unless alcohol, iron, Li^+, or ethylene glycol ingested.
- When pulling out tube, occlude its end (prevents aspiration of fluid remaining in the tube).

Haemodialysis This may be needed for poisoning from ethylene glycol, lithium, methanol, phenobarbital, salicylates, and sodium valproate.

Help on the web Healthcare providers in the UK can register for free toxological advice at www.toxbase.org or call 0344 892 0111 for Poisons Information Service.

Legal highs

Increasingly, 'designer' drugs, with chemical properties similar to illegal drugs (but yet sufficiently distinct to fall outside current legislation), are leading to acute poisoning and complications requiring admission. These drugs pose a difficult problem for the admitting physician, as the precise chemistry and mechanisms of action of both the active compound as well as any impurities are often unclear. Although many are legal, they can be as deadly as many well-known recreational drugs, leading to death or life-threatening complications such as rhabdomyolysis. Be aware that these drugs are out there, and ask specifically about legal highs when taking a history, as there are often no screening tools for these drugs.

Some specific poisons and their antidotes

Benzodiazepines Flumazenil (for respiratory arrest) 200mcg over 15s; then 100mcg at 60s intervals if needed. Usual dose range: 300-600mcg IV over 3-6min (up to 1mg; 2mg if on ICU). May provoke fits. Use only after expert advice.

β-blockers Severe bradycardia or hypotension. Try atropine up to 3mg IV. Give glucagon 2-10mg IV bolus + 5% glucose if atropine fails then infusion of 50mcg/kg/h. Also consider including phosphodiesterase inhibitor infusions (eg enoximone 5-20mcg/kg/min). If unresponsive, consider pacing.

Cyanide This fast-killing poison has affinity for Fe^{3+}, and inhibits the cytochrome system, ↓aerobic respiration (therefore patients are acidotic with raised lactate). Depending on degree of poisoning presentation can be:

- *Mild:* Dizziness, anxiety, tachycardia, nausea, drowsiness/confusion.
- *Moderate:* Vomiting, reduced consciousness, convulsions, cyanosis.
- *Severe:* Deep coma, fixed unreactive pupils, cardiorespiratory failure, arrhythmias, pulmonary oedema.

Treatment: ▸▸100% O_2, GI decontamination. If mild, supportive care is usually sufficient. If moderate/severe then specific treatment to bind cyanide is required. Give sodium nitrite/sodium thiosulfate, or dicobalt edetate 300mg IV over 1min, then 50mL 50% glucose IV (repeat once if no response after a minute); or hydroxocobalamin (Cyanokit®) 5g over 15min repeated once if required. *Get expert help.* See p847.

Carbon monoxide Despite hypoxaemia skin is pink (or pale), not blue, as carboxyhaemoglobin (COHb) displaces O_2 from Hb binding sites. For the same reasons SpO_2 from a pulse oximeter may be normal. Check ABG in a co-oximeter (ie ensure it measures haemoglobin, SaO_2, Meth-Hb and COHb) which will show low SaO_2 and high COHb (normal <5%). *Symptoms:* Headache, vomiting, ↑pulse, tachypnoea, and, if COHb >50%, fits, coma, and cardiac arrest.

Treatment: ▸▸Remove the source. Give 100% O_2 until COHb <10%. Metabolic acidosis usually responds to correction of hypoxia. If severe, anticipate cerebral oedema and give mannitol IVI (p831). Confirm diagnosis with an ABG quickly as levels may soon return to normal. Monitor ECG. If COHb >20%, patient has neurological or psychological features, or cardiovascular impairment, fails to respond to treatment, or is pregnant, consider hyperbaric O_2: discuss with the poisons service.

Digoxin *Symptoms:* ↓Cognition, yellow-green visual halos, arrhythmias, nausea, and anorexia. If serious arrhythmias are present, correct hypokalaemia, and inactivate with digoxin-specific antibody fragments (DigiFab®). If load or level is unknown, give 20 vials (800mg)—adult or child >20kg.

Heavy metals Enlist expert help.

Iron Desferrioxamine 15mg/kg/h IVI; max 80mg/kg/d. NB: gastric lavage if iron ingestion in last hour; consider whole-bowel irrigation.

Oral anticoagulants See p351. If major bleed, give vitamin K 5mg slow IV and prothrombin complex concentrate 50U/kg IV (or if unavailable, fresh frozen plasma 15mL/kg IVI). For abnormal INR with no (or minimal) bleeding, see *BNF*. If it is vital that anticoagulation continues, enlist expert help. Discuss with haematology. NB: coagulation defects may be delayed for 2-3d following ingestion.

Opiates (Many analgesics contain opiates.) Give naloxone, eg 0.4-2mg IV; repeat every 2min until breathing is adequate (it has a short $t½$, so it may need to be given often or IM; max ~10mg). Naloxone may precipitate features of opiate withdrawal—diarrhoea and cramps, which will normally respond to diphenoxylate and atropine (eg co-phenotrope). Sedate as needed (see p15). High-dose opiate misusers may need methadone (eg 10-30mg/24h PO) to combat withdrawal. Refer for help (*OHCS* p374).

Phenothiazine poisoning (Eg chlorpromazine.) No specific antidote. *Dystonia* (torticollis, retrocollis, glossopharyngeal dystonia, opisthotonus): try procyclidine, eg 5-10mg IM or IV. Treat shock by raising the legs (± plasma expander IVI, or inotropes if desperate). Restore body temperature. *Monitor ECG*. Use lorazepam IV for prolonged fits in the usual way (p826). *Neuroleptic malignant syndrome* consists of: hyperthermia, rigidity, extrapyramidal signs, autonomic dysfunction (labile BP, ↑HR, sweating, urinary incontinence), mutism, confusion, coma, ↑WCC, ↑CK; it may be treated with cooling. Dantrolene 1-2.5mg/kg IV (p572) (max 10mg/kg/day) can help, bromocriptine and amantadine are alternatives.

Carbon tetrachloride poisoning This solvent, used in many industrial processes, causes vomiting, abdominal pain, diarrhoea, seizures, coma, renal failure, and tender hepatomegaly with jaundice and liver failure. IV acetylcysteine may improve prognosis. Seek expert help.

Organophosphate insecticides Inactivate cholinesterase—the resulting increase in acetylcholine causes the **SLUD** response: **s**alivation, **l**acrimation, **u**rination, and **di**arrhoea. Also look for sweating, small pupils, muscle fasciculation, coma, respiratory distress, and bradycardia. *Treatment:* Wear gloves; remove soiled clothes. Wash skin. Take blood (FBC and serum cholinesterase activity). Give atropine IV 2mg every 10min till full atropinization (skin dry, pulse >70, pupils dilated). Up to 3d treatment may be needed. Also give pralidoxime 30mg/kg IVI over 20min, then 8mg/kg/h, max 12g in 24h. Even if fits are not occurring, diazepam 5-10mg IV slowly seems to help.

Paraquat poisoning (Found in weed-killers.) This causes D&V, painful oral ulcers, alveolitis, and renal failure. Diagnose by urine test. Give activated charcoal at once (100g followed by a laxative, then 50g/3-4h). ►*Get expert help.* Avoid O_2 early on (promotes lung damage).

Ecstasy poisoning Ecstasy is a semi-synthetic, hallucinogenic substance (MDMA, 3,4-methylenedioxymethamphetamine). Its effects range from nausea, muscle pain, blurred vision, amnesia, fever, confusion, and ataxia to tachyarrhythmias, hyperthermia, hyper/hypotension, water intoxication, DIC, ↑K^+, acute kidney injury (AKI), hepatocellular and muscle necrosis, cardiovascular collapse, and ARDS. There is no antidote and treatment is supportive. Management depends on clinical and lab findings, but may include:

- Administration of activated charcoal and monitoring of BP, ECG, and temperature for at least 12h (rapid cooling may be needed).
- Monitor urine output and U&E (AKI pp298-9), LFT, CK, FBC, and coagulation (DIC p352). Metabolic acidosis may benefit from treatment with bicarbonate.
- Anxiety: lorazepam 1-2mg IV as a slow bolus into a large vein. Repeat doses may be administered until agitation is controlled (see p826).
- Narrow complex tachycardias (p806) in adults: consider metoprolol 5mg IV.
- Hypertension can be treated with nifedipine 5-10mg PO or phentolamine 2-5mg IV. Treat hypotension conventionally (p790).
- Hyperthermia: attempt to cool, if rectal T° >39°C consider dantrolene 1mg/kg IV (may need repeating: discuss with your senior and a poisons unit). Hyperthermia with ecstasy is akin to serotonin syndrome, and propranolol, muscle relaxation, and ventilation may be needed.

Snakes (adders) *Anaphylaxis:* p794. *Signs of envenoming:* ↓BP (vasodilation, viper cardiotoxicity); D&V; swelling spreading proximally within 4h of bite; bleeding gums or venepuncture sites; anaphylaxis; ptosis; trismus; rhabdomyolysis; pulmonary oedema. *Tests:* ↑WCC; abnormal clotting; ↓platelets; U&E; ↑urine RBC; ↑CK; ↓P_aO_2, ECG. *Management:* Avoid active movement of affected limb (so use splints/slings). *Avoid incisions and tourniquets.* ►Get help from local/national poisons service. Is antivenom indicated (IgG from venom-immunized sheep)?—eg 10mL IV over 15min (adults *and* children) of *European Viper Antiserum* (from Monviato) for adder bites (see *BNF*);—20mL if severe envenoming have adrenaline to hand—p794. Monitor ECG. For non-UK endemic snakes, see *BNF*.

Paracetamol poisoning

12g (=24 tablets) or 150mg/kg in adults may be fatal. ►If the patient weighs >110kg, calculate ingested dose using a body weight of 110kg to avoid underestimating toxicity. If the patient is malnourished then 75mg/kg can kill.

Signs and symptoms None initially, or vomiting ± RUQ pain. Later: jaundice and encephalopathy from liver damage (the main danger) ± acute kidney injury (AKI).

Management *General measures:* See p838. GI decontamination is recommended in those presenting <4h after overdose: give activated charcoal 1g/kg (max 50g).

- Glucose, U&E, LFT, INR, ABG, FBC, HCO_3^-; blood paracetamol level at 4h post-ingestion.
- If <10-12h since overdose, not vomiting, and plasma paracetamol is above the line on the graph (see fig 19.26), start acetylcysteine.
- If >8-24h and suspicion of large overdose (>7.5g) err on the side of caution and start acetylcysteine, stopping it if level below treatment line and INR/ALT normal.
- If ingestion time is unknown, or it is staggered, or presentation is >15h from ingestion, treatment *may* still help. ►Get advice.

Acetylcysteine is given by IVI: 150mg/kg in 5% glucose over 15-60min; then 50mg/kg in 500mL of 5% glucose over 4h; then 100mg/kg/16h in 1L of 5% glucose. Rash is a common SE: treat with chlorphenamine + observe; do not stop unless anaphylatoid reaction with shock, vomiting, and wheeze (occur <10%). An alternative (if acetylcysteine unavailable) is methionine 2.5g/4h PO for 16h (total: 10g), but absorption is unreliable if vomiting.

Ongoing management

- Next day do INR, U&E, LFT. If INR rising, continue acetylcysteine until <1.4.
- If continued deterioration, discuss with the liver team. Don't hesitate to get help.
- Consider referral to specialist liver unit guided by eg King's College criteria (BOX, p275).

Salicylate poisoning

Aspirin is a weak acid with poor water solubility. It is present in many over-the-counter preparations. Uncoupling of oxidative phosphorylation leads to anaerobic metabolism and the production of lactate and heat. Effects are dose related and potentially fatal: •150mg/kg: mild toxicity. •250mg/kg: moderate •>500mg/kg: severe toxicity. Levels over 700mg/L are potentially fatal.

Signs and symptoms Unlike paracetamol, there are many early features:

- Vomiting, dehydration, hyperventilation, tinnitus, vertigo, sweating.
- Rarely ↓GCS, seizures, ↓BP and heart block, pulmonary oedema, hyperthermia.

Patients present initially with respiratory alkalosis due to a direct stimulation of the central respiratory centres and then develop a metabolic acidosis. Hyper- or hypoglycaemia may occur.

Management *General:* (pp838-9.) Correct dehydration. Keep patient on ECG monitor Give activated charcoal to all presenting ≤1h—consider even if delayed presentation, slow-release formations, or bezoar formation (can delay absorption): at least one dose of 1g/kg (max 50g). Consider repeat doses (two further doses of 50g, 4h apart).

1. *Bloods.* Paracetamol and salicylate level, glucose, U&E, LFT, INR, ABG, HCO_3^-, FBC Salicylate level may need to be repeated after 2h, due to continuing absorption if a potentially toxic dose has been taken. Monitor blood glucose 1-2hrly, beware hypoglycaemia, if severe poisoning, monitor salicylate levels, serum pH, and U&E
2. *Urine.* Check pH, consider catheterization to monitor output and pH.
3. *Correct acidosis.* If plasma salicylate level >500mg/L (3.6mmol/L) or severe metabolic acidosis, consider alkalinization of the urine, eg with 1.5L 1.26% sodium bicarbonate IV over 3h. Aim for urine pH 7.5-8. NB: monitor serum K^+ as hypokalaemia may occur, and should be treated (caution if AKI).
4. *Dialysis* may well be needed if salicylate level >700mg/L, and if AKI or heart failure, pulmonary or cerebral oedema, confusion or seizures, severe acidosis despite best medical therapy, or persistently ↑plasma salicylate. Contact nephrology early.

Discuss any serious cases with the local toxicological service or national poisons information service.

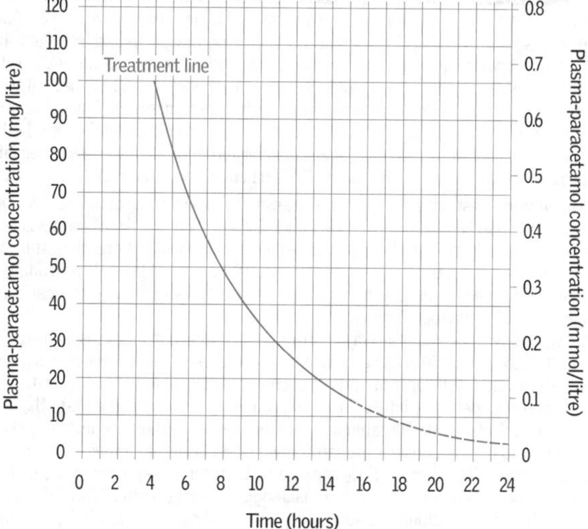

Fig 19.26 Plasma concentration of paracetamol vs time, see p844 for interpretation. The graph may mislead if HIV +ve (↓hepatic glutathione), or if long-acting paracetamol has been taken, or if pre-existing liver disease or induction of liver enzymes has occurred.

Reproduced from *Drug Safety Update* September 2012, vol 6, issue 2: A1 © Crown Copyright 2013.

►►Burns

Assessment *Burn size* is important to assess as it influences the size of the inflammatory response (vasodilation, increased vascular permeability) and thus fluid shift from the intravascular volume. Use Lund and Browder charts (see fig 19.27) or the *'rule of nines'* (arm: 9%; front of trunk 18%; head and neck 9%; leg 18%; back of trunk 18%; perineum 1%). Ignore erythema. *Burn depth* determines healing time/scarring; assessing this can be hard, even for the experienced. The big distinction is whether the burn is partial thickness (painful, red, and blistered) or full thickness (insensate/painless; grey-white). NB: burns can evolve, particularly over the first 48h.

Resuscitation Resuscitate and arrange transfer to specialist burns unit for all major burns (>25% partial thickness in adults and >20% in children). Assess site, size, and depth of burn (fig 19.27, to help calculate fluid requirements). Referral is still warranted in cases of full thickness burns >5%, partial thickness burns >10% in adults or >5% in children or the elderly, burns of special sites, chemical and electrical burns, and burns with inhalational injury.

- *Airway:* Beware of upper airway obstruction developing if hot gases inhaled. Suspect if history of fire in enclosed space, soot in oral/nasal cavity, singed nasal hairs or hoarse voice. A flexible laryngo/bronchoscopy is useful. Involve anaesthetists early and consider early intubation. Obstruction can develop in the first 24h.
- *Breathing:* Exclude life-threatening chest injuries (eg tension pneumothorax) and constricting burns—consider escharotomy if chest burns are impairing thorax excursion (*OHCS* p766). Give 100% O_2. Suspect carbon monoxide poisoning (p842) from history, cherry-red skin, and carboxyhaemoglobin level (COHb). With 100% O_2 $t½$ of COHb falls from 250min to 40min (consider hyperbaric O_2 if: pH<7.1; CNS signs; >25% COHb or >20% if pregnant). SpO_2 (oximetry) is unreliable in CO poisoning.
- *Circulation:* Partial thickness burns >10% in a child and >15% in adults require IV fluid resuscitation. Put up 2 large-bore (14G or 16G) IV lines. Do not worry if you have to put these through burned skin; intraosseous access is valuable in infants and can be used in adults (see *OHCS* p236). Secure them well: they are literally lifelines.

Use a *burns calculator* flow chart or a formula, eg: *Parkland formula* (popular): 4 × weight (kg) × % burn = mL Hartmann's solution in 24h, half given in 1st 8h. Replace fluid from the time of burn, not from the time first seen in hospital. *Formulae are only guides:* adjust IVI according to clinical response and urine output; aim for 0.5mL/kg/h (1mL/kg/h in children), ~50% more in electrical burns and inhalation injury. Monitor T° (core and surface); catheterize the bladder. Beware of over-resuscitation ('fluid creep') which can lead to complications such as abdominal compartment syndrome.

Treatment 'Cool the burn, warm the patient.' Do *not* apply cold water to extensive burns for long periods: this may intensify shock. Take care with circumferential full-thickness burns of the limbs as compartment syndrome may develop rapidly particularly after fluid resuscitation. Decompress (escharotomy and fasciotomy) as needed. If transferring to a burns unit, do not burst blisters or apply any special creams as this can hinder assessment. Simple saline gauze or paraffin gauze is suitable; cling film is useful as a temporary measure and relieves pain. Titrate morphine IV for good analgesia. Ensure tetanus immunity. Antibiotic prophylaxis is not routinely used.

Definitive dressings There are many dressings for partial thickness burns, eg biological (pigskin, cadaveric skin), synthetic, and silver sulfadiazine cream alone or with cerium nitrate as Flammacerium®; it forms a leathery eschar which resists infection. Major full-thickness burns benefit from early tangential excision and split-skin grafts as the burn is a major source of inflammatory cytokines and forms a rich medium for bacterial growth.

Smoke inhalation

Consider if:

- History of exposure to fire and smoke in an enclosed space
- Hoarseness or change in voice
- Harsh cough
- Stridor.
- Burns to face
- Singed nasal hairs
- Soot in saliva or sputum
- Inflamed oropharynx

Initially laryngospasm leads to hypoxia and straining (leading to petechiae), then hypoxic cord relaxation leads to true inhalation injury. Free radicals, cyanide compounds, and carbon monoxide (CO) accompany thermal injury. Cyanide (p842) compounds (generated, eg from burning plastics) stop oxidative phosphorylation, causing dizziness, headaches, and seizures. Tachycardia + dyspnoea soon give way to bradycardia + apnoea. CO is generated later in the fire as oxygen is depleted. NB: COHb levels do not correlate well with the severity of poisoning and partly reflect smoking status and urban life. Use nomograms to extrapolate peak levels.

►►100% O_2 is given to elute both cyanide and CO.

►►Involve ICU/anaesthetists early if any signs of airway obstruction or respiratory failure: early intubation and ventilation may be useful.

►►Enlist expert help in cyanide poisoning—see p842.

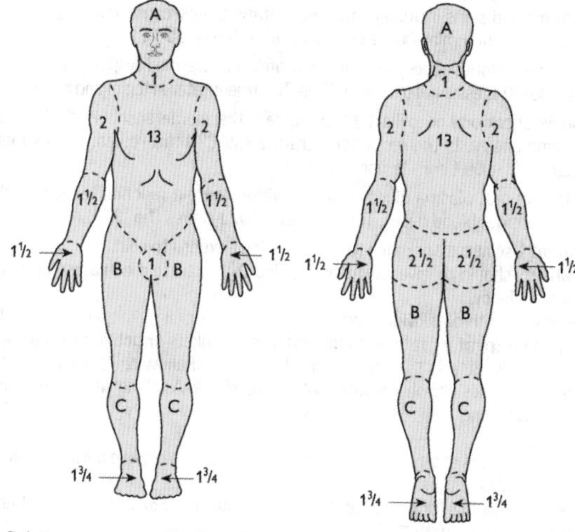

Relative percentage of body surface area affected by growth

Area	Age 0	1	5	10	15	Adult
A: half of head	9½	8½	6½	5½	4½	3½
B: half of thigh	2¾	3¼	4	4¼	4½	4¾
C: half of leg	2½	2½	2¾	3	3¼	3½

g 19.27 Lund and Browder charts.

knowledgement

: thank Professor Tor Chiu for help in preparing this topic.

Hypothermia

►*Have a high index of suspicion and a low-reading thermometer.* Most patients are elderly and do not complain of, or feel, cold—so they have not tried to warm up. In the young, hypothermia is usually from cold exposure (eg near-drowning), or is secondary to impaired consciousness (eg following excess alcohol or drug overdose).

Definition Hypothermia implies a core (rectal) temperature <35°C.

Causes In the elderly, hypothermia is often caused by a combination of factors:
- Impaired homeostatic mechanisms: usually age-related.
- Low room temperature: poverty, poor housing.
- Impaired thermoregulation: pneumonia, MI, heart failure.
- Reduced metabolism: immobility, hypothyroidism, diabetes mellitus.
- Autonomic neuropathy (p505); eg diabetes mellitus, Parkinson's.
- Excess heat loss: psoriasis and any other widespread dermatological diseases (ie TEN, erythrodermic eczema).
- ↓Cold awareness: dementia, confusion.
- Increased exposure to cold: falls, especially at night when cold.
- Drugs: major tranquillizers, antidepressants, diuretics, alcohol.

The patient
- If the patient is shivering then the hypothermia is mild, if they are not shivering despite temp <35°C then the hypothermia is severe.
- Symptoms and signs include confusion, agitation, ↓GCS, coma, bradycardia, hypotension and arrhythmias (AF, VT, VF), especially if temp <30°C.

There are many stories of people 'returning to life' when warmed despite absence of vital signs, see BOX. It is essential to rewarm (see 'Treatment' later in topic) and re-examine.

Diagnosis Check oral or axillary T°. If ordinary thermometer shows <36.5°C, use low-reading one PR. Is the rectal temperature <35°C? Infra-red ear thermometers can accurately reflect core temperature.

Tests Urgent U&E, plasma glucose, and amylase. Thyroid function tests; FBC; blood cultures. Consider blood gases. The ECG may show J-waves (fig 19.28).

Treatment Use ABCDE approach (p779)—but don't expose to cold.
- All patients should receive warm, humidified O_2; ventilate if comatose or respiratory insufficiency.
- Remove wet clothing, *slowly rewarm*, aiming for rise of ½°C/h (check temperature, BP, HR, and respiratory rate every 30min) using blankets or active external warming (hot air duvets). If T° rising too quickly stop and allow to cool slightly. Rapid rewarming causes peripheral vasodilation and shock. A falling BP can be a sign of too rapid warming.
- Warm IVI.
- Cardiac monitor is essential (AF, VF, and VT can occur at any time during rewarming or on stimulation).
- Consider antibiotics for the prevention of pneumonia (p166). Give these routinely to patients over 65yrs with T° <32°C.
- Consider urinary catheter (to monitor renal function).

NB: in sudden hypothermia from immersion or profound hypothermia with cardiovascular instability/cardiac arrest, the temperature needs to be raised rapidly. Options include warmed fluid lavage (intravesical, nasogastric, intrapleural, intraperitoneal) and intravascular warming (cardiopulmonary bypass, dialysis). In the event of cardiac arrest, defibrillation is usually unsuccessful if T° <30°C (consider amiodarone or bretylium). Resuscitation must continue until core T° >33°C (*OHCS* p786).

Complications Arrhythmias (if there is a cardiac arrest continue resuscitating until T° >33°C, as cold brains are less damaged by hypoxia); pneumonia; pancreatitis; A DIC. *Prognosis:* Depends on age and degree of hypothermia. If age >70yrs and <32°C then mortality >50%.

Before hospital discharge Anticipate problems. Will it happen again? What their network of support? Review medication (could you stop tranquillizers)? How progress to be monitored? Liaise with GP/social worker.

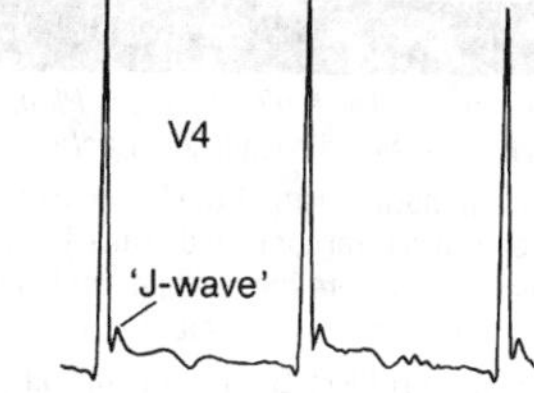

Fig 19.28 J-wave in hypothermia.
Courtesy of Dr R Luke and Dr E McLachlan.

'I did not die but nothing of life remained...'

Remember that death is a process not an event, and that in hypothermia, *all* processes are suspended: metabolism may slow to as much as 10% of baseline, drastically diminishing the oxygen requirements of all tissues. Perhaps this is what Dante had in mind for the last round of the 9th circle of *Hell*, in which those betraying their benefactors are encased in ice (*canto XXXIV*) 'Com'io divenni allor gelato e fioco...Io non mori e non rimasi vivo—How frozen I then became: I did not die but nothing of life remained'.

Human records: 13 month old Canadian Erica Nordby came to life 2 hours after her heart stopped (core T°: 16°C). Anna Bågenholm, a Swedish trainee orthopaedic surgeon, became trapped under freezing water covered by a layer of ice for 80 minutes following a skiing accident, suffering a cardiac arrest (core T°: 13.7°C). After resuscitation and 20 days in intensive care, she regained consciousness, suffering no permanent brain damage. She is now a radiologist. ►Do not declare anybody dead until they are warm and dead.

Major disasters

Planning All hospitals have a detailed *Major Incident Plan*, but additionally the tasks of key personnel can be distributed on individual *Action Cards*.

At the scene Call the police to notify them of the Major Incident and ask them to take command. They will set up a central command centre to assess and manage the incident, depending on casualty numbers they will inform multiple hospitals of the need to prepare for the imminent arrival of casualties.

Safety: Paramount—your own and others. Be visible (luminous monogrammed jacket) and wear protective clothing where appropriate (safety helmet; waterproofs; boots; respirator in chemical environment).

Triage: See OHCS p800. There are several commercial systems available to label patients so emergency personnel can see at a glance the scale of the incident. The key is to divide patients by the urgency of care/transfer to hospital:

1. Emergency (label **RED** = will die in a few minutes if no treatment)
2. Urgent (label YELLOW =will die in ~2h if no treatment)
3. Non-urgent (label **GREEN** = walking wounded/those who are stable and can wait)
4. Deceased (label **BLUE/WHITE**).

Communications: Essential; each emergency service will dispatch a control vehicle and will have a designated incident officer for liaison. Support medical staff from hospital report to the medical incident officer (MIO)—he or she is usually the first doctor on the scene. Their job is to assess then communicate to the receiving hospital the number + severity of casualties, to organize resupply of equipment and to replace fatigued staff. The MIO must resist temptation to treat casualties as this compromises their role.

Equipment: Must be portable and include: intubation and cricothyrotomy set; intravenous fluids (colloid); bandages and dressings; chest drain (+flutter valve); amputation kit (when used, ideally 2 doctors should concur); drugs—*analgesic:* morphine *anaesthetic:* ketamine 2mg/kg IV over >60s (0.5mg/kg is a powerful analgesic without respiratory depression); limb splints (may be inflatable); defibrillator/monitor ± pulse oximeter.

Evacuation: Remember that with immediate treatment on scene, the priority for evacuation may be reduced (eg a tension pneumothorax—**RED**—once relieved can wait for evacuation and becomes YELLOW), but those who may suffer by delay at the scene must go first. Send any severed limbs to the same hospital as the patient ideally chilled—but not frozen.

At the hospital A 'major incident' is declared. The *first receiving* hospital will take most of the casualties; the *support* hospital(s) will cope with overflow and may provide mobile teams so that staff are not depleted from the first hospital. A control room is established and the medical coordinator ensures staff have been summoned and informed of their roles, nominates a triage officer, and supervises the best use of inpatient beds and ICU/theatre resources.

Blast injuries

These may be caused by domestic (eg gas explosion) or industrial (eg mining) accidents, or by terrorist bombs. Death may occur without any obvious external injury. Injury occurs in a number of ways:

1. *Blast wave:* A transient (milliseconds) wave of overpressure expands rapidly producing cellular disruption, shearing forces along tissue planes (submucosal/subserosal haemorrhage) and re-expansion of compressed trapped gas—bowel perforation, fatal air embolism.
2. *Blast wind:* This can totally disrupt a body or cause avulsive amputations. Bodies can be thrown and sustain injuries on landing.
3. *Missiles:* Penetration or laceration from missiles are by far the commonest injuries. Missiles arise from the bomb or are secondary, eg glass.
4. *Flash burns:* These are usually superficial and occur on exposed skin.
5. *Crush injuries:* Beware sudden death or acute kidney injury from rhabdomyolysis after release.
6. *Contamination:* There is increasing concern about the use of biological or radioactive material in terrorist bombs. Even domestic or industrial blasts can scatter chemicals widely and cause both superficial and penetrating contamination. Consider the location and mechanism of the blast, and seek advice.
7. *Psychological injury:* Eg post-traumatic stress disorder (*OHCS* p353).

Treatment: Approach the same as any major trauma (*OHCS* p778). Rest and observe any suspected of exposure to significant blast but without other injury. Gun-shot injury: see *OHCS* p789. Major blast injuries, whatever the cause, should be reported to the police for investigation.

Contents

Chapter 1: Thinking about medicine

1 Davis K, Stremikis K, Squires D, *et al. Mirror, mirror on the wall: How the performance of the U healthcare system compares internationally*. New York: The Commonwealth Fund, 2014. http://www.com monwealthfund.org/publications/fund-reports/2014/jun/mirror-mirror
2 Appleby J. *Spending on health and social care over the next 50 years. Why think long term?* Lo don: The Kings Fund, 2013. https://www.kingsfund.org.uk/time-to-think-differently/publications/spendin health-and-social-care-over-next-50-years
3 Begley A, Pritchard-Jones K, Biriot\i M, *et al*. Listening to patients with cancer: using a literary-base research method to understand patient-focused care. *BMJ Open* 2014; 4(10):e005550. http://bmjopen.bm com/content/4/10/e005550
4 Francis R. *Report of the Mid-Staffordshire NHS Foundation Trust Public Enquiry*. London: The St tionery Office, 2013. http://webarchive.nationalarchives.gov.uk/20150407084003/http://www.midstaffspu licinquiry.com/home
5 Saunders J. Compassion. *Clin Med* 2015; 15:121–4. http://www.clinmed.rcpjournal.org/content/15/2/12 full.pdf+html
6 Mani N, Slevin N, Hudson A. What three wise men have to say about diagnosis. *BMJ* 2011; 343:d776 http://www.bmj.com/content/343/bmj.d7769
7 Klein JG. Five pitfalls in decisions about diagnosis and prescribing. *BMJ* 2005; 330:781–4. http://www.br com/content/330/7494/781
8 Schulz K. *Being wrong: Adventures in the margin of error*. London: Portobello Books, 2011
9 Berlinger N. *After harm: Medical error and the ethics of forgiveness*. Baltimore, MD: John Hopki University Press, 2005
10 Little P, White P, Kelly J, *et al*. Randomised control trial of a brief intervention targeting predominan non-verbal communication in general practice consultations. *Br J Gen Pract* 2015; 65(635):e351–6. http: bjgp.org/content/65/635/e351.long
11 Heath I. A wolf in sheep's clothing: a critical look at the ethics of drug taking. *BMJ* 2003; 327:856. http www.bmj.com/content/327/7419/856
12 Eley D, Wilkinson D, Cloninger CR. Physician understand thyself, and develop your resilience. *BMJ C reers* 2013; 18 April. http://careers.bmj.com/careers/advice/view-article.html?id=20011843
13 Academy of Royal Colleges. *A code of practice for the diagnosis and confirmation of death*. 20 http://www.aomrc.org.uk/publications/reports-guidance/ukdec-reports-and-guidance/code-practic diagnosis-confirmation-death/
14 Steinhauser KE, Christakis NA, Clipp EC, *et al*. Factors considered important at the end of life by p tients, family, physicians, and other care providers. *JAMA* 2000; 284(19):2476–82. http://jamanetwork.co journals/jama/fullarticle/193279
15 Ruegger J, Hodgkinson S, Field-Smith A, *et al*. Care of adults in the last days of life: summary of NI guidance. *BMJ* 2015; 351:h6631. http://www.bmj.com/content/351/bmj.h6631
16 Sokol DK. *Doing clinical ethics: A hands on guide for clinicians and others*. Amsterdam: Spring Netherlands, 2012
17 Sokol DK, McFadzean WA, Dickson WA, *et al*. Ethical dilemmas in the acute setting: a frame-work clinicians. *BMJ* 2011; 343:d5528. http://www.bmj.com/content/343/bmj.d5528.long

18 Huxtable R. For and against the four principles of biomedical ethics. *Clin Ethics* 2013; 8(2/3):39–43

19 NICE. *Depression: The treatment and management of depression in adults* [CG90]. 2009, updated 2016. https://www.nice.org.uk/guidance/CG90

20 NICE. *Violence and aggression: Short-term management in mental health, health and community setting* [NG10]. 2015. https://www.nice.org.uk/guidance/ng10

21 O'Mahony D, O'Sullivan D, Byrne S, *et al.* STOPP/START criteria for potentially inappropriate prescribing in older people: version 2. *Age Ageing* 2015; 44(2):213-8. https://academic.oup.com/ageing/article-lookup/doi/10.1093/ageing/afu145

22 Kurrle SE, Cameron ID, Geeves RB. A quick ward assessment of older patients by junior doctors. *BMJ* 2014: 350:h607. http://www.bmj.com/content/350/bmj.h607

23 NICE. *Falls in older people: Assessing risk and prevention* [CG161]. 2013. https://www.nice.org.uk/guidance/cg161

24 Knight M, Tuffnell D, Kenyon S, *et al.* (eds) on behalf of MBRRACE-UK. *Saving lives, improving mothers' care: surveillance of maternal deaths in the UK 2012-2014 and lessons learned to inform maternity care from the UK and Ireland. Confidential Enquiries into Maternal Deaths and Morbidity 2009-2014*. Oxford: National Perinatal Epidemiology Unit, University of Oxford, 2016

25 Greenhalgh T. *How to read a paper* (5th edn). Oxford: Blackwell Books, 2014

26 Greenland S, Senn SJ, Rothman KJ, *et al.* Statistical tests, P values, confidence intervals, and power: a guide to misinterpretations. *Eur J Epidemiol* 2016; 31:337–50

27 Greenhalgh T, Howick J, Maskrey N. Evidence based medicine: a movement in crisis? *BMJ* 2014; 348:g3725. http://www.bmj.com/content/348/bmj.g3725

Chapter 2: History and examination

Spence D. The world is round. *BMJ* 2008; 336:1134

Magilner D. Localized cervical pruritus as the presenting symptom of a spinal cord tumor. *Pediatr Emerg Care* 2006; 22(10):746–7

Mackowiak PA, Wasserman SS, Levine MM. A critical appraisal of 98.6 degrees F, the upper limit of the normal body temperature, and other legacies of Carl Reinhold August Wunderlich. *JAMA* 1992; 268(12):1578–80. http://jamanetwork.com/journals/jama/article-abstract/400116

Roghmann MC, Warner J, Mackowiak PA. The relationship between age and fever magnitude. *Am J Med Sci* 2001; 322(2):68–90. http://www.sciencedirect.com/science/article/pii/S0002962915346103

Diskin CJ. Towards an understanding of oedema. *BMJ* 1999; 318:1610. http://bmj.com/cgi/content/full/318/7198/1610

Cheung W, Yu PX, Little BM, *et al.* Anorexia and cachexia in renal failure—is leptin the culprit? Role of leptin and melanocortin signaling in uremia-associated cachexia. *J Am Soc Nephrol* 2005; 16:2245–50. http://www.jci.org/articles/view/22521

Rastogi V, Purohit P, Peters BP, *et al.* Pulmonary infection with *Serratia marcescens*. *Indian J Med Microbiol* 2002; 20:167–8. http://www.ijmm.org/text.asp?2002/20/3/167/6946

Koumbourlis AC. Pectus excavatum: pathophysiology and clinical characteristics. *Paediatr Respir Rev* 2009; 10(1):3–6. http://www.prrjournal.com/article/S1526-0542(08)00083-3/abstract

Anglin R, Yuan Y, Moayyedi P, *et al.* Risk of upper gastrointestinal bleeding with selective serotonin reuptake inhibitors with or without concurrent nonsteroidal anti-inflammatory use: a systematic review and meta-analysis. *Am J Gastroenterol* 2014; 109:811–19. http://www.nature.com/ajg/journal/v109/n6/full/ajg201482a.html

NICE. *Depression: The treatment and management of depression in adults* [CG90]. 2009, updated 2016. http://www.nice.org.uk/CG90

Ford AC, Marwaha A, Lim A, *et al.* What is the prevalence of clinically significant endoscopic findings in subjects with dyspepsia? Systematic review and meta-analysis. *Clin Gastroenterol Hepatol* 2010; 8(10):830–7. http://www.ncbi.nlm.nih.gov/pubmed?term=20541625

Hodkinson HM. Evaluation of a mental test score for assessment of mental impairment in the elderly. 1972. *Age and Ageing* 2012; 41 Suppl 3:iii35–40. http://ageing.oxfordjournals.org/content/41/suppl_3/iii35.long

NICE guidelines: Chest pain of recent onset: assessment and diagnosis. Updated Nov 2016. https://www.nice.org.uk/guidance/cg95/chapter/Recommendations#people-presenting-with-stable-chest-pain

Moore C. A functional neuroimaging study of the variables that generate category-specific object processing differences. *Brain* 1999; 122 (Pt 5):943–62. http://brain.oxfordjournals.org/content/122/5/943.long

Assié G, Bahurel H, Bertherat J, *et al.* The Nelson's syndrome... revisited. *Pituitary* 2004; 7:209-15. http://link.springer.com/article/10.1007/s11102-005-1403-y

Dickinson CJ, Martin JF. Megakaryocytes and platelet clumps as the cause of finger clubbing. *Lancet* 1987; 2(8573):1434–5. http://www.thelancet.com/journals/lancet/article/PIIS0140-6736(87)91132-9/abstract

Chapter 3: Cardiovascular medicine

Britton J. Bupropion: a new treatment for smokers. *BMJ* 2000; 321:65. http://www.bmj.com/cgi/content/full/321/7253/65

Hippisley-Cox J. Predicting cardiovascular risk in England and Wales. *BMJ* 2008; 336:1475. http://www.bmj.com/content/336/7659/1475

Josan K, Majumdar SR, McAlister FA. The efficacy and safety of intensive statin therapy: a meta-analysis of randomized trials. *CMAJ* 2008; 178(5):576–84. https://www.ncbi.nlm.nih.gov/pmc/articles/PMC2244680/

Capewell S. "Chest pain—please admit": is there an alternative? *BMJ* 2000; 320:951. http://www.bmj.com/cgi/content/full/320/7240/951

Berk W. Clinical implications of low QRS complex voltage. *J Emerg Med* 1987; 5:305–10

Herzog C, Zwerner PL, Doll JR, *et al.* Significant coronary artery stenosis: comparison on per-patient and per-vessel or per-segment basis at 64-section CT angiography. *Radiology* 2007; 244(1):112–20. http://radiology.rsna.org/con-tent/244/1/112.short

Aspirin for primary prevention of disease. http://www.nyrdtc.nhs.uk/docs/dud/DU_65_Aspirin.pdf

NICE. *Unstable angina and NSTEMI: Early management* [CG94]. 2010, updated 2013. https://www.nice.org.uk/guidance/cg94

9 Nattel S, Opie LH. Controversies in atrial fibrillation. *Lancet* 2006; 367:262. http://www.thelancet.com/journals/lancet/article/PIIS0140-6736(06)68037-9/abstract
10 Behr ER, Veysey MJ, Berry D, *et al.* Optimum dose of digoxin. *Lancet* 1997; 349(9068):1845 http://www.thelancet.com/journals/lancet/article/PIIS0140-6736(05)61735-7/fulltext
11 The Digitalis Investigation Group. The effect of digoxin on mortality and morbidity in patients with heart failure. *N Engl J Med* 1997; 336:525–33. http://www.nejm.org/doi/full/10.1056/NEJM199702203360801
12 NICE. General principles for treating people with stable angina. In *Stable angina: Management* [CG126] Chapter 1.3. 2011, updated 2016. https://www.nice.org.uk/guidance/cg126/chapter/1-Guidance#general-principles-for-treating-people-with-stable-angina
13 NICE. *Chest pain of recent onset: Assessment and diagnosis* [CG95]. 2010, updated 2016. http://www.nice.org.uk/guidance/CG95
14 Roffi M, Patrono C, Collet JP, *et al.* 2015 ESC Guidelines for the management of acute coronary syndromes in patients presenting without persistent ST-segment elevation. *Eur Heart J* 2016; 37(3):267–315 http://eurheartj.oxfordjournals.org/content/37/3/267.long
15 Task Force on the management of ST-segment elevation acute myocardial infarction of the European Society of Cardiology (ESC). ESC Guidelines for the management of acute myocardial infarction in patients presenting with ST-segment elevation. *Eur Heart J* 2012; 33(20):2569–619. http://eurheartj.oxfordjournals.org/content/33/20/2569.long
16 Junghans C. Risk assessment after acute coronary syndrome. *BMJ* 2006; 333:1080. http://www.bmj.com/content/333/7578/1079
17 Lichtman JH, Bigger JT, Blumenthal JA, *et al.* Depression and Coronary Heart Disease: Recommendations for Screening, Referral, and Treatment: A Science Advisory From the American Heart Association Prevention Committee of the Council on Cardiovascular Nursing, Council on Clinical Cardiology, Council on Epidemiology and Prevention, and Interdisciplinary Council on Quality of Care and Outcomes Research: Endorsed by the American Psychiatric Association. *Circulation* 2008; 118:1768–75. http://circ.ahajournals.org/content/118/17/1768.long
18 DVLA. *Cardiovascular disorders: Assessing fitness to drive*. March 2016. https://www.gov.uk/guidance/cardiovascular-disorders-assessing-fitness-to-drive
19 Gorenek B, Lundqvist C, Terradellas J, *et al.* Cardiac arrhythmias in acute coronary syndromes: position paper from the joint EHRA, ACCA, and EAPCI task force. *Eur Heart J Acute Cardiovasc Care* 2015; 4(4):38
20 Matteson EL, Kluge FJ. Think clearly, be sincere, act calmly: Adolf Kussmaul (February 22, 1822-May 2 1902) and his relevance to medicine in the 21st century. *Curr Opin Rheumatol* 2003; 15(1):29–34
21 Massimo M. Minimally invasive coronary surgery: fad or future? *BMJ* 1998; 316:88
22 NICE. *Off-pump coronary artery bypass grafting* [IPG377]. 2011. http://guidance.nice.org.uk/IPG377
23 Brown WR, Moody DM, Venkata R, Challa VR, *et al.* Longer duration of cardiopulmonary bypass is associated with greater numbers of cerebral microemboli. *Stroke* 2000; 31 707–13. http://stroke.ahajournals.org/content/31/3/707
24 Perez-Silva A, Merino J. Frequent ventricular extrasystoles: significance, prognosis and treatment. *ESC E-J Cardiol Pract* 2011; 9(17). http://www.escardio.org/Journals/E-Journal-of-Cardiology-Practice/Volume-9/Frequent-ventricular-extrasystoles-significance-prognosis-and-treatment
25 NICE. *Atrial fibrillation: Management*. 2014. https://www.nice.org.uk/guidance/cg180/chapter/Recommendations
26 Lubitz SA, Magnani JW, Ellinor PT, *et al.* Atrial fibrillation and death after myocardial infarction: risk marker or causal mediator? *Circulation* 2011; 123:2063–5. http://circ.ahajournals.org/content/123/19/20 abstract
27 Wyse DG, Waldo AL, DiMarco JP, *et al.* A comparison of rate control and rhythm control in patients with atrial fibrillation. *N Engl J Med* 2002; 347:1825–33. http://www.nejm.org/doi/full/10.1056/NEJMoa021328
28 Oral H. Circumferential pulmonary-vein ablation for chronic atrial fibrillation. *N Engl J Med* 20 354(9):934–41. http://www.nejm.org/doi/full/10.1056/NEJMoa050955
29 Phang R, Prutkin J, Ganz L. Overview of atrial flutter. *UpToDate*®. 2015. http://www.uptodate.com/contents/overview-of-atrial-flutter?source=search_result&search=atrial+flutter&selectedTit le=1-150
30 Mant J. Warfarin vs aspirin for stroke prevention in elderly with atrial fibrillation (the Birmingham Atrial Fibrillation Treatment of the Aged Study, BAFTA): a randomised controlled trial. *Lancet* 20 370:493–503. http://www.thelancet.com/journals/lancet/article/PIIS0140673607612331/abstract
31 Bristow M, Saxon L, Boehmer J, *et al.* Cardiac-resynchronization therapy with or without an implantable defibrillator in advanced chronic heart failure. *N Engl J Med* 2004; 350(21):2140–50. http://www.nejm.org/doi/full/10.1056/NEJMoa032423
32 NICE. *Implantable cardioverter defibrillators and cardiac resynchronisation therapy for arrhythmias and heart failure* [TA314]. 2014. https://www.nice.org.uk/guidance/ta314
33 NICE. *Chronic heart failure* [CG108]. 2010. https://www.nice.org.uk/guidance/cg108
34 Patient. *Palliative care of heart failure*. 2016. http://www.patient.co.uk/showdoc/40024526/
35 McKee PA, Castelli WP, McNamara PM, *et al.* The natural history of congestive heart failure: the Framingham study. *N Engl J Med* 1971; 285(26):1441–6. http://www.nejm.org/doi/full/10.1056/NEJM19711223285260
36 Dargie HJ, McMurray JJ. Diagnosis and management of heart failure. *BMJ* 1994; 308:321–8. https://www.ncbi.nlm.nih.gov/pmc/articles/PMC2539274/
37 Levenson JW, McCarthy EP, Lynn J, *et al.* The last six months of life for patients with congestive heart failure. *J Am Geriatr Soc* 2000; 48(5 Suppl):S101–9. http://onlinelibrary.wiley.com/doi/10.1111/j.1532-5415.20 tb03119.x/abstract
38 Cleland JG, McGowan J, Clark A, *et al.* The evidence for beta blockers in heart failure. *BMJ* 1999; 318:8 5. https://www.ncbi.nlm.nih.gov/pmc/articles/PMC1115260/
39 Fonarow GC, Abraham WT, Albert NM, *et al.* Influence of beta-blocker continuation or withdrawal on outcomes in patients hospitalized with heart failure: findings from the OPTIMIZE-HF program. *J Am Coll Cardiol* 2008; 52(3):190–9
40 Pitt B, Zannad F, Remme WJ, *et al.* The effect of spironolactone on morbidity and mortality in patients with severe heart failure. *N Engl J Med* 1999; 341:709–17. http://content.nejm.org/cgi/reprint/341/10/709.
41 Taylor AL, Ziesche S, Yancy C, *et al.* Combination of isosorbide dinitrate and hydralazine in blacks with heart failure. *N Engl J Med* 2004; 351(20):2049–57. http://content.nejm.org/cgi/content/full/351/20/2049

42 Stewart S, McMurray JJ. Palliative care for heart failure. Time to move beyond treating and curing to improving the end of life. *BMJ* 2002; 325(7370):915–16. https://www.ncbi.nlm.nih.gov/pmc/articles/PMC1124429/
43 Addington-Hall J. Dying from heart failure: lessons from palliative care. *BMJ* 1998; 317(7164):961–2. http://www.pubmedcentral.nih.gov/articlerender.fcgi?artid=1114039
44 NICE. *Hypertension in adults: Diagnosis and management* [CG127]. 2011, updated 2016. https://www.nice.org.uk/guidance/cg127
45 MacMahon S, Alderman MH, Lindholm LH, *et al*. Blood-pressure-related disease is a global health priority. *Lancet* 2008; 371:1480–2. http://www.thelancet.com/journals/lancet/article/PIIS0140-6736(08)60632-7/fulltext
46 Lewington S, Clarke R, Qizilbash N, *et al*. Age-specific relevance of usual blood pressure to vascular mortality: a meta-analysis of individual data for one million adults in 61 prospective studies. *Lancet* 2003; 361(9362):1060–13. http://www.ncbi.nlm.nih.gov/pubmed/12493255
47 Beckett NS, Peters R, Fletcher AE, *et al*. Treatment of hypertension in patients 80 years of age or older. *N Engl J Med* 2008; 58:1887–98. http://content.nejm.org/cgi/reprint/358/18/1887.pdf
48 Law M, Wald N, Morris J. Lowering blood pressure to prevent myocardial infarction and stroke: a new preventive strategy. *Health Technol Assess* 2003; 7(31):1–94. https://www.ncbi.nlm.nih.gov/pubmedhealth/PMH0015113/
49 SPRINT Research Group. A randomized trial of intensive versus standard blood-pressure control. *N Engl J Med* 2015; 373(22):2103–16
50 ALLHAT Officers and Coordinators for the ALLHAT Collaborative Research Group. The Antihypertensive and Lipid-Lowering Treatment to Prevent Heart Attack Trial. Major outcomes in high-risk hypertensive patients randomized to angiotensin-converting enzyme inhibitor or calcium channel blocker vs diuretic. *JAMA* 2002; 288:2981–97. http://jama.ama-assn.org/content/288/23/2981.full
51 van den Meiracker AH, Dees A. Hypertensive crisis: definition, pathophysiology and treatment. *Ned Tijdschr Geneeskd* 1999; 143(44):2185–90
52 Stollerman GH. Rheumatic carditis. *Lancet* 1995; 346:390–2
53 Albert D, Harel L, Karrison T. The treatment of rheumatic carditis: a review and meta-analysis. *Medicine* 1995; 74:1–12
54 Koudy Williams J, Vita JA, Manuck SB, *et al*. Psychosocial factors impair vascular responses of coronary arteries. *Circulation* 1991; 84:2146–53
55 Steptoe A, Molloy GJ. Personality and heart disease. *Heart* 2007; 93:783–4
56 Huffman JC, Celano CM, Beach SR, *et al*. Depression and cardiac disease: epidemiology, mechanisms, and diagnosis. *Cardiovasc Psychiatry Neurol* 2013; 2013:695925. https://www.ncbi.nlm.nih.gov/pmc/articles/PMC3638710/
57 Otto C. Aortic stenosis--listen to the patient, look at the valve. *N Engl J Med* 2000; 343:652–4. http://www.nejm.org/doi/full/10.1056/NEJM200008313430910
58 Chopra HL, Nanda N. *Textbook of Cardiology (A Clinical & Historical Perspective)*. New Delhi: Jaypee Brothers Medical Publishers, 2012; 667
59 Soutter H. The repair of mitral stenosis. *Br Med J* 1925; 2(3379):603–6
60 Ogur G. Variable clinical expression of Holt-Oram syndrome in three generations. *Turk J Pediatr* 1998; 40(4):613–18. https://www.ncbi.nlm.nih.gov/labs/articles/10028874/
61 British Heart Foundation. *Inflammation and your heart: Endocarditis, pericarditis and myocarditis*. 2015. https://www.bhf.org.uk/publications/heart-conditions/medical-information-sheets/inflammation-and-your-heart
62 Chambers J, Sandoe J, Ray S, *et al*. The infective endocarditis team: recommendations from an international working group. *Heart* 2014; 100(7):524–7. http://heart.bmj.com/content/100/7/524.long
63 Durack D, Lukes AS, Bright DK. New criteria for diagnosis of infective endocarditis: utilization of specific echocardiographic findings. Duke Endocarditis Service. *Am J Med* 1994; 96: 200–9.
64 Beeching N. *Infectious Diseases*. London: Wolfe, 1994; 136.
65 NICE. *Prophylaxis against infective endocarditis: antimicrobial prophylaxis against infective endocarditis in adults and children undergoing interventional procedures* [CG64]. 2008, updated 2016. https://www.nice.org.uk/Search?q=CG64
66 Habib G, Lancellotti P, Antunes MJ, *et al*. 2015 ESC Guidelines for the management of infective endocarditis. *Eur Heart J* 2015; 36(44):3075–128. http://eurheartj.oxfordjournals.org/content/36/44/3075.long
67 Caforio AL, Pankuweit S, Arbustini E, *et al*. Current state of knowledge on aetiology, diagnosis, management, and therapy of myocarditis: a position statement of the European Society of Cardiology Working Group on Myocardial and Pericardial Diseases. *Eur Heart J* 2013; 34:2636–48. http://eurheartj.oxfordjournals.org/content/34/33/2636.long
68 Adler Y, Charron P, Imazio M, *et al*. 2015 ESC Guidelines for the diagnosis and management of pericardial diseases. *BMJ* 2002; 325(7370):915–16. https://www.ncbi.nlm.nih.gov/pmc/articles/PMC1124429/
69 Baumgartner H, Bonhoeffer P, De Groot NM, *et al*. ESC Guidelines for the management of grown-up congenital heart disease (new version 2010). *Eur Heart J* 2010; 31(23):2915–57. http://eurheartj.oxfordjournals.org/content/31/23/2915.long
70 De Mozzi P, Longo UG, Galanti G, *et al*. Bicuspid aortic valve: a literature review and its impact on sport activity. *Br Med Bull* 2008; 85:63–85. http://bmb.oxfordjournals.org/content/85/1/63.long
71 NICE. *Transcatheter endovascular closure of perimembranous ventricular septal defect* [IPG336]. 2010. https://www.nice.org.uk/guidance/IPG336
72 Bashore TM. Adult congenital heart disease: right ventricular outflow tract lesions. *Circulation* 2007; 115(14):1933–47 http://circ.ahajournals.org/content/115/14/1933.long
73 Wang XM, Wu LB, Sun C, *et al*. Clinical application of 64-slice spiral CT in the diagnosis of the Tetralogy of Fallot. *Eur J Radiol* 2007; 64(2):296–301. http://www.ejradiology.com/article/S0720-048X(07)00103-9/abstract
74 Driver and Vehicle Licensing Agency. *Assessing fitness to drive - a guide for medical professionals*. 2016. https://www.gov.uk/government/publications/assessing-fitness-to-drive-a-guide-for-medical-professionals

References

1 Johnson DC. Importance of adjusting carbon monoxide diffusing capacity (DLCO) and carbon monoxide transfer coefficient (KCO) for alveolar volume. *Respir Med* 2000; 94(1):28-37. http://www.resmedjournal.com/article/S0954-6111(99)90740-0/abstract
2 Spira A. Airway gene expression; a novel diagnostic test for lung cancer in smokers. *Proc Amer Assoc Cancer Res* 2006; 47:242
3 Doerschuk C. Pulmonary alveolar proteinosis - is host defense awry? *N Engl J Med* 2007; 356: 547-9. http://www.nejm.org/doi/full/10.1056/NEJMp068259
4 NICE. *Pneumonia in adults: Diagnosis and management* [CG191]. 2014. https://www.nice.org.uk/guidance/cg191
5 Man SY, Lee N, Ip M, *et al*. Prospective comparison of three predictive rules for assessing severity of community-acquired pneumonia in Hong Kong. *Thorax* 2007 62:348-53. https://www.ncbi.nlm.nih.gov/pmc/articles/PMC2092476/
6 Lim WS. Severity assessment in community-acquired pneumonia: moving on. *Thorax* 2007; 62:287-8. https://www.ncbi.nlm.nih.gov/pmc/articles/PMC2092475/
7 Kumar S, Hammerschlag MR. Acute respiratory infection due to *Chlamydia pneumoniae*: current status of diagnostic methods. *Clin Infect Dis* 2007; 44(4):568-76. http://cid.oxfordjournals.org/content/44/4/568.long
8 Stringer JR, Beard CB, Miller RF, *et al*. A new name for Pneumocystis from humans and new perspectives on the host-pathogen relationship. *Emerg Infect Dis* 2002; 8(9):891-6.
9 Kaplan JE, Benson C, Holmes KT, *et al*. *Guidelines for prevention and treatment of opportunistic infections in HIV-infected adults and adolescents*. Atlanta, GA: CDC, 2009. http://www.cdc.gov/mmwr/preview/mmwrhtml/rr5804a1.htm
10 Hui DS. Review of clinical symptoms and spectrum in humans with influenza A/H5N1 infection. *Respirology* 2008; 13 Suppl 1:S10-3. http://www.ncbi.nlm.nih.gov/pubmed/18366521
11 The Writing Committee of the World Health Organization (WHO) Consultation on Human Influenza A/H5. Avian Influenza A (H5N1) Infection in Humans. *N Engl J Med* 2005; 353:1374-85. http://content.nejm.org/cgi/content/full/353/13/1374
12 Engin A. Influenza type A (H5N1) virus infection. *Mikrobiyol Bul* 2007; 41(3):485-94. http://www.ncbi.nlm.nih.gov/pubmed/17933264
13 Public Health England. *Avian influenza: guidance and algorithms for managing human cases*. 2014. https://www.gov.uk/government/publications/avian-influenza-guidance-and-algorithms-for-managing-human-cases
14 *Avian influenza guidance and algorithms*. http://www.hpa.org.uk/web/HPAweb&HPAwebStandard/HPAweb_C/1195733851442
15 British Thoracic Society. *Guidelines on severe acute respiratory syndrome*. 2004. http://www.brit-thoracic.org.uk/guidelines/severe-acute-respiratory-syndrome-guideline.aspx
16 Hui DS. An overview on severe acute respiratory syndrome (SARS). *Monaldi Arch Chest Dis* 2005; 63(3):149-57
17 Gumel AB, Nuño M, Chowell G. Mathematical assessment of Canada's pandemic influenza preparedness plan. *Can J Infect Dis Med Microbiol* 2008; 19(2):185-92. https://www.ncbi.nlm.nih.gov/pmc/articles/PMC2605860/
18 Pasteur MC, Bilton D, Hill AT, *et al*. British Thoracic Society guideline for non-CF bronchiectasis. *Thorax* 2010; 65 Suppl 1:i1-58. http://thorax.bmj.com/content/65/Suppl_1/i1.long
19 Ramsey BW, Davies J, McElvaney NG, *et al*. A CFTR potentiator in patients with cystic fibrosis and the G551D mutation. *N Engl J Med* 2011; 365(18):1663-72. https://www.ncbi.nlm.nih.gov/pmc/articles/PMC3230303/
20 Rehman A, Baloch NU, Janahi IA. Lumacaftor-ivacaftor in patients with cystic fibrosis homozygous for Phe508del CFTR. *N Engl J Med* 2015; 373(18):1783-4. http://www.nejm.org/doi/pdf/10.1056/NEJMc1510466
21 Alton EW, Armstrong DK, Ashby D, *et al*. Repeated nebulisation of non-viral CFTR gene therapy in patients with cystic fibrosis: a randomised, double-blind, placebo-controlled, phase 2b trial. *Lancet Respir Med* 2015; 3(9):684-91. https://www.ncbi.nlm.nih.gov/pmc/articles/PMC4673100/
22 NICE. *Guidance on the diagnosis and treatment of lung cancer*. 2011. http://guidance.nice.org.uk/CG121
23 Bertazzi PA. Descriptive epidemiology of malignant mesothelioma. *Med Lav* 2005; 96(4):287-303. http://www.ncbi.nlm.nih.gov/pubmed/16457426
24 Tsiouris A, Walesby RK. Malignant pleural mesothelioma: current concepts in treatment. *Nat Clin Pract Oncol* 2007; 4(6):344-52. http://www.nature.com/nrclinonc/journal/v4/n6/full/ncponc0839.html
25 NICE. *Lung cancer: Diagnosis and management* [CG121]. 2011. http://guidance.nice.org.uk/CG121
26 Agarwal R. Allergic bronchopulmonary aspergillosis. *Chest* 2009; 135:805-26. http://www.sciencedirect.com/science/article/pii/S0012369209602099
27 Graf K. Five-years surveillance of invasive aspergillosis in a university hospital. *BMC Infect Dis* 2011 11:163. https://www.ncbi.nlm.nih.gov/pmc/articles/PMC3128051/
28 Herbrecht R, Denning DW, Patterson TF, *et al*. Voriconazole versus amphotericin B for primary therapy of invasive aspergillosis. *N Engl J Med* 2002; 347:408-15. http://www.nejm.org/doi/full/10.1056/NEJMoa020191
29 Morfín-Maciel B, Barragán-Meijueiro Mde L, Nava-Ocampo AA. Individual and family household smoking habits as risk factors for wheezing among adolescents. *Prev Med* 2006; 43(2):98-100. http://www.sciencedirect.com/science/article/pii/S0091743506001538
30 Størdal K, Johannesdottir GB, Bentsen BS, *et al*. Acid suppression does not change respiratory symptoms in children with asthma and gastro-oesophageal reflux disease. *Arch Dis Child* 2005; 90(9):956-60 https://www.ncbi.nlm.nih.gov/pmc/articles/PMC1720585/
31 Douglas JD. If you want to cure their asthma, ask about their job. *Prim Care Respir J* 2005; 14(2):65-7. http://www.nature.com/articles/pcrj2004122
32 Holloway EA, West RJ. Integrated breathing and relaxation training (the Papworth Method) for adults with asthma in primary care: a randomised controlled trial. *Thorax* 2007; 62(12):1039-42. https://www.ncbi.nlm.nih.gov/pmc/articles/PMC2094294/

33 British Thoracic Society. *British guideline on the management of asthma*. 2016. https://www.brit-thoracic.org.uk/document-library/clinical-information/asthma/btssign-asthma-guideline-2016/
34 Cates CJ, Cates MJ, Lasserson TJ. Regular treatment with formoterol for chronic asthma: serious adverse events. *Cochrane Database Syst Rev* 2008; 4:CD006923. http://onlinelibrary.wiley.com/doi/10.1002/14651858.CD006923.pub2/abstract
35 Anon. Using beta 2-stimulants in asthma. *Drug Ther Bull* 1997; 35:1–4.
36 NICE. *Omalizumab for severe persistent allergic asthma* [TA133]. 2007. https://www.nice.org.uk/guidance/TA133
37 Hensley MJ. Use of inhaled corticosteroids was associated with the development of cataracts. *Evid Based Med* 1998; 3:24. http://ebm.bmj.com/content/3/1/24.full.pdf+html
38 Anon. Beyond the lungs—a new view of COPD. *Lancet* 2007; 370:713. http://www.thelancet.com/journals/lancet/article/PIIS0140-6736(07)61349-X/abstract
39 Wouters E. COPD: a chronic and overlooked pulmonary disease. *Lancet* 2007; 370:715–16. http://www.thelancet.com/journals/lancet/article/PIIS0140-6736(07)61352-X/abstract
40 Steiner M, Barton RL, Singh SJ, *et al*. Nutritional enhancement of exercise performance in chronic obstructive pulmonary disease: a randomised controlled trial. *Thorax* 200358(9):745–51. https://www.ncbi.nlm.nih.gov/pmc/articles/PMC1746806/
41 Poole PJ, Black PN. Mucolytic agents for chronic bronchitis or chronic obstructive pulmonary disease. *Cochrane Database Syst Rev* 2006; 3:CD001287. http://onlinelibrary.wiley.com/doi/10.1002/14651858.CD001287.pub2/abstract
42 Soriano JB, Lamprecht B, Ramírez AS, *et al*. Mortality prediction in chronic obstructive pulmonary disease comparing the GOLD 2007 and 2011 staging systems: a pooled analysis of individual patient data. *Lancet Respir Med* 2015; 3(6):443–50. http://www.thelancet.com/journals/lanres/article/PIIS2213-2600(15)00157-5/abstract
43 Tiotropium versus salmeterol for the prevention of exacerbations of COPD. *N Engl J Med* 2011; 364:1093–103. http://www.nejm.org/doi/full/10.1056/NEJMoa1008378
44 Nannini L, Cates CJ, Lasserson TJ, *et al*. Combined corticosteroid and long-acting beta-agonist in one inhaler versus separate components for COPD. *Cochrane Database Syst Rev* 2007; 4:CD003794. http://www.ncbi.nlm.nih.gov/pubmed/17943798
45 Bernard GR, Artigas A, Brigham KL, *et al*. The American-European Consensus Conference on ARDS. Definitions, mechanisms, relevant outcomes, and clinical trial coordination. *Am J Respir Crit Care Med* 1994; 149(3 Pt 1):818–24. http://www.atsjournals.org/doi/pdf/10.1164/ajrccm.149.3.7509706
46 Diaz-Reganon Valverde G, Fernández Rico R, Iribarren Sarrías JL, *et al*. The administration of 20 ppm of inhaled nitric oxide produces a faster response than the inhalation of 5 ppm in adult respiratory distress syndrome. *Rev Esp Anesthesiol Reanim* 2000; 47(2):57–62
47 Afshari A, Brok J, Møller AM, *et al*. Inhaled nitric oxide for acute respiratory distress syndrome (ARDS) and acute lung injury in children and adults. *Cochrane Database Syst Rev* 2010; 7:CD002787. http://onlinelibrary.wiley.com/doi/10.1002/14651858.CD002787.pub2/abstract
48 Lamontagne F, Briel M, Guyatt GH, *et al*. Corticosteroid therapy for acute lung injury, acute respiratory distress syndrome, and severe pneumonia: a meta-analysis of randomized controlled trials. *J Crit Care* 2010; 25(3):420–35. http://www.jccjournal.org/article/S0883-9441(09)00234-2/abstract
49 Deal EN, Hollands JM, Schramm GE, *et al*. Role of corticosteroids in the management of acute respiratory distress syndrome. *Clin Ther* 2008; 30(5):787–99. http://www.sciencedirect.com/science/article/pii/S0149291808001823
50 Davies C, Gleeson FV, Davies RJ, *et al*. BTS guidelines for the management of pleural infection. *Thorax* 2003; 58 Suppl 2:ii18–28. https://www.ncbi.nlm.nih.gov/pmc/articles/PMC1766018/
51 Peppard PE, Young T, Palta M, *et al*. Prospective study of the association between sleep-disordered breathing and hypertension. *N Engl J Med* 2000; 342:1378–84. http://www.nejm.org/doi/full/10.1056/NEJM200005113421901
52 NICE. *Continuous positive airway pressure for the treatment of obstructive sleep apnoea/hypopnoea syndrome* [TA139]. 2008. http://www.nice.org.uk/Guidance/TA139
53 Iannuzzi MC, Rybicki BA, Teirstein AS. Sarcoidosis. *N Engl J Med* 2007; 357(21):2153–65. http://www.nejm.org/doi/full/10.1056/NEJMra071714
54 Bradley B, Branley HM, Egan JJ, *et al*. Interstitial lung disease guideline: the British Thoracic Society in collaboration with the Thoracic Society of Australia and New Zealand and the Irish Thoracic Society. *Thorax* 2008; 63(Suppl V):v1–v58. http://thorax.bmj.com/content/63/Suppl_5/v1.long
55 Grönhagen-Riska C. Angiotensin-converting enzyme. I. Activity and correlation with serum lysozyme in sarcoidosis, other chest or lymph node diseases and healthy persons. *Scand J Respir Dis* 1979; 60(2):83–93
56 Iannuzzi MC, Sah BP. Sarcoidosis. In: *Merk Manual*. http://www.merckmanuals.com/professional/pulmonary_disorders/sarcoidosis/sarcoidosis.html
57 Evans M, Sharma O, LaBree L, *et al*. Differences in clinical findings between Caucasians and African Americans with biopsy-proven sarcoidosis. *Ophthalmology* 2007; 114(2):325–33. http://www.aaojournal.org/article/S0161-6420(06)00994-8/abstract
58 Bradley B, Branley HM, Egan JJ, *et al*. Interstitial lung disease guideline: the British Thoracic Society in collaboration with the Thoracic Society of Australia and New Zealand and the Irish Thoracic Society. *Thorax* 2008; 63:v1–v58 http://thorax.bmj.com/content/63/Suppl_5/v1.long
59 Watanabe N, Tanada S, Sasaki Y. Pulmonary clearance of aerosolized 99mTc-DTPA in sarcoidosis I patients. *Q J Nucl Med Mol Imaging* 2007; 51(1):82–90. http://www.minervamedica.it/en/journals/nuclear-med-molecular-imaging/issue.php?cod=R39Y9999N00
60 Bradley B, Branley HM, Egan JJ, *et al*. Interstitial lung disease guideline: the British Thoracic Society in collaboration with the Thoracic Society of Australia and New Zealand and the Irish Thoracic Society. *Thorax* 2008; 63(Suppl V):v1–v58. http://thorax.bmj.com/content/63/Suppl_5/v1.long
61 Fisher M, Nathan SD, Hill C, *et al*. Predicting life expectancy for pirfenidone in idiopathic pulmonary fibrosis. *J Manag Care Spec Pharm* 2017; 23(3):S17–S24.

Chapter 5: Endocrinology

1 Simpson RW, Shaw JE, Zimmet PZ. The prevention of type 2 diabetes—lifestyle change or pharmacotherapy? A challenge for the 21st century. *Diabetes Res Clin Pract* 2003; 59(3):165–80. http://www.ncbi.nlm.nih.gov/m/pubmed/12590013/
2 Cartwright RD. The role of sleep in changing our minds: a psychologist's discussion of papers on memory reactivation and consolidation in sleep. *Learn Mem* 2004; 11(6):660–3. https://www.ncbi.nlm.nih.gov/pmc/articles/PMC534693/
3 Weetman AP. Autoimmune thyroid disease: propagation and progression. *Eur J Endocrinol* 2003; 148(1):1–9. http://www.eje-online.org/content/148/1/1.long
4 Gale E. Is there really an epidemic of type 2 diabetes? *Lancet* 2003; 362:503–4. http://www.thelancet.com/journals/lancet/article/PIIS0140-6736(03)14148-7/abstract
5 Inoue K, Matsumoto M, Akimoto K. Fasting plasma glucose and HbA1c as risk factors for type 2 diabetes. *Diabet Med* 2008; 25(10):1157–63. http://onlinelibrary.wiley.com/doi/10.1111/j.1464-5491.2008.02572.x/abstract
6 Westman EC, Yancy WS Jr, Mavropoulos JC, *et al*. The effect of a low-carbohydrate, ketogenic diet versus a low-glycemic index diet on glycemic control in type 2 diabetes mellitus. *Nutr Metab (Lond)* 2008; 5:36. https://www.ncbi.nlm.nih.gov/pmc/articles/PMC2633336/
7 Hemmingsen B, Lund SS, Gluud C, *et al*. Intensive glycaemic control for patients with type 2 diabetes: systematic review with meta-analysis and trial sequential analysis of randomised clinical trials. *BMJ* 2011; 343:d6898. https://www.ncbi.nlm.nih.gov/pmc/articles/PMC3223424/
8 Zinman B, Lachin JM, Inzucchi SE. Empagliflozin, cardiovascular outcomes, and mortality in type 2 diabetes. *N Engl J Med* 2015; 373(22):2117–28. http://www.nejm.org/doi/full/10.1056/NEJMc1600827
9 Dose Adjustment For Normal Eating (DAFNE). http://www.dafne.uk.com/
10 The Diabetes Control and Complications Trial Research Group. The effect of intensive treatment of diabetes on the development and progression of long-term complications in insulin-dependent diabetes mellitus. *N Engl J Med* 1993; 329(14):977–86. http://www.nejm.org/doi/full/10.1056/NEJM199309303291401
11 Belch J. Aspirin does not help as primary prevention in DM. *BMJ* 2008; 337:a1840. http://www.bmj.com/cgi/content/full/337/oct16_2/a1840
12 Davidson MB, Wong A, Hamrahian AH, *et al*. Effect of spironolactone therapy on albuminuria in patients with type 2 diabetes treated with angiotensin-converting enzyme inhibitors. *Endocr Pract* 2008; 14(8):985–92. http://journals.aace.com/doi/abs/10.4158/EP.14.8.985
13 NICE. *Chronic kidney disease: Early identification and management of chronic kidney disease in adults in primary and secondary care* [CG73]. https://www.nice.org.uk/guidance/cg73
14 Murad MH, Coto-Yglesias F, Wang AT, *et al*. Clinical review: drug-induced hypoglycemia: a systematic review. *J Clin Endocrinol Metab* 2009; 94(3):741–5. http://press.endocrine.org/doi/pdf/10.1210/jc.2008-1416
15 Kapoor RR, James C, *et al*. Advances in the diagnosis and management of hyperinsulinemic hypoglycemia. *Nat Clin Pract Endocrinol Metab* 2009; 5(2):101–12. http://www.nature.com/nrendo/journal/v5/n2/full/ncpendmet1046.html
16 Geraghty M, Draman M, Moran D, *et al*. Hypoglycaemia in an adult male: a surprising finding in pursuit of insulinoma. *Surgeon* 2008; 6(1):57–60
17 Abraham P, Avenell A, Park CM, *et al*. A systematic review of drug therapy for Graves' hyperthyroidism. *Eur J Endocrinol* 2005; 153(4):489–98. http://www.eje-online.org/content/153/4/489.long
18 Kahaly GJ, Pitz S, Hommel G, *et al*. Randomized, single blind trial of intravenous versus oral steroid monotherapy in Graves' orbitopathy. *J Clin Endocrinol Metab* 2005; 90(9):5234–40. http://press.endocrine.org/doi/pdf/10.1210/jc.2005-0148
19 Hedback G, Odén A. Recurrence of hyperparathyroidism; a long-term follow-up after surgery for primary hyperparathyroidism. *Eur J Endocrinol* 2003; 148(4):413–21. http://www.eje-online.org/content/148/4/413.long
20 Hoff AO, Cote GJ, Gagel RF. Multiple endocrine neoplasias. *Annu Rev Physiol* 2000; 62:377. http://www.annualreviews.org/doi/pdf/10.1146/annurev.physiol.62.1.377
21 Renehan AG, Brennan BM. Acromegaly, growth hormone and cancer risk. *Best Pract Res Clin Endocrinol Metab* 2008; 22(4):639–57. http://pubmedhh.nlm.nih.gov/cgi-bin/abstract.cgi?id=18971124&from=cqsr
22 Etxabe J, Vazquez JA. Morbidity and mortality in Cushing's disease: an epidemiological approach. *Clin Endocrinol* 1994; 40:479–84. http://onlinelibrary.wiley.com/doi/10.1111/j.1365-2265.1994.tb02486.x/abstract
23 Brosnan CM, Gowing NF. Addison's disease. *BMJ* 1996; 312(7038):1085–7. https://www.ncbi.nlm.nih.gov/pmc/articles/PMC2350885/
24 State Coroner for Western Australia. *Failure to diagnose: Addison's disease*. 2007. http://www.racgp.org.au/afp/200710/200710bird.pdf
25 Boyle JG, Davidson DF, Perry CG, *et al*. Comparison of diagnostic accuracy of urinary free metanephrines, vanillyl mandelic acid, and catecholamines and plasma catecholamines for diagnosis of pheochromocytoma. *J Clin Endocrinol Metab* 2007; 92(12):4602–8. http://press.endocrine.org/doi/pdf/10.1210/jc.2005-2668
26 Herrmann HC, Chang G, Klugherz BD, *et al*. Hemodynamic effects of sildenafil in men with severe coronary artery disease. *N Engl J Med* 2000; 342(22):1622–6. http://www.nejm.org/doi/full/10.1056/NEJM200006013422201
27 Minniti G, Gilbert DC, Brada M. Modern techniques for pituitary radiotherapy. *Rev Endocr Metab Disord* 2009; 10(2):135–44. http://link.springer.com/article/10.1007%2Fs11154-008-9106-0
28 Chanson P. Acromegaly. *Presse Med* 2009; 38(1):92–102. https://www.ncbi.nlm.nih.gov/pubmed/19004612

Chapter 6: Gastroenterology

1 Al Moutran H. Microstomia. *Medscape*. 2015. http://www.emedicine.com/ent/topic148.htm
2 Batur P, Stewart WJ, Isaacson JH. Increased prevalence of aortic stenosis in patients with arteriovenous malformations of the gastrointestinal tract in Heyde syndrome. *Arch Intern Med* 2003; 163(15):1821–4 http://jamanetwork.com/journals/jamainternalmedicine/fullarticle/755859
3 Unlugenc H, Guler T, Gunes Y, Isik G. Comparative study of the antiemetic efficacy of ondansetron, propofol and midazolam in the early postoperative period. *Eur J Anaesthesiol* 2004; 21(1):60–5. http://pubmedhh.nlm.nih.gov/cgi-bin/abstract.cgi?id=14768925&from=cqsr

4 NICE. *Dyspepsia and gastro-oesophageal reflux disease* [CG184]. 2014. https://www.nice.org.uk/Guidance/cg184
5 NICE. *Acute upper gastrointestinal bleeding in over 16s: management* [CG141]. 2012. https://www.nice.org.uk/Guidance/cg141
6 NICE. *Suspected cancer: Recognition and referral* [NG12]. 2015. https://www.nice.org.uk/Guidance/ng12
7 European Crohn's and Colitis Organisation (ECCO). *ECCO Consensus on Surgery for Ulcerative Colitis*. 2016. https://www.ecco-ibd.eu/index.php/publications/ecco-guidelines-science/published-ecco-guidelines.html
8 European Crohn's and Colitis Organisation (ECCO). *ECCO Crohn's Disease (CD) Consensus Update (2016)*. 2016. https://www.ecco-ibd.eu/index.php/publications/ecco-guidelines-science/published-ecco-guidelines.html
9 Ludvigsson JF, Bai JC, Biagi F, *et al*. Diagnosis and management of adult coeliac disease: guidelines from the British Society of Gastroenterology. *Gut* 63(8):1210–28. https://www.ncbi.nlm.nih.gov/pmc/articles/PMC4112432/
10 Juturi JV, Maghfoor I, Doll DC, *et al*. A case of biliary carcinoid presenting with pancreatitis and obstructive jaundice. *Am J Gastroenterol* 2000; 95(10):2973–4. http://www.nature.com/ajg/journal/v95/n10/full/ajg20001463a.html
11 Hillbom M, Pieninkeroinen I, Leone M. Seizures in alcohol-dependent patients: epidemiology, pathophysiology and management. *CNS Drugs* 2003; 17(14):1013–30. https://www.ncbi.nlm.nih.gov/pubmed/14594442
12 European Association for the Study of the Liver (EASL). EASL-EASD-EASO Clinical Practice Guidelines for the management of non-alcoholic fatty liver disease. *J Hepatol* 2016; 64(6):1388–402. http://www.journal-of-hepatology.eu/article/S0168-8278(15)00734-5/fulltext

Chapter 7: Renal medicine

1 Scottish Intercollegiate Guidelines Network. *Management of suspected bacterial urinary tract infection in adults: a national clinical guideline* (SIGN 88). 2012. http://www.sign.ac.uk/pdf/sign88.pdf
2 Kidney Disease: Improving Global Outcomes (KDIGO) Acute Kidney Injury Work Group. KDIGO clinical practice guideline for acute kidney injury. *Kidney Int Suppl* 2012; 2:1–138. http://kdigo.org/home/guidelines/acute-kidney-injury/
3 London AKI Network. *Guidelines and pathways*. http://www.londonaki.net/clinical/guidelines-pathways.html
4 NICE. *Algorithms for IV fluid therapy in adults*. 2013. https://www.nice.org.uk/guidance/cg174/resources/intravenous-fluid-therapy-in-adults-in-hospital-algorithm-poster-set-191627821
5 UK Renal Association. *Clinical practice guidelines: treatment of acute hyperkalaemia in adults*. March 2014. http://www.renal.org/guidelines/joint-guidelines/treatment-of-acute-hyperkalaemia-in-adults#sthash.LACGYarj.dpbs
6 Kidney Disease: Improving Global Outcomes (KDIGO) CKD Work Group. KDIGO 2012 clinical practice guideline for the evaluation and management of chronic kidney disease. *Kidney Int Suppl* 2013; 3:1–150. http://kdigo.org/home/guidelines/ckd-evaluation-management/
7 Evans PD, Taal MW. Epidemiology and causes of chronic kidney disease. *Medicine* 2015; 43:450–3. http://www.medicinejournal.co.uk/article/S1357-3039(15)00117-6/fulltext
8 NICE. *Chronic kidney disease in adults: Assessment and management* [CG182]. Updated Jan 2015. https://www.nice.org.uk/guidance/cg182
9 Kidney Disease: Improving Global Outcomes (KDIGO) Glomerulonephritis Work Group. KDIGO clinical practice guideline for glomerulonephritis. *Kidney Int Suppl* 2012; 2:139–274. http://kdigo.org/home/glomerulonephritis-gn/
10 Molitch ME, Adler AI, Flyvbjerg A, *et al*. Diabetic kidney disease: a clinical update from Kidney Disease: Improving Global Outcomes. *Kidney Int* 2015; 87(1):20–30. http://www.kidney-international.theisn.org/article/S0085-2538(15)30004-1/abstract

Chapter 8: Haematology

1 van der Klooster JM. A medical mystery. Lead poisoning. *Singapore Med J* 2004; 45(10):497–9. http://pubmedhh.nlm.nih.gov/cgi-bin/abstract.cgi?id=15455173&from=cqsr
2 The Joint United Kingdom (UK) Blood Transfusion and Tissue Transplantation Services Professional Advisory Committee. *Transfusion handbook* (5th edn). 2014. Available free at: http://www.transfusionguidelines.org/transfusion-handbook
3 NICE. *Neutropenic sepsis: Prevention and management in people with cancer* [CG151]. 2012. https://www.nice.org.uk/guidance/cg151

Chapter 9: Infectious diseases

1 Laxminarayan R, Duse A, Wattal C, *et al*. Antibiotic resistance - the need for global solutions. *Lancet Infect Dis* 2013; 13(12):1057–98. http://www.thelancet.com/journals/laninf/article/PIIS1473-3099(13)70318-9/abstract
2 NICE. *Antimicrobial stewardship: systems and processes for effective antimicrobial medicine use* [NG15]. 2015. https://www.nice.org.uk/guidance/ng15
3 NICE. *Tuberculosis* [NG33]. 2016. https://www.nice.org.uk/guidance/ng33
4 Public Health England. *PHE guidance on the use of antiviral agents for the treatment and prophylaxis of seasonal influenza*. 2016. https://www.gov.uk/government/uploads/system/uploads/attachment_data/file/580509/PHE_guidance_antivirals_influenza_2016_2017.pdf
5 Goldacre B. What the Tamiflu saga tells us about drug trials and big pharma. *The Guardian* 2014; 10 April. https://www.theguardian.com/business/2014/apr/10/tamiflu-saga-drug-trials-big-pharma
6 British Association for Sexual Health and HIV. *BASHH guidelines*. https://www.bashh.org/guidelines [accessed September 2016]

7 British HIV Association. *British HIV Association guidelines for the treatment of HIV-1-positive adults with antiretroviral therapy 2015*. 2015. http://www.bhiva.org/documents/Guidelines/Treatment/2015/2015-treatment-guidelines.pdf
8 Loveday HP, Wilson JA, Pratt RJ, *et al*. epic3: National evidence based guidelines for preventing healthcare-associated infections in NHS hospitals in England. *J Hosp Infect* 2014; 86s1:s1-s70. https://www.his.org.uk/files/3113/8693/4808/epic3_National_Evidence-Based_Guidelines_for_Preventing_HCAI_in_NHSE.pdf
9 Johnson V, Stockley JM, Dockrell D, *et al*. Fever in returned travellers presenting in the United Kingdom: recommendations for investigation and initial management. *J Infect* 2009; 59(1):1-18. https://www.ncbi.nlm.nih.gov/pubmed/19595360
10 Lalloo DG, Shingadia D, Bell DJ. UK malaria treatment guidelines 2016. *J Infect* 2016; 72(6):635-49. http://www.journalofinfection.com/article/S0163-4453(16)00047-5/abstract
11 Sinclair D, Donegan S, Iba R, *et al*. Artesunate versus quinine for severe malaria. *Cochrane Database Syst Rev* 2012; 6:CD005967. http://onlinelibrary.wiley.com/doi/10.1002/14651858.CD005967.pub4/full
12 via World Health Organization. *Health topics*. http://www.who.int/topics/en/ [accessed September 2016]
13 Rasmussen SA, Jamieson DJ, Honein MA, *et al*. Zika virus and birth defects — reviewing the evidence for causality. *N Engl J Med* 2016; 374:1981-7. http://www.nejm.org/doi/full/10.1056/NEJMsr1604338#t=article
14 Medlock JM, Leach SA. Effect of climate change on vector borne disease in the UK. *Lancet Infect Dis* 2015; 15(6):721-30. http://www.thelancet.com/journals/laninf/article/PIIS1473-3099(15)70091-5/abstract
15 European concerted action on Lyme borreliosis (EUCALB). http://www.eucalb.com [accessed September 2016]
16 Sudarshi D, Brown M. Human African trypanosomiasis in non-endemic countries. *Clin Med* 2015; 15(1):70-3. http://www.clinmed.rcpjournal.org/content/15/1/70.full.pdf
17 Lambourne JR, Brooks T. Brucella and coxiella: if you don't look, you don't find. *Clin Med* 2015; 15(1):91-2. http://www.clinmed.rcpjournal.org/content/15/1/91.abstract
18 Forbes AE, Zochowski WJ, Dubrey SW, *et al*. Leptospirosis and Weil's disease in the UK. *QJM* 2012; 105(2):1151-62. http://qjmed.oxfordjournals.org/content/105/12/1151.long
19 World Health Organization. *Clinical management of patients with viral haemorrhagic fever: a pocket guide for front-line health workers: interim emergency guidance for country adaptation*. 2016. http://apps.who.int/iris/bitstream/10665/205570/1/9789241549608_eng.pdf?ua=1
20 Barrett J, Brown M. Traveller's diarrhoea. *BMJ* 2016; 353:i1937. http://www.bmj.com/content/353/bmj.i1937.long
21 Riddle MS, DuPont HL, Connor BA. ACG clinical guideline: diagnosis, treatment, and prevention of acute diarrheal infections in adults. *Am J Gastroenterol* 2016; 111:602-22. doi:10.1038/ajg.2016.126. http://gi.org/wp-content/uploads/2016/05/ajg2016126a.pdf
22 Beeching N, Dassanayake A. Tropical liver disease. *Medicine* 2011; 39(9):556-60. http://www.medicine-journal.co.uk/article/S1357-3039(11)00154-X/abstract
23 Rodrigo C, Fernando D, Rajapakse S. Pharmacological management of tetanus: an evidence based review. *Crit Care* 2014; 18:217. https://ccforum.biomedcentral.com/articles/10.1186/cc13797
24 Varghese GM, Trowbridge P, Doherty T. Investigating and managing pyrexia of unknown origin. *BMJ* 2010; 341:c5470. http://www.bmj.com/content/341/bmj.c5470.long

Chapter 10: Neurology

1 NICE. *Headaches in over 12s: Diagnosis and management* [CG150]. 2012. https://www.nice.org.uk/guidance/cg150
2 NICE. *Alteplase for treating acute ischaemic stroke* [TA264]. 2012. https://www.nice.org.uk/guidance/ta264
3 NICE. *Delirium: Prevention, diagnosis and management* [CG103]. 2010. https://www.nice.org.uk/guidance/cg103
4 Fong TG, Davis D, Growdon ME, *et al*. The interface between delirium and dementia in elderly adults. *Lancet Neurol* 2015; 14(8):823-32. https://www.ncbi.nlm.nih.gov/pmc/articles/PMC4535349/
5 NICE. *Dementia: Supporting people with dementia and their carers in health and social care* [CG42]. 2006, updated 2016. https://www.nice.org.uk/guidance/cg42
6 NICE. *Donepezil, galantamine, rivastigmine and memantine for the treatment of Alzheimer's disease* [TA217]. 2011. https://www.nice.org.uk/guidance/ta217
7 Berg AT, Berkovic SF, Brodie MJ, *et al*. Revised terminology and concepts for organization of seizures and epilepsies: report of the ILAE Commission on Classification and Terminology, 2005-2009. *Epilepsia* 2010; 51(4):676-85. https://www.ncbi.nlm.nih.gov/pubmed/20196795
8 NICE. *Multiple sclerosis in adults: Management* [CG186]. 2014. https://www.nice.org.uk/guidance/cg186

Chapter 11: Oncology and palliative care

1 Cancer Research. *UK statistics*. http://www.cancerresearchuk.org/health-professional/cancer-statistics [accessed September 2016]
2 National Cancer Institute. *Communication in cancer health: professional version*. http://www.cancer.gov/about-cancer/coping/adjusting-to-cancer/communication-hp-pdq#section/_9
3 Baile WF, Buckman R, Lenzi R, *et al*. SPIKES: a six-step protocol for delivering bad news: application to the patient with cancer. *Oncologist* 2000; 5(4):302-11. http://theoncologist.alphamedpress.org/content/5/4/302.long
4 National Cancer Institute. *The genetics of cancer*. 2015. https://www.cancer.gov/about-cancer/causes-prevention/genetics/overview-pdq
5 NICE. *Familial breast cancer: Classification, care and managing breast cancer and related risks in people with a family history of breast cancer* [CG164]. 2013, updated 2015. https://www.nice.org.uk/guidance/cg164
6 NICE. *Suspected cancer: Recognition and referral* [NG12]. 2015. https://www.nice.org.uk/guidance/ng12
7 Kerr DJ, Haller DG, Verweij J. Principles of chemotherapy. In Kerr DJ, Haller DG, van der Valde CJH, *et al.* (eds) *Oxford Textbook of Oncology* (3rd edn). Oxford: Oxford University Press; 2016:186-95

8 Pérez Fidalgo JA, García Fabregat L, Cervantes A, *et al*. Management of chemotherapy extravasation: ESMO-EONS Clinical Practice Guidelines. *Ann Oncol* 2012; 23(suppl 7): vii167–vii173. https://academic.oup.com/annonc/article/23/suppl_7/vii167/145139/Management-of-chemotherapy-extravasation-ESMO-EONS
9 Loren AW, Mangu PB, Beck LN, *et al*. Fertility preservation for patients with cancer: American Society of Clinical Oncology clinical practice guideline update. *J Clin Oncol* 2013; 31(19):2500–10. http://ascopubs.org/doi/full/10.1200/JCO.2013.49.2678
10 Ahmad SS, Duke S, Jena R, *et al*. Advances in radiotherapy. *BMJ* 2012; 345e7765. http://www.bmj.com/content/345/bmj.e7765.long
11 DeAngelo D, Alyea EP. Oncologic emergencies. In: Singh AK, Loscalzo J (eds) *The Brigham Intensive Review of Internal Medicine*. Oxford: Oxford University Press, 2014:159–67
12 Lee DLY, Anthoney A. Complications of systemic therapy - gut infections and acute diarrhoea. *Clin Med* 14(5):528–45. http://www.clinmed.rcpjournal.org/content/14/5/528.full.pdf+html
13 Pelosof LC, Gerber DE. Paraneoplastic syndromes: an approach to diagnosis and treatment. *Mayo Clin Proc* 2010; 85(9):838–54. http://www.mayoclinicproceedings.org/article/S0025-6196(11)60214-0/abstract
14 Sturgeon CM, Lai LC, Duffy MJ. Serum tumour markers: how to order and interpret them. *BMJ* 2009; 339:b3527. http://www.bmj.com/content/339/bmj.b3527.long
15 Schröder FH, Hugosson J, Roobol MJ, *et al*. Screening and prostate cancer mortality: results of the European Randomised Study of Screening for Prostate Cancer (ERSPC) at 13 years of follow up. *Lancet* 2014; 384(9959):2027–35. http://www.thelancet.com/journals/lancet/article/PIIS0140-6736(14)60525-0/abstract
16 Temel JS, Greer JA, Muzikansky A, *et al*. Early palliative care for patients with metastatic non-small-cell lung cancer. *N Engl J Med* 2010; 363:733–42. http://www.nejm.org/doi/full/10.1056/NEJMoa1000678
17 World Health Organization. *Analgesic ladder*. http://www.who.int/cancer/palliative/painladder/en/
18 NHS England. *NPSA safety alert: Risk of distress and death from inappropriate doses of naloxone in patients on long-term opioid/opiate treatment*. 2014. https://www.england.nhs.uk/wp-content/uploads/2014/11/psa-inappropriate-doses-naloxone.pdf
19 NHS Scotland. *Scottish palliative care guidelines*. 2014. http://www.palliativecareguidelines.scot.nhs.uk/
20 Universities of Hull, Staffordshire and Aberdeen. *Spiritual care at the end of life: A systematic review*. 2010. https://www.gov.uk/government/uploads/system/uploads/attachment_data/file/215798/dh_123804.pdf
21 Kaye P. Spiritual pain. In: *Notes on symptom control in hospice and palliative care*. Hospice Education Institute. 1990.
22 Ruegger J, Hodgkinson S, Field-Smith A, *et al*. Care of adults in the last days of life. *BMJ* 2015; 351:h6631. http://www.bmj.com/content/351/bmj.h6631
23 General Medical Council. *Treatment and care towards the end of life*. 2010. http://www.gmc-uk.org/static/documents/content/Treatment_and_care_towards_the_end_of_life_-_English_1015.pdf

Chapter 12: Rheumatology

1 Doherty M, Dacre J, Dieppe P, *et al*. The 'GALS' locomotor screen. *Ann Rheum Dis* 1992; 51:1165–9. https://www.ncbi.nlm.nih.gov/pmc/articles/PMC1012427/
2 Courtney P, Doherty M. Joint aspiration and injection. *Best Pract Res Clin Rheumatol* 2005; 19:345–69. http://www.bprclinrheum.com/article/S1521-6942(05)00010-0/abstract
3 Speed C. Low back pain. *BMJ* 2004; 328:1119–21. https://www.ncbi.nlm.nih.gov/pmc/articles/PMC406328/
4 NICE. *Low back pain in adults: Early management* [CG88]. 2009. https://www.nice.org.uk/guidance/cg88
5 Woolf AD, Pfleger B. Burden of major musculoskeletal conditions. *Bull World Health Organ* 2003; 81(9):646–56. https://www.ncbi.nlm.nih.gov/pmc/articles/PMC2572542/
6 Sowers M, Jannausch M, Stein E, *et al*. C-reactive protein as a biomarker of emergent osteoarthritis. *Osteoarthritis Cartilage* 2002; 10(8):595–601. https://www.ncbi.nlm.nih.gov/pubmed/12479380
7 NICE. *Osteoarthritis: Care and management* [CG177]. Available at: https://www.nice.org.uk/guidance/cg177
8 Bellamy N, Campbell J, Robinson V, *et al*. Viscosupplementation for the treatment of osteoarthritis of the knee. *Cochrane Database Syst Rev* 2006; 2:CD005321. http://onlinelibrary.wiley.com/doi/10.1002/14651858.CD005321.pub2/abstract
9 García-De La Torre I. Advances in the management of septic arthritis. *Rheum Dis Clin North Am* 2003; 29(1):61–75. https://www.ncbi.nlm.nih.gov/pubmed/12635500
10 Ross JJ, Saltzman CL, Carling P, *et al*. Pneumococcal septic arthritis: review of 190 cases. *Clin Infect Dis* 2003; 36(3):319–27. http://cid.oxfordjournals.org/content/36/3/319.long
11 Coakley G, Mathews C, Field M, *et al*. BSR & BHPR, BOA, RCGP and BSAC guidelines for management of the hot swollen joint in adults, 2006. *Rheumatology (Oxford)* 2006; 45(8):1039–41. http://rheumatology.oxfordjournals.org/content/45/8/1039.long
12 Mathews CJ, Kingsley G, Field M, *et al*. Management of septic arthritis: a systematic review. *Ann Rheum Dis* 2007; 66(4):440–5. https://www.ncbi.nlm.nih.gov/pmc/articles/PMC1856038/
13 Blizard Institute Clinical Effectiveness Group. *NSAIDs: Reducing the risk summary guidelines*. 2015. http://www.blizard.qmul.ac.uk/ceg-resource-library/clinical-guidance/clinical-guidelines.html
14 McGettigan P, Henry D. Cardiovascular risk with non-steroidal anti-inflammatory drugs: systematic review of population-based controlled observational studies. *PLoS Med* 2011; 8(9):e1001098. https://www.ncbi.nlm.nih.gov/pmc/articles/PMC3181230/
15 Scarpignato C, Lanas A, Blandizzi C, *et al*. Safe prescribing of non-steroidal anti-inflammatory drugs in patients with osteoarthritis - an expert consensus addressing benefits as well as gastrointestinal and cardiovascular risks. International NSAID Consensus Group. *BMC Med* 2015; 13:55. https://www.ncbi.nlm.nih.gov/pmc/articles/PMC4365808/
16 Chan F, Wong VW, Suen BY, *et al*. Combination of COX-2 and PPI for prevention of recurrent ulcer bleeding in patients at very high risk. *Lancet* 2007; 369:1621–6. http://www.thelancet.com/journals/lancet/article/PIIS0140-6736(07)60749-1/abstract
17 Calgüneri M, Ureten K, Akif Oztürk M, *et al*. Extra-articular manifestations of rheumatoid arthritis: results of a university hospital of 526 patients in Turkey. *Clin Exp Rheumatol* 2006; 24(3):305–8. http://www.clinexprheumatol.org/article.asp?a=2873

18 Young A, Koduri G. Extra-articular manifestations and complications of rheumatoid arthritis. *Best Pract Res Clin Rheumatol* 2007; 21(5):907–27. http://www.bprclinrheum.com/article/S1521-6942(07)00063-0/abstract

19 Farid SS, Azizi G, Mirshafiey A. Anti-citrullinated protein antibodies and their clinical utility in rheumatoid arthritis. *Int J Rheum Dis* 2013; 16(4):379–86. http://onlinelibrary.wiley.com/doi/10.1111/1756-185X.12129/abstract

20 Brown AK, Wakefield RJ, Conaghan PG, *et al*. New approaches to imaging early inflammatory arthritis. *Clin Exp Rheumatol* 2004; 22(5 Suppl 35): S18–25. http://www.clinexprheumatol.org/article.asp?a=2432

21 Szekanecz Z, Kerekes G, Dér H, *et al*. Accelerated atherosclerosis in rheumatoid arthritis. *Ann N Y Acad Sci* 2007; 1108:349–58. http://onlinelibrary.wiley.com/doi/10.1196/annals.1422.036/abstract

22 Aletaha D, Neogi T, Silman AJ, *et al*. 2010 Rheumatoid arthritis classification criteria: an American College of Rheumatology/European League Against Rheumatism collaborative initiative. *Arthritis Rheum* 2010; 62(9):2569–81. http://onlinelibrary.wiley.com/doi/10.1002/art.27584/abstract

23 O'Dell JR. Therapeutic strategies for rheumatoid arthritis. *N Engl J Med* 2004; 350:2591–602. http://www.nejm.org/doi/full/10.1056/NEJMra040226

24 British Society for Rheumatology. *National guidelines for the monitoring of second line drugs*. 2000. http://www.rheumatology.org.uk/includes/documents/cm_docs/2009/m/monitoring_second_line_drugs.pdf

25 NICE. *Adalimumab, etanercept and infliximab for the treatment of rheumatoid arthritis* [TA130]. 2007. https://www.nice.org.uk/guidance/ta130

26 NICE. *Adalimumab, etanercept, infliximab, rituximab and abatacept for the treatment of rheumatoid arthritis after the failure of a TNF inhibitor* [TA195]. 2010. https://www.nice.org.uk/guidance/ta195

27 NICE. *Tocilizumab for the treatment of rheumatoid arthritis* [TA247]. 2012. https://www.nice.org.uk/guidance/ta247

28 NICE. *Abatacept for the treatment of rheumatoid arthritis after the failure of conventional disease-modifying anti-rheumatic drugs* [TA234]. 2011. https://www.nice.org.uk/guidance/ta234

29 Ramiro S, Gaujoux-Viala C, Nam JL, *et al*. Safety of synthetic and biological DMARDs: a systematic literature review informing the 2013 update of the EULAR recommendations for management of rheumatoid arthritis. *Ann Rheum Dis* 2014; 73(3):529–35

30 Thompson A, Gandhi KK, Hochberg MC, *et al*. Incidence of malignancy in adult patients with rheumatoid arthritis: a meta-analysis. *Arthritis Res Ther* 2015; 17(1):212. https://www.ncbi.nlm.nih.gov/pmc/articles/PMC4536786/

31 Zhang W, Doherty M, Pascual E, *et al*. EULAR evidence based recommendations for gout. Part I: Diagnosis. Report of a task force of the Standing Committee for International Clinical Studies Including Therapeutics (ESCISIT). *Ann Rheum Dis* 2006; 65(10):1301–11. https://www.ncbi.nlm.nih.gov/pmc/articles/PMC1798330/

32 Sturrock R. Gout. Easy to misdiagnose. *BMJ* 2000; 320:132–3. https://www.ncbi.nlm.nih.gov/pmc/articles/PMC1128728/

33 Jordan KM, Cameron JS, Snaith M, *et al*. British Society for Rheumatology and British Health Professionals in Rheumatology guideline for the management of gout. *Rheumatology* 2007; 46(8):1372–4. http://rheumatology.oxfordjournals.org/content/46/8/1372.full

34 Cronstein BN, Terkeltaub R. The inflammatory process of gout and its treatment. *Arthritis Res Ther* 2006; 8 Suppl 1:S3. https://arthritis-research.biomedcentral.com/articles/10.1186/ar1908

35 Becker MA, Schumacher HR Jr, Wortmann RL, *et al*. Febuxostat compared with allopurinol in patients with hyperuricemia and gout. *N Engl J Med* 2005; 353(23):2450–61. http://www.nejm.org/doi/full/10.1056/NEJMoa050373

36 Zhang W, Doherty M, Bardin T, *et al*. EULAR recommendations for calcium pyrophosphate deposition. Part II: Management. *Ann Rheum Dis* 2011; 70:571–5. http://ard.bmj.com/content/70/4/571.full

37 Wanders A, Heijde DV, Landewe R, *et al*. Nonsteroidal antiinflammatory drugs reduce radiographic progression in patients with ankylosing spondylitis: a randomized clinical trial. *Arthritis Rheum* 2005; 52(6):1756–65. https://www.ncbi.nlm.nih.gov/pubmed/15934081

38 NICE. *Adalimumab, etanercept and infliximab for ankylosing spondylitis* [TA143]. 2008. https://www nice.org.uk/guidance/ta143

39 Hakim A, Clunie G, Haq I (eds). *Oxford handbook of rheumatology* (3rd edn). Oxford: Oxford University Press, 2011

40 Di Lorenzo AL. HLA-B27 syndromes. *Medscape*. 2015. http://emedicine.medscape.com/article/1201027-overview

41 Distler JH, Distler O. Tyrosine kinase inhibitors for the treatment of fibrotic diseases such as systemic sclerosis: towards molecular targeted therapies. *Ann Rheum Dis* 2010; 69 Suppl 1:i48–51. http://ard.bmj com/content/69/Suppl_1/i48.long

42 Gross WL, Reinhold-Keller E. [ANCA-associated vasculitis (Wegener's granulomatosis, Churg-Strauss syndrome, microscopic polyangiitis). 1. Systemic aspects, pathogenesis and clinical aspects.] *Z Rheumato* 1995; 54(5):279–90. https://www.ncbi.nlm.nih.gov/pubmed/8578884

43 Rahman A. Systemic lupus erythematosus. *N Engl J Med* 2008; 358:929–39. http://www.nejm.org/doi full/10.1056/NEJMra071297

44 NICE. *Final appraisal determination. Belimumab for treating active autoantibody-positive systemi lupus erythematosus*. 2016. https://www.nice.org.uk/guidance/GID-TAG273/documents/final-appraisal determination-document

45 Goral S, Ynares C, Shappell SB, *et al*. Recurrent lupus nephritis in renal transplant recipients revisited: is not rare. *Transplantation* 2003; 75(5):651–6. https://www.ncbi.nlm.nih.gov/pubmed/12640304

46 Baglin TP, Keeling DM, Watson HG. British Committee for Standards in Haematology. Guidelines on ora anticoagulation (warfarin): third edition - 2005 update. *Br J Haematol* 2006; 132(3):277–85. https://www ncbi.nlm.nih.gov/pubmed/16409292

47 Petri M, Orbai AM, Alarcón GS, *et al*. Derivation and validation of the Systemic Lupus Internationa Collaborating Clinics classification criteria for systemic lupus erythematosus. *Arthritis Rheum* 201 64(8):2677–86. https://www.ncbi.nlm.nih.gov/pmc/articles/PMC3409311/

48 Jennette JC, Falk RJ, Bacon PA, *et al*. 2012 Revised International Chapel Hill Consensus Conferenc Nomenclature of Vasculitides. *Arthritis Rheum* 2012; 65(1):1–11

49 Trejo-Gutierrez JF, Larson JM, Abril A. Shortness of breath, weak pulses, and a high ESR. *Lancet* 200 371:176. http://www.thelancet.com/pdfs/journals/lancet/PIIS0140-6736(08)60109-9.pdf

50 Dasgupta B, Borg FA, Hassan N, *et al.* BSR and BHPR guidelines for the management of GCA. *Rheumatology (Oxford)* 2010; 49(8):1594–7. http://rheumatology.oxfordjournals.org/content/49/8/1594.long
51 Dasgupta B, Giant Cell Arteritis Guideline Development Group. Concise guidance: diagnosis and management of giant cell arteritis. *Clin Med (Lond)* 2010; 10(4):381–6. https://www.ncbi.nlm.nih.gov/pubmed/20849016
52 Stephens RS, Brown C. Persistent lower abdominal and groin pain: what is the diagnosis? *Am J Med* 2005; 118(4):364–7. http://www.amjmed.com/article/S0002-9343(05)00088-4/abstract
53 Weiner SM, Peter HH. Neuropsychiatric involvement in systemic lupus erythematosus. Part 1: clinical presentation and pathogenesis. *Med Klin* 2002; 97(12):730–7. https://www.ncbi.nlm.nih.gov/pubmed/12491066
54 Reilly PA, Littlejohn GO. Peripheral arthralgic presentation of fibrositis/fibromyalgia syndrome. *J Rheum* 1992; 19:281–3 https://www.ncbi.nlm.nih.gov/pubmed/1629829
55 Richards SC, Scott DL. Prescribed exercise in people with fibromyalgia: parallel group randomised controlled trial. *BMJ* 2002; 325:185–9. https://www.ncbi.nlm.nih.gov/pmc/articles/PMC117444/
56 Busch AJ, Schachter CL, Overend TJ, *et al.* Exercise for fibromyalgia: a systematic review. *J Rheumatol* 2008; 35:1130–44. https://www.ncbi.nlm.nih.gov/pubmed/18464301
57 Goldenberg DL. Multidisciplinary modalities in the treatment of fibromyalgia. *J Clin Psychiatry* 2008; 69 Suppl 2:25–9. https://www.ncbi.nlm.nih.gov/pubmed/18537461
58 NICE. *Chronic fatigue syndrome/myalgic encephalomyelitis (or encephalopathy): Diagnosis and management* [CG53]. 2007. https://www.nice.org.uk/Guidance/cg53
59 New Zealand Guidelines Group. *New Zealand acute low back pain guide*. 2004. http://www.acc.co.nz/PRD_EXT_CSMP/groups/external_communications/documents/guide/prd_ctrb112930.pdf
60 Schneider M, Vernon H, Ko G, *et al.* Chiropractic management of fibromyalgia syndrome: a systematic review of the literature. *J Manipulative Physiol Ther* 2009; 32:25–40. https://www.ncbi.nlm.nih.gov/pubmed/19121462
61 Russell IJ, Orr MD, Littman B, *et al.* Elevated cerebrospinal fluid levels of substance P in patients with the fibromyalgia syndrome. *Arthritis Rheum* 1994; 37:1593–601. https://www.ncbi.nlm.nih.gov/pubmed/7526868
62 Russell IJ, Vaeroy H, Javors M, *et al.* Cerebrospinal fluid biogenic amine metabolites in fibromyalgia/fibrositis syndrome and rheumatoid arthritis. *Arthritis Rheum* 1992; 35:550–6. https://www.ncbi.nlm.nih.gov/pubmed/1374252
63 Wood PB, Schweinhardt P, Jaeger E, *et al.* Fibromyalgia patients show an abnormal dopamine response to pain. *Eur J Neurosci* 2007; 25:3576–82. https://www.ncbi.nlm.nih.gov/pubmed/17610577
64 Reichrath J, Bens G, Bonowitz A, *et al.* Treatment recommendations for pyoderma gangrenosum: an evidence-based review of the literature based on more than 350 patients. *J Am Acad Dermatol* 2005; 53(2):273–83. https://www.ncbi.nlm.nih.gov/pubmed/16021123

Chapter 13: Surgery

1 American Society of Anesthesiologists Committee. Practice guidelines for preoperative fasting and the use of pharmacologic agents to reduce the risk of pulmonary aspiration: application to healthy patients undergoing elective procedures: an updated report by the American Society of Anesthesiologists Committee on Standards and Practice Parameters. *Anesthesiology* 2011; 114(3):495–511. https://www.ncbi.nlm.nih.gov/pubmed/21307770
2 General Medical Council. *Consent: Patients and doctors making decisions together*. 2008. http://www.gmc-uk.org/guidance/ethical_guidance/consent_guidance_index.asp
3 BAPEN. *Screening & 'MUST'*. 2016. http://www.bapen.org.uk/screening-and-must/must
4 NICE. *Anticoagulation—oral* [Clinical Knowledge Summaries]. 2015. http://cks.nice.org.uk/anticoagulation-oral#!management
5 NIE. *Ipilimumab for previously treated advanced (unresectable or metastatic) melanoma* [TA268]. 2012. https://www.nice.org.uk/guidance/ta268
6 Hodi FS, O'Day SJ, McDermott DF, *et al.* Improved survival with ipilimumab in patients with metastatic melanoma. *N Engl J Med* 2010; 363(8):711–23. http://www.nejm.org/doi/full/10.1056/NEJMoa1003466
7 NICE. *Early and locally advanced breast cancer: Diagnosis and treatment* [CG80]. 2009. https://www.nice.org.uk/guidance/cg80
8 NICE. *Advanced breast cancer: Diagnosis and treatment* [CG81]. 2009, updated 2014. https://www.nice.org.uk/guidance/cg81
9 NICE. *Obesity: Identification, assessment and management* [CG189]. 2014. https://www.nice.org.uk/guidance/cg189.
10 Halpin V. Early cholecystectomy. *BMJ Best Practice*. http://bestpractice.bmj.com/best-practice/evidence/intervention/0411/0/sr-0411-i1.html
11 NICE. *Varicose veins: Diagnosis and management* [CG168]. 2013. https://www.nice.org.uk/guidance/cg168

Chapter 14: Clinical chemistry

1 NICE. *Intravenous fluid therapy in adults in hospital* [CG174]. 2013. https://www.nice.org.uk/Guidance/cg174
2 Levey A, Bosch JP, Lewis JB, *et al.* A more accurate method to estimate glomerular filtration rate from serum creatinine: a new prediction equation. Modification of Diet in Renal Disease Study Group. *Ann Intern Med* 1999; 130:461–70. https://www.ncbi.nlm.nih.gov/pubmed/10075613
3 Renneboog B, Musch W, Vandemergel X, *et al.* Mild chronic hyponatremia is associated with falls, unsteadiness, and attention deficits. *Am J Med* 2006; 119:71.e1–8. https://www.ncbi.nlm.nih.gov/pubmed/16431193
4 Robertson GL. Vaptan for the treatment of hyponatraemia. *Nat Rev Endocrinol* 2011; 7:151–61. http://www.nature.com/nrendo/journal/v7/n3/full/nrendo.2010.229.html
5 Smellie S. Spurious hypokalaemia. *BMJ* 2007; 334:693. http://www.bmj.com/content/334/7595/693
6 Thomas J, Doherty SM. HIV infection--a risk factor for osteoporosis. *J Acquir Immune Defic Syndr* 2003; 33(3):281–91. https://www.ncbi.nlm.nih.gov/pubmed/12843738

7 Patel AM, Goldfarb S. Got calcium? Welcome to the calcium-alkali syndrome. *J Am Soc Nephrol* 2010; 9:1440–3. http://jasn.asnjournals.org/content/21/9/1440.long
8 Berenson JR. Treatment of hypercalcemia of malignancy with bisphosphonates. *Semin Oncol* 2002; 29(6 Suppl 21):12–18. https://www.ncbi.nlm.nih.gov/pubmed/12584690
9 LeGrand SB, Leskuski D, Zama I. Narrative review: furosemide for hypercalcemia: an unproven yet common practice. *Ann Intern Med* 2008; 149:259–63. https://www.ncbi.nlm.nih.gov/pubmed/18711156
10 Robey RB, Lash JP, Arruda JA. Does furosemide have a role in the management of hypercalcemia? *Ann Intern Med* 2009; 150:146–7. https://www.ncbi.nlm.nih.gov/pubmed/19153420
11 Fitzpatrick LA. The hypocalcemic states. In: Favus M (ed) *Disorders of bone and mineral metabolism*. Philadelphia, PA: Lippincott Williams & Wilkins, 2002:568–88
12 Kramer HJ, Choi HK, Atkinson K, *et al*. The association between gout and nephrolithiasis in men: The Health Professionals' Follow-Up Study. *Kidney Int* 2003; 64:1022–6. https://www.ncbi.nlm.nih.gov/pubmed/12911552
13 Kanis JA, Johnell O, Oden A, *et al*. FRAX and the assessment of fracture probability in men and women from the UK. *Osteoporos Int* 2008; 19:385–97. https://www.ncbi.nlm.nih.gov/pmc/articles/PMC2267485/
14 NICE. *Alendronate, etidronate, risedronate, raloxifene and strontium ranelate for the primary prevention of osteoporotic fragility fractures in postmenopausal women* [TA160]. 2008, updated 2011. https://www.nice.org.uk/Guidance/ta160
15 Howe TE, Shea B, Dawson LJ, *et al*. Exercise for preventing and treating osteoporosis in postmenopausal women. *Cochrane Database Syst Rev* 2011; 7:CD000333. http://onlinelibrary.wiley.com/doi/10.1002/14651858.CD000333.pub2/abstract
16 Gillespie WJ. Hip protectors for preventing hip fractures in older people. *Cochrane Database Syst Rev* 2010; 10:CD001255. http://onlinelibrary.wiley.com/doi/10.1002/14651858.CD001255.pub4/abstract
17 Eberling P. Osteoporosis in men. *N Engl J Med* 2008; 358:1474–82. http://www.nejm.org/doi/full/10.1056/NEJMcp0707217
18 Vollbrecht J, Rao DS. Tumor-induced osteomalacia. *N Engl J Med* 2008; 358:1282. http://www.nejm.org/doi/full/10.1056/NEJMicm066066#t=article
19 Wermers RA, Tiegs RD, Atkinson EJ, *et al*. Morbidity and mortality associated with Paget's disease of bone: a population study. *J Bone Miner Res* 2008; 23:819–25. https://www.ncbi.nlm.nih.gov/pmc/articles/PMC2515478/
20 NICE. *Chronic kidney disease: Early identification and management of chronic kidney disease in adults in primary and secondary care* [CG73]. 2008. https://www.nice.org.uk/guidance/cg73
21 Anon. Randomised trial of cholesterol lowering in 4444 patients with coronary heart disease: the Scandinavian Simvastatin Survival Study (4S). *Lancet* 1994; 344:1383–9. https://www.ncbi.nlm.nih.gov/pubmed/7968073
22 Shepherd J, Cobbe SM, Ford I, *et al*. Prevention of coronary heart disease with pravastatin in men with hypercholesterolemia. West of Scotland Coronary Prevention Study Group. *N Engl J Med* 1995; 333:1301–8. http://www.nejm.org/doi/full/10.1056/NEJM199511163332001#t=article
23 Sacks FM, Pfeffer MA, Moye LA, *et al*. The effect of pravastatin on coronary events after myocardial infarction in patients with average cholesterol levels. Cholesterol and Recurrent Events Trial investigators. *N Engl J Med* 1996; 335:1001–9. http://www.nejm.org/doi/full/10.1056/NEJM199610033351401#t=article
24 Heart Protection Study Collaborative Group. MRC/BHF Heart Protection Study of cholesterol lowering with simvastatin in 20,536 high-risk individuals: a randomised placebo-controlled trial. *Lancet* 2002; 360:7–22. http://www.thelancet.com/journals/lancet/article/PIIS0140-6736(02)09327-3/abstract
25 Libby P. Inflammation in atherosclerosis. *Nature* 2002; 420:868–74. http://www.nature.com/nature/journal/v420/n6917/full/nature01323.html
26 Versmissen J, Oosterveer DM, Yazdanpanah M, *et al*. Efficacy of statins in familial hypercholesterolaemia: a long term cohort study. *BMJ* 2008; 337:a2423 https://www.ncbi.nlm.nih.gov/pmc/articles/PMC2583391/
27 NICE. *Cardiovascular disease: Risk assessment and reduction, including lipid modification* [CG181]. 2014, updated 2016. https://www.nice.org.uk/guidance/CG181
28 McKenney JM, Davidson MH, Jacobson TA, *et al*. Final conclusions and recommendations of the National Lipid Association Statin Safety Assessment Task Force. *Am J Cardiol* 2006; 8A:89C–94C. https://www.ncbi.nlm.nih.gov/pubmed/16581336
29 Robinson JG, Farnier M, Krempf M, *et al*. Efficacy and safety of alirocumab in reducing lipids and cardiovascular events. *N Engl J Med* 2015; 372(16):1489–99. http://www.nejm.org/doi/full/10.1056/NEJMoa1501031

Chapter 15: Eponymous syndromes

1 Todd J. The syndrome of Alice in Wonderland. *Can Med Assoc J* 1955; 73(9):701–4. https://www.ncbi.nlm.nih.gov/pmc/articles/PMC1826192/
2 Cau C. The Alice in Wonderland syndrome. *Minerva Med* 1999; 90(10):397–401. https://www.ncbi.nlm.nih.gov/pubmed/10767914
3 Fritschy D, Fasel J, Imbert JC, *et al*. The popliteal cyst. *Knee Surg Sports Traumatol Arthrosc* 2006; 14(7):623–8. https://www.ncbi.nlm.nih.gov/pubmed/16362357
4 Scheinfeld NS. Erythema induratum (nodular vasculitis). *Medscape*. 2016. http://emedicine.medscape.com/article/1083213-overview
5 Hakim A, Gavin Clunie G, Haq I. Behçet's disease. In: *Oxford Handbook of Clinical Rheumatology* (3rd edn). Oxford: Oxford University Press, 2011:490–1.
6 Mariotti AJ, Agrawal R, Hotaling AJ. The role of tonsillectomy in pediatric IgA nephropathy. *Arch Otolaryngol Head Neck Surg* 2009; 135(1):85–7. https://www.ncbi.nlm.nih.gov/pubmed/19153312
7 Fourcade G, Bengler C, Campello CH, *et al*. [Bickerstaff's syndrome presenting with coma, tetraplegia and blindness]. *Rev Neurol (Paris)* 2007; 163(2):231–4. https://www.ncbi.nlm.nih.gov/pubmed/17351542
8 Fitzgerald RC, di Pietro M, Ragunath K, *et al*. British Society of Gastroenterology guidelines on the diagnosis and management of Barrett's oesophagus. *Gut* 2014; 63(1):7–42. http://gut.bmj.com/content/63/1/7.long
9 Tham T. *Guidelines on the diagnosis and management of Barrett's oesophagus - an update 2015* [Online only] http://www.bsg.org.uk/clinical-guidelines/oesophageal/guidelines-on-the-diagnosis-and-management-of-barrett-s-oesophagus.html

10 Ambardekar AV, Krantz MJ. The Brugada syndrome: the perfect storm of genetics and environment? *Int J Cardiol* 2009; 141(1):108–9. https://www.ncbi.nlm.nih.gov/pubmed/19157599

11 Hedley PL, Jørgensen P, Schlamowitz S, *et al.* The genetic basis of Brugada syndrome: a mutation update. *Hum Mutat* 2009; 30(9):1256–66. https://www.ncbi.nlm.nih.gov/pubmed/19606473

12 Moon SJ, Lee JK, Kim TW, *et al.* Idiopathic transverse myelitis presenting as the Brown-Séquard syndrome. *Spinal Cord* 2008; 47(2):176–8. http://www.nature.com/sc/journal/v47/n2/full/sc200823a.html

13 Menon KV, Shah V, Kamath PS. The Budd-Chiari syndrome. *N Engl J Med* 2004; 350:578–85. http://www.nejm.org/doi/full/10.1056/NEJMra020282

14 Vaglio A, Moosig F, Zwerina J. Churg-Strauss syndrome: update on pathophysiology and treatment. *Curr Opin Rheumatol* 2012; 24(1):24–30. https://www.ncbi.nlm.nih.gov/pubmed/22089097

15 Liberski PP, Sikorska B, Hauw JJ, *et al.* Tubulovesicular structures are a consistent (and unexplained) finding in the brains of humans with prion diseases. *Virus Res* 2008; 132(1–2):226–8. https://www.ncbi.nlm.nih.gov/pubmed/18164506

16 CJD surveillance unit in Edinburgh. 2009. http://www.cjd.ed.ac.uk/documents/figs.pdf

17 Dorsey K, Zou S, Schonberger LB, *et al.* Lack of evidence of transfusion transmission of Creutzfeldt-Jakob disease in a US surveillance study. *Transfusion* 2009; 49(5):977–84. https://www.ncbi.nlm.nih.gov/pubmed/19170987

18 Iwasaki Y, Mimuro M, Yoshida M, *et al.* Clinical diagnosis of Creutzfeldt-Jakob disease: accuracy based on analysis of autopsy-confirmed cases. *J Neurol Sci* 2008; 277(1–2):119–23. https://www.ncbi.nlm.nih.gov/pubmed/19056094

19 Armstrong RA. Creutzfeldt-Jakob disease and vision. *Clin Exp Optom* 2006; 89(1):3–9. https://www.ncbi.nlm.nih.gov/pubmed/16430434

20 Zanusso G, Ferrari S, Cardone F, *et al.* Detection of pathologic prion protein in the olfactory epithelium in sporadic Creutzfeldt-Jakob disease. *N Engl J Med* 2003; 348:711–19. http://www.nejm.org/doi/full/10.1056/NEJMoa022043#t=article

21 Tatersall R, Turner B. Brown-Séquard and his syndrome. *Lancet* 2000; 356:61–3. http://www.thelancet.com/journals/lancet/article/PIIS0140-6736(00)02441-7/abstract

22 Goodall CA, Head MW, Everington D, *et al.* Raised CSF phospho-tau concentrations in variant Creutzfeldt-Jakob disease: diagnostic and pathological implications. *J Neurol Neurosurg Psychiatry* 2006; 77(1):89–91. https://www.ncbi.nlm.nih.gov/pmc/articles/PMC2117383/

23 Karazindiyanoglu S, Cayan S. The effect of testosterone therapy on lower urinary tract symptoms/bladder and sexual functions in men with symptomatic late-onset hypogonadism. *Aging Male* 2008; 11(3):146–9. https://www.ncbi.nlm.nih.gov/pubmed/18821291

24 Studd J. A comparison of 19th century and current attitudes to female sexuality. *Gynecol Endocrinol* 2007; 23(12):673–81. https://www.ncbi.nlm.nih.gov/pubmed/18075842

25 Cussons AJ, Bhagat CI, Fletcher SJ, *et al.* Brown-Séquard revisited: a lesson from history on the placebo effect of androgen treatment. *Med J Aust* 2002; 177(11–12):678–9. https://www.ncbi.nlm.nih.gov/pubmed/12463999

26 Bliss M. *Harvey Cushing: A life in surgery*. Toronto: University of Toronto Press, 2005

27 Liberski PP, Brown P. Kuru: its ramifications after fifty years. *Exp Gerontol* 2009; 44(1–2):63–9. https://www.ncbi.nlm.nih.gov/pubmed/18606515

28 Miller N. *The misfolding diseases unfold*. Beremans Limited. 2004 http://www.beremans.com/pdf/The_misfolding_diseases_unfold.pdf

29 Lepur D, Peterković V, Kalabrić-Lepur N. Neuromyelitis optica with CSF examination mimicking bacterial meningomyelitis. *Neurol Sci* 2009; 30(1):51–4. https://www.ncbi.nlm.nih.gov/pubmed/19145403

30 Kim SH, Kim W, Li XF, *et al.* Repeated treatment with rituximab based on the assessment of peripheral circulating memory B cells in patients with relapsing neuromyelitis optica over 2 years. *Arch Neurol* 2011; 68(11):1412–20. http://jamanetwork.com/journals/jamaneurology/fullarticle/1107915

31 Trauner M, Meier PJ, Boyer JL. Molecular pathogenesis of cholestasis. *N Engl J Med* 1998; 339:1217–27. http://www.nejm.org/doi/full/10.1056/NEJM199810223391707

32 Badalamente MA, Hurst LC. Efficacy and safety of injectable mixed collagenase subtypes in the treatment of Dupuytren's contracture. *J Hand Surg Am* 2007; 32(6):767–74. https://www.ncbi.nlm.nih.gov/pubmed/17606053

33 Wetter TC. Restless legs syndrome: a review for the renal care professionals. *EDTNA ERCA J* 2001; 27(1):42–6. https://www.ncbi.nlm.nih.gov/pubmed/12603074

34 Schaefer RM, Tylki-Szymaćska A, Hilz MJ. Enzyme replacement therapy for Fabry disease: a systematic review of available evidence. *Drugs* 2009; 69(16):2179–205. https://www.ncbi.nlm.nih.gov/pubmed/19852524

35 Narváez J, Domingo-Domenech E, Gómez-Vaquero C, *et al.* Biological agents in the management of Felty's syndrome: a systematic review. *Semin Arthritis Rheum* 2012; 41(5):658–68. https://www.ncbi.nlm.nih.gov/pubmed/22119104

36 Weinshenker BG. Neuromyelitis optica: what it is and what it might be. *Lancet* 2003; 361(9361):889–90. http://www.thelancet.com/journals/lancet/article/PIIS0140-6736(03)12784-5/abstract

37 Losacco T, Punzo C, Santacroce L. [Gardner syndrome: clinical and epidemiologic up to date]. *Clin Ter* 2005; 156(6):267–71. https://www.ncbi.nlm.nih.gov/pubmed/16463563

38 Okai T, Yamaguchi Y, Sakai J, *et al.* Case report: complete regression of colonic adenomas after treatment with sulindac in Gardner's syndrome: a 4-year follow-up. *J Gastroenterol* 2001; 36:778–82. https://www.ncbi.nlm.nih.gov/pubmed/11757751

39 Mignot E. Narcolepsy and the HLA system. *N Engl J Med* 2001; 344:692. http://www.nejm.org/doi/full/10.1056/NEJM200103013440918#t=article

40 Freeman RD, Zinner SH, Müller-Vahl KR, *et al.* Coprophenomena in Tourette syndrome. *Dev Med Child Neurol* 2009; 51(3):218–27. https://www.ncbi.nlm.nih.gov/pubmed/19183216

41 Turtle L, Robertson MM. Tics, twitches, tales: the experiences of Gilles de la Tourette's syndrome. *Am J Orthopsychiatry* 2008; 78(4):449–55. https://www.ncbi.nlm.nih.gov/pubmed/19123766

42 Himle MB, Woods DW, Piacentini JC, *et al.* Brief review of habit reversal training for Tourette syndrome. *J Child Neurol* 2006; 21(8):719–25. https://www.ncbi.nlm.nih.gov/pubmed/16970874

43 Hughes RA, Swan AV, Raphaël JC, *et al.* Immunotherapy for Guillain-Barré syndrome: a systematic review. *Brain* 2007; 130(Pt 9):2245–57. https://www.ncbi.nlm.nih.gov/pubmed/17337484

44 Nagayama H, Katayama Y. Nippon Rinsho. [Apheresis therapy in Guillain-Barré syndrome]. *Nihon Rinsho* 2008; 66(6):1195–9. https://www.ncbi.nlm.nih.gov/pubmed/18540370

45 McCusker EJ, Richards F, Sillence D, *et al*. Huntington's disease: neurological assessment of potential gene carriers presenting for predictive DNA testing. *Clin Neurosci* 2000; 7(1):38–41. https://www.ncbi.nlm.nih.gov/pubmed/10847649

46 Tranebjaerg L, Samson RA, Green GE. Jervell and Lange-Nielsen Syndrome. *GeneReviews®* 2002 July 29 [updated November 2014]. https://www.ncbi.nlm.nih.gov/books/NBK1405/

47 Bersudsky M, Rosenberg P, Rudensky B, *et al*. Lipopolysaccharides of a Campylobacter coli isolate from a patient with Guillain-Barré syndrome display ganglioside mimicry. *Neuromuscul Disord* 2000; 10:182–6. https://www.ncbi.nlm.nih.gov/pubmed/10734265

48 Janniger CK. Klippel-Trenaunay-Weber syndrome. *Medscape*. 2016. http://reference.medscape.com/article/1084257-overview

49 Vassalo R, Ryu JH, Colby TV, *et al*. Pulmonary Langerhans cell histiocytosis. *N Engl J Med* 2000 342:1969–78. http://www.nejm.org/doi/full/10.1056/NEJM200006293422607

50 Beyerbach DM. Lown-Ganong-Levine syndrome. *Medscape*. 2015. http://emedicine.medscape.com/article/160097-overview

51 Quinlivan R, Vissing J, Hilton-Jones D, *et al*. Physical training for McArdle disease. *Cochrane Database Syst Rev* 2011; 12:CD007931. http://onlinelibrary.wiley.com/doi/10.1002/14651858.CD007931.pub2/abstract

52 Quinlivan R, Martinuzzi A, Schoser B. Pharmacological and nutritional treatment for McArdle disease (glycogen storage disease type V). *Cochrane Database Syst Rev* 2010; 12:CD003458. http://onlinelibrary.wiley.com/doi/10.1002/14651858.CD003458.pub4/abstract

53 Ault J. Marchiafava-Bignami disease. *Medscape*. 2016. http://emedicine.medscape.com/article/1146086-overview

54 Parker C. Eculizumab for paroxysmal nocturnal haemoglobinuria. *Lancet* 2009; 373(9665):759–67. http://www.thelancet.com/journals/lancet/article/PIIS0140-6736(09)60001-5/abstract

55 Lambrecht NW. Ménétrier's disease of the stomach: a clinical challenge. *Curr Gastroenterol Rep* 2011; 13(6):513–17. https://www.ncbi.nlm.nih.gov/pubmed/21931998

56 Yamamoto M, Harada S, Ohara M, *et al*. Clinical and pathological differences between Mikulicz's disease and Sjögren's syndrome. *Rheumatology (Oxford)* 2005; 44(2):227–34. http://rheumatology.oxfordjournals.org/content/44/2/227.long

57 Asher RAJ. Munchausen's syndrome. *Lancet* 1951; 257:339–41. https://www.ncbi.nlm.nih.gov/pubmed/14805062

58 Ponec RJ, Saunders MD, Kimmey MB. Neostigmine for the treatment of acute colonic pseudo-obstruction. *N Engl J Med* 1999; 341:137–41. http://www.nejm.org/doi/full/10.1056/NEJM199907153410301#t=article

59 Hatzimouratidis K, Eardley I, Giuliano F, *et al*. EAU guidelines on penile curvature. *Eur Urol* 2012; 62(3):543–52. https://www.ncbi.nlm.nih.gov/pubmed/22658761

60 Kim ED. Local therapies to heal the penis: fact or fiction? *J Androl* 2008; 30(4):384–90. https://www.ncbi.nlm.nih.gov/pubmed/19023141

61 Aomar Millán IF, Candel Erenas JM, *et al*. [Up-date of the diagnosis and treatment of vasospastic angina]. *Rev Clin Esp* 2008; 208(2):94–6. https://www.ncbi.nlm.nih.gov/pubmed/18261397

62 Keller KB, Lemberg L. Prinzmetal's angina. *Am J Crit Care* 2004; 13(4):350–4. https://www.ncbi.nlm.nih.gov/pubmed/15293589

63 Wanders RJA, Waterham HR, Leroy BP. Refsum disease. *GeneReviews®* 2006 March 20 [updated June 11 2015]. https://www.ncbi.nlm.nih.gov/books/NBK1353/

64 Fox RI. Sjögren's syndrome. *Lancet* 2005; 366:321–31. https://www.ncbi.nlm.nih.gov/pubmed/16039337

65 Worswick S, Cotliar J. Stevens-Johnson syndrome and toxic epidermal necrolysis: a review of treatment options. *Dermatol Ther* 2011; 24(2):207–18. https://www.ncbi.nlm.nih.gov/pubmed/21410610

66 Jayne DRW. Conventional treatment and outcome of Wegener's granulomatosis and microscopic polyangiitis. *CCJM* 2002; 69(Suppl 2):SII110–5. http://www.ccjm.org/supplements/single-view/conventional-treatment-and-outcome-of-wegener-s-granulomatosis-and-microscopic-polyangiitis/0d8061df095[illegible]aa4829194e88a0a1ba6b.html

67 Kuo SH, Debnam JM, Fuller GN, *et al*. Wernicke's encephalopathy: an underrecognized and reversible cause of confusional state in cancer patients. *J Oncology* 2009; 76(1):10–8. https://www.karger.com/Article/Abstract/174951

68 Marth T, Raoult D. Whipple's disease. *Lancet* 2003; 361(9353):239–46. http://www.thelancet.com/journals/lancet/article/PIIS0140-6736(03)12274-X/abstract

69 Auernhammer CJ, Göke B. Medical treatment of gastrinomas. *Wien Klin Wochenschr* 2007; 119(19-20):609–15. https://www.ncbi.nlm.nih.gov/pubmed/17985097

70 Anon. Listening to patients with rare diseases. *Lancet* 2009; 373:868. http://www.thelancet.com/pdfs/journals/lancet/PIIS0140-6736(09)60519-5.pdf

Chapter 16: Radiology

No references for this chapter

Chapter 17: Reference intervals

No references for this chapter

Chapter 18: Practical procedures

1 Johnston AJ, Streater CT, Noorani R, *et al*. The effect of peripherally inserted central catheter (PICC) valve technology on catheter occlusion rates - The 'ELeCTRiC study. *J Vasc Access* 2012: 13(4):421–5. https://www.ncbi.nlm.nih.gov/pubmed/22505280

1 Hawkes C. Smart handles and red flags in neurological diagnosis. *Hosp Med* 2002; 63:732–42. https://www.ncbi.nlm.nih.gov/pubmed/12512200
2 NICE. *Sepsis: Recognition, diagnosis and early management* [NG51]. 2016. https://www.nice.org.uk/guidance/ng51
3 Task Force on the management of ST-segment elevation acute myocardial infarction of the European Society of Cardiology (ESC). ESC Guidelines for the management of acute myocardial infarction in patients presenting with ST-segment elevation. *Eur Heart J* 2012; 33(20):2569–619. http://eurheartj.oxfordjournals.org/content/33/20/2569.long
4 Roffi M, Patrono C, Collet JP, *et al*. 2015 ESC Guidelines for the management of acute coronary syndromes in patients presenting without persistent ST-segment elevation. *Eur Heart J* 2016; 37(3):267–315. http://eurheartj.oxfordjournals.org/content/37/3/267.long
5 NICE. *Ticagrelor for the treatment of acute coronary syndromes* [TA236]. 2011. https://www.nice.org.uk/guidance/ta236
6 Resuscitation Council (UK). *Advanced life support* (7th edn). London: Resuscitation Council (UK), 2016
7 Scottish Intercollegiate Guidelines Network. *British guideline on the management of asthma* (SIGN 141). 2014. https://www.brit-thoracic.org.uk/document-library/clinical-information/asthma/btssign-asthma-guideline-2014/
8 NICE. Management of exacerbations of COPD. In: *Chronic obstructive pulmonary disease in over 16s: Diagnosis and management* [CG101]. 2010. https://www.nice.org.uk/guidance/cg101/chapter/1-guidance#management-of-exacerbations-of-copd
9 MacDuff A, Arnold A, Harvey J, *et al*. Management of spontaneous pneumothorax: British Thoracic Society pleural disease guideline 2010. *Thorax* 2010; 65(Suppl 2):ii18–31. http://thorax.bmj.com/content/65/Suppl_2/ii18.long
10 Lim WS, Baudouin SV, George RC, *et al*. BTS guidelines for the management of community acquired pneumonia in adults: update 2009. *Thorax* 2009; 64(Suppl 3):iii1–55. http://thorax.bmj.com/content/64/Suppl_3/iii1.long
11 NICE. Recommendations. In: *Venous thromboembolic diseases: Diagnosis, management and thrombophilia testing* [CG141]. 2012. https://www.nice.org.uk/guidance/cg144/chapter/recommendations
12 NICE. *Acute upper gastrointestinal bleeding in over 16s: Management* [CG141]. 2012. https://www.nice.org.uk/guidance/cg141
13 McGill F, Heyderman R, Michael B, *et al*. The UK Joint Specialist Societies guideline on the diagnosis and management of acute meningitis and meningococcal sepsis in immunocompetent adults. *J Infect* 2016; 72:405–38. http://www.journalofinfection.com/article/S0163-4453(16)00024-4/abstract
14 NICE. *Epilepsies: Diagnosis and management* [CG137]. 2012, updated 2016. https://www.nice.org.uk/guidance/cg137
15 NICE. *Head injury: Assessment and early management* [CG176]. 2014. https://www.nice.org.uk/guidance/cg176
16 Joint British Diabetes Societies Inpatient Care Group. *The management of diabetic ketoacidosis in adults*. Second edition. Update: September 2013. https://www.diabetes.org.uk/Documents/About%20Us/What%20we%20say/Management-of-DKA-241013.pdf
17 Joint British Diabetes Societies Inpatient Care Group. *The management of the hyperosmolar hyperglycaemic state (HHS) in adults with diabetes*. August 2012. https://www.diabetes.org.uk/Documents/Position%20statements/JBDS-IP-HHS-Adults.pdf

Abbreviations: F indexes a notable figure or image; dis = disease; syn = syndrome.

A

C

E

I

M

N

O

P

Q

R

S

U

V

W

X

Y

Z

Early warning score

Early warning scores are scoring systems based on physiological parameters. The magnitude of the given score reflects how far the parameter varies from normal. The collated score from different parameters is used in:

- the assesssment of acute illness
- the detection of a clinical deterioration
- the initiation of a timely and competent clinical response.

A standardized National Early Warning Score (NEWS) is recommended for use across the NHS.[1] The components of the NEWS are detailed in fig A1. An appropriate clinical response to the aggregate score from fig A1 is outlined in fig A2.

PHYSIOLOGICAL PARAMETERS	3	2	1	0	1	2	3
Respiration Rate	≤8		9 - 11	12 - 20		21 - 24	≥25
Oxygen Saturations	≤91	92 - 93	94 - 95	≥96			
Any Supplemental Oxygen		Yes		No			
Temperature	≤35.0		35.1 - 36.0	36.1 - 38.0	38.1 - 39.0	≥39.1	
Systolic BP	≤90	91 - 100	101 - 110	111 - 219			≥220
Heart Rate	≤40		41 - 50	51 - 90	91 - 110	111 - 130	≥131
Level of Consciousness				A			V, P, or U

[*]The NEWS initiative flowed from the Royal College of Physicians' NEWSDIG, and was jointly developed and funded in collaboration with the Royal College of Physicians, Royal College of Nursing, National Outreach Forum and NHS Training for Innovation.

Fig A1 National Early Warning Score for adult patients.

1 Royal College of Physicians. *National Early Warning Scores (NEWS): standardising the assessment of acute illness severity in the NHS*. London: RCP, 2012.

NEWS SCORE	FREQUENCY OF MONITORING	CLINICAL RESPONSE
0	Minimum 12 hourly	• Continue routine NEWS monitoring with every set of observations
Total: 1-4	Minimum 4-6 hourly	• Inform registered nurse who must assess the patient; • Registered nurse to decide if increased frequency of monitoring and / or escalation of clinical care is required;
Total: 5 or more or 3 in one parameter	Increased frequency to a minimum of 1 hourly	• Registered nurse to urgently inform the medical team caring for the patient; • Urgent assessment by a clinician with core competencies to assess acutely ill patients; • Clinical care in an environment with monitoring facilities;
Total: 7 or more	Continuous monitoring of vital signs	• Registered nurse to **immediately** inform the medical team caring for the patient – this should be at least at Specialist Registrar level; • Emergency assessment by a clinical team with critical care competencies, which also includes a practitioner/s with advanced airway skills; • Consider transfer of Clinical care to a level 2 or 3 care facility, i.e. higher dependency or ITU;

Fig A2 Clinical response to NEWS triggers. © RCP 2012.

►Early warning scores are tools to aid assessment. They do not replace clinical judgement: use yours and respect the clinical opinion of others.

►Refer to local early warning scores where available.

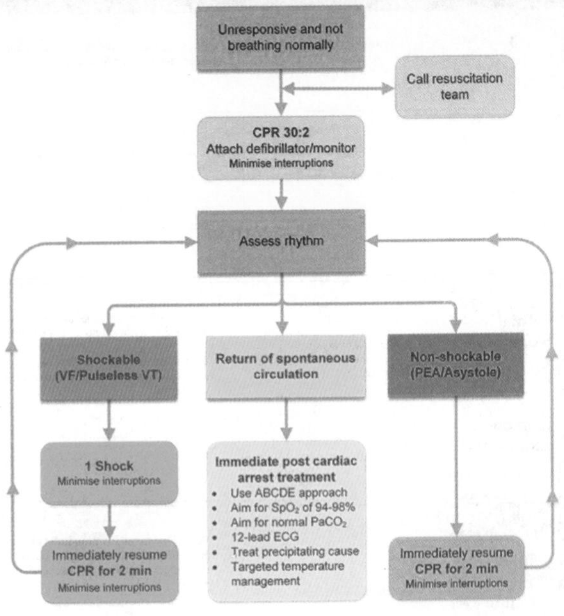

During CPR

- Ensure high quality chest compressions
- Minimise interruptions to compressions
- Give oxygen
- Use waveform capnography
- Continuous compressions when advanced airway in place
- Vascular access (intravenous or intraosseous)
- Give adrenaline every 3-5 min
- Give amiodarone after 3 shocks

Treat Reversible Causes

- Hypoxia
- Hypovolaemia
- Hypo-/hyperkalaemia/metabolic
- Hypothermia

- Thrombosis - coronary or pulmonary
- Tension pneumothorax
- Tamponade – cardiac
- Toxins

Consider

- Ultrasound imaging
- Mechanical chest compressions to facilitate transfer/treatment
- Coronary angiography and percutaneous coronary intervention
- Extracorporeal CPR

Fig A3 Cardiac arrest: advanced life support algorithm 2015.

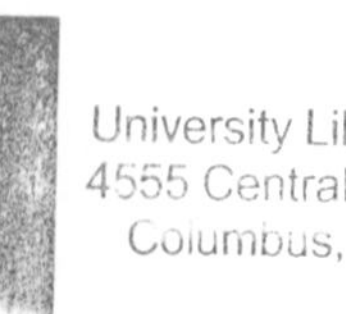

►►Cardiorespiratory arrest

►► Ensure the safety of the patient and yourself.

►► Confirm diagnosis: a patient who is unresponsive and not breathing properly is in cardiac arrest (a manual pulse check is inaccurate and not recommended).

Basic life support Shout for help. Ask someone to call the arrest team and bring the defibrillator. Note the time. ABC:

►► *Airway:* Head tilt (if no spine injury) and chin lift/jaw thrust.

►► *Breathing:* Look, listen, and feel for breathing for no more than 10 seconds. If there is any doubt whether breathing is normal, proceed to chest compressions.

►► *Chest compressions:* Place the heel of one hand on the centre of the chest (lower half of the stenum). Place your second hand on top and interlock fingers. Use straight arms. Give compressions at a rate of 100–120/min. Aim to compress the sternum 5–6cm. After 30 compressions give 2 rescue breaths. Do not interrupt compressions >10s. Continue with a ratio of 30:2 until defibrillator is available.

Advanced life support See algorithm fig A3.

- Continue chest compressions while adhesive defibrillation/monitoring pads are put in place. Plan all actions before pausing chest compressions.
- Stop chest compression for <5s to assess rhythm. Determine whether the rhythm is shockable (VF/pulseless VT) or non-shockable (asystole, pulseless electrical activity).

Shockable rhythm: VF/pulseless VT

►► A single person performs uninterrupted chest compressions while everyone else prepares for defibrillation: stand clear, move oxygen delivery device 1m away.

►► Select the appropriate energy on the defibrillator (150J or manufacturer's guidelines). When defibrillator is charged and safety check complete, the rescuer performing chest compressions stands clear and the shock is delivered.

►► CPR is resumed immediately (30:2). Reassess pulse/rhythm only after 2 minutes of CPR.

►► Repeat if shockable rhythm remains. Give drugs after 3 shocks (see Drugs, this topic).

Non-shockable rhythm: asystole/pulseless electrical activity (PEA)

►► Continue CPR 30:2. Obtain IV access and secure airway. Once airway secure switch to continuous compressions and ventilation. Give adrenaline 1mg IV.

►► Check rhythm every 2 minutes.

►► Consider reversible causes (4Hs and 4Ts: hypoxia, hypovolaemia, hyper/hypokalaemia/other metabolic derangement, hypothermia, thrombosis, tension pneumothorax, tamponade, toxins).

Drugs

- Give adrenaline 1mg IV every 3–5 mins for both shockable (from 3rd shock) and non-shockable rhythms. In practice this means at every other rhythm check or shock.[1]
- In shockable rhythms give amiodarone 300mg IV after 3 defibrillation attempts. Consider a further 150mg IV after 5 shocks. Lidocaine is an alternative.

Discontinuing resuscitation Needs clinical judgement: what is the likelihood of achieving a successful return of spontaneous circulation? If there is a shockable rhythm or a reversible cause then attempts are usually continued. It is reasonable to discontinue if asystole >20mins without a reversible cause. Ask for the opinion of others in the resuscitation team.

Resuscitation decisions Consider, discuss, and record CPR decisions:

- at the request of a patient with capacity
- as part of end-of-life care (p12, p536)
- in deteriorating, severe illness.

► Your patient should be involved in decisions about CPR (unless it would cause physical or psychological harm). Explain your clinical decision to them, including futility.

► Do not make judgements about the quality of life of others based on your own perception.

1 Meta-analysis fails to show that adrenaline increases survival to hospital discharge (http://www.ncbi.nlm.nih.gov/pubmed/24193240). RCT results are awaited (Paramedic 2: The Adrenaline Trial ISRCTN 73485024).

Useful doses for the new doctor

►These pages outline the typical adult doses of drugs that a foundation doctor will be called upon to prescribe. Refer to local guidelines first. If in any doubt, consult a drug formulary (eg British National Formulary www.bnf.org) especially if ↓eGFR or weight <50kg. Always check allergies before prescribing.

Drug	Dose and frequency	Notes
Analgesics		
Paracetamol	1g/6h PO/PR/IV, max. 4g/24h	Avoid if hepatic impairment.
Ibuprofen	400mg/8h PO, max 2.4g/24h	SE: gastritis; bronchospasm; AKI; fluid retention; hypersensitivity. CI: peptic ulcer; NSAID-induced asthma; coagulopathy; advanced CKD; heart failure.
Diclofenac sodium	50mg/8h PO/PR	
Codeine phosphate	30–60mg/4h PO/IM, max 240mg/24h	Chronic pain, eg malignancy, may require higher doses (see p536). Reduce dose if ↓eGFR. Care in head injury, as may hinder neurological assessment. SE: N&V; constipation; drowsiness; hypotension; respiratory depression, dependence. CI: respiratory depression.
Dihydrocodeine tartrate	30mg/4–6h PO, or 50mg/4–6h IM/SC	
Morphine	5–10mg/4h PO/IM	
Oxycodone	2.5–5mg/4h PO	
Tramadol	50–100mg/4h PO/IM/IV	
Antibiotics (refer to local guidelines)		
Phenoxymethylpenicillin	500mg/6h PO (max 4g/24h)	SE: rash; hypersensitivity and anaphylaxis; diarrhoea. CI: history of allergy.
Benzylpenicillin	0.6–1.2g/6h IV/IM	
Flucloxacillin	250–500mg/6h PO/IM 1g/6h IV	
Erythromycin	250–500mg/6h PO	IV only if oral treatment not possible. Beware of cytochrome P450 interactions (not azithromycin). SE: N&V; diarrhoea; cholestasis; QT prolongation; pancreatitis
Clarithromycin	250–500mg/6h PO	
Azithromycin	500mg/24h PO	
Doxycycline	200mg/24h PO as a single dose then 100mg/24h	SE: hypersensitivity; hepatotoxicity; may exacerbate myasthenia gravis and SLE. CI: pregnancy; age <12y.
Metronidazole	400mg/8h PO, or 500mg/8h IV, or 1g/8h PR	IV only if oral treatment not possible.
Gentamicin	5mg/kg/24h IV adjusted to serum concentration	Adjust dose for renal function. SE: nephrotoxicity (correct volume depletion); electrolyte disturbance; ototoxicity.
Trimethoprim	200mg/12h PO	CI: 1st trimester (folate antagonist).
Anti-emetics		
Cyclizine	50mg/8h PO/IM/IV	SE: drowsiness.
Metoclopramide	10mg/8h PO/IM/IV	SE: extrapyramidal SE, especially in young adults.
Ondansetron	4–8mg/8–12h PO/IV	SE: constipation; headache CI: long QT syndrome.